# Epithelial-Mesenchymal Plasticity in Cancer Metastasis

# Epithelial-Mesenchymal Plasticity in Cancer Metastasis

## Molecular Reprogramming, Cellular Adaptation, and Clinical Implications

Editors

**Mohit Kumar Jolly**
**Toni Celia-Terrassa**

MDPI • Basel • Beijing • Wuhan • Barcelona • Belgrade • Manchester • Tokyo • Cluj • Tianjin

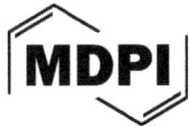

*Editors*
Mohit Kumar Jolly
Indian Institute of Science
India

Toni Celia-Terrassa
Hospital del Mar Medical Research Institute (IMIM)
Spain

*Editorial Office*
MDPI
St. Alban-Anlage 66
4052 Basel, Switzerland

This is a reprint of articles from the Special Issue published online in the open access journal *Journal of Clinical Medicine* (ISSN 2077-0383) (available at: https://www.mdpi.com/journal/jcm/special_issues/EMP).

For citation purposes, cite each article independently as indicated on the article page online and as indicated below:

LastName, A.A.; LastName, B.B.; LastName, C.C. Article Title. *Journal Name* **Year**, *Article Number*, Page Range.

**ISBN 978-3-03936-724-5 (Hbk)**
**ISBN 978-3-03936-725-2 (PDF)**

© 2020 by the authors. Articles in this book are Open Access and distributed under the Creative Commons Attribution (CC BY) license, which allows users to download, copy and build upon published articles, as long as the author and publisher are properly credited, which ensures maximum dissemination and a wider impact of our publications.

The book as a whole is distributed by MDPI under the terms and conditions of the Creative Commons license CC BY-NC-ND.

# Contents

**About the Editors** . . . . . . . . . . . . . . . . . . . . . . . . . . . . . . . . . . . . . . . . . . . . . . . . . . . . . . . . . . . . ix

**Mohit Kumar Jolly and Toni Celia-Terrassa**
Insights into the Multi-Dimensional Dynamic Landscape of Epithelial–Mesenchymal Plasticity through Inter-Disciplinary Approaches
Reprinted from: *J. Clin. Med.* **2020**, *9*, 1624, doi:10.3390/jcm9061624 . . . . . . . . . . . . . . . . . 1

**Branislava Ranković, Nina Zidar, Margareta Žlajpah and Emanuela Boštjančič**
Epithelial-Mesenchymal Transition-Related MicroRNAs and Their Target Genes in Colorectal Cancerogenesis
Reprinted from: *J. Clin. Med.* **2019**, *8*, 1603, doi:10.3390/jcm8101603 . . . . . . . . . . . . . . . . . 5

**Vishal Singh, Keshav Kumar Jha, Jyothsna K. M, Rekha V. Kumar, Varun Raghunathan and Ramray Bhat**
Iduronate-2-Sulfatase-Regulated Dermatan Sulfate Levels Potentiate the Invasion of Breast Cancer Epithelia through Collagen Matrix
Reprinted from: *J. Clin. Med.* **2019**, *8*, 1562, doi:10.3390/jcm8101562 . . . . . . . . . . . . . . . . . 27

**Tamasa De, Shina Goyal, Gowri Balachander, Kaushik Chatterjee, Prashant Kumar, Govind Babu K. and Annapoorni Rangarajan**
A Novel Ex Vivo System Using 3D Polymer Scaffold to Culture Circulating Tumor Cells from Breast Cancer Patients Exhibits Dynamic E-M Phenotypes
Reprinted from: *J. Clin. Med.* **2019**, *8*, 1473, doi:10.3390/jcm8091473 . . . . . . . . . . . . . . . . . 43

**Sugandha Bhatia, James Monkman, Tony Blick, Pascal HG Duijf, Shivashankar H. Nagaraj and Erik W. Thompson**
Multi-Omics Characterization of the Spontaneous Mesenchymal–Epithelial Transition in the PMC42 Breast Cancer Cell Lines
Reprinted from: *J. Clin. Med.* **2019**, *8*, 1253, doi:10.3390/jcm8081253 . . . . . . . . . . . . . . . . . 57

**Binita Nath, Anil P. Bidkar, Vikash Kumar, Amaresh Dalal, Mohit Kumar Jolly, Siddhartha S. Ghosh and Gautam Biswas**
Deciphering Hydrodynamic and Drug-Resistant Behaviors of Metastatic EMT Breast Cancer Cells Moving in a Constricted Microcapillary
Reprinted from: *J. Clin. Med.* **2019**, *8*, 1194, doi:10.3390/jcm8081194 . . . . . . . . . . . . . . . . . 89

**Yan-Jiun Huang, Yi-Hua Jan, Yu-Chan Chang, Hsing-Fang Tsai, Alexander TH Wu, Chi-Long Chen and Michael Hsiao**
ATP Synthase Subunit Epsilon Overexpression Promotes Metastasis by Modulating AMPK Signaling to Induce Epithelial-to-Mesenchymal Transition and Is a Poor Prognostic Marker in Colorectal Cancer Patients
Reprinted from: *J. Clin. Med.* **2019**, *8*, 1070, doi:10.3390/jcm8071070 . . . . . . . . . . . . . . . . . 105

**Vimalathithan Devaraj and Biplab Bose**
Morphological State Transition Dynamics in EGF-Induced Epithelial to Mesenchymal Transition
Reprinted from: *J. Clin. Med.* **2019**, *8*, 911, doi:10.3390/jcm8070911 . . . . . . . . . . . . . . . . . . 119

**Sugandha Bhatia, James Monkman, Tony Blick, Cletus Pinto, Mark Waltham, Shivashankar H Nagaraj and Erik W Thompson**
Interrogation of Phenotypic Plasticity between Epithelial and Mesenchymal States in Breast Cancer
Reprinted from: *J. Clin. Med.* **2019**, *8*, 893, doi:10.3390/jcm8060893 . . . . . . . . . . . . . . . . . 137

**Menghan Liu, Sarah E Hancock, Ghazal Sultani, Brendan P Wilkins, Eileen Ding, Brenna Osborne, Lake-Ee Quek and Nigel Turner**
Snail-Overexpression Induces Epithelial-mesenchymal Transition and Metabolic Reprogramming in Human Pancreatic Ductal Adenocarcinoma and Non-tumorigenic Ductal Cells
Reprinted from: *J. Clin. Med.* **2019**, *8*, 822, doi:10.3390/jcm8060822 . . . . . . . . . . . . . . . . . 161

**Barnali Deb, Vinuth N. Puttamallesh, Kirti Gondkar, Jean P. Thiery, Harsha Gowda and Prashant Kumar**
Phosphoproteomic Profiling Identifies Aberrant Activation of Integrin Signaling in Aggressive Non-Type Bladder Carcinoma
Reprinted from: *J. Clin. Med.* **2019**, *8*, 703, doi:10.3390/jcm8050703 . . . . . . . . . . . . . . . . . 179

**Swapnil C. Kamble, Arijit Sen, Rahul D. Dhake, Aparna N. Joshi, Divya Midha and Sharmila A. Bapat**
Clinical Stratification of High-Grade Ovarian Serous Carcinoma Using a Panel of Six Biomarkers
Reprinted from: *J. Clin. Med.* **2019**, *8*, 330, doi:10.3390/jcm8030330 . . . . . . . . . . . . . . . . . 201

**Shengnan Xu, Kathryn E. Ware, Yuantong Ding, So Young Kim, Maya U. Sheth, Sneha Rao, Wesley Chan, Andrew J. Armstrong, William C. Eward, Mohit Kumar Jolly and Jason A. Somarelli**
An Integrative Systems Biology and Experimental Approach Identifies Convergence of Epithelial Plasticity, Metabolism, and Autophagy to Promote Chemoresistance
Reprinted from: *J. Clin. Med.* **2019**, *8*, 205, doi:10.3390/jcm8020205 . . . . . . . . . . . . . . . . . 219

**Mohit Kumar Jolly and Toni Celià-Terrassa**
Dynamics of Phenotypic Heterogeneity Associated with EMT and Stemness during Cancer Progression
Reprinted from: *J. Clin. Med.* **2019**, *8*, 1542, doi:10.3390/jcm8101542 . . . . . . . . . . . . . . . . . 235

**Tatiana S. Gerashchenko, Nikita M. Novikov, Nadezhda V. Krakhmal, Sofia Y. Zolotaryova, Marina V. Zavyalova, Nadezhda V. Cherdyntseva, Evgeny V. Denisov and Vladimir M. Perelmuter**
Markers of Cancer Cell Invasion: Are They Good Enough?
Reprinted from: *J. Clin. Med.* **2019**, *8*, 1092, doi:10.3390/jcm8081092 . . . . . . . . . . . . . . . . . 255

**Timothy M. Thomson, Cristina Balcells and Marta Cascante**
Metabolic Plasticity and Epithelial-Mesenchymal Transition
Reprinted from: *J. Clin. Med.* **2019**, *8*, 967, doi:10.3390/jcm8070967 . . . . . . . . . . . . . . . . . 273

**Sagar S. Varankar and Sharmila A. Bapat**
Uncoupling Traditional Functionalities of Metastasis: The Parting of Ways with Real-Time Assays
Reprinted from: *J. Clin. Med.* **2019**, *8*, 941, doi:10.3390/jcm8070941 . . . . . . . . . . . . . . . . . 297

**Josep Baulida, Víctor M. Díaz and Antonio García de Herreros**
Snail1: A Transcriptional Factor Controlled at Multiple Levels
Reprinted from: *J. Clin. Med.* **2019**, *8*, 757, doi:10.3390/jcm8060757 . . . . . . . . . . . . . . . . . 319

**Xiang Nan, Jiang Wang, Haowen Nikola Liu, Stephen T.C. Wong and Hong Zhao**
Epithelial-Mesenchymal Plasticity in Organotropism Metastasis and Tumor Immune Escape
Reprinted from: *J. Clin. Med.* **2019**, *8*, 747, doi:10.3390/jcm8050747 .................. 341

**Dongya Jia, Xuefei Li, Federico Bocci, Shubham Tripathi, Youyuan Deng, Mohit Kumar Jolly, José N. Onuchic and Herbert Levine**
Quantifying Cancer Epithelial-Mesenchymal Plasticity and its Association with Stemness and Immune Response
Reprinted from: *J. Clin. Med.* **2019**, *8*, 725, doi:10.3390/jcm8050725 .................. 357

**Patricia G. Santamaría, Gema Moreno-Bueno and Amparo Cano**
Contribution of Epithelial Plasticity to Therapy Resistance
Reprinted from: *J. Clin. Med.* **2019**, *8*, 676, doi:10.3390/jcm8050676 .................. 389

**Gray W. Pearson**
Control of Invasion by Epithelial-to-Mesenchymal Transition Programs during Metastasis
Reprinted from: *J. Clin. Med.* **2019**, *8*, 646, doi:10.3390/jcm8050646 .................. 413

**Snahlata Singh and Rumela Chakrabarti**
Consequences of EMT-Driven Changes in the Immune Microenvironment of Breast Cancer and Therapeutic Response of Cancer Cells
Reprinted from: *J. Clin. Med.* **2019**, *8*, 642, doi:10.3390/jcm8050642 .................. 427

**Patricia G. Santamaría, María J. Mazón, Pilar Eraso and Francisco Portillo**
UPR: An Upstream Signal to EMT Induction in Cancer
Reprinted from: *J. Clin. Med.* **2019**, *8*, 624, doi:10.3390/jcm8050624 .................. 447

**Hsiao-Chen Chiu, Chia-Jung Li, Giou-Teng Yiang, Andy Po-Yi Tsai and Meng-Yu Wu**
Epithelial to Mesenchymal Transition and Cell Biology of Molecular Regulation in Endometrial Carcinogenesis
Reprinted from: *J. Clin. Med.* **2019**, *8*, 439, doi:10.3390/jcm8040439 .................. 465

**Alice Conigliaro and Carla Cicchini**
Exosome-Mediated Signaling in Epithelial to Mesenchymal Transition and Tumor Progression
Reprinted from: *J. Clin. Med.* **2019**, *8*, 26, doi:10.3390/jcm8010026 .................. 483

# About the Editors

**Mohit Kumar Jolly** is the leader of the Cancer Systems Biology laboratory and an Assistant Professor at the Centre for BioSystems Science and Engineering, Indian Institute of Science, since 2018. He has made seminal contributions to decoding the emergent dynamics of epithelial-mesenchymal plasticity (EMP) in cancer metastasis, through mathematical modeling of regulatory networks implicated in EMP. His work has featured on the cover of the *Journal of Clinical Medicine, Cancer Research, and Molecular and Cellular Biology*, and he won the 2016 iBiology Young Scientist Seminar Series—a coveted award for communicating one's research to a diverse audience. Currently, his lab focuses on decoding mechanisms and implications of non-genetic heterogeneity in cancer metastasis and therapy resistance, with a specific focus on mechanism-based and data-based mathematical modeling in close collaboration with experimental cancer biologists and clinicians.

**Toni Celia-Terrassa** is the Group Leader of the Cancer Stem Cells & Metastasis Lab since 2018. He has made remarkable contributions to the mammary stem cell, cancer stem cell, and the metastasis colonization research fields. His studies have revealed groundbreaking concepts about the implications of the epithelial-to-mesenchymal transition (EMT) and its reversion during the metastatic colonization of distant tissues. In addition, he has contributed with novel insights about the different dynamics of EMT and the functional consequences during metastasis. Currently, his lab focuses on achieving a better understanding of EMT–MET dynamics during the late stages of metastasis.

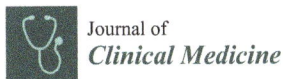 

*Editorial*

# Insights into the Multi-Dimensional Dynamic Landscape of Epithelial–Mesenchymal Plasticity through Inter-Disciplinary Approaches

**Mohit Kumar Jolly [1],\* and Toni Celia-Terrassa [2],\***

1. Centre for BioSystems Science and Engineering, Indian Institute of Science, Bangalore 560012, India
2. Cancer Research Program, IMIM (Hospital del Mar Medical Research Institute), 08003 Barcelona, Spain
\* Correspondence: mkjolly@iisc.ac.in (M.K.J.); acelia@imim.es (T.C.-T.)

Received: 25 May 2020; Accepted: 26 May 2020; Published: 27 May 2020

Epithelial–mesenchymal transition (EMT), first described by Dr. Elizabeth (Betty) Hay in the 1980s during vertebrate embryonic development [1], has important implications in cancer aggressiveness [2]. EMT is a cellular biological process in which cells lose their epithelial characteristics such as cell polarity and cell–cell adhesion and gain traits of the mesenchymal phenotype such as invasive and migratory abilities [3]. Recent in vitro, in vivo and in silico investigations have highlighted that EMT is a continuum of many hybrid states with various combinations of epithelial and mesenchymal markers and traits, associated with high phenotypic plasticity, demonstrated by dynamic reversible transitions as well as the gain of stemness, drug resistance and metabolic adaptability [4,5]. This revised perspective has led to EMT and its reverse process mesenchymal to epithelial transition (MET) being referred to as epithelial–mesenchymal plasticity (EMP). Classically, the EMP status of a cell has been characterized by molecular markers associated with epithelial (E-cadherin and cytokeratin) and mesenchymal (vimentin, N-cadherin and fibronectin) phenotypes. However, EMP characterization based only on molecular markers is not sufficient. Thus, new recent methods of characterizing EMP based on cellular morphology, biophysical traits, and functional properties (such as response to drugs) has been proven to be useful to understand EMP from a multi-dimensional dynamic perspective.

In this Special Issue, the authors discuss the implications of the EMP seen in stemness, drug resistance [6], immune-suppression [7–9], metabolic reprograming and the interaction of cancer cells with the tumor microenvironment. We have diverse topics related to the transcriptional and microRNA-mediated control of EMP networks [10,11], the multi-omics [12,13] and morphological mapping of EMP [14], integrative approaches to link EMP with metabolic reprogramming and/or autophagy [15,16], and the designing of novel ex vivo systems such as microfluidic setups and 3D polymer scaffolds to visualize the dynamics and heterogeneity of EMP in cancer cells [17,18]. This Special Issue, through a collection of review and research articles, represents the emerging inter-disciplinary approaches being taken to elucidate the nonlinear dynamics of EMP and their differential contributions to disease aggressiveness.

Phenotypic plasticity can often lead to non-mutational heterogeneity, thus further increasing the "fitness" of cells in dynamic environments [5]. Such heterogeneity was seen in EMP as well in a study with single cell-derived clonal progenies from established subpopulations in PMC42 breast cancer cells. These progenies showed clonal diversity and intrinsic plasticity with varied functional traits such as proliferation, stemness, therapy response, migration and invasion [19]. The migration and invasion traits are not only cell-autonomous; instead, they can be affected by the effects of cancer cells on the extracellular matrix (ECM) by degrading ECM proteins. Singh et al. showed how increased dermatan sulphate (DS) in breast cancer cells can facilitate invasion and morphological changes by remodeling the fibrillar matrix microenvironment [20]. Thus, cancer cells exhibiting varying degrees of EMP may exhibit individual and/or cooperative cell migration; different relative levels of biomarkers for these different migration modes were shown to be associated with aggressive cancer progression [16,21].

EMP has also been shown to cross paths with metabolic reprograming—an important hallmark of cancer [4]. Here, Liu et al. showed how Snail—a well-known EMT-inducer—can reduce the oxidative metabolism of pancreatic cancer cells and increase glucose uptake and lactate production, thus increasing glucose metabolism [22]. In another study by Huang et al. in colorectal cancer, ATP synthase subunit ε was found to be upregulated and promote metastasis by inducing EMT [23].

Overall, this collection of articles represents the diversity of experimental and computational tools and approaches, academic backgrounds and contributions that have been made by experts who have contributed to our understanding of the mechanisms and implications of EMP in cancer progression. We sincerely hope that this collection will serve as a valuable resource, enabling the cross-fertilization of ideas, with the goal of characterizing the dynamics of EMP and their contribution to disease burden.

**Conflicts of Interest:** The authors declare no conflict of interest.

## References

1. Hay, E.D. An overview of epithelio-mesenchymal transformation. *Cells Tissues Organs* **1995**, *154*, 8–20. [CrossRef] [PubMed]
2. Nieto, M.A.; Huang, R.Y.; Jackson, R.A.; Thiery, J.P. EMT: 2016. *Cell* **2016**, *166*, 21–45. [CrossRef] [PubMed]
3. De Craene, B.; Berx, G. Regulatory networks defining EMT during cancer initiation and progression. *Nat. Rev. Cancer* **2013**, *13*, 97–110. [CrossRef] [PubMed]
4. Thomson, T.M.; Balcells, C.; Cascante, M. Metabolic plasticity and epithelial-mesenchymal transition. *J. Clin. Med.* **2019**, *8*, 967. [CrossRef] [PubMed]
5. Jolly, M.K.; Celia-Terrassa, T. dynamics of phenotypic heterogeneity associated with EMT and stemness during cancer progression. *J. Clin. Med.* **2019**, *8*, 1542. [CrossRef]
6. Santamaria, P.G.; Moreno-Bueno, G.; Cano, A. Contribution of epithelial plasticity to therapy resistance. *J. Clin. Med.* **2019**, *8*, 676. [CrossRef]
7. Singh, S.; Chakrabarti, R. Consequences of EMT-driven changes in the immune microenvironment of breast cancer and therapeutic response of cancer cells. *J. Clin. Med.* **2019**, *8*, 642. [CrossRef]
8. Nan, X.; Wang, J.; Liu, H.N.; Wong, S.T.C.; Zhao, H. epithelial-mesenchymal plasticity in organotropism metastasis and tumor immune escape. *J. Clin. Med.* **2019**, *8*, 747. [CrossRef]
9. Jia, D.; Li, X.; Bocci, F.; Tripathi, S.; Deng, Y.; Jolly, M.K.; Onuchic, J.N.; Levine, H. quantifying cancer epithelial-mesenchymal plasticity and its association with stemness and immune response. *J. Clin. Med.* **2019**, *8*, 725. [CrossRef]
10. Baulida, J.; Díaz, V.M.; García de Herreros, A. Snail1: A transcriptional factor controlled at multiple levels. *J. Clin. Med.* **2019**, *8*, 757. [CrossRef] [PubMed]
11. Ranković, B.; Zidar, N.; Žlajpah, M.; Boštjančič, E. Epithelial-mesenchymal transition-related microRNAs and their target genes in colorectal cancerogenesis. *J. Clin. Med.* **2019**, *8*, 1603. [CrossRef]
12. Bhatia, S.; Monkman, J.; Blick, T.; Duijf, P.H.; Nagaraj, S.H.; Thompson, E.W. Multi-omics characterization of the spontaneous mesenchymal–epithelial transition in the PMC42 breast cancer cell lines. *J. Clin. Med.* **2019**, *8*, 1253. [CrossRef]
13. Deb, B.; Puttamallesh, V.N.; Gondkar, K.; Thiery, J.P.; Gowda, H.; Kumar, P. Phosphoproteomic profiling identifies aberrant activation of integrin signaling in aggressive non-type bladder carcinoma. *J. Clin. Med.* **2019**, *8*, 703. [CrossRef]
14. Devaraj, V.; Bose, B. Morphological state transition dynamics in EGF-induced epithelial to mesenchymal transition. *J. Clin. Med.* **2019**, *8*, 911. [CrossRef]
15. Xu, S.; Ware, K.; Ding, Y.; Kim, S.; Sheth, M.; Rao, S.; Chan, W.; Armstrong, A.; Eward, W.; Jolly, M.; et al. An integrative systems biology and experimental approach identifies convergence of epithelial plasticity, metabolism, and autophagy to promote chemoresistance. *J. Clin. Med.* **2019**, *8*, 205. [CrossRef]
16. De, T.; Goyal, S.; Balachander, G.; Chatterjee, K.; Kumar, P.; Babu, K.G.; Rangarajan, A. A novel ex vivo system using 3D polymer scaffold to culture circulating tumor cells from breast cancer patients exhibits dynamic E-M phenotypes. *J. Clin. Med.* **2019**, *8*, 1473. [CrossRef]

17. Nath, B.; Bidkar, A.P.; Kumar, V.; Dalal, A.; Jolly, M.K.; Ghosh, S.S.; Biswas, G. Deciphering hydrodynamic and drug-resistant behaviors of metastatic EMT breast cancer cells moving in a constricted microcapillary. *J. Clin. Med.* **2019**, *8*, 1194. [CrossRef]
18. Bhatia, S.; Monkman, J.; Blick, T.; Pinto, C.; Waltham, M.; Nagaraj, S.H.; Thompson, E.W. Interrogation of phenotypic plasticity between epithelial and mesenchymal states in breast cancer. *J. Clin. Med.* **2019**, *8*, 893. [CrossRef]
19. Singh, V.; Jha, K.K.; M, J.K.; Kumar, R.V.; Raghunathan, V.; Bhat, R. Iduronate-2-sulfatase-regulated dermatan sulfate levels potentiate the invasion of breast cancer epithelia through collagen matrix. *J. Clin. Med.* **2019**, *8*, 1562. [CrossRef]
20. Kamble, S.; Sen, A.; Dhake, R.; Joshi, A.; Midha, D.; Bapat, S. Clinical stratification of high-grade ovarian serous carcinoma using a panel of six biomarkers. *J. Clin. Med.* **2019**, *8*, 330. [CrossRef]
21. Pearson, G.W. control of invasion by epithelial-to-mesenchymal transition programs during metastasis. *J. Clin. Med.* **2019**, *8*, 646. [CrossRef]
22. Liu, M.; Hancock, S.E.; Sultani, G.; Wilkins, B.P.; Ding, E.; Osborne, B.; Quek, L.-E.; Turner, N. Snail-overexpression induces epithelial-mesenchymal transition and metabolic reprogramming in human pancreatic ductal adenocarcinoma and non-tumorigenic ductal cells. *J. Clin. Med.* **2019**, *8*, 822. [CrossRef]
23. Huang, Y.-J.; Jan, Y.-H.; Chang, Y.-C.; Tsai, H.-F.; Wu, A.T.; Chen, C.-L.; Hsiao, M. ATP synthase subunit epsilon overexpression promotes metastasis by modulating AMPK signaling to induce epithelial-to-mesenchymal transition and is a poor prognostic marker in colorectal cancer patients. *J. Clin. Med.* **2019**, *8*, 1070. [CrossRef] [PubMed]

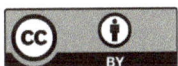

© 2020 by the authors. Licensee MDPI, Basel, Switzerland. This article is an open access article distributed under the terms and conditions of the Creative Commons Attribution (CC BY) license (http://creativecommons.org/licenses/by/4.0/).

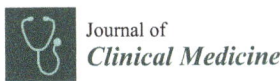

*Article*

# Epithelial-Mesenchymal Transition-Related MicroRNAs and Their Target Genes in Colorectal Cancerogenesis

Branislava Ranković, Nina Zidar, Margareta Žlajpah and Emanuela Boštjančič *

Faculty of Medicine, Institute of Pathology, University of Ljubljana, Korytkova 2, 1000 Ljubljana, Slovenia; branislava.rankovic@mf.uni-lj.si (B.R.); nina.zidar@mf.uni-lj.si (N.Z.); margareta.zlajpah@mf.uni-lj.si (M.Ž.)
* Correspondence: emanuela.bostjancic@mf.uni-lj.si; Tel.: +386-15437195

Received: 16 August 2019; Accepted: 27 September 2019; Published: 3 October 2019

**Abstract:** MicroRNAs of the *miR-200* family have been shown experimentally to regulate epithelial-mesenchymal transition (EMT). Although EMT is the postulated mechanism of development and progression of colorectal cancer (CRC), there are still limited and controversial data on expression of *miR-200* family and their target genes during CRC cancerogenesis. Our study included formalin-fixed paraffin-embedded biopsy samples of 40 patients (10 adenomas and 30 cases of CRC with corresponding normal mucosa). Expression of *miR-141*, *miR-200a/b/c* and *miR-429* and their target genes (*CDKN1B*, *ONECUT2*, *PTPN13*, *RND3*, *SOX2*, *TGFB2* and *ZEB2*) was analysed using quantitative real-time PCR. Expression of E-cadherin was analysed using immunohistochemistry. All miRNAs were down-regulated and their target genes showed the opposite expression in CRC compared to adenoma. Down-regulation of the *miR-200* family at the invasive front in comparison to the central part of tumour was observed as well as a correlation of expression of *miR-200b*, *CDKN1B*, *ONECUT2* and *ZEB2* expression to nodal metastases. Expression of the *miR-200* family and *SOX2* also correlated with E-cadherin staining. These results suggest that the *miR-200* family and their target genes contribute to progression of adenoma to CRC, invasive properties and development of metastases. Our results strongly support the postulated hypotheses of partial EMT and intra-tumour heterogeneity during CRC cancerogenesis.

**Keywords:** colorectal adenoma; colorectal carcinoma; metastases; intra-tumour heterogeneity; epithelial-mesenchymal transition; *miR-200* family; target genes

## 1. Introduction

Colorectal cancer (CRC) is one of the most common cancers worldwide. Five-year survival for patients with early CRC is approximately 90%, while for patients with advanced CRC, survival drops to 8%–12%. The prognosis can improve significantly with the introduction of population screening programs; however, 40%–50% of CRC patients still develop metastases [1,2]. Cancerogenesis of CRC is divided into well-established discrete stages, from normal mucosa to invasive carcinoma. The majority of CRC develops from precursor lesions—adenomas. The molecular pathways that are responsible for transformation of normal mucosa to adenoma and CRC are well understood and include stepwise accumulation of mutations (microsatellite instability or MSI pathway; chromosome instability or CIN pathway), epigenetic changes (CpG island methylator phenotype, CIMP) and changes in gene expression [3,4]. The majority of events occur before the formation of adenoma. Despite extensive research, the role of epithelial-mesenchymal transition (EMT) remains one of the controversial aspects of CRC development from normal mucosa to adenoma and carcinoma. EMT is believed to be one of the key processes in development of metastases in CRC, being responsible for the increased motility of cancer cells at the invasive front [5–7].

EMT is one of the crucial processes in embryonal development, being essential for morphogenesis and organ development [5]. In adult life, it contributes to physiological and pathological processes, such as wound healing, tissue regeneration, organ fibrosis and development and progression of malignant tumours. During EMT, epithelial cells undergo extensive changes that lead to separation of cells, re-organization of the extracellular matrix and an increase in cell motility, and invasion [6–9].

EMT is difficult to observe at a molecular level due to the reversible nature of changes, present only in a minority of cells [6,7,9]. Several markers of EMT have been described since its postulated contribution to cancer development [5–10]. Besides up-regulation of transcriptional factors of EMT, several miRNAs have been found to be involved in EMT regulation, the most frequent finding being down-regulation of the *miR-200* family (*miR-200a, miR-200b, miR-200c, miR-141, miR-429*), which is an important feature of EMT [2,6]. Transcription factors of EMT and their regulators are thought to support all cancer stages: from tumour initiation, establishment of precancerous lesion, accumulation of genetic alterations and escape from tumour surveillance and development of metastases [11].

Despite numerous publications suggesting that EMT might be responsible for metastases development in CRC [2,10,12], there is limited data about the involvement of EMT, including the *miR-200* family and their target genes [13], at early stages of CRC cancerogenesis. There is also limited data on differential expression of the *miR-200* family in different parts of the tumour, i.e., at the invasive front of CRC in comparison to the central part of the tumour, suggesting intra-tumour heterogeneity (ITH). ITH has emerged as an important phenomenon in cancer and it is related to different morphologic and phenotypic profiles of tumour cell in various parts of the tumour, including cellular morphology, gene expression and (epi)genetic/genomic aberrations, as well as metastatic potential. It is believed to contribute to cancer progression, resistance to therapy and recurrences [14]. ITH of the *miR-200* family might contribute to a lower expression of epithelial markers and gain of mesenchymal markers at the invasive front [13].

We therefore hypothesized that EMT in CRC might be responsible for malignant transformation of adenoma to carcinoma, development of metastases to the regional lymph nodes and ITH. Our aim was to investigate expression of the *miR-200* family and their target genes in CRC cancerogenesis from normal mucosa to adenoma and carcinoma without and those with nodal metastases. To the best of our knowledge, there has been no research systematically exploring the involvement of the *miR-200* family and their target genes in all stages of CRC development.

## 2. Experimental Section

### 2.1. Tissue Samples

Tissue samples from 40 patients with adenoma and CRC were included in the study. For routine histopathologic examination, tissue samples were fixed in 10% buffered formalin and embedded in paraffin (FFPE). CRC specimens were evaluated according to standard procedures and after histopathologic examination, pTNM (pathologic Tumour Node Metastasis) classification was assessed on the basis of the depth of invasion and extent of the primary tumour, the number of lymph nodes with metastases, and the presence of distant metastases [15]. Samples were collected retrospectively from the archives of the Institute of Pathology, Faculty of Medicine, University of Ljubljana. For all patients, tumour samples and samples of normal mucosa (if available) were included. Patients treated either by radiotherapy, chemotherapy or biologic drugs prior to surgery were excluded from the study. On the basis of clinical and histopathological features, samples were divided into three groups: patients with adenoma ($n = 10$), patients with carcinoma without nodal metastases (CRC N0, $n = 13$), patients with carcinoma with nodal metastases (CRC N+, $n = 17$).

In all cases, EMT was evaluated based on the expression of E-cadherin, *miR-200* family and miRNAs target genes. For the purpose of the study, adenomas were compared to carcinoma and normal colon mucosa. Carcinoma with regional lymph node metastases were compared to those without lymph node metastases. ITH was analysed comparing the invasive front of the tumour and the centre of the tumour in both CRC N0 and CRC N+ groups.

The investigation was carried out following the rules of the Declaration of Helsinki. The study was approved by the National Medical Ethics Committee (Republic of Slovenia, Ministry of Health).

*2.2. Immunohistochemistry*

FFPE tissue samples were cut at 4 µm for immunohistochemistry. All reagents were from Ventana Medical Systems Inc. (Tuscon, AZ, USA) except where otherwise indicated. Commercially available antibodies against E-cadherin (Dako Agilent, Santa Clara, CA, USA, M3612, clone NC4-38, dilution 1:10) were used. Deparaffinization, antigen retrieval and staining were performed in an automatic immunostainer (Benchmark XT, Ventana, Tuscon, AZ, USA) using horseradish peroxidase (iVIEW DAB Detection Kit, Roche, Basel, Switzerland) for colour development. The sections were then counterstained with haematoxylin.

*2.3. RNA Isolation from Formalin-Fixed Paraffin Embedded (FFPE) Tissue Samples*

2.3.1. RNA Isolation from FFPE Tissue Slides

Tissue samples were cut at 10 µm from FFPE tissue blocks and four sections were used for the isolation procedure. Total RNA isolation was performed using an AllPrep DNA/RNA FFPE kit (Qiagen, Hilden, Germany) according to the manufacturer's protocol. The concentration and quality of the isolates were assessed with a spectrophotometer ND-1000 (Nanodrop, Thermo Fisher Scientific, Waltham, MA, USA) at wavelengths 260, 280 and 230 nm.

2.3.2. RNA Isolation from FFPE Tissue Cores (Punched) Samples

For analysis of ITH, tumour samples were punched from FFPE tissue blocks (from invasive front and central part of tumour) using a 600 µm needle. For the isolation procedure, 3 punches were used from each tumour region. Total RNA isolation was performed using a MagMax FFPE DNA/RNA Ultra kit (Applied Biosystems, Foster City, CA, USA) according to the manufacturer's protocol with one modification. Protease digestion was performed overnight at 56 °C with shanking for 15 s at 300 rpm every 4 min. The concentration and quality of the isolates were assessed with a spectrophotometer ND-1000 (Nanodrop, Thermo Fisher Scientific, Waltham, MA, USA) at the wavelengths 260, 280 and 230 nm.

2.3.3. RNA Quality Assessment

Reverse transcription (RT) followed by amplification of the *GAPDH*, a housekeeping gene (100 base pairs), using quantitative real-time PCR (qPCR) and Sybr Green technology, was used as quality control. All of the samples included in the study had passed amplification of *GAPDH* (initially quality control) and those that did not amplify were not included in the study (we isolated at least twice as many samples as are included within this manuscript). Second, for selected genes, we chose TaqMan primers and probes that amplify and detect PCR products less than 100 bp long (Table 1).

*2.4. Analysis of Expression of Family miR-200 and miR-205*

miRNAs family *miR-200* was analysed using qPCR based on the TaqMan methodology (Thermo Fisher Scientific, Waltham, MA, USA). A pre-designed mixture of probes and primers specific for target miRNAs expression was used. Prior to qPCR, three pools of RNA samples were created, obtained from normal mucosa, adenomas and advanced CRC. After RT, the cDNA was diluted in five steps, ranging from 4-point dilution to 1024-point dilution, and the probes were tested for qPCR efficiency. All the qPCR efficiency reactions were performed on a RotorGene Q (Qiagen, Hilden, Germany) in triplicate.

**Table 1.** Probes used for miRNAs and mRNAs quantification using quantitative real-time PCR (qPCR).

| Probe Name | Probe ID Number | Length of PCR Product (bp [1]) |
|---|---|---|
| B2M | Hs 99999907_m1 | 75 |
| CDKN1B | Hs00153277_m1 | 71 |
| IPO8 | Hs 00183533_m1 | 71 |
| ONECUT2 | Hs00191477_m1 | 57 |
| PTPN13 | Hs01106214_m1 | 65 |
| RND3 | Hs01003594_m1 | 91 |
| SOX2 | Hs04234836_s1 | 86 |
| TGFB2 | Hs01555416_m1 | 67 |
| WAVE3 | Hs00903488_m1 | 57 |
| ZEB1 | Hs03680599_m1 | 63 |
| ZEB2 | Hs01095318_m1 | 58 |
| RNU6B | ID 001093 | Nd [2] |
| miR-141 | ID 000463 | nd |
| miR-200a | ID 000502 | nd |
| miR-200b | ID 002251 | nd |
| miR-200c | ID 002300 | nd |
| miR-205 | ID 000509 | nd |
| miR-429 | ID 001024 | nd |
| miR-1274b | ID 002884 | nd |

[1] bp, base pair; [2] nd, not defined.

2.4.1. Reverse Transcription (RT)

Looped primers for specific reverse transcription (RT) of miRNAs and a MicroRNA TaqMan RT kit (Applied Biosystems, Foster City, CA, USA) were utilized following the manufacturer's protocol. *RNU6B* and *miR-1247b* were used as reference genes (RGs). MicroRNAs, *miR-141*, *miR-200a*, *miR-200b*, *miR-200c* and *miR-429* were tested relative to the geometric mean of expression of *RNU6B* and *miR-1247b* (Table 1). Briefly, a 10 µL RT reaction master mix was performed with 10 ng of total RNA sample, 1.0 µL of MultiScribe Reverse Transcriptase (50 U/µL), 1.0 µL of Reverse Transcription Buffer (10×), 0.1 µL of dNTP (100 mM), 0.19 µL RNAase inhibitor (20 U/µL), and 2.0 µL of RT primer (5×). The reaction conditions were: 16 °C for 30 min, 42 °C for 30 min, 85 °C for 5 min.

2.4.2. Quantitative Real-Time PCR (qPCR)

qPCR for miRNAs was carried out in a 10 µL PCR master mix containing 5.0 µL TaqMan 2× FastStart Essential DNA Probe Master (Roche, Basel, Switzerland), 0.5 µL TaqMan assay and 4.5 µL RT products diluted 100-fold. The qPCR reactions were performed on a RotorGene Q (Qiagen, Hilden, Germany) in duplicate, as follows: initial denaturation at 95 °C for 10 min, 40 cycles for 15 s at 95 °C (denaturation) and for 60 s at 60 °C (primers annealing and elongation). The signal was collected at the endpoint of every cycle.

*2.5. Analysis of Expression of miR-200 Family Target Genes*

mRNA expression of protein-coding genes was analysed using qPCR based on the TaqMan methodology (Thermo Fisher Scientific, Waltham, MA, USA). A pre-designed mixture of probes and primers specific for target mRNAs expression was used. Prior to qPCR, four pools of RNA samples were created, obtained from normal mucosa, adenomas, advanced CRC without and CRC with nodal metastases. After RT and PreAmp, the pre-amplified cDNA was diluted in four steps, ranging from 5-point dilution to 625-point dilution, and the probes were tested for qPCR efficiency. All the qPCR efficiency reactions were performed on a RotorGene Q (Qiagen, Hilden, Germany) in triplicate.

2.5.1. Reverse Transcription (RT)

Target mRNAs of the *miR-200* family, *CDKN1B, ONECUT2, PTPN13, RND3, SOX2, TGFB2, WAVE3, ZEB1* and *ZEB2* (Table 1), were analysed relatively to the geometric mean of RGs, *IPO8* and *B2M*. mRNAs were reverse transcribed using a OneTaq RT-PCR Kit (New England Biolabs, Ipswich, MA, USA) using random primers according to the manufacturer's instructions. Reverse transcription reactions were started with 3.0 μL (60 ng) of total RNA and 1.0 μL of Random Primer Mix incubated at 70 °C for 5 min. The 10 μL RT master mix included 5.0 μL of M-MuLV Reaction Mix, 1.0 μL of M-MuLV reverse transcriptase and 4.0 μL of reaction mix after random priming. The reaction conditions were: 25 °C for 5 min, t 42 °C for 60 min and 80 °C for 4 min.

2.5.2. Pre-Amplification and Quantitative Real-Time PCR (qPCR)

Following RT, pre-amplification was performed using a TaqMan PreAmp Master Mix (Applied Biosystems, Foster City, CA, USA) in 10 μL according to the manufacturer's protocol. The resulting PreAmp reaction was diluted 5-fold and 4.5 μL was used in a 10 μL reaction volume with a 5.0 μL of 2x FastStart Essential DNA Probe Master Mix (Roche, Basel, Switzerland) and 0.5 μL of TaqMan probe. Thermal conditions were applied as follows: 50 °C for 2 min, initial denaturation at 95 °C for 10 min and 40 cycles of denaturation at 95 °C for 15 s and annealing at 60 °C for 1 min. All qPCR analyses were performed on a Rotor Gene Q (Qiagen, Hilden, Germany) in duplicate. The signal was collected at the endpoint of each cycle.

*2.6. Statistical Analysis of Experimental Data*

The results were presented as relative gene expression. All Cqs were corrected for PCR efficiencies and the expression of the gene of interest (GOI, $Cq_{GOI}$) was calculated relative to a geometric mean of RGs ($Cq_{RG}$), named $\Delta Cq$. In CRC samples, mRNAs and miRNAs expression differences were compared between tumours and adjacent normal tissue using $\Delta Cq$ and the Willcoxon Rank test. For comparison of relative quantification of mRNA and miRNA between independent groups of samples (i.e., adenomas and normal mucosa), $\Delta Cq$ and the Mann-Whitney test were used. The same test was used for comparison of tumours with nodal metastases to those without nodal metastases, except that $\Delta\Delta Cq$ was used. For all correlations/associations, Spearman rank-order correlation was used. Statistical analysis of data was performed using SPSS version 24 (SPSS Inc., Chicago, IL, USA). Differences were considered to be significant at $p < 0.05$.

## 3. Results

*3.1. Patients and Tissue Samples*

The group of adenomas included 10 patients, the group of CRC without lymph node metastases (CRC N0) included 13 patients and the group of CRC with lymph node metastases (CRC N+) included 17 patients. As a control group, microscopically normal colon mucosa from surgical margins from 30 patients with CRC N0 and CRC N+ was used. Sex, age and location for each group are presented in Table 2. Only cases with a clear-cut biopsy diagnosis were included. In the group of adenomas, there were four tubular adenomas with high grade dysplasia, four tubulovillous adenomas with high grade dysplasia and two tubulovillous adenomas with low grade dysplasia.

All tissue samples were fixed for 24 h in 10% buffered formalin prior to paraffin embedding. After fixation and embedding, tissues were cut into 3–4 μm slides and stained with haematoxylin and eosin for routine histopathological examination. For the purposes of our study, representative paraffin blocks were collected from the archives of the Institute of Pathology, Faculty of Medicine, University of Ljubljana.

Table 2. Patients' characteristics and results of immunohistochemistry for E-cadherin.

| Group | Age (Mean ± SD) | Gender (Male:Female) | pTNM [1] | No. of Cases with Weak or Focal Loss of Staining of E-Cadherin |
|---|---|---|---|---|
| Adenoma (n = 10) | 61.00 ± 10.99 | 10:0 | - | 4 <br> 40.0% |
| CRC N0 (n = 13) | 74.62 ± 11.09 | 4:9 | pT1N0 (n = 1) <br> pT2N0 (n = 2) <br> pT3N0 (n = 8) <br> pT4N0 (n = 2) | 7 <br> 53.9% |
| CRC N+ (n = 17) | 70.88 ± 13.87 | 8:9 | pT3N1 (n = 6) <br> pT4N1 (n = 4) <br> pT4N2 (n = 7) | 9 <br> 52.9% |

[1] pathologic Tumor Node Metastasis classification [15].

*3.2. Immunohistochemistry and Expression of E-Cadherin*

E-cadherin staining was preserved in the normal colon mucosa and mostly in adenomas and carcinomas. However, in a proportion of samples of adenoma and carcinoma, we observed focal loss or weak staining of E-cadherin at the periphery of the lesion or the invasive front. All four cases of adenoma with decreased E-cadherin staining showed high-grade dysplasia. The staining of E-cadherin was also decreased in seven of 13 cases with CRC N0 and in nine of 17 cases with CRC N+. The results are summarized in Figures 1 and 2 and Table 2.

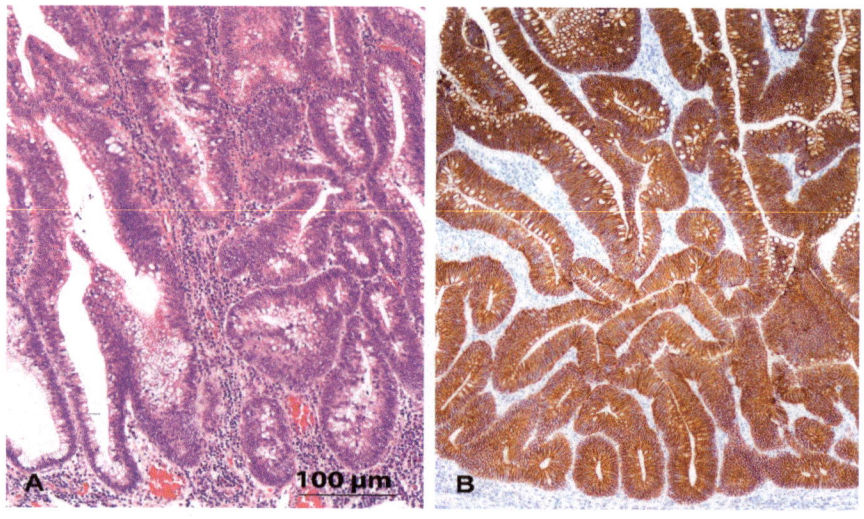

**Figure 1.** (**A**) Tubular adenoma. HE, orig. magnification 100×; (**B**) Immunohistochemistry for E-cadherin in adenoma (n = 10): diffuse, strong membranous reaction. Orig. magnification 100×.

Microscopic analysis of the CRCs and adenomas showed that all cases retained an epithelioid morphology, even those with a decreased expression of E-cadherin. No spindle cell morphology was found in any case of adenoma or CRC, either in the central parts or at the invasive front (Figures 1 and 2).

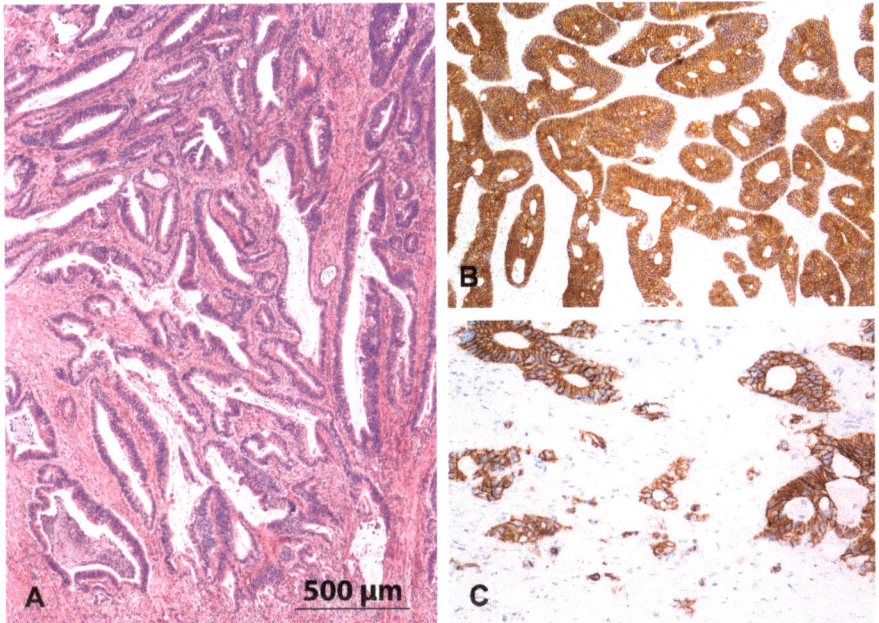

**Figure 2.** (**A**) Moderately differentiated adenocarcinoma. HE, orig. magnification 40×; (**B**,**C**) Immunohistochemistry for E-cadherin in adenocarcinoma ($n = 30$): strong membranous reaction in central part of the tumour (**B**) and focally reduced staining at the invasive tumour front (**C**). Orig. magnification 100×.

*3.3. Undetectable Expression of Markers of EMT*

The expression level of *miR-205*, *ZEB1* (target of *miR-200* family) and *WAVE3* (target of *miR-200b*) was beyond the detection limit when analysing the amplification efficiency on pooled samples. These EMT markers were therefore omitted from further analysis. Expression of *miR-205*, *ZEB1* and *WAVE3* was beyond the limit of detection in all groups, i.e., normal mucosa, adenoma, CRC N0 and CRC N+.

*3.4. Expression of the miR-200 Family and Its Target Genes in Adenoma Compared to Normal Colon Mucosa*

The geometric mean of expression of RGs for miRNA was comparable between adenoma and normal mucosa of patients with CRC N0, but different from the geometric mean of expression in normal mucosa of patients with CRC N+. All the comparisons of adenoma to normal mucosa were therefore performed only with normal mucosa of CRC N0. We also observed a statistical difference for four out of five investigated miRNAs when comparing normal mucosa of CRC N0 with normal mucosa of CRC N+. This observation further supported our selection of normal mucosa samples for comparison of miRNAs and mRNAs expression to that in adenoma.

The expression of all miRNAs was up-regulated in adenoma compared to normal mucosa of CRC N0. Up-regulation was statistically significant in the case of *miR-141* (~12.2-fold, $p = 0.001$), *miR-200b* (~14.3-fold, $p < 0.001$), *miR-200c* (~23.4-fold, $p < 0.001$) and *miR-429* (~33.2-fold, $p < 0.001$). Results are summarized in Figure 3a.

All investigated and expressed target genes, *CDKN1B*, *PTPN13*, *RND3*, *SOX2* and *ZEB2*, were down-regulated in adenoma compared to normal mucosa of CRC N0, except *ONECUT2* and *TGFB2*, which were up-regulated. Moreover, *PTPN13*, *SOX2* and *ZEB2* were expressed only in two out of 10 samples of adenoma, so a calculation of statistical significance would not be appropriate.

To summarize, down-regulation reached statistical significance only in the case of *CDKN1B* (~2.3-fold, $p = 0.015$) and *RND3* (~5.9-fold, $p < 0.001$), both targets of *miR-200b*. Results are summarized in Figure 3b.

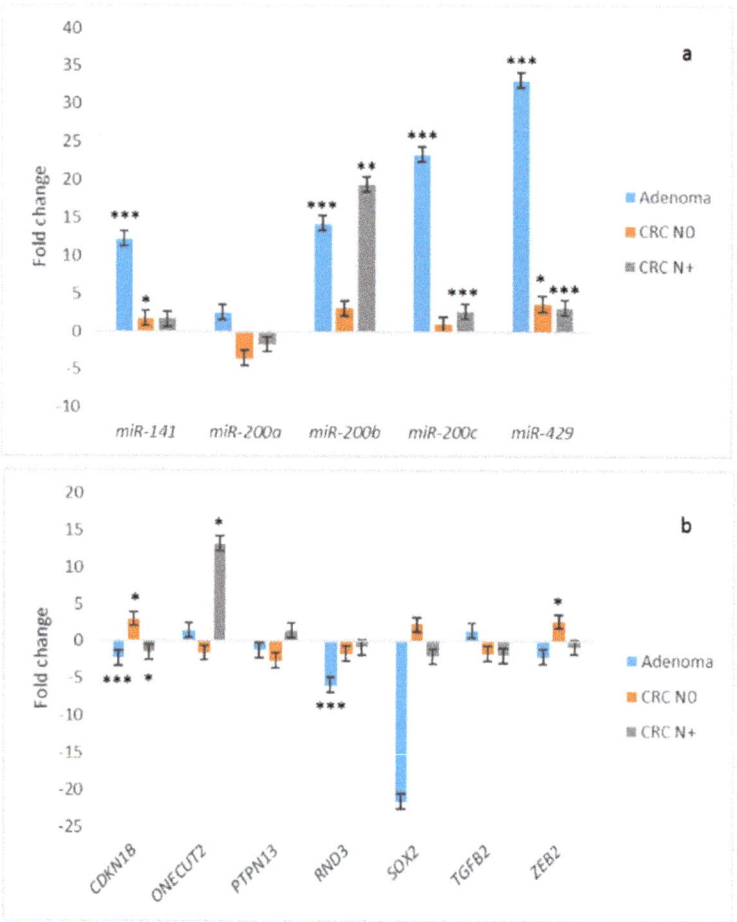

**Figure 3.** Expression of *miR-200* family and their target genes in adenoma ($n = 10$), CRC N0 ($n = 13$) and CRC N+ ($n = 17$) in comparison with normal mucosa ($n = 13$, $n = 13$ and $n = 17$, respectively): (**a**) Expression of *miR-200* family; (**b**) expression of target genes of *miR-200* family. Legend: CRC, colorectal carcinoma; N0, without nodal metastases; N+, with nodal metastases; * $p \leq 0.05$; ** $p \leq 0.01$; *** $p \leq 0.001$.

We also observed a statistically significant strong negative correlation between the expression of *CDKN1B* and *miR-200a* ($r_s = -0.648$, $p = 0.043$) in adenomas.

*3.5. Expression of the miR-200 Family and Its Target Genes in Carcinoma without Nodal Metastasis Compared to Normal Mucosa*

Expression of all miRNAs was up-regulated in CRC N0 compared to corresponding normal mucosa, except *miR-200a*, which was down-regulated. Up-regulation was statistically significant in the case of *miR-141* (~1.7-fold, $p = 0.019$) and *miR-429* (~3.7-fold, $p = 0.041$). Results are summarized in Figure 3a.

In contrast to adenoma, investigated target genes *CDKN1B*, *PTPN13*, *RND3*, *SOX2* and *ZEB2* were up-regulated in CRC N0, except *ONECUT2* and *TGFB2*, which were down-regulated. Statistically significant up-regulation was observed for *CDKN1B* (~3.0-fold, $p = 0.015$) and for *ZEB2* (~2.7-fold, $p = 0.011$). Results are summarized in Figure 3b.

The Spearman coefficient of correlation showed that in CRC N0, expression of *miR-200a* was in correlation with the expression of *TGFB2* ($r_s = 0.900$, $p = 0.037$), *CDKN1B* was in correlation with *miR-141* ($r_s = 0.683$, $p = 0.042$) and *RND3* to *miR-200c* ($r_s = 0.867$, $p = 0.002$). All correlations were positive and strong or very strong. Results are presented in Figure 4.

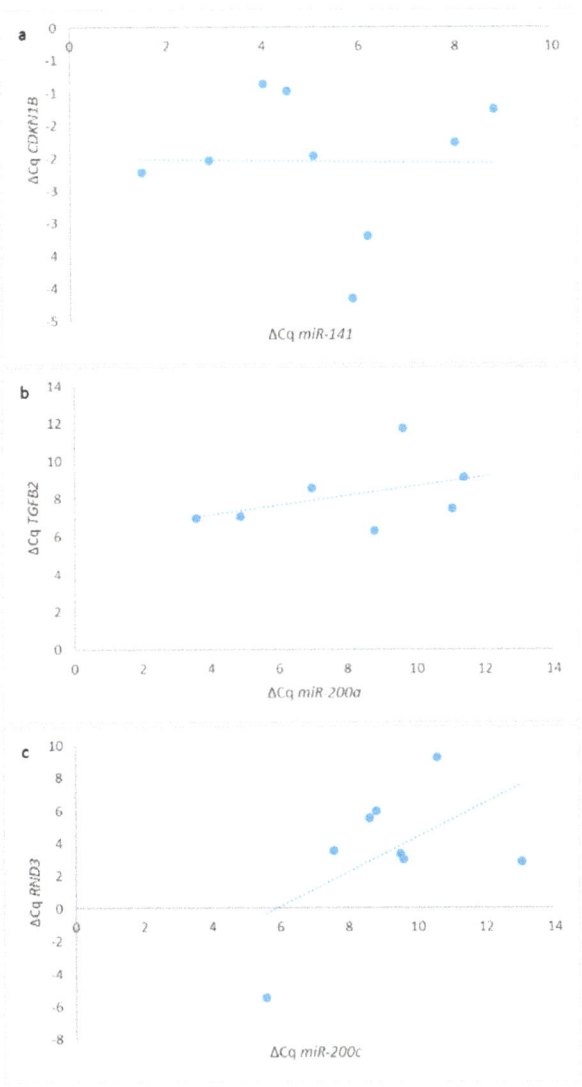

**Figure 4.** Correlations of expression of *miR-200* family and their target genes in CRC N0 ($n = 10$): (**a**) correlation between *miR-141* and *CDKN1B*; (**b**) correlation between *miR-200a* and *TGFB2*; (**c**) correlation between *miR-200c* and *RND3*.

### 3.6. Expression of the miR-200 Family and Its Target Genes in Carcinoma with Nodal Metastasis Compared to Normal Mucosa

The expression of all miRNAs, except *miR-200a*, was up-regulated in CRC N+ compared to corresponding normal mucosa; up-regulation was statistically significant in the case of *miR-200b* (~19.4-fold, $p < 0.001$), *miR-200c* (~2.7-fold, $p = 0.003$) and *miR-429* (~3.2-fold, $p = 0.006$). Results are summarized in Figure 3a.

Expression of miRNAs' targets was more heterogeneous in CRC N+ than in adenoma and CRC N0. *PTPN13*, *ONECUT*, *SOX2* and *RND3* were up-regulated, and *TGFB2*, *ZEB2* and *CDKN1B* showed down-regulation in CRC N+ compared to its corresponding normal mucosa. Statistical significance was reached only in the case of *CDKN1B* (~1.5-fold, $p = 0.017$) and *ONECUT* (~13.1-fold, $p = 0.018$). Results are summarized in Figure 3b.

The Spearman coefficient of correlation showed that *miR-200a*, *miR-200c* and *miR-141* were expressed in negative correlation with *TGFB2* in CRC N+ ($r_s = -0.841$, $p = 0.005$; $r_s = -0.765$, $p = 0.016$; $r_s = -0.668$, $p = 0.049$; respectively).

### 3.7. Expression of miRNAs and Their Target Genes in Adenomas Compared to Carcinomas

We observed a statistically significant difference in the expression patterns of *miR-200* family and their target genes when adenomas were compared to CRC N0 or CRC N+. Four miRNAs were differentially expressed between adenomas and either CRC N0 or CRC N+ (*miR-200a*, $p = 0.026$ and $p < 0.001$, respectively; *miR-200c*, $p = 0.001$ and $p < 0.001$, respectively; *miR-141*, $p = 0.007$ and $p < 0.001$, respectively; *miR-429*, $p = 0.011$ and $p < 0.001$, respectively); *miR-200b* was differentially expressed only between adenomas and CRC N+ ($p = 0.003$). Results are summarized in Figure 5a.

In contrast to miRNA, the only miRNAs target gene that was differentially expressed between adenomas and both CRC N0 and CRC N+ was *CDKN1B* ($p < 0.001$ and $p = 0.001$, respectively). In adenomas, differential expression in comparison with CRC N0 was also observed for *ZEB2* ($p = 0.034$) and *SOX2* ($p = 0.046$), and in comparison with CRC N+, *ONECUT2* ($p = 0.006$) and *RND3* ($p < 0.001$). Results are summarized in Figure 5b.

### 3.8. Comparison of Expression of miRNAs and Its Target Genes in Carcinoma with Nodal Metastases to Carcinoma without Nodal Metastasis

Expression in each carcinoma sample was normalized to its corresponding normal mucosa. Groups of CRC N0 and CRC N+ were then compared with each other. It was shown that there was no significant change in expression of investigated miRNAs between CRC N+ compared with CRC N0, except for *miR-200b*. Results are summarized in Figure 6a.

Target genes of the *miR-200* family, *ONECUT2* showed up-regulation in CRC N+ compared with CRC N0 ($p = 0.028$), whereas *ZEB2* and *CDKN1B* showed down-regulation in CRC N+ compared with CRC N0 ($p = 0.038$ and $p = 0.001$, respectively). Results are summarized in Figure 6b.

### 3.9. Tumour Heterogeneity-Expression of the miR-200 Family in the Central Parts of Carcinoma Compared to the Invasive Front

In a subset of CRC N0 ($n = 7$) and CRC N+ samples ($n = 8$), there was enough material to obtain tissue cores from the central parts and invasive front of the tumour. All miRNAs were mainly down-regulated at the invasive front compared with central part of the tumour.

In the case of CRC N0, four out of seven samples showed down-regulation at the invasive front compared with the central part of tumour, with no statistically significant change in expression. In CRC N+, seven out of eight samples showed down-regulation at the invasive front compared with the central part, with certain miRNA expression being absent, i.e., *miR-200c*. A statistically significant difference in expression between the invasive front and central parts of the tumour was observed for *miR-200b* ($p = 0.028$) and *miR-429* ($p = 0.028$).

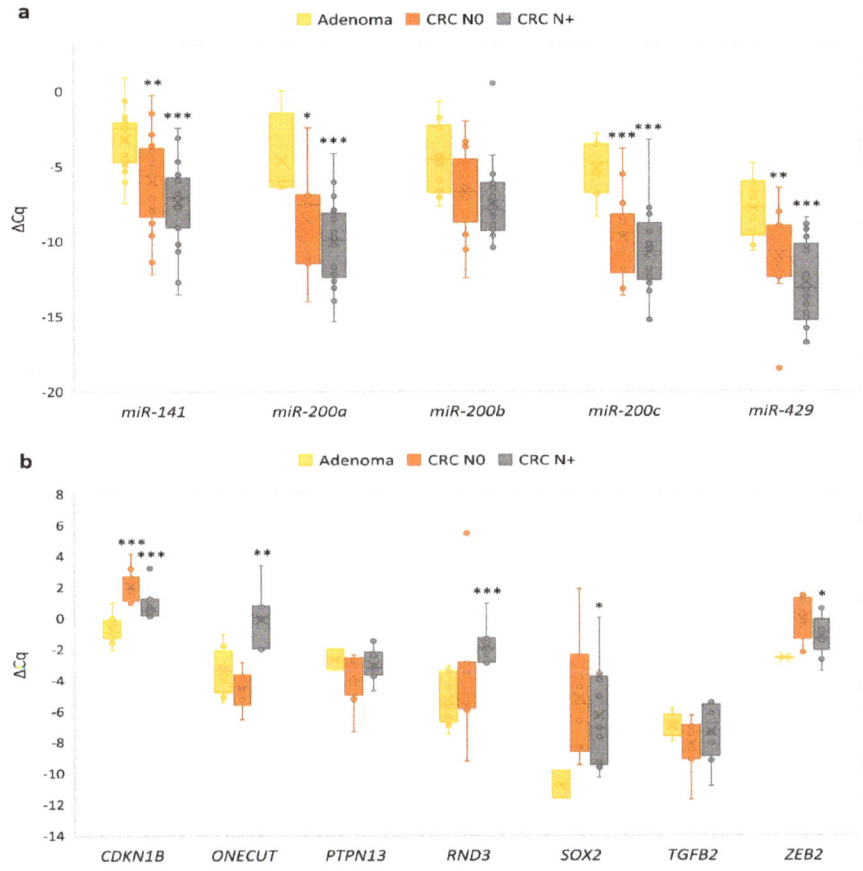

**Figure 5.** Expression of the *miR-200* family and their target genes in adenoma ($n = 10$) in comparison with CRC N0 ($n = 13$) and CRC N+ ($n = 17$): (**a**) expression of the *miR-200* family; (**b**) expression of *miR-200* family target genes. Legend: CRC, colorectal carcinoma; ΔCq, delta quantitation cycle; N0, without nodal metastases; N+, with nodal metastases; * $p \le 0.05$; ** $p \le 0.01$; *** $p \le 0.001$.

Additionally, the expression of *miR-200b* was significantly differentially expressed when invasive front (normalized to the central parts of the tumour) was compared between CRC N0 and CRC N+ ($p = 0.046$).

Results are presented in Figure 7 as a heat-map of FC between invasive front and central parts for each sample.

*3.10. Expression of E-Cadherin and Correlation of Its Expression to the Expression of miRNAs and mRNAs*

All miRNAs showed down-regulation and all their target genes showed up-regulation in samples of CRC when comparing those with focal or weak E-cadherin staining with those with preserved staining. A statistically significant change in expression was observed in the case of all miRNAs ($p = 0.036$ for *miR-141*, $p = 0.003$ for *miR-200a*, $p = 0.014$ for *miR-200b*, $p = 0.003$ for *miR-200c*, $p = 0.034$ for *miR-429*) and in the case of SOX2 ($p = 0.05$). Results are summarized in Figure 8a,b.

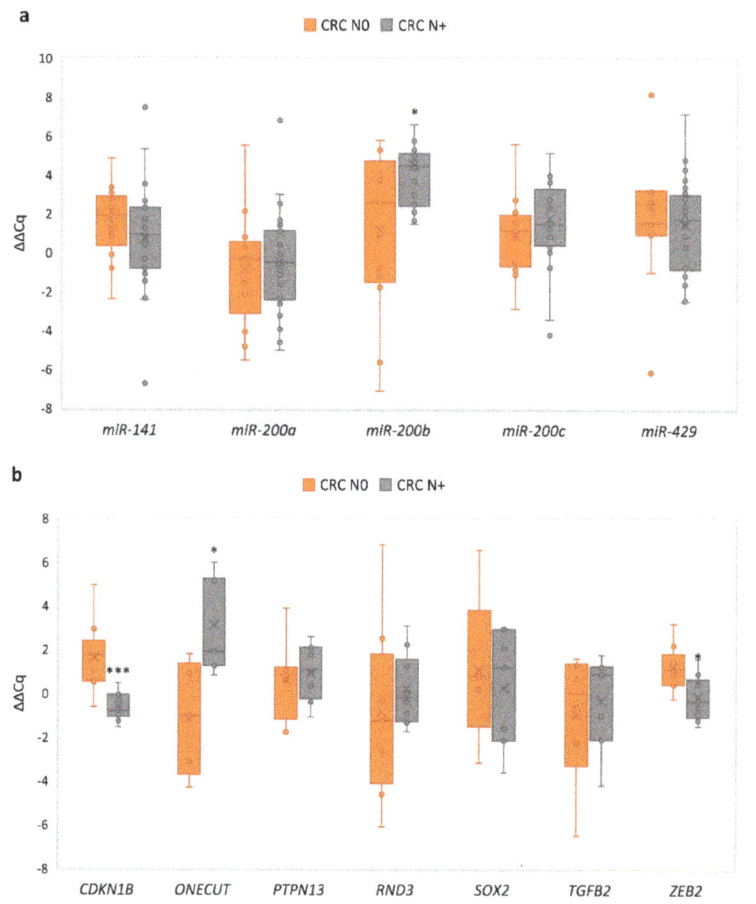

**Figure 6.** Expression of the *miR-200* family and their target genes in CRC N0 (*n* = 13) in comparison with CRC N+ (*n* = 17): (**a**) expression of the *miR-200* family; (**b**) expression of *miR-200* family target genes. Legend: CRC, colorectal carcinoma; ΔΔCq, delta quantitation cycle; N0, without nodal metastases; N+, with nodal metastases; * $p \leq 0.05$; *** $p \leq 0.001$.

| Sample Number | CRC | FC_miR-141 | FC_miR-200a | FC_miR-200b | FC_miR-200c | FC_miR-429 |
|---|---|---|---|---|---|---|
| 1 | CRC N0 | 0.46 | 0.27 | 0.56 | 0.59 | 0.29 |
| 2 | CRC N0 | 0.24 | 0.45 | 0.41 | 0.36 | 0.41 |
| 3 | CRC N0 | 0.18 | 0.11 | 0.14 | 0.12 | 0.11 |
| 4 | CRC N0 | 0.44 | 0.36 | 1.20 | 0.44 | 0.43 |
| 5 | CRC N0 | 1.88 | 2.91 | 3.81 | 2.41 | 2.23 |
| 6 | CRC N0 | 2.96 | 1.74 | 2.04 | 1.37 | 2.38 |
| 7 | CRC N0 | 1.69 | 1.54 | 1.84 | 2.01 | 1.15 |
| 8 | CRC N+ | 1.60 | 0.12 | No exp in C | No exp in C | 0.31 |
| 9 | CRC N+ | 0.02 | No exp at IF | 0.52 | No exp at IF and in C | No exp at IF |
| 10 | CRC N+ | 0.04 | 0.37 | 0.01 | No exp at IF and in C | 0.11 |
| 11 | CRC N+ | 0.18 | 0.61 | 0.14 | 0.27 | No exp in C |
| 12 | CRC N+ | 0.65 | 0.09 | 0.84 | No exp in C | 0.27 |
| 13 | CRC N+ | 1.62 | 9.49 | No exp in C | No exp in C | 0.85 |
| 14 | CRC N+ | 0.30 | 0.16 | 0.18 | 0.51 | 0.15 |
| 15 | CRC N+ | 0.12 | 0.24 | 0.29 | 0.52 | 0.27 |

**Figure 7.** Heat-map of *miR-200* family expression at the invasive front in comparison with central parts of the CRC. Legend: C, central part of the tumour; CRC, colorectal cancer; exp, expression; FC, fold change; IF invasive front; N0, without nodal metastases; N+, with nodal metastases.

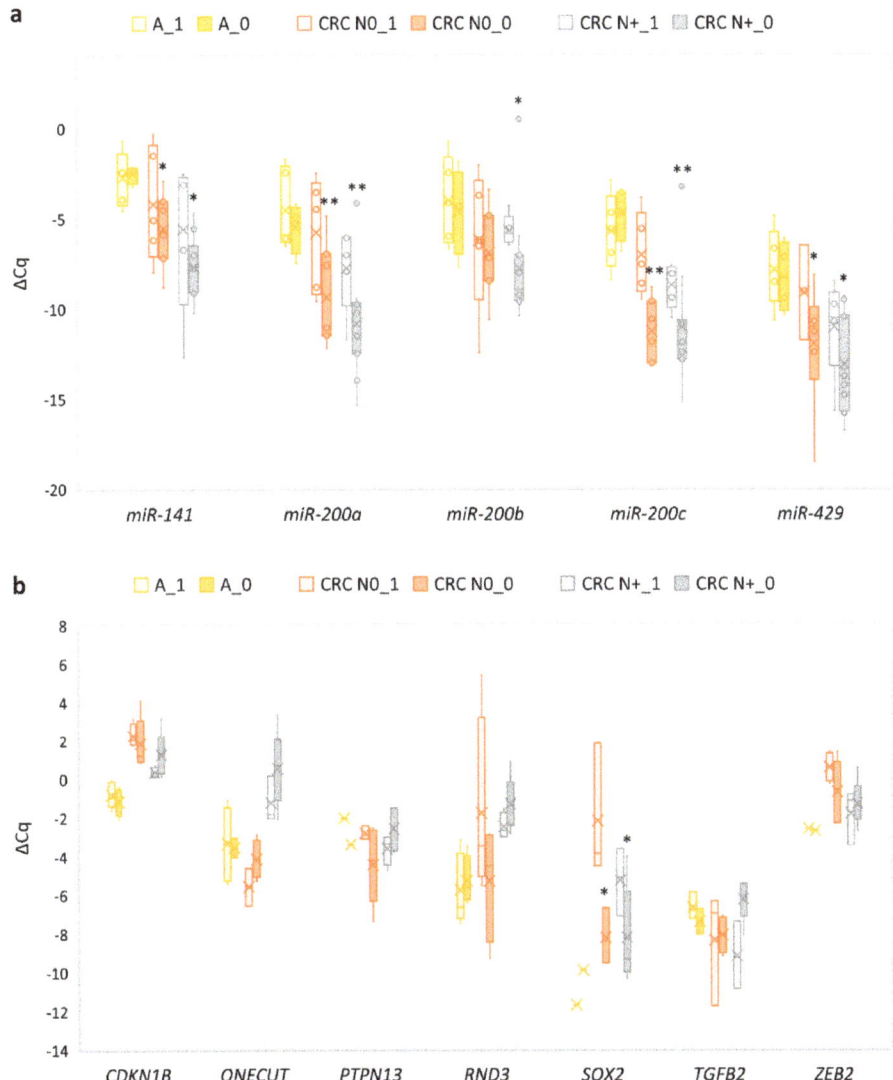

**Figure 8.** Expression of *miR-200* family and their target genes in adenoma, CRC N0 and CRC N+ based on E-cadherin expression: (**a**) expression of *miR-200* family; (**b**) expression of target genes of *miR-200* family. Legend: CRC, colorectal carcinoma; N0, without nodal metastases; N+, with nodal metastases; 1, preserved expression of E-cadherin ($n = 6$, $n = 6$ and $n = 8$ for adenoma, CRC N0 and CRC N+, respectively); 0, weak or focal loss of E-cadherin ($n = 4$, $n = 7$ and $n = 9$ for adenoma, CRC N0 and CRC N+, respectively); * $p \leq 0.05$; ** $p \leq 0.01$.

*3.11. Correlations between miRNAs and Their Target Genes across All Samples*

Numerous correlations were observed between the expression of miRNAs and the expression of their target genes. Surprisingly, correlations between the expression of certain miRNAs and genes that are not yet functionally validated as targets for that particular miRNA, were also observed. All observed correlations are summarized in table (Table 3).

**Table 3.** Statistically significant correlations between expression of *miR-200* family and their target genes and association with E-cadherin staining.

| Correlations | CDKN1B | ONECUT2 | PTPN13 | RND3 | SOX2 | TGFB2 | ZEB2 | E-Cadherin |
|---|---|---|---|---|---|---|---|---|
| *miR-200a* | −0.360 | −0.395 | / | −0.325 | / | / | / | 0.474 |
| *miR-200b* | / | / | / | −0.384 | / | / | / | 0.400 |
| *miR-200c* | −0.503 | / | / | −0.337 | / | / | / | 0.484 |
| *miR-141* | / | / | / | −0.351 | / | / | / | 0.355 |
| *miR-429* | / | / | / | −0.347 | / | / | / | 0.363 |
| E-cadherin | / | / | / | / | 0.521 | / | / | 1 |

Additionally, the expression of *miR-200b* ($r_s = -0.499$, $p < 0.001$) and *miR-429* ($r_s = -0.287$, $p = 0.014$) were in negative correlation with the severity of the disease (normal mucosa, adenoma, CRC N0 and CRC N+). When samples were divided into only three groups (normal mucosa, adenoma and CRC), a correlation of the severity of the disease was observed with the expression of a higher number of miRNAs and their target genes, namely *miR-200b* ($r_s = -0.620$, $p < 0.001$), *miR-200c* ($r_s = -0.401$, $p < 0.001$), *miR-141* ($r_s = -0.420$, $p < 0.001$), *miR-429* ($r_s = -0.522$, $p < 0.001$), and *CDKN1B* ($r_s = 0.377$, $p = 0.007$), *PTPN13* ($r_s = -0.426$, $p = 0.006$), and *RND3* ($r_s = 0.467$, $p = 0.016$).

## 4. Discussion

EMT has emerged as an important mechanism in cancerogenesis but its role in CRC remains only partially understood. Full EMT is usually observed only in well-controlled experimental conditions, e.g., in cell lines, but it is rarely observed in human tumours [11,16]. We therefore hypothesized that partial EMT, but not full EMT, is induced during CRC cancerogenesis. Our previous studies showed that the use of a single or a few epithelial or mesenchymal markers as a tool for following EMT as a whole is not appropriate [16]. We therefore used several EMT markers (E-cadherin, *miR-200* family and their target genes) in correlation with morphology. Our results support the hypothesis that EMT plays an important role in CRC, both in its development and progression, but only as partial EMT. Our analysis was performed on normal mucosa, adenoma, and carcinoma, including CRC cases with and without nodal metastases, and a comparison between the invasive front and central part of the tumours.

We first analysed the expression of members of the *miR-200* family, which have been demonstrated as one of the key regulators of EMT in various experimental and human studies [11,16,17]. We found that all five investigated miRNAs were significantly down-regulated in CRC in comparison with adenoma. Both *miR-200a* and *miR-200b* down-regulation have already been described in CRC samples [18–20]. However, the results on *miR-141*, *miR-200c* and *miR-429* expression in previous studies are controversial. Whereas, one study described decreased expression of *miR-141* in CRC tissue [21], another study reported up-regulation in CRC compared with adjunct normal mucosa [22]. Similarly, *miR-200c* was observed as up-regulated in some studies [23–25] but down-regulated in others [26]. Furthermore, *miR-429* has previously been described as both down-regulated [27] and up-regulated in CRC tissue [28,29]. Our study also showed that all members of the *miR-200* family were up-regulated in adenomas and all, except *miR-200a*, in CRC compared with normal mucosa. In contrast to CRC, there are limited data in the literature on expression of the *miR-200* family in colorectal adenomas and rare published studies have reported that *miR-200a* and *miR-200c* were not significantly changed in adenoma tissue when compared with normal mucosa [30].

The finding of a partial EMT induction is further supported by immunohistochemical analysis of E-cadherin, showing focal loss or weak expression in a proportion of adenoma and CRC, and its correlation with down-regulation of all members of the *miR-200* family. Similarly to previously reported studies on E-cadherin expression [31], we found that staining was preserved in all cases of CRC and adenoma, with prevailing membranous immunoreactivity. However, in contrast to our results, a previous study reported that there was no difference between protein expression in tumours and normal mucosa. Another study reported a similar observation as in our study, i.e., E-cadherin expression in all colorectal adenomas and CRC, although it presented with reduced expression in half of them [32]. It has been previously described that *miR-200a* is down-regulated in cells with a reduced expression of E-cadherin protein [18], whereas *miR-200b* decline was not statistically associated with expression of E-cadherin [33]. However, there are limited data about the expression of other members of the *miR-200* family in correlation with E-cadherin protein expression. Our study thus suggests that EMT is induced during CRC cancerogenesis through down-regulation of the *miR-200* family, resulting in a focal loss or weak expression of E-cadherin that might be often observed in partial EMT, in which cells transiently acquire the maximum plasticity and attain hybrid epithelial/mesenchymal phenotype [34].

Though these results strongly suggest induction of EMT in CRC, one criterion for full EMT was not fulfilled, i.e., morphology. When we performed microscopic analysis of CRC and adenoma in comparison with E-cadherin immunohistochemistry, we found that all cases retained an epithelioid morphology, even those with decreased expression of E-cadherin. No spindle cell morphology was found in any case of adenoma or CRC, either in the central parts or at the invasive front. Cell–cell junctions connect epithelial cells, they are polarized, differentiating epithelia from other tissues. In contrast, mesenchymal cells are not polarized and do not possess cell–cell junctions. They are therefore able to migrate through the extracellular matrix, invade and resist apoptosis. During full EMT, epithelial cells undergo extensive changes, they lose polarity, cell–cell junctions (i.e., loss of functional E-cadherin) and reorganize their cytoskeleton, resulting in spindle shaped cells. All these changes lead to a separation of cells and an increase in cell motility at the invasive front [2,5–12].

Interestingly, when we compared *miR-200* family expression in the central parts of the tumours and the invasive front, we found their down-regulation at the invasive front in 73% of cases. However, the difference was significant only for *miR-200b*. This finding further supports the concept of ITH even on the level of miRNAs [14]. *miR 200b* was found to be down-regulated in tumour budding cells at the invasive front in 71% of cases [33] and is believed to have a tumour-promoting role in CRC by targeting *RND3* and *CDKN1B* [35]. In addition to *miR-200b*, several published data also described decreased expression of *miR-200c* at the invasive front of the tumour in metastatic CRC cases [36–38]. Additionally, *miR-200a/b/c* were also found to be down-regulated at the invasive front of CRC cases with degraded basement membrane [39] but there is limited data in the literature about the expression of *miR-141* and *miR-429* at the invasive front. Down-regulation of the *miR-200* family is believed to be correlated with the loss of the epithelial and gain of the mesenchymal-like phenotype at the invasive front, resulting in increased invasiveness of the CRC tumour cells, thus contributing to migration through the extracellular matrix, colonization of the lymph node and metastatic potential [40]. There is limited data on the expression of coding and/or non-coding genes at the invasive front in comparison with the tumour centre. Previous studies [38,39] and our findings indicate an expression gradient of the *miR-200* family related to ITH. However, recent publications have reported ITH mainly in the context of mutation, copy number variation and methylation status [41–43]. ITH includes spatial and temporal ITH, morphological ITH, clonal ITH (derived from genomic instability), and non-clonal ITH (derived from microenvironment interactions). Since ITH is believed to be closely related to cancer progression, resistance to therapy, and recurrence, it is important to consider different types of ITH when investigating mechanisms of cancer progression, prognosis and treatment opportunities [14].

One of the most important aspects of CRC is its metastatic capacities. We therefore analysed the contribution of EMT to the development of nodal metastases. Since invasive properties and metastatic potential are not equivalent functional terms [44], we compared CRC cases without with those witht nodal metastases. We found statistically significant up-regulation of *miR-200b* in CRC with compared with CRC without nodal metastases, implicating miRNAs and possibly EMT in the progression of CRC. This observation and the observed potential invasive role of *miR-200b* in CRC suggest a contribution of *miR-200b* to the invasive and metastatic properties of CRC. Expression of *miR-200b* and *miR-429* were also in correlation with the pTNM stage of CRC, further suggesting a role not only of *miR-200b* but also *miR-429* in CRC progression. It has already been reported that both *miR-200b* and *miR-429* might contribute to the metastatic potential of CRC [20,29,45] and moreover, that up-regulation of *miR-141* contributes to the development of distant metastases in breast cancer [46].

We also investigated target genes (*CDKN1B*, *ONECUT2*, *PTPN13*, *RND3*, *SOX2*, *TGFB2*, *WAVE3*, *ZEB1* and *ZEB2*) of the *miR-200* family. Interestingly, only *CDKN1B*, *ONECUT2* and *ZEB2* were differentially expressed in CRC without nodal metastases compared with CRC with nodal metastases. *ZEB2* and *CDKN1B* are targets of *miR-200b* and *ONECUT2* is a target of *miR-429*. Our observation in relation to *CDKN1B* is in accordance with a previously reported study showing that reduced expression of *CDKN1B* is correlated with a poor prognosis for patients with CRC [47]. Using experimental models, it has been shown that *miR-429* reverses TGF-β-induced EMT by interfering with ONECUT2 in CRC cells [26]. However, to the best of our knowledge, this is the first report of ONECUT2 involvement in the human metastatic potential of CRC. In contrast, it has already been reported that ZEB2, which is one of the first identified *miR-200* family targets, promotes tumour metastatic potential and correlates with a poor prognosis for human CRC [48–50]. We observed an inverse expression of *miR-200b* and *ZEB2* in CRC with nodal metastases compared with CRC without nodal metastases, further supporting the postulated ZEB/miR-200 interaction in CRC cancerogenesis [50].

In addition to metastatic potential, all target genes were differentially expressed in CRC compared with normal mucosa. Interestingly, this finding is opposite to that observed in adenoma compared with normal mucosa. The majority of target genes (*CDKN1B*, *PTPN13*, *RND3*, *SOX2* and *ZEB2*) were down-regulated in adenoma compared to normal mucosa. Moreover, *PTPN13*, *SOX2* and *ZEB2* showed detectable expression only in two out of 10 adenoma cases, whereas *ONECUT2* and *TGFB2* were up-regulated. There is limited data on the expression of target genes of the *miR-200* family in colorectal adenoma and, to the best of our knowledge, only *CDKN1B* and *SOX2* have so far been investigated, excluding studies on dysplastic lesions in inflammatory bowel diseases. Immunohistochemistry for *SOX2* has shown that it is expressed in a minority of adenoma cases and all of them were with high-grade dysplasia [51,52]. Similarly, both of our cases that showed expression of *SOX2* (also showing expression of *PTPN13* and *ZEB2*) were adenomas with high-grade dysplasia. Our results thus suggest that an inverse expression of the *miR-200* family and *SOX2* might contribute to the differentiation/proliferation of cells also during CRC cancerogenesis, as already described in neurons [53]. *CDKN1B* was expressed in all cases of adenoma, however, limited published data have reported that *CDKN1B* is not expressed in approx. 20% of adenomas and carcinomas [54] and that its expression does not significantly change during the adenoma–carcinoma sequence/progression of CRC [55]. The only gene that was in correlation to all investigated miRNAs was *RND3*, also known as *RHOE*. *RND3* plays a critical role in arresting cell cycle distribution, inhibiting cell growth and inducing apoptosis and differentiation, and is implicated in processes such as proliferation and migration through cytoskeletal rearrangement. Although it appears that this protein is differently altered according to the tumour context, it has been demonstrated that aberrant *RND3* expression may be the leading cause of tumour metastasis and chemotherapy resistance with a pro-tumourigenic role [56,57]. Accordingly, in tumour and adjacent normal tissues from 202 patients with CRC, including 80 nodal metastases, Rnd3 expression using immunohistochemistry was analysed. Its expression was significantly correlated with depth of invasion, lymph node metastasis and distant metastasis. Most importantly, disease-free and overall survivals were significantly poorer for patients with Rnd3-positive tumours than for those with Rnd3-negative [58].

We were not able to detect expression of certain EMT markers. First, we were not able to detect expression of *miR-205* in the tissue samples of normal colon mucosa, adenoma or CRC. Although there are some published studies on *miR-205* expression in experimental models of CRC, only a few of them have described expression in tissue specimens of patients with CRC [59–61]. In all of them, *miR-205* was down-regulated, detected on fresh frozen tissues. Members of the *miR-200* family have been observed not only as regulators of EMT but also of EMT-transcriptional factors (EMT-TF), e.g., *ZEB1* and *ZEB2*. However, *ZEB1* was below the detection limit in our samples, whereas *ZEB2* was expressed. In the case of EMT-TFs, there is a possible difference in spatiotemporal expression, depending on the tissue context and tumour type [11]. Members of the same EMT-TF family can even have antagonistic functions. Furthermore, it has been demonstrated that activation of any single EMT-TF is sufficient to induce partial/incomplete EMT and an absence of specific EMT-TF cannot be considered to be proof of the absence of EMT [44]. We were also not able to detect a target gene of *miR-200b*, *WAVE3*, involved in actin cytoskeleton remodelling, participating in the control of cell shape [13].

One of the limitations of our study is a different comparison between adenomas and CRC, and normal mucosa. In excised adenomas (because of endoscopic removal), normal mucosa is often not present, or it is present in very small amounts. In contrast, in patients with CRC, the colon was resected and all resected specimens contained normal mucosa. Each CRC sample was therefore compared to its corresponding normal mucosa as paired tissue samples, using the Wilcoxon Rank test. In contrast, adenomas were compared with normal mucosa samples of CRC resected samples as independent groups of samples, using the Mann–Whitney test. The difference in genetic background, which should be eliminated when comparing paired tissue samples, could lead to overestimation of changes in expression in adenomas in comparison to normal mucosa. Another limitation is related to "normal" samples, which very often present a significant problem in human research. As healthy colon is not resected, truly normal mucosa cannot be obtained. In our study, "normal" samples were taken at least 20 cm away from the tumour and they showed no microscopic abnormalities. However, genetic and protein aberrations may also be present in morphologically normal mucosa [62], although it seems highly unlikely that EMT is activated in such samples. We therefore believe that, despite certain limitations, these samples may be used as corresponding control samples to overcome differences in the genetic background. Moreover, in addition to tumours, various inflammatory diseases, infarction etc. are also an indication for colon surgery. However, when studying EMT, these resection specimens are not suitable for "normal" control, since EMT can also be activated in these diseases.

## 5. Conclusions

Comparing the expression of the *miR-200* family and their target genes in adenoma and CRC with and without nodal metastases showed three patterns. The first pattern was observed in adenoma in comparison with normal mucosa. The second, and opposite to the first, was observed in CRC compared with adenoma and the third pattern was observed in cases of CRC with nodal metastases. Interestingly, all investigated miRNAs were down-regulated in cases with a reduced E-cadherin expression and were mainly down-regulated at the invasive front in comparison with central parts of the tumour. Our results strongly support the postulated hypothesis of partial EMT and ITH during CRC cancerogenesis.

**Author Contributions:** Conceptualization, N.Z. and E.B.; methodology, M.Ž. and E.B.; software, E.B. and M.Ž.; validation, M.Ž., B.R. and E.B.; formal analysis, M.Ž., B.R. and E.B.; investigation, M.Ž., and B.R.; resources, N.Z. and B.R.; writing—original draft preparation, B.R. and E.B.; writing—review and editing, E.B. and N.Z.; visualization, M.Ž.; supervision, E.B. and N.Z. Authorship must be limited to those who have contributed substantially to the work reported.

**Funding:** This research was funded by Slovenian Research Agency, grant number J3-1754 and P3-0054.

**Conflicts of Interest:** The authors declare no conflict of interest.

## References

1. Balch, C.; Ramapuram, J.B.; Tiwari, A.K. The epigenomics of embryonic pathway signaling in colorectal cancer. *Front. Pharmacol.* **2017**, *8*, 267. [CrossRef] [PubMed]
2. Cao, H.; Xu, E.; Liu, H.; Wan, L.; Lai, M. Epithelial-mesenchymal transition in colorectal cancer metastasis: A system review. *Pathol. Res. Pract.* **2015**, *211*, 557–569. [CrossRef] [PubMed]
3. Nazemalhosseini Mojarad, E.; Kuppen, P.J.; Aghdaei, H.A.; Zali, M.R. The CpG island methylator phenotype (CIMP) in colorectal cancer. *Gastroenterol. Hepatol. Bed Bench* **2013**, *6*, 120–128. [PubMed]

4. Kudryavtseva, A.V.; Lipatova, A.V.; Zaretsky, A.R.; Moskalev, A.A.; Fedorova, M.S.; Rasskazova, A.S.; Shibukhova, G.A.; Snezhkina, A.V.; Kaprin, A.D.; Alekseev, B.Y.; et al. Important molecular genetic markers of colorectal cancer. *Oncotarget* **2016**, *7*, 53959–53983. [CrossRef] [PubMed]
5. Goossens, S.; Vandamme, N.; Van Vlierberghe, P.; Berx, G. EMT transcription factors in cancer development re-evaluated: Beyond EMT and MET. *Biochim. Biophys. Acta Rev. Cancer* **2017**, *1868*, 584–591. [CrossRef] [PubMed]
6. Iwatsuki, M.; Mimori, K.; Yokobori, T.; Ishi, H.; Beppu, T.; Nakamori, S.; Baba, H.; Mori, M. Epithelial-mesenchymal transition in cancer development and its clinical significance. *Cancer Sci.* **2010**, *101*, 293–299. [CrossRef]
7. Prieto-Garcia, E.; Diaz-Garcia, C.V.; Garcia-Ruiz, I.; Agullo-Ortuno, M.T. Epithelial-to-mesenchymal transition in tumor progression. *Med. Oncol.* **2017**, *34*, 122. [CrossRef]
8. Acloque, H.; Thiery, J.P.; Nieto, M.A. The physiology and pathology of the EMT. Meeting on the epithelial-mesenchymal transition. *EMBO Rep.* **2008**, *9*, 322–326. [CrossRef]
9. Bryant, D.M.; Mostov, K.E. From cells to organs: Building polarized tissue. *Nat. Rev. Mol. Cell Biol.* **2008**, *9*, 887–901. [CrossRef]
10. Gurzu, S.; Silveanu, C.; Fetyko, A.; Butiurca, V.; Kovacs, Z.; Jung, I. Systematic review of the old and new concepts in the epithelial-mesenchymal transition of colorectal cancer. *World J. Gastroenterol.* **2016**, *22*, 6764–6775. [CrossRef]
11. Stemmler, M.P.; Eccles, R.L.; Brabletz, S.; Brabletz, T. Non-redundant functions of EMT transcription factors. *Nat. Cell Biol.* **2019**, *21*, 102–112. [CrossRef] [PubMed]
12. Findlay, V.J.; Wang, C.; Watson, D.K.; Camp, E.R. Epithelial-to-mesenchymal transition and the cancer stem cell phenotype: Insights from cancer biology with therapeutic implications for colorectal cancer. *Cancer Gene Ther.* **2014**, *21*, 181–187. [CrossRef] [PubMed]
13. Humphries, B.; Yang, C. The microRNA-200 family: Small molecules with novel roles in cancer development, progression and therapy. *Oncotarget* **2015**, *6*, 6472–6498. [CrossRef] [PubMed]
14. Stanta, G.; Bonin, S. Overview on clinical relevance of intra-tumor heterogeneity. *Front. Med. (Lausanne)* **2018**, *5*, 85. [CrossRef] [PubMed]
15. Brierley, J.D.; Gospodarowicz, M.K.; Wittekind, C. (Eds.) *TNM Classification of Malignant Tumours*, 8th ed.; Wiley Blackwell: Oxford, UK, 2017.
16. Zidar, N.; Bostjancic, E.; Gale, N.; Kojc, N.; Poljak, M.; Glavac, D.; Cardesa, A. Down-regulation of microRNAs of the miR-200 family and miR-205, and an altered expression of classic and desmosomal cadherins in spindle cell carcinoma of the head and neck–hallmark of epithelial-mesenchymal transition. *Hum. Pathol.* **2011**, *42*, 482–488. [CrossRef] [PubMed]
17. Zidar, N.; Bostjancic, E.; Jerala, M.; Kojc, N.; Drobne, D.; Stabuc, B.; Glavac, D. Down-regulation of microRNAs of the miR-200 family and up-regulation of Snail and Slug in inflammatory bowel diseases—Hallmark of epithelial-mesenchymal transition. *J. Cell. Mol. Med.* **2016**, *20*, 1813–1820. [CrossRef]
18. Pichler, M.; Ress, A.L.; Winter, E.; Stiegelbauer, V.; Karbiener, M.; Schwarzenbacher, D.; Scheideler, M.; Ivan, C.; Jahn, S.W.; Kiesslich, T.; et al. MiR-200a regulates epithelial to mesenchymal transition-related gene expression and determines prognosis in colorectal cancer patients. *Br. J. Cancer* **2014**, *110*, 1614–1621. [CrossRef]
19. Liang, W.C.; Fu, W.M.; Wong, C.W.; Wang, Y.; Wang, W.M.; Hu, G.X.; Zhang, L.; Xiao, L.J.; Wan, D.C.; Zhang, J.F.; et al. The lncRNA H19 promotes epithelial to mesenchymal transition by functioning as miRNA sponges in colorectal cancer. *Oncotarget* **2015**, *6*, 22513–22525. [CrossRef]
20. Lv, Z.; Wei, J.; You, W.; Wang, R.; Shang, J.; Xiong, Y.; Yang, H.; Yang, X.; Fu, Z. Disruption of the c-Myc/miR-200b-3p/PRDX2 regulatory loop enhances tumor metastasis and chemotherapeutic resistance in colorectal cancer. *J. Transl. Med.* **2017**, *15*, 257. [CrossRef]
21. Feng, L.; Ma, H.; Chang, L.; Zhou, X.; Wang, N.; Zhao, L.; Zuo, J.; Wang, Y.; Han, J.; Wang, G. Role of microRNA-141 in colorectal cancer with lymph node metastasis. *Exp. Ther. Med.* **2016**, *12*, 3405–3410. [CrossRef]
22. Ding, L.; Yu, L.L.; Han, N.; Zhang, B.T. miR-141 promotes colon cancer cell proliferation by inhibiting MAP2K4. *Oncol. Lett.* **2017**, *13*, 1665–1671. [CrossRef]

23. Wang, M.; Zhang, P.; Li, Y.; Liu, G.; Zhou, B.; Zhan, L.; Zhou, Z.; Sun, X. The quantitative analysis by stem-loop real-time PCR revealed the microRNA-34a, microRNA-155 and microRNA-200c overexpression in human colorectal cancer. *Med. Oncol.* **2012**, *29*, 3113–3118. [CrossRef] [PubMed]
24. Chen, J.; Wang, W.; Zhang, Y.; Hu, T.; Chen, Y. The roles of miR-200c in colon cancer and associated molecular mechanisms. *Tumour Biol.* **2014**, *35*, 6475–6483. [CrossRef] [PubMed]
25. Roh, M.S.; Lee, H.W.; Jung, S.B.; Kim, K.; Lee, E.H.; Park, M.I.; Lee, J.S.; Kim, M.S. Expression of miR-200c and its clinicopathological significance in patients with colorectal cancer. *Pathol. Res. Pract.* **2018**, *214*, 350–355. [CrossRef] [PubMed]
26. Lu, Y.X.; Yuan, L.; Xue, X.L.; Zhou, M.; Liu, Y.; Zhang, C.; Li, J.P.; Zheng, L.; Hong, M.; Li, X.N. Regulation of colorectal carcinoma stemness, growth, and metastasis by an miR-200c-Sox2-negative feedback loop mechanism. *Clin. Cancer Res.* **2014**, *20*, 2631–2642. [CrossRef]
27. Sun, Y.; Shen, S.; Liu, X.; Tang, H.; Wang, Z.; Yu, Z.; Li, X.; Wu, M. MiR-429 inhibits cells growth and invasion and regulates EMT-related marker genes by targeting Onecut2 in colorectal carcinoma. *Mol. Cell. Biochem.* **2014**, *390*, 19–30. [CrossRef]
28. Li, J.; Du, L.; Yang, Y.; Wang, C.; Liu, H.; Wang, L.; Zhang, X.; Li, W.; Zheng, G.; Dong, Z. MiR-429 is an independent prognostic factor in colorectal cancer and exerts its anti-apoptotic function by targeting SOX2. *Cancer Lett.* **2013**, *329*, 84–90. [CrossRef]
29. Han, Y.; Zhao, Q.; Zhou, J.; Shi, R. miR-429 mediates tumor growth and metastasis in colorectal cancer. *Am. J. Cancer Res.* **2017**, *7*, 218–233.
30. Wang, X.; Chen, L.; Jin, H.; Wang, S.; Zhang, Y.; Tang, X.; Tang, G. Screening miRNAs for early diagnosis of colorectal cancer by small RNA deep sequencing and evaluation in a Chinese patient population. *Onco Targets Ther.* **2016**, *9*, 1159–1166. [CrossRef]
31. Bezdekova, M.; Brychtova, S.; Sedlakova, E.; Langova, K.; Brychta, T.; Belej, K. Analysis of Snail-1, E-cadherin and claudin-1 expression in colorectal adenomas and carcinomas. *Int. J. Mol. Sci.* **2012**, *13*, 1632–1643. [CrossRef]
32. Kroepil, F.; Fluegen, G.; Totikov, Z.; Baldus, S.E.; Vay, C.; Schauer, M.; Topp, S.A.; Esch, J.S.; Knoefel, W.T.; Stoecklein, N.H. Down-regulation of CDH1 is associated with expression of SNAI1 in colorectal adenomas. *PLoS ONE* **2012**, *7*, e46665. [CrossRef] [PubMed]
33. Knudsen, K.N.; Lindebjerg, J.; Nielsen, B.S.; Hansen, T.F.; Sorensen, F.B. MicroRNA-200b is downregulated in colon cancer budding cells. *PLoS ONE* **2017**, *12*, e0178564. [CrossRef] [PubMed]
34. Jolly, M.K.; Mani, S.A.; Levine, H. Hybrid epithelial/mesenchymal phenotype(s): The 'fittest' for metastasis? *Biochim. Biophys. Acta Rev. Cancer* **2018**, *1870*, 151–157. [CrossRef] [PubMed]
35. Fu, Y.; Liu, X.; Zhou, N.; Du, L.; Sun, Y.; Zhang, X.; Ge, Y. MicroRNA-200b stimulates tumour growth in TGFBR2-null colorectal cancers by negatively regulating p27/kip1. *J. Cell. Physiol.* **2014**, *229*, 772–782. [CrossRef] [PubMed]
36. Hur, K.; Toiyama, Y.; Takahashi, M.; Balaguer, F.; Nagasaka, T.; Koike, J.; Hemmi, H.; Koi, M.; Boland, C.R.; Goel, A. MicroRNA-200c modulates epithelial-to-mesenchymal transition (EMT) in human colorectal cancer metastasis. *Gut* **2013**, *62*, 1315–1326. [CrossRef] [PubMed]
37. Muto, Y.; Suzuki, K.; Kato, T.; Tsujinaka, S.; Ichida, K.; Takayama, Y.; Fukui, T.; Kakizawa, N.; Watanabe, F.; Saito, M.; et al. Heterogeneous expression of zinc-finger E-box-binding homeobox 1 plays a pivotal role in metastasis via regulation of miR-200c in epithelial-mesenchymal transition. *Int. J. Oncol.* **2016**, *49*, 1057–1067. [CrossRef] [PubMed]
38. Jepsen, R.K.; Novotny, G.W.; Klarskov, L.L.; Christensen, I.J.; Hogdall, E.; Riis, L.B. Investigating intra-tumor heterogeneity and expression gradients of miR-21, miR-92a and miR-200c and their potential of predicting lymph node metastases in early colorectal cancer. *Exp. Mol. Pathol.* **2016**, *101*, 187–196. [CrossRef]
39. Paterson, E.L.; Kazenwadel, J.; Bert, A.G.; Khew-Goodall, Y.; Ruszkiewicz, A.; Goodall, G.J. Down-regulation of the miRNA-200 family at the invasive front of colorectal cancers with degraded basement membrane indicates EMT is involved in cancer progression. *Neoplasia* **2013**, *15*, 180–191. [CrossRef]
40. Davalos, V.; Moutinho, C.; Villanueva, A.; Boque, R.; Silva, P.; Carneiro, F.; Esteller, M. Dynamic epigenetic regulation of the microRNA-200 family mediates epithelial and mesenchymal transitions in human tumorigenesis. *Oncogene* **2012**, *31*, 2062–2074. [CrossRef]

41. Naxerova, K.; Reiter, J.G.; Brachtel, E.; Lennerz, J.K.; van de Wetering, M.; Rowan, A.; Cai, T.; Clevers, H.; Swanton, C.; Nowak, M.A.; et al. Origins of lymphatic and distant metastases in human colorectal cancer. *Science* **2017**, *357*, 55–60. [CrossRef]
42. Saito, T.; Niida, A.; Uchi, R.; Hirata, H.; Komatsu, H.; Sakimura, S.; Hayashi, S.; Nambara, S.; Kuroda, Y.; Ito, S.; et al. A temporal shift of the evolutionary principle shaping intratumor heterogeneity in colorectal cancer. *Nat. Commun.* **2018**, *9*, 2884. [CrossRef] [PubMed]
43. Uchi, R.; Takahashi, Y.; Niida, A.; Shimamura, T.; Hirata, H.; Sugimachi, K.; Sawada, G.; Iwaya, T.; Kurashige, J.; Shinden, Y.; et al. Integrated multiregional analysis proposing a new model of colorectal cancer evolution. *PLoS Genet.* **2016**, *12*, e1005778. [CrossRef] [PubMed]
44. Brabletz, T.; Kalluri, R.; Nieto, M.A.; Weinberg, R.A. EMT in cancer. *Nat. Rev. Cancer* **2018**, *18*, 128–134. [CrossRef] [PubMed]
45. Sun, Y.; Shen, S.; Tang, H.; Xiang, J.; Peng, Y.; Tang, A.; Li, N.; Zhou, W.; Wang, Z.; Zhang, D.; et al. miR-429 identified by dynamic transcriptome analysis is a new candidate biomarker for colorectal cancer prognosis. *OMICS* **2014**, *18*, 54–64. [CrossRef] [PubMed]
46. Debeb, B.G.; Lacerda, L.; Anfossi, S.; Diagaradjane, P.; Chu, K.; Bambhroliya, A.; Huo, L.; Wei, C.; Larson, R.A.; Wolfe, A.R.; et al. miR-141-mediated regulation of brain metastasis from breast cancer. *J. Natl. Cancer Inst.* **2016**, *108*. [CrossRef] [PubMed]
47. Li, J.Q.; Miki, H.; Wu, F.; Saoo, K.; Nishioka, M.; Ohmori, M.; Imaida, K. Cyclin A correlates with carcinogenesis and metastasis, and p27(kip1) correlates with lymphatic invasion, in colorectal neoplasms. *Hum. Pathol.* **2002**, *33*, 1006–1015. [CrossRef] [PubMed]
48. Sreekumar, R.; Harris, S.; Moutasim, K.; DeMateos, R.; Patel, A.; Emo, K.; White, S.; Yagci, T.; Tulchinsky, E.; Thomas, G.; et al. Assessment of nuclear ZEB2 as a biomarker for colorectal cancer outcome and TNM risk stratification. *JAMA Netw. Open* **2018**, *1*, e183115. [CrossRef]
49. Li, M.Z.; Wang, J.J.; Yang, S.B.; Li, W.F.; Xiao, L.B.; He, Y.L.; Song, X.M. ZEB2 promotes tumor metastasis and correlates with poor prognosis of human colorectal cancer. *Am. J. Transl. Res.* **2017**, *9*, 2838–2851.
50. Brabletz, S.; Brabletz, T. The ZEB/miR-200 feedback loop–a motor of cellular plasticity in development and cancer? *EMBO Rep.* **2010**, *11*, 670–677. [CrossRef]
51. Talebi, A.; Kianersi, K.; Beiraghdar, M. Comparison of gene expression of SOX2 and OCT4 in normal tissue, polyps, and colon adenocarcinoma using immunohistochemical staining. *Adv. Biomed. Res.* **2015**, *4*, 234. [CrossRef]
52. Miller, T.J.; McCoy, M.J.; Hemmings, C.; Iacopetta, B.; Platell, C.F. Expression of PD-L1 and SOX2 during rectal tumourigenesis: Potential mechanisms for immune escape and tumour cell invasion. *Oncol. Lett.* **2018**, *16*, 5761–5768. [CrossRef] [PubMed]
53. Pandey, A.; Singh, P.; Jauhari, A.; Singh, T.; Khan, F.; Pant, A.B.; Parmar, D.; Yadav, S. Critical role of the miR-200 family in regulating differentiation and proliferation of neurons. *J. Neurochem.* **2015**, *133*, 640–652. [CrossRef] [PubMed]
54. Arber, N.; Hibshoosh, H.; Yasui, W.; Neugut, A.I.; Hibshoosh, A.; Yao, Y.; Sgambato, A.; Yamamoto, H.; Shapira, I.; Rosenman, D.; et al. Abnormalities in the expression of cell cycle-related proteins in tumors of the small bowel. *Cancer Epidemiol. Biomark. Prev.* **1999**, *8*, 1101–1105.
55. Ohuchi, M.; Sakamoto, Y.; Tokunaga, R.; Kiyozumi, Y.; Nakamura, K.; Izumi, D.; Kosumi, K.; Harada, K.; Kurashige, J.; Iwatsuki, M.; et al. Increased EZH2 expression during the adenoma-carcinoma sequence in colorectal cancer. *Oncol. Lett.* **2018**, *16*, 5275–5281. [CrossRef] [PubMed]
56. Jie, W.; Andrade, K.C.; Lin, X.; Yang, X.; Yue, X.; Chang, J. Pathophysiological functions of Rnd3/RhoE. *Compr. Physiol.* **2015**, *6*, 169–186. [CrossRef] [PubMed]
57. Paysan, L.; Piquet, L.; Saltel, F.; Moreau, V. Rnd3 in Cancer: A Review of the evidence for tumor promoter or suppressor. *Mol. Cancer Res.* **2016**, *14*, 1033–1044. [CrossRef]
58. Zhou, J.; Yang, J.; Li, K.; Mo, P.; Feng, B.; Wang, X.; Nie, Y.; Fan, D. RhoE is associated with relapse and prognosis of patients with colorectal cancer. *Ann. Surg. Oncol.* **2013**, *20*, 175–182. [CrossRef]
59. Orang, A.V.; Safaralizadeh, R.; Hosseinpour Feizi, M.A.; Somi, M.H. Diagnostic and prognostic value of miR-205 in colorectal cancer. *Asian Pac. J. Cancer Prev.* **2014**, *15*, 4033–4037. [CrossRef]
60. Li, P.; Xue, W.J.; Feng, Y.; Mao, Q.S. MicroRNA-205 functions as a tumor suppressor in colorectal cancer by targeting cAMP responsive element binding protein 1 (CREB1). *Am. J. Transl. Res.* **2015**, *7*, 2053–2059.

61. Boulagnon-Rombi, C.; Schneider, C.; Leandri, C.; Jeanne, A.; Grybek, V.; Bressenot, A.M.; Barbe, C.; Marquet, B.; Nasri, S.; Coquelet, C.; et al. LRP1 expression in colon cancer predicts clinical outcome. *Oncotarget* **2018**, *9*, 8849–8869. [CrossRef]
62. Polley, A.C.; Mulholland, F.; Pin, C.; Williams, E.A.; Bradburn, D.M.; Mills, S.J.; Mathers, J.C.; Johnson, I.T. Proteomic analysis reveals field-wide changes in protein expression in the morphologically normal mucosa of patients with colorectal neoplasia. *Cancer Res.* **2006**, *66*, 6553–6562. [CrossRef] [PubMed]

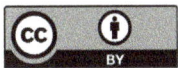

© 2019 by the authors. Licensee MDPI, Basel, Switzerland. This article is an open access article distributed under the terms and conditions of the Creative Commons Attribution (CC BY) license (http://creativecommons.org/licenses/by/4.0/).

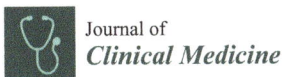 

*Article*

# Iduronate-2-Sulfatase-Regulated Dermatan Sulfate Levels Potentiate the Invasion of Breast Cancer Epithelia through Collagen Matrix

Vishal Singh [1], Keshav Kumar Jha [2], Jyothsna K. M [2], Rekha V. Kumar [3], Varun Raghunathan [2] and Ramray Bhat [1,*]

1. Department of Molecular Reproduction Development and Genetics, Indian Institute of Science, Bangalore 560012, India
2. Department of Electrical Communications and Engineering, Indian Institute of Science, Bangalore 560012 India
3. Department of Pathology, Kidwai Memorial Institute of Oncology, Bangalore 560029, India
* Correspondence: ramray@iisc.ac.in

Received: 7 July 2019; Accepted: 27 August 2019; Published: 30 September 2019

**Abstract:** Cancer epithelia show elevation in levels of sulfated proteoglycans including dermatan sulfates (DS). The effect of increased DS on cancer cell behavior is still unclear. We hypothesized that decreased expression of the enzyme Iduronate-2-sulfatase (IDS) can lead to increased DS levels, which would enhance the invasion of cancer cells. Breast cancer sections shows depleted IDS levels in tumor epithelia, when compared with adjacent untransformed breast tissues. IDS signals showed a progressive decrease in the non-transformed HMLE, transformed but non-invasive MCF-7 and transformed and invasive MDA-MB-231 cells, respectively, when cultured on Type 1 collagen scaffolds. DS levels measured by ELISA increased in an inverse-association with IDS levels. Knockdown of IDS in MCF-7 epithelia also increased the levels of DS. MCF-7 cells with depleted IDS expression, when imaged using two photon-excited fluorescence and second harmonic generation microscopy, exhibited a mesenchymal morphology with multiple cytoplasmic projections compared with epithelioid control cells, interacted with their surrounding matrix, and showed increased invasion through Type 1 collagen matrices. Both these traits were phenocopied when control MCF-7 cells were cultivated on Type 1 collagen gels polymerized in the presence of DS. In monolayer cultures, DS had no effect on MCF-7 migration. In the context of our demonstration that DS enhances the elastic modulus of Type 1 collagen gels, we propose that a decrease of IDS expression leads to accumulation within cancer epithelia of DS: the latter remodels the collagen around cancer cells leading to changes in cell shape and invasiveness through fibrillar matrix milieu.

**Keywords:** dermatan sulfate; breast cancer; iduronate-2-sulfatase

## 1. Introduction

Breast cancer is the most common cancer occurring among women all over the world. Upon transformation, malignant epithelial cells breach their basement membrane and migrate through their surrounding stromal microenvironment [1]. The latter consists of resident cells such as fibroblasts and macrophages and a complex mixture of extracellular matrix proteins, which are primarily fibrillar, such as Type 1 collagen and elastin [2,3].

Migration may involve remodeling and degradation of collagen fibers by diffusible matrix metalloproteinases secreted by cancer epithelia or by active motility, which involves attachment to, and movement of cells along, matrix fibers with appropriate rearrangements of their microfilament cytoskeleton [4,5]. Such distinct mechanisms lead to diversity in the morphology of cancer cell migrations, from unicellular amoeboid or mesenchymal to collective multicellular modes [6]. In addition to negotiating their way through such collagen-rich matrices, cancer epithelia are able to effect changes in the pattern and arrangement of their surrounding collagen-rich matrices. This has been characterized historically by histopathologists as desmoplasia and consists of the alteration in the fibrillar patterns of existent, and freshly synthesized, collagen [7,8].

Rearrangement of collagen fibers by cancer cells may take place through distinct mechanisms. One such mechanism involves upregulation within cancer cells of lysyl oxidase (LOX), an enzyme that catalyzes cross-linking of collagen with elastin fibers [9–11]. Expression of LOX is a strong predictor for both migration and metastasis [10,12–15].

A second mechanism that cancer cells use to remodel their surrounding microenvironment is the expression of sulfated proteoglycans (PGs), proteins with one or more variable linear chains of repeating disaccharide units, known as glycosaminoglycans (GAGs) [16,17]. PGs are known to be elevated in, and are under active investigation as biomarkers for, cancer progression [18]. PGs have the ability to (re)constitute extracellular architecture through binding multiple proteins: both ligands and receptors that regulate cancer growth. They critically regulate the tumor cell motile phenotype by affecting their adhesive/migratory abilities and thus contribute to the metastatic cascade [18]. When cells are cultured in 3D matrix scaffolds, dermatan sulfate proteoglycans (DSPGs) are predominantly upregulated [19]. Dermatan sulfates, a type of GAG, have a unique disaccharide motif: N-Acetyl Galactosamine (GalNAc) and Iduronic Acid (IdoA), with potential sites for sulfation on either monosaccharide [20]. Decorin, one of the best studied DSPGs, binds to collagen through its protein core. The highly charged polysaccharide chains influence the material properties of the matrix by creating hydrogels through attraction of water through their high negative charge. Alterations in sulfation and proportion of GAGs such as chondroitin sulfate (CS) and dermatan sulfate (DS) have been reported in tumor transformation and progression [21], suggesting a possible mechanism by which CS/DS influences cancer progression. In contrast with CS, a potential role of DS in tumor progression is poorly understood.

DS GAGs get degraded in the lysosomes: the first step of degradation (hydrolysis of the C2-sulfate ester bond at the non-reducing end of 2-O-sulfo-$\alpha$-L-iduronic acid residues) is mediated by the enzyme iduronate-2-sulfatase (IDS) through removal of sulfate groups from the glycan chain [22]. IDS belongs to the family of arylsulfatases, evolutionarily related enzymes that can hydrolyze sulfate esters of a variety of substrates such as sulfated GAGs, sulfo-lipids and -proteins, and steroids [23,24]. Mutations in the gene encoding IDS manifests as an X-linked lysosomal storage disease called mucopolysaccharidosis type II, also known as Hunter syndrome [25]. Deficiency in IDS leads to accumulation of DS in the tissues leading to an exaggeration of their ability to remodel Type 1 collagen [26].

In this manuscript, we begin by asking whether DS are elevated in breast cancer epithelia compared with untransformed breast cells, when cultivated in three-dimensional collagen scaffolds. Upon confirming the same, we show that this may occur through the downregulation of the DS degrading enzyme IDS, which in turn is elevated in non-cancerous epithelia located adjacently to tumor tissue wherein, its levels are low. This is consistent with the emerging evidence on the misregulation of several arylsulfatases upon malignant transformation of cells. Using a series of assays involving epifluorescence- and two-photon- and second-harmonic generation microscopy, we show how the deficiency of IDS in the cell line MCF-7 and the resultant accumulation of DS alters the interaction between Type 1 collagen and cancer cells promotes the invasion of the latter through stiffer fibrillar matrix environments.

## 2. Experimental Section

### 2.1. Antibodies and Reagents

The antibodies and reagents used in the study along with their source are as follows: goat polyclonal Iduronate 2-sulfatse (IDS) antibody (AF2449, R&D, Minneapolis, MN, USA) (used for immunocytochemistry (ICC) and immunohistochemistry), Mouse Anti-LAMP2 antibody (ab25631,

Abcam, Cambridge, UK, used for ICC), Alcian blue 8GX (RM471) dye (HiMedia, Bangalore, India), Dulbecco's modified Eagle medium (DMEM) (HiMedia, Bangalore, India), Fetal Bovine Serum (FBS) (Life Technologies, New York, NY, USA), penicillin-streptomycin (HiMedia, Bangalore, India), trypsin (HiMedia, Bangalore, India), paraformaldehyde (Merck, Bangalore, India), Triton X-100 (HiMedia, Bangalore, India), anti-goat antibody conjugated with Cy3 (Invitrogen, New York, NY, USA), anti-mouse antibody conjugated with Alexa fluor488 (Invitrogen, New York, NY, USA), DAPI (4′,6-Diamidine-2′-phenylindole dihydrochloride) (Invitrogen, New York, NY, USA), Phalloidin conjugated with Alexa fluor 488 and 660 (Invitrogen, New York, NY, USA), BSA (HiMedia, Bangalore, India), Type I collagen (Gibco, New York, NY, USA), Propidium iodide (HiMedia, Bangalore, India), TRIzol™ reagent (Invitrogen, New York, NY, USA), Turbofect (Thermo Fischer Scientific, Waltham, MA, USA), Dermatan sulfatase (Sigma, New York, NY, USA), Papain from papaya latex (P3125, Sigma, New York, NY, USA), 1,9-Dimethyl-Methylene Blue zinc chloride double salt (DMMB, 341088, Sigma, New York, NY, USA), and Iodoacetic acid (I4386, Sigma, New York, NY, USA).

*2.2. Cell Culture*

Human breast cancer cells MDA-MB-231 (transformed, triple negative, invasive) and MCF-7 (transformed non-invasive) were grown and maintained in DMEM supplemented with 10% FBS and 1X penicillin-streptomycin at 37 °C and 5% $CO_2$ atmosphere. MDA-MB-231 culture media was also had Ham's F-12 medium. Non-transformed HMLE cells were cultured in DMEM:F12 media (1:1) supplemented with insulin, EGF and hydrocortisone. 3D Type I collagen-rich extracellular matrix on-top and embedded cultures were prepared by seeding the trypsinized cells over and within a thin layer of 1 mg/mL Type 1 collagen. Type-1 collagen scaffolds were prepared by adding 8 volumes of acid-extracted unpolymerized Type 1 collagen (Gibco, USA) along with 1 volume of 10× DMEM and an appropriate volume of 0.1 N sodium hydroxide to bring the final concentration of polymerizing collagen to 1 mg/mL (pH: 7). The scaffolds were polymerized by incubating at 37 °C for 30 min in $CO_2$ incubator. Subsequently, trypsinized cells were added on top or embedded in Type I collagen scaffolds and then cultured for 2 days in serum-free defined medium. 293FT cells (Invitrogen), used for lentivirus production, were grown and maintained in DMEM supplemented with 10% heat-inactivated FBS.

*2.3. Lentiviral Vector Production and Transduction*

Lentiviral Iduronate 2 sulfatase (IDS) shRNA vectors (TRCN0000051543-7) for IDS knockdown and scrambled control shRNA were purchased from Sigma, USA. All lentiviral vectors were produced in 293FT cells by cotransfection of the IDS or scrambled control shRNA lentiviral vectors along with packaging plasmids (pLP1, pLP2, and VSVG, Addgene, Watertown, NY, USA) using Turbofect reagent (Thermo Fisher Scientific, Waltham, MA, USA) according to manufacturer instructions. The supernatant was collected 48 h and 72 h post-transfection and was centrifuged for 15 min at 3000× $g$ and 4 °C to remove cell debris, and then passed through a 0.2-μm filter. Vector supernatants were concentrated 10–100 folds by using lenti-X concentrator (Takara Bio Inc., Kusatsu, Shiga, Japan) and centrifugation at 1500 g for 45 min at 4 °C. The pellet was dissolved in media and frozen at −80 °C. IDS shRNA stable cell lines were established by transducing MCF-7 cells with the purified virus, and stable pools of cells were selected with 1 μg/mL puromycin.

*2.4. RT-qPCR*

RNA from the cell lines (MDA-MB-231, MCF-7, HMLE, MCF-7 transduced with shRNA #1, #2 and scrambled) grown in 3D matrix of Type 1 collagen (1 mg/mL) for 48 h were isolated using TRIzol™ reagent (Thermo Fisher Scientific, USA) as per manufacturer's protocol. Isolated RNA was quantified using UV-visible spectrophotometer (NanoDrop™). RNA (1μg) was reverse transcribed using Verso™ cDNA synthesis kit (Thermo Fisher Scientific AB-1453). All samples were processed at the same time and resulting cDNA was diluted 1:10. Real time PCR with SYBR green detection system (Thermo Fisher Scientific) was performed using StepOne Plus™ real-time PCR system (ABI) and IDS primers: Forward

5′-CGCGTTTCTTTCCTCACTGG-3′ and Reverse 5′-CCGACATGGTCACATAGCCA-3′ (Annealing temperature: 60 °C). Appropriate no-RT and no template controls were included in each biological repeat. 18S rRNA was used as internal control gene for normalization.

### 2.5. Alcian Blue Staining of Breast Tissues and Cell Lines

Adjacent breast and tumor sections were de-paraffinized and hydrated with distilled water. Sections were then incubated in Alcian Blue (1%, pH 1.0) for 1 h, washed in running tap water and then rinsed in distilled water. Finally, the sections were dehydrated through graded alcohols, cleared, mounted and photographs were captured using Olympus Ix81 microscope equipped with a digital camera. Pixel quantification of the Alcian blue stain was done using Image J software. For this, the captured images were first converted to grayscale, inverted and then equal area was selected in the luminal epithelia of healthy breast, and cancer epithelia for the comparison of Alcian blue pixels. Similarly, HMLE, MCF-7, and MCF-7 cells transduced with lentiviral IDS shRNAs and scrambled control vectors and MDA-MB-231 were grown on Type I collagen (300 µg/mL) for 48 h, fixed with 4% formaldehyde, washed with PBS and stained with Alcian blue (1%, pH 1.0) overnight. Thereafter, cells were washed with PBS, investigated for autofluorescence from the dye (green in color) through laser scanning confocal microscopy using a LSM 880 with Airyscan (Carl Zeiss, Oberkochen, Germany) microscope and analyzed by ZEN 2.1 (blue edition, Carl Zeiss, Oberkochen, Germany) software. Thereafter, pixel quantification of the autofluorescence from Alcian blue stain was done in the captured images using Image J 1.52a (National Institutes of Health, Rockville, USA) software. Scatter plots of pixel intensity in the case of tissue and cell lines were plotted using GraphPad 5.0 (GraphPad Software Inc, San Diego, USA) software.

### 2.6. Immunocytochemistry

About $5 \times 10^3$ cells (MDA-MB-231, MCF-7, HMLE, MCF-7 cells transduced with IDS shRNA #1 or shRNA #2 or scrambled shRNA) were seeded on the top of Type I collagen scaffolds (1 mg/mL) per well of 8-well chamber slide (Eppendorf, New York, NY, USA). After 48 h, the cells were washed with phosphate-buffered saline (PBS) twice, fixed with 4% paraformaldehyde (for 20 min) and permeabilized using 0.1% Triton-X100 (15 min) at room temperature (RT). The cells were then washed 3 times with PBS and incubated with the blocking solution (1% BSA in PBS) for 1 h at RT. The cells were then incubated with the primary antibodies, anti-IDS at 1 µg/mL and anti-LAMP2 at 1/100 dilution, for overnight at 4 °C, washed 3 times with PBS plus 0.1% Tween-20 thereafter for 15 min, and incubated with secondary antibodies (Alexa561-tagged anti-goat and Alex488-tagged anti-mouse) and phalloidin conjugated with Alexa 633 (each at 1/500 dilution) for 1 h at RT. Thereafter, cells were washed with PBS three times and incubated with DAPI (1 µg/mL) and fluorophore-conjugated phalloidin for 10 min at RT, followed by rinsing with PBS. The images of 3D cultures were obtained by laser scanning confocal microscopy using a LSM 880 with Airyscan (Carl Zeiss, Oberkochen, Germany) microscope and analyzed by ZEN 2.1 (blue edition, Carl Zeiss, Oberkochen, Germany) software.

### 2.7. Immunohistochemistry

The 5-µm-thick tissue sections were made from paraffin embedded blocks of breast cancer patients from Kidwai Memorial Institute of Oncology with informed consent of the patients. The slides were first deparaffinized and were then subjected to antigen retrieval using citrate buffer. Thereafter, the tissue sections were immunostained with goat anti-IDS antibody (1 µg/mL) overnight at 4 °C. The sections were then incubated with Alexa 561-tagged anti goat secondary antibody at 1/500 dilution for an hour at RT. Thereafter, cells were washed with PBS three times and incubated with DAPI (1 µg/mL) for 10 min at RT, followed by rinsing with PBS and mounted with glycerol. All sections were photographed using epifluorescence microscope (Olympus IX81, Center Valley, USA) and identical exposure times.

## 2.8. In Vitro Invasion Assay

The membrane on the top chamber (12-well insert; pore size 8 µm, HiMedia, Bangalore, India) was coated with a mixture of 200 µg/mL of Type I collagen and allowed to polymerize in absence or presence of 50 µg/mL of dermatan sulfate (Sigma, New York, NY, USA), overnight in $CO_2$ incubator. In the inserts where Type I collagen was polymerized in absence of dermatan sulfate (DS), $3 \times 10^4$ of MCF-7 cells transduced with IDS shRNA or scrambled shRNA were seeded on the top chamber in medium without serum and medium with serum was placed in lower chamber as a chemoattractant. Similarly, in the inserts where Type 1 collagen was polymerized in presence of DS, $3 \times 10^4$ of wild type MCF-7 cells were seeded. Appropriate controls were also maintained in each experiment. The cells were incubated for 48 h and non-invasive cells were removed by cotton swab. The invasive cells were fixed, stained for DAPI and analyzed using epifluorescence microscope (Olympus IX81, Center Valley, USA). The number of invaded cells on each whole membrane was counted.

## 2.9. ELISA for DS Estimation

The in vitro quantitative determination of DS concentrations in lysates of HMLE, MDA-MB-231, MCF-7 cells, MCF-7 cells transduced with IDS shRNA or scrambled shRNA, cultured in 3D matrix of Type I collagen (1 mg/mL), was carried out using ELISA kit (Elabscience, Houston, TX, USA). The micro ELISA plate provided in this kit was pre-coated with an antibody specific to Human DS and its estimation was done according to manufactures recommendation. Briefly, a standard solution of DS ranging from 20 ng/mL to 0.31 ng/mL was prepared. Next, 100 µL of standard or cell lysate (prepared by digesting 3D collagen culture using papain and hence representing the microenvironmental sGAG consisting of both intracellular and matrix-sequestered sGAGs) were added to each well of ELISA plate and incubated for 90 min at 37 °C. Thereafter, liquid was removed and 100 µL of biotinylated detection antibody were added to each well which was incubated for 1 h at 37 °C. Then, liquid was aspirated, and washing was done 3 times with wash buffer. Next, 100 µL of HRP conjugate were added and incubated for 30 min at 37 °C. After aspirating and washing 5 times with wash buffer, 90 µL of substrate reagent was added and incubation was done for 15 min at 37 °C. After this, 50 µL of stop solution was added and the color that developed was read at 450 nm immediately (Tecan infinite M200 Pro™, Mannedorf, Switzerland). The four-parameter logistic (4PL) curve model was used to analyze and quantify the DS levels. The DS levels were normalized to total protein as quantified using Bradford assay.

## 2.10. Scratch Assay

The effect of DS on migration capacities of MCF-7 cells was assessed by in vitro wound healing or scratch assay. Approximately $2 \times 10^4$ cells were seeded per well of an 8-well chamber slide and grown to a confluence of 80–90% at 37 °C in an atmosphere of 5% $CO_2$:95% air. A wound was created by scraping the cells with a sterile 200 µL pipette tip in the middle of the culture well. After removing cellular debris with sterile PBS, cells were incubated with 50 µg/mL of DS for 48 h. An untreated control was also maintained. Thereafter, cells were stained with DAPI and wound closure photographs were captured using Olympus Ix81 epifluorescence microscope equipped with a digital camera and analyzed using Image J software.

## 2.11. Dimethylmethylene Blue (DMMB) Assay

Sulfated GAGs can be measured directly by use of a metachromatic dye, 1,9-Dimethylmethylene blue (DMMB, 341088, Sigma, New York, NY, USA). The GAG-dye complex results in an absorption spectrum shift that can be measured at between 515 and 530 nm, which is directly proportional to the amount of sulfated GAGs. HMLE, MDA-MB-231 and MCF-7 cells cultured in 3D matrix of Type I collagen (1 mg/mL) for 48 h were digested with papain (300 µg/mL) at 60 °C for 3 h. Thereafter, iodoacetic acid was added to a final concentration of 10mM. A standard curve of chondroitin 4 sulfate ranging 0–10 µg/mL was also prepared. Then, 50 µL of lysate or standard were added to 50 µL of DMMB dye in a microplate well and the plate was read at 525 nm in a microplate reader (Tecan infinite M200 Pro™).

*2.12. Experimental Setup for Two Photon Microscopy and Image Analysis*

A mode-locked fiber laser (Coherent Fidelity HP) with operational wavelength 1040 nm, pulse width of 140 fs and repetition rate of 80 MHz was used as the fundamental excitation to acquire second harmonic generation (SHG) and two photon emission fluorescence (TPEF) images of the samples. The incident beam was scanned using a galvo-scanner (GVS001, Thorlabs, Newton, MA, USA) with the beam focused on the sample using a 60× water immersion objective (NA 1.2, Olympus, Shinjuku, Japan). The SHG emission signal from the collagen and TPEF images from the cell of the same field of view were collected separately using photomultiplier tube (R3896, Hamamatsu, Japan) in epi-detection using two different filter sets with wavelength range of 520 nm ± 20 nm and 605 nm ± 55 nm, respectively. The incident power at the focus for cell and collagen was 2.5 mW and 7.5 mW, respectively. The optical resolution of the multi-photon imaging was estimated to be ~600 nm. Four different field of views of 50 × 50 microns size of cell and collagen surrounding the cell along and two different field of views of the collagen far away from the cell were imaged.

*2.13. Atomic Force Microscopy (AFM)*

For AFM measurements, Type 1 collagen polymerized in the absence or presence of 50 µg/mL was freshly prepared and incubated in PBS until acquisition. The apparent modulus of elasticity of the cells was measured using an Atomic Force Microscope (XE Bio from Park Systems, Suwon, Korea). We used a V-shaped cantilever with a spherical bead of diameter 5.2 mm made of silicon dioxide attached to its bottom (AppNano HYDRA6V-200NG-TL; AppNano, Mountain View, CA, USA). The stiffness of the cantilever was measured using a thermal tuning method available with the AFM and was found to be 0.041 N/m. The relation between the deformation of the cantilever and the voltage on the photodetector (A-B sensitivity) was calibrated by indenting the cantilever on the petri dish. The calibration was done whenever the laser position on the cantilever was adjusted. We used a cantilever speed of 0.8 mm/s while approaching as well as retracting from the cell. The point was designated as the modulus of the cell. For obtaining the elastic modulus and the point of contact from the F-d curves, we used the Hertzian contact model as follows. First, the approach region of the F-d curve when the cantilever is not in contact with the cell is identified, and the force in this region is corrected to zero. In this region, the F-d curve is linear and almost flat. A straight line is fitted to this region, and this line is subtracted from the F-d curve to correct for the baseline force. The elastic modulus and contact point are now obtained from the baseline-corrected F-d curve by fitting a Hertzian contact model for the region between 0.2 and 2 nN.

*2.14. Statistical Analysis*

Data are presented as mean ± standard error of mean. Unpaired $t$-test was used to compare between groups and one-way ANOVA with Tukey's post-hoc test was used for comparison of more than two groups. $p < 0.05$ was considered significant. All statistical analyses and graphs were plotted using GraphPad Prism 5.0 (GraphPad Software Inc., San Diego, CA, USA).

## 3. Results

*3.1. Sulfated Proteoglycans Are Elevated in Breast Cancer Epithelia in Vivo and in Culture*

To assess the levels of sulfated proteoglycans (sPGs) between normal and malignant breast epithelia, we stained five sets of sections of breast cancer and patient-matched adjacent tissue with Alcian blue, a dye that specifically binds to sulfated mucopolysaccharides at pH = 1.0 [27]. The tumor cells were found to stain to a greater extent for sPGs than the cells that constituted the normal acinar architectures in the adjacent areas (Figure 1A–C; blue represents sPGs). To confirm that the sPGs were being secreted by cancer cells, the untransformed HMLE cells, non-invasive MCF-7 cells and the triple-negative invasive MDA-MB-231 cells were cultured on top of Type I collagen matrix scaffolds, fixed and stained with Alcian blue. When compared to HMLE, MCF-7 and to a greater extent MDA-MB-231 cells showed significantly higher signals for sPGs (Figure 1D, E; green fluorescence represents sPGs (see Figure S1), results with another dye staining sGAGs, DMMB, are shown in Figure S2, and a plot of individual cell autofluorescent signals is shown in Figure S3). Alteration in material properties of the tumor microenvironment has been shown to profoundly affect cancer invasion [28]; moreover, among sPGs, DS is increasingly shown to alter the fibrillar properties of collagenous microenvironments and is also preferentially upregulated within 3D cultures [19]. Therefore, we next asked whether the enzymes regulating the levels of DS were responsible for the elevated levels of sPGs.

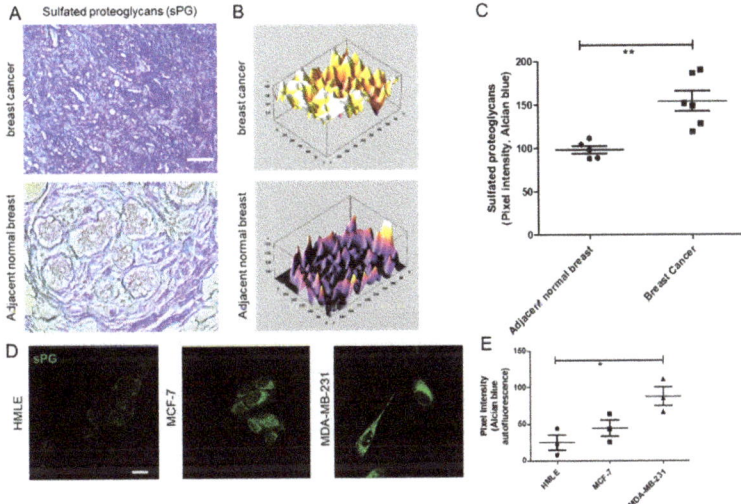

**Figure 1.** Sulfated proteoglycans are elevated in breast cancer epithelia in vivo and in culture. (**A**) Breast cancer (top) and patient-matched adjacent non-transformed (bottom) breast tissue sections were stained with Alcian blue dye (blue), which detects sulfated proteoglycans (sPGs) at pH 1. Scale bar = 50 μm. (**B**) 3D profile plots representing sPGs levels in tissue sections of breast cancer (top) and adjacent normal breast (bottom) with bright colored peaks showing higher staining for Alcian blue in breast cancer tissues (blue-low; white-high). (**C**) Scatter plot showing pixel intensities of Alcian blue staining in breast cancer and adjacent normal breast tissue sections ($n = 5$). (**D**) Confocal micrographs of Alcian blue autofluorescence (green signal) in stained immortalized breast epithelial cells HMLE (left), non-invasive malignant MCF-7 (middle) and the triple negative invasive MDA-MB-231 cells cultured on top of 1 mg/mL Type 1 collagen gels. Scale bar = 20 μm. (**E**) Scatter plot showing pixel intensities of Alcian blue autofluorescence in stained HMLE, MCF-7 and MDA-MB-231 cells cultured on top of 1 mg/mL Type 1 collagen gels (lines in graphs represents mean ± SE of three independent experiments). Significance was measured using one-way ANOVA (* $p < 0.05$) and student's $t$ test (** $p < 0.01$).

## 3.2. Decreased IDS Expression and High DS Levels in Cancer Epithelia

To ascertain whether DS were being secreted by cancer cells to a greater extent than untransformed cells, ELISA was performed on the lysates of 3D Type I collagen cultures of HMLE, MCF-7 and MDA-MB-231 cells. DS levels, normalized to total proteins were highest in MDA-MB-231, followed by MCF-7 and lowest in HMLE lysates (Figure 2A).

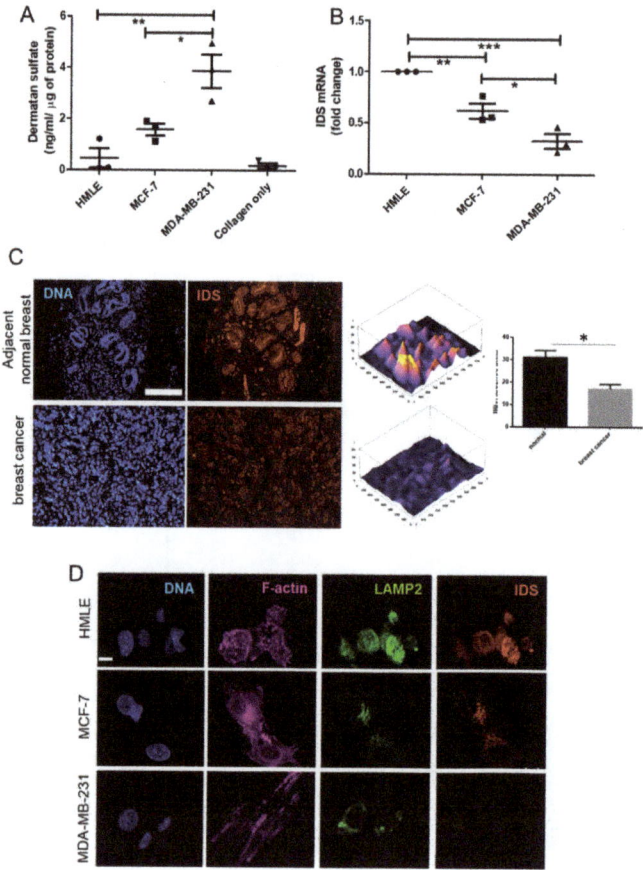

**Figure 2.** Levels of iduronate-2 sulfatase (IDS) are decreased in cancer epithelia in vivo and in culture. (**A**) Scatter plot of dermatan sulfate (DS) levels normalized to total protein measured using ELISA in HMLE, MCF-7 and MDA-MB-231 cells cultured in 3D Type 1 collagen scaffolds. (**B**) Scatter plot of IDS mRNA levels in HMLE, MCF-7 and MDA-MB-231 cells cultured in 3D Type 1 collagen scaffolds, as determined by real time PCR with 18S rRNA as internal control. (**C**) (left) Epifluorescence micrographs of matched normal breast sections (top) and breast cancer tissues (bottom) stained for DNA (using DAPI; blue), and IDS (using antibody; red), scale = 200 µm. (middle) 3D profile plots of IDS levels in normal (top) and cancer (bottom) sections with bright colored peaks showing higher staining for IDS in nontransformed cells. (right) Bar graph showing a statistically significant decrease in IDS levels in breast cancer tissues compared with adjacent breast epithelial cells (50 cells, 5 fields, 2 sample sets). (**D**) Confocal micrographs of HMLE, MCF-7 and MDA-MB-231 cells cultured on top of Type 1 collagen scaffolds and stained for DNA (with DAPI; blue), F-actin (with phalloidin; pink), acidic compartment (with antibody against LAMP2; green), and for IDS (antibody; red), scale = 20 µm. Significance was measured using one-way ANOVA and student's $t$ test (* $p < 0.05$, ** $p < 0.01$, *** $p < 0.001$).

IDS mediates the first step of the degradation of DS, through hydrolysis of sulfate ester bonds at the non-reducing end of 2-O-sulfo-α-L-iduronic acid [25]. Hypothesizing that the accumulation of DS could be explained by a decrease in expression of IDS (based on reported decrease in mRNA levels in human breast tissues with increased stage of cancer progression, specific histopathological types, and increased lymph node metastasis in The Cancer Genome Atlas, Figure S4), we assessed the transcript levels of IDS in breast cells cultured in Type 1 collagen scaffolds, using quantitative real-time PCR (qRTPCR): mRNA levels were highest in HMLE, followed by MCF-7 and lowest in MDA-MB-231 (Figure 2B). The relatively higher levels of IDS have been earlier reported in the context of non-invasive MCF-7 and T47D breast cancer cell lines [29]. We then performed immunohisto- and cyto-chemical analysis to assess IDS protein levels in breast cancer epithelia in cancer tissues and 3D collagen cultures of cell lines, respectively. We found that IDS protein was highly expressed in non-cancerous acinar epithelia with very sparse staining in cancer cells within the sections (Figure 2C). In fixed and stained 3D cell cultures, HMLE showed highest levels of IDS, followed by MCF-7, with sparse staining in case of MDA-MB-231. Given the known canonical localization of IDS in lysosomes, we stained the acidic compartments of cells using LAMP-2. In both HMLE and MCF-7, the IDS signals were colocalized with LAMP-2 (Figure 2D; no-primary antibody control for IDS staining is shown in Figure S5). We then asked whether depletion of IDS within the non-invasive MCF-7 cells would affect their morphological phenotype.

*3.3. IDS Knockdown Leads to Higher DS Levels*

Stable repression of IDS expression was carried out using cognate shRNA (two distinct clones), through lentiviral transduction in MCF-7 cells. IDS knockdown was assessed using qRTPCR, which showed that considerably lower mRNA levels in MCF-7 cells transduced for both shRNA clones compared with control MCF-7 transduced with a scrambled shRNA in 3D Type I collagen cell cultures (Figure 3A). Using immunocytochemistry, we also found a decrease in IDS protein levels in MCF-7 cells transduced with either of the IDS shRNA clones, as compared to scrambled shRNA controls, when the cells were cultured in Type I collagen (Figure 3B). It is pertinent to point out that we also noticed a difference in cell shape concomitant with IDS perturbation: compared with the typical polygonal shape of MCF-7 cells cultured on top of Type 1 collagen, IDS-depleted cells had a more spindle-like appearance typical of mesenchymal cells. We then asked whether a decrease in IDS levels increases sPG levels. IDS-depleted MCF-7 cells grown on Type 1 collagen, fixed and stained with Alcian blue, showed significantly higher levels of sPGs, compared to scrambled shRNA transduced MCF-7 cells (Figure 3C,D). We first assessed whether IDS knockdown also resulted in increased DS levels within MCF-7 cells. This was confirmed using ELISA, in lysates of IDS-depleted MCF-7 cells compared with scrambled shRNA controls when the cells were grown in 3D Type 1 collagen scaffolds (Figure 3E).

*3.4. IDS Downregulation Increases Invasion of Mesenchymal MCF-7 Cells through Collagen Matrices*

We next examined the effect of IDS depletion on the shape of MCF-7 cells cultured in 3D collagen scaffold in greater detail using two-photon excitation fluorescence (TPEF) microscopy accompanied by second harmonic generation (SHG) imaging with the help of F-actin stained cells. IDS-depleted cells had numerous cytoplasmic projections from their surface which was found to be seen rarely in the case of the polygonal control MCF-7 cells. In addition, collagen fibers, well organized around control MCF-7, were found to be spatially coincident with cells upon IDS knockdown indicative of greater cell-matrix interaction (Figure 4A). To further probe such interactive behavior, we cultured cells within transwells coated with Type 1 collagen and assessed their propensity for invasion. IDS shRNA-transduced MCF-7 cells showed significantly greater invasion compared to scrambled shRNA-transduced MCF-7 cells (Figure 4B). Kaplan–Meier plots for risk-free and overall survival showed that higher IDS levels correlated with better prognosis among patients whose expression levels were curated within GEO, EGA and TCGA databases [30] (Figure 4C,D).

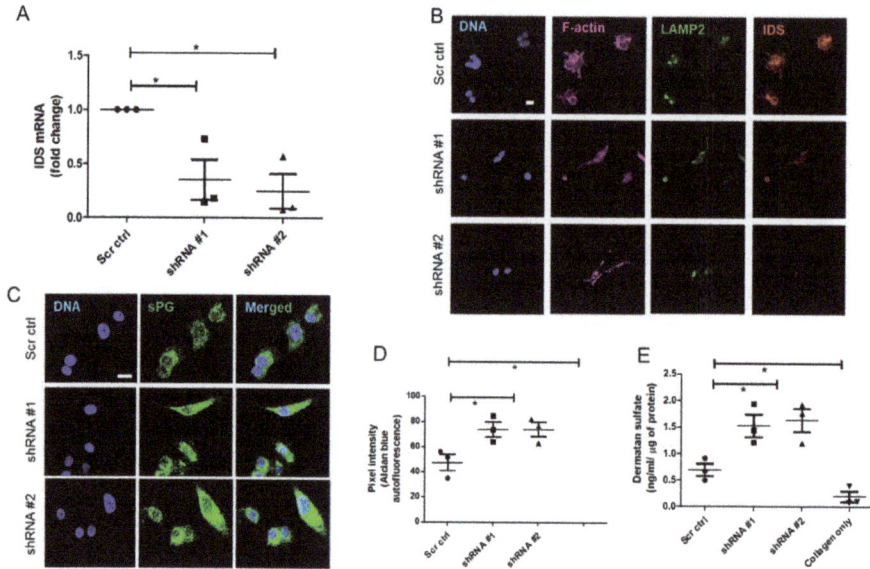

**Figure 3.** Decrease in IDS levels increases DS levels and alters the shape of MCF-7 cells. (**A**) Graphical representation showing a downregulation of IDS mRNA levels in MCF-7 cells upon lentiviral transduction of 2 shRNA clones, compared with scrambled control shRNA transduction, using qRT-PCR. 18S rRNA was used as an internal control. (**B**) Confocal micrographs of MCF-7 cells with scrambled- and IDS-specific shRNA transduction, stained for DNA (using DAPI, blue), F-actin (using phalloidin, pink), acidic compartment (using anti-LAMP-2 antibody, green) and IDS (using anti-IDS antibody, red). Depletion of IDS is accompanied with change in shape of MCF-7 cells from polyhedral to a spindle-like morphology, scale = 10 µm. (**C**) Confocal micrographs of MCF-7 cells with scrambled- and IDS-specific shRNA transduction, stained for DNA (using DAPI, blue), and sulfated proteoglycans (using Alcian Blue, green), scale = 20 µm. (**D**) Scatter plot representation of the pixel intensities of autofluorescent signals from Alcian Blue staining from 3C. (**E**) Scatter plot representation depicting dermatan sulfate (DS) levels in control and IDS knockdown MCF-7 cells when cultured in 3D Type 1 collagen scaffolds, analyzed using ELISA. Levels are represented as scatter plots (mean ± SE of three independent experiments). Significance was measured using one-way ANOVA (* $p < 0.05$).

### 3.5. DS-Type 1 Collagen Scaffolds Increase Invasion of Mesenchymal MCF-7 Cells

To assess whether the increased invasiveness of mesenchymal MCF-7 was a direct result of elevated DS, or an indirect effect of the latter on Type 1 collagen polymerization, scratch assays were performed wherein the ability of MCF-7 cells to fill a scratch were assessed in the presence or absence of 50 µg/mL of DS added to the medium. In both cases, MCF-7 cells were unable to fill the scratch (Figure 5A). On the other hand, in transwells coated with Type 1 collagen, which was polymerized in the presence of 50 µg/mL of DS, MCF-7 cells showed greater invasion compared with controls (Figure 5B,C). Assessed with TPEF microscopic imaging of F-actin, MCF-7 cells grown on top of DS-spiked Type 1 collagen scaffolds also exhibited a more mesenchymal phenotype with several cytoplasmic protrusions (Figure 5D).

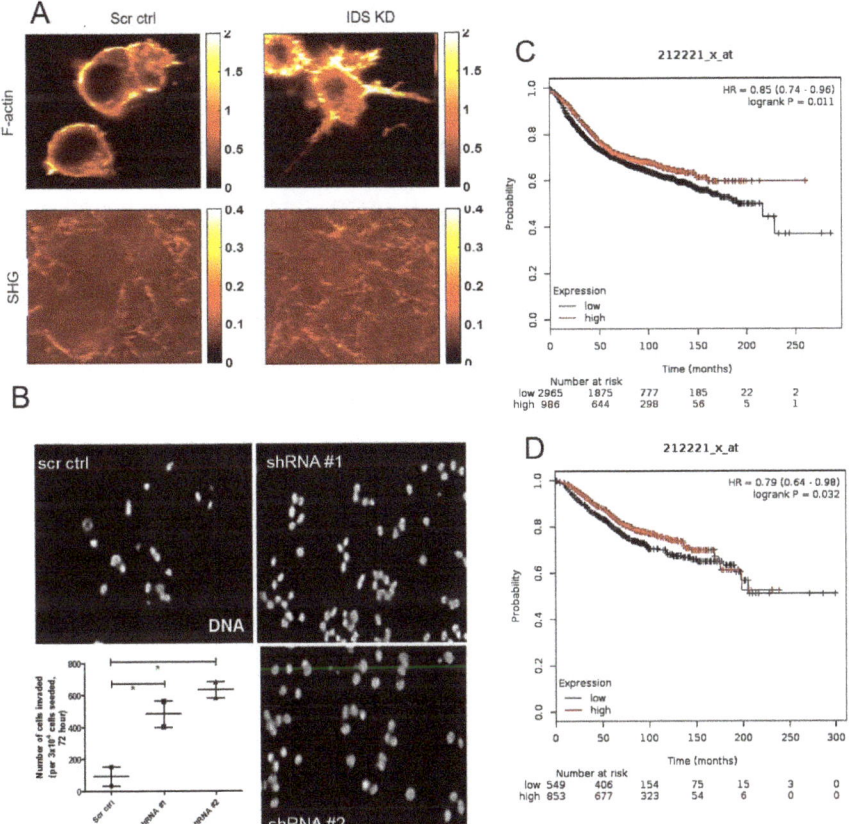

**Figure 4.** Low levels of IDS increase invasion of MCF-7 and correlate with poorer prognosis of breast cancer patients. (**A**) Two photon micrographs of MCF-7 control cells (left) and with IDS knockdown (right) showing phalloidin staining of actin cytoskeleton (top) and second harmonic generation signals (bottom), scale = 10 μm. (**B**) Epifluorescence micrographs of the invasion of MCF-7 cells stained for DNA (using DAPI), lentivirally transduced with scrambled shRNA and 2 shRNA clones against IDS through transwells coated with Type 1 collagen. DAPI was used as indicator of invaded cells. Graphical representation of the number of invaded cells shown in 4B. (**C,D**) Kaplan–Meier plots of risk-free survival and overall survival, respectively, reveal a significant correlation between higher IDS expression and better survival (lines in graphs represent mean ± SE of 2–3 independent experiments). Significance was measured using one-way ANOVA (* $p < 0.05$).

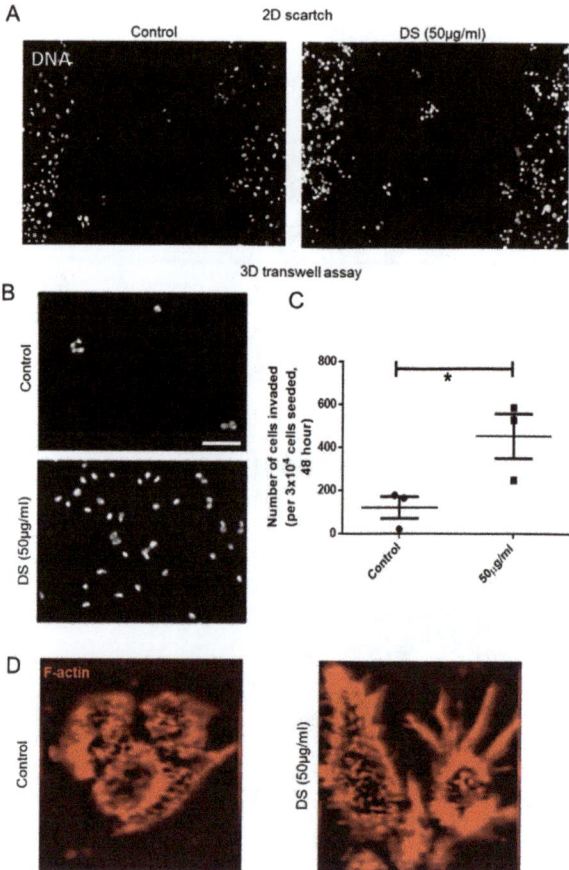

**Figure 5.** Increase in DS levels phenocopies IDS depletion and increases MCF-7 invasion. (**A**) Epifluorescence micrographs showing lack of migration of MCF-7 within scratches made in monolayers (left, control; right, upon treatment with 50 µg/mL Dermatan Sulfate (DS)). The cells were visualized by staining DNA using DAPI. (**B**) Epifluorescence micrographs showing invasion of MCF-7 through Type 1 collagen-coated transwells (top, control; bottom, transwells coated with Type 1 collagen scaffold polymerized in the presence of 50 µg/mL DS). The cells were visualized by using DNA stain DAPI. (**C**) Scatter plot showing the number of invaded cells in 5B. (**D**) Two-photon micrographs of MCF-7 cells cultured in 3D Type 1 collagen scaffold (left) and in 3D Type 1 collagen scaffolds polymerized in the presence of 50 µg/mL DS (right) showing F-actin staining (using phalloidin, red) (lines in graphs represent mean ± SE of three independent experiments). Significance was measured using Student's $t$ test (* $p < 0.05$).

## 4. Discussion

The last decade has seen unprecedented advances in our understanding of the mechanical cues exchanged between cancer epithelia and their matrix microenvironments [31]. Malignantly transformed cells mount a complex response on their surrounding matrix glycoproteins that are part of the basement membranes and the surrounding collagen-rich stroma. The response consists of direct degradation of protein and glycan molecules through upregulation of proteases (such as MMPs) and glycosidases (such as heparanases) [32,33]. Degradation may also be mediated through the activation of tissue-resident fibroblasts which can remodel the matrix within the cancer niche [34,35].

Distinct from degradation, cancer cells and activated fibroblasts also secrete unique matrix proteins into their surrounding milieu. The proteins are referred to as the cancer matrisome and may serve as unique signatures for diagnosis and prognosis of cancer [36,37]. The cancer matrisome differs from untransformed cell secreted matrices not just in their proteomic composition but also in their glycan content. The latter in turn alters the patterning and linkages between matrix proteins resulting in specific mechanical changes in the cancer microenvironment [38]. What is the nature of such glycans and how are they upregulated?

To address these questions, we examined the effect of a specific GAG: dermatan sulfate in tumor environments. The rationale for choosing DS was twofold: Firstly, proteoglycans bearing DS such as decorin alter collagen fiber patterns. Secondly, unlike heparan sulfates, the role of DS still remains ill-understood in the context of carcinomatosis. In consonance with our hypothesis, the expression levels of DS-degrading enzyme IDS were depleted in all histological types of cancers when examined in the TCGA database and observed to be decreased in invasive malignant epithelia compared with non-invasive or untransformed breast epithelia. This was concomitant with an increase in DS levels within the extracellular milieu. The decrease in levels of IDS in non-invasive MCF-7 cells not only increased their invasion, but also the shape of these cells on collagen matrices, polygonal in control cells, underwent a change to a more mesenchymal type with cytoplasmic protrusions. The incorporation of GAGs has been elegantly shown to alter cell-ECM interactions and induce the acquisition of mesenchymal phenotype [39]. The transformation in cellular phenotype is therefore, likely the consequence of the upregulation in DS levels and its alteration in polymerization pattern of Type 1 collagen. This is because MCF-7 cells cultured in Type 1 collagen that was polymerized in the presence of DS, also showed an increase in cell invasion and mesenchymal cell shape. To examine the effect of DS on collagen polymerization, we examined the control and IDS-depleted MCF-7 cells grown on Type 1 collagen scaffolds using SHG microscopy. We detected a clear separation between control MCF-7 cells and surrounding collagen fibers. On the other hand, SHG signals of fibers were intermingled with cells that had depletion of IDS, suggesting greater interaction between cells and extracellular matrix (ECM). Our findings suggest that the presence of DS in Type I collagen changes the rheological properties, making it more permissive to better cell-matrix adhesion and invasion. In line with this, preliminary observations using atomic force microscopy indicate an increase in stiffness of DS-spiked Type 1 collagen matrix when compared with unspiked control matrix (Figure S6).

Our observations suggest that DS secreted by transformed cells can alter the mechanical properties and polymeric arrangement of surrounding collagen fibers leading to enhanced cell matrix interaction and mesenchymal migration. Our findings raise several important questions. Does the alteration in collagen polymer patterning as a result of increased DS further feedback on IDS expression? Important observations by workers in the field show that fibroblasts grown in 3D embedded in collagen make more DS than HS, with the latter bound to the collagen fibers [19]. However, it is not known if this increase in DS is through the downregulation of IDS.

Second, in what way does DS alter the patterns of Type 1 collagen in order to bring about an increase in invasiveness of cancer epithelia? DS consists of iduronic acid, which, being inherently more flexible than glucuronic acid, can bind to its cognate binding partners much more strongly [40,41]. DS is known to bind to growth factors [42]. Therefore, high levels of DS in the collagenous milieu may also enhance the sequestration of growth factors in the vicinity of cells leading to better availability of these ligands for cell proliferation and migration.

Finally, we asked how the presence of DS in the collagen allows the cells to stretch and change its shape. It is possible that DS, while increasing stiffness of Type 1 collagen scaffold, also alters the interfacial tension between the cells and matrices allowing for a greater optimal contact between the cell and their surrounding fibers. The increase in sulfation of GAGs in concurrence with epithelial to mesenchymal transition (EMT) has previously been reported. Maupin and coworkers, using a diverse set of pancreatic cancer cell lines and Alcian blue, found that mesenchymal cancer cells show increased sulfation. Inducing EMT in Panc-1 mesenchymal-like cell line with TGFβ also led to a significant increase in overall levels of sulfation by altering the expression of sulfotransferases [43]. Our study is complimentary to these efforts in demonstrating that not only the increase in sulfotransferases, but also a depletion of sulfatases may lead to EMT. Future experimentations will be devoted to elucidation of the mechanochemical effect of DS on collagen fibrillogenesis as well as investigating the effects of DS on expression of cell adhesion molecules and cytoskeletal elements that determine cell shape change.

## 5. Conclusions

We conclude by proposing that the progression towards invasiveness of transformed breast epithelia is associated with an appropriate decrease in desulfation of dermatan sulfate (DS) proteoglycans leading to their accumulation within their surrounding stromal collagen-rich matrix. The accumulated DS modifies Type 1 collagen and potentiates the invasion of breast cancer cells. Therefore, our findings potentially open a new window for therapeutic targeting of dermatan sulfates in order to decrease the burden of cancer metastasis and invasion.

**Supplementary Materials:** The following are available online at http://www.mdpi.com/2077-0383/8/10/1562/s1, Figure S1: Bright field (left) and laser confocal (right) micrographs of the same field of Alcian blue-stained MCF-7 cells cultured on top of 1 mg/mL Type 1 collagen gels. Images show that the levels of green autofluorescence signals correspond to the intensity of Alcian blue staining in the brightfield. Scale bar = 50 µm, Figure S2: Scatter plot of DMMB assay depicting levels of sulfated glycosaminoglycans (GAGs) in HMLE, MCF-7 and MDA-MB-231 cells grown in 3D Type-I collagen scaffolds. (Data is mean ± SE of three independent experiments). Significance was measured using one-way ANOVA (* $p < 0.05$, ** $p < 0.01$), Figure S3: Scatter plot showing pixel intensities of Alcian blue autofluorescence in stained HMLE, MCF-7 and MDA-MB-231 cells cultured on top of 1 mg/mL Type 1 collagen gels. Each spot represents autofluorescent signal from single cells from all three independent experiments. Significance was measured using student's $t$-test (** $p < 0.01$, (*** $p < 0.001$), Figure S4: Graphs of stage-specific, histotype-specific, and lymph node-metastasis-specific mRNA levels of IDS in breast cancer patients from TCGA presented in its graphical user interface UALCAN, Figure S5: Confocal micrographs of MCF-7 cells with no primary antibody (negative control) grown on Type 1 collagen scaffolds and stained for F-actin and DNA, Scale = 20 µm, Figure S6: Graph showing median elastic modulus of Type 1 collagen measured by atomic force microscopy and its interquartile distribution, when polymerized without and in the presence of 50 µg/mL dermatan sulfate (DS).

**Author Contributions:** Conceptualization, V.S. and R.B.; data curation, V.S. and R.B.; formal analysis, V.S., K.K.J., J.K.M., V.R. and R.B.; funding acquisition, V.S., V.R. and R.B.; investigation, V.S., K.K.J., J.K.M., V.R. and R.B.; methodology, V.S., K.K.J., J.K.M., R.V.K., V.R. and R.B.; resources, V.S., R.V.K., R.B.; validation, V.S., K.K.J., J.K.M., V.R. and R.B.; visualization, V.S., V.R. and R.B.; writing—original draft preparation, V.S. and R.B.; writing—review and editing, V.S., K.K.J., J.K.M, R.V.K., V.R. and R.B.; supervision, V.R. and R.B.; and project administration, R.B.

**Funding:** R.B. would like to acknowledge funding support from SERB ECR fellowship (DSTO1586) and CSIR (1671) and the DBT-IISc partnership program (BT/PR27952/INF/22/212/2018). V.S. would like to acknowledge support from DST SERB NPDF fellowship (DSTO1751). V.R. would like to acknowledge financial support from DST Indo-Korea joint research project (INT/Korea/P-44).

**Acknowledgments:** We also like to thank the Divisional Bioimaging Facility, Biological Science Division at IISc.

**Conflicts of Interest:** The authors declare no conflict of interest. The funders had no role in the design of the study; in the collection, analyses, or interpretation of data; in the writing of the manuscript, or in the decision to publish the results.

## References

1. Bissell, M.J.; Radisky, D.C.; Rizki, A.; Weaver, V.M.; Petersen, O.W. The organizing principle: Microenvironmental influences in the normal and malignant breast. *Differentiation* **2002**, *70*, 537–546. [CrossRef] [PubMed]
2. Bhat, R.; Bissell, M.J. Of plasticity and specificity: Dialectics of the microenvironment and macroenvironment and the organ phenotype. Wiley interdisciplinary reviews. *Wiley Interdisc. Rev. Dev. Biol.* **2014**, *3*, 147–163. [CrossRef] [PubMed]
3. Hynes, R.O. The extracellular matrix: Not just pretty fibrils. *Science* **2009**, *326*, 1216–1219. [CrossRef] [PubMed]
4. Wolf, K.; Friedl, P. Molecular mechanisms of cancer cell invasion and plasticity. *Br. J. Dermatol.* **2006**, *154*, 11–15. [CrossRef] [PubMed]

5. Friedl, P.; Wolf, K. Tube travel: The role of proteases in individual and collective cancer cell invasion. *Cancer Res.* **2008**, *68*, 7247–7249. [CrossRef]
6. Friedl, P.; Locker, J.; Sahai, E.; Segall, J.E. Classifying collective cancer cell invasion. *Nat. Cell Biol.* **2012**, *14*, 777–783. [CrossRef] [PubMed]
7. Walker, R.A. The complexities of breast cancer desmoplasia. *Breast Cancer Res.* **2001**, *3*, 143–145. [CrossRef]
8. DeClerck, Y.A. Desmoplasia: A response or a niche? *Cancer Discov.* **2012**, *2*, 772–774. [CrossRef]
9. Perryman, L.; Erler, J.T. Lysyl oxidase in cancer research. *Future Oncol.* **2014**, *10*, 1709–1717. [CrossRef]
10. Lee, Y.S.; Park, Y.; Kwon, M.; Roh, J.L.; Choi, S.H.; Nam, S.Y.; Kim, S.Y. Expression of Lysyl Oxidase Predictive of Distant Metastasis of Laryngeal Cancer. *Otolaryngol. Head Neck Surg.* **2017**, *156*, 489–497. [CrossRef]
11. Johnston, K.A.; Lopez, K.M. Lysyl oxidase in cancer inhibition and metastasis. *Cancer Lett.* **2018**, *417*, 174–181. [CrossRef] [PubMed]
12. Helleman, J.; Jansen, M.P.; Ruigrok-Ritstier, K.; van Staveren, I.L.; Look, M.P.; Meijer-van Gelder, M.E.; Sieuwerts, A.M.; Klijn, J.G.; Sleijfer, S.; Foekens, J.A.; et al. Association of an extracellular matrix gene cluster with breast cancer prognosis and endocrine therapy response. *Clin. Cancer Res.* **2008**, *14*, 5555–5564. [CrossRef] [PubMed]
13. Sodek, K.L.; Ringuette, M.J.; Brown, T.J. Compact spheroid formation by ovarian cancer cells is associated with contractile behavior and an invasive phenotype. *Int. J. Cancer.* **2009**, *124*, 2060–2070. [CrossRef] [PubMed]
14. Liu, Y.; Wang, G.; Liang, Z.; Mei, Z.; Wu, T.; Cui, A.; Liu, C.; Cui, L. Lysyl oxidase: A colorectal cancer biomarker of lung and hepatic metastasis. *Thorac. Cancer* **2018**, *9*, 785–793. [CrossRef] [PubMed]
15. Peng, C.; Liu, J.; Yang, G.; Li, Y. Lysyl oxidase activates cancer stromal cells and promotes gastric cancer progression: Quantum dot-based identification of biomarkers in cancer stromal cells. *Int. J. Nanomed.* **2018**, *13*, 161–174. [CrossRef]
16. Iozzo, R.V.; Sanderson, R.D. Proteoglycans in cancer biology, tumour microenvironment and angiogenesis. *J. Cell Mol. Med.* **2011**, *15*, 1013–1031. [CrossRef]
17. Varki, A. *Essentials of Glycobiology*, 3rd ed.; Cold Spring Harbor Laboratory Press: New York, NY, USA, 2017; p. 823.
18. Nikitovic, D.; Berdiaki, A.; Spyridaki, I.; Krasanakis, T.; Tsatsakis, A.; Tzanakakis, G.N. Proteoglycans-Biomarkers and Targets in Cancer Therapy. *Front. Endocrinol.* **2018**, *9*, 69. [CrossRef]
19. Lee, P.H.; Trowbridge, J.M.; Taylor, K.R.; Morhenn, V.B.; Gallo, R.L. Dermatan sulfate proteoglycan and glycosaminoglycan synthesis is induced in fibroblasts by transfer to a three-dimensional extracellular environment. *J. Biol. Chem.* **2004**, *279*, 48640–48646. [CrossRef]
20. Trowbridge, J.M.; Gallo, R.L. Dermatan sulfate: New functions from an old glycosaminoglycan. *Glycobiology* **2002**, *12*, 117R–125R. [CrossRef]
21. Kozma, E.M.; Wisowski, G.; Latocha, M.; Kusz, D.; Olczyk, K. Complex influence of dermatan sulphate on breast cancer cells. *Exp. Biol. Med.* **2014**, *239*, 1575–1588. [CrossRef]
22. Coronado-Pons, I.; Novials, A.; Casas, S.; Clark, A.; Gomis, R. Identification of iduronate-2-sulfatase in mouse pancreatic islets. *Am. J. Physiol. Endocrinol. Metab.* **2004**, *287*, 983–990. [CrossRef] [PubMed]
23. Parenti, G.; Meroni, G.; Ballabio, A. The sulfatase gene family. *Curr. Opin. Genet. Dev.* **1997**, *7*, 386–391. [CrossRef]
24. Diez-Roux, G.; Ballabio, A. Sulfatases and human disease. *Annu. Rev. Genom. Hum. Genet.* **2005**, *6*, 355–379. [CrossRef] [PubMed]
25. Demydchuk, M.; Hill, C.H.; Zhou, A.; Bunkoczi, G.; Stein, P.E.; Marchesan, D.; Deane, J.E.; Read, R.J. Insights into Hunter syndrome from the structure of iduronate-2-sulfatase. *Nat. Commun.* **2017**, *8*, 15786. [CrossRef] [PubMed]
26. Laoharawee, K.; Podetz-Pedersen, K.M.; Nguyen, T.T.; Evenstar, L.B.; Kitto, K.F.; Nan, Z.; Fairbanks, C.A.; Low, W.C.; Kozarsky, K.F.; McIvor, R.S. Prevention of Neurocognitive Deficiency in Mucopolysaccharidosis Type II Mice by Central Nervous System-Directed, AAV9-Mediated Iduronate Sulfatase Gene Transfer. *Hum. Gene Ther.* **2017**, *28*, 626–638. [CrossRef] [PubMed]
27. Fisher, M.; Solursh, M. Glycosaminoglycan localization and role in maintenance of tissue spaces in the early chick embryo. *Development* **1977**, *42*, 195–207.
28. Gkretsi, V.; Stylianopoulos, T. Cell Adhesion and Matrix Stiffness: Coordinating Cancer Cell Invasion and Metastasis. *Front. Oncol.* **2018**, *8*, 145. [CrossRef] [PubMed]

29. Bhattacharyya, S.; Tobacman, J.K. Steroid sulfatase, arylsulfatases A and B, galactose-6-sulfatase, and iduronate sulfatase in mammary cells and effects of sulfated and non-sulfated estrogens on sulfatase activity. *J. Steroid Biochem. Mol. Biol.* **2007**, *103*, 20–34. [CrossRef] [PubMed]
30. Gyorffy, B.; Lanczky, A.; Eklund, A.C.; Denkert, C.; Budczies, J.; Li, Q.; Szallasi, Z. An online survival analysis tool to rapidly assess the effect of 22,277 genes on breast cancer prognosis using microarray data of 1,809 patients. *Breast Cancer Res. Treat.* **2010**, *123*, 725–731. [CrossRef]
31. Wolfenson, H.; Yang, B.; Sheetz, M.P. Steps in Mechanotransduction Pathways that Control Cell Morphology. *Annu. Rev. Physiol.* **2019**, *81*, 585–605. [CrossRef]
32. Alcaraz, J.; Mori, H.; Ghajar, C.M.; Brownfield, D.; Galgoczy, R.; Bissell, M.J. Collective epithelial cell invasion overcomes mechanical barriers of collagenous extracellular matrix by a narrow tube-like geometry and MMP14-dependent local softening. *Integr. Biol.* **2011**, *3*, 1153–1166. [CrossRef] [PubMed]
33. Arvatz, G.; Shafat, I.; Levy-Adam, F.; Ilan, N.; Vlodavsky, I. The heparanase system and tumor metastasis: Is heparanase the seed and soil? *Cancer Metastasis Rev.* **2011**, *30*, 253–268. [CrossRef] [PubMed]
34. Erdogan, B.; Ao, M.; White, L.M.; Means, A.L.; Brewer, B.M.; Yang, L.; Washington, M.K.; Shi, C.; Franco, O.E.; Weaver, A.M.; et al. Cancer-associated fibroblasts promote directional cancer cell migration by aligning fibronectin. *J. Cell Biol.* **2017**, *216*, 3799–3816. [CrossRef] [PubMed]
35. Erdogan, B.; Webb, D.J. Cancer-associated fibroblasts modulate growth factor signaling and extracellular matrix remodeling to regulate tumor metastasis. *Biochem. Soc. Trans.* **2017**, *45*, 229–236. [CrossRef] [PubMed]
36. Naba, A.; Clauser, K.R.; Lamar, J.M.; Carr, S.A.; Hynes, R.O. Extracellular matrix signatures of human mammary carcinoma identify novel metastasis promoters. *eLife* **2014**, *3*, e01308. [CrossRef] [PubMed]
37. Socovich, A.M.; Naba, A. The cancer matrisome: From comprehensive characterization to biomarker discovery. *Semin. Cell Dev. Biol.* **2018**, *89*, 157–166. [CrossRef] [PubMed]
38. Paszek, M.J.; DuFort, C.C.; Rossier, O.; Bainer, R.; Mouw, J.K.; Godula, K.; Hudak, J.E.; Lakins, J.N.; Wijekoon, A.C.; Cassereau, L.; et al. The cancer glycocalyx mechanically primes integrin-mediated growth and survival. *Nature* **2014**, *511*, 319–325. [CrossRef] [PubMed]
39. Dahal, S.; Huang, P.; Murray, B.T.; Mahler, G.J. Endothelial to mesenchymal transformation is induced by altered extracellular matrix in aortic valve endothelial cells. *J. Biomed. Mater. Res. A* **2017**, *105*, 2729–2741. [CrossRef]
40. Bartolini, B.; Thelin, M.A.; Svensson, L.; Ghiselli, G.; van Kuppevelt, T.H.; Malmstrom, A.; Maccarana, M. Iduronic acid in chondroitin/dermatan sulfate affects directional migration of aortic smooth muscle cells. *PLoS ONE* **2013**, *8*, e66704. [CrossRef]
41. Thelin, M.A.; Bartolini, B.; Axelsson, J.; Gustafsson, R.; Tykesson, E.; Pera, E.; Oldberg, A.; Maccarana, M.; Malmstrom, A. Biological functions of iduronic acid in chondroitin/dermatan sulfate. *FEBS J.* **2013**, *280*, 2431–2446. [CrossRef]
42. Mizumoto, S.; Yamada, S.; Sugahara, K. Molecular interactions between chondroitin-dermatan sulfate and growth factors/receptors/matrix proteins. *Curr. Opin. Struct. Biol.* **2015**, *34*, 35–42. [CrossRef] [PubMed]
43. Maupin, K.A.; Sinha, A.; Eugster, E.; Miller, J.; Ross, J.; Paulino, V.; Keshamouni, V.G.; Tran, N.; Berens, M.; Webb, C.; et al. Glycogene expression alterations associated with pancreatic cancer epithelial-mesenchymal transition in complementary model systems. *PLoS ONE* **2010**, *5*, e13002. [CrossRef] [PubMed]

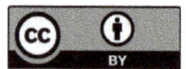

© 2019 by the authors. Licensee MDPI, Basel, Switzerland. This article is an open access article distributed under the terms and conditions of the Creative Commons Attribution (CC BY) license (http://creativecommons.org/licenses/by/4.0/).

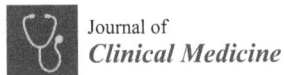 

Article

# A Novel Ex Vivo System Using 3D Polymer Scaffold to Culture Circulating Tumor Cells from Breast Cancer Patients Exhibits Dynamic E-M Phenotypes

Tamasa De [1], Shina Goyal [2], Gowri Balachander [3,4], Kaushik Chatterjee [3,5], Prashant Kumar [6,7,*], Govind Babu K. [2,*] and Annapoorni Rangarajan [1,3,*]

1. Department of Molecular Reproduction, Development and Genetics, Indian Institute of Science, Bangalore 560012, India; tamasade@iisc.ac.in
2. Department of Medical Oncology, Kidwai Memorial Institute of Oncology, Bangalore 560029, India; shina.goyal@gmail.com
3. Center for Biosystems Science and Engineering, Indian Institute of Science, Bangalore 560012, India; phsgmb@nus.edu.sg (G.B.); kchatterjee@iisc.ac.in (K.C.)
4. Department of Physiology, Yong Loo Lin School of Medicine, National University Health System, MD9-04-11, 2 Medical Drive, Singapore 117593, Singapore
5. Department of Materials Engineering, Indian Institute of Science, Bangalore 560066, India
6. Institute of Bioinformatics, International Technology Park, Bangalore 560066, India
7. Manipal Academy of Higher Education (MAHE), Manipal 576104, Karnataka, India
* Correspondence: prashant@ibioinformatics.org (P.K.); kgblaugh@gmail.com (G.B.K.); anu@iisc.ac.in (A.R.); Tel.: +91-80-28416140 (P.K.); +91-98-45072940 (G.B.K.); +91-80-22933263 (A.R.); Fax: +91-80-28416132 (P.K.); +91-80-23600999 (A.R.)

Received: 13 July 2019; Accepted: 9 August 2019; Published: 16 September 2019

**Abstract:** The majority of the cancer-associated deaths is due to metastasis—the spread of tumors to other organs. Circulating tumor cells (CTCs), which are shed from the primary tumor into the circulation, serve as precursors of metastasis. CTCs have now gained much attention as a new prognostic and diagnostic marker, as well as a screening tool for patients with metastatic disease. However, very little is known about the biology of CTCs in cancer metastasis. An increased understanding of CTC biology, their heterogeneity, and interaction with other cells can help towards a better understanding of the metastatic process, as well as identify novel drug targets. Here we present a novel ex vivo 3D system for culturing CTCs from breast cancer patient blood samples using porous poly(ε-caprolactone) (PCL) scaffolds. As a proof of principle study, we show that ex vivo culture of 12/16 (75%) advanced stage breast cancer patient blood samples were enriched for CTCs identified as CK+ (cytokeratin positive) and CD45− (CD45 negative) cells. The deposition of extracellular matrix proteins on the PCL scaffolds permitted cellular attachment to these scaffolds. Detection of Ki-67 and bromodeoxyuridine (BrdU) positive cells revealed proliferating cell population in the 3D scaffolds. The CTCs cultured without prior enrichment exhibited dynamic differences in epithelial (E) and mesenchymal (M) composition. Thus, our 3D PCL scaffold system offers a physiologically relevant model to be used for studying CTC biology as well as for individualized testing of drug susceptibility. Further studies are warranted for longitudinal monitoring of epithelial–mesenchymal transition (EMT) in CTCs for clinical association.

**Keywords:** circulating tumor cells (CTCs); breast cancer; 3D culture; epithelial-mesenchymal heterogeneity

## 1. Introduction

Most of the cancer-related mortality is caused due to metastasis—the spread of cancer to secondary vital organs [1,2]. This is a complex phenomenon involving dissemination of cells from the primary site, intravasation into the circulatory system followed by extravasation, and finally successful colonization in secondary tumor sites such as liver, lung, bone and brain [1,2]. Cancer that is diagnosed at the primary site is relatively easier to manage compared to those with metastatic lesions. Circulating tumor cells (CTCs) derived from either the primary or metastatic tumors serve as precursors of metastasis [3]. To begin to understand the biology of CTCs and their role in the metastatic process, it is important to culture CTCs in a suitable microenvironment that recapitulates their physiological features.

CTCs represent an extraordinarily rare population in the milieu of billions of blood cells, and hence, their identification and isolation pose critical impediments to their characterization [4]. In the past decade or so, several technologies have come up to isolate and detect CTCs. Broadly CTC detection is done by two methods, one involving pre-enrichment with markers, and the other without enrichment, which is also known as direct detection of CTCs. The reported technologies for direct detection include (1) line-confocal microscopy and (2) surface-enhanced Raman scattering nanoparticles (SERS) [5,6]. On the other hand, marker-based pre-enrichment methods include several techniques, for example, Cell Search™, Dynabeads® CD45, EPISPOT (EPithelial ImmunoSPOT), ClearCell® FX1 System, Herringbone CTC-Chip, CTC-iChip, DEPArray™ System, etc. [4,7–9]. However, pre-enrichment results in the loss of CTCs that do not express the chosen markers. Further, several detection techniques involve cell-fixation which does not allow subsequent CTC expansion for biological characterization including stemness, drug resistance, etc. In addition, most of these methods detect only low numbers of CTCs (<20%) [10]. Hence, there is an unmet need to establish a robust method with improved efficiency for CTC enrichment to enable a better understanding of their biology.

Conventional two-dimensional (2D) culture system suffers from major limitations in terms of altered cellular morphology, motility, polarity and other functional aspects. When grown on a 2D substrate, cells lose their in vivo morphology and importantly their cell–cell and cell–matrix interactions. Further, stiffness of materials typically used for 2D cell cultures, such as tissue culture polystyrene (TCPS) and glass, are several orders of magnitude (GigaPascals) higher than the stiffness of human tissues (kiloPascals) [11]. In addition, studies have also demonstrated altered signaling in cancer cells when cultured in 2D platforms [12]. Therefore, we sought to develop a three-dimensional (3D) culture system to enrich and expand the rare population of CTCs.

Three-dimensional culture systems have been widely explored to study breast cancer over the past three decades. A variety of 3D gel-based matrices like collagen, Matrigel, laminin-rich extracellular matrix (lrECM), fibrin, etc., have been routinely used to mimic cell-basement membrane interactions. However, the abundance of ECM already present in these matrices reduces the secretion of native ECM molecules by cancer cells [12,13]. To overcome these limitations, we recently developed a 3D porous scaffold synthesized using a synthetic biomaterial, poly(ε-caprolactone) (PCL) that better mimics the architecture and stiffness of breast tumors, and enables deposition of native ECM [13]. Our 3D culture system showed improved cell–cell and cell–matrix interactions. Furthermore, global microarray analysis revealed that cancer cells cultured in this 3D scaffold are able to maintain increased stemness and epithelial–mesenchymal transition (EMT) properties, and show closer association to in vivo tumor growth than conventional 2D cultures on TCPS [13]. Thus, this 3D porous PCL scaffold system offers a superior model system to mimic the native tumor microenvironment.

In this study, we have exploited the 3D porous PCL scaffold to enrich CTCs derived from breast cancer patient blood samples without any prior enrichment. We have previously shown that culture of patient blood cells under hypoxic conditions for 14 days in laser ablated microwells helps in the enrichment of CTC subpopulation from RBC lysed nucleated cell fraction [14] Using various lineage-specific markers, we further showed gradual depletion of other blood cell lineages with time [14] More recently, we used a similar strategy to expand CTCs in agar-microwells [15]. However, being inert, agar does not allow deposition of extracellular matrix. Therefore, here, we established a 3D

PCL scaffold-based method, which better mimics the native cellular in vivo environment and allows ECM deposition, for culturing CTCs from RBC-depleted nucleated cell pellets of advanced breast cancer patient samples under hypoxic conditions. We detected CK-positive and CD45-negative CTCs in 12/16 patient samples using this culture method. We detected the deposition of thread-like and sheet-like ECM on the scaffold providing a substratum for cells to adhere and proliferate. Our study shows intra-patient and inter-patient heterogeneity with respect to the epithelial (E) and mesenchymal (M) characteristics suggesting a dynamic EMT spectrum in CTCs. Thus, we established a unique model system by creating in vivo-like functionality to culture CTCs from whole blood samples without prior enrichment. Our model may provide a versatile system for studying CTC biology as well as in the use of a number of downstream exciting applications for the clinical utility of CTCs.

## 2. Materials and Methods

### 2.1. Patients Sample, Blood Collection and Processing

Blood samples were collected from 16 chemo-naïve metastatic breast cancer patients. This study was approved by the institutional review board at Indian Institute of Science (IISc) and at the Kidwai Memorial Institute of Oncology (KMIO/MEC/017/23.March.2017, KMIO/MEC/018/23.March.2017, KMIO/MEC/011.November.2016). All patients gave their informed consent for the completion of the study. Among 16 patients (median age of breast cancer patients = 50.5), 31 patients were ER/PR positive (81.25%), 2 patients were triple negative (12.5%), and 8 patients were HER-2 positive (50%). Out of all these 16 patients with breast cancer, 1 patient had only brain metastasis (6.25%), 14 patients had liver, lung and bone metastasis (87.5%), and 3 patient had contralateral axillary and lymph node metastasis along with lung/liver/bone metastasis (Supplementary Table S1). Clinicopathological information was recorded for each patient. Blood sample (~10 mL) was collected at a single draw in chemo-naïve conditions. All the samples were collected in sterile EDTA-coated vacutainer tubes (BD) and maintained at 4 °C until processing.

Blood samples were processed within 3–6 h of withdrawal to avoid blood clotting and to maintain cell viability. In order to isolate nucleated cells, plasma and blood cells were separated from whole blood by centrifuging at 1200 rpm for 10 min. Blood cells were then treated with chilled red blood cell (RBC) lysis buffer (154 mM $NH_4Cl$, 10 mM $KHCO_3$, 0.1 mM EDTA) at a ratio of 1:5 with a gentle-mixing followed by incubation at room temperature (25 °C) for 15 min. Next, the whole content was centrifuged at 1200 rpm for 10 min at room temperature to remove lysed RBC fragments. The leftover, largely nucleated cells following RBS lysis were resuspended in fresh Dulbecco's modified Eagle's medium (DMEM; Sigma-Aldrich, Saint Louis, MO, USA) supplemented with 10% fetal bovine serum (FBS, Gibco, Invitrogen, Carlsbad, CA, USA) containing antibiotics streptomycin sulphate and benzylpenicillin at final concentrations of 100 µg/mL and 100 U/mL, respectively. Each processed sample was split into multiple wells of a 96-well plate (~10 mL RBC-lysed blood was distributed into 5 or 6 wells).

### 2.2. Preparation of 3D Scaffold System

Fabrication of 3D PCL porous scaffolds is mentioned in detail elsewhere [13]. Briefly, sodium chloride (Fisher scientific, Hampton, Hampshire, USA) crystals of a defined size range of 250–425 µm were used as the porogen. PCL (average molecular weight $M_n$ = 80,000 g/mol; Sigma) was dissolved in chloroform and added on to the salt bed in 96 polypropylene plate. Finally, it was vacuum dried, and the salt was leached in $dH_2O$ for three consecutive days with daily change of water to completely leach the salt. Subsequently, the morphology, pore size and pore interconnectivity were confirmed by scanning electron microscopy (SEM). Finally, scaffolds were made sterile using 70% ethanol wash followed by UV exposure for 30 min before using for tissue culture.

## 2.3. Culture of CTCs in 3D PCL Scaffolds

The RBC-lysed nucleated cells were seeded in scaffolds and maintained at 37 °C in 5% ($v/v$) $CO_2$ and 1.1% $O_2$ under humidified conditions. Each processed sample was split into multiple wells of a 96-well plate (~10 mL RBC-lysed blood was distributed into 5 or 6 wells). The culture medium (DMEM + 10% FBS) was changed after 72 h the first time after seeding, followed by every alternative day up to 14 days.

## 2.4. Immunophenotyping of Cells

Cells and scaffolds were fixed with 3.7% formaldehyde for 15 min and permeabilized with 0.2% Triton X-100 for maximum 10 min followed by three washes with PBST (0.05% Tween 20 in 1× PBS) each for 5 min. Blocking was done with blocking buffer (0.2% fish skin gelatin: FSG, 0.01% Tween 20, 0.2% sodium azide: $NaN_3$) for 45 min. Primary antibodies were used at 1:200 dilutions for overnight at 4 °C. Excess antibodies were removed by giving three washes with PBST each for 5 min. Secondary antibodies were used at 1:200 dilutions and incubated at dark for 2 h at room temperature. In some studies, Phalloidin conjugated with Alexa Fluor™ 488 and Alexa Fluor™ 546 were used for 2 h in dark. Counterstaining for nucleus with Hoechst 33342 was done by incubating for 5 min in dark. All the samples were imaged using epifluorescence (Olympus IX71) or confocal laser (Olympus FV10i/Olympus FV3000/Leica SP8) microscope. Image processing was performed by ImageJ software.

## 2.5. Study of Cell Morphology by Scanning Electron Microscopy (SEM)

RBC-depleted nucleated cells from patient blood sample cultured in scaffolds were fixed with 2.5% glutaraldehyde for 12 h at 4 °C. The cell-laden scaffolds were then dehydrated in a gradient of ethanol, 30, 50, 70, 90, and 100%, each for a period of 10 min. The samples were completely air-dried and gold-coated by means of sputtering apparatus before observation to avoid charging under the electron beam. The samples were analyzed using SEM microscopy (JEOL SEM, Peabody, MA, USA).

## 2.6. Bromodeoxyuridine (BrdU) Assay for Cell Proliferation in 3D PCL Scaffolds

### 2.6.1. Immunofluorescence-Based BrdU Assay

For immunostaining, RBC-depleted nucleated cells cultured in 3D PCL scaffolds (at day 7, day 14) were permeabilized with 0.2% Triton X-100 on ice for 90 sec followed by fixation with 3.7% formaldehyde at RT. Cells were denatured with denaturing solution (2N HCl, 0.5% Triton X-100) for 30 min at RT, followed by blocking (0.5% BSA, 0.5% Triton X-100) for 30 min at RT. Primary anti-BrdU was used at 1:1000 dilution for 2 h at RT. Excess antibodies were removed by washing thrice with PBST. Secondary antibody was used at 1:200 dilution for 1 h at RT in dark, followed by three washes with PBST. Finally, counterstaining for nucleus was done with Sytox green (Invitrogen, Carlsbad, CA, USA) for 5 min at RT in dark. Imaging was done in Leica SP8 confocal laser microscope. Images were processed with ImageJ software.

### 2.6.2. Colorimetry-Based BrdU Assay

RBC-depleted nucleated cells from blood samples of breast cancer patients were cultured in 3D PCL scaffolds for different day points (day 3, day 7, day 14) under hypoxic condition. MDA-MB-231 cells were cultured under a similar condition which was taken as control. Further, similar cells were cultured in 2D culture system for 24 h under normoxia which was taken as the 2D control. On the particular day point, BrdU label (1:2000 dilution in tissue culture media) was added and left for 48 h for incubation inside the incubator. Scaffolds containing cells were then fixed and denatured using fixative or denaturing solution (Calbiochem QIA58) by incubating for 30 min at room temperature (RT). Primary anti-BrdU antibody was used at 1:100 dilutions for 1 h at RT. Excess antibody was removed by using 1× wash buffer, provided with the kit. HRP conjugated secondary antibody was used at 1:1000 dilution for 30 min at RT followed by three washes with wash buffer. Wells were flooded with ddH$_2$O. Next, the substrate (TMB-tetramethylbenzidine) was added in the well and was incubated in dark for 15 min at 37 °C which resulted in a change of color of the solution to blue. Finally, stop solution was added which turns the solution yellow colored. Absorbance was measured at dual wavelengths, 450 nm and 595 nm, within 30 min of adding stop solution.

## 3. Results

### 3.1. Culture of Breast Cancer Patient-Derived Cells in 3D PCL Scaffolds

In an attempt to establish CTC culture in 3D porous PCL scaffolds, blood samples were collected from 16 chemo-naïve breast cancer patients clinically diagnosed with brain, liver or lung metastases (Supplementary Table S1). Three-dimensional PCL scaffolds were fabricated as per the standardized protocol [13] (Supplementary Figure S1A). Following the separation of plasma from blood cells and RBC lysis, the nucleated cell pellet was resuspended in media and seeded in 3D PCL scaffolds (schematic in Figure 1A). After 14 days, the scaffold culture was stained and imaged. Fluorescence micrographs showed positivity for nucleus and F-actin, revealing the presence of nucleated cells (Supplementary Figure S1B). These observations were corroborated with scanning electron microscopy with SEM micrographs showing the presence of fewer cells after 3 days and 7 days of culture (Figure 2Ai,ii), which gradually increased by 14 days of culture (Figure 2Aiii,iv). We also observed the presence of cells attached to scaffolds by day 7 of culture (yellow arrow, Figure 2Aii) and the presence of cell clusters by day 14 of culture in 3D PCL scaffolds (blue arrow, Figure 2Aiii) as well as intercellular connections (red arrow, Figure 2Aiv). Interestingly, we noted the deposition of thread-like (Figure 2Bi) and sheet-like (Figure 2Bii) extracellular matrix (ECM) in the scaffold culture. Immunostaining for the ECM protein laminin confirmed ECM deposition by cells on the PCL scaffold (Figure 2C). These observations suggested the significant capture and expansion of nucleated cells from the blood in 3D PCL scaffolds.

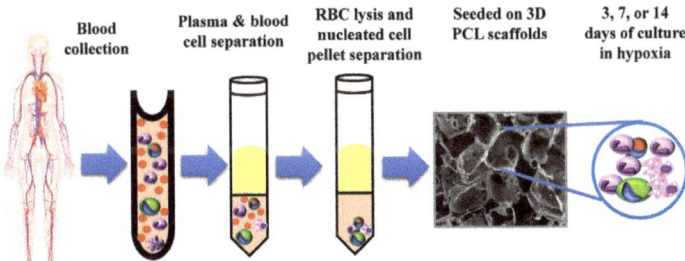

**Figure 1.** Workflow of culturing breast cancer patient blood-derived cells in 3D poly(ε-caprolactone) (PCL) scaffolds. Schematic showing the culture method of breast cancer patient blood samples for culturing circulating tumor cells (CTCs).

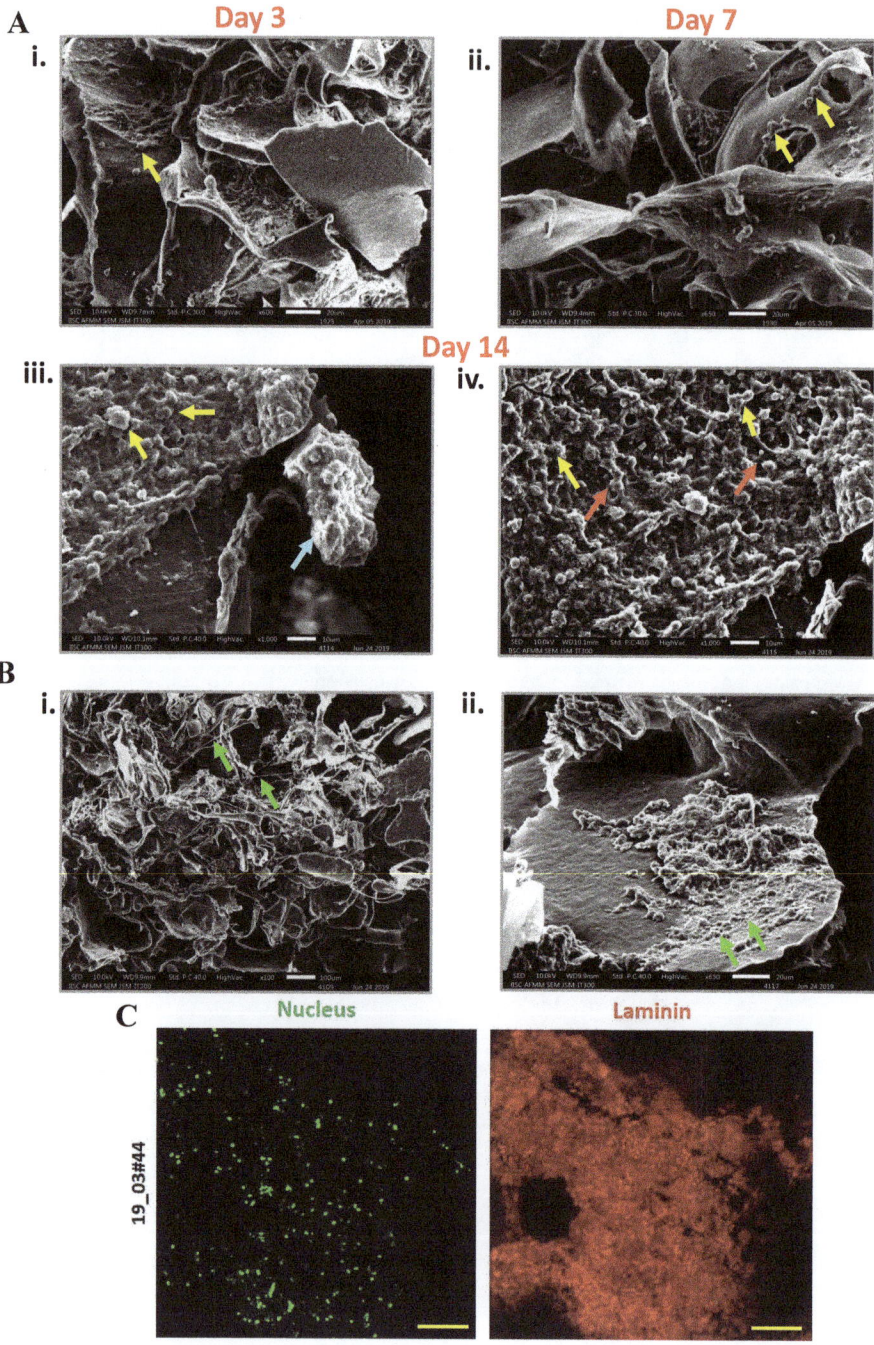

**Figure 2.** Detection of cell clusters and extracellular matrix (ECM) deposition in 3D PCL scaffolds. (**Ai–iv**) SEM micrographs showed the presence of increasing numbers of cells in day 3, day 7 and day 14 cultures of red blood cell (RBC)-depleted nucleated cell pellet of patient samples cultured in 3D PCL scaffold (yellow arrows). Formation of clusters (**iii**) (blue arrow) and the presence of intercellular

contacts (**iv**) (red arrows) was detected after 14 days of culture. Scale bar represents 20 µm. Images are representative of 6 patient samples. (**B**) Scanning electron microscopy analysis revealed the deposition of thread-like (**i**) and sheet-like (**ii**) ECM (green arrows). Images are representative of 4 patient samples. (**C**) Cells were immunostained for ECM protein Laminin (red); nucleus counterstained with Hoechst 33342 (pseudocoloured green). Imaging was performed using confocal microscope and maximum intensity projections are shown. Scale bar represents 100 µm. Minus primary antibody served as negative control and did not show staining; data not shown.

## 3.2. Detection of CK-Positive and CD45-Negative Cells in 3D Scaffold Cultures

CTCs immunocaptured by epithelial cell adhesion molecule (EpCAM) antibodies in devices including FDA-approved CellSearch are often identified as cytokeratin (CK)-positive and CD45-negative cells [16–18]. Therefore, we sought to identify CK+/CD45− cells in 3D PCL scaffolds by dual staining. We undertook immunostaining for panCK and CD45 concomitant with a nuclear counterstain (Hoechst 33342). Confocal microscopy confirmed the presence of panCK-positive and CD45-negative cells derived from blood samples of breast cancer patients (Figure 3). Thus, the detection of CK-positive and CD45-negative cells confirmed the presence of breast cancer patient-derived CTCs in the 3D PCL scaffolds. In addition, we also observed CK+ cells surrounded by CD45+ cell.

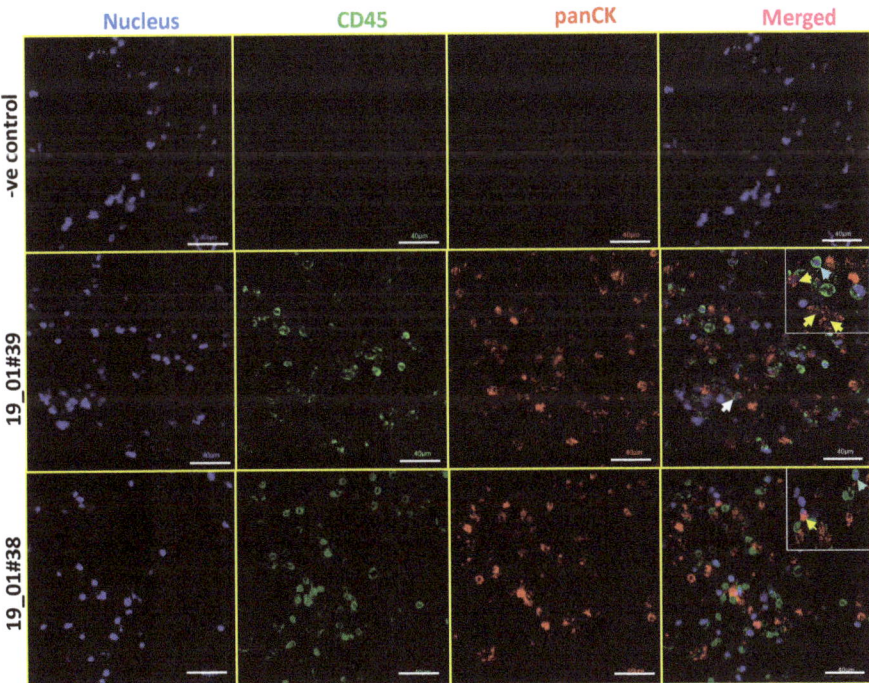

**Figure 3.** Identification of CK-positive and CD45-negative CTCs in breast cancer patient blood samples cultured in 3D PCL scaffold. Immunostaining shows the presence of panCK+/CD45− CTCs in day 14 cultures of patient blood samples cultured in 3D PCL scaffolds. Top panel shows negative control (minus primary antibody). Middle and bottom panels show immunostaining done on two different patient samples. Yellow arrows indicate panCK+ and CD45 negative CTCs while blue arrows indicate CD45 positive leucocyte lineage cells. White arrow shows CK+ cells surrounded by CD45+ cells. Imaging was performed using confocal microscope, and maximum intensity projections are shown. Inset shows higher magnification. Scale bar represents 40 µm. Images are representative of 7 independent patient samples.

## 3.3. Cell Proliferation in 3D PCL Scaffolds

After establishing a novel 3D system to culture CTCs from patient-blood derived nucleated cells, we tested whether this culture system facilitates cell proliferation. After testing the expression of Ki-67, a proliferative marker, in actively dividing MDA-MB-231 cells as a positive control (Supplementary Figure S2A,B) we checked the expression of Ki-67 in the RBC-depleted nucleated cells cultured in the PCL scaffolds for 14 days. Fluorescence images revealed distinct nuclear localization of Ki-67 (Figure 4A), suggesting that these cells are actively proliferating in 3D PCL scaffolds. This observation was confirmed in 2 independent breast cancer patient samples cultured in the scaffolds.

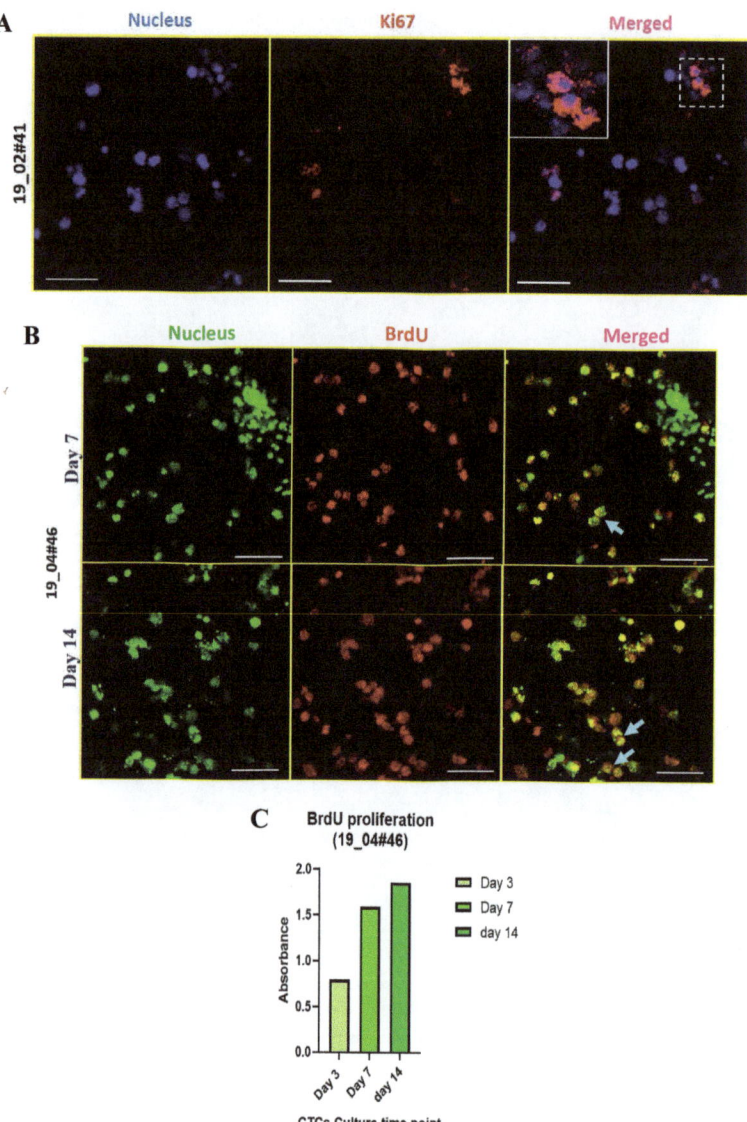

**Figure 4.** Active cell proliferation in breast cancer patient-derived cells cultured in 3D PCL scaffolds. (**A**) Fluorescence images of Ki-67 positive patient blood cells harvested after 14 days of culture in 3D

PCL scaffolds. Cells were stained for nucleus (Hoechst 33342, blue), Ki-67 (red). Images are representative of 2 independent patient samples. (**B**) Patient-derived cells were exposed to a single pulse of 50 µM BrdU on day 7 and day 14 of culture and harvested after 48 h for immunostaining for BrdU incorporation. Fluorescence images show BrdU-positive cells (red), stained for nucleus (Sytox green); blue arrows show the merge. Imaging was performed using confocal microscope and maximum intensity projections are shown. Scale bar represents 40 µm (**A**,**B**). (**C**) Graph shows BrdU incorporation in patient-derived cells over time (day 3, day 7, day 14) in culture as measured by colorimetry. Images are representative of 2 independent patient samples.

To further confirm active cell proliferation, we performed BrdU-based cell proliferation assay. After exposing day 7 and day 14 cultures to BrdU for 48 h, we did immunostaining using anti-BrdU-specific antibodies. We detected around 10 out of 30 cells (per field) as BrdU-positive cells (blue arrows) by 7 days of culture, whereas approximately 20 out of 30 cells were BrdU-positive by 14 days of culture (Figure 4B). Further, we performed a colorimetry-based assay to validate the fluorescence-based observation of BrdU incorporation. We exposed cells cultured in the 3D scaffold to BrdU label for 48 h at different time points, including day 3, day 7 and day 14. The graph revealed a gradual increase in BrdU incorporation (based on relative absorbance) (Figure 4C). Together, these data revealed active cell proliferation in 3D PCL scaffolds.

### 3.4. Epithelial (E) and Mesenchymal (M) Heterogeneity in Patient-Derived CTCs

Since our CTC culture strategy did not involve a prior enrichment with epithelial markers such as EpCAM, we exploited this system to investigate whether CTC subsets enriched by growing in 3D PCL scaffold showed the presence of epithelial (E) and mesenchymal (M)-type cells. For this, we analyzed the expression of sets of epithelial and mesenchymal markers. We selected a series of epithelial (panCK/CK18/ZO-1/E-cad) and mesenchymal marker (N-cad/Vimentin) markers which were first confirmed across breast cancer cell lines (Supplementary Figure S3A,B). Immunostaining of CTCs cultured in PCL scaffolds for the aforementioned markers revealed the presence of differential expression of both E- and M-type markers within the same patient, as well as across different patients (Figure 5). The result showed dual expression of both epithelial and mesenchymal markers suggesting the existence of intermediate EMT phenotype (Figure 5). Notably, M-type marker expression was more in most of the patient samples, suggestive of an intermediate mesenchymal phenotype, which well correlated with our earlier observation where we saw intermediate mesenchymal scores for the breast CTCs [19].

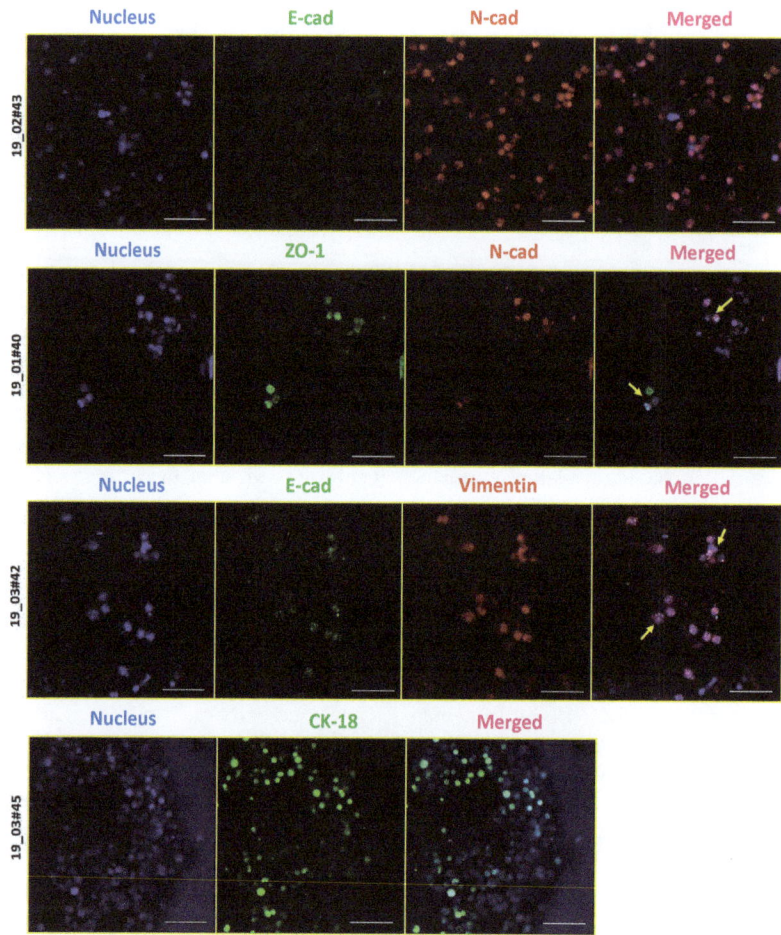

**Figure 5.** E-M characterization of CTCs derived from blood samples of breast cancer patients. Immunostaining revealed the presence of epithelial (E)-type CTCs expressing E-cad, ZO-1, or CK18 (green), and mesenchymal (M)-type CTCs expressing vimentin or N-cad (red). Cells were stained for nucleus (Hoechst 33342, blue). Imaging was performed using confocal microscope and maximum intensity projections are shown. Scale bar represents 40 µm. Images are representative of 4 independent patient samples.

To further address E-M heterogeneity, we first confirmed the dual expression of a combination of E (pan-CK)- and M (vimentin)-type markers across breast cancer cell lines MCF 7 and MDA MB 231 (Supplementary Figure S4). Dual immunofluorescence of panCK and vimentin on day 14 cultures of patient-derived CTCs showed the presence of heterogeneous expression of E and M markers (Figure 6A). A detailed analysis of the images revealed 5 categories of cells ranging from E (exclusively), E > M, E = M, M > E, M (exclusively) (Figure 6B) suggesting dynamic changes in epithelial and mesenchymal composition, similar to a recent report [20]. This dynamic E-M heterogeneity and the existence of intermediate/hybrid cells is supported by recent literature [21,22].

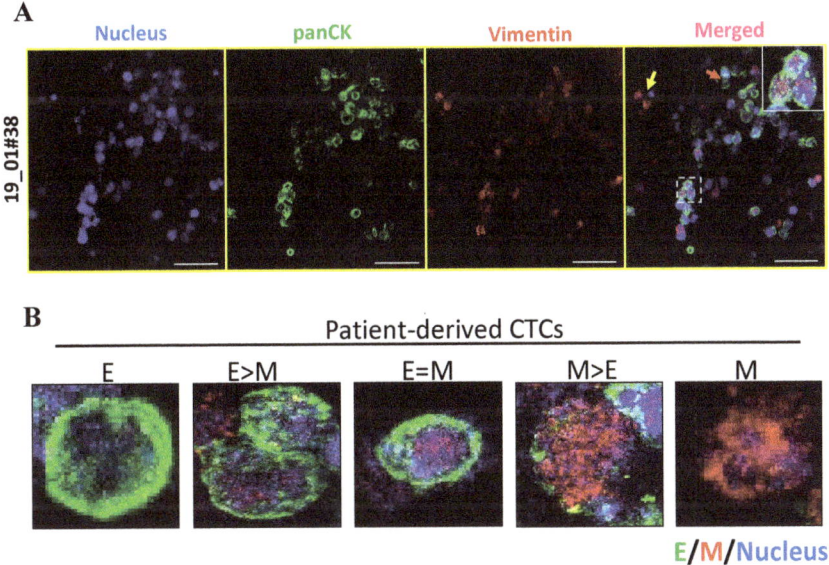

**Figure 6.** E-M heterogeneity and intermediate phenotypes in breast cancer patient-derived CTCs. (**A**) Co-staining for panCK and vimentin in patient-derived CTCs revealed the presence of marked heterogeneity with respect to E and M marker expression. (**B**) Representative fluorescence images of 5 different types of CTCs: E (exclusively), E > M, E = M, M > E and M (exclusively). Cells were counterstained for nucleus (Hoechst 33342, blue), E-type markers (green), and M-type markers (red). Imaging was performed using confocal microscope and maximum intensity projections are shown. Scale bar represents 40 μm (**A**). Images are representative of 2 independent patient samples.

## 4. Discussion

CTCs are considered as surrogate markers for monitoring and evaluating patient treatment responses. Current advances in technology have enabled us to isolate these rare CTC populations. However, the real challenge lies in the successful expansion of these cells in culture conditions. Our group has previously established laser-ablated microwells-based method for the rapid expansion of CTCs [14]. Recently, we improvised the method using agar rather than tapered microwells to culture these cells [15]. However, 2D culture methods are incompetent to mimic natural structural organization. They also exhibit compromised morphology and differentiation. Also, deposition of the extracellular matrix is critical for proper attachment and proliferation. Several 3D scaffolds either use a material like agar, which fails to allow ECM deposition, or matrigel, which has an abundant ECM that might not mimic the environment faced by CTCs at the secondary site. To overcome these concerns, we developed a 3D culture method using 3D porous PCL scaffolds which allowed deposition of ECM from the cells derived from patient samples and enabled the culture of CTCs.

When RBC-depleted nucleated cell pellets from whole blood from breast cancer patient samples were cultured in the 3D porous PCL scaffolds, we observed cell clusters which were positive for F actin. Our SEM micrographs revealed the presence of ECM deposition on the PCL scaffolds. This observation was confirmed by immunostaining for Laminin protein, a component of the extracellular matrix. In this study, SEM micrographs have revealed the formation of inter-cellular connections and tumor like masses or tumoroids derived from nucleated patient-blood samples. CTCs are typically identified based on the expression of epithelial markers such as keratins, EpCAM and the absence of common leukocyte marker CD45 [23]. In accordance with this, we noted the presence of pan-cytokeratin positive and CD45 negative cells in our 3D cultures. We cannot rule out the possibility that these are epithelial tumor cells engulfed by fibroblasts and macrophages; further characterization needs to be done to rule this out. However, recent reports have suggested the existence of E-M heterogeneity based on the expression of both epithelial and mesenchymal markers [24]. We further characterized the epithelial and mesenchymal properties of CTCs in 3D PCL scaffolds. Our results indicated dual expression of both epithelial (pan CK) and mesenchymal markers (vimentin), revealing the presence of intermediate/hybrid EMT phenotype. Moreover, we also observed differential expression holds true for several other markers including E-cadherin, ZO-1, N cadherin and vimentin as well. Further investigation is required to validate the same with various histological subtypes of breast cancers (based on ER/PR/HER2 status).

The breast cancer patient-derived CTCs effectively reflect inter- and intra-patient heterogeneity in terms of E or M markers expression. Additionally, cell proliferation assays confirmed the expansion of viable nucleated cells in 3D culture system. Although our data showed proliferating cell population, and we have previously demonstrated the gradual depletion of other lineage cells [14], it still remains to be confirmed if CTCs are indeed proliferating in these scaffolds by undertaking a co-staining staining for Pan-CK, CD45, and Ki67. The proliferating cells as observed by Ki67 and BrdU positivity in our study could include both CTCs as well as other cell types, such as cancer associated fibroblasts and macrophages, which may provide a suitable microenvironment for the enrichment of CTCs. Nevertheless, our study revealed visualization of viable cytokeratin positive/CD45 negative cells, and the detection of ZO-1 alone and ZO-1/N-cad double positive cells in these scaffolds by the end of 14 days in culture. Thus, our study shows that culture of RBC-lysed, nucleated cells from patient blood in 3D-PCL scaffold can serve as a novel system for culturing CTCs. Taken together, our study has demonstrated an easy but effective 3D culture method for in vitro culture and possible expansion of CTCs. Hence, this could serve as an excellent platform for a deeper study of CTC biology and metastasis. Taken together, we conclude that our novel ex vivo 3D culture system would provide a more reliable system for future personalized drug-screening for cancer patients.

**Supplementary Materials:** The following are available online at http://www.mdpi.com/2077-0383/8/9/1473/s1, Figure S1: 3D PCL scaffolds exhibit good porosity and pore inter-connectivity, and show the presence of cells, Figure S2: Active cell proliferation in breast cancer cell line (MDA-MB-231), Figure S3: Expression of epithelial (E) and mesenchymal (M) markers across breast cancer cell lines, Figure S4: E-M heterogeneity in breast cancer cell lines. Table S1: Clinical parameters of breast cancer patients (Invasive ductal carcinoma (IDC) analyzed in this study.

**Author Contributions:** T.D., A.R., G.B.K. and P.K. designed methodology; T.D. standardized and performed all experiments and collected all data; S.G., G.B.K. helped with patient selection, and collection of blood samples and patient data; T.D., S.G., G.B., P.K., G.B.K. and A.R. analyzed the data; T.D. drafted the manuscript; A.R., G.B.K, G.B., K.C. and P.K. reviewed and edited the manuscript; all the authors read and approved the final version of the manuscript.

**Funding:** This work was funded primarily by a joint grant from Rajiv Gandhi University of Health Science, Bangalore (RGUHS) to A.R., G.B.K. and P.K., and in part by an Indo-Israel Joint Research Grant (UGC) to A.R. A.R. is a recipient of the Welcome Trust/DBT India Alliance Fellowship. P.K. is a recipient of the Ramanujan Fellowship awarded by Department of Science and Technology (DST), Government of India. T.D. is a recipient of research fellowship from the University Grants Commission (UGC), New Delhi, India.

**Acknowledgments:** A.R. acknowledges DBT-IISc partnership programme, and support from DST-FIST and UGC, Govt. of India, to the department of MRDG, IISc. Authors sincerely thank the central confocal facility and SEM facility at IISc.

**Conflicts of Interest:** The authors declare no conflict of interest.

## References

1. Chaffer, C.L.; Weinberg, R.A. A perspective on cancer cell metastasis. *Science* **2011**, *331*, 1559–1564. [CrossRef] [PubMed]
2. Fidler, I.J. The pathogenesis of cancer metastasis: The'seed and soil'hypothesis revisited. *Nat. Rev. Cancer* **2003**, *3*, 453. [CrossRef] [PubMed]
3. Micalizzi, D.S.; Maheswaran, S.; Haber, D.A. A conduit to metastasis: Circulating tumor cell biology. *Genes Dev.* **2017**, *31*, 1827–1840. [CrossRef]

4. Yu, M.; Stott, S.; Toner, M.; Maheswaran, S.; Haber, D.A. Circulating tumor cells: Approaches to isolation and characterization. *J. Cell Biol.* **2011**, *192*, 373–382. [CrossRef] [PubMed]
5. Schiro, P.G.; Zhao, M.; Kuo, J.S.; Koehler, K.M.; Sabath, D.E.; Chiu, D.T. Sensitive and high-throughput isolation of rare cells from peripheral blood with ensemble-decision aliquot ranking. *Angew. Chem. Int. Ed.* **2012**, *51*, 4618–4622. [CrossRef] [PubMed]
6. Wang, X.; Qian, X.; Beitler, J.J.; Chen, Z.G.; Khuri, F.R.; Lewis, M.M.; Shin, H.J.C.; Nie, S.; Shin, D.M. Detection of circulating tumor cells in human peripheral blood using surface-enhanced Raman scattering nanoparticles. *Cancer Res.* **2011**, *71*, 1526–1532. [CrossRef] [PubMed]
7. Miller, M.C.; Doyle, G.V.; Terstappen, L.W. Significance of circulating tumor cells detected by the CellSearch system in patients with metastatic breast colorectal and prostate cancer. *J. Oncol.* **2010**, *2010*. [CrossRef] [PubMed]
8. Alix-Panabières, C. EPISPOT assay: Detection of viable DTCs/CTCs in solid tumor patients. In *Minimal Residual Disease and Circulating Tumor Cells in Breast Cancer*; Springer: Berlin/Heidelberg, Germany, 2012; pp. 69–76.
9. Vishnoi, M.; Peddibhotla, S.; Yin, W.; Scamardo, A.T.; George, G.C.; Hong, D.S.; Marchetti, D. The isolation and characterization of CTC subsets related to breast cancer dormancy. *Sci. Rep.* **2015**, *5*, 17533. [CrossRef]
10. Pantel, K.; Brakenhoff, R.H.; Brandt, B. Detection, clinical relevance and specific biological properties of disseminating tumour cells. *Nat. Rev. Cancer* **2008**, *8*, 329. [CrossRef]
11. Paszek, M.J.; Zahir, N.; Johnson, K.R.; Lakins, J.N.; Rozenberg, G.I.; Gefen, A.; Reinhart-King, C.A.; Margulies, S.S.; Dembo, M.; Boettiger, D. Tensional homeostasis and the malignant phenotype. *Cancer Cell* **2005**, *8*, 241–254. [CrossRef]
12. Riedl, A.; Schlederer, M.; Pudelko, K.; Stadler, M.; Walter, S.; Unterleuthner, D.; Unger, C.; Kramer, N.; Hengstschläger, M.; Kenner, L. Comparison of cancer cells in 2D vs 3D culture reveals differences in AKT–mTOR–S6K signaling and drug responses. *J Cell Sci* **2017**, *130*, 203–218. [CrossRef] [PubMed]
13. Balachander, G.M.; Balaji, S.A.; Rangarajan, A.; Chatterjee, K. Enhanced metastatic potential in a 3D tissue scaffold toward a comprehensive in vitro model for breast cancer metastasis. *Acs Appl. Mater. Interfaces* **2015**, *7*, 27810–27822. [CrossRef] [PubMed]
14. Khoo, B.L.; Lee, S.C.; Kumar, P.; Tan, T.Z.; Warkiani, M.E.; Ow, S.G.; Nandi, S.; Lim, C.T.; Thiery, J.P. Short-term expansion of breast circulating cancer cells predicts response to anti-cancer therapy. *Oncotarget* **2015**, *6*, 15578. [CrossRef] [PubMed]
15. Balakrishnan, A.; Koppaka, D.; Anand, A.; Deb, B.; Grenci, G.; Viasnoff, V.; Thompson, E.W.; Gowda, H.; Bhat, R.; Rangarajan, A. Circulating Tumor Cell cluster phenotype allows monitoring response to treatment and predicts survival. *Sci. Rep.* **2019**, *9*, 7933. [CrossRef] [PubMed]
16. Nagrath, S.; Sequist, L.V.; Maheswaran, S.; Bell, D.W.; Irimia, D.; Ulkus, L.; Smith, M.R.; Kwak, E.L.; Digumarthy, S.; Muzikansky, A. Isolation of rare circulating tumour cells in cancer patients by microchip technology. *Nature* **2007**, *450*, 1235. [CrossRef] [PubMed]
17. Stott, S.L.; Hsu, C.-H.; Tsukrov, D.I.; Yu, M.; Miyamoto, D.T.; Waltman, B.A.; Rothenberg, S.M.; Shah, A.M.; Smas, M.E.; Korir, G.K. Isolation of circulating tumor cells using a microvortex-generating herringbone-chip. *Proc. Natl. Acad. Sci. USA* **2010**, *107*, 18392–18397. [CrossRef] [PubMed]
18. Farace, F.; Massard, C.; Vimond, N.; Drusch, F.; Jacques, N.; Billiot, F.; Laplanche, A.; Chauchereau, A.; Lacroix, L.; Planchard, D. A direct comparison of CellSearch and ISET for circulating tumour-cell detection in patients with metastatic carcinomas. *Br. J. Cancer* **2011**, *105*, 847. [CrossRef] [PubMed]
19. Yadavalli, S.; Jayaram, S.; Manda, S.; Madugundu, A.; Nayakanti, D.; Tan, T.; Bhat, R.; Rangarajan, A.; Chatterjee, A.; Gowda, H. Data-driven discovery of extravasation pathway in circulating tumor cells. *Sci. Rep.* **2017**, *7*, 43710. [CrossRef] [PubMed]
20. Yu, M.; Bardia, A.; Wittner, B.S.; Stott, S.L.; Smas, M.E.; Ting, D.T.; Isakoff, S.J.; Ciciliano, J.C.; Wells, M.N.; Shah, A.M. Circulating breast tumor cells exhibit dynamic changes in epithelial and mesenchymal composition. *Science* **2013**, *339*, 580–584. [CrossRef]
21. Agnoletto, C.; Corrà, F.; Minotti, L.; Baldassari, F.; Crudele, F.; Cook, W.J.J.; Di Leva, G.; d'Adamo, A.P.; Gasparini, P.; Volinia, S. Heterogeneity in circulating tumor cells: The relevance of the stem-cell subset. *Cancers* **2019**, *11*, 483. [CrossRef]
22. Jolly, M.K.; Boareto, M.; Huang, B.; Jia, D.; Lu, M.; Ben-Jacob, E.; Onuchic, J.N.; Levine, H. Implications of the hybrid epithelial/mesenchymal phenotype in metastasis. *Front. Oncol.* **2015**, *5*, 155. [CrossRef] [PubMed]

23. Maheswaran, S.; Haber, D.A. Circulating tumor cells: A window into cancer biology and metastasis. *Curr. Opin. Genet. Dev.* **2010**, *20*, 96–99. [CrossRef] [PubMed]
24. Bednarz-Knoll, N.; Alix-Panabières, C.; Pantel, K. Clinical relevance and biology of circulating tumor cells. *Breast Cancer Res.* **2011**, *13*, 228. [CrossRef] [PubMed]

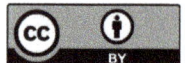

© 2019 by the authors. Licensee MDPI, Basel, Switzerland. This article is an open access article distributed under the terms and conditions of the Creative Commons Attribution (CC BY) license (http://creativecommons.org/licenses/by/4.0/).

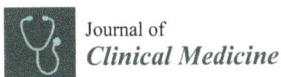

*Article*

# Multi-Omics Characterization of the Spontaneous Mesenchymal–Epithelial Transition in the PMC42 Breast Cancer Cell Lines

Sugandha Bhatia [1,2,3,*], James Monkman [1,2,3], Tony Blick [1,2,3], Pascal HG Duijf [1,3,4], Shivashankar H. Nagaraj [1,2,3] and Erik W. Thompson [1,2,3,*]

1. Institute of Health and Biomedical Innovation, Queensland University of Technology, Brisbane, QLD 4059, Australia
2. School of Biomedical Sciences, Faculty of Health, Queensland University of Technology, Brisbane, QLD 4000, Australia
3. Translational Research Institute, Brisbane, QLD 4102, Australia
4. University of Queensland Diamantina Institute, The University of Queensland, Woolloongabba, QLD 4102, Australia
* Correspondence: sugandha.bhatia@hdr.qut.edu.au (S.B.); e2.thompson@qut.edu.au (E.W.T.)

Received: 10 July 2019; Accepted: 15 August 2019; Published: 19 August 2019

**Abstract:** Epithelial–mesenchymal plasticity (EMP), encompassing epithelial–mesenchymal transition (EMT) and mesenchymal–epithelial transition (MET), are considered critical events for cancer metastasis. We investigated chromosomal heterogeneity and chromosomal instability (CIN) profiles of two sister PMC42 breast cancer (BC) cell lines to assess the relationship between their karyotypes and EMP phenotypic plasticity. Karyotyping by GTG banding and exome sequencing were aligned with SWATH quantitative proteomics and existing RNA-sequencing data from the two PMC42 cell lines; the mesenchymal, parental PMC42-ET cell line and the spontaneously epithelially shifted PMC42-LA daughter cell line. These morphologically distinct PMC42 cell lines were also compared with five other BC cell lines (MDA-MB-231, SUM-159, T47D, MCF-7 and MDA-MB-468) for their expression of EMP and cell surface markers, and stemness and metabolic profiles. The findings suggest that the epithelially shifted cell line has a significantly altered ploidy of chromosomes 3 and 13, which is reflected in their transcriptomic and proteomic expression profiles. Loss of the TGFβR2 gene from chromosome 3 in the epithelial daughter cell line inhibits its EMT induction by TGF-β stimulus. Thus, integrative 'omics' characterization established that the PMC42 system is a relevant MET model and provides insights into the regulation of phenotypic plasticity in breast cancer.

**Keywords:** copy number variations (CNV); epithelial–mesenchymal transition (EMT); karyotyping; mesenchymal–epithelial transition (MET); metabolism; proteomics; RNA-sequencing; seahorse extracellular flux analyser; whole exome sequencing

---

## 1. Introduction

Breast cancer, a leading cause of cancer death in women, is recognized as a molecularly heterogeneous disease [1,2]. Breast cancer cell culture systems and patient-derived xenografts (PDX) recapitulate many of the intrinsic molecular subtypes of breast cancer [3]. Various experimental techniques have been employed in these models, such as exome sequencing, copy-number analysis, whole-transcriptome, epigenome and methylome analyses, and identification of biomarkers that were mapped simultaneously to the genotypic and/or phenotypic behaviour in relevance to breast cancer subtypes or mammary gland development [4–15]. The compendium of molecular profiles defining up to 90 different breast cancer cell lines provides a valuable resource and has been studied extensively [10–13,15], not only for the discovery of new breast cancer genes [10], but also for investigations of their subtype-specific pathobiology, cancer stem cell biology, biomarkers, and response to different drug therapies [16]. Thus, cell culture systems provide important models for studying the molecular mechanisms of neoplastic transformation and are extremely useful in translational research.

Epithelial–mesenchymal plasticity (EMP), which encompasses epithelial–mesenchymal transition (EMT) and its reversal (mesenchymal–epithelial transition; MET), including hybrid states within this spectrum, is considered an important hallmark of cancer that drives metastasis [17–19]. EMT provides carcinoma cells with the ability to undergo cellular morphogenesis, allowing clusters of epithelial cells to form independent motile mesenchymal-like cells that can disseminate. MET is thought to subsequently reinstate proliferation and allow collective outgrowth at the metastatic site. The genetic and phenotypic heterogeneity of carcinoma cells across the EMP axis also has importance in therapy-resistance seen after EMT [20–23]. The molecular and cellular analyses of EMT features in breast cancer cell lines have also been analysed thoroughly and scoring tools have been developed to quantify the extent of EMT [24–29].

EMP studies in cancer cell lines have been widely reported. Therein, EMP is either induced by external stimuli, such as hypoxia [30], TGF-β [31], EGF [32], FGF [33], or by inducible expression or repression of EMT-inducing transcription factors [34,35]. Transformed breast cancer cells obtained by introducing oncogenes or cancer-associated genes into normal primary human mammary epithelial cells, such as HMLE and D492 cells, have also been remodelled as HMLER and D492M, respectively, to study cancer development including EMT [36–39]. To our knowledge, the PMC42 system is the only breast cancer cell line model where a spontaneous MET event has led to a new stable variant [40]. In this regard, the PMC42 system provides a unique case study to investigate the molecular and phenotypic characteristics of a stable MET in carcinoma without the use of external stimuli or genetic manipulation.

The relationships between different levels of regulation (genomic, transcriptomic, metabolomic, etc.) in the intrinsic endogenous plasticity (i.e., not exogenously induced) seen in several EMP systems has not been systematically studied, although each has separately been implicated in EMP regulation. Here, we interrogate and integrate the molecular portrait of PMC42, a unique human breast carcinoma cell line originally established from the pleural effusion of a breast cancer patient in 1983 [41]. Original cultures of PMC42 cells were reported to be heterogeneous, with at least eight different morphological types identified by phase contrast and electron microscopy [41,42]. In earlier studies, PMC42 cells were shown to grow both as a monolayer and as cords in suspension, and have shown features of myoepithelial cells [41,43,44]. PMC42 cells obtained from Dr. Robert Whitehead [41,42] were subsequently annotated as PMC42-ET. PMC42-ET exhibits a 'Basal B' (mesenchymal) transcriptome (E Tomaskovic-Crook and T Blick, unpublished observation) [30] and PMC42-LA cells were a spontaneous derivative cell line from PMC42-ET developed by Dr. Leigh Ackland [40,45]. Although epithelially shifted to the extent that they can produce a functional epithelium in 3-dimensional (3D) cultures [45], they still cluster transcriptomically with PMC42-ET cells (E Tomaskovic-Crook and T Blick, unpublished observation) [30]. This makes these cell lines an ideal system to study MET. Comparison of the karyotype, exome, transcriptome, proteome and metabolic phenotype of PMC42-ET and its epithelial "daughter" cell line PMC42-LA were performed to gain insights into the dynamic events that contributed to this spontaneous MET, in reference to EMP studies.

## 2. Materials and Methods

### 2.1. Cell Lines and Cell Culture

Cells (BT-549, Hs578T, MCF-7, T47D, MDA-MB-157, MDA-MB-231, MDA-MB-468, SUM-159) were obtained from the American Type Culture Collection (Manassas, VA, USA). PMC42-ET and the derivative PMC42-LA cell line were derived from a breast cancer pleural effusion with appropriate institutional ethics clearance (Institutional Review Board of the Peter MacCallum Hospital, Melbourne) [41–43,45].

Cell lines were cultured in Dulbecco's modified Eagle's medium (DMEM) containing glucose (4.5 g/L), L-Glutamine (0.5 g/L) and sodium pyruvate (0.1 g/L) (Corning, Catalog number 10-013-CVR), and supplemented with 10% foetal bovine serum (FBS; Gibco™, Thermo Fischer Scientific, Waltham, MA, USA) and antibiotics penicillin and streptomycin (Gibco™, Life Technologies, NY, USA; Catalog number 15140122), and maintained at 37 °C, 5% $CO_2$, and 95% humidity. Cells were routinely tested and were negative for *Mycoplasma*.

*2.2. Preparation of Metaphase Spread and Karyotyping*

After 60%–70% of confluency was achieved in 60 mm dishes, cells were treated with 10 µL of demecolcine (10 µg/mL) for 3–4 h. Cells were harvested using trypsin (Corning™ 25053CI) and the pellet was gently treated with hypotonic solution (75 mM KCl) for 40–60 min at 37 °C and fixed in cold methanol/acetic acid (3:1). Two or three drops of suspended cells were applied to glass slides and chromosomes were stained with DAPI and imaged by confocal microscopy (Olympus Fluoview FV1200 Confocal Laser Scanning Microscope, Olympus Australia Pty. Ltd., Melbourne, Victoria, Australia). Counting was performed manually in ImageJ. Karyotype assessment via G-band analysis was performed by a commercial genotyping service (StemCore Facility, Brisbane, QLD, Australia) and 50 metaphases were analysed per cell line.

*2.3. DNA Extraction, Whole Exome Sequencing and Processing of Sequencing Data*

Genomic DNA was extracted from cells using Bioline Isolate II Genomic DNA kit (Cat: BIO-52067) as per the manufacturer's instructions. After quantifying the DNA and checking the purity, DNA samples were shipped to GENEWIZ (Suzhou, China) for whole exome sequencing (WES) and subsequent analysis.

Genewiz, Inc. (Suzhou, China) performed initial quality control assessments and subsequent exome capture using the SureSelectXT HS Target enrichment kit (Agilent). All samples were paired-end multiplex sequenced (2 × 150 base pairs) on the Illumina Hiseq 2500 platform to a median target depth of over 50× WES data have been deposited at NCBI under BioProject ID PRJNA557326.

Paired-end reads underwent quality control before alignment to the reference human genome (hg19) using Burrows-Wheeler alignment (BWA, version 0.7.12-r1039) [46] and SAMtools (version 1.6) [47]. Realignment and recalibration were performed using the Genome Analysis Toolkit (GATK, version 3.5) [48]. Single nucleotide variants (SNVs) and insertions and deletions (indels) were called using GATK with default settings. Annotation of variants (SNP and indels) was performed using ANNOVAR [49,50]. Control-FREEC v 10.6 was used for detecting and filtering the CNV [51].

CRAVAT (Cancer-Related Analysis of Variants Toolkit), a tool specifically tailored to analyze cancer-specific variants [52], was used for identification and prioritization of genes with a possible role in cancer tumorigenesis in the PMC42 cell lines. Identification and annotation of cancer-specific driver missense mutations was performed using CHASM (Cancer-specific High-throughput Annotation of Somatic Mutations) [53,54]. To identify and prioritize pathogenic missense mutations, VEST (Variant Effect Scoring Tool), a supervised machine learning-based classifier [55], was also applied. Both CHASM and VEST computational scores are integrated in the CRAVAT suite.

*2.4. RNA Extraction, cDNA Synthesis and RT-qPCR*

Total RNA was extracted from cells using TRIzol (Life Technologies) and subsequent reactions were carried out as per the Bioline Isolate II RNA Micro kit manufacturer's instructions, and cDNA was synthesized using SensiFAST™ cDNA Synthesis kit from Bioline. Real time-quantitative PCR (RT-qPCR) was performed using the SYBR Green Master Mix in a ViiA7 Real-Time PCR system (Applied Biosystems) and analysis performed using the Quantstudio™ Real-Time PCR software v1.1 (Applied Biosystems, Life Technologies). The primers sequences are listed in Supplementary Table S1.

Hierarchical clustering of transcriptional profiles was performed using the Morpheus online tool [56]. Data were normalized against the overall mean expression of all measured genes [57].

*2.5. Whole Transcriptome Sequencing and Analysis of PMC42 Cell Lines*

mRNA transcript abundances for PMC42 cell lines were measured using RNA-seq as previously reported [30]; data have been deposited at NCBI under bioproject ID PRJNA322427. Sequence alignment to the hg19 reference genome was performed using TopHat [58] with default parameters. Differential expression analysis was performed using CuffDiff [58] with default parameters. RNA sequencing results were re-analysed for interrogation of fold changes across the two PMC42 cell lines with respect to the chromosome number. Gene Set Enrichment Analysis [59] was also applied to identify enrichment of gene signatures contained in the Molecular Signatures Database (MSigDB). The filtered gene lists with $p < 0.01$ were also examined by Ingenuity Pathway Analysis®(IPA) for functional annotation and gene network analysis. The GSVA method from the GSVA R/Bioconductor package was also applied on the gene expression data for the PMC42-ET and PMC42-LA cell lines to score samples against the TGFβ-EMT signature.

*2.6. Data-Independent Acquisition (DIA) Mass Spectrometry of PMC42 Cell Lines*

Cells were washed with ice-cold phosphate buffered saline (PBS), and lysed directly in cell lysis buffer containing 4% (w/v) SDS, 10 mM dithiothreitol (DTT), 10 mM Tris-HCl along with Roche compete protease and phosphatase inhibitors (Roche, Rotkreuz, Switzerland). Lysates were sonicated to shear DNA, and protein concentration was quantified using the Pierce™ BCA Protein Assay Kit (Thermo Scientific, Rockford, IL, USA). On the basis of protein quantifications, each experimental sample was aliquoted into 25 µg samples for processing using the FASP method [60]. Digestion was performed overnight using Trypsin/Lys-C (Promega) mix in 1:50 of protein. Fragmented peptides were then dissolved in 0.1% formic acid and processed for a final clean-up step using C18 Zip-Tips (Millipore; Billerica, MA, USA).

Protein Pilot (V 4.1) software from SCIEX was used for peptide identification. The human protein library was built using the UniProt database (release 2018_05, [61]) with the following settings: Sample Type, identification; Cysteine alkylation, acrylamide; Instrument, TripleT of 5600; Species, human; ID focus, Biological modification; Enzyme, trypsin; Search effort, thorough ID. False discovery rate (FDR) was calculated within ProteinPilot software and peptides identified with greater than 99% and a local FDR of 1% was applied for the peptide identification. PeakView Software was employed to measure the peptide abundance with standard parameters [62] and manual inspection was carried out to confirm the accuracy of the spectra. Six peptides per protein were used to measure the protein abundance. The differences in protein abundance between PMC42-ET and -LA were calculated based on the significance and fold-changes. MSstats was used to calculate protein level significance by applying a linear mixed-effects model [63]. The model combines quantitative measures for a targeted protein across peptides, charge states, transitions, samples, and conditions; the system detects proteins that change in abundance among conditions more systematically than would be expected by random chance, while controlling the FDR. In house scripts in Python and R were developed for further analysis.

*2.7. Fluorescence Activated Cell Sorting (FACS)*

Cells were lifted with Accutase®(Corning, Catalog # 25-058-CI) and stained with anti-human CD44-FITC (BD Pharmingen) and anti-human CD24-PB (Exbio) antibodies at manufacturer's recommended dilutions in 0.1% BSA (Bovine serum albumin, Sigma) diluted in DPBS for 1 h in a rotary shaker at room temperature. Cells were analysed in the presence of propidium iodide (1 µg/mL) using a BD LSRFortessa (BD Biosciences). After doublet discrimination and compensation for spectral overlap, data were analysed by using FlowJo Software (BD Biosciences). For TGFβR2 surface expression, cells were stained with primary antibody (RandD Systems, Cat# AF-241-NA) as per manufacture recommended dilutions for 1 h and then with secondary goat antibody for 1 h.

## 2.8. Immunocytochemistry

The cell lines were seeded at a density of 10,000 cells/well in 48-well plates (Thermo Scientific Nunclon™ Delta Surface-150687). During immunocytochemistry, the growth medium was discarded, and cells were washed thrice gently with Dulbecco's modified PBS (DPBS; pH 7.5). Briefly, cells were fixed in 4% paraformaldehyde ± 0.1% Triton X-100 (depending on the desired permeabilization conditions), rinsed with DPBS, and incubated with primary antibodies at 4 °C overnight. After rinsing again in DPBS, cells were incubated with an appropriate fluorescence-conjugated secondary antibody (Supplementary Table S2) and with diamidino phenyl indole (DAPI) as a nuclear stain (diluted to a final concentration of 1 µg/mL) for 2 h at room temperature in the dark with gentle rotary shaking. The plates were then washed thrice with DPBS and images were captured on a high-content imaging platform (Cytell Cell Imaging System (GE Healthcare) or IN Cell Analyser 6000 (GE Healthcare, Buckinghamshire, UK), as indicated), with approximately 6–9 fields of view taken per well. Images were further analysed and quantified using the IN Cell Investigator software v1.0 (GE Healthcare).

## 2.9. Seahorse Metabolic Analyser

Collagen (Rat tail, type 1, Cat 354236, BD Biosciences)-coated Seahorse cell culture plates (Seahorse *Bioscience*, 102601-100) were seeded at a density of 20,000 cells per well (XFe96 cell culture microplate; Seahorse Biosciences, North Billerica, MA, USA). The cells were allowed to grow for 24–48 h at 37 °C in 5% $CO_2$, after which the cells were washed and replaced with assay media (unbuffered DMEM or RPMI supplemented with 10 mM glucose, 1 mM sodium pyruvate, 2mM L-glutamine, no sodium bicarbonate at pH 7.4). The cells were incubated for 1 h at 37 °C in a non-$CO_2$ incubator. Mitochondrial complex inhibitors (1.2 µM oligomycin, 1.2 µM carbonyl cyanide p-(trifluoromethoxy)-phenyl-hydrazone (FCCP) and combined 1 µM rotenone with 1 µM antimycin A) were preloaded in the injection ports. For basal rate measurements, ECAR (Extra Cellular Acidification Rate) and OCR (Oxygen Consumption Rate) measurements were assessed. Experiments were performed in triplicates and the data were normalized by cell number.

## 2.10. Statistical Analysis

All experiments were carried out at least three times unless otherwise indicated. Data were analysed using GraphPad Prism version 7 statistical software (GraphPad Software, La Jolla, CA, USA).

## 3. Results

### 3.1. Comparison of PMC42 Cell Lines with Other BC Cell Lines (Luminal, Basal A and Basal B)

Hierarchical clustering of RT-qPCR data of the 9 breast cell lines for EMP markers, inducers and regulators, along with the BC clinically relevant *ESR1*, *PGR* and *ERBB2* gene products, showed substantial variation across the cell lines and revealed two major branches (Figure 1A). Luminal cell lines MCF-7 and T47D, along with the Basal A MDA-MB-468 cell line formed one cluster, whereas the PMC42 cell lines were more closely associated with the other cluster of four Basal B cell lines (BT-549, SUM-159, MDA-MB-157, HS578T). Interestingly, when the heat map was computed on the basis of $log_2$ fold difference in expression of each gene with respect to PMC42-ET cells, the PMC42-LA cell line clustered more closely with luminal MCF-7, T47D cells and Basal A MDA-MB-468 cells (Figure 1B). This further illustrates that PMC42-LA has more predominant epithelial markers as compared to its parental PMC42-ET cell line. Interestingly, we also observed the complete absence of expression of the FoxA1 gene in PMC42-ET cell line.

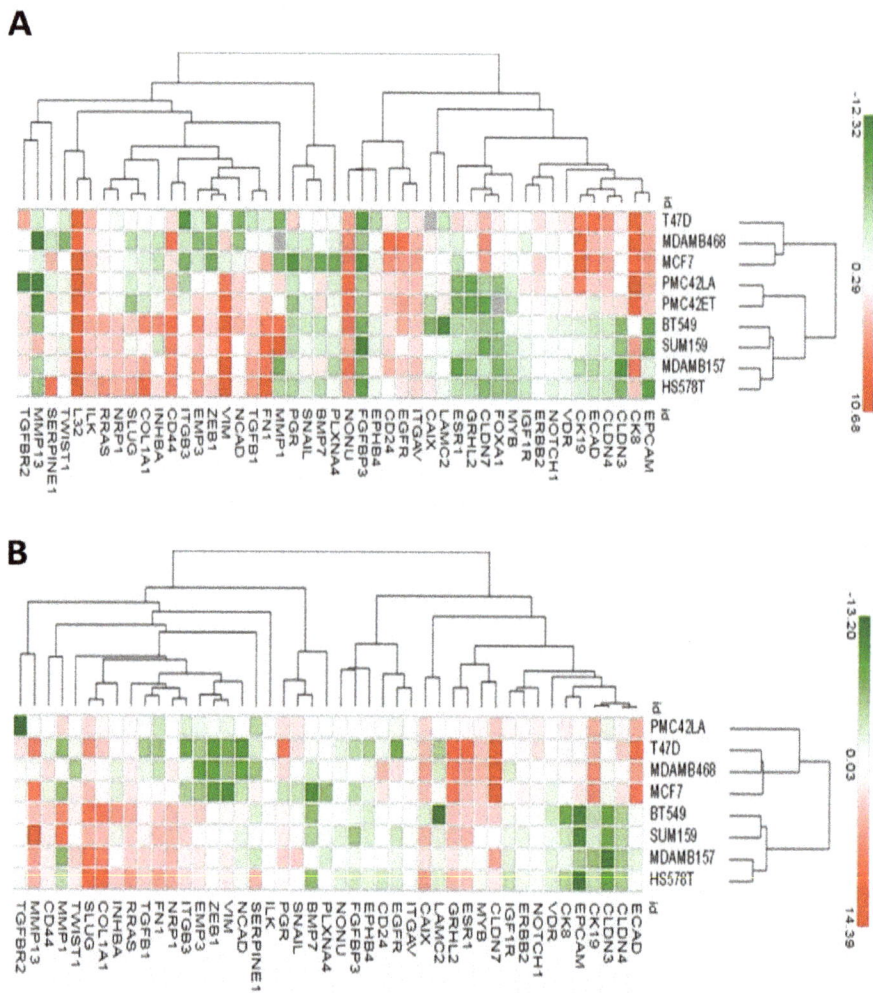

**Figure 1.** Gene expression heatmaps of selected breast cancer cell lines. (**A**) The normalized mRNA expression values of the breast cancer cell lines obtained against the overall mean expression of all measured genes were subjected to unsupervised hierarchical clustering using Morpheus (Gene-E tool). In the average-linkage cluster algorithm, Pearson correlation was used to measure dissimilarity. (**B**) Unsupervised cluster analysis of the relative expression values of breast cancer cell lines with respect to PMC42-ET.

### 3.2. CD44$^+$CD24$^{-/low}$ Phenotype Association with Breast Molecular Subtypes and Other EMT Markers

The CD44$^{high}$/CD24$^{low}$ profile is a putative marker of cancer stemness and is also associated with EMT phenotype [25]. The proportions of CD44$^{+/high}$/CD24$^{-/low}$ cell populations across the PMC42 cell lines were compared with five other breast cancer cell lines (MCF-7, T47D, MDA-MB-468, MDA-MB-231 and SUM-159) and the expression of these surface markers was simultaneously assessed by FACS analysis (Figure 2A,B). Surprisingly, PMC42-LA cells were remarkably stem-like in relation to these markers, as predominantly all cells gated within the CD44$^{high}$/CD24$^{low}$ subpopulation, similar to MDA-MB-231 and SUM-159 cells representing the most mesenchymal Basal-B subgroup [25], whereas

75.2% of the more mesenchymal PMC42-ET cells were in the CD44$^{high}$/CD24$^{low}$ state. In agreement with previous reports [64], MCF-7 cultures (Luminal subgroup; [25]), had a small population of CD24$^{-/low}$/CD44$^+$ cells (~20%) and the MDA-MB-468 cell line (Basal-A subgroup; [25]), had higher expression of both CD44 and CD24 markers (96.4% of cells gated in CD44$^{high}$/CD24$^{high}$ state). Compared to MCF-7 and T47D, all other cell lines were mainly constituted by cells with high levels of CD44, and except MDA-MB-468 also showed lower proportions of CD24 expression, consistent with their mesenchymal subgrouping (Figure 2A,B).

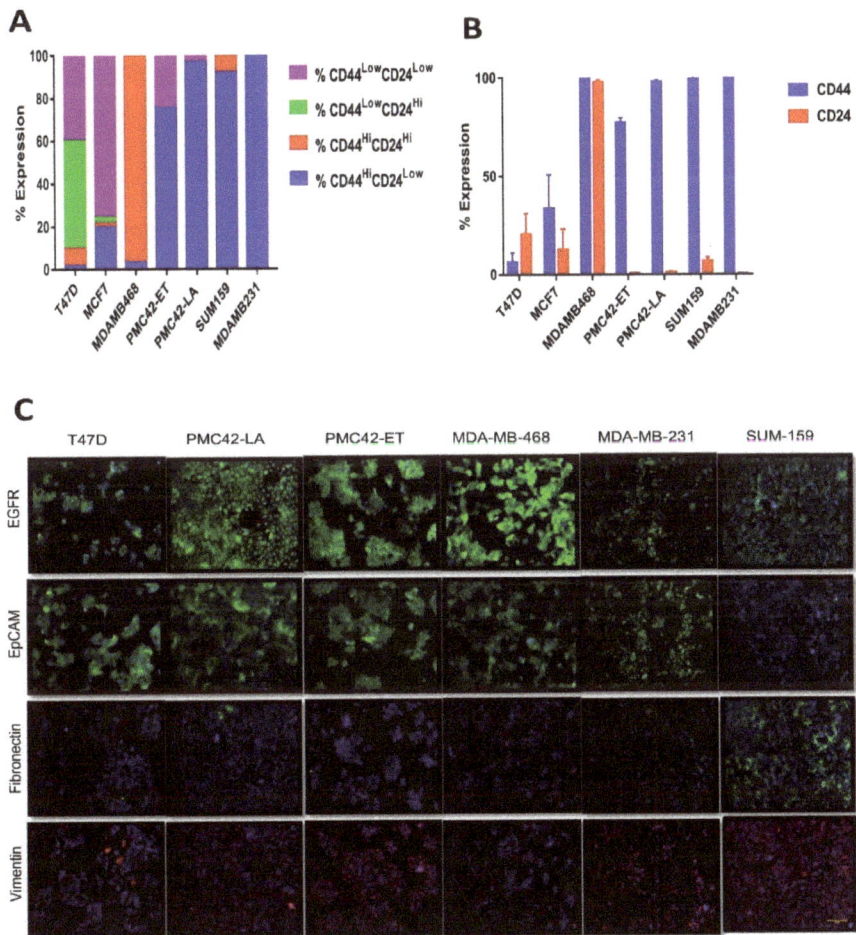

**Figure 2.** Assessment of stemness and other EMP markers. (**A**) Proportions of the subpopulations defined by the combination of the stem cell markers CD44 and CD24 in PMC42 cell lines and a panel of breast cancer cell lines. (**B**) The relative expression of the stem cell markers CD44 and CD24 in a panel of breast cancer cell lines representative of different molecular subtypes by flow cytometry. Mean ± SD of three independent experiments is shown. (**C**) Immunofluorescence microscopy analysis of EMT marker proteins. Cell lines were stained with antibodies against the epithelial marker EpCAM and against the mesenchymal markers EGFR, vimentin and fibronectin. Scale bar, 100 µm.

The CD44$^{+/high}$/CD24$^{-/low}$ cell populations across PMC42-ET, PMC42-LA, MCF-7 and MDA-MB-468 were also assessed after stimulation of the cells with EGF or TGF-β for 72 h. Both MCF-7 and MDA-MB-468 cell lines exhibited a 10%–20% increase in their $CD44^{high}/CD24^{low}$ proportions after treatment with EGF, but not with TGF-β. PMC42-ET cells, however, could be made potentially stem-enriched with 93%–94% population of cells in $CD44^{high}/CD24^{low}$ state after stimulation with either EGF or TGF-β, which was due to increased CD44 expression (Supplementary Figure S1).

EMT-associated markers EGFR, EpCAM, fibronectin and vimentin were also evaluated using immunofluorescence for the six breast cancer cell lines (Figure 2C). EGFR expression was highest for MDA-MB-468 cells, in which EGFR is known to be amplified [65]. EpCAM expression at cellular junctions was observed for T47D, PMC42-LA and MDA-MB-468 cell lines, and fibronectin expression was only observed for SUM-159 cells. Vimentin expression was universally positive in SUM-159, MDA-MB-231 and PMC42-ET cells, whereas on an average 10% and 20% of the cells were positive for vimentin expression in MDA-MB-468 and PMC42-LA cells, respectively, as quantified using IN Cell Investigator software, which is consistent with previous reports [39,40,66].

### 3.3. Comparative RNA-seq Analysis of PMC42 Cell Lines

RNA-seq results obtained previously for the EGF-induced EMT studies in PMC42 system [30] were re-analysed to study the transcriptional differences between the two PMC42 cell lines. Comparative analysis was investigated using the "Hallmark" geneset collection within the MSigDB of GSEA and IPA. Negative enrichment for signatures related to EMT ($p < 0.001$, NES = −1.73), TNFA signalling via NFκb ($p = 0.007$, NES = −1.55), inflammatory response signature ($p = 0.004$, NES = −1.52) and hypoxia signature ($p = 0.016$, NES = −1.41) were observed in PMC42-LA with respect to its parental cell line PMC42-ET using GSEA (Figure 3A). Using IPA for the comparative RNA-seq analysis, the top-five significant upstream regulators we identified were focused on the inhibition of TNF, TGFβ-1, EGFR and JNK gene in PMC42-LA, whereas estrogen receptor gene was considered an activated regulator in PMC42-LA. IPA also reported a significant gene network indicating the importance of TWIST2 downregulation and SPDEF upregulation in the epithelial PMC42-LA cells (Supplementary Figure S2A).

### 3.4. Comparative Proteome Quantification of Alterations in the PMC42 Cell Line System

We next performed comparative proteomics and subjected protein extracts from the two PMC42 cell lines to mass spectrometry. Among a total of 2460 identified and annotated proteins in the PMC42 cell lines, 244 proteins were expressed at significantly different levels in the two cell lines (adjusted $p$ value < 0.01). Of these, 73 proteins were significantly upregulated, and 61 proteins were significantly downregulated by a factor of 2-fold or more in the epithelial PMC42-LA cells. KEGG pathway analysis indicated that differentially regulated proteins were involved in glycolysis/gluconeogenesis (ALDH1A3, ALDH3A1, ALDOC) ($p = 0.00073$), proteasome (PSB3, PSB6, PSB7, PSMD1-4) ($p = 6.06 \times 10^{-8}$), protein processing in endoplasmic reticulum ($p = 3.06 \times 10^{-6}$) and carbon metabolism (ALDOC, SUCA, G6PD, HXK1, DLDH) ($p = 0.00039$), respectively. The volcano plot that shows the difference in protein levels between PMC42-ET and PMC42-LA also highlights several EMT markers, among which mesenchymal markers, such as VIM and EGFR, were upregulated by 4-fold ($p < 2.51 \times 10^{-5}$) and 2-fold ($p < 5.83 \times 10^{-5}$), respectively, in PMC42-ET cells (Figure 3B). Epithelial markers, such as KRT19 and F11R (Junctional adhesion molecule A), were significantly upregulated in PMC42-LA by 4.75-fold ($p < 0.00066$) and 4.6-fold ($p < 00093$), respectively. IPA also deduced glycolysis (with a z-score of 3.5), aryl hydrocarbon receptor signalling (with a z-score of 3.1) and ILK signalling (with a z-score of 1.6) as significantly upregulated canonical pathways in the epithelial PMC42-LA cell line. Gene network enrichment plot from proteomics analysis indicated a possible role of NFκb complex dysregulation in PMC42-LA cells (Supplementary Figure S2B), which is also in agreement with the similar GSEA findings from RNA-seq analysis.

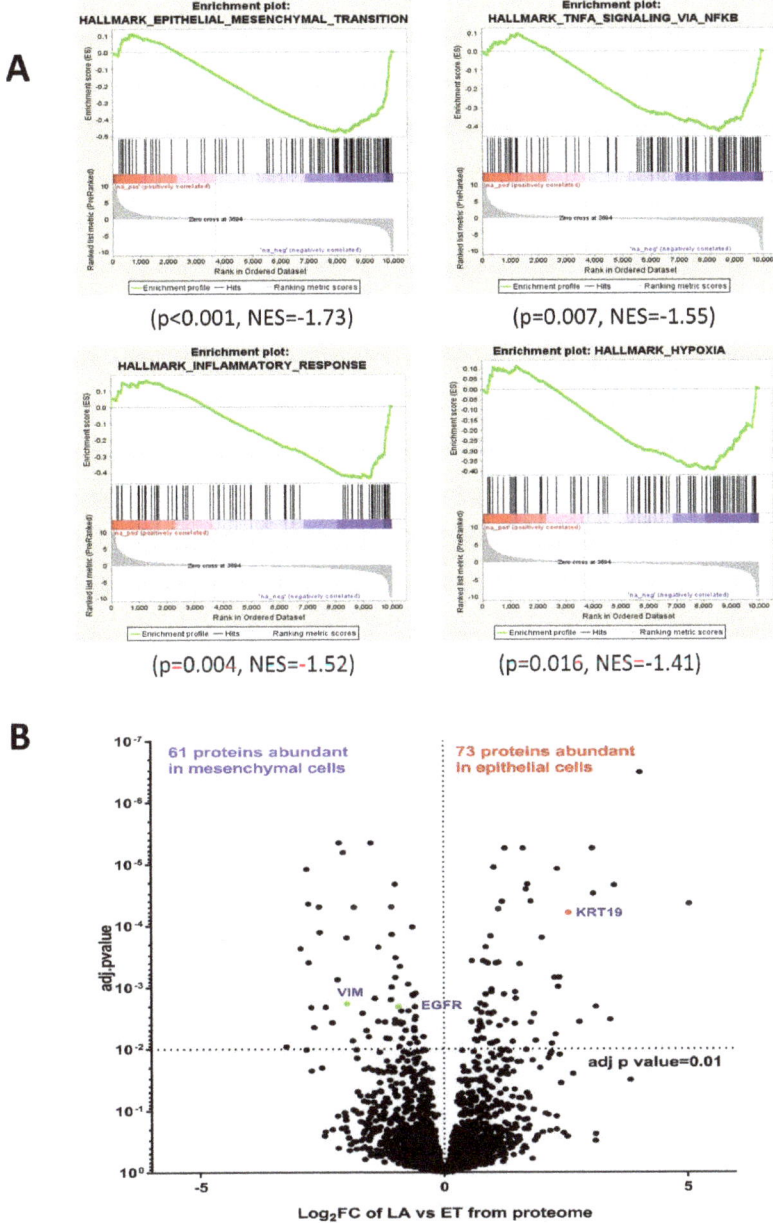

**Figure 3.** Comparative analysis of transcriptomic and proteomic data from PMC42 cell lines. (**A**) Results from representative enrichment plots from Gene Set Enrichment Analysis (GSEA) ($p < 0.05$) are shown from comparative transcriptome analysis. These data revealed a significant negative enrichment for gene sets involved in EMT in PMC42-LA. (**B**) Quantitative proteome analysis of PMC42-LA in comparison to PMC42-ET reflected in volcano plot shows that 73 proteins were significantly upregulated, and 61 proteins were significantly downregulated.

## 3.5. Karyotypic Heterogeneity Exists within and across the Sister Breast Cancer Cell Lines PMC42-ET and PMC42-LA

Chromosomal instability (CIN), including numerical CIN (resulting in aneuploidy) and structural CIN (resulting in partial chromosomal gains and losses and translocations) are inherent in cancer and underpin many of the phenotypic manifestations that contribute to cancer progression. Hence, in order to assess their possible contributions to the spontaneous MET seen in the PMC42 system, we explored whether karyotype differences existed in the PMC42 cell lines using metaphase spreads and karyotypic G-banding.

First, we determined the copy number status per chromosome. Chromosomal counts from individual cells in each PMC42 cell line were plotted as a heatmap, where PMC42-ET and PMC42-LA cells clearly are seen as two separate clusters (Figure 4A). CIN, and resulting aneuploidy, is a hallmark of cancer, and despite this strong partition into 2 clusters, variable ploidy distribution was also reflected within each of the PMC42 cell lines. We identified copy number differences of individual chromosomes (Figure 4A). Significant differences in the ploidy levels between the cell lines are represented in Table 1, where eight chromosomes show high chromosomal number differences across the two cell lines. Tetrasomy was observed more often for chromosomes 3, 5, 7, 19 and 22 in PMC42-ET, whereas in PMC42-LA, tetrasomy was observed for chromosomes 7 and 19. Loss of chromosome 22 was found in 100% of PMC42-LA cells, as only a single copy was present in each of 50 cells assessed for karyotyping. The patterns of positive and negative chromosomal correlation with regards to their ploidy were also studied for individual cells in the two PMC42 cell lines, where no strongly significant association was confirmed for PMC42-LA, but positive correlations were observed between chromosomes 9 and 14, and 17 and 20, respectively ($r^2 = 0.67$ and $0.59$, Pearson correlation) (p-value of $7.64 \times 10^{-8}$ and $6.37 \times 10^{-6}$), and a negative correlation ($r^2 = -0.51$) (p-value of 0.0001) was found between chromosomes 9 and 12, in the PMC42-ET cell line (Supplementary Tables S3 and S4). Overall, PMC42-ET was primarily comprised of near-triploid karyotypes with a modal number of 68 chromosomes (range 59–75), whereas PMC42-LA was primarily comprised of near-triploid karyotypes with a modal chromosome number of 63 (range 52–64) (Figure 4B). The total chromosome numbers in the two cell lines are significantly different ($p < 0.0001$) (Figure 4C). Two observations suggest an increased level of CIN in PMC42-ET compared to PMC42-LA. First, PMC42-ET cells show a broader range of chromosome numbers, 17, compared to 13 in PMC42-LA cells and more individual chromosome numbers deviate from the modal number (Supplementary Figure S3A,B). Second, GSEA on our RNA-seq data shows a significant depletion in the expression of 70 genes that are part of the well-established CIN70 signature [67] in PMC42-LA cells compared to PMC42-ET cells ($p = 0.027$; Figure 4D). This suggests that CIN may have promoted the transition from PMC42-ET to PMC42-LA.

Next, as expected, karyotyping revealed that the PMC42-LA derivative cell line harbours some of the major structural rearrangements seen in the parental PMC42-ET cells. For example, one of the arms of each of chromosomes 2, 3 and 8 is shorter or truncated, the p-arm of chromosome 9 is fused with the long arm of chromosome 10, and chromosome 21 has a third copy of its p-arm fused with the long arm of chromosome 7 (Figure 5A,B). Some characteristics, such as truncated arms of chromosomes 2 and 3, trisomy 1 and trisomy 20, and a modal chromosomal number of 66, were consistent with initial reports in 1983 [42]. In PMC42-LA cells only, we also observed a few (in the range of 1–4) marker chromosomes whose derivative chromosomal origins cannot be recognized via karyotyping (Figure 5B, marked as 'mar' and Figure 5C, marked as 'UNC'). Ploidy distributions of each chromosome from 50 karyotyped cells of each cell line also reflect the dynamics of copy number alterations at the chromosomal level (Figure 5C).

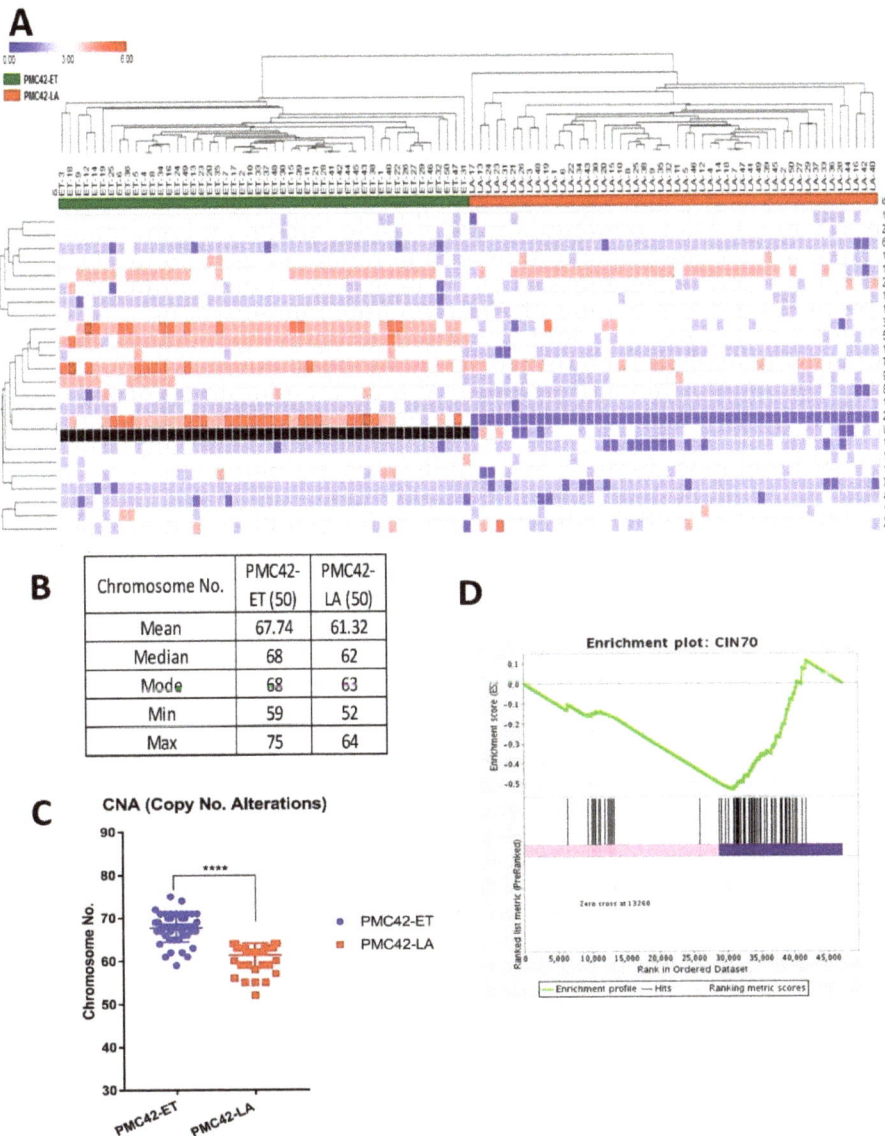

**Figure 4.** Chromosomal ploidy distribution of PMC42 cell lines. (**A**) Heatmap for copy number distribution of chromosomes deciphered from 50 karyotypes from each of the PMC42-ET and PMC42-LA cell lines *(UNC: Unidentified Chromosome)*. (**B**) Distribution of chromosome numbers of PMC42-ET and PMC42-LA cell lines. (**C**) Chromosome numbers analysed from PMC42-ET and PMC42-LA for a total of 50 cells were compared for each cell line. Significance was determined by an unpaired *t* test with Welch's correction, with **** $p < 0.0001$. (**D**) CIN70 enrichment plot following Gene Set Enrichment Analysis.

**Table 1.** Ploidy alterations of 50 single cells from PMC42-ET and PMC42-LA were compared using *t*-test.

| Chromosome No. | *p*-Value across ET vs. LA |
| --- | --- |
| 22 | $5.28847 \times 10^{-45}$ |
| 5 | $1.50398 \times 10^{-28}$ |
| 13 | $7.71473 \times 10^{-23}$ |
| 11 | $9.42164 \times 10^{-20}$ |
| 3 | $3.33503 \times 10^{-18}$ |
| 7 | $8.49205 \times 10^{-14}$ |
| 8 | $3.73987 \times 10^{-8}$ |
| 9 | $1.08547 \times 10^{-6}$ |
| 10 | 0.012162341 |
| X | 0.0151172 |
| 14 | 0.022502942 |
| 18 | 0.083804992 |
| 12 | 0.260603283 |
| 1 | 0.278286015 |
| 15 | 0.531258862 |
| 2 | 0.678929758 |
| 6 | 0.717332498 |
| 16 | 0.748135128 |
| 4 | 0.75812698 |
| 17 | 0.771687988 |
| 20 | 0.814301536 |
| 21 | 0.823855275 |
| 19 | 0.928168854 |

Taken together, these results indicate that numerical chromosomal heterogeneity exists between and within the PMC42 cell lines. In addition, PMC42-ET cells show features of CIN and PMC42-LA cells harbour some specific structural abnormalities not observed in PMC42-ET cells. These changes could underpin the transition of PMC42-ET cells to a more epithelial phenotype.

*3.6. Cancer Driver Mutations in PMC42 Cell Lines*

WES was performed to probe more deeply the genetic aberrations in the PMC42 system. After applying selective filters for delineating deleterious mutations within exons, we identified 465 SNVs in PMC42-ET and 475 SNVs in PMC42-LA (Figure 6A,B). We considered missense, non-sense, frame-shift and splice site mutations that involve structural and functional alteration of the protein products as deleterious. The number of Indels present in PMC42-ET were 83 and in PMC42-LA were 85. Approximately 75.4% of the somatic mutations and 60% of the Indels were shared between the parental and derivative cell line (Figure 6C,D). The results of deleterious SNV and Indels identified using WES across PMC42-ET and PMC42-LA cells are shown in the supplementary document (Supplementary Tables S5 and S6 for PMC42-ET and Tables S7 and S8 for PMC42-LA). CHASM score was computed for all the missense mutations identified in the PMC42 cell lines to identify driver mutations. The top 9 potential drivers that were common between the two PMC42 cell lines were *TP53, MERTK, DNMT3A, CPZ, PPM1H, PPIP5K2, C10orf76, DNAH7, CFTR* (Figure 6E). We also compared the driver mutations identified in the PMC42 cell lines with the TCGA mutations dataset using the CRAVAT interface (Figure 6F). The TP53 mutation site (H36R) was reported earlier in the TCGA dataset, whereas the other top 4 driver missense mutation locations identified were considered novel, as they were not reported in the TCGA dataset (as observed from the CRAVAT interface). The deleterious genes identified in the PMC42 cell lines were also stratified in a gene-family matrix according to their known role in cancers using the Broad Institute's GSEA analysis. We identified three commonly mutated tumour suppressor genes between two PMC42 cell lines (*NF2 (attaining stop gain function), TP53, TSC2*) and an additional mutated tumour suppressor gene *ATM* in PMC42-ET only. Eight commonly mutated oncogenes (*ARNT (TF), EML4, GNAS, NTRK3 (PK), PER1 (TF), TCL1A (TF), TLX1, TTL*) and 2 additional mutated oncogenes *TAL1 and IL6ST* in PMC42-ET only were also identified for their role in tumorigenesis (Table 2; Table 3). Interestingly, the gene-family matrix derived for the deleterious genes in the PMC42-LA cell line in reference to parental PMC42-ET cell line identifies mutations in 2 significant EMT-promoting transcription factors, *SNAI2* (K188N) and *SOX3* (R22P) (Supplementary Tables S9 and S10) and other EMT genes, such as *GSN (R397W), WNT1 (T363K), ITGA4 (R565W) and NID2 (G426E)* (Supplementary Table S7). In addition to that, the EMT-associated splice variation regulator *ESRP2* (R248S) was found to be mutated in the parental PMC42-ET cell line.

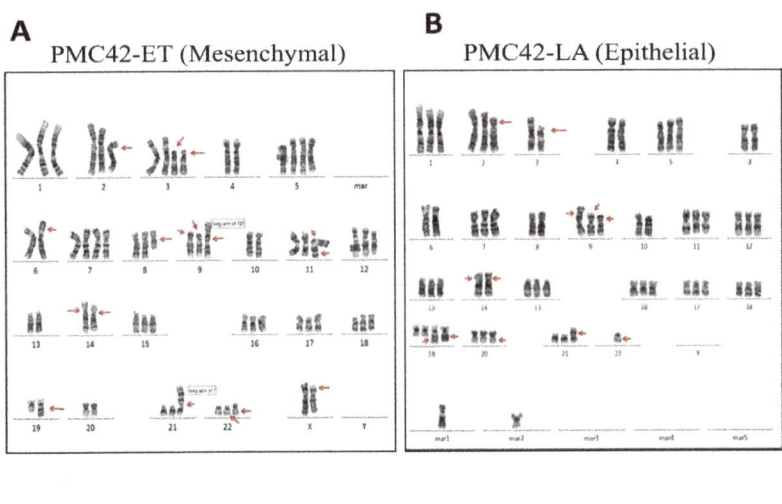

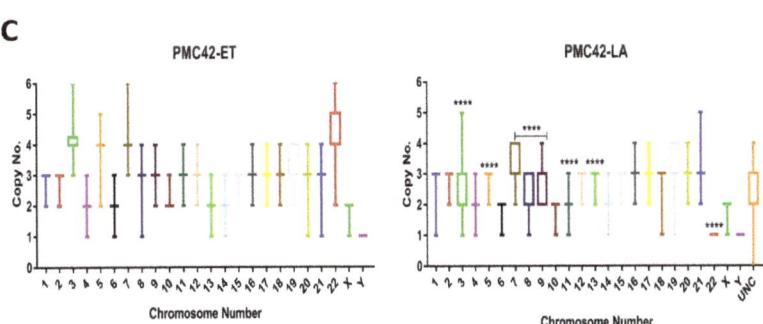

**Figure 5.** Karyotypic analysis of PMC42 cell lines. (**A**) A representative G-banded karyotype of the near-triploid cell line PMC42-ET, showing structural and numerical changes. (**B**) A representative G-banded karyotype of the cell line PMC42-LA. *Arrows* point to main chromosomal alterations. *Mar$_n$* marker chromosome (**C**) Ploidy distribution of each chromosome is presented for PMC42-ET and PMC42-LA from 50 karyotyped cells. *P*-values are indicated (as described in Table 1 using Student's *t*-test), and data presented in box (median, first and third quartiles) and whisker (extreme value) plots (*UNC: Unidentified Chromosome*).

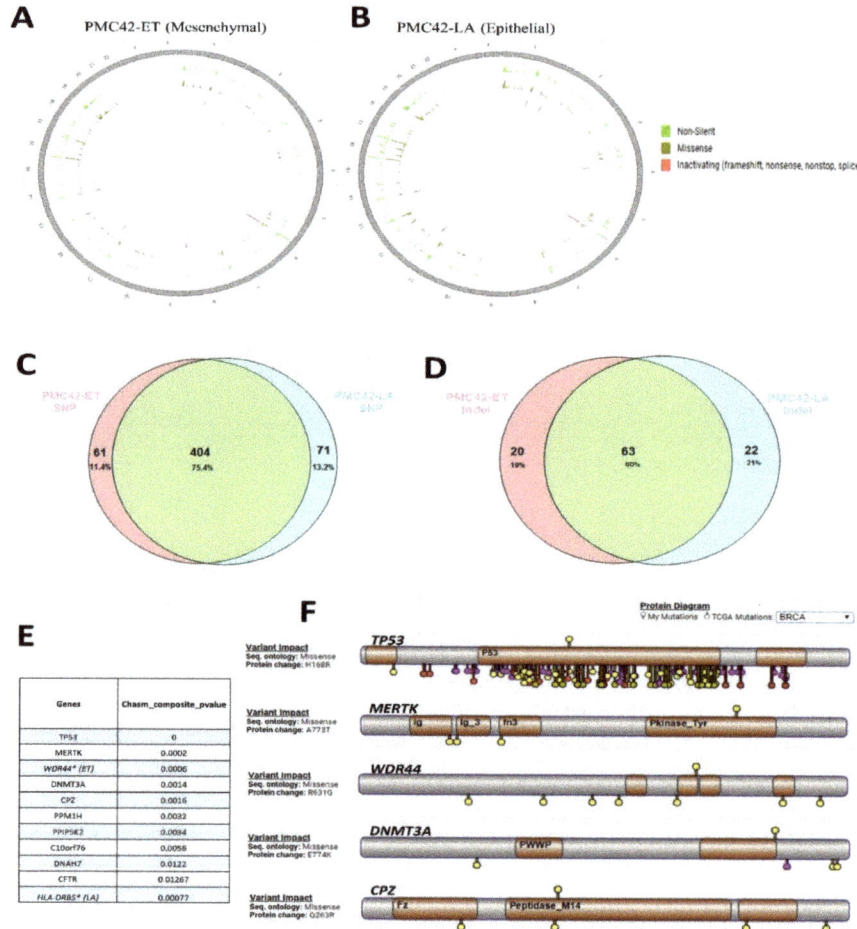

**Figure 6.** Assessment of whole-exome sequencing (WES) from PMC42 cell lines. Chromosome-specific distribution of non-silent, missense, and inactivating mutations are displayed on Circos plots for PMC42-ET (**A**) and the derivative PMC42-LA (**B**) cell lines, respectively. Representation of shared and unique (**C**) SNVs and (**D**) indels discovered by WES for PMC42-ET and PMC42-LA. (**E**) CHASM score was computed and (**F**) the top 10 potential driver mutations for PMC42-ET and PMC42-LA were determined. The top 5 potential driver mutations for PMC42-ET and PMC42-LA were annotated for their presence within protein sequences (indicated on the top of each gene) and compared for somatic mutations identified in TCGA dataset (indicated on the bottom of each gene) for the same protein sequences, using the software CRAVAT [68].

Table 2. Gene set enrichment analysis (GSEA) for genes with deleterious mutations (SNV and Indels) identified in PMC42-ET.

| | Cytokines and Growth Factors (CGF) | Transcription Factor (TF) | Homeodomain Proteins (HP) | Cell Differentiation Markers (CM) | Protein Kinases (PK) | Translocated Cancer Genes (TCG) | Oncogenes | Tumour Suppressors |
|---|---|---|---|---|---|---|---|---|
| Tumour suppressors | 0 | 1 | 0 | 0 | 1 | 0 | 0 | 4* |
| Oncogenes | 1 | 4 | 1 | 1 | 1 | 8 | 10& | |
| Translocated cancer genes | 0 | 4 | 1 | 0 | 1 | 8* | | |
| Protein kinases | 0 | 0 | 0 | 0 | 17# | | | |
| Cell differentiation markers | 2 | 0 | 0 | 8! | | | | |
| Homeodomain proteins | 0 | 4 | 4@ | | | | | |
| Transcription factor | 0 | 28$ | | | | | | |
| Cytokines and Growth Factors | 6^ | | | | | | | |

Note: (4* tumour suppressor genes are ATM (PK), NF2, TP53 (TF), TSC2 8$ translocated cancer genes/oncogenes are ARNT (TF), EML4, NTRK3 (PK), PER1 (TF), TAL1 (TF), TCL1A (TF), TLX1, TTL and 2& additional oncogenes are GNAS, IL6ST (CM and CGF) 17# protein kinases are ANKK1, ATM, AURKB, CSNK1G2, FRK, LRRK2, MAP3K9, MAST4, MERTK, NRBP2, NTRK3, PASK, PKMYT1, PRKDC, ROCK2, SLK, TTN 8! cell differentiation markers are CR1, CR2, FCGR3A, IGLL1, IL6ST, LILRB5, MSR1, SEMA7A 4@ homeodomain proteins are HOMEZ, IRX3, TLX1, ZEB2 28$ transcription factors are ARNT, CEBPZ, CHD4, E2F1, ESR1, EYA3, FOXI1, HOMEZ, IRX3, MED21, NEUROD4, NRI12, PER1, PRDM2, RFX5, RREB1, RRN3, SP1, SRA1, SUPT5H, TAL1, TFDP3, TLX1, TP53, UHRF1, ZEB2, ZNF160, ZNF91 6^ cytokines and growth factors are C5, CMTM2, CYR61, IL6ST, SEMA6D, SEMA7A) (Green colour denotes mutations unique to this cell line).

**Table 3.** Gene set enrichment analysis (GSEA) for genes with deleterious mutation (SNV and Indels) identified in PMC42-LA.

| | Cytokines and Growth Factors | Transcription Factor | Homeodomain Proteins | Cell Differentiation Markers | Protein Kinases | Translocated Cancer Genes | Oncogenes | Tumour Suppressors |
|---|---|---|---|---|---|---|---|---|
| **Tumour suppressors** | 0 | 1 | 0 | 0 | 0 | 0 | 0 | 3* |
| **Oncogenes** | 0 | 3 | 1 | 0 | 1 | 7 | 8& | |
| **Translocated cancer genes** | 0 | 3 | 1 | 0 | 1 | 7* | | |
| **Protein kinases** | 0 | 0 | 0 | 0 | 15# | | | |
| **Cell differentiation markers** | 1 | 0 | 0 | 6! | | | | |
| **Homeodomain proteins** | 0 | 3 | 3@ | | | | | |
| **Transcription factor** | 0 | 24$ | | | | | | |
| **Cytokines and Growth Factors** | 5ˆ | | | | | | | |

Note: (3* **tumour suppressor genes** are NF2, TP53 (TF), TSC2. 7* **translocated cancer genes/oncogenes** are ARNT (TF), EML4, NTRK3 (PK), PER1 (TF), TCL1A (TF), TLX1, TTL and 1& additional oncogene is GNAS, 15# **protein kinases** are ANKK1, AURKB, CSNK1G2, FRK, MAP3K9, MAST4, MERTK, NRBP2, NTRK3, PASK, PKMYT1, RIPK2, ROCK2, RPS6KA5, STK16 6! **cell differentiation markers** are CR1, CR2, FCGR3A, JGLL1, LILRB5, SEMA7A 3@ **homeodomain proteins** are HOMEZ, TLX1, ZEB2 24$ **transcription factors** are ARNT, CEBPZ, CHD4, E2F1, ESR1, FOXI1, HOMEZ, MED21, NEUROD4, NR1I2, PER1, PRDM2, RFX5, RREB1, RRN3, SP1, SRA1, SUPT5H, TLX1, TP53, UHRF1, ZEB2, ZNF160, ZNF318 5ˆ **cytokines and growth factors** are C5, CMTM2, CYR61, SEMA6D, SEMA7A (Green color denotes mutations unique to this cell line).

## 3.7. Inference of CNV from Exome Sequencing Data

The estimated copy number ratios of chromosomal segments for PMC42-ET relative to PMC42-LA are shown in Figure 7. Control-FREEC was used to determine the copy number ratio profiles and to identify regions with significant amplification or loss. The copy number profiles deduced from WES resulted in a total of 166 gain and 34 loss segments in PMC42-ET, relative to PMC42-LA. The most significant losses are from 5p, 20p, Xq and whole chromosome 13, while the major gains are in chromosomes 3, 5q, 7q, 10q, 11q, 20q and 21. The identified genomic regions of amplification or loss were also consistent with our karyotyping studies. Copy number changes of the regions (i.e., amplification of chromosomes 3, 5, 7, 9,11, 22 and loss of chromosomes 13 in PMC42-ET relative to PMC42-LA) detected in the WES study were also identified in karyotyping. Additionally, WES data reflects amplification in chromosomes 10q and 21, which might be due to nonreciprocal translocation events of an additional chromosome 9 with chromosome 10q and chromosome 21 with 7q as shown in karyotype analysis. WES helps in revealing the amplifications/losses at the gene level, whereas karyotyping reflects the overall ploidy distribution better (as reflected in Figure 5), as it is a representation of single cells. The amplified/lost regions from WES data for PMC42-ET with respect to PMC42-LA is also provided in additional Supplementary Table S11.

## 3.8. TGFBR2 Ablation and Influence on EMT Induction in PMC42-LA

When analyzing the segments of genes that were completely lost in either of the PMC42 cell lines, we identified two regions from PMC42-LA that were completely missing. The chromosome 1 region carrying genes *FOXD2, FOXE3* and the chromosome 3 region containing genes *GADL1, RBMS3, TGFBR2* were completely lost from the PMC42-LA cell line. The specific functions of *FOXD2* and *FOXE3* genes are yet to be determined, however the role of *TGFBR2* in EMT induction is well established [27,69,70]. The surface expression of TGFβR2 in the PMC42 system was analysed in comparison with several other cell lines (T47D, MDA-MB-468, SUM-159 and MDA-MB-231) using FACS (Figure 8A). High TGFβR2 surface expression was seen in almost all the cells for Basal B cell lines SUM-159 and MBA-MB-231, whereas only 40% of PMC42-ET cells expressed TGFβR2 on their surface, and TGFβR2 expression was completely absent on PMC42-LA cells, which is in concordance with our WES-deduced results. The surface expression of TGFBR2 on T47D cells was also negligible, consistent with their low EMT-associated TGF-β enrichment score (TES) [27]. RNA-seq analysis of the PMC42 cell lines was also interrogated using the algorithms as described [27] to obtain their TES values and identify any evidence of intrinsic TGF-β-induced EMT. The PMC42-ET had a TES value of 0.594 which is relatively high compared to the PMC42-LA TES value of −0.015. The low/negative TES value of PMC42-LA is also in concordance with the previously deduced TES values from Luminal and Basal A cell lines (MCF7: −0.58977; T47D: −0.69277; MDAMB468: −0.66892), whereas Basal B cell lines have relatively higher TES values (MDA-MB-231 0.130999; SUM159PT: 0.430126). TES values for the various breast cancer cell lines are taken from Supplementary data file S10 of [27].

PMC42-ET and PMC42-LA cell lines were also tested for their EMT induction with EGF, TGF-β and combined treatments using RT-qPCR (Figure 8B). E-cadherin was significantly downregulated with combined EGF and TGF-β growth factor treatments in the PMC42-ET cell line compared to either EGF or TGFβ alone, suggesting that TGF-β augments the previously reported EGF-induced EMT [30]. There was significant upregulation of mesenchymal markers vimentin, Slug and CD44 in both the cell lines with EGF, and with combined EGF and TGF-β treatment in PMC42-ET cells, however there were no effects of TGF-β treatments on PMC42-LA cells (Figure 8B,C). At an individual factor level, assessed via transcriptomics, several modulators or mediators of TGF-β signalling were impacted across PMC42 cell lines (e.g., AGR2, RhoA, TGFB1, CTNNB1, JUNB) were significantly downregulated in PMC42-LA. Thus, the PMC42-LA cell line did not display any predisposition to undergo EMT-like changes in mesenchymal gene expression with TGF-β treatment.

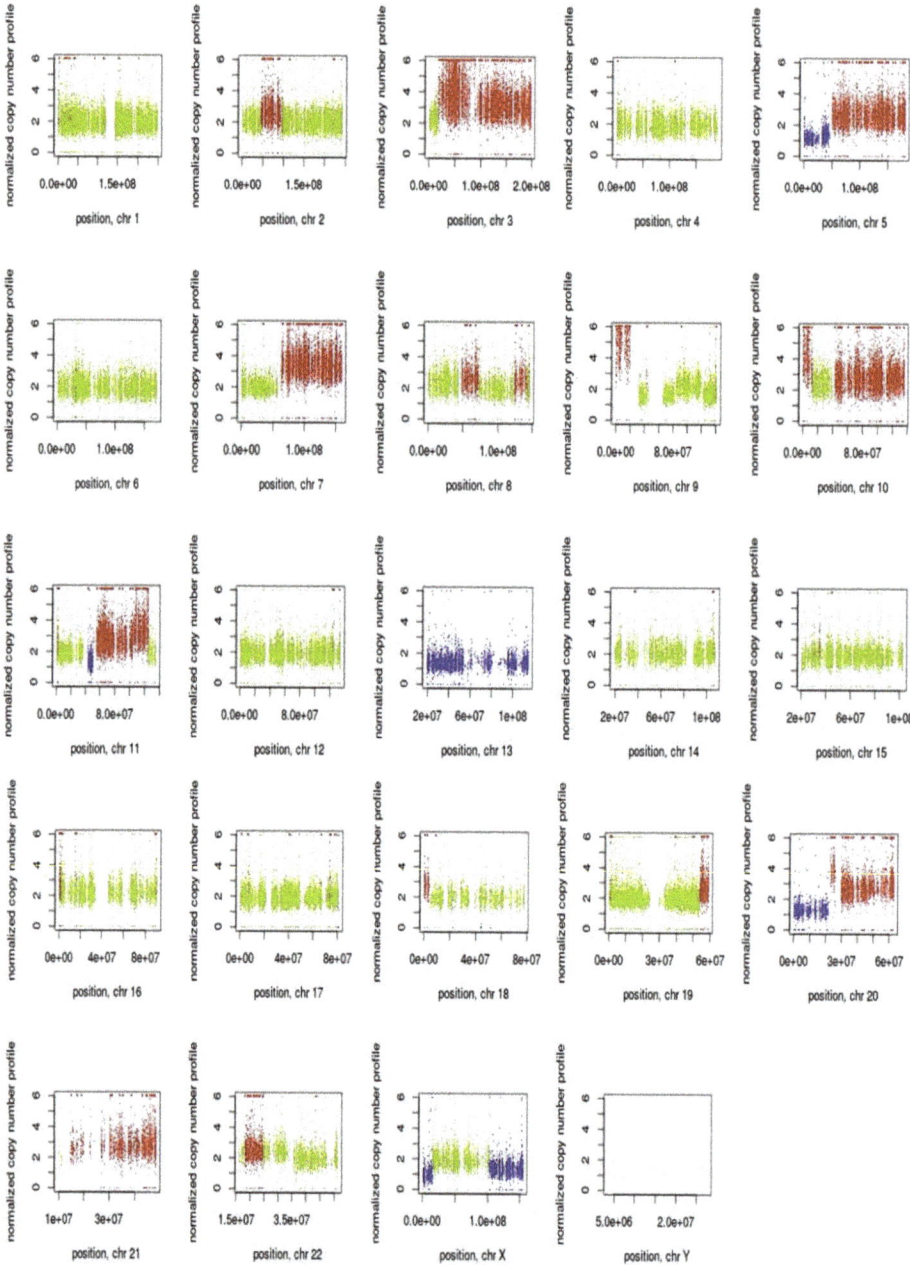

**Figure 7.** Visualization of Control-FREEC v 6.0 output from PMC42 cell lines exome sequencing data (Illumina HiSeq 2000). Copy number profiles for all chromosomes are shown of PMC42-ET in comparison to PMC42-LA, normal copy number status is shown in green, copy number gains are reflected in red and copy number losses are shown in blue.

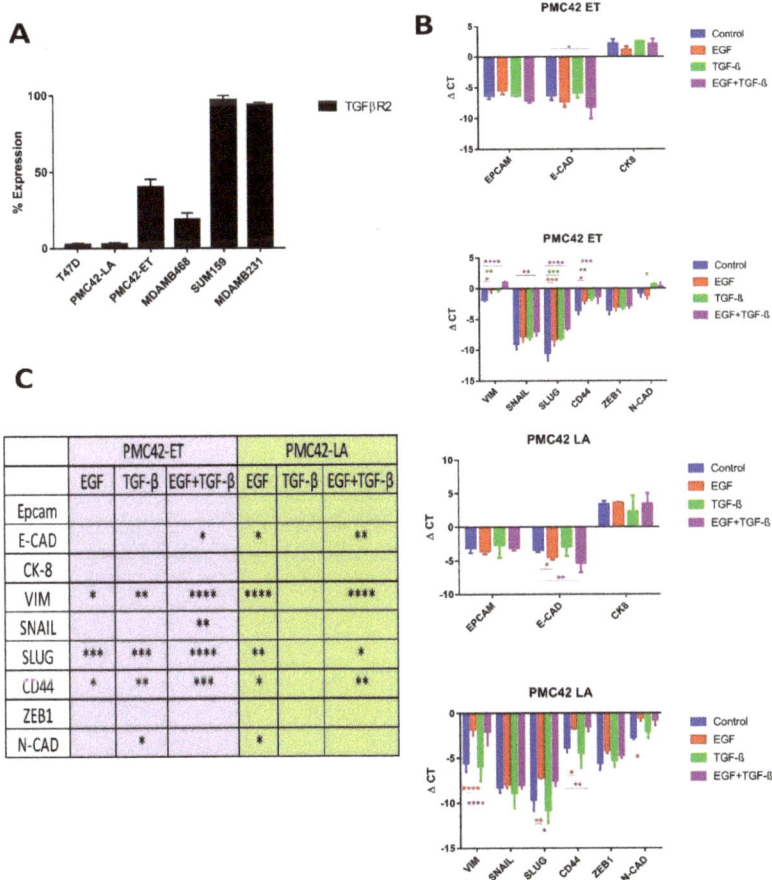

**Figure 8.** TGFBR2 ablation and influence on EMT induction in PMC42-LA. (**A**) Cell surface expression levels of TGFβR2 in a panel of breast cancer cell lines representative of distinct molecular subtypes. (**B**) PMC42-ET and PMC42-LA cells were treated for 5 days with 10 ng/mL EGF, 10 ng/mL TGF-β and combined 10 ng/mL of EGF and TGF-β. qPCR analysis of epithelial and mesenchymal markers were tested after EMT induction for 6 days with growth factor treatments. dCt values normalized against L32 and as an average from triplicates are shown. Statistical method applied is a two-way ANOVA with * indicating a $p$-value $< 0.1$, ** $p$-value $< 0.01$, *** $p$-value $< 0.001$ and **** $p$-value $< 0.0001$. (**C**) $p$-values calculated using 2-way ANOVA against each gene expression are tabulated.

### 3.9. Inter-Data Relationships from CNV and RNA-seq with Proteome Data

Correlations were assessed between protein expression and gene expression, and between protein expression and copy number variation, after applying the filter to only those proteins ($n = 244$) that were significantly dysregulated. For the RNAseq-to-proteome comparison, the Spearman correlation coefficient was 0.748 (Figure 9A), whereas the correlation was only 0.39 for CNV deciphered from WES at the gene level compared to the proteome (Figure 9B). Assessment of impact of CNV changes at whole differential RNA expression level reflects a Spearman's correlation coefficient of $r = 0.002805$, with a non-significant $p$ value of 0.77 (Supplementary Figure S4). Undoubtedly, some of the gene expression levels are influenced by changes in amplification or depletion of gene dosage at allele level, but this is probably masked by the likelihood that gene expression can be significantly modulated by other factors, such as epigenetics or transcription factors. Interestingly, when extrapolating RNA-seq and proteome results for the 244 differential expressed proteins, AGR2 shows relatively very high gene expression in PMC42-LA compared to PMC42-ET. An essential role of induced AGR2 in re-acquisition of epithelial markers has been reported [71], where activated Smad and Erk signalling cascades were identified as mutually complementary pathways responsible for TGF-β-mediated inhibition of AGR2. Since TGFBR2 expression is absent in PMC42-LA, AGR2 may be playing a crucial role in maintaining the epithelial phenotype of PMC42-LA cells. This is consistent with a strong enrichment of ARG2 expression in the Luminal subgroup of breast cancer cell lines, and some enrichment in Basal A, compared to Basal B (Supplementary Figure S3C).

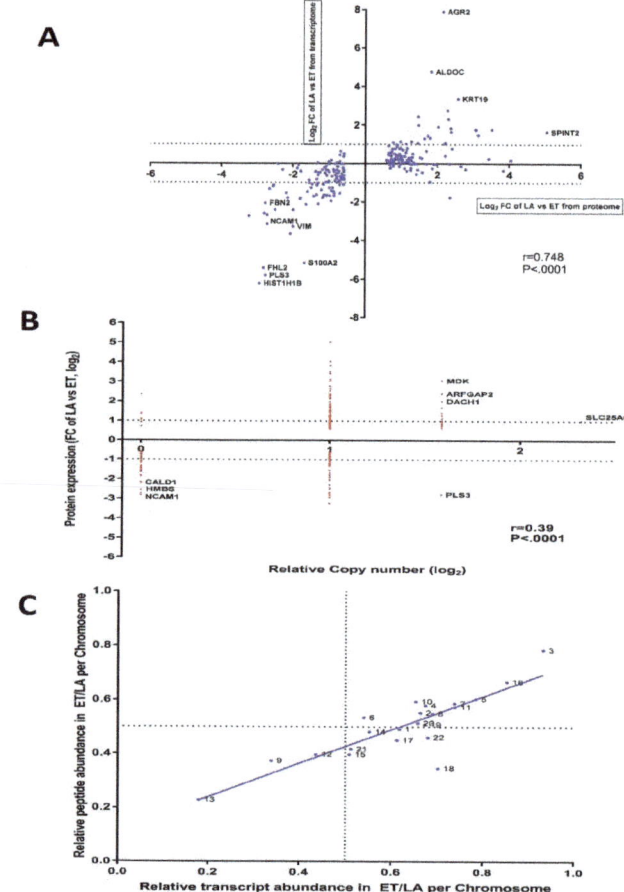

**Figure 9.** Inter-data relationships from CNV, RNA-seq and proteome studies in PMC42 cell lines. (**A**) Log$_2$ fold change of mRNA and protein expression levels of 244 significantly differential expressed proteins for PMC42-LA vs PMC42 ET were computed. Spearman's correlation coefficient ($r$ with $p$-value) between log$_2$ fold change of protein and mRNA expression is indicated at the bottom right. Dotted horizontal bars indicate 2-fold upregulation and downregulation on the log$_2$ scale for mRNA expression. (**B**) Log$_2$ fold change of 244 significantly differential expressed proteins were linked to the genomic copy number and spearman's correlation coefficient ($r$ with $p$-value) is indicated at the bottom right. (**C**) Correlation between relative peptide and transcriptome abundance in PMC42-ET vs. PMC42-LA per genomic coordinate. Correlation analysis was performed in GraphPad Prism with $R^2$ value of 0.7361 ($p < 0.0001$).

## 3.10. The Differences in PMC42 Karyotypes are Reflected in Their Transcriptome and Proteome Ratios

The significant genomic differences in the PMC42 cell lines led us to ask whether the changes in chromosome content mediated changes in transcriptome and proteome that could influence phenotype determination. The relative transcriptome and proteome abundance for a given chromosome across the two PMC42 cell lines were computed from $\log_2$-transformed fold changes of each transcript and proteome. To reduce the noise from the transcriptomic abundance, transcripts that were not expressed or for which normalized values were less than 10 in both the cell lines were discarded. The results show remarkable concordance between the chromosome copy number content and the corresponding transcript and protein abundance from chromosome 3 and chromosome 13 (Figure 9C). PMC42-ET cells have four copies of chromosome 3 on average, whereas PMC42-LA cells have an average of 2 copies, while PMC42-LA cells have three copies of chromosome 13 on average, whereas two copies are present in PMC42-ET. Apart for chromosome 3, transcript and proteome abundance from chromosomes 5, 7, 10 and 16 is also higher in PMC42-ET relative to PMC42-LA, which also corresponds to their higher ploidy distribution in PMC42-ET, except for chromosome 16. Strikingly, the discriminant gene analysis performed for chromosomes 13 and 3 also identified specific genes on chromosome 13 (*DNAJC15, SPG20, SLITRK6* and *DACH1*) that had significant overlap in GSEA with genes down-regulated in TMX2-28 cells (breast cancer) which do not express ESR1 [Gene ID = 2099] compared to the parental MCF-7 cells, which do [72], ($p$-value $1.6 \times 10^{-5}$). Therefore, we hypothesised that the gain in chromosome 13 upregulated the expression of various genes that drives the signalling mechanism of ER in PMC42-LA, causing it to be represented as an upstream regulator in our comparative IPA findings. The results show a high degree of concordance between the relative transcript and proteome abundance across the PMC42 cell lines ($r^2 = 0.736$).

## 3.11. Bioenergetic Profiles of PMC42 Cells in Comparison with Other Breast Cancer Cell Lines

Since glycolysis was one of the significantly attenuated pathways identified in proteome analysis, we also evaluated the mitochondrial bioenergetic profiles of PMC42 cell lines by measuring their oxygen consumption and glycolysis rates in comparison with the other four breast cancer cell lines: MCF-7, T47D (Luminal), MDA-MB-468 (Basal A) and MDA-MB-231, SUM-159 (Basal B). The extracellular acidification rate (ECAR) and oxygen consumption rate (OCR), as indicators of lactic acid production during glycolysis and mitochondrial respiration during OXPHOS, respectively, were measured (Figure 10). Interestingly, the baseline ECAR status of PMC42-LA was lower than all other cell lines evaluated (Figure 10A). Basal B/mesenchymal MDA-MB-231 and SUM-159 cell lines exhibited higher ECAR as compared to all other cell lines. The higher OCR was seen in luminal MCF-7 and T47D cell lines (Figure 10B).

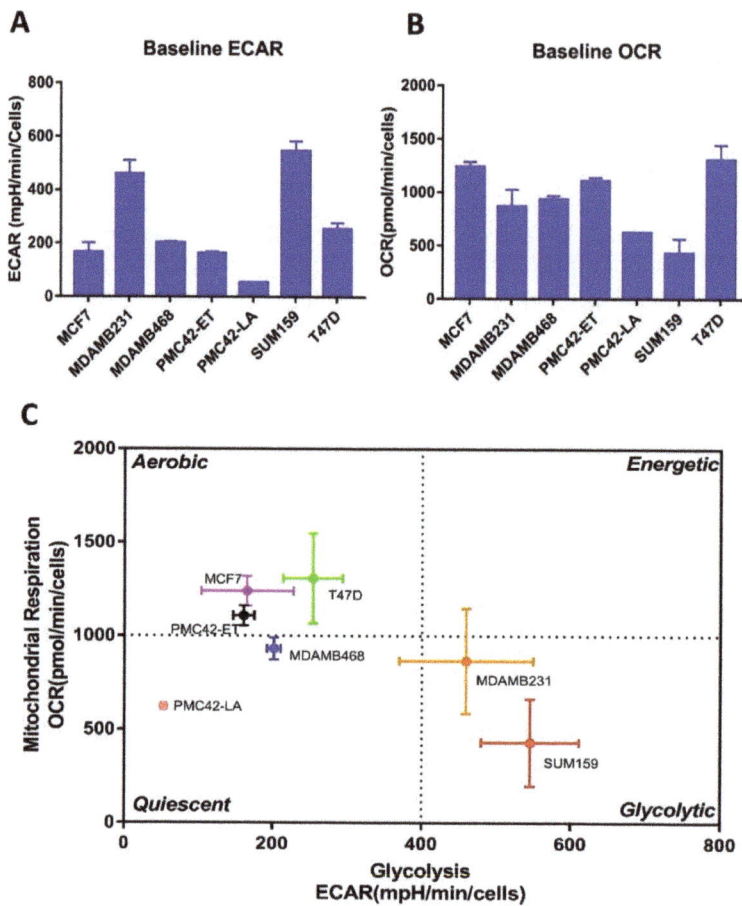

**Figure 10.** Metabolic profile of PMC42-ET, PMC42-LA and a panel of breast cancer cell lines representative of distinct molecular subtypes. (**A**) Extracellular acidification rate (ECAR) and (**B**) Basal oxygen consumption rate (OCR) measurements. (**C**) OCR: ECAR quadrant showing the bioenergetics phenotype of cell lines using Seahorse analyser (data presented as mean ± s.d., $n = 3$).

## 4. Discussion

Although the requirement of MET in metastasis is somewhat controversial [21,73–75], the transition of mesenchymally orientated cancer cells to a more epithelial state has been shown to allow cancer cells to survive and seed in distant sites prior to development of a metastatic lesion [18,68,76–78]. The comprehensive integrated analysis of the PMC42 system enhances our understanding of the regulation of molecular events relevant to MET change in the context of breast cancer. In this study, utilization of several omics (exome, transcriptome, proteome) platforms, along with karyotyping and metabolic status, has allowed integrative insights not possible with isolated studies (Figure 11). The PMC42 cell line model system comprises a mesenchymal, parental PMC42-ET cell line and an epithelial derivative PMC42-LA cell line that exhibits profound morphological changes [40], decreased cellular proliferation, distinct karyotype, depletion of TGFBR2 gene, distinct pathways mediated by TNF-alpha signalling, and decreased metabolic bioenergetics.

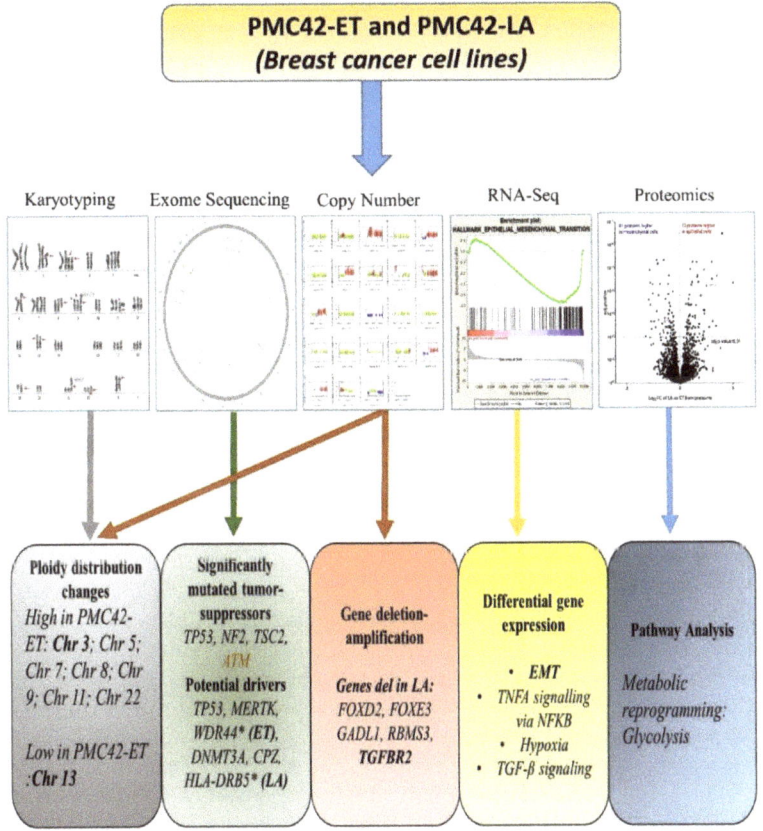

**Figure 11.** Graphical abstract reflecting the multiple outcomes from the comprehensive and integrative—omics characterization and karyotyping of the PMC42 model system.

Our study identified common canonical driver mutations in TP53, MERTK and DNMT3A in the PMC42 system, as well as a number of unique molecular alterations in the PMC42-ET and PMC42-LA genes that are mutated (Supplementary Tables S5–S8) and have thus potentially impacted the phenotypic heterogeneity seen. Some of the allelic heterogeneous mutations detected in PMC42-LA have also been associated with EMT drivers or markers; we identified novel mutations in *GSN (R397W), WNT1 (T363K), SNAI2 (K188N), ITGA4 (R565W), SOX3 (R22P) and NID2 (G426E)* (Supplementary Table S7). SNAI2-null mice are reported to have retarded epithelial migration rates [79], and SOX3 has been implicated in the malignant behaviour of glioblastoma [80], EMT, and in the promotion of migration and invasion of osteosarcoma cells [81,82]. A N161K mutation in SOX3 was found associated with progression of SCLC along with other mutated SOX members [83]. The implications of genomic variants for these other markers have not been studied or reported in context of EMT. These identified mutations in EMT drivers evaluated at differential gene expression level reflected complete absence of expression of WNT1 and 6-fold downregulation of ITGA4 in PMC42-LA cells.

Comparison of transcriptome and proteome analyses across PMC42 cell lines, combined with GSEA and IPA, were performed to gain insights into the biological processes dysregulated within our model system. In our transcriptome studies, the expression of forkhead box A1 (FOXA1) gene, which acts to control transcription of estrogen receptor-regulated genes and repress the basallike features of breast cancer cells [84–87], was observed only in PMC42-LA. We observed upregulation in the expression of several specific genes that favour the MET in PMC42-LA, including AGR2 and GRHL2. The most prominent feature of GSEA analysis was the strong down-regulation of EMT in PMC42-LA ($p$-value of < 0.001) (Figure 3). These results indicate that this model system is highly appropriate for studies of EMP [40]. Interestingly, the combined analysis of both transcriptome and proteome across PMC42 cell lines using IPA also indicated that EGFR and ER may be common upstream regulators that are dysregulated between the two cell lines. The ability of EGFR signalling to drive EMT is widely reported in literature [88–90] and is also considered an important driver of MDA-MB-231 invasion leading to formation of brain metastasis [91]. Studies from GSEA and IPA also highlighted an involvement of the TNF-α pathway, mediated by NFKB ($p$-value 0.007), as a major attenuated pathway between PMC42 cell lines. Significant assessment from in vitro studies have highlighted the significance of various cytokines, such as TNF-α [92,93] and growth factors such as EGF and TGF-β in mediating EMT changes, and how these targets can have therapeutic implications in combating EMP [20,93,94].

Furthermore, our recent published work also investigated the dynamic interconversions observed between the transitional epithelial and mesenchymal subpopulations delineated by EpCAM profiling in the predominantly epithelial PMC42-LA breast cancer cells. The subtleties of this transition vary in proportion of epithelial and mesenchymal phenotypes as determined from single cells clonal propagation. Differences observed in the functional attributes of the single cell-derived clones further explains the stochastic nature and the intrinsic cellular plasticity in PMC42-LA. Interestingly, the implementation of whole exome sequencing across the EpCAM-high and -low subpopulation indicates that observed intrinsic phenotypic plasticity in PMC42-LA was not attributable to chromosomal instability [66]. Moreover, the PMC42-LA subline derived from PMC42-ET and remaining phenotypically stable over two decades has maintained distinct karyotype with reduced number of chromosomes and significant ploidy disparity reflected for eight of the chromosomes.

In this pattern of karyotypic differences reflected in the genomic copy number alterations across the two cell lines, we observed that the allele fractions had significantly deviated in the PMC42-LA daughter cell line ($p$-value < 0.0001). PMC42-ET has the higher chromosome number, consistent with a relative increase of its transcriptome and proteome abundance (Figure 9C), a broader range of chromosome numbers, and a higher CIN70 score (Figures 4 and 5). The gain of chromosome 13 and the loss of chromosome 3 in PMC42-LA were the most prominent changes reflected in both the transcriptome and proteome (Figure 9C). Strikingly, the locus of TGFBR2 gene is also on chromosome 3. Notably, we observe a potential link between the deletion affecting the TGF-β receptor gene TGFBR2 in PMC42-LA and its negative TES scores assessed from transcriptome analysis. Moreover, the aberration of TGFBR2 also made PMC42-LA cell line non-responsive to TGF-β1 stimulus for EMT mediated changes (Figure 8C). Thus, changes in specific chromosomes in PMC42-ET, with the acquisition of new mutations and genetic deletion of TGFBR2, may have contributed to the derivation of the MET observed in the PMC42-LA cells. The assessment of the impact of copy number variations at single-gene level across the whole differential mRNA analysis did not yield a significant association (Supplementary Figure S4). Differential gene expression instead of solely based on amplification of gene copies can also be modulated by other factors, such as gene epigenetics or transcription factors. Indeed, Ohshima et al. had associated the gene expression level of various oncogenes with copy number and found that the R value varied between 0.06 and 0.53 across different cancer datasets [95].

CD44 and CD24 are considered putative stem cell markers [96,97] and expression profiling of selected breast cancer cell lines in this study correlates well with previously performed studies on the same cell lines [64,98,99]. Expression of CD24 was equally low or negligible in both the PMC42 cell lines and interestingly, we find higher expression of CD44 in PMC42-LA than anticipated. Many studies have confirmed the CD44$^{high}$/CD24$^{low}$ profile as a reflection of a mesenchymal state [25,39,100]. However, the epithelially shifted PMC42-LA reflected the increase in CD44$^{high}$/CD24$^{low}$ profile as compared to the parental PMC42-ET cells. There are other reports of ambiguity regarding functional aspects of these markers [101], suggesting that further investigations of stemness and the regulatory factors in this cell system are required.

Understanding the mechanistic basis of metabolic alterations and their role in tumorigenesis is currently an area of intense research interest [102–106]. Despite glycolysis being one of the significantly attenuated pathways in PMC42-LA cells identified through proteomics analysis, Seahorse experiments indicated decreases in both oxidative metabolism and glycolysis in PMC42-LA cells relative to PMC42-ET. This suggests that the observed metabolic alterations may be attributable to differences in mitochondrial number, rather than proteome differences in metabolic genes required for glycolysis: *ALDH1A3*, *ALDH3A1* and *ALDOC* between cell lines. The analysis of metabolic phenotypes emphasises the importance of using bioenergetics profiles to decipher phenotype assessment, rather than drawing conclusions solely from mutational profiling, RNA-seq and/or proteome data [107,108].

## 5. Conclusions

In conclusion, the data we have presented herein underscore profound differences in the PMC42 system by allowing for a comprehensive integration of whole exome sequencing, RNA-seq, proteomics and karyotyping data. The identification of novel somatic mutations and indels provide insights into the differences between the two cell lines at genetic scale that potentially drive the phenotypic differences from the genomic level. The loss of *TGFBR2* gene from the derivative PMC42-LA cell line contributes to a reduction in intrinsic TGFB signalling, and these cells are also refractory to TGF-β-induced EMT, however this pathway did not emerge from GSEA analysis. Comparative RNA-seq also demonstrated the PMC42 system to be an authentic MET model. The inter-data relationships illustrate a high degree of concordance between the relative transcript and proteome abundance and chromosome copy number variations across the PMC42 cell lines and identified putative targets to reverse MET. The novel findings provide mechanistic insights into how genomic instability and karyotypic variations have led to acquisition of new autonomous clonal karyotype and phenotype, which is still related to, but distinct from the parental cell line. However, further metabolomics and epigenetics studies might be more compelling to add into the paradigm to determine implications for mesenchymal to epithelial plasticity changes. Overall, this investigation provides an example of the heterogenous changes that may occur in expanding cancer populations and provides evidence for the levels on which these changes occur to affect their phenotypic properties.

**Supplementary Materials:** The following are available online at http://www.mdpi.com/2077-0383/8/8/1253/s1.

**Author Contributions:** S.B., E.W.T., S.H.N. designed the experiments. S.B., J.M. performed the experiments. S.B., T.B., P.H.G.D., E.W.T. analysed the data. Genewiz personnel performed and analysed the whole exome sequencing data. S.B. wrote the manuscript. E.W.T., P.H.G.D., J.M. refined and edited the manuscript. S.H.N., E.W.T. supervised the study.

**Funding:** This work was supported in part by the National Breast Cancer Foundation (CG-10-04) to EWT.

**Acknowledgments:** This work was supported in part by the National Breast Cancer Foundation (CG-10-04) to E.W.T. We would like to thank FACS core facility and Microscopy core facility based at TRI for their technical assistance. Proteomics work was done at QUT CARF Facility. The Translational Research Institute receives support from the Australian Government. During the course of the study, S.B. was supported by QUTPRA scholarship. We would also like to thank Peiru Chen for her help in proteomics assessment, Jennifer Gunter for helping with seahorse analyser and Momeneh Foroutan for deriving and providing TES values for PMC42 cell lines.

**Conflicts of Interest:** The authors declare they have no competing financial interests in relation to the work described.

## References

1. Turashvili, G.; Brogi, E. Tumor Heterogeneity in Breast Cancer. *Front. Med.* **2017**, *4*, 227. [CrossRef] [PubMed]
2. Rivenbark, A.G.; O'Connor, S.M.; Coleman, W.B. Molecular and cellular heterogeneity in breast cancer: challenges for personalized medicine. *Am. J. Pathol.* **2013**, *183*, 1113–1124. [CrossRef] [PubMed]
3. Saunus, J.M.; Smart, C.E.; Kutasovic, J.R.; Johnston, R.L.; Kalita-de Croft, P.; Miranda, M.; Rozali, E.N.; Vargas, A.C.; Reid, L.E.; Lorsy, E.; et al. Multidimensional phenotyping of breast cancer cell lines to guide preclinical research. *Breast Cancer Res. Treat.* **2018**, *167*, 289–301. [CrossRef] [PubMed]
4. Keller, P.J.; Lin, A.F.; Arendt, L.M.; Klebba, I.; Jones, A.D.; Rudnick, J.A.; DiMeo, T.A.; Gilmore, H.; Jefferson, D.M.; Graham, R.A.; et al. Mapping the cellular and molecular heterogeneity of normal and malignant breast tissues and cultured cell lines. *Breast Cancer Res.* **2010**, *12*, R87. [CrossRef] [PubMed]
5. Hollestelle, A.; Nagel, J.H.; Smid, M.; Lam, S.; Elstrodt, F.; Wasielewski, M.; Ng, S.S.; French, P.J.; Peeters, J.K.; Rozendaal, M.J.; et al. Distinct gene mutation profiles among luminal-type and basal-type breast cancer cell lines. *Breast Cancer Res. Treat.* **2010**, *121*, 53–64. [CrossRef] [PubMed]
6. Lehmann, B.D.; Bauer, J.A.; Chen, X.; Sanders, M.E.; Chakravarthy, A.B.; Shyr, Y.; Pietenpol, J.A. Identification of human triple-negative breast cancer subtypes and preclinical models for selection of targeted therapies. *J. Clin. Investig.* **2011**, *121*, 2750–2767. [CrossRef] [PubMed]
7. Neve, R.M.; Chin, K.; Fridlyand, J.; Yeh, J.; Baehner, F.L.; Fevr, T.; Clark, L.; Bayani, N.; Coppé, J.-P.; Tong, F.; et al. A collection of breast cancer cell lines for the study of functionally distinct cancer subtypes. *Cancer Cell* **2006**, *10*, 515–527. [CrossRef] [PubMed]
8. Prat, A.; Parker, J.S.; Karginova, O.; Fan, C.; Livasy, C.; Herschkowitz, J.I.; He, X.; Perou, C.M. Phenotypic and molecular characterization of the claudin-low intrinsic subtype of breast cancer. *Breast Cancer Res.* **2010**, *12*, R68. [CrossRef]
9. Smart, C.E.; Morrison, B.J.; Saunus, J.M.; Vargas, A.C.; Keith, P.; Reid, L.; Wockner, L.; Amiri, M.A.; Sarkar, D.; Simpson, P.T.; et al. In Vitro Analysis of Breast Cancer Cell Line Tumourspheres and Primary Human Breast Epithelia Mammospheres Demonstrates Inter- and Intrasphere Heterogeneity. *PLoS ONE* **2013**, *8*, e64388. [CrossRef]
10. Kao, J.; Salari, K.; Bocanegra, M.; Choi, Y.-L.; Girard, L.; Gandhi, J.; Kwei, K.A.; Hernandez-Boussard, T.; Wang, P.; Gazdar, A.F.; et al. Molecular Profiling of Breast Cancer Cell Lines Defines Relevant Tumor Models and Provides a Resource for Cancer Gene Discovery. *PLoS ONE* **2009**, *4*, e6146. [CrossRef]
11. Daemen, A.; Griffith, O.L.; Heiser, L.M.; Wang, N.J.; Enache, O.M.; Sanborn, Z.; Pepin, F.; Durinck, S.; Korkola, J.E.; Griffith, M.; et al. Modeling precision treatment of breast cancer. *Genome Boil.* **2013**, *14*, R110. [CrossRef]
12. Barretina, J.; Caponigro, G.; Stransky, N.; Venkatesan, K.; Margolin, A.A.; Kim, S.; Wilson, C.J.; Lehár, J.; Kryukov, G.V.; Sonkin, D.; et al. Addendum: The Cancer Cell Line Encyclopedia enables predictive modelling of anticancer drug sensitivity. *Nature* **2012**, *492*, 290. [CrossRef]
13. Subramanian, A.; Narayan, R.; Corsello, S.M.; Peck, D.D.; Natoli, T.E.; Lu, X.; Gould, J.; Davis, J.F.; Tubelli, A.A.; Asiedu, J.K.; et al. A Next Generation Connectivity Map: L1000 platform and the first 1,000,000 profiles. *Cell* **2017**, *171*, 1437–1452. [CrossRef]
14. Cope, L.M.; Fackler, M.J.; Lopez-Bujanda, Z.; Wolff, A.C.; Visvanathan, K.; Gray, J.W.; Sukumar, S.; Umbricht, C.B. Do Breast Cancer Cell Lines Provide a Relevant Model of the Patient Tumor Methylome? *PLoS ONE* **2014**, *9*, e105545. [CrossRef]
15. Jiang, G.; Zhang, S.; Yazdanparast, A.; Li, M.; Pawar, A.V.; Liu, Y.; Inavolu, S.M.; Cheng, L. Comprehensive comparison of molecular portraits between cell lines and tumors in breast cancer. *BMC Genom.* **2016**, *17*, 1079. [CrossRef]
16. Heiser, L.M.; Sadanandam, A.; Kuo, W.L.; Benz, S.C.; Goldstein, T.C.; Ng, S.; Gibb, W.J.; Wang, N.J.; Ziyad, S.; Tong, F.; et al. Subtype and pathway specific responses to anticancer compounds in breast cancer. *Proc. Natl. Acad. Sci. USA* **2012**, *109*, 2724–2729. [CrossRef]
17. Hugo, H.; Ackland, M.L.; Blick, T.; Lawrence, M.G.; Clements, J.A.; Williams, E.D.; Thompson, E.W. Epithelial—mesenchymal and mesenchymal—epithelial transitions in carcinoma progression. *J. Cell. Physiol.* **2007**, *213*, 374–383. [CrossRef]
18. Nieto, M.A.; Huang, R.Y.J.; Jackson, R.A.; Thiery, J.P. EMT: 2016. *Cell* **2016**, *166*, 21–45. [CrossRef]

19. Jolly, M.K.; Tripathi, S.C.; Jia, D.; Mooney, S.M.; Celiktas, M.; Hanash, S.M.; Mani, S.A.; Pienta, K.J.; Ben-Jacob, E.; Levine, H. Stability of the hybrid epithelial/mesenchymal phenotype. *Oncotarget* **2016**, *7*, 27067–27084. [CrossRef]
20. Bhatia, S.; Monkman, J.; Toh, A.K.L.; Nagaraj, S.H.; Thompson, E.W. Targeting epithelial–mesenchymal plasticity in cancer: clinical and preclinical advances in therapy and monitoring. *Biochem. J.* **2017**, *474*, 3269–3306. [CrossRef]
21. Fischer, K.R.; Durrans, A.; Lee, S.; Sheng, J.; Li, F.; Wong, S.T.; Choi, H.; El Rayes, T.; Ryu, S.; Troeger, J.; et al. Epithelial-to-mesenchymal transition is not required for lung metastasis but contributes to chemoresistance. *Nature* **2015**, *527*, 472–476. [CrossRef]
22. Zheng, X.; Carstens, J.L.; Kim, J.; Scheible, M.; Kaye, J.; Sugimoto, H.; Wu, C.C.; LeBleu, V.S.; Kalluri, R. Epithelial-to-mesenchymal transition is dispensable for metastasis but induces chemoresistance in pancreatic cancer. *Nature* **2015**, *527*, 525–530. [CrossRef]
23. Redfern, A.D.; Spalding, L.J.; Thompson, E.W. The Kraken Wakes: induced EMT as a driver of tumour aggression and poor outcome. *Clin. Exp. Metastasis* **2018**, *35*, 285–308. [CrossRef]
24. Blick, T.; Widodo, E.; Hugo, H.; Waltham, M.; Lenburg, M.E.; Neve, R.M.; Thompson, E.W. Epithelial mesenchymal transition traits in human breast cancer cell lines. *Clin. Exp. Metastasis* **2008**, *25*, 629–642. [CrossRef]
25. Blick, T.; Hugo, H.; Widodo, E.; Waltham, M.; Pinto, C.; Mani, S.A.; Weinberg, R.A.; Neve, R.M.; Lenburg, M.E.; Thompson, E.W. Epithelial Mesenchymal Transition Traits in Human Breast Cancer Cell Lines Parallel the $CD_{44}^{hi}/CD_{24}^{lo/-}$ Stem Cell Phenotype in Human Breast Cancer. *J. Mammary Gland. Boil. Neoplasia* **2010**, *15*, 235–252. [CrossRef]
26. Tan, T.Z.; Miow, Q.H.; Miki, Y.; Noda, T.; Mori, S.; Huang, R.Y.-J.; Thiery, J.P. Epithelial-mesenchymal transition spectrum quantification and its efficacy in deciphering survival and drug responses of cancer patients. *EMBO Mol. Med.* **2014**, *6*, 1279–1293. [CrossRef]
27. Foroutan, M.; Cursons, J.; Hediyeh-Zadeh, S.; Thompson, E.W.; Davis, M.J. A Transcriptional Program for Detecting TGFbeta-Induced EMT in Cancer. *Mol. Cancer Res.* **2017**, *15*, 619–631. [CrossRef]
28. Foroutan, M.; Bhuva, D.D.; Lyu, R.; Horan, K.; Cursons, J.; Davis, M.J. Single sample scoring of molecular phenotypes. *BMC Bioinform.* **2018**, *19*, 404. [CrossRef]
29. George, J.T.; Jolly, M.K.; Xu, S.; Somarelli, J.A.; Levine, H. Survival outcomes in cancer patients predicted by a partial EMT gene expression scoring metric. *Cancer Res.* **2017**, *77*, 6415–6428. [CrossRef]
30. Cursons, J.; Leuchowius, K.-J.; Waltham, M.; Tomaskovic-Crook, E.; Foroutan, M.; Bracken, C.P.; Redfern, A.; Crampin, E.J.; Street, I.; Davis, M.J.; et al. Stimulus-dependent differences in signalling regulate epithelial-mesenchymal plasticity and change the effects of drugs in breast cancer cell lines. *Cell Commun. Signal.* **2015**, *13*, 26. [CrossRef]
31. Buonato, J.M.; Lan, I.S.; Lazzara, M.J. EGF augments TGFβ-induced epithelial–mesenchymal transition by promoting SHP2 binding to GAB1. *J. Cell Sci.* **2015**, *128*, 3898–3909. [CrossRef]
32. Hugo, H.J.; Wafai, R.; Blick, T.; Thompson, E.W.; Newgreen, D.F. Staurosporine augments EGF-mediated EMT in PMC42-LA cells through actin depolymerisation, focal contact size reduction and Snail1 induction—A model for cross-modulation. *BMC Cancer* **2009**, *9*, 235. [CrossRef]
33. Kurimoto, R.; Iwasawa, S.; Ebata, T.; Ishiwata, T.; Sekine, I.; Tada, Y.; Tatsumi, K.; Koide, S.; Iwama, A.; Takiguchi, Y. Drug resistance originating from a TGF-beta/FGF-2-driven epithelial-to-mesenchymal transition and its reversion in human lung adenocarcinoma cell lines harboring an EGFR mutation. *Int. J. Oncol.* **2016**, *48*, 1825–1836. [CrossRef]
34. Tiwari, N.; Tiwari, V.K.; Waldmeier, L.; Balwierz, P.J.; Arnold, P.; Pachkov, M.; Meyer-Schaller, N.; Schübeler, D.; Van Nimwegen, E.; Christofori, G. Sox4 Is a Master Regulator of Epithelial-Mesenchymal Transition by Controlling Ezh2 Expression and Epigenetic Reprogramming. *Cancer Cell* **2013**, *23*, 768–783. [CrossRef]
35. Yamamoto, M.; Sakane, K.; Tominaga, K.; Gotoh, N.; Niwa, T.; Kikuchi, Y.; Tada, K.; Goshima, N.; Semba, K.; Inoue, J. Intratumoral bidirectional transitions between epithelial and mesenchymal cells in triple-negative breast cancer. *Cancer Sci.* **2017**, *108*, 1210–1222. [CrossRef]
36. Taube, J.H.; Herschkowitz, J.I.; Komurov, K.; Zhou, A.Y.; Gupta, S.; Yang, J.; Hartwell, K.; Onder, T.T.; Gupta, P.B.; Evans, K.W.; et al. Core epithelial-to-mesenchymal transition interactome gene-expression signature is associated with claudin-low and metaplastic breast cancer subtypes. *Proc. Natl. Acad. Sci. USA* **2010**, *107*, 15449–15454. [CrossRef]

37. Morel, A.-P.; Lièvre, M.; Thomas, C.; Hinkal, G.; Ansieau, S.; Puisieux, A. Generation of Breast Cancer Stem Cells through Epithelial-Mesenchymal Transition. *PLoS ONE* **2008**, *3*, e2888. [CrossRef]
38. Briem, E.; Ingthorsson, S.; Traustadottir, G.A.; Hilmarsdottir, B.; Gudjonsson, T. Application of the D492 Cell Lines to Explore Breast Morphogenesis, EMT and Cancer Progression in 3D Culture. *J. Mammary Gland. Boil. Neoplasia* **2019**, *24*, 139–147. [CrossRef]
39. Mani, S.A.; Guo, W.; Liao, M.-J.; Eaton, E.N.; Ayyanan, A.; Zhou, A.Y.; Brooks, M.; Reinhard, F.; Zhang, C.C.; Shipitsin, M.; et al. The epithelial-mesenchymal transition generates cells with properties of stem cells. *Cell* **2008**, *133*, 704–715. [CrossRef]
40. Hugo, H.J.; Kokkinos, M.I.; Blick, T.; Ackland, M.L.; Thompson, E.W.; Newgreen, D.F. Defining the E-Cadherin Repressor Interactome in Epithelial-Mesenchymal Transition: The PMC42 Model as a Case Study. *Cells Tissues Organs* **2011**, *193*, 23–40. [CrossRef]
41. Whitehead, R.H.; Bertoncello, I.; Webber, L.M.; Pedersen, J.S. A new human breast carcinoma cell line (PMC42) with stem cell characteristics. I. Morphologic characterization. *J. Natl. Cancer Inst.* **1983**, *70*, 649–661.
42. Whitehead, R.H.; Webber, L.M.; Bertoncello, I.; Vitali, A.A.; Monaghan, P. A New Human Breast Carcinoma Cell Line (PMC42) With Stem Cell Characteristics. II. Characterization of Cells Growing as Organoids. *J. Natl. Cancer Inst.* **1983**, *71*, 1193–1203.
43. Whitehead, R.H.; Quirk, S.J.; Vitali, A.A.; Funder, J.W.; Sutherland, R.L.; Murphy, L.C. A new human breast carcinoma cell line (PMC42) with stem cell characteristics. III. Hormone receptor status and responsiveness. *J. Natl. Cancer Inst.* **1984**, *73*, 643–648.
44. Ackland, M.L.; Newgreen, D.F.; Fridman, M.; Waltham, M.C.; Arvanitis, A.; Minichiello, J.; Price, J.T.; Thompson, E.W. Epidermal Growth Factor-Induced Epithelio-Mesenchymal Transition in Human Breast Carcinoma Cells. *Lab. Investig.* **2003**, *83*, 435–448. [CrossRef]
45. Ackland, M.; Michalczyk, A.; Whitehead, R. PMC42, A Novel Model for the Differentiated Human Breast. *Exp. Cell Res.* **2001**, *263*, 14–22. [CrossRef]
46. Li, H.; Durbin, R. Fast and accurate short read alignment with Burrows–Wheeler transform. *Bioinformatics* **2009**, *25*, 1754–1760. [CrossRef]
47. Li, H.; Handsaker, B.; Wysoker, A.; Fennell, T.; Ruan, J.; Homer, N.; Marth, G.; Abecasis, G.; Durbin, R. The Sequence Alignment/Map format and SAMtools. *Bioinformatics* **2009**, *25*, 2078–2079. [CrossRef]
48. McKenna, A.; Hanna, M.; Banks, E.; Sivachenko, A.; Cibulskis, K.; Kernytsky, A.; Garimella, K.; Altshuler, D.; Gabriel, S.; Daly, M.; et al. The Genome Analysis Toolkit: A MapReduce framework for analyzing next-generation DNA sequencing data. *Genome Res.* **2010**, *20*, 1297–1303. [CrossRef]
49. Wang, K.; Li, M.; Hakonarson, H. ANNOVAR: functional annotation of genetic variants from high-throughput sequencing data. *Nucleic Acids Res.* **2010**, *38*, e164. [CrossRef]
50. ANNOVAR. Available online: http://openbioinformatics.org/annovar/ (accessed on 30 January 2019).
51. Boeva, V.; Popova, T.; Bleakley, K.; Chiche, P.; Cappo, J.; Schleiermacher, G.; Janoueix-Lerosey, I.; Delattre, O.; Barillot, E. Control-FREEC: A tool for assessing copy number and allelic content using next-generation sequencing data. *Bioinformatics* **2012**, *28*, 423–425. [CrossRef]
52. Douville, C.; Carter, H.; Kim, R.; Niknafs, N.; Diekhans, M.; Stenson, P.D.; Cooper, D.N.; Ryan, M.; Karchin, R. CRAVAT: cancer-related analysis of variants toolkit. *Bioinformatics* **2013**, *29*, 647–648. [CrossRef]
53. Carter, H.; Samayoa, J.; Hruban, R.H.; Karchin, R. Prioritization of driver mutations in pancreatic cancer using cancer-specific high-throughput annotation of somatic mutations (CHASM). *Cancer Boil. Ther.* **2010**, *10*, 582–587. [CrossRef]
54. Carter, H.; Chen, S.; Isik, L.; Tyekucheva, S.; Velculescu, V.E.; Kinzler, K.W.; Vogelstein, B.; Karchin, R. Cancer-specific High-throughput Annotation of Somatic Mutations: computational prediction of driver missense mutations. *Cancer Res.* **2009**, *69*, 6660–6667. [CrossRef]
55. Carter, H.; Douville, C.; Stenson, P.D.; Cooper, D.N.; Karchin, R. Identifying Mendelian disease genes with the Variant Effect Scoring Tool. *BMC Genom.* **2013**, *14*, S3. [CrossRef]
56. Morpheus. Available online: https://software.broadinstitute.org/morpheus/ (accessed on 25 Febrary 2019).
57. Mar, J.C.; Kimura, Y.; Schroder, K.; Irvine, K.M.; Hayashizaki, Y.; Suzuki, H.; Hume, D.; Quackenbush, J. Data-driven normalization strategies for high-throughput quantitative RT-PCR. *BMC Bioinform.* **2009**, *10*, 110. [CrossRef]

58. Trapnell, C.; Roberts, A.; Goff, L.; Pertea, G.; Kim, D.; Kelley, D.R.; Pimentel, H.; Salzberg, S.L.; Rinn, J.L.; Pachter, L. Differential gene and transcript expression analysis of RNA-seq experiments with TopHat and Cufflinks. *Nat. Protoc.* **2012**, *7*, 562–578. [CrossRef]
59. GSEA. Available online: http://www.broad.mit.edu/gsea (accessed on 24 April 2019).
60. Wiśniewski, J.R.; Zougman, A.; Nagaraj, N.; Mann, M. Universal sample preparation method for proteome analysis. *Nat. Methods* **2009**, *6*, 359–362. [CrossRef]
61. UniProt. Available online: https://www.uniprot.org/ (accessed on 25 November 2018).
62. PeakView Software. Available online: https://sciex.com/products/software/peakview-software (accessed on 25 November 2018).
63. Clough, T.; Thaminy, S.; Ragg, S.; Aebersold, R.; Vitek, O. Statistical protein quantification and significance analysis in label-free LC-MS experiments with complex designs. *BMC Bioinform.* **2012**, *13*, S6. [CrossRef]
64. Ricardo, S.; Vieira, A.F.; Gerhard, R.; Leitão, D.; Pinto, R.; Cameselle-Teijeiro, J.F.; Milanezi, F.; Schmitt, F.; Paredes, J. Breast cancer stem cell markers CD44, CD24 and ALDH1: expression distribution within intrinsic molecular subtype. *J. Clin. Pathol.* **2011**, *64*, 937–946. [CrossRef]
65. Matalkah, F.; Martin, E.; Zhao, H.; Agazie, Y.M. SHP2 acts both upstream and downstream of multiple receptor tyrosine kinases to promote basal-like and triple-negative breast cancer. *Breast Cancer Res.* **2016**, *18*, 25. [CrossRef]
66. Bhatia, S.; Monkman, J.; Blick, T.; Pinto, C.; Waltham, M.; Nagaraj, S.H.; Thompson, E.W. Interrogation of Phenotypic Plasticity between Epithelial and Mesenchymal States in Breast Cancer. *J. Clin. Med.* **2019**, *8*, 893. [CrossRef]
67. Carter, S.L.; Eklund, A.C.; Kohane, I.S.; Harris, L.N.; Szallasi, Z. A signature of chromosomal instability inferred from gene expression profiles predicts clinical outcome in multiple human cancers. *Nat. Genet.* **2006**, *38*, 1043–1048. [CrossRef]
68. Gunasinghe, N.P.A.D.; Wells, A.; Thompson, E.W.; Hugo, H.J. Mesenchymal–epithelial transition (MET) as a mechanism for metastatic colonisation in breast cancer. *Cancer Metastasis Rev.* **2012**, *31*, 469–478. [CrossRef]
69. Tsubakihara, Y.; Moustakas, A. Epithelial–mesenchymal Transition and Metastasis under the Control of Transforming Growth Factor beta. *Int. J. Mol. Sci.* **2018**, *19*, 3672. [CrossRef]
70. Pino, M.S.; Kikuchi, H.; Zeng, M.; Herraiz, M.T.; Sperduti, I.; Berger, D.; Park, D.Y.; Iafrate, A.J.; Zukerberg, L.R.; Chung, D.C. Epithelial to mesenchymal transition is impaired in colon cancer cells with microsatellite instability. *Gastroenterology* **2010**, *138*, 1406–1417. [CrossRef]
71. Sommerova, L.; Ondrouskova, E.; Vojtesek, B.; Hrstka, R. Suppression of AGR2 in a TGF-β-induced Smad regulatory pathway mediates epithelial-mesenchymal transition. *BMC Cancer* **2017**, *17*, 546. [CrossRef]
72. Gozgit, J.M.; Pentecost, B.T.; Marconi, S.A.; Ricketts-Loriaux, R.S.J.; Otis, C.N.; Arcaro, K.F. PLD1 is overexpressed in an ER-negative MCF-7 cell line variant and a subset of phospho-Akt-negative breast carcinomas. *Br. J. Cancer* **2007**, *97*, 809–817. [CrossRef]
73. Ye, X.; Brabletz, T.; Kang, Y.; Longmore, G.D.; Nieto, M.A.; Stanger, B.Z.; Yang, J.; Weinberg, R.A. Upholding a role for EMT in breast cancer metastasis. *Nature* **2017**, *547*, E1–E3. [CrossRef]
74. Fischer, K.R.; Altorki, N.K.; Mittal, V.; Gao, D. Fischer et al. reply. *Nature* **2017**, *547*, E5. [CrossRef]
75. Brabletz, T.; Kalluri, R. EMT in cancer. *Nat. Rev. Cancer* **2018**, *18*, 128–134. [CrossRef]
76. Beerling, E.; Seinstra, D.; De Wit, E.; Kester, L.; Van Der Velden, D.; Maynard, C.; Schäfer, R.; Van Diest, P.; Voest, E.; Van Oudenaarden, A.; et al. Plasticity between Epithelial and Mesenchymal States Unlinks EMT from Metastasis-Enhancing Stem Cell Capacity. *Cell Rep.* **2016**, *14*, 2281–2288. [CrossRef]
77. Brabletz, T. To differentiate or not—Routes towards metastasis. *Nat. Rev. Cancer* **2012**, *12*, 425–436. [CrossRef]
78. van Denderen, B.J.; Thompson, E.W. Cancer: The to and fro of tumour spread. *Nature* **2013**, *493*, 487–488. [CrossRef]
79. Savagner, P.; Kusewitt, D.F.; Carver, E.A.; Magnino, F.; Choi, C.; Gridley, T.; Hudson, L.G. Developmental transcription factor slug is required for effective re-epithelialization by adult keratinocytes. *J. Cell. Physiol.* **2005**, *202*, 858–866. [CrossRef]
80. Vicentic, J.M.; Drakulic, D.; Garcia, I.; Vukovic, V.; Aldaz, P.; Puskas, N.; Nikolic, I.; Tasic, G.; Raicevic, S.; Garros-Regulez, L.; et al. SOX3 can promote the malignant behavior of glioblastoma cells. *Cell Oncol.* **2019**, *42*, 41–54. [CrossRef]
81. Guo, Y.; Yin, J.; Tang, M.; Yu, X. Downregulation of SOX3 leads to the inhibition of the proliferation, migration and invasion of osteosarcoma cells. *Int. J. Oncol.* **2018**, *52*, 1277–1284. [CrossRef]

82. Qiu, M.; Chen, D.; Shen, C.; Shen, J.; Zhao, H.; He, Y. Sex-determining region Y-box protein 3 induces epithelial-mesenchymal transition in osteosarcoma cells via transcriptional activation of Snail1. *J. Exp. Clin. Cancer Res.* **2017**, *36*, 46. [CrossRef]
83. Rudin, C.M.; Durinck, S.; Stawiski, E.W.; Poirier, J.T.; Modrusan, Z.; Shames, D.S.; Bergbower, E.A.; Guan, Y.; Shin, J.; Guillory, J.; et al. Comprehensive genomic analysis identifies SOX2 as a frequently amplified gene in small-cell lung cancer. *Nat. Genet.* **2012**, *44*, 1111–1116. [CrossRef]
84. Badve, S.; Turbin, D.; Thorat, M.A.; Morimiya, A.; Nielsen, T.O.; Perou, C.M.; Dunn, S.; Huntsman, D.G.; Nakshatri, H. FOXA1 Expression in Breast Cancer Correlation with Luminal Subtype A and Survival. *Clin. Cancer Res.* **2007**, *13*, 4415–4421. [CrossRef]
85. Rangel, N.; Fortunati, N.; Osella-Abate, S.; Annaratone, L.; Isella, C.; Catalano, M.G.; Rinella, L.; Metovic, J.; Boldorini, R.; Balmativola, D.; et al. FOXA1 and AR in invasive breast cancer: new findings on their co-expression and impact on prognosis in ER-positive patients. *BMC Cancer* **2018**, *18*, 703. [CrossRef]
86. Fu, X.; Jeselsohn, R.; Pereira, R.; Hollingsworth, E.F.; Creighton, C.J.; Li, F.; Shea, M.; Nardone, A.; De Angelis, C.; Heiser, L.M.; et al. FOXA1 overexpression mediates endocrine resistance by altering the ER transcriptome and IL-8 expression in ER-positive breast cancer. *Proc. Natl. Acad. Sci. USA* **2016**, *113*, E6600–E6609. [CrossRef]
87. Bernardo, G.M.; Bebek, G.; Ginther, C.L.; Sizemore, S.T.; Lozada, K.L.; Miedler, J.D.; Anderson, L.A.; Godwin, A.K.; Abdul-Karim, F.W.; Slamon, D.J.; et al. FOXA1 represses the molecular phenotype of basal breast cancer cells. *Oncogene* **2013**, *32*, 554–563. [CrossRef]
88. Al Moustafa, A.-E.; Ala-Eddin, A.M. EGF-receptor signaling and epithelial-mesenchymal transition in human carcinomas. *Front. Biosci.* **2012**, *4*, 671–684. [CrossRef]
89. Lo, H.-W.; Hsu, S.-C.; Xia, W.; Cao, X.; Shih, J.-Y.; Wei, Y.; Abbruzzese, J.L.; Hortobagyi, G.N.; Hung, M.-C. Epidermal Growth Factor Receptor Cooperates with Signal Transducer and Activator of Transcription 3 to Induce Epithelial-Mesenchymal Transition in Cancer Cells via Up-regulation of TWIST Gene Expression. *Cancer Res.* **2007**, *67*, 9066–9076. [CrossRef]
90. Mizumoto, A.; Yamamoto, K.; Nakayama, Y.; Takara, K.; Nakagawa, T.; Hirano, T.; Hirai, M. Induction of epithelial–mesenchymal transition via activation of epidermal growth factor receptor contributes to sunitinib resistance in human renal cell carcinoma cell lines. *J. Pharmacol. Exp. Ther.* **2015**, *355*, 152–158. [CrossRef]
91. Nie, F.; Yang, J.; Wen, S.; An, Y.-L.; Ding, J.; Ju, S.-H.; Zhao, Z.; Chen, H.-J.; Peng, X.-G.; Wong, S.T.C.; et al. Involvement of epidermal growth factor receptor overexpression in the promotion of breast cancer brain metastasis. *Cancer* **2012**, *118*, 5198–5209. [CrossRef]
92. Tang, D.; Tao, D.; Fang, Y.; Deng, C.; Xu, Q.; Zhou, J. TNF-Alpha Promotes Invasion and Metastasis via NF-Kappa B Pathway in Oral Squamous Cell Carcinoma. *Med Sci. Monit. Basic Res.* **2017**, *23*, 141–149. [CrossRef]
93. Li, C.W.; Xia, W.; Huo, L.; Lim, S.O.; Wu, Y.; Hsu, J.L.; Chao, C.H.; Yamaguchi, H.; Yang, N.K.; Ding, Q.; et al. Epithelial–mesenchymal transition induced by TNF-alpha requires NF-kappaB-mediated transcriptional upregulation of Twist1. *Cancer Res.* **2012**, *72*, 1290–1300. [CrossRef]
94. Marcucci, F.; Stassi, G.; De Maria, R. Epithelial–mesenchymal transition: a new target in anticancer drug discovery. *Nat. Rev. Drug Discov.* **2016**, *15*, 311–325. [CrossRef]
95. Ohshima, K.; Hatakeyama, K.; Nagashima, T.; Watanabe, Y.; Kanto, K.; Doi, Y.; Ide, T.; Shimoda, Y.; Tanabe, T.; Ohnami, S.; et al. Integrated analysis of gene expression and copy number identified potential cancer driver genes with amplification-dependent overexpression in 1,454 solid tumors. *Sci. Rep.* **2017**, *7*, 1546. [CrossRef]
96. Hurt, E.M.; Kawasaki, B.T.; Klarmann, G.J.; Thomas, S.B.; Farrar, W.L. CD44+ CD24− prostate cells are early cancer progenitor/stem cells that provide a model for patients with poor prognosis. *Br. J. Cancer* **2008**, *98*, 756–765. [CrossRef]
97. Klonisch, T.; Wiechec, E.; Hombach-Klonisch, S.; Ande, S.R.; Wesselborg, S.; Schulze-Osthoff, K.; Los, M. Cancer stem cell markers in common cancers—Therapeutic implications. *Trends Mol. Med.* **2008**, *14*, 450–460. [CrossRef]
98. Li, W.; Ma, H.; Zhang, J.; Zhu, L.; Wang, C.; Yang, Y. Unraveling the roles of CD44/CD24 and ALDH1 as cancer stem cell markers in tumorigenesis and metastasis. *Sci. Rep.* **2017**, *7*, 13856. [CrossRef]
99. Fillmore, C.M.; Kuperwasser, C. Human breast cancer cell lines contain stem-like cells that self-renew, give rise to phenotypically diverse progeny and survive chemotherapy. *Breast Cancer Res.* **2008**, *10*, R25. [CrossRef]

100. Bane, A.; Viloria-Petit, A.; Pinnaduwage, D.; Mulligan, A.M.; O'Malley, F.P.; Andrulis, I.L. Clinical–pathologic significance of cancer stem cell marker expression in familial breast cancers. *Breast Cancer Res. Treat.* **2013**, *140*, 195–205. [CrossRef]
101. Jaggupilli, A.; Elkord, E. Significance of CD44 and CD24 as Cancer Stem Cell Markers: An Enduring Ambiguity. *Clin. Dev. Immunol.* **2012**, *2012*, 1–11. [CrossRef]
102. Jones, N.P.; Schulze, A. Targeting cancer metabolism—Aiming at a tumour's sweet-spot. *Drug Discov. Today* **2012**, *17*, 232–241. [CrossRef]
103. Heiden, M.G.V. Targeting cancer metabolism: a therapeutic window opens. *Nat. Rev. Drug Discov.* **2011**, *10*, 671–684. [CrossRef]
104. Meijer, T.W.; Peeters, W.J.; Dubois, L.J.; Van Gisbergen, M.W.; Biemans, R.; Venhuizen, J.-H.; Span, P.N.; Bussink, J. Targeting glucose and glutamine metabolism combined with radiation therapy in non-small cell lung cancer. *Lung Cancer* **2018**, *126*, 32–40. [CrossRef]
105. Chao, T.-K.; Huang, T.-S.; Liao, Y.-P.; Huang, R.-L.; Su, P.-H.; Shen, H.-Y.; Lai, H.-C.; Wang, Y.-C. Pyruvate kinase M2 is a poor prognostic marker of and a therapeutic target in ovarian cancer. *PLoS ONE* **2017**, *12*, e0182166. [CrossRef]
106. Shackelford, D.B.; Abt, E.; Gerken, L.; Vasquez, D.S.; Seki, A.; Leblanc, M.; Wei, L.; Fishbein, M.C.; Czernin, J.; Mischel, P.S.; et al. LKB1 inactivation dictates therapeutic response of non-small cell lung cancer to the metabolism drug phenformin. *Cancer Cell* **2013**, *23*, 143–158. [CrossRef]
107. Hardie, R.-A.; Van Dam, E.; Cowley, M.; Han, T.-L.; Balaban, S.; Pajic, M.; Pinese, M.; Iconomou, M.; Shearer, R.F.; McKenna, J.; et al. Mitochondrial mutations and metabolic adaptation in pancreatic cancer. *Cancer Metab.* **2017**, *5*, 7. [CrossRef]
108. Pelicano, H.; Zhang, W.; Liu, J.; Hammoudi, N.; Dai, J.; Xu, R.-H.; Pusztai, L.; Huang, P. Mitochondrial dysfunction in some triple-negative breast cancer cell lines: role of mTOR pathway and therapeutic potential. *Breast Cancer Res.* **2014**, *16*, 434. [CrossRef]

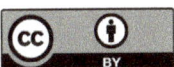

© 2019 by the authors. Licensee MDPI, Basel, Switzerland. This article is an open access article distributed under the terms and conditions of the Creative Commons Attribution (CC BY) license (http://creativecommons.org/licenses/by/4.0/).

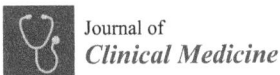 

Article

# Deciphering Hydrodynamic and Drug-Resistant Behaviors of Metastatic EMT Breast Cancer Cells Moving in a Constricted Microcapillary

**Binita Nath [1,†], Anil P. Bidkar [2,†], Vikash Kumar [1], Amaresh Dalal [1], Mohit Kumar Jolly [3], Siddhartha S. Ghosh [2] and Gautam Biswas [1,4,*]**

1. Department of Mechanical Engineering, Indian Institute of Technology Guwahati, Guwahati 781 039, India
2. Department of Biosciences and Bioengineering, Indian Institute of Technology Guwahati, Guwahati 781 039, India
3. Centre for BioSystems Science and Engineering, Indian Institute of Science Bangalore, Bangalore 560 012, India
4. Department of Mechanical Engineering, Indian Institute of Technology Kanpur, Kanpur 208 016, India
* Correspondence: gtm@iitg.ac.in; Tel.: +91-512-259-7656
† The authors contributed equally to this article.

Received: 5 July 2019; Accepted: 7 August 2019; Published: 9 August 2019

**Abstract:** Epithelial to mesenchymal transition (EMT) induces cell migration, invasion, and drug resistance, and consequently, contributes to cancer metastasis and disease aggressiveness. This study attempted to address crucial biological parameters to correlate EMT and drug-treated cancer cells traversing through microcapillaries, reminiscent of metastatic conditions. MDA-MB-468 breast cancer cells induced to undergo EMT by treatment with 20 ng/mL of epidermal growth factor (EGF) were initially passed through several blockages and then through a constricted microchannel, mimicking the flow of invasive metastatic cells through constricted blood microcapillaries. EMT cells acquired enhanced migratory properties and retained 50% viability, even after migration through wells 10–15 µm in size and a constricted passage of 7 µm and 150 µm in length at a constant flow rate of 50 µL/h. The hydrodynamic properties revealed cellular deformation with a deformation index, average transit velocity, and entry time of 2.45, 12.3 mm/s, and 31,000 µs, respectively for a cell of average diameter 19 µm passing through one of the 7 µm constricted sections. Interestingly, cells collected at the channel outlet regained epithelial character, undergoing reverse transition (mesenchymal to epithelial transition, MET) in the absence of EGF. Remarkably, real-time polymerase chain reaction (PCR) analysis confirmed increases of 2- and 2.7-fold in the vimentin and fibronectin expression in EMT cells, respectively; however, their expression reduced to basal level in the MET cells. A scratch assay revealed the pronounced migratory nature of EMT cells compared with MET cells. Furthermore, the number of colonies formed from EMT cells and paclitaxel-treated EMT cells after passing through a constriction were found to be 95 ± 10 and 79 ± 4, respectively, confirming that the EMT cells were more drug resistant with a concomitant two-fold higher expression of the multi-drug resistance (MDR1) gene. Our results highlight the hydrodynamic and drug-evading properties of cells that have undergone an EMT, when passed through a constricted microcapillary that mimics their journey in blood circulation.

**Keywords:** metastasis; constricted microchannel; hydrodynamic parameters; breast cancer cells; epithelial to mesenchymal transition; EMT; mesenchymal to epithelial transition; MET; cell viability

## 1. Introduction

Epithelial to mesenchymal transition (EMT) is a physiological phenotypic shift of epithelial to mesenchymal cells, where the breakdown of cell–cell and cell–extracellular matrix connections permits the migration of cells to distant locations [1]. The role of EMT is well documented in normal embryonic development, tissue regeneration, organ fibrosis, and wound healing [2]. Furthermore, EMT is involved in tumor progression with metastatic expansion and the generation of tumor cells with stem cell properties that play a major role in resistance to cancer treatment. Although mesenchymal cells possess increased migratory capacity, invasiveness, and greater resistance to apoptosis [3], the dynamics of EMT during invasion are yet to be fully elucidated to resolve the mystery of cancer metastasis. On the other hand, the reverse transition, i.e., mesenchymal to epithelial transition (MET), is attributed to the migrating mesenchymal cells once they reach their destination [4]. MET is thought to be crucial for the colonization of a metastatic niche by disseminated tumor cells. EMT and MET are not binary phenomena, and tumor cells can be in multiple hybrid states and express both epithelial and mesenchymal genes [5,6]. Such hybrid cells can move collectively as clusters and may be stem-like and metastatic compared with cells with a complete EMT phenotype [7,8]. Experimentally, EMT can be induced by adding growth factors such as epidermal growth factor (EGF), transforming growth factor beta (TGF-β), and hepatocyte growth factor (HGF); EGF and TGF-β induce EMT via Smad2/3 and ERK1/2 pathways [9,10]. Various processes are involved in initiating an EMT, including activation of transcription factor, expression of specific cell-surface proteins, re-formation and expression of cytoskeletal proteins, creation of extracellular matrix (ECM)-degrading enzymes, and changes in the expression of specific microRNAs [11]. The epithelial cells that undergo EMT and invade the bloodstream from the primary site often display alterations in gene expression and lose some epithelial characteristics, such as apical–basal polarity [12]. Important characteristics of EMT include downregulation of epithelial markers including E-cadherin, occludin, and claudin. Contrarily, increases in the levels of mesenchymal markers such as N-cadherin, vimentin, and fibronectin have been associated with EMT. The expression pattern of these genes can be tracked to study the behavior of the cells while transitioning from epithelial to mesenchymal or vice versa.

In most previous studies, the morphology and characteristics of cells undergoing EMT and MET have been studied under static conditions [13,14]. Hence, the physiological conditions in which the EMT cells traverse through the blood vessels or microcapillaries and undergo reverse transition at the secondary site are a very important area of investigation. An attempt to find the percentage viability and metastatic potency of the EMT cells after transiting through microcapillaries would reveal important information that could address many of the questions related to the complex phenomenon of cancer metastasis. Moreover, a detailed investigation of the treatment of cancer cells with drugs at different stages of their flow from the primary site to a secondary site undergoing EMT to MET transitions (through the capillaries) would be crucial for designing future theranostic devices aiming at curative or palliative treatment. Hence the dynamics of the motion, deformation, and behavioral changes of EMT cancer cells passing through microcapillaries still seem to be underexplored and require further attention.

In this work, we attempted to address some of the questions related to the motion of EMT cancer cells through microcapillaries. For this purpose, a 2.85 mm long microchannel was fabricated using polydimethylsiloxane (PDMS), with an overall width of 184 µm. At a distance of 700 µm from the inlet, four 30 µm square blockages were inserted, varying the gap between the blockages in the range 10–15 µm. This complex configuration of the blocks and gaps helped us to mimic the broken basement membrane via which cancer cells invade the blood capillaries. Further, at a distance of 1000 µm from the blockages, a network of constricted channels each of width 7 µm, which mimic the blood microcapillaries, were introduced. The motion of the EMT cells through this complex network allowed the investigation of some hydrodynamic parameters along with some crucial biological assays. The deformation index, entry time, and transit velocity of the cells at different stages provide an understanding of the behavior of cells in microcapillaries. The EMT cells at the inlet, and the cells that were collected from the outlet and regrown (MET), were examined by analyzing several protein expressions, real-time polymerase chain reaction (PCR) analysis, and flow cytometric analysis. The viability of the cells was calculated using dye staining assays. A comparison between the migrating ability of EMT cells and epithelial cells was made by performing a scratch assay. Moreover, the metastatic potency of the EMT cells passing through the constricted channel was observed by performing colony formation assays. Whereas paclitaxel treatment resulted in decreased viability ($IC_{50}$ = 98 nM) and colony formation ability of epithelial cells, paclitaxel-treated EMT cells showed a lower response to drug treatment. Furthermore, a thorough investigation to identify the effectiveness of drug treatment during various stages of cancer cell flow through microcapillaries was undertaken, which may prove very beneficial for scientists, oncologists, and cancer therapeutics. Figure 1 shows a graphical representation of the objectives of the present study.

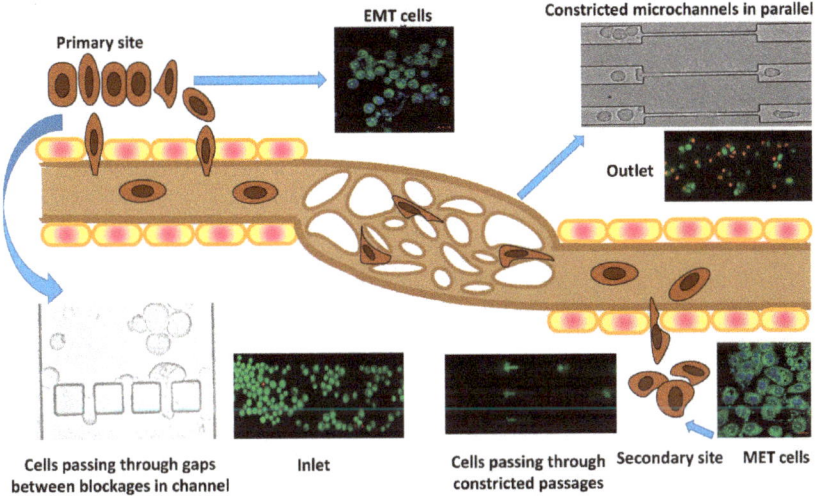

**Figure 1.** Schematic representation of the motion of metastatic cancer cells from the primary site to a distant secondary site through microcapillaries.

## 2. Experimental Section

### 2.1. Cell Culture

Breast cancer (MDA-MB-468) cells were obtained from National Centre for Cell Science, Pune, India. These cells were maintained in a $CO_2$ incubator (5% $CO_2$) with humidified air. Cells were cultured in DMEM (Dulbecco's modified Eagle's medium) containing 10% FBS (fetal bovine serum) and antibiotic solution (penicillin and streptomycin). MTT (3-(4,5-dimethylthiazol-2-yl)-2,5-diphenyltetrazolium bromide), hEGF (human epidermal growth factor), and a GenElute Mammalian Total RNA Miniprep Kit were purchased from Sigma Aldrich. A cDNA synthesis kit and the cyanine dye SYBR Green were purchased from BioRad Laboratories. Alexafluor 488-tagged anti-vimentin antibody was obtained from Abcam.

### 2.2. EMT Induction in MDA-MB-468 Cells

Nearly confluent MDA-MB-468 cells were washed with phosphate-buffered saline (PBS), trypsinized, and counted in a Countess cell counter (Thermo Fisher Scientific). Cells were seeded in a six-well plate at a density of $2 \times 10^5$ cells per well in 2 mL of medium (10% FBS). The six-well plates were incubated in a $CO_2$ incubator for 24 h for complete attachment of the MDA-MB-468 cells. After 24 h, the medium in each well was replaced with a serum-free medium and the cells were again incubated for 12 h. Subsequently, the cells were treated with EGF at 10, 20, and 40 ng/mL in a serum-free medium. The morphology of the untreated and EGF-treated cells was monitored and images were captured in a microscope (Nikon Eclipse Ti-U). These EGF treated cells (MDA-MB-468 cells) are henceforth referred to as EMT cells.

## 2.3. Fabrication of Microchannels

An Su8 master silicon wafer was prepared in the CeNSE Department of IISc Bangalore, India, having imprints for 12 channels in the single master. All the channels were fabricated based on the design shown in Figure 2A. PDMS solution was prepared by mixing SYLGARD 184 silicone elastomer with a cross-linker in a ratio of 10:1. A nylon ring of inner diameter equal to the width of the Su8 master was used to make the mold. PDMS solution was poured over the Su8 master bounded by the nylon ring. Upon solidification of the PDMS layer, it was gently peeled off and individual channels were cut out using a surgical blade. The inlet and outlet were punched out using a punching tool. The open channels were then sealed by placing them over a glass slide after treatment with oxygen plasma.

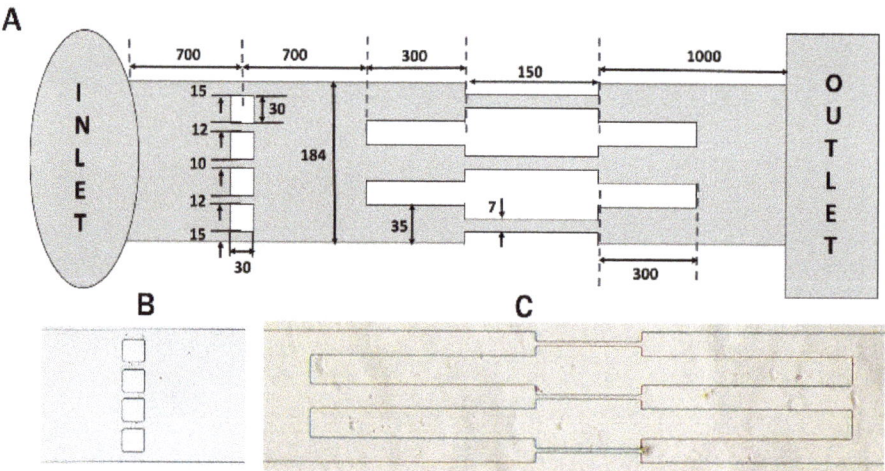

**Figure 2.** Design of the microchannel. (**A**) Schematic representation of the microchannel (not to scale); (**B**) magnified view of the 30 µm blockages; (**C**) magnified view of the series of constricted channels. All dimensions in µm.

## 2.4. Experimental Setup

Semi-rigid polyethylene tubing of outer diameter 1.09 mm and inner diameter 0.38 mm (Prolab Marketing, New Delhi, India) was connected to the inlet and outlet of the microchannel. The cells suspended in DMEM were filled into a syringe from an Eppendorf tube and the syringe was fitted in a syringe pump. The microscope and pump were connected to a power source. With activation of the syringe pump, the cells and the suspending medium started to fill the connecting tube and flow through the microchannel. In general, the average velocity of blood (usually measured in cm/s) varies from 0.03 to 40 cm/s as the blood flows through the vena cava, capillaries, and aorta [15]. The cells suspended in the medium were allowed to flow pass at a constant flow rate of 50 µL/h. The motion of the cells were observed and recorded at a high frame rate of 30,000–50,000 fps using the video module of Phantom PCC 2.8 software, manufactured by Vision Research (Wayne, NJ, USA). The videos were then deconvoluted to obtain images at required time instants. The supplementary videos are shown at a reduced speed of 200 fps for clarity.

## 2.5. Flow Cytometry for Vimentin Expression

MDA-MB-468 cells were seeded in a six-well plate at a density of $2 \times 10^5$ cells per well. After EMT induction, the cells were washed with PBS, trypsinized, and collected in 1.5 mL tubes. The cells were fixed with 1 mL of formaldehyde (4% in PBS) at room temperature for 15 min. Thereafter, the cells were centrifuged and washed with PBS. Subsequently, permeabilization of the cell membranes was achieved by adding chilled methanol (90%) on ice. After 30 min of incubation on ice, the cells were centrifuged and washed with PBS. Alexafluor 488-tagged anti-vimentin antibody was added to the cells in 4% bovine serum albumin (BSA) solution, and then the cells were incubated for 30 min in the dark. Subsequently, the cells were washed with ice-cold PBS, resuspended in PBS, and analyzed immediately in a flow cytometer (Cytoflex, Beckman Coulter, Indianapolis, IN, USA).

## 2.6. Real-time Polymerase Chain Reaction (RT-PCR)

Vimentin and fibronectin are two important markers for mesenchymal transitions. The expression of vimentin and fibronectin was examined using quantitative real-time PCR (qPCR) for MDA-MB-468, EMT, and MET cells. The cells were collected at different stages of the experimental procedure, such as at the inlet and outlet of the microchannel. For obtaining MET cells, the EMT cells that passed through the channel were collected at the outlet and regrown. The cells were then lysed and total RNA was isolated using an RNA isolation kit. Total RNA (1 µg) was then used to prepare cDNA using a cDNA synthesis kit. qPCR was performed using the primers for vimentin, fibronectin, MDR1 (ABCB1), and GAPDH (Table S1, Supplementary Information). SYBR Green was used as a reporter dye in a Rotor-Gene Q (Qiagen) instrument. The relative expressions of vimentin and fibronectin were calculated by the $\Delta\Delta C_t$ method using glyceraldehyde-3-phosphate dehydrogenase (GAPDH) as the endogenous control.

## 2.7. Dual Staining

Trypan blue dye is used to stain membrane-compromised or dead cells, whereas live cells exclude the dye. MDA-MB-468 cells were seeded in a 60 mm cell culture dish in the presence of DMEM and treated with 20 ng/mL of EGF for 24 h. The EMT cells were then washed with PBS, trypsinized, and suspended in DMEM in an Eppendorf tube. Equal volumes of trypan blue dye (10 µL) and the cells were mixed and loaded in the counting chamber. The viable cells (%) were counted using a Countess automated cell counter (Invitrogen). The images highlighting the live and dead cells were also captured using the same instrument. The viability results represented data of triplicate experiments. Acridine orange and ethidium bromide (AO/EtBr) staining was performed to study the viability of the cells passing through the constricted microchannel at four different locations, i.e., at the inlet (1st), while the cells flow through the blockages (2nd), followed by the 7 µm constricted microchannels (3rd), and at the outlet (4th). Briefly, EGF-treated cells were stained with a mixture of AO (100 µg/mL) and EtBr (100 µg/mL) in DMEM for 15 min. After washing with PBS, the cells were trypsinized, mixed with AO/EtBr solution, and passed through the microchannel. When the cells had reached the outlet, the flow pump was stopped and images of the cells at the above-mentioned sites were captured using a Nikon Eclipse Ti-U microscope.

## 2.8. Confocal Imaging to Study the Morphology of Induced EMT Cells

Briefly, $2 \times 10^5$ cells were seeded in a 35 mm dish fitted with a coverslip. After attachment, the serum-free medium was added. The cells were treated with 20 ng/mL of EGF for 24 h, then calcein-AM staining was performed. Subsequently, the cells were fixed with 4% formaldehyde and the nuclei were stained with DAPI (4′,6-diamidino-2-phenylindole). Images were obtained in the confocal microscope.

## 2.9. Scratch Assay for Invasion Study

A scratch assay is generally used to observe interactions and migrations among cells. A scratch is marked on a monolayer of cells and subsequent cell migration is captured microscopically at regular time intervals. For this assay, MDA-MB-468 (parental) EMT cells were seeded on 35 mm Petri dishes, whereas EMT cells were treated with 20 ng/mL hEGF. These culture dishes were then scratched with a sterile pipette tip to create a 'wound' in the respective dishes. Cell debris was removed by washing with PBS and the plates were kept in an incubator at 37 °C under humidified conditions with 5% $CO_2$ for 48 h. The images of the fresh wounds, and also the healing of the wounds, were examined under a Nikon Eclipse Ti-U microscope at 24 and 48 h, respectively, and the corresponding images were examined to differentiate their migration ability.

### 2.10. Cell Viability Assay

To study the viability of the paclitaxel-treated cells, MTT assays were carried out. MDA-MB-468 cells were seeded in a 96-well plate at a density of 5000 cells per well, then the cells were treated with different concentrations of paclitaxel (0–200 nM) for 48 h. After completion of the treatment, the cells were incubated with MTT solution (0.25 µg/mL) in PBS for 2 h. Finally, the MTT solution was aspirated and 150 µL of dimethyl sulfoxide (DMSO) were added to each well. The absorbance of MTT was recorded in a multiplate reader at 570 nm. The cell viability of the treated samples was calculated assuming 100% viability in untreated wells. The results were represented accumulating data from three sets of experiments.

### 2.11. Colony Formation Assay

The colony formation study was performed to investigate whether the EMT cells retained their metastatic ability after passing through the channel. The experiment was designed in such a way that we could compare the number of colonies of the epithelial, EMT, and MET cells along with their paclitaxel-treated counterparts. Epithelial and MET cells were treated with 100 nM paclitaxel for 48 h and a total of 200 cells were seeded for colony formation. In the case of EMT and paclitaxel-treated (EMT + PTX) cells, the cells were treated with EGF or EGF + 100 nM paclitaxel, respectively, for 48 h. After completion of the treatment, the cells were passed through the channel and collected in an Eppendorf tube. The collected cells were counted and dispersed in DMEM in a 12-well plate at a density of 200 cells per well. The plates were incubated for 10 days at 37 °C in an incubator, then the grown colonies of the cells in each well were fixed with 100% methanol and stained with crystal violet. The colonies from each well were counted at 10× magnification under a bright-field microscope (Nikon Eclipse Ti-U, Tokyo, Japan). The results were accumulated based on triplicate experiments.

## 3. Results

### 3.1. Experimental Setup

The basic layout of the microchannel is shown in Figure 2A. The channel was 2.85 mm long between the inlet and outlet sections and its width was 184 µm. At a distance of 700 µm from the inlet, four square blockages of width 30 µm were present. The blockages were unequally spaced along the width of the channel, creating unequal gaps. The gap between the walls of the channel and the first blockage, from either side was 15 µm and the next two blockages were at a distance of 12 µm from the first blockage, leaving a gap of 10 µm between the two center blockages.

At a distance of 700 µm from the blockages, the channel diverged into three parallel channels of width 35 µm and length 300 µm, each of which further reduced to constricted microchannels of width 7 µm and length 150 µm. The channel outlet was at a distance of 1 mm from the constricted channels. Magnified views of the blockage section and the constricted channel section are shown in Figure 2B,C, respectively. The motion of the cells through the blockage section represented their invasiveness through the network of several capillaries. The locomotion of the cells through the entire channel (from inlet to outlet) has been shown in Supplementary video S1.

### 3.2. EGF Induced EMT Transition in MDA-MB-468 Cells

EGF induced EMT transition of MDA-MB-468 cells can be monitored by overexpression of the vimentin and N-cadherin that helps in the migration of EMT cells [16,17]. In our experiments, we used

EGF to induce EMT to mimic the in vivo conditions. To study the amount of EGF required to convert cells to the mesenchymal state, MDA-MB-468 cells were treated with 10, 20, and 40 ng/mL EGF. After treatment for 24 h, the cells were observed under a microscope for morphological changes. It was observed that untreated cells were in tight contact with each other, but after EGF treatment the cells became rounded losing their contacts (Figure 3A,D). After confirming the morphological changes, a flow cytometric assay was performed to study vimentin expression (for details, see the Experimental section). The cells showed increased expression of vimentin when treated with EGF at 10, 20, and 40 ng/mL (Figure 3B), confirming an EMT. In addition, the viability of these EGF-treated cells was studied using trypan blue staining. From microscopic observations, it was found that cell death was higher in the case of 40 ng/mL EGF treatment.

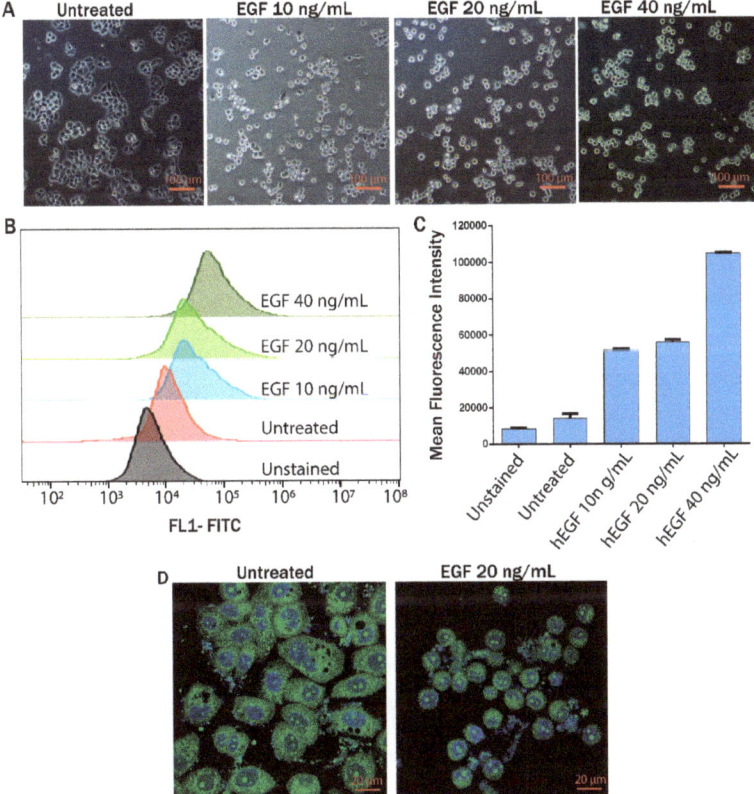

**Figure 3.** Epithelial to mesenchymal transition (EMT) induction in MDA-MB-468 cells. (**A**) Changes in the morphology of cells treated with increasing concentrations of epidermal growth factor (EGF); (**B,C**) histograms from flow cytometry for vimentin expression (**B**), with corresponding mean fluorescence intensity shown in a bar plot (**C**); (**D**) alteration in the cytoplasmic and nuclear morphology studied by calcein-AM DAPI (4′,6-diamidino-2-phenylindole) staining.

Therefore, although the maximum vimentin expression was observed at 40 ng/mL EGF, we chose 20 ng/mL of EGF for further experiments. Wound healing assays revealed a greater migratory ability of EMT cells than the untreated cells (referred to as 'epithelial cells') (Figure S1).

## 3.3. Flow Dynamics of EMT Cells

Figure 4 shows the flow dynamics of the EMT cells when they pass through the gaps of various sizes between the 30 µm blockages. Figure 4A illustrates the various time instants recorded during the experiments while the cells passed through any gap. Time $t_1$ was taken at the instant when the cell was just about to enter the gap (the cell front touches the entry line). This was followed by time $t_2$, which is the instant when the entire cell had entered the gap (the rear of the cell touched the entry line). Finally, we recorded time $t_3$ when the cell was about to exit from the gap (the front of the cell touched the exit line). Based on the values of $t_1$, $t_2$, and $t_3$, the deformation index, entry time, and transit velocity of the cell, while moving through the gaps, were calculated.

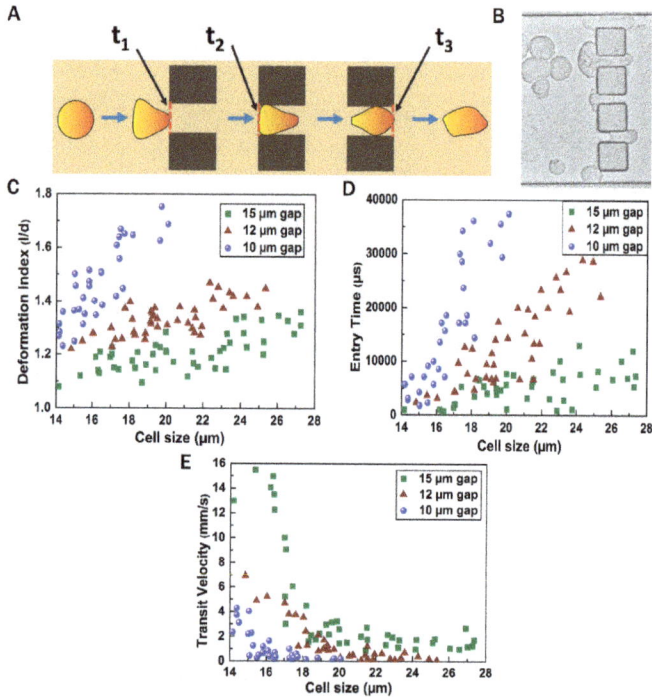

**Figure 4.** Flow dynamics of cells through blockages. (**A**) Stepwise motion of the cell through a blockage; (**B**) microscopic view of invasion of cells through the gaps between blockages (**C–E**) deformation index, entry time, and transit velocity of the cells through the gaps of varying sizes between blockages, respectively.

A microscopic image of the cells passing through the gaps between the blockages is shown in Figure 4B. Figure 4C shows the deformation index of the cells while passing through the gaps. The cell sizes varied in the range of 14–28 µm diameter and the gap sizes varied as 10, 12, and 15 µm. Figure 4D shows the entry time required for the cells of different sizes to enter the gap, and the velocity with which the cells transit through the gaps has been shown in Figure 4E. It was observed that through the 10 µm gap, comparatively smaller cells (size less than ~20 µm) tended to pass through and, owing to increased confinement, the deformation index and entry time of the cells passing through the 10 µm gap were very high compared with the 12 and 15 µm gaps. The gaps of 12 and 15 µm allowed more cells to pass through. For any particular cell size, the deformation index and entry time were minimum, and the transit velocity was maximum in the 15 µm gap. Supplementary video S2 depicts the motion of the EMT cells through the gaps between the blockages in the channel. It was observed that a cell of diameter 20 µm (approx) exhibited deformation index of 1.69, 1.31, and 1.21 with the corresponding entry time of 37,428, 14,334, and 7667 µs, and possessed transit velocity of 0.227, 0.326, and 1.47 mm/s, while traversing through the 10, 12, and 15 µm gap, respectively.

As mentioned earlier (Figure 2), each of the three constricted passages were of equal length (150 µm) and width (7 µm). Figure 5 shows the flow dynamics of the cells through the constricted 7 µm microchannels. Time instants $t_4$, $t_5$, and $t_6$ were observed when a cell passed through any of the constricted paths. As shown in Figure 5A, $t_4$ is the time instant when the cell front touched the entry point in any channel, $t_5$ is the time instant when the entire cell has just entered the constricted passage and its rear touched the entry point, and $t_6$ is the time instant when the deformed cell's front touched the exit point. The entry time was calculated by subtracting $t_4$ from $t_5$. The ratio of the maximum elongation length ($l$) to the undeformed cell diameter ($d$) was calculated as the deformation index. The average transit velocity was obtained by dividing the distance travelled (150 µm) by the time taken ($t_6-t_4$). A microscopic view of the cells flowing through the constricted channels is shown in Figure 5B. Figure 5C shows the deformation index of the cells through the constricted 150 µm long passage. The cell sizes varied in the range of 14–28 µm. It was observed that the large cells underwent enhanced elongation compared with small cells. The transit velocity and entry time of the cells are shown in Figure 5D,E, respectively. It is noted that large cells took more time to accommodate themselves inside the constricted passage, exhibiting an enhanced entry time and a lower transit velocity.

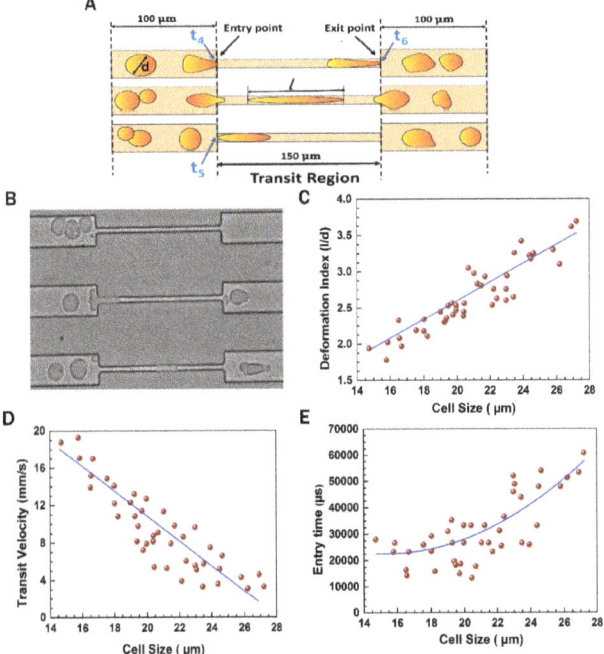

**Figure 5.** Flow dynamics of cells through a constricted 7 µm channel. (**A**) Stepwise motion of the cells through the constricted channel; (**B**) microscopic image of cells passing through constricted microchannel; (**C–E**) deformation index, entry time, and transit velocity of the cells through the 7 µm constricted passage, respectively.

A typical cell of size 19 µm diameter showed a deformation index of 2.45, transit velocity of 12.3 mm/s, and entry time of 31,000 µs, while moving through one of the constricted sections of the channel. The blue lines in the plots depict the general trend of the nature of the cells. These are the best fitted curves obtained from the data points in the graph. Supplementary video S3 depicts the motion of the cancer cells through the constricted microchannels.

### 3.4. Epithelial to Mesenchymal and Mesenchymal to Epithelial Transitions

Epithelial cells possess tight contacts with neighboring cells, and thus express proteins required for adherence (E-cadherin, occludin), whereas EMT-transformed cells become loosely attached, gaining migratory properties. In our experiments, we used vimentin as a standard EMT marker to confirm the epithelial or mesenchymal status of the cells [18]. The presence of EMT in MDA-MB-468 cells, and also the viability of the cells at the outlet, can be used to study the behavior of these cells in blood vessels.

EMT was induced in presence of EGF. However, in the absence of EGF during movement, downregulation of vimentin and fibronectin were observed in the cells collected at the outlet, which defines possible reverse transition to MET. Therefore, EMT-induced cells were collected at the outlet of the microchannel (referred to as MET cells) and studied for possible MET characteristics. From gene expression studies (Figure 6), it was confirmed that EGF-treated cells showed a 2.7–fold higher expression of vimentin protein compared with untreated epithelial cells, confirming the epithelial to mesenchymal transition of MDA-MB-468 cells. Similarly, fibronectin expression also increased two-fold (Figure 6A) [12]. These events are similar to those that occur at the primary site of the tumor, where the expression of the epithelial marker decreases and mesenchymal marker protein expression increases simultaneously during EMT [19]. We isolated these mesenchymal cells and passed them through the microchannel, which mimicked the entry and movement of the mesenchymal cells in blood vessels. In general, when the mesenchymal cells reach the bloodstream, they travel to different parts of the body and start to be converted into the epithelial state. Hence, in our experiments, cells passing through the microchannel were collected at the outlet and were grown to study their MET characteristics. Surprisingly, vimentin and fibronectin expression reached its basal level as in epithelial cells, confirming the complete mesenchymal to epithelial transition.

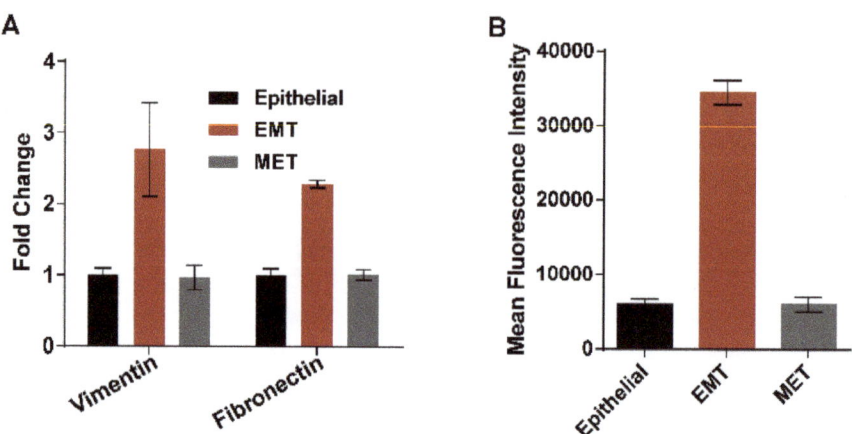

**Figure 6.** Gene expression studies by real-time PCR and flow cytometry. (**A**) Comparison of expression of vimentin and fibronectin genes in epithelial, EMT, and mesenchymal to epithelial transition (MET) cells; (**B**) vimentin expression studied at the protein level using anti-vimentin antibody in flow cytometry.

### 3.5. Viability of EMT Cells

As mentioned previously, the microchannel consisted of several obstructions, and the cells passing through the channel underwent deformation and pronounced morphological changes, decreasing the percentage of viable cells at the outlet [20]. Mesenchymal transformed MDA-MB-468 cells were collected by trypsinization before starting the experiment. The fluorescent images in Figure 3D confirmed the membrane integrity of EMT cells. For studying the viability, we performed AO/EtBr staining. Figure 7A shows the qualitative images of the cells at different sections of the channel. At the inlet, all of the cells were evenly stained with AO, with a few red dots indicating EtBr fluorescence due to dead cells. On passing the gaps of 10, 12, and 15 µm (between blockages), the cells were observed to be mostly alive. However, once the cells had passed through the 7 µm constriction and reached the outlet, almost 50% of the cells took up EtBr, confirming cell death. Similar events resulting in cell apoptosis have been observed during migration and invasion through blood capillaries smaller than their own diameter [21,22]. Quantitative estimation of the cell death during the flow was estimated by trypan blue staining, which further confirmed the presence of live cells at the outlet of the channel. Figure 7B indicates that around 50% of the cells were alive at the outlet.

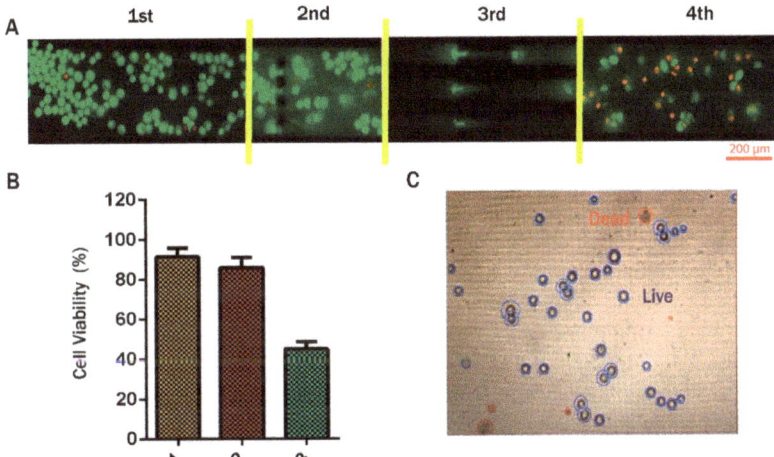

**Figure 7.** Cell viability assessment. (**A**) Acridine orange and ethidium bromide (AO/EtBr)-stained images at different sections of the channel; (**B**) comparison of the percentage of EMT cells viable after passing through the constriction with the initial conditions and with cells maintained in the same environment for the same period of time but not passed through the constriction. Cell condition 1 refers to the initial EMT cells, cell condition 2 refers to mock experimental control EMT cells kept in the same environment without passing through the channel, and cell condition 3 refers to the cells collected from the outlet of the microchannel; (**C**) image of stained cells obtained from the Countess automated cell counter.

### 3.6. Clonogenicity of EMT Cells

The ability of a single cell to grow and form colonies was studied by clonogenic or colony formation assay. Initially, MDA-MB-468 (epithelial) cells were treated with different concentrations of paclitaxel (PTX) to study the antiproliferative properties of the PTX. From the MTT assay results for 48 h treatment (Figure 8A), it was observed that PTX was able to inhibit the proliferation of the cells in a dose-dependent manner and the $IC_{50}$ of the PTX was found to be 98 ± 4 nM. Next, epithelial, EMT, and MET cells were treated with PTX and an equal number of cells were seeded to form colonies. All the cells treated with EGF, i.e., EMT and EMT treated with PTX, were passed through the channel and seeded for colony formation. Epithelial and MET cells, and also their drug-treated counterparts, were not passed through the microchannel. It was observed from Figure 8B,C that a total of 150 ± 3 colonies were formed from untreated epithelial cells, whereas epithelial cells treated with PTX showed 78 ± 5 colonies, confirming the antiproliferative effect of the PTX. Surprisingly, the number of colonies formed in EMT cells induced by EGF was 95 ± 10, whereas EMT cells treated with PTX formed 79 ± 4 colonies. Similarly, untreated MET cells formed 131 ± 6 colonies, whereas

MET cells treated with PTX developed 80 ± 8 colonies. From the results, it was concluded that both epithelial and MET cells treated with PTX showed a decreased number of colonies due to the effect of the drug. In contrast, EMT cells treated with PTX did not show a significant reduction in colony formation. Early reports suggested that EMT cells become drug resistant by acquiring increased drug efflux pumps, leading to a smaller amount of the drug being available for therapeutic action inside the cells [23]. In this regard, we analyzed the expression of the MDR1 in the epithelial, EMT, and EMT cells. MDR1 protein forms drug efflux pumps in the cell membrane to avoid cell death from therapeutic drugs. The results of the real-time PCR analysis in Figure 8D show that the EMT cells possess 2-fold higher expression of the MDR1 as compared to epithelial cells. The expression remains similar for MET cells. Hence, the increased number of colonies in EMT cells after PTX treatment may be attributed to the acquired resistance of the EMT cells due to increased MDR1 expression. To the best of our knowledge, this is the first report in which the hydrodynamic behavior of EMT cells is correlated with drug-resistant metastatic phenomena of breast cancer cells.

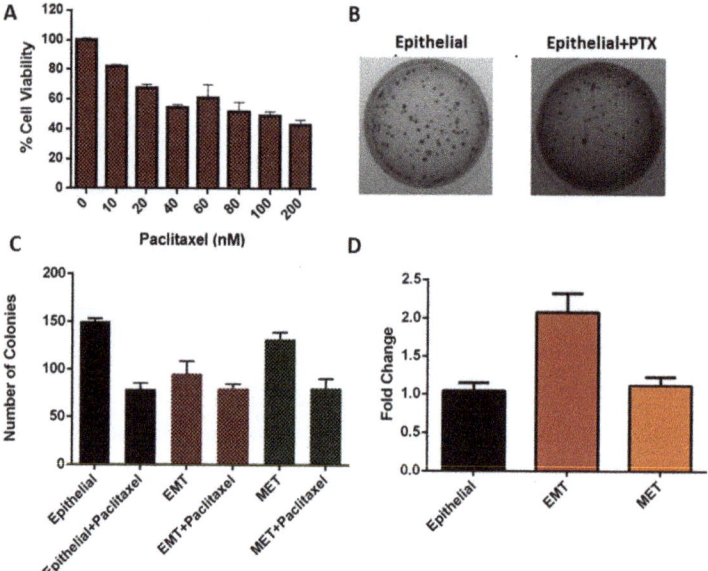

**Figure 8.** (**A**) MTT (3-(4,5-dimethylthiazol-2-yl)-2,5-diphenyltetrazolium bromide) assay results of the paclitaxel treatment of MDA-MB-468 cells for 48 h; (**B**) representative photograph of the colony formation assay of epithelial and drug-treated epithelial cells; (**C**) comparison of the number of colonies formed by the paclitaxel-treated epithelial, EMT, and MET cells with their respective controls; (**D**) real-time PCR assay results showing MDR-1 expression in epithelial, EMT, and MET cells.

## 4. Discussion

The motion of the cells through the blockage section of the microchannel represents invasive behavior of the cells through the basement membrane to enter the bloodstream. On the other hand, the motion of the cells through the constricted channels represents their motion through the network of blood capillaries. Our experimental design of microchannels and working protocols showed stepwise movements of EMT cells similar to that of in vivo metastatic cells (Figure 5). Starting from standardization of EGF dose (20 ng/mL), induction of EMT and susbsequent gene expression profiling of vimentin and fibronectin were perfomed systematically (Figures 3 and 6) before conducting the flow experiments. The scratch assays (Figure S1) supported the migratory ability of EGF induced EMT cells, as evident from other reports [24]. It is to be mentioned here that during the initial stages of

EMT, biochemical changes inside the cells cause alterations in the morphology of the cells, which was observed in Figure 3 [25]. Normally, epithelial cells are tightly attached to the basement membrane; however, during EMT, cells lose their contact with the attached surface and undergo migration and invasion. Both the migratory and invasive properties are associated with the expression of the genes from the signaling pathways involved. Certain epithelial marker proteins such as E-cadherin, claudin, and occludin are downregulated in the mesenchymal state, whereas mesenchymal markers (N-cadherin, vimentin, Snail) are upregulated [26]. Such alterations in vimentin and fibronectin expression confirmed EMT formation (Figure 6). Interestingly, these EMT cells passing through the gaps of various blockages and the constricted capillaries revealed some important hydrodynamic parameters, like deformaton index and transit velocities, as depicted in Figures 4 and 5. Such parameters are important to understand the ability of metastatic cells to move through several hindrances while reaching the distant secondary site from the primary origin. It is quite intriguing that the cells undergo deformation several times during such movement through microcapillaries. In reality, the cancer cells pass through several such hindrances (as demonstrated in Figures 4B and 5B) while moving from a primary site to reach a secondary site during metastasis. Such cancer cells get deformed on multiple occasions during their movement through a system of capillaries. Importantly, having been deformed some cells still remain viable for spreading cancer. Our experimental design has explained deformability and survival behavior of EMT while passing through several barriers and constricted portion of microchannel.

A significant population of EMT cells retained viability to spread cancer, as evident from the trypan blue staining experiment (Figure 7). When the disseminated mesenchymal cells reach a secondary site (site of metastases) by traversing the network of blood capillaries, they may undergo a reverse transition (MET) as metastases largely recapitulate an epithelial-like pathology similar to the corresponding primary tumor [27]. It is very important to understand that the environment faced by the cells at the secondary site completely differs from the cells at primary site. In our microchannel, we considered the outlet as a secondary site. This experimental design led us to analyze the morphology and properties of the cells collected from the outlet. The real-time PCR and flow cytometry results for vimentin and fibronectin expression described in Section 3.4 (Figure 6) have shown that the cells collected from outlet completely returned back to the epithelial state after incubation in a growth factor-free medium. As such, there was no evidence that some of the cells are residing at mesenchymal state. Similarly, the MDR-1 expression of the MET cells also reached the basal levels, indicating the complete mesenchymal to epithelial transition. The MTT assay provided the required drug concentration for treating cells in various transition phages. The $IC_{50}$ value of PTX treated MDA-MB-468 cells was obtained by this assay. The same dose of PTX was further used to treat EMT and MET cells (cells collected at the outlet). Finally, EMT alone, and EMT and MET treated with PTX separately, were compared for their colony formation abilities. Virulence of EMT with increased number of colonies and resistance to PTX treatment with high MDR1 expression (Figure 8) deciphered drug-resistant behavior of metastatic EMT cells passing through microchannel. The strength of our study is not only limited to movement of EMT cells mimicking in vivo conditions, but it also deciphers the drug resistant properties of EMT, as well as reverse transition phenotype, in terms of gene expressions.

## 5. Conclusions

This paper describes the flow of EMT cells in constricted microcapillaries while retaining their metastatic potential. The EMT induced MDA-MB-468 cells regained their epithelial nature with potential ability to grow and divide after passing through the microchannel traversing through several barriers. During such migration, the cells undergo deformation and transitions that were established experimentally. Higher expression of EMT markers such as vimentin and fibronectin and enhanced migratory ability of the cells, confirmed by the scratch assay, described their metastatic behaviors. While exhibiting metastasis, cells invade through surrounding tissue layers to enter the blood circulation. These aspects of the cell migration were studied in microchannels possessing barriers in the form of blockages and constricted passages to mimic in vivo conditions. In experimental setup, hydrodynamic properties of the moving EMT cells were evaluated, which revealed pronounced deformability of the cells. Surprisingly, the viable cells collected at the outlet were transformed into MET with the ability to form colonies, similar to a condition for formation of secondary tumor in metastasis. Further, the effect of a chemotherapeutic drug (paclitaxel) on the cells revealed higher expression of the multidrug resistance MDR-1 gene in EMT cells, which possibly enhanced their drug resistance, than epithelial and MET cells. Our experimental findings provide insight into flow dynamics of EMT cells and their drug resistant behaviors during the progress of metastasis. The current information, resembling migration properties of metastatic cells through tissues and blood vessels in vivo, would be beneficial to devise therapeutic strategies in future.

**Supplementary Materials:** The following are available online at http://www.mdpi.com/2077-0383/8/8/1194/s1. Table S1: Primer sequences used for real-time PCR study. Figure S1: Wound healing assay results revealing migration of the EGF treated cells. Supplementary video S1 shows the flow of cells in the entire channel from the inlet to the outlet reservoir. Supplementary video S2 shows the motion of cells through the gaps between the blockages in the channel. Supplementary video S3 shows the motion of cells through the constricted passages in the channel.

**Author Contributions:** B.N. fabricated the channels; B.N. and A.P.B. performed the experiments, interpreted the data, prepared the figures, and the manuscript; V.K. assisted in videography of flow experiments and analyzing the data; A.D. provided scientific inputs on flow experiments; M.K.J. delivered critical inputs regarding cell transitions; S.S.G. monitored and discussed the experimental processes and results; G.B. conceptualized, mentored, and coordinated the whole project.

**Funding:** This research received no external funding.

**Acknowledgments:** The authors acknowledge financial support from the Department of Biotechnology Programme Support (BT/PR13560/COE/34/44/2015) and the Department of Biotechnology (BT/PR 25095/NER/95/1011/2017). Partial support of the Meity project No. 5(9)/2012-NANO (Vol. II) is also acknowledged. The authors are grateful to the Centre for Nanotechnology and Central Instruments Facility (CIF) and IIT Guwahati for providing instrument facilities. The authors gratefully acknowledge the generous help received from. Rudra Pratap and Prosenjit Sen of the Centre for Nano Science and Engineering, Indian Institute of Science, Bangalore, India. One of us (G.B.) expresses his gratitude for a J.C. Bose National Fellowship of DST, India.

**Conflicts of Interest:** The authors declare no conflict of interest.

## References

1. Yilmaz, M.; Christofori, G. EMT, the cytoskeleton, and cancer cell invasion. *Cancer Metastasis Rev.* **2009**, *28*, 15–33. [CrossRef] [PubMed]
2. Kim, D.; Xing, T.; Yang, Z.; Dudek, R.; Lu, Q.; Chen, Y.H. Epithelial mesenchymal transition in embryonic development, tissue repair and cancer: A comprehensive overview. *J. Clin. Med.* **2017**, *7*, 1. [CrossRef] [PubMed]
3. Kalluri, R.; Neilson, E.G. Epithelial-mesenchymal transition and its implications for fibrosis. *J. Clin. Investig.* **2003**, *112*, 1776–1784. [CrossRef] [PubMed]
4. Radisky, D.C.; LaBarge, M.A. Epithelial-mesenchymal transition and the stem cell phenotype. *Cell Stem Cell* **2008**, *2*, 511–512. [CrossRef] [PubMed]
5. Jolly, M.K.; Ware, K.E.; Gilja, S.; Somarelli, J.A.; Levine, H. EMT and MET: Necessary or permissive for metastasis? *Mol. Oncol.* **2017**, *11*, 755–769. [CrossRef] [PubMed]
6. Jolly, M.K.; Somarelli, J.A.; Sheth, M.; Biddle, A.; Tripathi, S.C.; Armstrong, A.J.; Hanash, S.M.; Bapat, S.A.; Rangarajan, A.; Levine, H. Hybrid epithelial/mesenchymal phenotypes promote metastasis and therapy resistance across carcinomas. *Pharmacol. Ther.* **2018**, *194*, 161–184. [CrossRef]
7. Kröger, C.; Afeyan, A.; Mraz, J.; Eaton, E.N.; Reinhardt, F.; Khodor, Y.L.; Thiru, P.; Bierie, B.; Ye, X.; Burge, C.B.; et al. Acquisition of a hybrid E/M state is essential for tumorigenicity of basal breast cancer cells. *Proc. Natl. Acad. Sci. USA* **2019**, *116*, 7353–7362. [CrossRef]
8. Pastushenko, I.; Blanpain, C. EMT transition states during tumor progression and metastasis. *Trends Cell Biol.* **2018**, *29*, 212–226. [CrossRef]
9. Wendt, M.K.; Allington, T.M.; Schiemann, W.P. Mechanisms of the epithelial–mesenchymal transition by TGF-β. *Future Oncol.* **2009**, *5*, 1145–1168. [CrossRef]

10. Kim, J.; Kong, J.; Chang, H.; Kim, H.; Kim, A. EGF induces epithelial-mesenchymal transition through phospho-Smad2/3-Snail signaling pathway in breast cancer cells. *Oncotarget* **2016**, *7*, 85021–85032. [CrossRef]
11. Kalluri, R.; Weinberg, R.A. The basics of epithelial-mesenchymal transition. *J. Clin. Investig.* **2010**, *120*, 1786. [CrossRef]
12. Thiery, J.P. Epithelial–mesenchymal transitions in tumour progression. *Nat. Rev. Cancer* **2002**, *2*, 442–454. [CrossRef] [PubMed]
13. Gregory, P.A.; Bracken, C.P.; Smith, E.; Bert, A.G.; Wright, J.A.; Roslan, S.; Morris, M.; Wyatt, L.; Farshid, G.; Lim, Y.Y.; et al. An autocrine TGF-β/ZEB/miR-200 signaling network regulates establishment and maintenance of epithelial-mesenchymal transition. *Mol. Boil. Cell* **2011**, *22*, 1686–1698. [CrossRef]
14. Stylianou, N.; Lehman, M.L.; Wang, C.; Fard, A.T.; Rockstroh, A.; Fazli, L.; Jovanovic, L.; Ward, M.; Sadowski, M.C.; Kashyap, A.S.; et al. A molecular portrait of epithelial–mesenchymal plasticity in prostate cancer associated with clinical outcome. *Oncogene* **2018**, *38*, 2436. [CrossRef] [PubMed]
15. Tortora, G.J.; Derrickson, B. The cardiovascular system: Blood vessels and hemodynamics. In *Principles of Anatomy and Physiology*, 9th ed.; John Wiley and Sons: Hoboken, NJ, USA, 2012; pp. 610–635.
16. Shih, W.; Yamada, S. N-cadherin-mediated cell–cell adhesion promotes cell migration in a three-dimensional matrix. *J. Cell Sci.* **2012**, *125*, 3661–3670. [CrossRef] [PubMed]
17. Battaglia, R.A.; Delic, S.; Herrmann, H.; Snider, N.T. Vimentin on the move: New developments in cell migration. *F1000Research* **2018**, *7*, 1796. [CrossRef]
18. Mendez, M.G.; Kojima, S.-I.; Goldman, R.D. Vimentin induces changes in cell shape, motility, and adhesion during the epithelial to mesenchymal transition. *FASEB J.* **2010**, *24*, 1838–1851. [CrossRef]
19. Kim, A.Y.; Kwak, J.H.; Je, N.K.; Lee, Y.H.; Jung, Y.S. Epithelial-mesenchymal transition is associated with acquired resistance to 5-fluorouracil in HT-29 colon cancer cells. *Toxicol. Res.* **2015**, *31*, 151–156. [CrossRef]
20. Nath, B.; Raza, A.; Sethi, V.; Dalal, A.; Ghosh, S.S.; Biswas, G. Understanding flow dynamics, viability and metastatic potency of cervical cancer (HeLa) cells through constricted microchannel. *Sci. Rep.* **2018**, *8*, 17357. [CrossRef]
21. Au, S.H.; Storey, B.D.; Moore, J.C.; Tang, Q.; Chen, Y.L.; Javaid, S.; Sarioglu, A.F.; Sullivan, R.; Madden, M.W.; O'Keefe, R.; et al. Clusters of circulating tumor cells traverse capillary-sized vessels. *Proc. Natl. Acad. Sci. USA* **2016**, *113*, 4947–4952. [CrossRef]
22. Le Bot, N. Entosis: Cell death by invasion. *Nat. Cell Boil.* **2007**, *9*, 1346. [CrossRef] [PubMed]
23. Singh, A.; Settleman, J. EMT, cancer stem cells and drug resistance: An emerging axis of evil in the war on cancer. *Oncogene* **2010**, *29*, 4741–4751. [CrossRef] [PubMed]
24. Kyra, C. Collective Cell Migration and Metastases Induced by an Epithelial-to-Mesenchymal Transition in *Drosophila* Intestinal Tumors. *Nat. Commun.* **2019**, *10*, 2311.
25. Savagner, P. Epithelial–mesenchymal transitions: From cell plasticity to concept elasticity. In *Current Topics in Developmental Biology*; Elsevier Academic Press: Cambridge, MA, USA, 2015; Volume 112, pp. 273–300.
26. Davis, F.M.; Azimi, I.; Faville, R.A.; Peters, A.A.; Jalink, K.; Putney, J.W., Jr.; Goodhill, G.J.; Thompson, E.W.; Roberts-Thomson, S.J.; Monteith, G.R. Induction of epithelial–mesenchymal transition (EMT) in breast cancer cells is calcium signal dependent. *Oncogene* **2014**, *33*, 2307–2316. [CrossRef] [PubMed]
27. Yao, D.; Dai, C.; Peng, S. Mechanism of the Mesenchymal-Epithelial Transition and Its Relationship with Metastatic Tumor Formation. *Mol. Cancer Res.* **2011**, *9*, 1608–1620. [CrossRef] [PubMed]

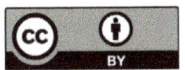

© 2019 by the authors. Licensee MDPI, Basel, Switzerland. This article is an open access article distributed under the terms and conditions of the Creative Commons Attribution (CC BY) license (http://creativecommons.org/licenses/by/4.0/).

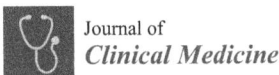

Article

# ATP Synthase Subunit Epsilon Overexpression Promotes Metastasis by Modulating AMPK Signaling to Induce Epithelial-to-Mesenchymal Transition and Is a Poor Prognostic Marker in Colorectal Cancer Patients

Yan-Jiun Huang [1,2,†], Yi-Hua Jan [3,†], Yu-Chan Chang [3,†], Hsing-Fang Tsai [3], Alexander TH Wu [4,5,‡], Chi-Long Chen [6,7,‡] and Michael Hsiao [3,4,8,*]

1. Division of Colorectal Surgery, Department of Surgery, Taipei Medical University Hospital, Taipei Medical University, Taipei 110, Taiwan
2. Department of Surgery, College of Medicine, Taipei Medical University, Taipei 110, Taiwan
3. Genomics Research Center, Academia Sinica, Taipei 115, Taiwan
4. The PhD Program for Translational Medicine, College of Medical Science and Technology, Taipei Medical University, Taipei 110, Taiwan
5. Graduate Institute of Medical Sciences, National Defense Medical Center, Taipei 114, Taiwan
6. Department of Pathology, Taipei Medical University Hospital, Taipei Medical University, Taipei 110, Taiwan
7. Department of Pathology, College of Medicine, Taipei Medical University, Taipei 110, Taiwan
8. Department of Biochemistry, College of Medicine, Kaohsiung Medical University, Kaohsiung 807, Taiwan
* Correspondence: mhsiao@gate.sinica.edu.tw; Tel.: +886-2-27871243; Fax: +886-2-27899931
† These authors contributed equally to this work
‡ These authors are senior authors and contribute equally to this study.

Received: 7 June 2019; Accepted: 16 July 2019; Published: 21 July 2019

**Abstract:** Metastasis remains the major cause of death from colon cancer. We intend to identify differentially expressed genes that are associated with the metastatic process and prognosis in colon cancer. ATP synthase epsilon subunit (*ATP5E*) gene was found to encode the mitochondrial $F_0F_1$ ATP synthase subunit epsilon that was overexpressed in tumor cells compared to their normal counterparts, while other genes encoding the ATP synthase subunit were repressed in public microarray datasets. CRC cells in which ATP5E was silenced showed markedly reduced invasive and migratory abilities. ATP5E inhibition significantly reduced the incidence of distant metastasis in a mouse xenograft model. Mechanistically, increased ATP5E expression resulted in a prominent reduction in E-cadherin and an increase in Snail expression. Our data also showed that an elevated *ATP5E* level in metastatic colon cancer samples was significantly associated with the AMPK-AKT-hypoxia-inducible factor-1α (HIF1α) signaling axis; silencing ATP5E led to the degradation of HIF1α under hypoxia through AMPK-AKT signaling. Our findings suggest that elevated ATP5E expression could serve as a marker of distant metastasis and a poor prognosis in colon cancer, and ATP5E functions via modulating AMPK-AKT-HIF1α signaling.

**Keywords:** ATP5E; AMPK; EMT; Metastasis; Colorectal Cancer

## 1. Introduction

Colorectal cancer (CRC) is one of the leading causes of morbidity and mortality worldwide, with about 1.4 million new cases reported in 2012 [1]. There was a global increase in CRC mortality, rising from an estimated 608,700 deaths in 2008 to almost 700,000 deaths in 2012 [1,2]. As a major clinical and public health concern, it is the third most commonly diagnosed cancer and the second leading cause of cancer-related deaths in both genders in the United States. Mortality resulting from CRC is associated with the disease stage, more-advanced grade, and the presence of obstruction [3]. Among these prognostic indicators, metastasis to distant organs (e.g., lung metastasis) is one of the most critical causes related to mortality [4]. Approximately 50% of patients develop distant metastases within 2 years after surgery and have a poor prognosis. Identifying a reliable diagnostic marker could serve to improve the management of patients with metastatic CRC.

Distant metastasis is one of the hallmarks of cancer and is comprised of a series of complex and interconnected cellular signaling networks. The so-called epithelial-to-mesenchymal transition (EMT) was shown to be the initiating and prerequisite cellular process for cancer cells to gain the ability to metastasize. The EMT is characterized by cancer cells' transformation from an epithelial phenotype to a mesenchymal phenotype, often reflected by increased vimentin (a mesenchymal marker) expression with a concomitant decrease in E-cadherin (an epithelial marker) expression [5,6]. Accumulating evidence suggests a close link between initiation of the EMT and metabolic reprogramming within cancer cells [7,8].

Bioenergetic proteins within mitochondria were found to possess the potential to be prognostic markers associated with cancer progression [9,10]. Among the metabolic pathways, adenosine monophosphate-activated protein kinase (AMPK) is considered a crucial energy sensor for regulating and adapting to hypoglycemic states [11,12]. To curb catabolic activity in the setting of energy depletion, phosphorylated (p)-AMPK interferes with Akt signaling through direct inhibition [13]. Furthermore, inhibiting the phosphorylation of Akt activates glycogen synthase kinase-3β (GSK3β) and consequently destabilizes Snail, which induces the expression of E-cadherin [14].

The Warburg effect is when cancer cells mainly generate their energy by glycolysis instead of oxidative phosphorylation; it is utilized by normal cells due to impaired mitochondrial function [15]. In line with Warburg's hypothesis, reports have shown that the β-catalytic subunit of H+-adenosine triphosphate (ATP) synthase is downregulated in renal and colon carcinomas along with the upregulation of glycolytic glyceraldehyde 3-phosphate dehydrogenase (GAPDH); the metabolic phenotype in these cells is considered a tumor progression marker with prognostic value for early-stage patients [16]. In addition, significant increases in ATP synthase α- and δ-subunits expressions were observed in primary tumors compared to the normal mucosa, while downregulation of the α- and δ-subunits led to decreased invasion in vitro in liver metastasis of primary CRC [17,18]. Based on these premises, we hypothesized that metastasis is an energy-demanding process that prompts cancer cells to acquire extra energy by upregulating energy-producing machinery. Increased ATP and ATP synthase hence appear to be potential targets for cancer therapy [19,20]. As one of the major mitochondrial enzymes, ATP synthase produces ATP and provides energy by driving phosphorylation of adenosine diphosphate (ADP) through a transmembrane proton gradient [21]. The enzyme includes an F0 sector composed of hydrophobic subunits for energy transduction, as well as an F1 sector composed of hydrophilic α-, β-, γ-, δ-, and ε-subunits for its catalytic function [22,23]. As to the roles of ATP synthase subunits in cancer development, little is known about the ε-subunit, which is encoded by the human ATP synthase epsilon subunit (*ATP5E*) gene and is located in the stalk region of the F1 sector [24,25]. A mutation in *ATP5E* leads to an isolated ATP synthase deficiency and mitochondrial disease, while the ε-subunit seems to be linked to incorporation of the c-subunit [26]. Knockdown of *ATP5E* inhibited the biogenesis of ATP synthase, reduced the ATP synthase complex, produced an insufficient ATP phosphorylating capacity, elevated the mitochondrial membrane potential, and caused unexpected c-subunit accumulation [27]. In addition, ATP5E was proven to be required for normal spindle orientation during embryonic divisions in *Drosophila* [28].

To date, the roles of *ATP5E* in CRC tumor development and disease progression remain unclear. Therefore, we investigated the relationship among ATP5E expression, disease stage, and survival in CRC patients. Moreover, we also investigated functional consequences of *ATP5E* alterations in CRC tumor cells, and the signaling axis that causes the EMT.

## 2. Experimental Section

### 2.1. Reagents, Cell Lines, and Lentiviral Transduction

Human CRC HCT116 and H3347 cells were obtained from American Type Culture Collection (Manassas, VA, USA) and grown in Dulbecco's modified Eagle medium (DMEM) and RPMI medium supplemented with 10% fetal bovine serum (FBS). As previously described, stable knockdown clones of HCT116 and H3347 cells were generated using short hairpin (sh)RNA directed against the *ATP5E* gene constructed in a pGIPZ-puro vector obtained from OpenBiosystems (Huntsville, AL, USA) [29]. A plasmid carrying a non-silencing (NS) control sequence was used to create control cells. Puromycin for stable clone selection was purchased from Sigma-Aldrich (St. Louis, MO, USA).

### 2.2. CRC Sample Selection and Immunohistochemical Analysis

The studied tissues were retrieved from the Department of Pathology, Taipei Municipal Wan Fang Hospital (Taipei, Taiwan) with Institutional Review Board approval (TMU-IRB 99049). Surgical specimens had been fixed in 10% buffered neutral formalin and embedded in paraffin. The histological diagnosis, tumor size, tumor invasiveness, and lymph node status of all cases were reviewed and confirmed by two pathologists (CLF and CLC). The final disease stages were determined according to the Cancer Staging System of the American Joint Committee of Cancer (AJCC). Clinical data, including the follow-up period, overall survival period, and disease-free survival period, were retrospectively collected from the medical record of each patient. Patients were followed-up for up to 152 months. Patients who died of postoperative complications within 30 days after surgery were excluded from the survival analysis.

A tissue microarray (TMA) was used for the IHC analysis of ATP5E expression in this study. A TMA containing CRC tissues and corresponding adjacent non-cancerous colon tissues was prepared, as described previously [30]. Three 1 mm cores from different areas of a tumor tissue in a paraffin block containing the tumor were selected in each case. If available, two 1-mm cores of adjacent non-cancerous normal colon mucosa were also selected in each case. In total, 243 archival CRC samples were assembled in the TMA. Antibodies used for IHC staining included anti-human ATP5E (1:100) (Abnova, Taipei, Taiwan), p-AMPKα thr-172 (1:50) (Cell Signaling Technology, Danvers, MA, USA), and E-cadherin (1:200) (BD Biosciences, Piscataway, NJ, USA). Immuno-detection was performed with an EnVision dual-link system-horseradish peroxidase (HRP) detection kit (DAKO, Glostrup, Denmark).

A four-point staining-intensity scoring system was devised to determine ATP5E expression in CRC TMA specimens, and staining-intensity scores ranged from 0 (no expression) to 3 (high expression). The results were classified into two groups according to the intensity and extent of staining: In the low-expression group, either no staining was present (staining intensity score = 0) or positive staining was detected in fewer than 10% of cells (staining intensity score = 1); and in the high-expression group, positive immunostaining was present in 10%–30% (staining intensity score = 2) or more than 30% of cells (staining intensity score = 3). All of the IHC staining results were reviewed and independently scored by two pathologists.

### 2.3. Animal Study

All animal work was conducted in accordance with a protocol approved by the Academia Sinica Institutional Animal Care and Utilization Committee. Age-matched severe combined immune-deficiency mutation and interleukin-2 receptor gamma chain deficiency (NOD SCID gamma) female mice (6–8 weeks old) originally from Jackson Laboratory (Farmington, CT, USA) were used. For the experimental tumorigenesis assay, $5 \times 10^6$ HCT 116 cells were re-suspended in 0.1 mL of phosphate-buffered saline (PBS) and subcutaneously injected into the backs of SCID mice. Tumor volumes were measured every week. If tumor masses occurred, they were harvested at the end of week 3. For the experimental metastasis assays, $10^6$ HCT 116 cells were re-suspended in 0.1 mL of PBS and injected into the lateral tail vein of SCID mice. Mouse lungs were harvested at 2.5 weeks after the injection. The number of lung metastatic nodules was measured, and the intensity of green fluorescence was quantified using a noninvasive bioluminescence system (IVIS-Spectrum, PerkinElmer, MA, USA). Tissues were fixed in 10% buffered neutral formalin and embedded in paraffin. Sections of 4 µm in thickness were stained with hematoxylin and eosin (H&E) for the histopathological analysis.

### 2.4. Western Blot Analysis

A Western blot analysis was performed with the primary antibodies anti-ATP5E (1:1000) (cat. no.: H00000514-M01, Abnova, Taipei, Taiwan), anti-pAkt ser 473 (1:1000) (cat. no.: 4060, Cell Signaling Technology), anti-Akt (1:2000) (cat. no.: 4691, Cell Signaling Technology), anti-pGSK3β (1:1000) (cat. no.: 9336, Cell Signaling Technology), anti-GSK3β (1:1000) (cat. no.: 9332, Cell Signaling Technology), anti-Snail (1:1000) (cat. no.: 3879, Cell Signaling Technology), anti-E-cadherin (1:1000) (cat. no.: 610182, BD Biosciences), and anti-α-tubulin ($1:10^4$) (Sigma-Aldrich, St. Louis, MO, USA).

### 2.5. Measurements of Intracellular ATP Levels

HCT116 and H3347 cells were cultured as described above before being trypsinized and washed twice with PBS for the ATP analysis. Cells ($8 \times 10^4$) were applied to each well of white-wall 96-well plates (Greiner Bio One, Frickenhausen, Germany). Intracellular ATP levels were quantified using a CellTiterGlo Assay (Promega, Madison, WI, USA) and a Victor3 plate reader (PerkinElmer Life Science, Waltham, MA, USA) following the manufacturer's instructions.

### 2.6. Invasion and Migration Analyses

For the invasion assay, polycarbonate filters were pre-coated with human fibronectin on the lower side and Matrigel on the upper side. Medium containing 10% FBS was added to each well of the lower compartment of the chamber. Cells were re-suspended in serum-free medium containing 0.1% bovine serum albumin and added to each well of the upper compartment. Cells were incubated for 16 h at 37 °C in 5% $CO_2$. At the end of incubation, cells were counted under a light microscope (200×, ten random fields from each well). All experiments were performed in quadruplicate. For the migration assay, wounds were created in confluent cells using a pipette tip and then rinsed with PBS to remove any free-floating cells and debris. Wound healing was measured at 0, 12, 24, and 36 h under a light microscope (100×).

### 2.7. Statistical Analysis

All observations were confirmed by at least three independent experiments. Data are presented as the mean ± standard deviation (SD). An analysis of variance (ANOVA) was used to evaluate the statistical significance of mean values. A Cox proportional hazards regression was used to test the prognostic significance of factors in univariate and multivariate models. The Kaplan-Meier method was used for the survival analysis. All statistical tests were two-sided, and $p < 0.05$ was considered significant.

## 3. Results

This section may be divided by subheadings. It should provide a concise and precise description of the experimental results, their interpretation, as well as the experimental conclusions that can be drawn.

### 3.1. Overexpression of ATP5E in CRC Is Associated with Distal Metastasis

We first analyzed expressions of ATP synthase subunits in the GSE23878 dataset containing 36 CRC tissues and 24 non-cancerous colon tissues. A hierarchical clustering analysis showed that expression profiles of genes coding ATP synthase subunits were suppressed in tumor tissues compared to normal tissues (Figure 1a). Interestingly, we found that *ATP5E*, which encodes the ATP synthase epsilon subunit, was uniquely overexpressed in tumor tissues compared to normal tissues (Figure 1b).

Next, we analyzed *ATP5E* expression in another microarray dataset from GSE41258 containing a panel of CRC samples that progressed from normal colon to polyps, primary tumors, and metastatic tumors. Surprisingly, *ATP5E* expression was significantly upregulated in primary tumors and increasingly upregulated in liver metastasis and lung metastasis (Figure 1c). To validate our findings, we performed an RT-PCR to detect mRNA expression levels of *ATP5E* in normal versus tumor tissues. In eight of nine CRC samples (88%), its expression in the tumor portion was markedly higher than that of the normal part (Figure 1d). We also performed an IHC analysis to examine ATP5E expression in 60 NT-paired CRC specimens. Staining results revealed a significant trend of higher expression of ATP5E in tumor tissues compared to normal tissues (Figure 1e,f, $p < 0.01$). To further determine the prognostic role of ATP5E, we performed an IHC analysis of 243 CRC patients with known clinical follow-up information. Among these patients (with median follow-up of 70 months for censored patients), there were 127 deaths, and demographic information is shown in Supplemental Table S1. Figure 1g illustrates representative scores for quantitating ATP5E expression based on its staining intensity. The Kaplan-Meier survival analysis showed that high levels of ATP5E were significantly correlated with worse overall survival and disease-free survival (Figure 1h,i, $p < 0.01$). Relationships of ATP5E expression levels with clinicopathological characteristics of CRC are summarized in Supplemental Table S1. Furthermore, univariate and multivariate COX regression analyses, including ATP5E scores, the tumor status, lymph node involvement, metastasis, stage, and recurrence, showed that ATP5E is indeed an independent marker of a poor prognosis in CRC patients (Supplemental Table S2).

*3.2. ATP5E Regulates Migration and Invasion In Vitro and In Vivo*

Based on the finding that ATP5E expression is associated with distant metastasis, we then hypothesized that ATP5E expression may affect the invasiveness of colon cancer cells. Figure 2a shows the endogenous expression of ATP5E in six colon cancer cell lines. To test whether ATP5E can modulate the invasive/migratory abilities of colon cancer cells, we silenced ATP5E expression in HCT116 and H3347 cells using a shRNA lentivirus (Figure 2b). A wound-healing assay showed that knockdown of *ATP5E* resulted in a ~40% reduction of the migratory ability of HCT116 and H3347 cells (Figure 2c). In addition, knockdown of ATP5E also diminished the migratory and invasive abilities of both cell lines as evaluated by a Boyden chamber assay (Figure 2d,e). To evaluate the effects of ATP5E expression on tumor metastasis in vivo, we intravenously injected HCT116 NS control cells and *shATP5E* cells into NOD-SCID mice. As shown in Figure 2f, the number of lung tumor nodules in the *shATP5E* group was 2.5-times lower than that in NS control mice ($p = 0.0002$). Furthermore, fluorescence microscopy and photon counts also displayed significant differences between the NS control and *shATP5E* mice (Figure 2g). A histopathological examination showed further evidence of decreased distant metastases of HCT116 *shATP5E* cells compared to HCT116 NS control cells (Figure 2h).

*3.3. ATP5E Expression Induces the EMT*

Since repression of ATP5E inhibited cancer cell migration and invasion *in vitro* and *in vivo*, we further investigated the possible mechanism that regulates CRC cell motility and invasiveness. According to the literature, metastatic cancer cells often acquire a mesenchymal phenotype through the EMT. To test whether ATP5E expression can modulate the EMT, we performed a Western blot analysis to detect E-cadherin and Snail expressions upon ATP5E suppression or ATP5E overexpression. Figure 3a shows that Snail expression decreased with concurrent induction of E-cadherin expression upon ATP5E silencing. Complementarily, overexpression of ATP5E in CX-1 cells upregulated Snail and resulted in E-cadherin suppression (Figure 3a). The IHC analysis in serial sections of CRC specimens also showed this inverse correlation between ATP5E and E-cadherin (Figure 3b). To confirm mRNA expression patterns of ATP5E and E-cadherin during CRC progression, we analyzed expressions of both genes from normal colon specimens to polyps, primary tumors, liver metastatic tumors, and lung metastatic tumors in the GSE41258 dataset. Interestingly, E-cadherin expression was frequently downregulated with concurrent upregulation of ATP5E in metastatic tumors compared to primary tumors (Figure 3c).

## 3.4. ATP5E Upregulation Connects the AMPK-AKT-HIF1a Signaling Axis to the EMT Phenotype in Lung Metastatic Tumors

To elucidate the possible signaling pathways for EMT induction, we extracted differentially expressed genes in lung metastatic tumors, which were predominately expression patterns of ATP5E high/E-cadherin low, from the GSE41258 dataset and subjected them to an IPA Upstream Regulator Analysis. With this approach, we found that the AKT-HIF1-α signaling axis was predicted to be activated (Figure 4a). Moreover, downstream targets of AKT and HIF1α, including fibronectin and E-cadherin, were differentially regulated (Figure 4b). While AMPK was not predicted to be activated but based on the negative regulatory relationship between AMPK and AKT, we hypothesized that phosphorylation of AMPK at thr-172 would be inhibited. To test this hypothesis, we performed a Western blot analysis to detect the phosphorylation status of AMPK and AKT. Data showed that AMPK was activated with concurrent inhibition of AKT activity upon ATP5E knockdown in HCT116 and H3347 cells (Figure 4c). Moreover, ATP5E knockdown of HCT116 cells abolished stabilization of the HIF1α protein in hypoxia (Figure 4d).

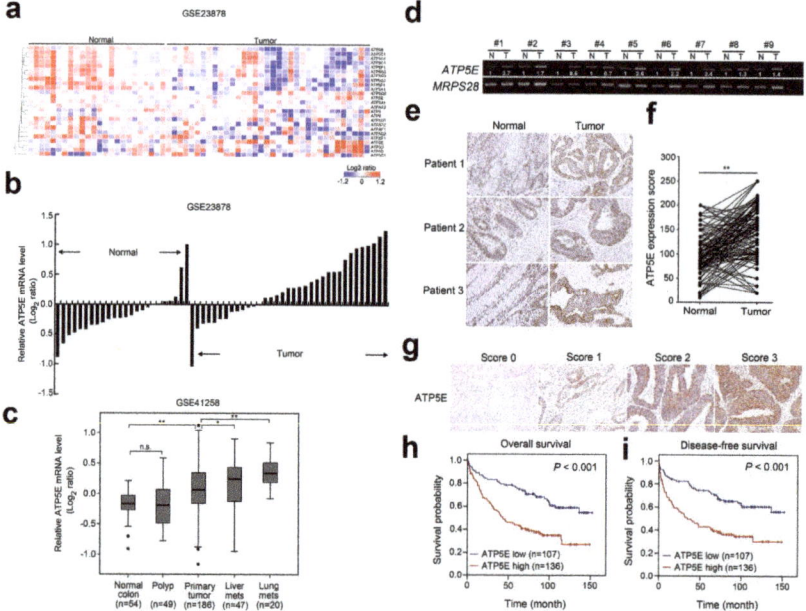

**Figure 1.** Overexpression of the ATP synthase epsilon subunit (ATP5E) in colorectal cancer (CRC) is associated with distal metastasis and a poor prognosis. (**a**) Microarray expression patterns of genes encode for ATP synthase in the GSE23878 dataset containing 36 CRC tissues and 24 non-cancerous colorectal tissues. (**b**) Relative expression of the *ATP5E* gene in the GSE23878 dataset ranked from lowest to highest. (**c**) Microarray expression patterns of the *ATP5E* gene were compared among 54 normal colon tissues, 49 polyp tissues, 186 primary tumors, 20 lung metastatic tumors, and 47 liver metastatic tumors in the GSE41258 dataset. (**d**) RT-PCR analysis of *ATP5E* levels in normal colon tissues (N) and tumor tissues (T) derived from nine patients. Data were normalized to the corresponding *MRPS28* level. (**e**) Representative IHC staining of ATP5E levels in normal colon and primary CRC tissues. (**f**) Distribution of immunoreactivity scores in normal colon and primary CRC tissues ($n = 60$). The scores were determined by the staining intensity x percentage of positive cells. (**g**) Representative scores for ATP5E IHC staining in CRC patients. (**h**) Kaplan-Meier plot of overall survival for 243 CRC patients, stratified by the ATP5E level. (**i**) Kaplan-Meier plot of disease-free survival for 243 CRC patients, stratified by the ATP5E level.

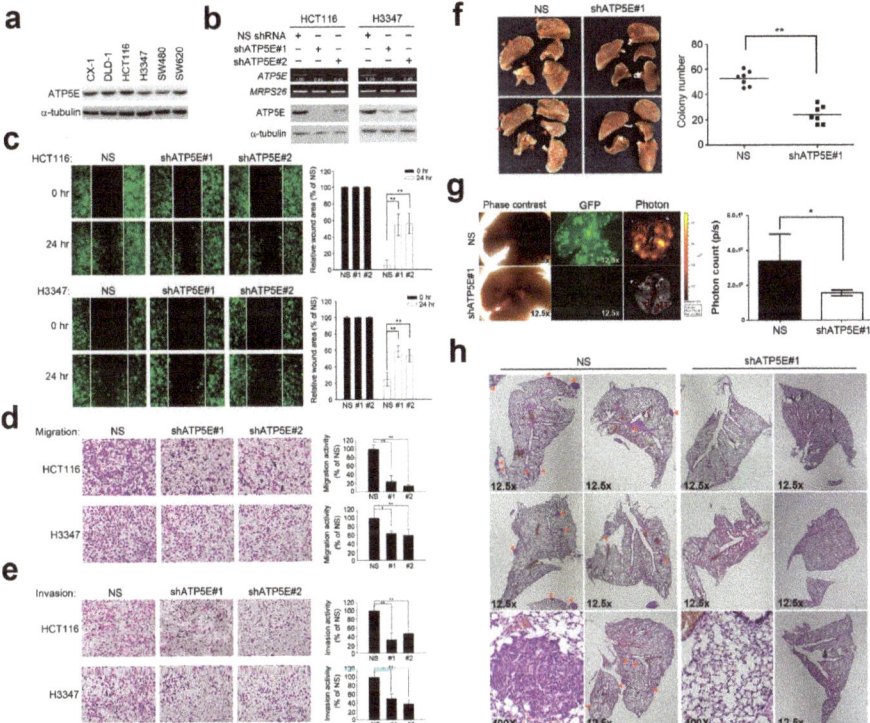

**Figure 2.** ATP synthase epsilon subunit (ATP5E) silencing inhibited invasion and migration *in vitro* and distal metastasis in vivo. (**a**) Endogenous ATP5E protein expression in six colorectal cancer cell lines. (**b**) Knockdown of ATP5E expression in HCT116 and H3347 cells by ATP5E shRNAs. The knockdown efficiency was determined by an RT-PCR and Western blot analyses. (**c**) Wound-healing assay carried out on HCT116 and H3347 cells. Relative wounded areas were compared between the non-silencing (NS) control and *shATP5E* cells at 24 h. (**d**) Migration assay for the NS control and *shATP5E* cells of the HCT116 and H3347 cell lines using Boyden chambers. (**e**) Invasion assay for the NS control and *shATP5E* cells of the HCT116 and H3347 cell lines using Boyden chambers pre-coated with Matrigel shown in the lower panel. (**f**) Representative lung images of mice injected with the NS control and *shATP5E* cells are shown in the left panel. Total numbers of lung metastatic nodules in individual mice 2.5 weeks after a tail vein injection of HCT116 NS control or *shATP5E* cells are shown in the right panel. (**g**) Green fluorescence and photon images of the lungs of mice injected with HCT116 NS control or *shATP5E* cells. The color bar represents the fluorescence intensity. (**h**) Representative H&E staining of lung sections at 12.5× and 400×. Red arrows indicate metastatic nodules.

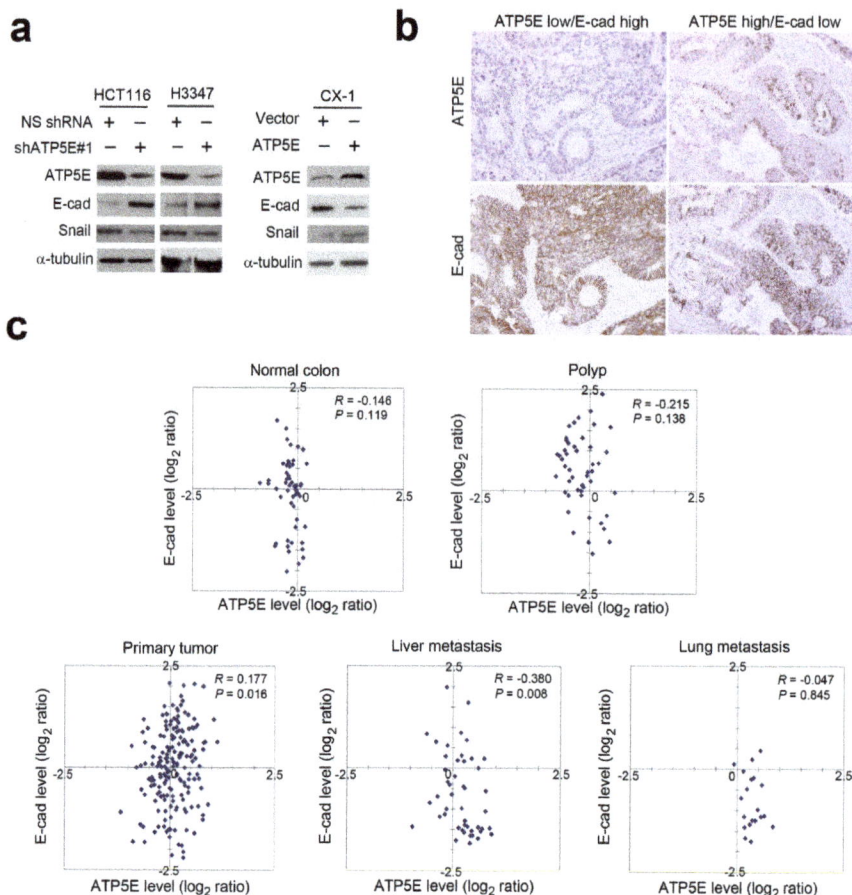

**Figure 3.** ATP synthase epsilon subunit (ATP5E) expression induces the epithelial-to-mesenchymal transition. (**a**) Western blot analysis of E-cadherin and Snail expressions upon ATP5E knockdown and overexpression. (**b**) IHC staining of ATP5E and E-cadherin in serial sections of colon cancer specimens. (**c**) ATP5E and E-cadherin expression profiles of normal colon, polyp, primary colon tumor, liver metastatic tumor, and lung metastatic tumor tissues in the GSE41258 microarray dataset.

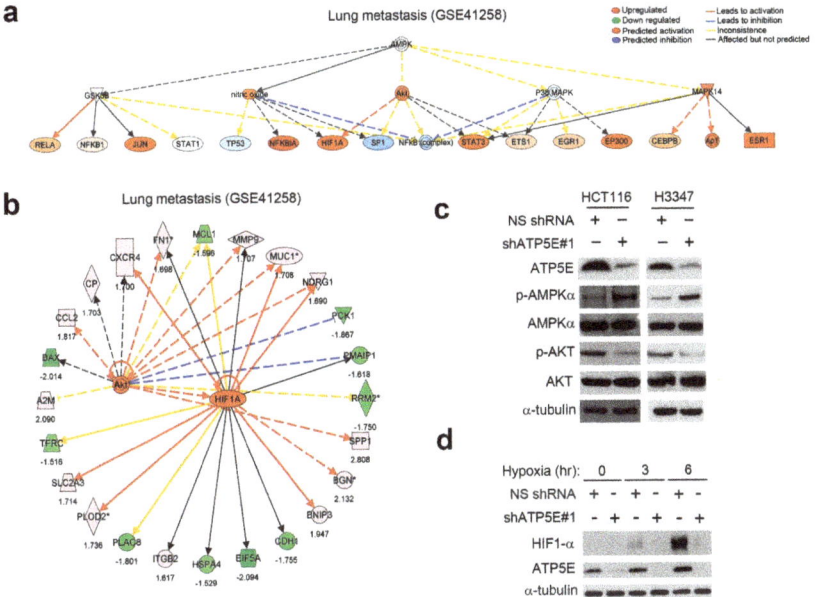

**Figure 4.** ATP synthase epsilon subunit (ATP5E) upregulation connects the adenosine monophosphate-activated protein kinase (AMPK)-AKT-hypoxia-inducible factor-1α (HIF1a) signaling axis to the epithelial-to-mesenchymal transition (EMT) phenotype in lung metastatic tumors. (**a**) Upstream regulator analysis of differentially expressed genes in lung metastatic tumors from the GSE41258 dataset. The orange circle indicates predicted activation, while the blue circle indicates predicted inhibition. (**b**) Differentially expressed genes downstream of AKT and HIF1a extracted from the GSE41258 dataset. (**c**) Western blot analysis of the phosphorylation status of AMPK and AKT upon ATP5E inhibition in HCT116 and H3347 cells. (**d**) Western blot analysis of the HIF1a protein upon ATP5E inhibition in hypoxia.

## 4. Discussion

In the present study, we determined the prognostic role of ATP5E expression in CRC patients and the functional consequences of ATP5E in two colon cancer cell lines *in vitro* and *in vivo*. To our knowledge, no previous investigation has determined the prognostic role of the *ATP5E* gene in human CRC. We concluded that the ATP5E expression status was significantly associated with both disease-free survival and overall survival. It was also inversely correlated with p-AMPK and E-cadherin expression statuses in terms of patient survival.

The role of F0/F1-ATP synthase in human cancer was evaluated in recent studies [7,16,17,31,32]. Nevertheless, most studies demonstrated that expression of the b-subunit of F0F1-ATP synthase is repressed in human cancer cells of the liver, colon, kidneys, lungs, breast, stomach, and esophagus compared to their corresponding normal tissues, whereas proteins (genes) involved in glycolysis are upregulated in most human tumors [16,31]. On the basis of these findings, it was hypothesized that the metabolic phenotype of tumor cells shifts from oxidative phosphorylation to glycolysis. However, results were obtained from a limited number of normal or tumor samples. Originally, Warburg hypothesized that cancer cells develop a defect in mitochondria that leads to impaired aerobic respiration and a subsequent strain on glycolytic metabolism, and these were supported by a number of reports [7,15,16,31,32]. However, subsequent work showed that mitochondrial function is not impaired in most cancers [33,34]. In addition, Shin et al. reported that downregulation of F0F1-ATP synthase induces an increase in 5-fluororuracil resistance [35]. Notwithstanding, F0F1-ATP synthase is overexpressed in liver metastasis of CRC, and higher expression of the b-subunit in breast cancer is related to poor outcomes for those patients [17,32]. In addition, ATP5A expression is upregulated in metastasized tumors and liver metastasis compared to primary tumors and normal cells in the colon [36]. High expression levels of ATP synthase 6 and the d-subunit of F0F1-ATP synthase were also, respectively, found in tumor samples of thyroid papillary carcinomas and lung adenocarcinomas [37]. Overexpression of the a- and b-subunits of F0F1-ATP synthase were correlated with metastasis in melanoma cell lines and lung and lymph node metastases related to primary tumors [38]. The major interpretation of these results is the direct impacts of increases in ATP synthase subunits on cellular energy transduction, which may obscure an extra contribution to the apoptotic potential resulting from the increase in mitochondrial oxidative phosphorylation. To accomplish the multistep cascade of metastasis, tumor cells may need an active supply of energy. Additionally, tumor cells have high levels of ATP and ATP synthase for their energy sources.

The role of F1F0-ATP synthase in cancer progression or metastasis has not yet been well characterized. In previous reports on clinical cancer samples, decreased expression of the b-subunit in colon and lung cancers was correlated with a poorer prognosis [7,16]. Data were reported in limited samples of the early stage, pT1+pT2, lung adenocarcinomas, and Duke's stage B2+B3 colon adenocarcinomas. Those results were contrary to our findings. Our results demonstrated that high expression of ATP5E was correlated with a poor prognosis in our pool of all subjects. Also, highly significant differences in overall survival and disease-free survival appeared between subjects in AJCC stages 3+4 and in stages 1+2 with higher ATP5E expression and those with lower ATP5E expression (Supplemental online Figure S1). Our findings concurred with the concept that cancer cells require more energy to trigger metastasis. Especially, Eukaryotic translation initiation factor 4E–binding protein 1 (4E-BP1) is a key downstream effector of mTOR complex 1 (mTORC1), which regulates mitochondrial activity and improves metabolic homeostasis [39,40]. Therefore, we observed the phosphorylation status of 4E-BP1 has been reduced in ATP5E knockdown stable cells (Supplemental online Figures S2 and S3). Recent studies focused on ATP and ATP synthase as targets for anticancer therapies in animal and cell line models [19,20]. Combined all evidences, we hypothesized that ATP5E dysfunction in colon tumorigenesis is correlated with ATP production, mitochondrial function, and then interacts with several oncogenic pathways

AMPK is a member of a protein kinase family that is activated during energy deficiencies in order to restore ATP levels [12]. Increasing the AMP/ATP ratio induces phosphorylation of AMPK by LKB1. However, p-AMPK expression (negative or positive) is not associated with survival in CRC. Only after combining with the p-MAPK3/1 status did the prognostic effect of p-AMPK significantly differ. Notably, p-AMPK expression is associated with superior CRC-specific survival among p-MAPK3/1-positive cases [37]. According to our findings, the high expression level of p-AMPK was significantly associated with good overall survival ($p = 0.041$) and disease-free survival ($p = 0.049$) (Supplemental online Figure S1). The Akt signaling pathway was also interfered with by activated AMPK with a direct interaction, which might result in a reduction of glycolysis through decreases in both hexokinase activity and transcription of glycolytic enzymes [13]. Since activation of the Akt pathway was implicated in induction of the EMT, we hypothesized that silencing of *ATP5E* and increasing the AMP/ATP ratio should induce activation of AMPK to inhibit Akt, which resulted in downregulation of Snail and subsequent upregulation of E-cadherin (Supplemental online Figure S4) [14]. Accordingly, we found that reducing expression of the *ATP5E* gene induced activation of AMPK, and thereby inhibited Akt and GSK3β phosphorylation. This signaling gave rise to decreased stability of Snail and subsequently increased the E-cadherin expression level (Figure 4B). In addition, patients with low ATP5E expression and high E-cadherin expression had better survival than those with high ATP5E expression and low E-cadherin expression. These results suggested that ATP5E is crucial for CRC prognosis.

Many cancer cells maintain a high level of anaerobic carbon metabolism in the presence of oxygen, which is a manifestation of the Warburg effect [15]. Macrolide inhibitors, such as oligomycin, of mitochondrial F0F1-ATP synthase selectively kill metabolically active tumor cells that do not fit in the

Warburg effect phenomenon. Oligomycin A has also been used to inhibit mitochondrial F0F1-ATP synthase in cancer metabolism research. Taken together with our results, the phenomenon of the Warburg effect still remains to be established in detail.

F0F1-ATP synthase (F0F1) synthesizes ATP in mitochondria coupled with proton flow driven by the Protonmotive force (PMF) across membranes. Based on previously studies, ATPase inhibitory factor 1 (ATPIF1, IF1) inhibits ATPase activity of mitochondrial F0F1-ATP synthase [41]. Under aerobic conditions, ATPIF1 make ATP from ADP and phosphate using a PMF generated by respiration, as a source of energy to drive their rotary mechanism. On the other hand, IF1-deficinet cells can maintain ATP after PMF loss by glycolysis. Therefore, we screened the expression between ATPIF1 and ATP5E in the TCGA clinical cohort (TCGA_COAD). The results showed that ATP5E was highly expressed in tumor part compared with normal adjacent tissues. In contrast, ATPIF1 is reduced in the tumor part than in the normal group. ATPIF1 and ATP5E form a significant negative correlation in clinical patients (Supplemental online Figure S5). However, extrinsic conditions influence (pH, ion concentration, etc.) the self-association and structure of IF1 [42]. In further experimental design, we will evaluate the mitochondrial membrane potential ($\triangle \Psi m$) and identify the detailed interplay between ATP5E and ATPIF1.

## 5. Conclusions

We showed that a high ATP5E expression level was associated with a poor prognosis, including disease recurrence, overall survival, and disease-free survival in CRC. Additionally, we used CRC cell lines to investigate the roles of ATP5E in tumor growth and metastasis both in vitro and in vivo. These findings point out the potential therapeutic implications, as they indicate that mitochondrial ATP synthase inhibitors may enhance the anticancer efficacy of metabolic drugs.

**Supplementary Materials:** The following are available online at http://www.mdpi.com/2077-0383/8/7/1070/s1, Table S1: The demography of patients with Colorectal Cancer; Table S2: The relationship between ATP5E expression and the clinical-pathological characteristics of colorectal cancer; Figure S1: Kaplan-Meier analysis of overall and disease-free survival in stage I-II and stage III-IV colon cancer patients, stratified by ATP5E expression; Figure S2: Relative intracellular ATP level upon ATP5E knockdown in HCT116 and H3347; Figure S3: Kaplan-Meier analysis of overall and disease-free survival in combination with ATP5E status and E-cadherin status; Figure S4: Kaplan-Meier analysis of overall and disease-free survival in combination with ATP5E status and E-cadherin status; Figure S5: A negative correlation between ATP5E and ATPIF1 (A) Heat-map showed the expression of ATP5A1, ATP5E and ATPIF1 in the TCGA colon adenocarcinoma clinical cohort. (B) Quantitation the expression level of ATP5E and ATPIF1 in normal adjacent tissues and primary tumor group, respectively. (C) Correlation plot performed the significant negative association between ATP5E with ATPIF1."

**Author Contributions:** M.H., C.L.C., and A.T.W. conceived and designed the study. C.L.C. and Y.C.H. collected CRC. samples and clinical information. Y.H.J., Y.C.C., and H.F.T. performed the experiments and acquired the result data. M.H., Y.H.J., C.L.C. and Y.C.H. reviewed the statistical analysis. Y.C.H., Y.H.J., Y.J.H. and Y.C.C. drafted the manuscript. M.H., C.L.C., and A.T.W. critically revised the manuscript and supervised the study. All authors read and approved the final manuscript.

**Funding:** This research was supported by Academia Sinica (AS-SUMMIT-108) to Michael Hsiao and Ministry of Science and Technology (MOST106-2320-B-038-035-MY3) to Chi-Long Chen. Yan-Jiun Huang was supported by TMU106-AE1-B47.

**Acknowledgments:** We would also like to thank the Genomics Research Center Instrument Core Facilities for their support for the Affymetrix microarray, IVIS spectrum, and Aperio digital pathology analyses.

**Conflicts of Interest:** The authors declare no conflict of interest.

## References

1. Ferlay, J.; Soerjomataram, I.; Dikshit, R.; Eser, S.; Mathers, C.; Rebelo, M.; Parkin, D.M.; Forman, D.; Bray, F. Cancer incidence and mortality worldwide: Sources, methods and major patterns in GLOBOCAN 2012. *Int. J. Cancer* **2015**, *136*, E359–E386. [CrossRef] [PubMed]
2. Jemal, A.; Bray, F.; Center, M.M.; Ferlay, J.; Ward, E.; Forman, D. Global cancer statistics. *CA Cancer J. Clin.* **2011**, *61*, 69–90. [CrossRef] [PubMed]
3. Griffin, M.R.; Bergstralh, E.J.; Coffey, R.J.; Beart, R.W., Jr.; Melton, L.J., 3rd. Predictors of survival after curative resection of carcinoma of the colon and rectum. *Cancer* **1987**, *60*, 2318–2324. [CrossRef]

4. Sargent, D.J.; Patiyil, S.; Yothers, G.; Haller, D.G.; Gray, R.; Benedetti, J.; Buyse, M.; Labianca, R.; Seitz, J.F.; O'Callaghan, C.J.; et al. End Points for Colon Cancer Adjuvant Trials: Observations and Recommendations Based on Individual Patient Data from 20,898 Patients Enrolled Onto 18 Randomized Trials from the ACCENT Group. *J. Clin. Oncol.* **2007**, *25*, 4569–4574. [CrossRef] [PubMed]
5. Bates, R.C.; Mercurio, A.M. The epithelial-mesenchymal transition (EMT) and colorectal cancer progression. *Cancer Biol. Ther.* **2005**, *4*, 365–370.
6. Thiery, J.P. Epithelial–mesenchymal transitions in tumour progression. *Nat. Rev. Cancer* **2002**, *2*, 442–454. [CrossRef] [PubMed]
7. Cuezva, J.M.; Ortega, Á.D.; Willers, I.; Sánchez-Cenizo, L.; Aldea, M.; Sánchez-Aragó, M. The tumor suppressor function of mitochondria: Translation into the clinics. *Biochim. Biophys. Acta Mol. Basis Dis.* **2009**, *1792*, 1145–1158. [CrossRef]
8. Ward, P.S.; Thompson, C.B. Metabolic Reprogramming: A Cancer Hallmark Even Warburg Did Not Anticipate. *Cancer Cell* **2012**, *21*, 297–308. [CrossRef]
9. Moreno-Sanchez, R.; Rodriguez-Enriquez, S.; Saavedra, E.; Marin-Hernandez, A.; Gallardo-Perez, J.C. The bioenergetics of cancer: Is glycolysis the main ATP supplier in all tumor cells? *BioFactors* **2009**, *35*, 209–225. [CrossRef]
10. Zu, X.L.; Guppy, M. Cancer metabolism: Facts, fantasy, and fiction. *Biochem. Biophys. Res. Commun.* **2004**, *313*, 459–465. [CrossRef]
11. Bujak, A.L.; Crane, J.D.; Lally, J.S.; Ford, R.J.; Kang, S.J.; Rebalka, I.A.; Green, A.E.; Kemp, B.E.; Hawke, T.J.; Schertzer, J.D.; et al. AMPK Activation of Muscle Autophagy Prevents Fasting-Induced Hypoglycemia and Myopathy during Aging. *Cell Metab.* **2015**, *21*, 883–890. [CrossRef]
12. Hardie, D.G.; Carling, D.; Carlson, M. The AMP-Activated/SNF1 Protein Kinase Subfamily: Metabolic Sensors of the Eukaryotic Cell? *Annu. Rev. Biochem.* **1998**, *67*, 821–855. [CrossRef]
13. Daignan-Fornier, B.; Pinson, B. 5-Aminoimidazole-4-carboxamide-1-beta-D-ribofuranosyl 5'-Monophosphate (AICAR), a Highly Conserved Purine Intermediate with Multiple Effects. *Metabolites* **2012**, *2*, 292–302. [CrossRef]
14. Zhou, B.P.; Deng, J.; Xia, W.; Xu, J.; Li, Y.M.; Gunduz, M.; Hung, M.C. Dual regulation of Snail by GSK-3beta-mediated phosphorylation in control of epithelial-mesenchymal transition. *Nat. Cell Biol.* **2004**, *6*, 931–940. [CrossRef]
15. Warburg, O. On the origin of cancer cells. *Science* **1956**, *123*, 309–314. [CrossRef]
16. Cuezva, J.M.; Chen, G.; Alonso, A.M.; Isidoro, A.; Misek, D.E.; Hanash, S.M.; Beer, D.G. The bioenergetic signature of lung adenocarcinomas is a molecular marker of cancer diagnosis and prognosis. *Carcinogenesis* **2004**, *25*, 1157–1163. [CrossRef]
17. Chang, H.J.; Lee, M.R.; Hong, S.-H.; Yoo, B.C.; Shin, Y.-K.; Jeong, J.Y.; Lim, S.-B.; Choi, H.S.; Jeong, S.-Y.; Park, J.-G. Identification of mitochondrial FoF1-ATP synthase involved in liver metastasis of colorectal cancer. *Cancer Sci.* **2007**, *98*, 1184–1191. [CrossRef]
18. Moreno-Sanchez, R.; Rodriguez-Enriquez, S.; Marin-Hernandez, A.; Saavedra, E. Energy metabolism in tumor cells. *FEBS J.* **2007**, *274*, 1393–1418. [CrossRef]
19. Geschwind, J.-F.H.; Ko, Y.H.; Torbenson, M.S.; Magee, C.; Pedersen, P.L. Novel therapy for liver cancer: Direct intraarterial injection of a potent inhibitor of ATP production. *Cancer Res.* **2002**, *62*, 3909–3913.
20. Gong, Y.; Sohn, H.; Xue, L.; Firestone, G.L.; Bjeldanes, L.F. 3,3'-Diindolylmethane is a novel mitochondrial H(+)-ATP synthase inhibitor that can induce p21(Cip1/Waf1) expression by induction of oxidative stress in human breast cancer cells. *Cancer Res.* **2006**, *66*, 4880–4887. [CrossRef]
21. Mitchell, P. Coupling of Phosphorylation to Electron and Hydrogen Transfer by a Chemi-Osmotic type of Mechanism. *Nature* **1961**, *191*, 144–148. [CrossRef]
22. Walker, J.; Fearnley, I.; Gay, N.; Gibson, B.; Northrop, F.; Powell, S.; Runswick, M.; Saraste, M.; Tybulewicz, V. Primary structure and subunit stoichiometry of F1-ATPase from bovine mitochondria. *J. Mol. Biol.* **1985**, *184*, 677–701. [CrossRef]
23. Walker, J.E.; Lutter, R.; Dupuis, A.; Runswick, M.J. Identification of the subunits of F1F0-ATPase from bovine heart mitochondria. *Biochemistry* **1991**, *30*, 5369–5378. [CrossRef]
24. Gabellieri, E.; Strambini, G.B.; Baracca, A.; Solaini, G. Structural mapping of the epsilon-subunit of mitochondrial H(+)-ATPase complex (F1). *Biophys. J.* **1997**, *72*, 1818–1827. [CrossRef]

25. Tu, Q.; Yu, L.; Zhang, P.; Zhang, M.; Zhang, H.; Jiang, J.; Chen, C.; Zhao, S. Cloning, characterization and mapping of the human *ATP5E* gene, identification of pseudogene *ATP5EP1*, and definition of the *ATP5E* motif. *Biochem. J.* **2000**, *347*, 17–21. [CrossRef]
26. Mayr, J.A.; Havlickova, V.; Zimmermann, F.; Magler, I.; Kaplanova, V.; Jesina, P.; Pecinova, A.; Nuskova, H.; Koch, J.; Sperl, W.; et al. Mitochondrial ATP synthase deficiency due to a mutation in the *ATP5E* gene for the F1 epsilon subunit. *Hum. Mol. Genet.* **2010**, *19*, 3430–3439. [CrossRef]
27. Havlíčková, V.; Kaplanová, V.; Nůsková, H.; Drahota, Z.; Houštěk, J. Knockdown of F1 epsilon subunit decreases mitochondrial content of ATP synthase and leads to accumulation of subunit c. *Biochim. Biophys. Acta Gen. Subj.* **2010**, *1797*, 1124–1129. [CrossRef]
28. Kidd, T.; Abu-Shumays, R.; Katzen, A.; Sisson, J.C.; Jimenez, G.; Pinchin, S.; Sullivan, W.; Ish-Horowicz, D. The epsilon-subunit of mitochondrial ATP synthase is required for normal spindle orientation during the Drosophila embryonic divisions. *Genetics* **2005**, *170*, 697–708. [CrossRef]
29. Chen, M.-W.; Hua, K.-T.; Kao, H.-J.; Chi, C.-C.; Wei, L.-H.; Johansson, G.; Shiah, S.-G.; Chen, P.-S.; Jeng, Y.-M.; Cheng, T.-Y.; et al. H3K9 Histone Methyltransferase G9a Promotes Lung Cancer Invasion and Metastasis by Silencing the Cell Adhesion Molecule Ep-CAM. *Cancer Res.* **2010**, *70*, 7830–7840. [CrossRef]
30. El-Rehim, D.M.A.; E Pinder, S.; Paish, C.E.; Bell, J.; Blamey, R.; Robertson, J.F.; Nicholson, R.I.; Ellis, I.O. Expression of luminal and basal cytokeratins in human breast carcinoma. *J. Pathol.* **2004**, *203*, 661–671. [CrossRef]
31. Isidoro, A.; Martínez, M.; Fernández, P.L.; Ortega, Á.D.; Santamaría, G.; Chamorro, M.; Reed, J.C.; Cuezva, J.M. Alteration of the bioenergetic phenotype of mitochondria is a hallmark of breast, gastric, lung and oesophageal cancer. *Biochem. J.* **2004**, *378*, 17–20. [CrossRef]
32. Isidoro, A.; Casado, E.; Redondo, A.; Acebo, P.; Espinosa, E.; Alonso, A.M.; Cejas, P.; Hardisson, D.; Vara, J.A.F.; Belda-Iniesta, C.; et al. Breast carcinomas fulfill the Warburg hypothesis and provide metabolic markers of cancer prognosis. *Carcinogenesis* **2005**, *26*, 2095–2104. [CrossRef]
33. Fantin, V.R.; St-Pierre, J.; Leder, P. Attenuation of LDH-A expression uncovers a link between glycolysis, mitochondrial physiology, and tumor maintenance. *Cancer Cell* **2006**, *9*, 425–434. [CrossRef]
34. Weinhouse, S. The Warburg hypothesis fifty years later. *J. Cancer Res. Clin. Oncol.* **1976**, *87*, 115–126. [CrossRef]
35. Shin, Y.-K.; Yoo, B.C.; Chang, H.J.; Jeon, E.; Hong, S.-H.; Jung, M.-S.; Lim, S.-J.; Park, J.-G. Down-regulation of mitochondrial F1F0-ATP synthase in human colon cancer cells with induced 5-fluorouracil resistance. *Cancer Res.* **2005**, *65*, 3162–3170. [CrossRef]
36. Yamasaki, M.; Takemasa, I.; Komori, T.; Watanabe, S.; Sekimoto, M.; Doki, Y.; Matsubara, K.; Monden, M. The gene expression profile represents the molecular nature of liver metastasis in colorectal cancer. *Int. J. Oncol.* **2007**, *30*, 129–138. [CrossRef]
37. Baba, Y.; Nosho, K.; Shima, K.; Meyerhardt, J.A.; Chan, A.T.; Engelman, J.A.; Cantley, L.C.; Loda, M.; Giovannucci, E.; Fuchs, C.S.; et al. Prognostic significance of AMP-activated protein kinase expression and modifying effect of MAPK3/1 in colorectal cancer. *Br. J. Cancer* **2010**, *103*, 1025–1033. [CrossRef]
38. Katagata, Y.; Kondo, S. Keratin expression and its significance in five cultured melanoma cell lines derived from primary, recurrent and metastasized melanomas. *FEBS Lett.* **1997**, *407*, 25–31. [CrossRef]
39. Morita, M.; Gravel, S.P.; Chenard, V.; Sikstrom, K.; Zheng, L.; Alain, T.; Gandin, V.; Avizonis, D.; Arguello, M.; Zakaria, C.; et al. mTORC1 controls mitochondrial activity and biogenesis through 4E-BP-dependent translational regulation. *Cell Metab.* **2013**, *18*, 698–711. [CrossRef]
40. Tsai, S.; Sitzmann, J.M.; Dastidar, S.G.; Rodriguez, A.A.; Vu, S.L.; McDonald, C.E.; Academia, E.C.; O'Leary, M.N.; Ashe, T.D.; La Spada, A.R.; et al. Muscle-specific 4E-BP1 signaling activation improves metanolic parameters durign agin and obesity. *J. Clin. Investig.* **2015**, *125*, 2952–2964. [CrossRef]
41. Fujikawa, M.; Imamura, H.; Nakamura, J.; Yoshida, M. Assessing actual contribution of IF1, inhibitor of mitochondrial FoF1, to ATP homeostasis, cell growth, mitochondrial morphology, and cell viability. *J. Biol. Chem.* **2015**, *287*, 18781–18787. [CrossRef]
42. Boreikaite, V.; Wicky, B.I.M.; Watt, I.N.; Clarke, J.; Walker, J.E. Extrinsic conditions influence the self-association and structure of $IF_1$, the regulatory protein of mitochondrial ATP synthase. *Proc. Natl. Acad. Sci. USA* **2019**, *116*, 10354–10359. [CrossRef]

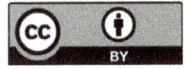

© 2019 by the authors. Licensee MDPI, Basel, Switzerland. This article is an open access article distributed under the terms and conditions of the Creative Commons Attribution (CC BY) license (http://creativecommons.org/licenses/by/4.0/).

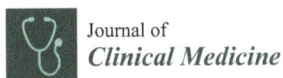

Article

# Morphological State Transition Dynamics in EGF-Induced Epithelial to Mesenchymal Transition

Vimalathithan Devaraj and Biplab Bose *

Department of Biosciences and Bioengineering, Indian Institute of Technology Guwahati, Guwahati 781039, India
* Correspondence: biplabbose@iitg.ac.in; Tel.: +91-361-2582216

Received: 18 April 2019; Accepted: 20 May 2019; Published: 26 June 2019

**Abstract:** Epithelial to Mesenchymal Transition (EMT) is a multi-state process. Here, we investigated phenotypic state transition dynamics of Epidermal Growth Factor (EGF)-induced EMT in a breast cancer cell line MDA-MB-468. We have defined phenotypic states of these cells in terms of their morphologies and have shown that these cells have three distinct morphological states—cobble, spindle, and circular. The spindle and circular states are the migratory phenotypes. Using quantitative image analysis and mathematical modeling, we have deciphered state transition trajectories in different experimental conditions. This analysis shows that the phenotypic state transition during EGF-induced EMT in these cells is reversible, and depends upon the dose of EGF and level of phosphorylation of the EGF receptor (EGFR). The dominant reversible state transition trajectory in this system was cobble to circular to spindle to cobble. We have observed that there exists an ultrasensitive on/off switch involving phospho-EGFR that decides the transition of cells in and out of the circular state. In general, our observations can be explained by the conventional quasi-potential landscape model for phenotypic state transition. As an alternative to this model, we have proposed a simpler discretized energy-level model to explain the observed state transition dynamics.

**Keywords:** epithelial to mesenchymal transition; morphology; phenotypic state transition; quantitative imaging; mathematical modeling; ultrasensitive switch; quasi-potential landscape

## 1. Introduction

Epithelial to Mesenchymal Transition (EMT) is a phenomenon in which epithelial cells lose contact between neighboring cells and become semi-adherent, thereby acquiring migratory mesenchymal phenotype [1,2]. EMT is one of the possible mechanisms of cancer metastasis [3–5]. During EMT, cells switch between multiple phenotypes [6–9]. In general, change in the phenotype of a cell is considered as a transition of the cell from one state to another [10]. Cues from external signals [11,12] and the noise in the cellular system [13] can drive cellular state transition.

The metaphor of Waddington's epigenetic landscape [14] is widely used to understand the directional state transition during differentiation [15]. In the generalized landscape model, cells move through a quasi-potential landscape with basins of attractions. The attractors are at lower potentials and are the preferred destination of cells. Each of those attractors is a particular phenotypic state [15].

The concept of potential landscape has been used to understand the phenotypic state transition dynamics of EMT [10,16]. Several authors have developed dynamical models of gene regulatory networks involved in EMT and created the potential landscape models based on those networks [17–19]. These studies have shown that the potential landscape of EMT has multiple attractors indicating that EMT is a multi-state transition process.

Cellular state transition studies also help us to understand the lineages of different phenotypes. Gupta et al. [13] investigated phenotypic heterogeneity in a breast cancer cell line and had shown that stem-like cells emerge from non-stem-like cells through stochastic state transition. Su et al. [20] investigated the state transition dynamics in drug-induced resistance in melanoma. Using single-cell gene expression study, Mojtahedi et al. [12] showed that differentiation of progenitor cells to erythroid or myeloid lineage involves critical state transition. Hormoz et al. [21] used single-cell analysis to infer state transition paths in mouse embryonic stem cells and showed that these cells go through stochastic and reversible transitions along a linear chain of states.

Cellular states are commonly defined in terms of expression of molecular markers [13,20,22] or genome-wide expression profile [23]. Zhang et al. [9] have shown that TGF-β1-induced EMT in MCF10A cells involves transitions between three states defined by the relative expression of E-cadherin and Vimentin. Several other authors have also categorized phenotypic states during EMT in terms of expression of molecular markers and have developed mathematical models of multi-stable systems to explain the emergence of these phenotypes [6–8]. Here, the assumption is that the levels of expression of molecules reflect the phenotypic state of a cell. However, the state of a cell can also be defined by quantitative phenotypic features. For example, Kimmel et al. [24] used cell motility to define phenotypic states and investigated state transition behaviors in mouse cells.

In the present work, we have used the morphology of a cell to define its phenotypic state and investigated the dynamics of morphological state transition during Epidermal Growth Factor (EGF)-induced EMT. The key phenotypic signatures of EMT in cell culture-based models are the loss of cell-cell contact, change in morphology, scattering, and migration of cells [1,25]. These phenotypic features can be measured quantitatively and can be used to study phenotypic state transition [26–28].

We induced EMT in MDA-MB-468 cells using EGF. MDA-MB-468 is a triple-negative adenocarcinoma cell line of basal A type [29,30]. EGF-induced EMT of MDA-MB-468 cell is a well-established model for EMT [31–36]. We observed three distinct cell states based on the morphology of MDA-MB-468 cells. We call these cell states as cobblestone, spindle, and circular. We show that the spindle and the circular cells are the migratory cells. We have used quantitative image analysis to measure the population distributions of cells in these three states during EMT and estimated the state transition paths using a population dynamic model. Our model and estimation strategy can be used for any state transition system with aggregate data at discrete time points. We show that the state transition paths followed by MDA-MB-468 cells depend upon the dose of EGF and a critical state transition decision is controlled by an ultrasensitive on/off switch. As an alternative to the quasi-potential landscape model, we propose a discretized energy-level model to explain the observed state transition dynamics.

## 2. Methods

### 2.1. Cell Lines and Culture Conditions

Human breast cancer cell line MDA-MB-468 was procured from National Center for Cell Sciences, Pune, India and cultured in Dulbecco's modified eagle medium (DMEM, Himedia, Mumbai, India) supplemented with 10% fetal bovine serum (Thermo Fisher Scientific, Waltham, MA, USA) at 37 °C in a humidified incubator with 5% $CO_2$. For experiments with EGF (Shenandoah biotechnology 100-26, Warwrick, PA, USA) treatment, cells were maintained in reduced serum media (0.5% FBS in DMEM) for 12 h, followed by treatment in reduced serum media.

### 2.2. Phalloidin-FITC Staining

Cells were grown in 96 well plates. After EGF treatment, cells were fixed with 4% paraformaldehyde for 10 min at room temperature. Cell membrane was permeabilized using 0.1% Triton X-100 in PBS, and the cells were stained with 0.1 μM of FITC Phalloidin conjugate in PBS for 1 h. Cells were counterstained with 30 μM DAPI in PBS for 5 min at room temperature. Cells were washed twice with PBS followed by imaging using an Epi-fluorescence microscope (Nikon Eclipse Ti-U, Nikon Instruments Europe BV, Amsterdam, The Netherlands).

## 2.3. Immunofluorescence

Cells were grown in 12 well glass chamber slide (Ibidi 81201, Grafelfing, Germany). After treatment, cells were fixed with ice-cold methanol and acetone in 1:1 ratio at −20 °C for 10 min. Cells were incubated with permeabilization buffer for 10 min at room temperature, followed by incubation with blocking buffer (1% BSA, 0.3 M glycine in PBS containing 0.1% Tween20) for 30 min at room temperature. Cells were stained overnight with fluorophore-conjugated primary antibody at 4 °C. Cells were washed twice in PBS followed by imaging using a confocal microscope (Zeiss LSM 880, Carl Zeiss Microscopy, LLC, Thornwood, NY, USA). Details of the antibodies used are given in Supplementary Table S3b.

## 2.4. Quantitative PCR

RNA was isolated using TRI reagent (Sigma, St. Louis, MO, USA) followed by Turbo DNAse (Thermo Fisher Scientific, Waltham, MA, USA) treatment to get rid of genomic DNA contamination. RNA was reverse transcribed using Verso cDNA synthesis kit (Thermo Fisher Scientific, Waltham, MA, USA). qPCR was performed using Quantifast SYBR Green (Rotor-Gene Q, QIAGEN, Hilden, Germany). All experiments were done in triplicates and normalized to cyclophilin A. Data analysis was done using LinRegPCR [37]. Primers used in qPCR are listed in Supplementary Table S4.

## 2.5. Quantitative Image Analysis

Cells were grown in 96 well plates. After treatment, cells were fixed with 4% paraformaldehyde for 10 min at room temperature. Cell membrane was permeabilized using 0.1% Triton X-100 in PBS, and the cells were stained with HCS cell mask red dye (Thermo Fisher Scientific, Waltham, MA, USA) at a final concentration of 0.001 µg/µL for 1 h. Cells were imaged using Epi-fluorescence microscope (Nikon Eclipse Ti-U, Nikon Instruments Europe BV, Amsterdam, The Netherlands). Ten non-overlapping fields of view were taken for each experimental condition. Image segmentation, object identification, and extraction of geometric features were accomplished using CellProfiler [38]. Classification of cells was carried out using CellProfiler Analyst through machine learning algorithm provided with it [39]. A set of rules was generated by training the tool with images that contain all possible cell types. Using those rules the experimental images were classified. Supplementary Figure S11 shows the quality of the training and the accuracy of the predictions from the trained data set.

## 2.6. Migration Assay

Cells were grown in transwell inserts in 24 well plates (Polycarbonate cell culture inserts with 8-micron pore size, Thermo Fisher Scientific, Waltham, MA, USA) with reduced serum media in both the insert as well as the plate. After 24 h of EGF treatment, transwell inserts were placed in a fresh plate with reduced serum media. After 6 h, cells lying within the insert were removed using a cotton swab and cells that had migrated to the other side of the membrane were fixed with 100% ice-cold methanol. Cells were stained with HCS cell mask red dye (Thermo Fisher Scientific, Waltham, MA, USA), and the migrated cells were imaged using a confocal microscope (Zeiss LSM 880, Carl Zeiss Microscopy, LLC, Thornwood, NY, USA).

## 2.7. Western Blotting

Cells were grown in 35 mm dishes. MDA-MB-468 cells were treated with different doses of EGF for different time points as mentioned in the results section. Whenever required, cells were treated with pathway inhibitor Gefitinib (Abcam ab142052, Cambridge, UK). After treatment, cells were lysed in RIPA buffer containing PMSF (1 mM), sodium orthovanadate (1 mM), sodium fluoride (50 mM) and EDTA (1 mM). Total protein was estimated by Lowry's method [40]. An equal amount of lysate from each sample was resolved by SDS PAGE and transferred to PVDF membrane by wet transfer. The membrane was blocked by 3% BSA in TBST for 2 h, followed by overnight incubation with primary antibody at 4 °C. Target proteins were detected by chemiluminescence (SuperSignal West Dura kit,

Thermo Fisher Scientific, Waltham, MA, USA) using HRP conjugated secondary antibody. Developed blots were imaged using a gel documentation system (ChemiDoc XRS+, BioRad, Hercules, CA, USA). Detected bands were quantified by densitometry using ImageJ [41]. Target proteins were normalized with respect to loading control. Details on the antibodies used are provided in Supplementary Table S3a.

## 2.8. Flow Cytometry

Cells grown in 35 mm dishes were treated with different doses of EGF for different time points as mentioned in the results section. Cells were trypsinized and re-suspended in PBS followed by methanol fixation (final concentration of 80% methanol). Fixed cells were kept in −20 °C for 15 min. Cells were incubated with blocking buffer (0.5% FBS in PBS) for 2 h at room temperature. The cells were stained overnight with primary antibody at 4 °C. Subsequently, the cells were stained with the Alexa Fluor 488 conjugated secondary antibody and analyzed in CytoFLEX (Beckman Coulter, Brea, CA, USA). The positive population was estimated by Overton histogram subtraction. Cells stained with only secondary antibody was used as a control in histogram subtraction. Data analysis was done using FCS Express 5 (De Novo Software, Glendale, CA, USA). Details of the antibodies used are given in Supplementary Table S3c.

## 2.9. Live and Dead Cell Estimation

We have used the method developed by Dengler et al. [42] and Wan et al. [43]. Cells were grown in 96 well plates. After treatment, propidium iodide (PI) was added at a final concentration of 1 µg/mL into each well without removing the media. Cells were incubated at 37 °C for 10 min. Dead cells with compromised membrane would take up PI. Fluorescence was measured using a microplate reader (Infinite M200 PRO, Tecan, Mannerdorf, Switzerland) at $\lambda_{ex}$ = 530 nm and $\lambda_{em}$ = 620 nm. Fold change in dead cells was estimated with respect to time $t = 0$ sample. Similarly, the change in the total cell population was also estimated. After treatment, staining solution (final concentration: 30 µg/mL of PI, 0.1 M EDTA, 0.5% Triton X-100) was added into each well without removing the media. Cells were incubated for 6 h at room temperature followed by fluorescence measurement. Percentage live and dead cells were estimated from this data. A standard curve was plotted to check the linear regime of the assay (Supplementary Figure S12).

## 2.10. Cell Viability Assay

MDA-MB-468 cells were seeded in 96 well plates. Cells were treated with different doses of Gefitinib for different time points. Subsequently, the viability of the cells was measured by 3-(4,5-dimethylthiazol-2yl)-2,5-diphenyltetrazolium bromide (MTT) assay [44]. DMSO was used as a solvent for Gefitinib. The percentage of cell viability was calculated relative to cells treated with an equivalent amount of DMSO in media (without Gefitinib).

## 2.11. Mathematical Model

A state transition model was developed to understand the dynamics in EGF-induced cell state transition. Experimental observations of cell state distribution and fold change in total cell population upon EGF treatment were used as input to the model. From the model we estimated the fraction of cells moving from one state to another state in a particular time interval. Details of the model and the estimation procedure are given in the Supplementary Text (Section S1 to S3). Parameter estimation and analysis of the model were done using MATLAB 2018a. The estimated parameters are given in Supplementary Tables S1 and S2.

## 2.12. Data Analysis

SigmaPlot was used to generate graphs and for statistical analyses. Mean of multiple data points are plotted with error bars representing standard deviations. Wherever applicable, suitable statistical tests were performed and are mentioned in respective figure legends/text.

## 3. Results

### 3.1. EGF-Induced EMT

We treated MDA-MB-468 cells with different doses of EGF to induce EMT. Cells were stained with Phalloidin to visualize the change in F-actin distribution and cell morphology. MDA-MB-468 cells grow as a monolayer of cobblestone-shaped cells attached to each other. Upon EGF treatment, the morphology of these cells changed, and they lost cell-cell contacts (Figure 1a).

Quantitative PCR showed that EGF-treated cells had higher expression of Vimentin, Fibronectin, Snail1, and Zeb1 (Figure 1b). Immunofluorescence imaging confirmed the increased expression of Vimentin and Snail1 post-EGF-treatment (Figure 1c). Our observations in changes in morphology and gene expression are in accordance with earlier reports of EGF-induced EMT in MDA-MB-468 cells [32,34,45].

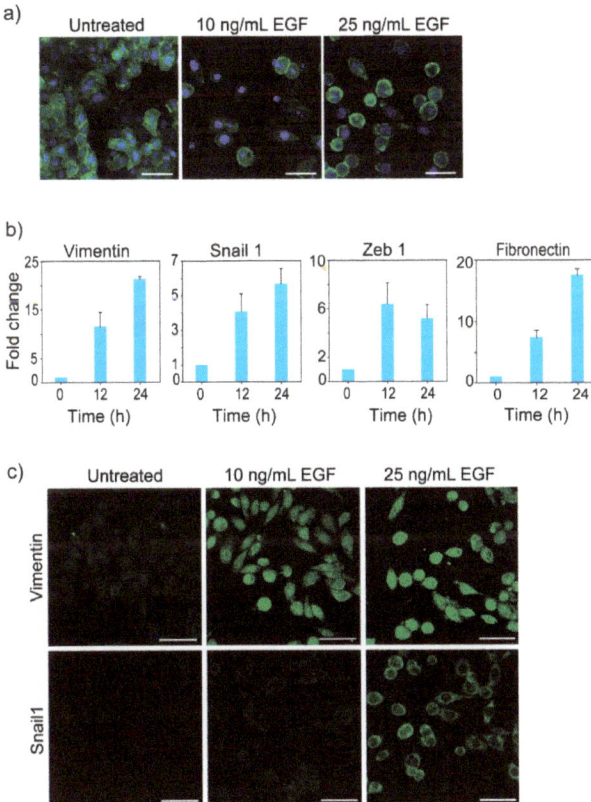

**Figure 1.** EGF induces EMT in MDA-MB-468 cells. (**a**) Cytoskeletal reorganization and change in morphology. After 24 h treatment with different doses of EGF, cells were stained with Phalloidin and DAPI. Green and blue colors represent the cytoskeleton and DNA content respectively. (**b**) Expression profile of EMT related genes. Cells were treated with 10 ng/mL of EGF and the fold change in expression was measured by qPCR. Averages of three measurements are shown with error bar representing standard deviation. Observed changes in expression of all the genes were statistically significant (Kruskal-Wallis analysis of variance, $p < 0.01$). (**c**) Immunofluorescence imaging of Vimentin and Snail1. Cells were treated with different doses of EGF for 24 h and stained with Fluorescent-dye conjugated anti-Vimentin and anti-Snail1 antibodies. Scale bar in images: 50 µm.

## 3.2. Morphological States of MDA-MB-468 Cells

Cells were stained with HCS cell mask red dye and imaged using a fluorescence microscope to observe EGF-dependent change in morphology (Figure 2a). We observed that in our experimental system, MDA-MB-468 cells had three distinct morphologies. We call these cells cobblestone, spindle, and circular cells (Figure 2b). Cobblestone cells were polygonal with cell-to-cell contact. Spindle cells and circular cells were scattered and loosely adhered. All these three cell types were in monolayer, and none of them were floating over the medium.

Through image analysis, we estimated the percentage of each cell types in a population. It was observed that the population distribution of these cells changed with the dose of EGF (Figure 2c). We considered these three morphologies as three phenotypic states.

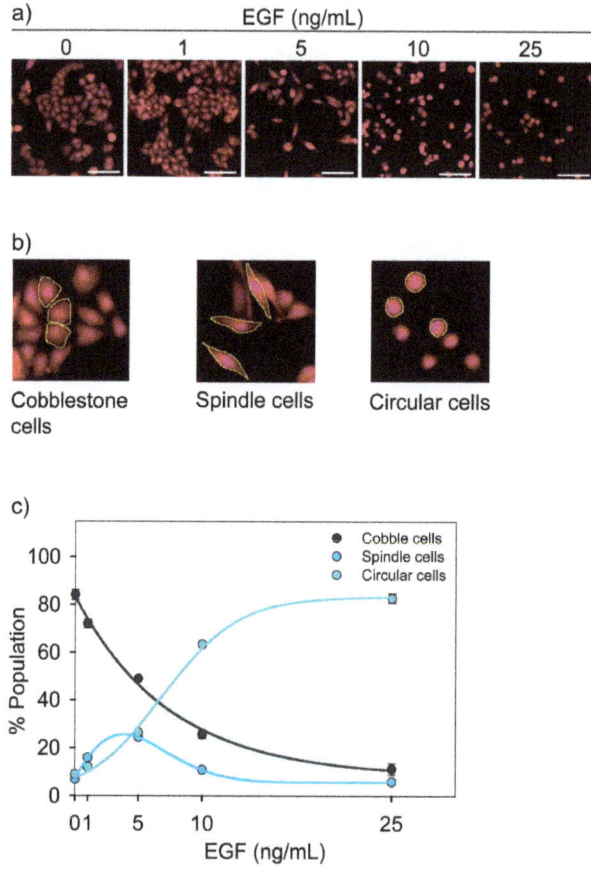

**Figure 2.** EGF-induced change in morphology of MDA-MB-468 cells. Cells were treated with different doses of EGF for 24 h, and the change in morphology was imaged by fluorescence microscopy. (**a**) Representative images for each dose of EGF show the dose-dependent effect of EGF on the morphology. Scale bar: 100 μm. (**b**) Cells with three distinct morphologies were observed. These are named as cobblestone, spindle and circular. Typical cell types in each category are highlighted by the yellow line. (**c**) EGF-induced change in population distribution. The graph represents quantitative data from image analysis. Each data point represents the mean of three independent experiments and error bars indicate standard deviation.

## 3.3. Functional Characterization of Three Cell States

We have done experiments to categorize the cell types based on their physiological functions. Through image analysis, we quantified the extent of scattering of cells upon EGF treatment. For each cell, we measured the number of nearest neighbors. For scattered cells, the number of nearest neighbors would be lesser than that of cells in a cluster. As shown in Supplementary Figure S2, the number of nearest neighbors for circular and spindle cells were lesser than that of cobble cells. The circular cells were found to be more scattered than spindle cells. The median number of nearest neighbors for the spindle and circular cells were one and zero, respectively.

We checked the migratory potential of these cells using the Boyden Chamber assay (Supplementary Figure S3). In the absence of EGF, very few cells migrated to the other side of the membrane, and they were spindle and circular. This shows that spindle and circular cells are inherently migratory phenotypes. We performed the same experiment in the presence of different doses of EGF. As shown earlier (Figure 2c), EGF treatment favored the formation of circular and spindle cells. In the Boyden Chamber assay for EGF-treated cells, a large number of cells migrated to the other side and they were again circular and spindle types. Therefore, circular and spindle cell states are the migratory phenotypes, while cobble cell state is a non-migratory phenotype.

Franchi et al. [46] have earlier shown that membrane filters used as inserts in cell culture experiments affects the morphology of MCF-7 cells. However, we did not observe such an effect of membrane insert on the morphology of the cells in our Boyden chamber assay.

## 3.4. Dose-Dependent Temporal Dynamics of State Transition

The time-dependent changes in the distribution of cells in three morphological states for different doses of EGF are shown in Figure 3. The population of cells remained in a steady state distribution in the absence of EGF (Figure 3a). The steady state distribution had the majority of cobble cells (79% ± 4%) and a minor proportion of spindle (13% ± 2%) and circular (8% ± 2%) cells.

At moderate doses of EGF (5 and 10 ng/mL), we observed reversible population dynamics with an initial rise in circular cells, followed by an increase in spindle cells and eventually the population distribution returned towards the initial state (Figure 3c,d). However, at a lower dose of EGF (1 ng/mL), a marginal increase in the spindle cell population was observed, but changes in population distribution were not statistically significant (ANOVA, $p > 0.01$). At a high dose (25 ng/mL EGF), cells mostly remained in the circular state till 60 h (Figure 3e).

## 3.5. Trajectories of Cell State Transition

The population dynamics observed in our experiments can emerge when cells jump from one phenotypic state to another depending upon the external cue. We used a mathematical model to estimate the state transition trajectories from the imaging data. Usually, cell state transition models are time-homogenous steady-state models that do not consider the death and birth of cells [13,20,47]. However, we have observed that our experimental system was not conserved and there was a change in the total number of cells with time (Supplementary Figure S4a). Further, reversible change in population distribution observed in our experiments ruled out the assumption of steady-state and time homogeneity.

We created a discrete-time population dynamics model that considers all possible state transitions along with birth and death of cells (Supplementary Text S1–S3). This is a generic model that can be used for any experimental system where aggregate population data is collected at discrete time intervals. We estimated the cell state transition parameters for each time interval by fitting the model to image analysis data (Supplementary Tables S1 and S2).

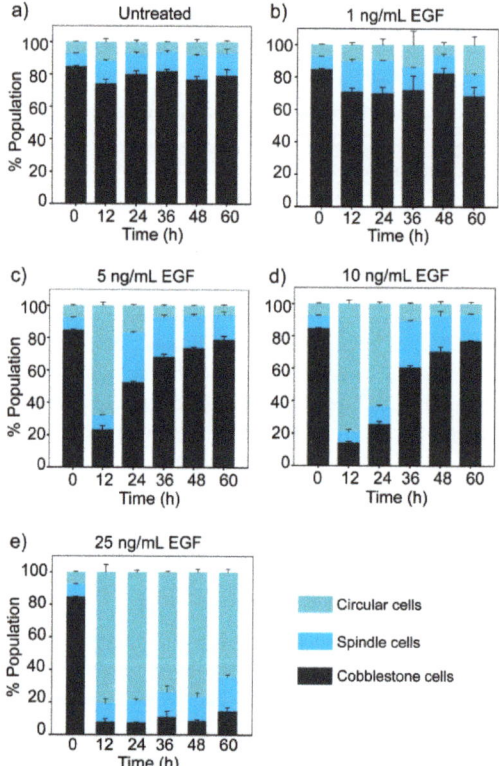

**Figure 3.** Dose- and time-dependent effect of EGF on population distribution. MDA-MB-468 cells were treated with different doses of EGF for different durations, and cells were imaged by fluorescence microscopy. The graph represents quantitative data from image analysis. Each data point represents the mean of three independent experiments and error bars indicate standard deviation. (**a**) In the absence of EGF; (**b**) 1 ng/mL EGF; (**c**) 5 ng/mL EGF; (**d**) 10 ng/mL EGF; (**e**) 25 ng/mL EGF.

Figure 4a shows the state transition diagram for cells treated with 10 ng/mL of EGF. From the estimated state transition parameters, we have calculated the normalized flux of cells through each path at each time intervals. Normalized flux represents the fraction of live cells moving through a particular path in a particular time interval. As shown in Figure 4a, the main flux of cells was in the cobble → circular → cobble path (solid black arrow).

For cells treated with 10 ng/mL of EGF, a substantial increase in the population of spindle cells was observed at 36 h (Figure 3d). The state transition model shows that this increase was due to the transition of some cells from the circular state to the spindle state in the interval of 24 h to 36 h (Figure 4a, blue line) and contributions of other state transition paths were minor.

The 24 to 36 h time interval is crucial as two branching processes were observed in this interval—circular → cobblestone and circular → spindle. To further investigate, we had additional observations at three hour intervals in this period (Supplementary Figure S5).

The state transition diagram for this expanded time interval is shown in Figure 4b. At 24 h, the majority of cells were in the circular state. At subsequent time intervals, a portion of these cells moved to spindle state. These cells in the spindle state followed two paths - either they stayed in the same state or moved to cobblestone state. Therefore, the reversal from circular to cobblestone state had a transition through the spindle state.

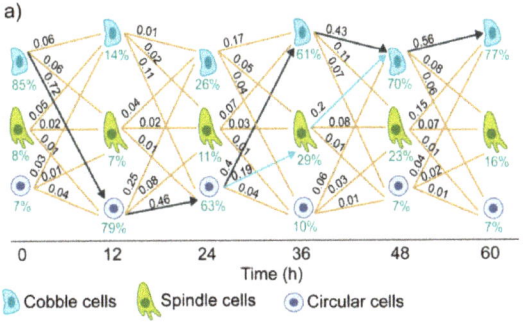

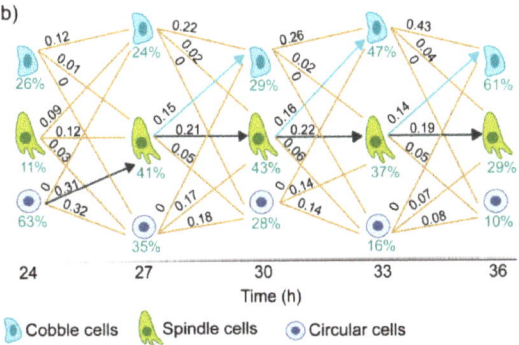

**Figure 4.** Cell state transition diagram of MDA-MB-468 cells treated with 10 ng/mL of EGF. Each line represents one state transition path. State transition parameters were estimated from the quantitative imaging data. Numerical values over the lines indicate the normalized flow of cells through those paths. Pointed black arrows show the dominant transition path and pointed blue arrows indicate the next dominant transition path. (a) State transition trajectories for observations at 12 h intervals till 60 h post-EGF treatment and (b) State transition trajectories for observations at 3 h intervals in the period of 24 to 36 h.

The key inferences from this state transition analysis are—(a) cell state transition in EGF-induced EMT of MDA-MB-468 cells is reversible, (b) the dominant state transition path for cells treated with a moderate dose of EGF is cobble → circular → spindle → cobble, and (c) spindle cells are predominantly formed from circular cells. Therefore, the emergence of spindle cells requires the transition of cells from cobblestone to circular state.

We also constructed the state transition diagram for cells treated with 25 ng/mL of EGF (Supplementary Figure S6). At this high dose of EGF, the dominant state transition path was cobble → circular. Since there was no reversal to cobble state, we did not observe any substantial increase in the spindle cell population in this experiment.

Our state transition model considered all possible paths of state transition along with cell death and birth. However, it can be hypothesized that the observed changes in the population distribution were due to preferential death and birth of cells in specific states and there was no cell state transition. To check the validity of this alternative hypothesis, we created a null model that consider birth and death of cells, but do not consider any cell state transition (Supplementary text, Section S3).

The estimates from this model for the change in cell number and the extent of cell death did not match with our experimental observations (Supplementary Figure S7). Instead, this model predicted very high and unrealistic cell death (Supplementary Figure S7a). Therefore, we rejected the null model.

## 3.6. Dynamics of EGF Signaling Drives the State Transition

The signal given by EGF gets encoded first in the temporal dynamics of phosphorylation of its receptor EGFR. In MDA-MB-468 cells, EGF induced a transient change in phosphorylation of EGFR, with a very fast rise followed by a gradual decline (Figure 5a). It was observed that the level of EGFR phosphorylation and the rate of its decay depend upon the dose of EGF.

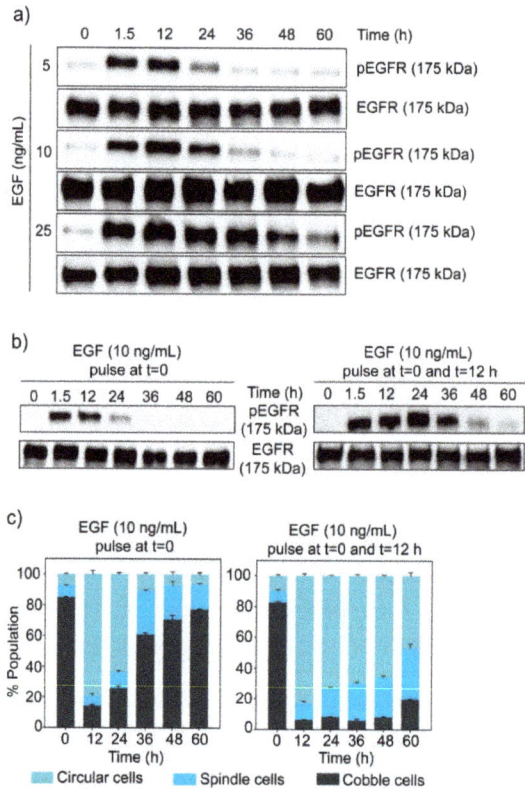

**Figure 5.** Temporal dynamics of phospho-EGFR in EGF treated MDA-MB-468 cells. (**a**) Cells were treated with different doses of EGF and phosphorylation of EGFR was measured at different time points by Western blotting. The experiment has been repeated three times and images of a representative experiment are shown. (**b**) MDA-MB-468 cells were given two pulses of EGF, and phospho-EGFR levels at different time points were measured by Western blotting. (**c**) Population distribution of MDA-MB-468 cells treated with two pulses of EGF. The graph represents data from quantitative image analysis. Each data point represents the mean of three independent experiments and error bars indicate standard deviation.

We also used flow cytometry to detect phosphorylation of EGFR. The temporal dynamics of EGFR phosphorylation observed in this experiment was similar to the results of Western blot experiments (Supplementary Figure S8). In all cases, the distributions of cells were broad but unimodal, indicating the absence of any distinct subpopulation. With EGF treatment, the whole population of cells moved to a higher level of EGFR phosphorylation and then with time, shifted back to a lower level.

In our experiments, we have observed that the circular and spindle cells were scattered and migratory. Lu et al. [48] have shown that EGF signaling promotes cell invasion and metastasis through dephosphorylation of Focal Adhesion Kinase (FAK), a key molecule involved in cell adhesion to the extracellular matrix [49–51]. In untreated MDA-MB-468 cells, phosphorylation of FAK was high (Supplementary Figure S9). In EGF-treated cells, phospho-FAK declined and returned to its high level only when the phospho-EGFR level dropped (compare Supplementary Figure S9 with Figure 5a). Therefore, the temporal dynamics of phospho-FAK was correlated with the temporal dynamics of phospho-EGFR and the population dynamics of cells.

From the observations of phospho-EGFR dynamics and the population distribution data, we can hypothesize that the cells move to circular state only when phospho-EGFR shoots very high. On the other hand, the transition to spindle cell state happens in the decay phase of phospho-EGFR dynamics. Subsequently, most of the cells return to the cobblestone state when phospho-EGFR reaches the basal level. In case of prolonged phospho-EGFR activation (like in 25 ng/mL EGF treated cells), cells remain stuck in the circular state for a longer duration.

To further understand the relationship between the dynamics of phospho-EGFR and cell state transition, we treated cells with two pulses of 10 ng/mL of EGF (at $t = 0$ and $t = 12$ h). In comparison to one dose of EGF, two pulses of EGF generated a higher phospho-EGFR level for a longer duration (Figure 5b). Similarly, when two pulses of EGF were given, most of the cells stayed in the circular state for a much longer duration than one dose of EGF (Figure 5c). These observations strengthened our hypothesis that high phospho-EGFR level is required to move cells to circular state and to keep those in that state.

### 3.7. An Ultrasensitive Switch-Like Response in State Transition

To further substantiate the hypothesis that the level of phospho-EGFR controls the cell state transition, we have plotted proportion of the circular cells against the level of phospho-EGFR in different experimental conditions (Figure 6). This figure resembles an ultrasensitive on/off switch wherein a small change in the input signal triggers a drastic change in the response [52]. The grey shaded region in Figure 6 represents the ultrasensitive region, where a slight shift in phosphorylation of EGFR will have a large impact on the circular cell population.

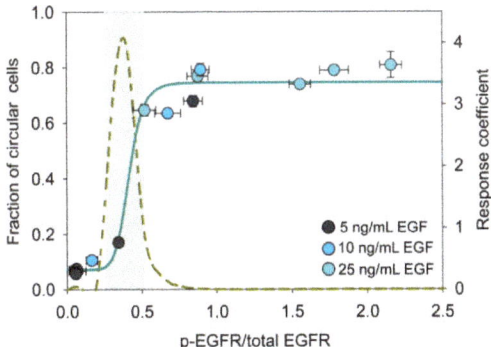

**Figure 6.** Ultrasensitive switch-like response during state transition. The plot shows the relation between the fraction of cells in circular state and phosphorylation of EGFR. Normalized level of phospho-EGFR was estimated by densitometry of Western blot images. Data were fitted to the Hill function (Hill coefficient $t = 8.6$). Ultrasensitive systems have a Hill coefficient greater than one. The dashed line represents the response coefficient [53]. The gray shaded region represents the ultrasensitive region where the response coefficient is greater than 1.

We perturbed this on/off switch using Gefitinib, an EGFR inhibitor. First, we treated cells with a high dose of EGF (25 ng/mL), which induced the phosphorylation of EGFR, thereby turning the switch ON. After 12 h, we added Gefitinib (0.2 µM) and turned the switch OFF. The dose of Gefitinib was much below its $IC_{50}$ value (Supplementary Figure S10).

On EGF treatment, most cells initially became circular (Figure 7c). However, when Gefitinib was added at 12 h, cells started to revert from the circular state to the spindle and cobblestone state (Figure 7a). Additionally, phosphorylation of EGFR dropped, and Phospho-FAK increased immediately after Gefitinib treatment (Figure 7a). These observations confirmed that there exists an ON/OFF switch involving phospho-EGFR that decides whether a cell will be in the circular state or not.

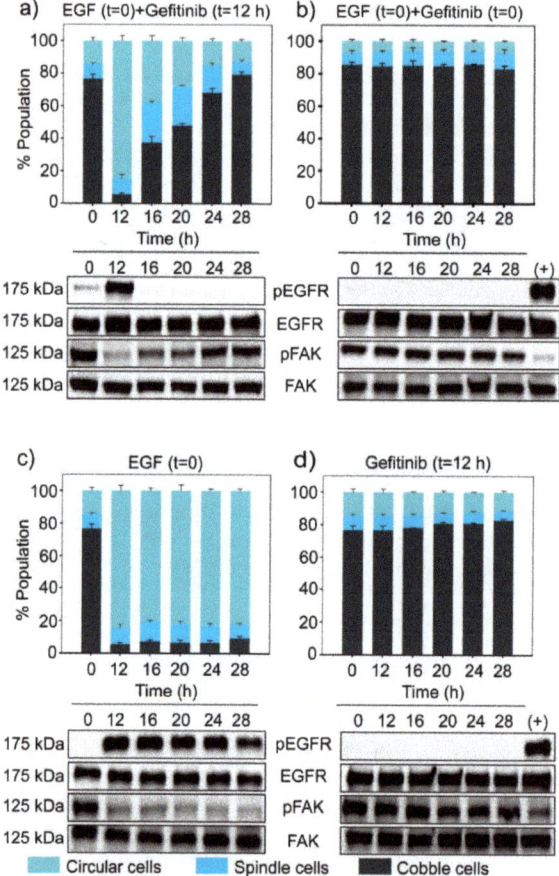

**Figure 7.** Blocking EGFR turns the ultrasensitive switch OFF. MDA-MB-468 cells were treated with different experimental conditions—(a) EGF (25 ng/mL) at $t = 0$ and Gefitinib (0.2 µM) at $t = 12$ h, (b) EGF (25 ng/mL) and Gefitinib (0.2 µM) together at $t = 0$, (c) only EGF (25 ng/mL) at $t = 0$, and (d) only Gefitinib (0.2 µM) at $t = 12$ h. For all the experimental conditions, EGFR, phospho-EGFR, FAK and phospho-FAK were measured by Western blotting and the corresponding population distribution was estimated through quantitative image analysis. EGF treated samples were used as positive control for phospho-EGFR in (b) and (d). The bar graph represents quantitative data from image analysis. Each data point represents the mean of three independent experiments and error bars indicate standard deviation.

## 4. Discussion

Epithelial to mesenchymal transition involves the transition of cells through multiple phenotypic states. In this work, we have identified state transition trajectories in an in vitro model system for EMT using quantitative imaging and mathematical modeling. We used EGF to induce EMT in our experiments and have elucidated the link between the temporal dynamics of EGFR phosphorylation and the cellular state transition dynamics.

Phenotypic state transition happens through two mechanisms—by stochastic fluctuation and by the instruction of an external cue [12,54,55]. Both of these are understood in terms of a quasi-potential landscape with multiple attractors representing distinct phenotypic states. In the first mechanism, cells move from one phenotypic state to another due to stochastic fluctuation [13]. This leads to a steady state distribution of cells in different phenotypic states. In our work, we have categorized cells in three morphological states. In untreated condition, the relative proportions cells in these three states remained almost constant throughout our observations.

An external cue changes the potential landscape pushing cells from one state to another [12,56]. This gives directionality to state transition and deviates the population distribution way from the steady-state distribution. For a time-varying input signal, the changes in the landscape will depend both on the strength of the signal and time.

In our experiments, we have observed both of these time- and dose-dependent effects. For moderate doses of EGF, activation of EGFR was short, leading to a reversible population dynamics. On the other hand, a high dose of EGF caused prolonged activation of EGFR and cells followed the unidirectional path cobble → circular.

We have observed that the spindle cells emerged primarily from the circular ones during the decay phase of EGFR phosphorylation. During this phase, the dominant course of state transition was circular → spindle → cobble; whereas, during the activation phase of EGFR, the path was cobble → circular. This means that the changes in the quasi-potential landscape during EGFR activation phase is different from that in the decay phase. The idea of signal-dependent change in the quasi-potential landscape and associated population dynamics is further substantiated in our experiments where two pulses of EGF were given, and cells were treated with an EGFR-inhibitor.

We have observed that transitions in and out of the circular state are linked with the phosphorylation status of EGFR and the relation is ultrasensitive. An ultrasensitive switch helps a cell in making all or none decision [57,58]. One of the canonical pathways activated by EGF is the MAPK pathway. MAPK pathway is known to have ultrasensitive switch-like behavior [59]. Melen et al. [60] have shown that during embryonic development of Drosophila cell state change triggered through EGFR activation has ultrasensitive behavior.

As discussed above, our observations on the state transition dynamics in EGF-induced EMT in MDA-MB-468 cells are in accordance with the concept of the quasi-potential landscape for phenotypic states. However, our observations can be explained by another formulation of state transition. In this, let us consider the phenotypic states as discrete, and each of those corresponds to a discrete energy level. We have observed that, in the absence of EGF, cells had at an apparent steady-state distribution of states– Cobble: Spindle: Circular = 0.79:0.13:0.08. In quasi-potential models, the steady state probability of a cell being in particular state is linked to the potential of that state according to the relation $U = -\ln(p)$, where $U$ and $p$ are the dimensionless potential and steady state probability respectively [15,18,61]. Therefore, we can calculate the potential for each of the cellular states in our experimental system as $U_i = -\ln(f_i)$, where $f_i$ is the fraction of cells in the $i^{th}$ state at steady state, $i$ = cobble, spindle, circular [62]. This allows us to draw a state diagram with phenotypic states arranged vertically as per their potentials (blue horizontal lines in Figure 8). This diagram is similar to the Jablonski diagram [63] used to represent state transition in molecular spectroscopy.

EGF treatment causes rapid activation of EGFR. During this fast activation, cells move to the circular state that has the highest potential (green arrow Figure 8). This is equivalent to transition from the ground state to an excited state in the Jablonski diagram. On the other hand, the decay of phospho-EGFR is a slow process, and the relaxation in the energy level of a cell is also slow. Therefore, a cell at the circular state does not jump directly to the lowest potential, but first jumps to spindle state that has the second highest potential (red arrows Figure 8).

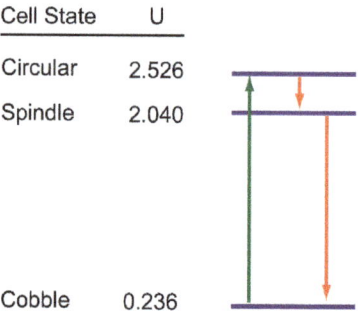

**Figure 8.** State diagram to understand state transition dynamics. Each morphological state corresponds to a specific discrete energy level in this diagram. These energy levels are shown by blue horizontal lines. Corresponding potentials (U) were calculated from the steady-state population distribution of cells in different states. State transitions are probabilistic and only the dominant state transition paths are shown here using green and red lines. All these state transitions were observed within 60 h of observations in cells treated with 10 ng/mL of EGF.

All state transitions are still probabilistic. The dose of EGF decides the probability of transition of a cell from the lowest potential to the highest one and the rate of relaxation. For a low dose of EGF, cells fail to move to the circular state; whereas a moderate to high dose of EGF forces most of the cells to the circular state. Similarly, the dose of EGF controls the rate of decay of phospho-EGFR and in turn, controls the speed of relaxation of cells from circular state to the lower potential states. Therefore, within 60 h, we have observed the circular → spindle → cobble transition in cells treated with 10 ng/mL of EGF, but have not observed the same for 25 ng/mL EGF treatment.

This formulation of discrete energy states has certain advantages over the conventional potential landscape model. Cell-based experiments like those in this paper never give complete empirical information about the shape of the potential landscape. Therefore, understanding the changes in the potential landscape with time and external cues is difficult. Generating a potential landscape is difficult when discrete states are defined using structural or functional aspects of a cell rather than the expression of specific markers. Our formulation does not have these limitations. As shown, one can calculate the potentials corresponding to discrete phenotypic states from steady-state data and then draw the state diagram that can be used to explain state transition trajectories. Further, this model is much simpler than the landscape model and readily amenable to stochastic modeling to explain the state transition behaviors.

Most of the previous studies on state transition in EMT were focused on specific molecular networks. Accordingly, cellular states were defined in terms of expression of specific molecular markers. Even though EMT is a complex process involving a large number of molecules, such studies on specific networks involving a handful of molecules are essential for understanding EMT. However, irrespective of our focus on a particular molecular network, EMT involves specific phenotypic changes in cells. These phenotypic changes can be measured quantitatively, and the measurement techniques can be scaled up for high-throughput experiments. In our work, we have used morphologies of cells to define phenotypic states. We have shown that quantitative image analysis can be used to study the dynamics of morphological state transition in an in vitro experiment. One can implement a similar strategy to study EMT in terms of other phenotypic features of EMT like migration potential of cells. Such studies involving direct characterization of quantitative phenotypic traits would augment molecular marker-based investigations.

**Supplementary Materials:** The following are available online at http://www.mdpi.com/2077-0383/8/7/911/s1, Methods S1–S3: Detailed information about the cell state transition mathematical model, Table S1: Fractional cell division values estimated from the model, Table S2: Fractional state transition values estimated from the model, Table S3: Information about various antibodies used in the experiments, Table S4: Sequences of the primers used in Real-time PCR, Figure S1: Schematic representation of the state transition model, Figure S2: Number of nearest neighboring cells to each cell type, Figure S3: Migration assay, Figure S4: Effect of EGF on cell viability and cell death, Figure S5: Population distribution of cells estimated at 3 h interval in the period of 24 to 36 h post EGF treatment, Figure S6: State transition trajectories of cells treated with 25 ng/mL EGF, Figure S7: Results of the null model for 10 ng/mL EGF treated cells, Figure S8: Dynamics of phospho-EGFR and total EGFR measured by Flow cytometry, Figure S9: Temporal dynamics of phospho-FAK, Figure S10: Effect of gefitinib on cell viability, Figure S11: Efficiency of cell type classification through machine learning, Figure S12: Standard curve to determine the linear regime of fluorescence-based plate reader assay, Figure S13: Pareto front and the objective function distribution of the state transition model for 10 ng/mL EGF treated cells, Figure S14: Fractions of each cell type predicted by the state transition model for 10 ng/mL EGF treated cells.

**Author Contributions:** V.D.: Designed and executed experiments, performed mathematical modeling and analysis, written manuscript; B.B.: Conceptualized and coordinated the project, designed experiments, performed mathematical modeling, and written manuscript.

**Funding:** We thank the Indian Council of Medical Research, Government of India, for financial support through Project No. 55/5/2012-BMS (pt III). We are thankful to the DBT Programme Support Facility, at IIT Guwahati, funded by Department of Biotechnology, Government of India (Project No. BT/PR13560/COE/34/44/2015) for resources and facilities for conducting experiments.

**Conflicts of Interest:** The authors declare no conflict of interest.

## References

1. Lamouille, S.; Xu, J.; Derynck, R. Molecular mechanisms of epithelial-mesenchymal transition. *Nat. Rev. Mol. Cell Biol.* **2014**, *15*, 178–196. [CrossRef]
2. Xu, J.; Lamouille, S.; Derynck, R. TGF-beta-induced epithelial to mesenchymal transition. *Cell Res.* **2009**, *19*, 156–172. [CrossRef]
3. Lo, H.C.; Zhang, X.H. EMT in Metastasis: Finding the Right Balance. *Dev. Cell* **2018**, *45*, 663–665. [CrossRef]
4. Mittal, V. Epithelial Mesenchymal Transition in Tumor Metastasis. *Annu. Rev. Pathol.* **2018**, *13*, 395–412. [CrossRef] [PubMed]
5. Tsai, J.H.; Yang, J. Epithelial-mesenchymal plasticity in carcinoma metastasis. *Genes Dev.* **2013**, *27*, 2192–2206. [CrossRef]
6. Hong, T.; Watanabe, K.; Ta, C.H.; Villarreal-Ponce, A.; Nie, Q.; Dai, X. An Ovol2-Zeb1 Mutual Inhibitory Circuit Governs Bidirectional and Multi-step Transition between Epithelial and Mesenchymal States. *PLoS Comput. Biol.* **2015**, *11*, e1004569. [CrossRef] [PubMed]
7. Jolly, M.K.; Tripathi, S.C.; Jia, D.; Mooney, S.M.; Celiktas, M.; Hanash, S.M.; Mani, S.A.; Pienta, K.J.; Ben-Jacob, E.; Levine, H. Stability of the hybrid epithelial/mesenchymal phenotype. *Oncotarget* **2016**, *7*, 27067–27084. [CrossRef] [PubMed]
8. Jolly, M.K.; Tripathi, S.C.; Somarelli, J.A.; Hanash, S.M.; Levine, H. Epithelial/mesenchymal plasticity: How have quantitative mathematical models helped improve our understanding? *Mol. Oncol.* **2017**, *11*, 739–754. [CrossRef]
9. Zhang, J.; Tian, X.J.; Zhang, H.; Teng, Y.; Li, R.; Bai, F.; Elankumaran, S.; Xing, J. TGF-beta-induced epithelial-to-mesenchymal transition proceeds through stepwise activation of multiple feedback loops. *Sci. Signal* **2014**, *7*, ra91. [CrossRef]
10. Jia, D.; Jolly, M.K.; Kulkarni, P.; Levine, H. Phenotypic Plasticity and Cell Fate Decisions in Cancer: Insights from Dynamical Systems Theory. *Cancers* **2017**, *9*, 70. [CrossRef]
11. Marr, C.; Zhou, J.X.; Huang, S. Single-cell gene expression profiling and cell state dynamics: Collecting data, correlating data points and connecting the dots. *Curr. Opin. Biotechnol.* **2016**, *39*, 207–214. [CrossRef]
12. Mojtahedi, M.; Skupin, A.; Zhou, J.; Castano, I.G.; Leong-Quong, R.Y.; Chang, H.; Trachana, K.; Giuliani, A.; Huang, S. Cell Fate Decision as High-Dimensional Critical State Transition. *PLoS Biol.* **2016**, *14*, e2000640. [CrossRef]
13. Gupta, P.B.; Fillmore, C.M.; Jiang, G.; Shapira, S.D.; Tao, K.; Kuperwasser, C.; Lander, E.S. Stochastic state transitions give rise to phenotypic equilibrium in populations of cancer cells. *Cell* **2011**, *146*, 633–644. [CrossRef]

14. Waddington, C.H. *The Strategy of the Genes: A Discussion of Some Aspects of Theoretical Biology*; Allen & Unwin: London, UK, 1957.
15. Wang, J.; Zhang, K.; Xu, L.; Wang, E. Quantifying the Waddington landscape and biological paths for development and differentiation. *Proc. Natl. Acad. Sci. USA* **2011**, *108*, 8257–8262. [CrossRef] [PubMed]
16. Sha, Y.; Haensel, D.; Gutierrez, G.; Du, H.; Dai, X.; Nie, Q. Intermediate cell states in epithelial-to-mesenchymal transition. *Phys. Boil.* **2019**, *16*, 021001. [CrossRef] [PubMed]
17. Li, C.; Balazsi, G. A landscape view on the interplay between EMT and cancer metastasis. *NPJ Syst. Biol. Appl.* **2018**, *4*, 34. [CrossRef] [PubMed]
18. Li, C.; Hong, T.; Nie, Q. Quantifying the landscape and kinetic paths for epithelial-mesenchymal transition from a core circuit. *Phys. Chem. Chem. Phys.* **2016**, *18*, 17949–17956. [CrossRef]
19. Biswas, K.; Jolly, M.K.; Ghosh, A. Stability and mean residence times for hybrid epithelial/mesenchymal phenotype. *Phys. Biol.* **2019**, *16*, 025003. [CrossRef]
20. Su, Y.; Wei, W.; Robert, L.; Xue, M.; Tsoi, J.; Garcia-Diaz, A.; Homet Moreno, B.; Kim, J.; Ng, R.H.; Lee, J.W.; et al. Single-cell analysis resolves the cell state transition and signaling dynamics associated with melanoma drug-induced resistance. *Proc. Natl. Acad. Sci. USA* **2017**, *114*, 13679–13684. [CrossRef]
21. Hormoz, S.; Singer, Z.S.; Linton, J.M.; Antebi, Y.E.; Shraiman, B.I.; Elowitz, M.B. Inferring Cell-State Transition Dynamics from Lineage Trees and Endpoint Single-Cell Measurements. *Cell Syst.* **2016**, *3*, 419–433.e418. [CrossRef] [PubMed]
22. Pisco, A.O.; Brock, A.; Zhou, J.; Moor, A.; Mojtahedi, M.; Jackson, D.; Huang, S. Non-Darwinian dynamics in therapy-induced cancer drug resistance. *Nat. Commun.* **2013**, *4*, 2467. [CrossRef] [PubMed]
23. Jang, S.; Choubey, S.; Furchtgott, L. Dynamics of embryonic stem cell differentiation inferred from single-cell transcriptomics show a series of transitions through discrete cell states. *eLife* **2017**, *6*. [CrossRef]
24. Kimmel, J.C.; Chang, A.Y.; Brack, A.S.; Marshall, W.F. Inferring cell state by quantitative motility analysis reveals a dynamic state system and broken detailed balance. *PLoS Comput. Biol.* **2018**, *14*, e1005927. [CrossRef] [PubMed]
25. Moreno-Bueno, G.; Peinado, H.; Molina, P.; Olmeda, D.; Cubillo, E.; Santos, V.; Palacios, J.; Portillo, F.; Cano, A. The morphological and molecular features of the epithelial-to-mesenchymal transition. *Nat. Protoc.* **2009**, *4*, 1591–1613. [CrossRef] [PubMed]
26. Marklein, R.A.; Lam, J.; Guvendiren, M.; Sung, K.E.; Bauer, S.R. Functionally-Relevant Morphological Profiling: A Tool to Assess Cellular Heterogeneity. *Trends Biotechnol.* **2018**, *36*, 105–118. [CrossRef]
27. Leggett, S.E.; Sim, J.Y.; Rubins, J.E.; Neronha, Z.J.; Williams, E.K.; Wong, I.Y. Morphological single cell profiling of the epithelial-mesenchymal transition. *Integr. Biol.* **2016**, *8*, 1133–1144. [CrossRef]
28. Mandal, M.; Ghosh, B.; Anura, A.; Mitra, P.; Pathak, T.; Chatterjee, J. Modeling continuum of epithelial mesenchymal transition plasticity. *Integr. Biol.* **2016**, *8*, 167–176. [CrossRef] [PubMed]
29. Neve, R.M.; Chin, K.; Fridlyand, J.; Yeh, J.; Baehner, F.L.; Fevr, T.; Clark, L.; Bayani, N.; Coppe, J.P.; Tong, F.; et al. A collection of breast cancer cell lines for the study of functionally distinct cancer subtypes. *Cancer Cell* **2006**, *10*, 515–527. [CrossRef]
30. Chavez, K.J.; Garimella, S.V.; Lipkowitz, S. Triple negative breast cancer cell lines: One tool in the search for better treatment of triple negative breast cancer. *Breast Dis.* **2010**, *32*, 35–48. [CrossRef] [PubMed]
31. Davis, F.M.; Parsonage, M.T.; Cabot, P.J.; Parat, M.-O.; Thompson, E.W.; Roberts-Thomson, S.J.; Monteith, G.R. Assessment of gene expression of intracellular calcium channels, pumps and exchangers with epidermal growth factor-induced epithelial-mesenchymal transition in a breast cancer cell line. *Cancer Cell Int.* **2013**, *13*, 76. [CrossRef]
32. Bonnomet, A.; Syne, L.; Brysse, A.; Feyereisen, E.; Thompson, E.W.; Noël, A.; Foidart, J.-M.; Birembaut, P.; Polette, M.; Gilles, C. A dynamic in vivo model of epithelial-to-mesenchymal transitions in circulating tumor cells and metastases of breast cancer. *Oncogene* **2012**, *31*, 3741. [CrossRef] [PubMed]
33. Lo, H.W.; Hsu, S.C.; Xia, W.; Cao, X.; Shih, J.Y.; Wei, Y.; Abbruzzese, J.L.; Hortobagyi, G.N.; Hung, M.C. Epidermal growth factor receptor cooperates with signal transducer and activator of transcription 3 to induce epithelial-mesenchymal transition in cancer cells via up-regulation of TWIST gene expression. *Cancer Res.* **2007**, *67*, 9066–9076. [CrossRef]
34. Davis, F.M.; Azimi, I.; Faville, R.A.; Peters, A.A.; Jalink, K.; Putney, J.W., Jr.; Goodhill, G.J.; Thompson, E.W.; Roberts-Thomson, S.J.; Monteith, G.R. Induction of epithelial–mesenchymal transition (EMT) in breast cancer cells is calcium signal dependent. *Oncogene* **2014**, *33*, 2307. [CrossRef] [PubMed]

35. Davis, F.M.; Peters, A.A.; Grice, D.M.; Cabot, P.J.; Parat, M.O.; Roberts-Thomson, S.J.; Monteith, G.R. Non-stimulated, agonist-stimulated and store-operated Ca2+ influx in MDA-MB-468 breast cancer cells and the effect of EGF-induced EMT on calcium entry. *PLoS ONE* **2012**, *7*, e36923. [CrossRef] [PubMed]
36. Verma, N.; Keinan, O.; Selitrennik, M.; Karn, T.; Filipits, M.; Lev, S. PYK2 sustains endosomal-derived receptor signalling and enhances epithelial-to-mesenchymal transition. *Nat. Commun.* **2015**, *6*, 6064. [CrossRef]
37. Ramakers, C.; Ruijter, J.M.; Deprez, R.H.; Moorman, A.F. Assumption-free analysis of quantitative real-time polymerase chain reaction (PCR) data. *Neurosci. Lett.* **2003**, *339*, 62–66. [CrossRef]
38. Kamentsky, L.; Jones, T.R.; Fraser, A.; Bray, M.A.; Logan, D.J.; Madden, K.L.; Ljosa, V.; Rueden, C.; Eliceiri, K.W.; Carpenter, A.E. Improved structure, function and compatibility for CellProfiler: Modular high-throughput image analysis software. *Bioinformatics* **2011**, *27*, 1179–1180. [CrossRef]
39. Jones, T.R.; Carpenter, A.E.; Lamprecht, M.R.; Moffat, J.; Silver, S.J.; Grenier, J.K.; Castoreno, A.B.; Eggert, U.S.; Root, D.E.; Golland, P.; et al. Scoring diverse cellular morphologies in image-based screens with iterative feedback and machine learning. *Proc. Natl. Acad. Sci. USA* **2009**, *106*, 1826–1831. [CrossRef]
40. Lowry, O.H.; Rosebrough, N.J.; Farr, A.L.; Randall, R.J. Protein measurement with the Folin phenol reagent. *J. Biol. Chem.* **1951**, *193*, 265–275.
41. Schneider, C.A.; Rasband, W.S.; Eliceiri, K.W. NIH Image to ImageJ: 25 years of image analysis. *Nat. Methods* **2012**, *9*, 671–675. [CrossRef]
42. Dengler, W.A.; Schulte, J.; Berger, D.P.; Mertelsmann, R.; Fiebig, H.H. Development of a propidium iodide fluorescence assay for proliferation and cytotoxicity assays. *Anticancer Drugs* **1995**, *6*, 522–532. [CrossRef]
43. Wan, C.P.; Sigh, R.V.; Lau, B.H. A simple fluorometric assay for the determination of cell numbers. *J. Immunol. Methods* **1994**, *173*, 265–272. [CrossRef]
44. Mosmann, T. Rapid colorimetric assay for cellular growth and survival: Application to proliferation and cytotoxicity assays. *J. Immunol. Methods* **1983**, *65*, 55–63. [CrossRef]
45. Davis, F.M.; Kenny, P.A.; Soo, E.T.L.; van Denderen, B.J.W.; Thompson, E.W.; Cabot, P.J.; Parat, M.-O.; Roberts-Thomson, S.J.; Monteith, G.R. Remodeling of purinergic receptor-mediated Ca2+ signaling as a consequence of EGF-induced epithelial-mesenchymal transition in breast cancer cells. *PLoS ONE* **2011**, *6*, e23464. [CrossRef] [PubMed]
46. Franchi, M.; Masola, V.; Bellin, G.; Onisto, M.; Karamanos, K.A.; Piperigkou, Z. Collagen Fiber Array of Peritumoral Stroma Influences Epithelial-to-Mesenchymal Transition and Invasive Potential of Mammary Cancer Cells. *J. Clin. Med.* **2019**, *8*, 213. [CrossRef] [PubMed]
47. Buder, T.; Deutsch, A.; Seifert, M.; Voss-Bohme, A. CellTrans: An R Package to Quantify Stochastic Cell State Transitions. *Bioinform. Biol. Insights* **2017**, *11*. [CrossRef]
48. Lu, Z.; Jiang, G.; Blume-Jensen, P.; Hunter, T. Epidermal growth factor-induced tumor cell invasion and metastasis initiated by dephosphorylation and downregulation of focal adhesion kinase. *Mol. Cell. Biol.* **2001**, *21*, 4016–4031. [CrossRef]
49. Matsumoto, K.; Ziober, B.L.; Yao, C.C.; Kramer, R.H. Growth factor regulation of integrin-mediated cell motility. *Cancer Metastasis Rev.* **1995**, *14*, 205–217. [CrossRef] [PubMed]
50. Turner, C.E. Paxillin and focal adhesion signalling. *Nat. Cell Biol.* **2000**, *2*, E231–E236. [CrossRef]
51. Clark, E.A.; Brugge, J.S. Integrins and signal transduction pathways: The road taken. *Science* **1995**, *268*, 233–239. [CrossRef]
52. Kholodenko, B.N.; Hoek, J.B.; Westerhoff, H.V.; Brown, G.C. Quantification of information transfer via cellular signal transduction pathways. *FEBS Lett.* **1997**, *414*, 430–434.
53. Goldbeter, A.; Koshland, D.E. Sensitivity amplification in biochemical systems. *Q. Rev. Biophys.* **1982**, *15*, 555–591. [CrossRef]
54. Chang, H.H.; Hemberg, M.; Barahona, M.; Ingber, D.E.; Huang, S. Transcriptome-wide noise controls lineage choice in mammalian progenitor cells. *Nature* **2008**, *453*, 544–547. [CrossRef] [PubMed]
55. Chen, J.Y.; Lin, J.R.; Cimprich, K.A.; Meyer, T. A two-dimensional ERK-AKT signaling code for an NGF-triggered cell-fate decision. *Mol. Cell* **2012**, *45*, 196–209. [CrossRef] [PubMed]
56. Moris, N.; Pina, C.; Arias, A.M. Transition states and cell fate decisions in epigenetic landscapes. *Nat. Rev. Genet.* **2016**, *17*, 693–703. [CrossRef] [PubMed]
57. Ferrell, J.E., Jr.; Machleder, E.M. The biochemical basis of an all-or-none cell fate switch in Xenopus oocytes. *Science* **1998**, *280*, 895–898. [CrossRef]

58. Narula, J.; Devi, S.N.; Fujita, M.; Igoshin, O.A. Ultrasensitivity of the Bacillus subtilis sporulation decision. *Proc. Natl. Acad. Sci. USA* **2012**, *109*, E3513–E3522. [CrossRef]
59. Huang, C.Y.; Ferrell, J.E., Jr. Ultrasensitivity in the mitogen-activated protein kinase cascade. *Proc. Natl. Acad. Sci. USA* **1996**, *93*, 10078–10083. [CrossRef]
60. Melen, G.J.; Levy, S.; Barkai, N.; Shilo, B.Z. Threshold responses to morphogen gradients by zero-order ultrasensitivity. *Mol. Syst. Biol.* **2005**, *1*. [CrossRef]
61. Wang, J.; Li, C.; Wang, E. Potential and flux landscapes quantify the stability and robustness of budding yeast cell cycle network. *Proc. Natl. Acad. Sci. USA* **2010**, *107*, 8195–8200. [CrossRef]
62. Sisan, D.R.; Halter, M.; Hubbard, J.B.; Plant, A.L. Predicting rates of cell state change caused by stochastic fluctuations using a data-driven landscape model. *Proc. Natl. Acad. Sci. USA* **2012**, *109*, 19262–19267. [CrossRef] [PubMed]
63. Atkins, P.; de Paula, J. *Atkin's Physical Chemistry*, 8th ed.; W. H. Freeman and Company: New York, NY, USA, 2006.

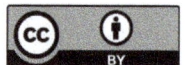

© 2019 by the authors. Licensee MDPI, Basel, Switzerland. This article is an open access article distributed under the terms and conditions of the Creative Commons Attribution (CC BY) license (http://creativecommons.org/licenses/by/4.0/).

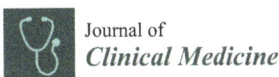

Article

# Interrogation of Phenotypic Plasticity between Epithelial and Mesenchymal States in Breast Cancer

Sugandha Bhatia [1,2,3,*], James Monkman [1,2,3], Tony Blick [1,2,3], Cletus Pinto [4,5], Mark Waltham [4,5], Shivashankar H Nagaraj [1,2,3] and Erik W Thompson [1,2,3,4,*]

1. Institute of Health and Biomedical Innovation, Queensland University of Technology, Brisbane, QLD 4059, Australia; james.monkman@qut.edu.au (J.M.); blick_tony@yahoo.com.au (T.B.); shiv.nagaraj@qut.edu.au (S.H.N.)
2. School of Biomedical Sciences, Faculty of Health, Queensland University of Technology, Brisbane, QLD 4000, Australia
3. Translational Research Institute, Brisbane, QLD 4102, Australia
4. Invasion and Metastasis Unit, St. Vincent's Institute, Melbourne, VIC 3065, Australia; cletusp136@gmail.com (C.P.); mwaltham@unimelb.edu.au (M.W.)
5. Department of Surgery, University of Melbourne, St. Vincent's Hospital, Melbourne, VIC 3065, Australia
* Correspondence: sugandha.bhatia@hdr.qut.edu.au (S.B.); e2.thompson@qut.edu.au (E.W.T.)

Received: 28 May 2019; Accepted: 20 June 2019; Published: 21 June 2019

**Abstract:** Dynamic interconversions between transitional epithelial and mesenchymal states underpin the epithelial mesenchymal plasticity (EMP) seen in some carcinoma cell systems. We have delineated epithelial and mesenchymal subpopulations existing within the PMC42-LA breast cancer cell line by their EpCAM expression. These purified but phenotypically plastic states, EpCAM$^{High}$ (epithelial) and EpCAM$^{Low}$ (mesenchymal), have the ability to regain the phenotypic equilibrium of the parental population (i.e., 80% epithelial and 20% mesenchymal) over time, although the rate of reversion in the mesenchymal direction (epithelial-mesenchymal transition; EMT) is higher than that in the epithelial direction (mesenchymal-epithelial transition; MET). Single-cell clonal propagation was implemented to delineate the molecular and cellular features of this intrinsic heterogeneity with respect to EMP flux. The dynamics of the phenotypic proportions of epithelial and mesenchymal states in single-cell generated clones revealed clonal diversity and intrinsic plasticity. Single cell-derived clonal progenies displayed differences in their functional attributes of proliferation, stemness marker (CD44/CD24), migration, invasion and chemo-sensitivity. Interrogation of genomic copy number variations (CNV) with whole exome sequencing (WES) in the context of chromosome count from metaphase spread indicated that chromosomal instability was not influential in driving intrinsic phenotypic plasticity. Overall, these findings reveal the stochastic nature of both the epithelial and mesenchymal subpopulations, and the single cell-derived clones for differential functional attributes.

**Keywords:** copy number variations (CNV); epithelial-mesenchymal transition (EMT); intratumoral heterogeneity; mesenchymal-epithelial transition (MET); phenotypic plasticity; single cell-derived clones; whole exome sequencing

## 1. Introduction

Cellular heterogeneity within and among cancers is the subject of considerable research, with evidence of genetic and phenotypic heterogeneity in both normal and neoplastic cells across different tissue types [1–4]. The proportion of cancer cells in distinct states is often correlated with tumor type and grade [5–9]. The degree of heterogeneity (whether inter-tumoral or intra-tumoral) is also considered as a significant predictor of metastatic potential [10–12]. In breast cancer, molecular profiling of patient tumors led to the identification of transcriptional breast cancer subtypes, categorized as Basal,

Luminal A, Luminal B, Her2+, Claudin-low and Normal-like [13–16], with further sub-classification of the triple negative breast cancers (TNBC) into 10 distinct groups [17]. Cancer cells in these differing phenotypic states exhibit important differences in their functional properties and clinical course [18–20].

Cellular plasticity allowing lineage transition is generally silenced in adult tissues except in undifferentiated stem cells [21]. Epithelial mesenchymal plasticity (EMP) is not restricted to transition across binary epithelial and mesenchymal states. In fact, cancer cell plasticity can be described as the continuum that exists between the forward process, epithelial-mesenchymal transition (EMT), as well as the reverse process, mesenchymal-epithelial transition (MET; reviewed in [22,23]). The activation of plasticity programmes in cancers arises as a pathological consequence of genetic and epigenetic changes in the tumor cells, and/or in response to exogenous stimuli including inflammation, hypoxia, or paracrine signaling ligands, such as transforming growth factor-β (TGF-β) and epidermal growth factor (EGF), that are primarily secreted by the tumor-associated stroma. Within individual tumors, carcinoma cells often exhibit a spectrum of phenotypic states along the EMP axis, or can often adopt a hybrid epithelial/mesenchymal (E/M) phenotype [22,24,25].

EMP-specific cellular phenotypes can be isolated using EpCAM, Integrin-β4 or CD44/CD24 expression in basal-like cell lines representing TNBC [26–29], or by using E-cadherin in mammary carcinoma in mouse PyMT models [30]. Similar work has also shown that basal, luminal and stem-like cancer cell subpopulations, isolated from different breast cancer cell lines, can stably retain intra-tumoral heterogeneity, and that all three populations of cells are able to initiate tumor formation in vivo [29]. The different pathological subtypes of breast and oral cancer cells have also been observed to transition between these states; non-cancer stem cells (CSCs) in the tumor tissue can spontaneously undergo EMT and dedifferentiate into new CSCs, thereby gaining tumorigenic potential [28,29,31,32]. Therefore, this plasticity has the capability to alter the whole cancer landscape, attenuate the oncogenic signaling networks, lead to acquisition of anti-apoptotic features, defend against chemotherapeutics, and reprogram angiogenic and immune cell functions [31,33–36].

Phenotypic diversity in cancer, attributed to both genetic and non-genetic dysregulation, also obscures many of the fundamentally important facets of cancer. Publicly-available cancer datasets, such as TCGA, Geo, ICGC and other resources, carry data obtained from high-throughput transcriptomic analyses, such as microarray, and RNA sequencing performed on whole cancer tissue biopsies. This provides population averages of gene expression levels, which limits its use for quantitatively investigating changes within the heterogeneous cellular subpopulations, highlighting the paramount importance of single cell analysis in these studies.

Studies have been performed at the single-cell level to evaluate gene-expression and genomic sequencing of distinct cell populations present within varying neoplasms in the breast, liver, kidney, and colon [37–40], allowing insight into the dynamics of clonal evolution in cancers [41]. The divergent modes of cancer spread were deduced through whole genome and single-nucleus sequencing of 68 samples from 7 high-grade serous ovarian cancers to infer the phylogenetic clades of the purified clones [42]. Population-wide, barcoded, single-cell RNA-sequencing data are emerging and herald a major refinement of our understanding of heterogeneity and plasticity [43–45]. Further studies are ongoing to investigate different cancer subtypes at the single-cell level. Variation in phenotypic plasticity within sub-clones has also been studied in breast cancer cell lines utilizing DNA barcode labeling [46], as well as in primary glioblastoma through estimation of copy-number variation of single cells obtained from single-cell RNA sequencing [47]. Dynamics of single cell transitions were also studied in breast cancer cells subjected to paclitaxel treatment to discern specific transcriptional variants responsible for the cell survival, as well as for the ability of cells to recover to their original state [48].

We have employed the PMC42-LA breast cancer cell model, an epithelial subline derived from its mesenchymal parental line, PMC42-ET [49–52]. The phenotypic heterogeneity that exists along the epithelial–mesenchymal axis was examined and validated in vitro, as well as in a mouse xenograft model. We performed clonal propagation of single cells and interrogated the phenotypically distinct clonal progenies for differential facets of plasticity along the EMP axis in a number of assays. We investigated whether the intrinsic plasticity observed is due to genomic/chromosomal instability through whole exome sequencing of sorted epithelial and mesenchymal states in PMC42-LA. Understanding the cellular dynamics of phenotypic states and how they transition within carcinomas is of particular significance in tumor pathobiology and could provide insights into the predictions of clinical outcomes, such as response to therapies and patient survival.

## 2. Materials and Methods

### 2.1. Cell Lines and Cell Culture

PMC42-ET (ET) cells were derived from a breast cancer pleural effusion by Dr. Robert Whitehead, Ludwig Institute for Cancer Research, Melbourne, Australia, with appropriate institutional ethics clearance (Institutional review board of the Peter MacCallum Hospital, Melbourne) and patient consent [53–55]. The PMC42-LA (LA) subline was derived further from the parental PMC42-ET cells by Dr. Leigh Ackland, Deakin University, Melbourne, Australia, [49,53–55] and was found to have more epithelial features than the parental PMC42-ET [51,56].

PMC42 cell lines were maintained in Dulbecco's modified Eagle's medium (DMEM) containing glucose (4.5 g/L), L-Glutamine (0.5 g/L) and sodium pyruvate (0.1 g/L) (Corning, Catalog number—10-013-CVR), and supplemented with 10% fetal bovine serum (FBS; Gibco$^{TM}$, Thermo, Victoria, Australia) and antibiotics, penicillin and streptomycin (Gibco$^{TM}$, Life Technologies Catalog number—15140122). Cell number and viability was determined by 0.4% trypan blue dye exclusion and loaded onto the TC20$^{TM}$ Automated Cell counter (Bio-Rad). Cells were routinely confirmed negative for *Mycoplasma* (MycoAlert$^{TM}$ mycoplasma detection kit, Lonza Catalog number LT07-318). Morphological assessment was performed using an Olympus CKX41 inverted microscope and by Crystal Violet staining [57].

### 2.2. Fluorescence Activated Cell Sorting (FACS) and Flow Cytometry

Cells were harvested with Accutase®(Corning, Catalog # 25-058-CI) and stained with anti-human CD44-FITC (BD Pharmingen), anti-human CD24-PB (Exbio) and anti-human EpCAM-APC (Biolegend) antibodies, as per manufacturer-recommended dilutions for 1 h at room temperature on a rotary shaker. Cells were analyzed in the presence of propidium iodide (1 µg/mL) using a BD LSR Fortessa (BD Biosciences). After doublet discrimination and compensation for spectral overlap, samples were analyzed using FlowJo Software v10.0.7 (BD Biosciences). For sorting, anti-human EpCAM-PerCP/Cy5.5 (Biolegend) antibody was used and cells were sorted using a BD FACS Aria IIu sorter (BD Biosciences).

### 2.3. Single Cell Cloning

Single cell sorting was carried out in 96-well plates from the whole population as well as after selecting the subpopulations (10%) of cells with the lowest and highest expression of EpCAM respectively, across PMC42-LA on the Astrios flow sorting machine (Beckman Coulter) (Figure 3). The wells were microscopically examined to ensure only single cells were seeded per well across three 96-well plates. Wells were propagated to generate single cell clones in equal proportions of media with PMC42-LA cell-conditioned media. Conditioned media was sourced from 1-week old cultured PMC42-LA cells and was double-filtered prior to its use.

Plates were maintained at 37 °C in a 5% (v/v) $CO_2$-humidified atmosphere and were examined every week for the presence of single colonies. After 4 weeks, 36 (12 selected from each 96-well plate) clones were transferred from the 96-well plates into 12-well plates via Passage 1, and then into T25 flasks via Passage 2, and subsequently profiled for EpCAM. The phenotypic stability of four selected clones was monitored throughout the study using EpCAM profiling by flow cytometry.

## 2.4. RNA Extraction, cDNA Synthesis and Reverse Transcriptase-quantitative PCR (RT-qPCR)

Total RNA was extracted from cells using TRIzol (Life Technologies) and subsequent reactions were carried out as per the Bioline Isolate II RNA Micro kit manufacturer's instructions. cDNA was synthesized using the SensiFAST™ cDNA Synthesis kit from Bioline. RT-qPCR was performed using the SYBR Green Master Mix in a ViiA7 Real-Time PCR system (Applied Biosystems, Carlsbad, CA, USA) and analysis performed using Quantstudio™ Real-Time PCR software v1.1 (Applied Biosystems, Life Technologies). The primer sequences are listed in Supplementary Table S1.

## 2.5. Western Blotting

Total cell lysates were prepared for each of the EpCAM subpopulations, the four selected PMC42-LA clones, and and parental PMC42-LA cell line by lysing the cells in the presence of RIPA Buffer (10 mM Tris-HCl pH 7.6, 10 mM NaCl, 3mM MgCl2, 1% nonidet P-40, 1 X Protease Inhibitor tablet (Roche)) on ice. Next, protein levels were quantified using the Pierce™ BCA Protein Assay Kit (Sigma) and 30 µg of total protein from each sample was prepared with sample reducing buffer (2 M Urea, 2% SDS (sodium dodecyl sulfate), 0.125 M Tris HCl, 0.1M DTT (dithiothreitol) and bromophenol blue) at a ratio of 3:1 (lysate: reducing buffer) and resolved on an SDS gel with Tris/Glycine/SDS gel running buffer. The samples were subsequently transferred onto nitrocellulose membranes (BioTrace NT, Pall Life Sciences, New York, NY, USA) using a Transblot apparatus (Bio-Rad) and blocked using 1:1 Odyssey®blocking buffer (LI-COR): 1X PBS prior to probing with mouse anti-E-cadherin mAb (clone 36/e-cad, BD Biosciences), mouse anti-vimentin mAb (clone V9, Dako), and mouse Pan-actin mAb (clone ACTN05, Thermo Scientific). Membranes were then scanned on the Odyssey imaging system (Li-Cor, Lincoln, NE, USA) to obtain a visual representation of the amount of protein present in the samples.

## 2.6. Immunocytochemistry

The EpCAM sorted subpopulation, parental PMC42-LA cells and the single cell-derived clones were seeded at a density of 10,000 cells/well in 48-well plates (Thermo Scientific Nunclon™ Delta Surface-150687). During immunocytochemistry, the growth medium was discarded, and cells were washed thrice gently with Dulbecco's modified phosphate-buffered saline (DPBS; pH 7.5). Briefly, cells were fixed in 4% paraformaldehyde ± 0.1% Triton X-100 (depending on the desired permeabilization conditions), rinsed with DPBS, and incubated with the designated primary antibodies at 4 °C overnight. After rinsing in DPBS, cells were incubated for 2 h at room temperature in the dark on a gentle rotary shaker with appropriate fluorescence-conjugated secondary antibody (Supplementary Table S2) and with diamidino phenyl indole (DAPI) as a nuclear stain (diluted to a final concentration of 1 µg/mL). The plates were then washed thrice with DPBS and images captured on a high-content imaging platform (Cytell Cell Imaging System (GE Healthcare, Buckinghamshire, UK), IN Cell Analyzer 6000 (GE Healthcare, Buckinghamshire, UK) or PerkinElmer Operetta®(PerkinElmer, Waltham, MA, USA) as indicated) with approximately 9 fields of view taken per well. Images were analyzed and merged using the respective software; IN Cell Investigator software v1.0 (GE Healthcare) or Harmony®v4.8 (PerkinElmer).

## 2.7. Cell Viability Assays

Cells were seeded at 5000 cells/well in a 96-well plate. After overnight incubation, the culture media was changed to include predetermined concentrations of selected drugs (doxorubicin, docetaxel, eribulin) for 72 h. For proliferation rate assessment with and without growth factor EGF, the cells were cultured, and readings were obtained every consecutive 3 days using MTT 3-(4,5-dimethylthiazol-2-yl)-2,5-diphenyl tetrazolium bromide) (Promega) assay. Cell viability for the drug assays was assessed by the resazurin-based Alamar Blue assay (#R7017, Sigma-Aldrich, St. Louis, MO, USA) and the florescence intensity in each well was measured after 1 h using a top-reading florescent plate reader (FLUO Star Omega, BMG LABTECH) with excitation at 544 nm and emission at 590 nm. Untreated cells served as a negative control. The experiments were performed in triplicate.

### 2.8. Incucyte®Migration and Invasion Assay

The cells were seeded in 96-well Essen ImageLock plates (Essen BioScience) to achieve a confluent density ($\sim 5 \times 10^5$ per well). After 24 h, cells were treated with mitomycin C (Roche Catalog # 10107409001) for 3 h and scratch wounds were made simultaneously in all culture wells using an Essen WoundMaker. For the Invasion assay using Incucyte, wells were coated with 100 µg/mL basement membrane extract (Cultrex, Trevigen-3433-010-01) in DMEM overnight before cell seeding and, after wound creation, wells were washed to remove dislodged cells and 50 µL of 1 mg/mL of reduced growth factor basement membrane extract diluted in culture mediamedium was added to fill the wound with extra cellular matrix (ECM). The plate was placed in a 37 °C humidified incubator for 1 h to allow the basement membrane to settle, then 50 µL of culture media ±20 ng/mL EGF was added so that the final concentration added was 10 ng/mL. The plates were scanned in the IncuCyte live-cell imaging system (Essen BioScience) at 2-h intervals for 72 h. The data were analyzed with the IncuCyte scratch wound assay software module (Cat No. 9600-0012) and version 2014A.

### 2.9. In Vivo Tumorigenesis

Severe combined immunodeficiency (SCID) mice (eight–ten weeks of age), were purchased from the Animal Resource Centre (ARC, Perth) through the Bio Resources Centre (BRC), St. Vincent's Hospital, Melbourne, Australia. The in vivo experiments were conducted at the BRC facility. PMC42-LA cells were transduced with the BL2T vector (modified by Dr Bryce van Denderen, St. Vincent Institute (SVI) from L2T clone containing the firefly luciferase 2 and tomato fluorescent gene [58]. The L2T clone was kindly provided by Dr. Michael F. Clarke, Stanford University, CA, USA). Approximately $2 \times 10^6$ BL2T PMC42-LA cells were injected into the mammary fat pad of three SCID mice. Nine months post-inoculation, mice were euthanized and the tumors were extracted, mounted with optimal cutting temperature compound (OCT; TissueTek, Sakura Finetek US), snap-frozen in liquid nitrogen-cooled 2-butanol, and stored at −80 °C prior to cryostat sectioning. Before sectioning the tumors onto glass slides, the specimens were processed from OCT to be formalin-fixed, paraffin-embedded. Standard histopathological assessment of the xenografts was performed by haematoxylin and eosin (H&E) staining, and double immunofluorescence staining for EpCAM and vimentin was performed in the Histology core facility at Translational Research Institute, Brisbane, Australia using the BenchMark®ULTRA automated slide stainer (Ventana Medical Systems, Inc., Tucson, AZ, USA). In order to avoid murine stromal contamination in the implanted tumors, all the sections were stained with human-specific V9 mouse monoclonal antibody against vimentin (Roche).

### 2.10. Preparation of Metaphase Spread

After 60%–70% cellular confluency was achieved in 60 mm dishes under standard culture conditions, cells were treated with 10 µL of demecolcine (stock: 10 µg/mL) for 3–4 h. Cells were harvested using trypsin (Corning™ 25053CI) and the cell pellet was gently treated with hypotonic solution (75 mM KCl) for 40–60 min at 37 °C and fixed in cold methanol/acetic acid (3:1). Two or three drops of suspended cells were applied to glass slides and chromosomes were stained with DAPI and counted using confocal microscopy (Olympus Fluoview FV1200 Confocal Laser Scanning Microscope, Olympus, Japan).

### 2.11. DNA Extraction, Whole Exome Sequencing and Processing of Sequencing Data

Genomic DNA was extracted from FACS-sorted EpCAM$^{High}$ and EpCAM$^{Low}$ PMC42-LA subpopulations using the Bioline Isolate II Genomic DNA Kit (Cat: BIO-52067), as per the manufacturer's instructions. After quantifying the DNA and checking the purity, DNA samples were shipped to GeneWiz, Inc. (Suzhou, China) for whole exome sequencing and subsequent analysis. They performed initial quality control assessments and subsequent exome capture using the SureSelectXT HS Target enrichment kit (Agilent Technologies, Santa Clara, CA, USA). All samples were paired-end multiplex sequenced (2 × 150) on the Illumina Hiseq 2500 platform to a median target depth of over 50×. Paired-end reads underwent quality control before alignment to the reference human genome (hg19) using Burrows-Wheeler alignment (BWA, version 0.7.12-r1039) [59] and SAMtools (version 1.6) [60]. Realignment and recalibration were performed using the Genome Analysis Toolkit (GATK, version 3.5) [61]. Single nucleotide variants (SNVs) and indels were called using GATK with default settings. Annotation of variants (SNP and Indels) was performed using ANNOVAR (http://www.openbioinformatics.org/annovar/) [62]. Control-FREEC v 10.6 was used for detecting and filtering the copy number variations (CNV) [63].

## 2.12. Statistical Analysis

All experiments were carried out at least three times unless otherwise indicated. Data were analyzed using GraphPad Prism version 7 statistical software (GraphPad Software, La Jolla, CA, USA).

## 3. Results

### 3.1. EpCAM Expression is Downregulated in Mesenchymal Cells

EpCAM expression as determined by publicly available gene array data is significantly lower in Basal B human breast cancer cell lines, which exhibit enhanced mesenchymal-like features, than in the Luminal and Basal A subgroups (Figure 1A) [64,65]. In the PMC42 system, which clusters with the Basal B cell lines (Eva Tomascovic-Crook, SVI, personal communication), the epithelially shifted PMC42-LA subline has significantly higher expression of EpCAM than the more mesenchymal, parental PMC42-ET cell line (Figure 1B). We found that the PMC42-LA subline comprises an $EpCAM^{Low}$ (mesenchymal) subpopulation in a discrete ratio of 20:80. The presence of an $EpCAM^{Low}$ population suggests an inherent and stable heterogeneity in this subline, which we further characterized on the basis of molecular and phenotypic characteristics and plasticity. $EpCAM^{High}$ and $EpCAM^{Low}$ subpopulations were isolated and analyzed for morphology and expression of epithelial and mesenchymal markers (Figure 1D,E and Supplementary Figure S1D). Crystal violet staining of single cell-seeded, sparsely cultured colonies emphasized their distinct morphology. The $EpCAM^{Low}$ subpopulation cells displayed distinct spindle-like shapes compared to the cobblestone colonies observed in the $EpCAM^{High}$ subpopulation (Figure 1C). Unsupervised hierarchical clustering of the ΔCt values from RT-qPCR of representative epithelial and mesenchymal markers revealed that the $EpCAM^{High}$ population aligned more closely with its parental population, and showed $EpCAM^{Low}$ to be a distinct subpopulation with more mesenchymal features (Figure 1D). The $EpCAM^{Low}$ cells expressed mesenchymal transcripts including vimentin, fibronectin, Notch1 and Neuropilin-1 with concomitant low levels of epithelial transcripts; E-cadherin, claudin-3, claudin-4 and CD24 in $EpCAM^{Low}$ cells were 2-fold lower as compared to parental PMC42-LA cells (Figure 1E). Higher expression of Snail, Slug and Zeb1 was also confirmed in the $EpCAM^{Low}$ subpopulation (Figure 1E). No significant difference was found in mRNA expression of the proliferation marker transcripts despite mesenchymal cell cultures expanding much more slowly than epithelial cells, as shown by the proliferative rate assessment in $EpCAM^{High}$ and $EpCAM^{Low}$ subpopulations, respectively. An initial lag was also observed in the proliferative rate of the $EpCAM^{Low}$ subpopulation (Figure 1F). These results led us to ask further whether isolated epithelial and mesenchymal states proliferate and remain in their purified phenotypic states, or whether the two phenotypes each have the capability to transition back towards the PMC42-LA mixed phenotype.

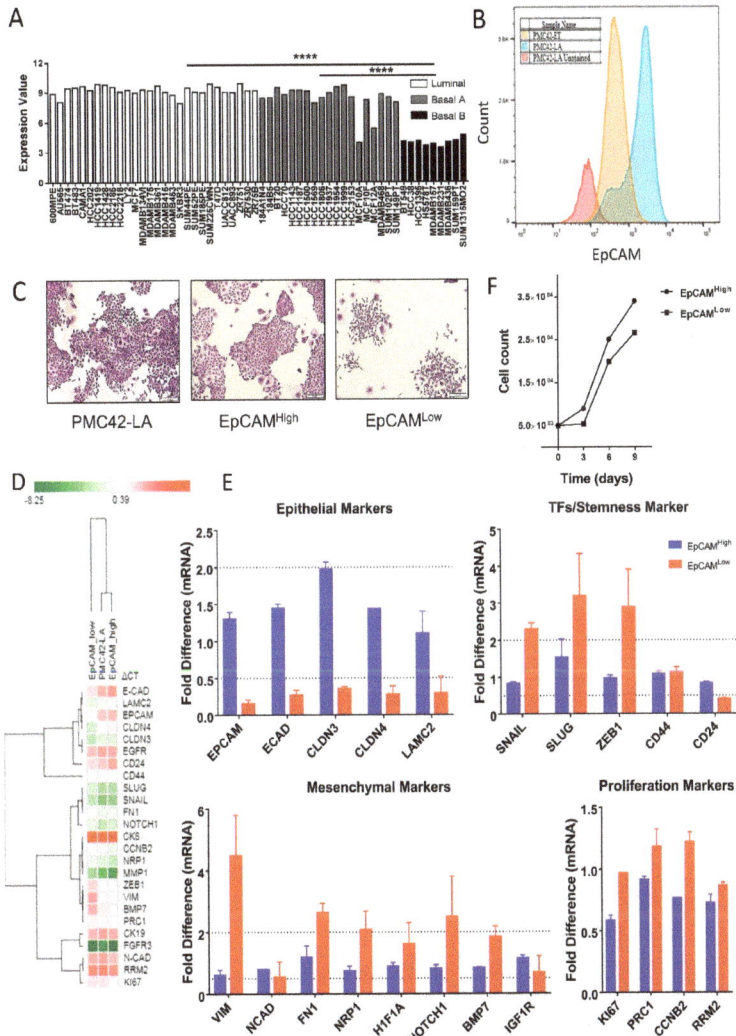

**Figure 1.** (**A**) EpCAM assessment in gene expression data of 50 breast cancer cell lines and five non-malignant breast cell lines, including three subtypes of luminal, basal A and basal B/mesenchymal. Data are from Array Express (accession no. E-MTAB-181) (Heiser et al., 2012) and are normalized log2-transformed values; **** $P < 0.0001$ (one-way ANOVA, with Tukey's multiple comparisons). (**B**) Histogram plots depicting differences in the surface levels of EpCAM protein across PMC42-ET and PMC42-LA cell lines. Negative control represents PMC42-LA unstained cells. The EpCAM expression is markedly low in the PMC42-ET parental cell line and the PMC42-LA cell line showed 15%–20% proportion of the population as EpCAM$^{Low}$. (**C**) Crystal violet staining of the colony images of PMC42 LA population and its subpopulations to emphasize the distinct mesenchymal phenotype of the EpCAM$^{Low}$ subpopulation when grown sparsely. (**D**) Hierarchical clustering performed using the Morpheus (Gene-E tool) of the normalized (ΔCt) values. (**E**) Gene expression analysis of 22 genes related to EMT markers and proliferation marker in EpCAM sorted subpopulations relative to expression in the parental (unsorted) PMC42-LA cell line. Data are represented as the mRNA fold difference ± standard error of the mean (SEM) (Results are from $n = 3$ independent biological experiments). (**F**) Proliferation rate for EpCAM$^{Low}$ and EpCAM$^{High}$ subpopulations were evaluated by MTT assay (data are representative of $n = 3$ independent biological experiments).

## 3.2. Cell-State Dynamics in PMC42-LA Breast Cancer Subpopulations

Following isolation of subpopulations of cells that were validated to show distinct epithelial and mesenchymal characteristics, respectively, we sought to determine the potential involvement of EMT and MET in the persistence of these two subpopulations in PMC42-LA cultures. FACS-sorted EpCAM$^{High}$ and EpCAM$^{Low}$ PMC42-LA subpopulations exhibited an average profile of 80:20, respectively. The outlying 10% of the cells in each direction were selected, resulting in subpopulations which were 98%–99% pure, based on post-sort quality control assessment. Sequential EpCAM profiling using FACS was performed every two weeks for eight weeks to evaluate the proportions of epithelial and mesenchymal cells as determined by their EPCAM expression status. For the EpCAM$^{High}$ subpopulation, we observed a rapid progression toward parental equilibrium within two–three weeks. In contrast, the time taken for a return to equilibrium for the EpCAM$^{Low}$ subpopulation was more than eight weeks (Figure 2A). PMC42-LA parental cells and the EpCAM-sorted subpopulations were also imaged for vimentin expression after two passages using immunocytochemistry and high-content imaging, with representative images collated and analyzed using Harmony software (Figure 2B). In the EpCAM$^{Low}$ subpopulation, ~57% of cells were positive for vimentin expression, compared to 18%–21% vimentin-positive cells in both the PMC-42 LA parental and EpCAM$^{High}$ populations (Figure 2C), which validated the results obtained using FACS (Figure 2A). These data revealed that this cell system tends to show a reversion to the parental phenotype transition; hence, single cell sorting and clonal propagation was then performed to gain insight into the dynamics of such inherent cellular plasticity and to investigate the subtleties of this transition beginning from a single cell (Figure 3).

## 3.3. PMC42-LA Tumors Exhibit Small Proportion of EMP

We also looked for evidence of plasticity in the PMC42-LA cells in vivo. Standard histopathological assessment of PMC42-LA xenografts was performed initially by H&E staining. The tumor was composed of a large central necrotic area surrounded by viable tissue at the periphery of the tumor (Figure 4A). To assess whether PMC42-LA derived tumors also display a similar proportion of epithelial mesenchymal heterogeneity as found in vitro, a xenograft tumor was immunostained for both EpCAM (red) and vimentin (green) (Figure 4B). Consistent expression of EpCAM was observed across the cell junctions. Overall, quantification from differential staining revealed 3.6% of the cells were vimentin-positive. Vimentin-positive cells (green), which indicate EMT, were clearly seen as clusters in distinct areas of the tumor, specifically at the tumor periphery and at inter-tumoral regions along the tumor-necrosis border. Use of the human-specific V9 anti-vimentin antibody clearly distinguishes the presence of EMT in cancer cells from surrounding mouse stroma.

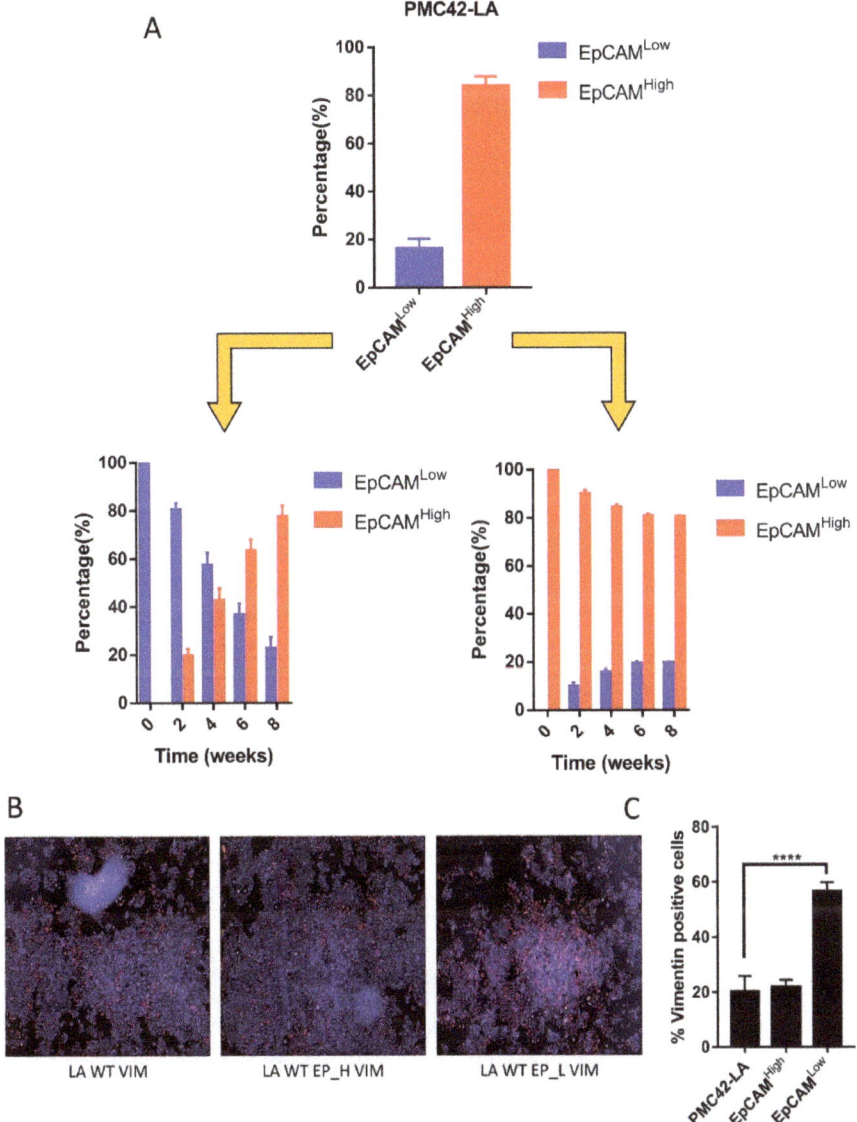

**Figure 2.** (**A**) Bar charts showing the proportion of cells in EpCAM$^{low}$ and EpCAM$^{high}$ state as intermittently assessed by FACS every two weeks from in vitro culture of FACS isolated EpCAM low and high subpopulations. Data analyzed using repeated measures ANOVA for temporal dynamics signify $P = 0.0001$ for EpCAM high transitions and $P < 0.0001$ for EpCAM Low transitions. (**B**) Immunofluorescence images captured on Operetta high-content imaging system and clustering of nine images at 10× resolution from the center of the well for vimentin expression. (**C**) Bar graph quantifying the number of cells positive for Vimentin expression across PMC42-LA parental and EpCAM sorted subpopulations using Operetta Harmony software. Significant differences were calculated using a paired *t*-test, **** $P < 0.0001$.

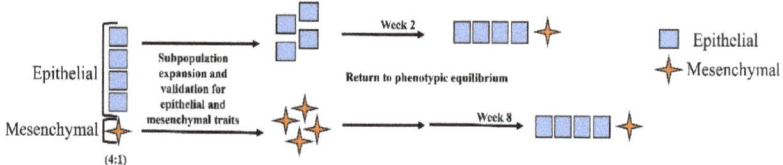

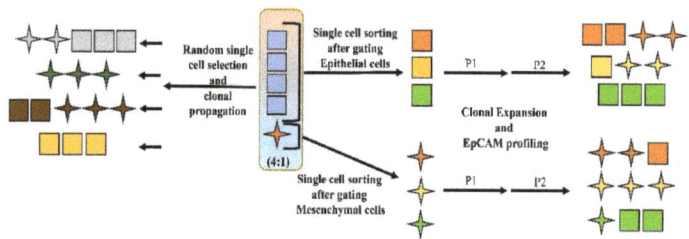

**Figure 3.** (**A**) Schematic depicting the results of phenotypic equilibrium achieved across sorted and passaged EpCAM subpopulations. (**B**) FACS based single cell sorting and clonal propagation to examine the proportion of epithelial and mesenchymal cells using EpCAM profiling. Single cells were randomly selected across the whole cell population, as well as after gating for epithelial and mesenchymal selection, and seeded in 96-well plates. The progeny of the cells were EpCAM profiled after Passage 2 to identify variation across phenotypic plasticity.

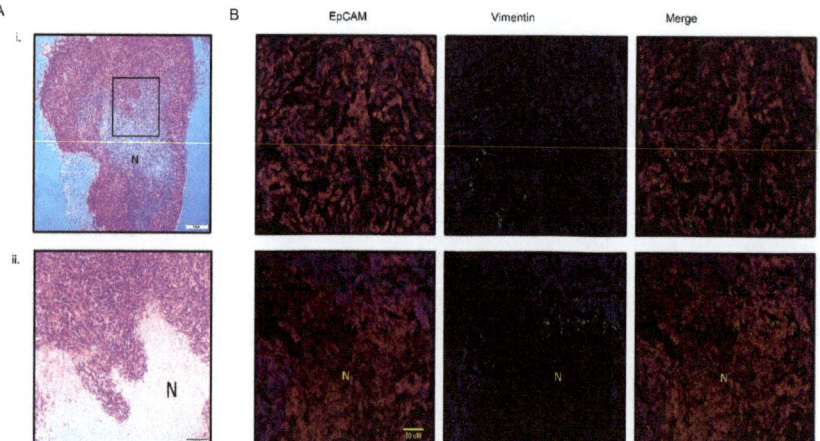

**Figure 4.** (**A**) Hematoxylin and eosin staining of xenograft PMC42-LA tumor; (*i*) low magnification at 4× (*ii*) high magnification at 10×. (**B**) Representative images (20×) of EpCAM (red), Vimentin (green), and nucleus (blue) staining in PMC42-LA derived tumor from mice. Ubiquitous expression of EpCAM was observed across the cell junctions whereas ~4% vimentin-positive cells were distributed randomly across the whole tumor sectioned slide as well as being present around the necrotic area of tumor. N, necrotic area. Scale bar, 50 µM.

*3.4. Generation of Single Cell Clones*

Phenotypic Plasticity Exists across Single Cell-Derived Clones

After three weeks in culture, a number of single cell clones were selected, fixed and co-stained for EpCAM and vimentin. Interestingly, in clones derived from the parental PMC42-LA population, differential intrinsic E/M plasticity was observed, with some clones exhibiting spontaneous EMT as evidenced by vimentin staining (Figure 5A). Single-cell clones also demonstrated morphological diversity, with some exhibiting tightly associated cell junctions and tight cobblestone morphology consistent with an epithelial phenotype, while others exhibited spindle-like and elongated features, consistent with a mesenchymal phenotype. Some of the single-cell clones derived from PMC42-LA parental cells also exhibited mixed morphologies, where colonies of both tight clusters and elongated cells could be observed (Figure 5B).

Clones derived from the EpCAM$^{Low}$ subpopulations were validated as having a mesenchymal phenotype when compared to their parental PMC42-LA line, proving the EpCAM profiling by FACS to be a robust method to distinguish and isolate cells along the EMP axis for temporal propagation. Twelve random clones were selected for EpCAM profiling, where 33% of the clones displayed an epithelial phenotype, 25% of the clones displayed a mesenchymal-enriched phenotype, and the remaining 42% of the clones retained a heterogeneous mixture phenotype (Figure 5C). All clones displayed EpCAM profiles that were distinct from the parental population (80:20), highlighting the phenotypic plasticity and stochastic EMP processes that exist in subpopulations of cancer cells.

*3.5. Characterization of the Four Selected Clones across EMP Axis*

Four clones (Clones A–D) selected according to their differential EpCAM proportions (Figure 5D,E) were further assessed for their intrinsic phenotypes along the EMP axis. Two clones were selected based on predominant EpCAM$^{High}$ (epithelial) and EpCAM$^{Low}$ (mesenchymal) phenotype (Clone A and Clone B), while an additional two were selected due to their mixed nature, containing 75:25 (Clone C) and 60:40 (Clone D) of EpCAM$^{High}$ and EpCAM$^{Low}$ states, respectively. The expression level of 18 EMT marker genes was assessed to score the selected clones according to their EMP status (Figure 6A). Hierarchical clustering for EMP markers reflected the close alignment of Clones A and C with the PMC42-LA parental line, while Clones D and B clustered as a separate clade, exhibiting differential levels of plasticity features at the transcriptomic level with regard to their EMP status. The expression levels of mesenchymal markers were significantly higher for Clone B. Clone C and Clone D display intermediate/mixed phenotypes (consistent with their EpCAM profiling, Figure 5D). PMC42-LA cells are responsive to EGF stimulation for proliferation and EMT induction [57], so clones were also evaluated for the effect of EGF. EGF treatment induced a transcriptionally measurable EMT in Clones A, C and D, but not Clone B, which exhibits a high basal expression of mesenchymal genes, suggesting EGF cannot drive the EMT beyond this point in this system (Supplementary Table S3). Clones were assayed for their proliferation rates and the mesenchymal phenotype Clone B demonstrated significantly lower proliferation rates compared to parental PMC42-LA cells. With EGF stimulation, increases in proliferation were observed for parental and the clonal progenies except for Clone A (Figure 6B).

Immunofluorescence staining revealed a marked difference in the spatial localization and expression of markers for EMP status across the different clones. PMC42-LA and Clone A possessed a predominantly epithelial morphology with segments of EpCAM and E-cadherin expression on the cell junctions, which were missing from Clone B. Each clone, as well as a parental cell line has vimentin-positive cells, however the percentage varies for each clone (Figure 6D). The number and intensity of vimentin-positive cells was higher for Clone B (also supported by Western blot analysis (Figure 6C)) whereas Clone D showed constitutively higher expression of N-cadherin on the cell junctions as compared to parental and other clones. There were subtle differences between the parental PMC42-LA cells and the clones in the cytoskeletal arrangement and focal adhesion formation of the cells clustered in colonies as depicted by phalloidin and paxillin staining, respectively (Figure 6D).

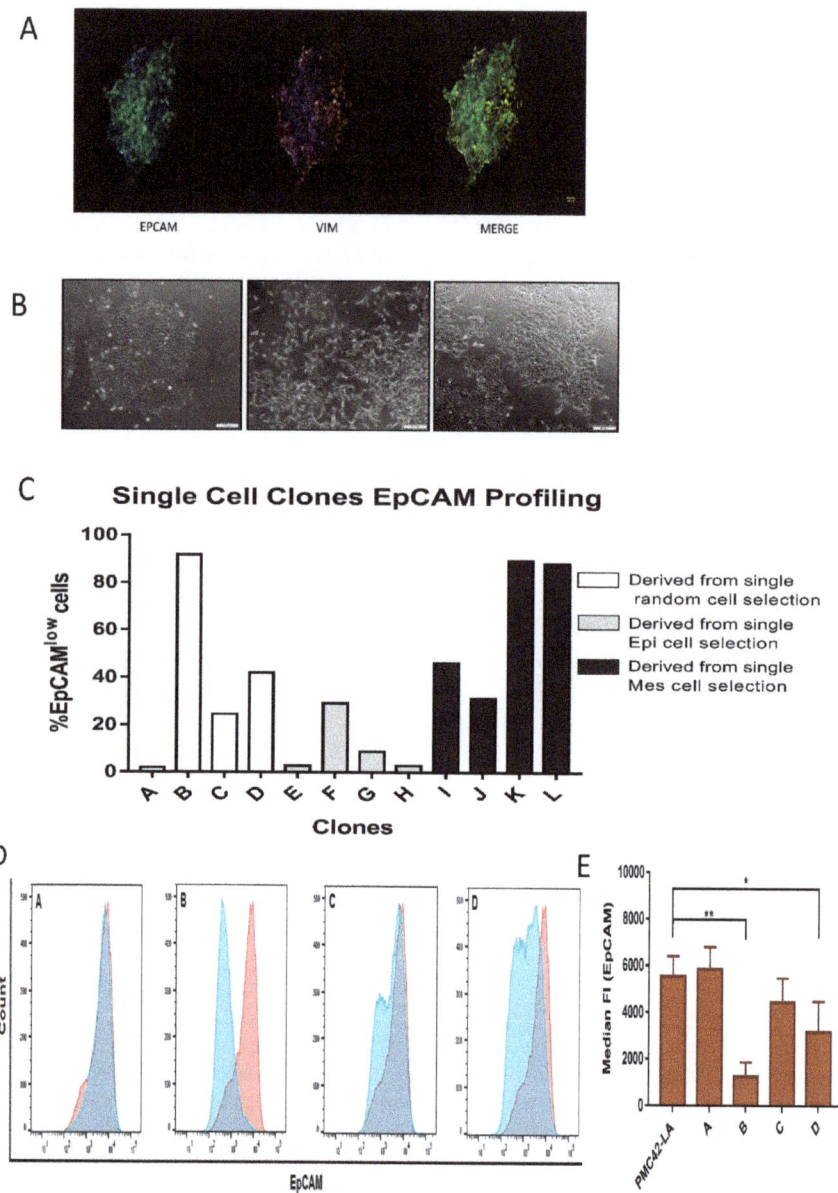

**Figure 5.** (**A**) EpCAM expression on the cellular junctions and concomitant vimentin-positive cells growing out from an individual cell derived clone (pictures were taken after three weeks of single-cell clonal propagation). (**B**) Morphological assessment of epithelial clustered colony, mesenchymal segregated cells, and mixed epithelial and elongated colonies obtained from clonal propagation of single cells after gating for EpCAM$^{low}$ and EpCAM$^{high}$ cells after the first passage. Scale bar, 200 µM. (**C**) FACS profiling for EpCAM results in distribution of EpCAM low and high cells at variable ratios across various single cell-derived clones. (**D**) Histograms depicting the proportion of EpCAM high and EpCAM low cells in the four selected clones as overlap with parental EpCAM profile (red). (**E**) Staining intensity of EpCAM for the clones and parental PMC42-LA cells assessed by median fluorescence intensity unit ($n = 4$). Significant differences were calculated by one-way ANOVA and nonparametric Dunnett's multiple comparisons test. * $P < 0.05$, ** $P < 0.01$.

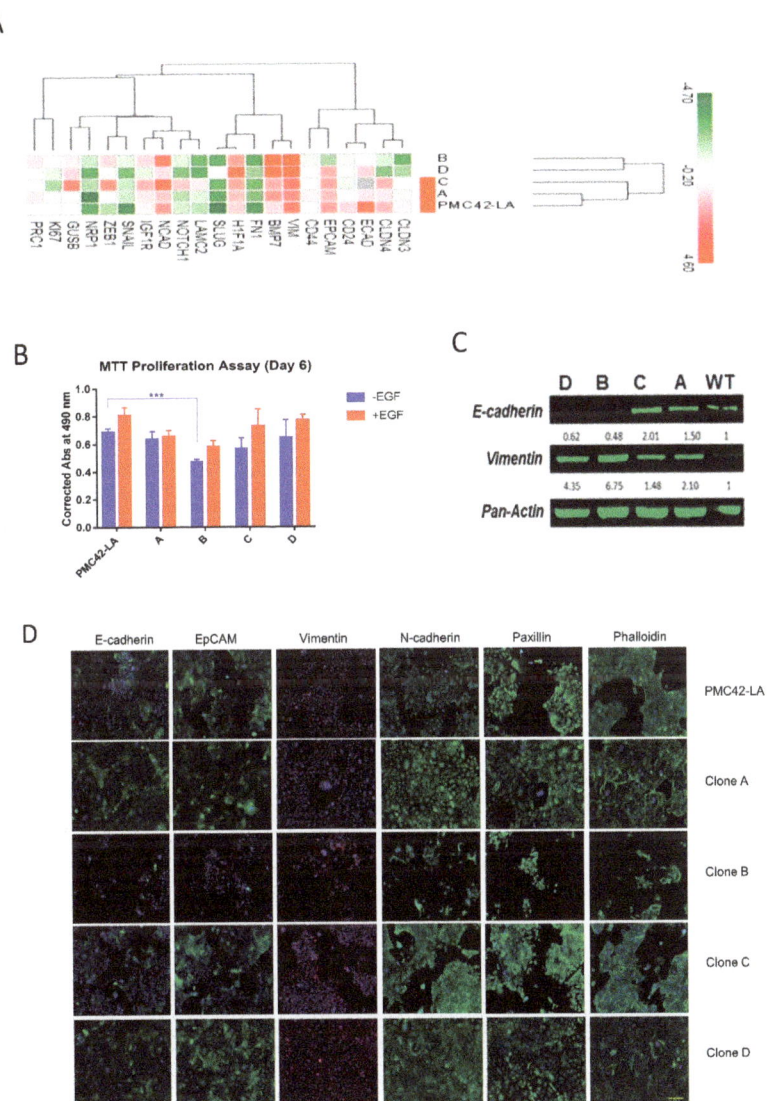

**Figure 6.** (**A**) Hierarchical clustering of the ΔCt values for the transcriptome data with epithelial-mesenchymal transition (EMT) marker genes for the four clones and PMC42-LA cell line. (**B**) Proliferation rate assessment for the selected clones and parental PMC42-LA with and without epidermal growth factor (EGF) stimulation ($n = 3$). Significant differences were calculated by two-way ANOVA and Sidak's multiple comparisons test. *** $P < 0.001$ (**C**) The expression of E-cadherin and vimentin as determined by immunoblotting for the clones and parental PMC42-LA cells. Pan Actin was used as the loading control. (**D**) Immunofluorescence microscopy analysis of changes in the localization and expression levels of EMT influencing marker proteins. Selected clones and parental PMC42-LA subline were stained with antibodies against the epithelial markers E-cadherin and EpCAM, against the mesenchymal marker Vimentin and N-cadherin, against paxillin to detect focal adhesion plaques, and with phalloidin to visualize the actin cytoskeleton. Scale bar, 100 μm.

## 3.6. Clone D Demonstrates Enhanced Migratory and Invasive Capacity Compared to Other Clones, but Similar to the Parental Cell Line

Analyzing collective cell migration in a scratch wound assay, we found that Clone D migrated comparably to the parental cell line, whereas Clones B and C were significantly slower to repair the wound. Only the parental PMC42-LA cells and Clone D showed an increased rate of wound closure with EGF treatment relative to their unstimulated counterparts (Figure 7A,B). At the end time point of the assay, i.e., after three days, cells were fixed and stained with vimentin antibody. Vimentin-positive cells were observed along the wound edge of all the clones and the parental PMC42-LA cells (Supplementary Figure S2A). Interestingly, Clone B with high endogenous vimentin expression did not possess a strong migratory phenotype in this assay. Using Matrigel to mimic invasion through the basement membrane and into ECM, the parental cell line PMC42-LA and Clone D displayed the strongest invasive phenotype, and only clone D and the parental PMC42-LA cells were more invasive after EGF stimulation compared to untreated cells. The invasive capacity was thus similar for the clones and parental cell line compared to that of the migratory phenotype, despite a drastic reduction in the extent of wound closure after 72 h (reduced by ~20% in the absence of EGF) (Figure 7C).

## 3.7. Variation in Stemness Traits across the Clones and PMC42-LA

Next, the parental cell line and its derivative clone were assessed for their stemness properties using CD44 and CD24 markers. Interestingly, a biphasic population distribution for CD24 expression was observable for the PMC42 parental line but not in any of the sub-clones. The median fluorescence intensity of CD44 was lower for Clones B, C and D compared to the parental line and Clone A (Figure 7D). Low CD24 expression also correlated positively with lower EpCAM expression in Basal B cell lines (Supplementary Figure S1C) [65]. Clone B, with the lowest EpCAM expression showed 73.3% of cells within the CD24 low fraction, whereas the remaining clones possessed a CD24 low fraction (Q1: representing CD44 high, CD24 low) of less than 25% (Figure 7D). The EpCAM$^{Low}$ subpopulation also had a marked increase (~10%) in their CD44$^{High}$/CD24$^{Low}$ "stem-like" population relative to the parental cell line (Supplementary Figure S1A,B), and is consistent with RT-qPCR results showing consistent CD44 expression but 2-fold downregulation in CD24 expression compared to parental PMC42-LA cells (Figure 1E).

## 3.8. Variable Drug Resistance of Single Cell-Derived Clones of PMC42-LA

The chemotherapeutic sensitivity of PMC42-LA and sub-clones was also investigated with doxorubicin, eribulin and docetaxel. The half maximal inhibitory concentration (IC50) of parental PMC42-LA and the selected clones was determined using serial 3-fold dilutions of each drug, followed by Alamar Blue assay. The IC50 of parental PMC42-LA was calculated as 98.94 nM for doxorubicin, 0.83 nM for eribulin and 0.79 nM for docetaxel (Supplementary Figure S2). The sub-clones showed variable response to the different chemo-treatments (Figure 8A). This assay revealed that Clone D was significantly more resistant than the other clones and the parental cell line across all three drug treatments. These data demonstrate that in this cell system, the epithelial or mesenchymal enriched sub-clones were surpassed by Clone D (with mixed phenotype states of 60 epithelial: 40 mesenchymal cells) in their chemo-resistance phenotype.

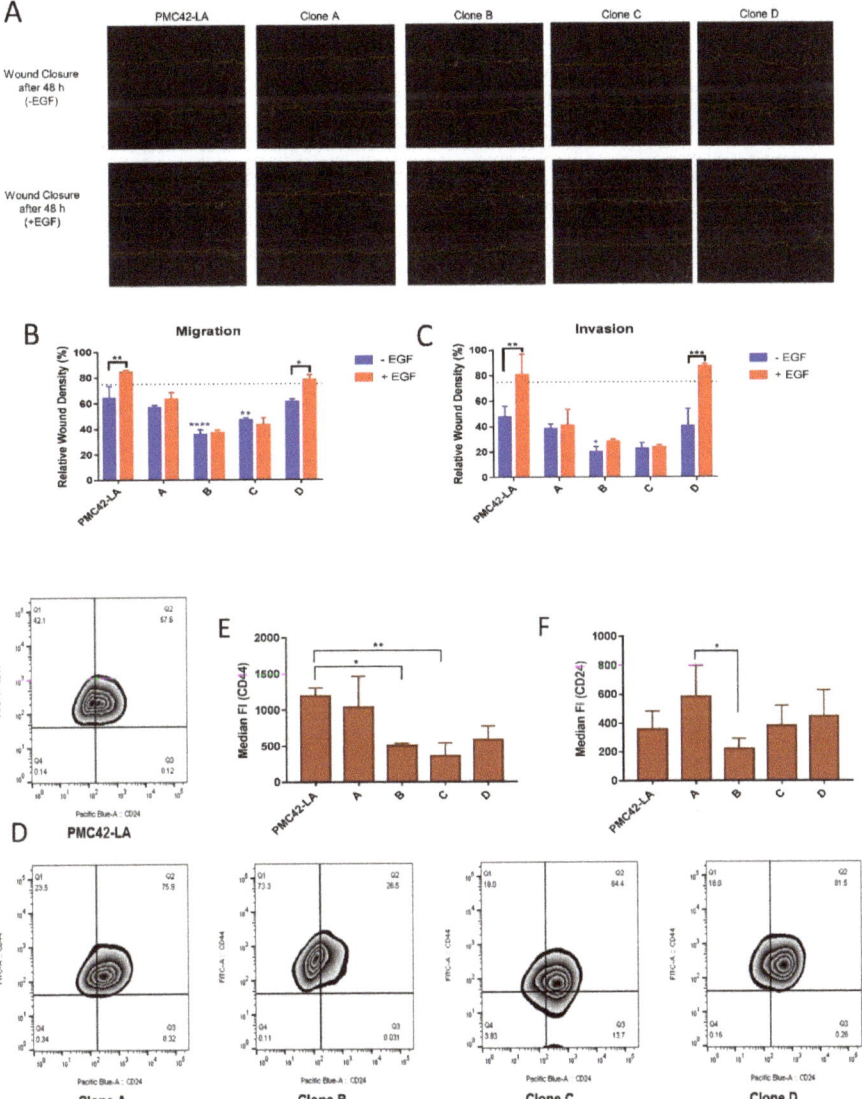

**Figure 7.** (**A**) In vitro migration capacity of PMC42-LA cells and clone cell lines. The capacity to migrate with and without EGF treatment was measured by live cell imaging in a scratch wound healing assay (IncuCyte ZOOM). Microscope images of migrated PMC42-LA cells and clones are shown after 48 h. Yellow lines denote the original scratch wound. The variation in the density of wound closure with and without EGF treatment is clearly depicted across clones. (**B**) Percentage of relative wound density obtained from IncuCyte™ Scratch Wound Cell Migration. (**C**) Invasion assay after 48 h represented as bar graph. Data are presented as the mean ± std dev of three independent experiments. Significant differences were calculated by two-way ANOVA and Sidak's multiple comparisons test. * $P < 0.05$, ** $P < 0.01$, *** $P < 0.001$, **** $P < 0.0001$ (**D**) Zebra plot showing the flow cytometry surface staining of CD44 and CD24 expression markers on parental and clonal progenies of PMC42-LA. (**E**) Staining intensity of CD44 assessed by median fluorescence intensity unit ($n = 4$). (**F**) Staining intensity of CD24 assessed by median fluorescence intensity unit ($n = 4$). Significant differences were calculated by one-way ANOVA and nonparametric Dunnett's multiple comparisons test. * $P < 0.05$, ** $P < 0.01$.

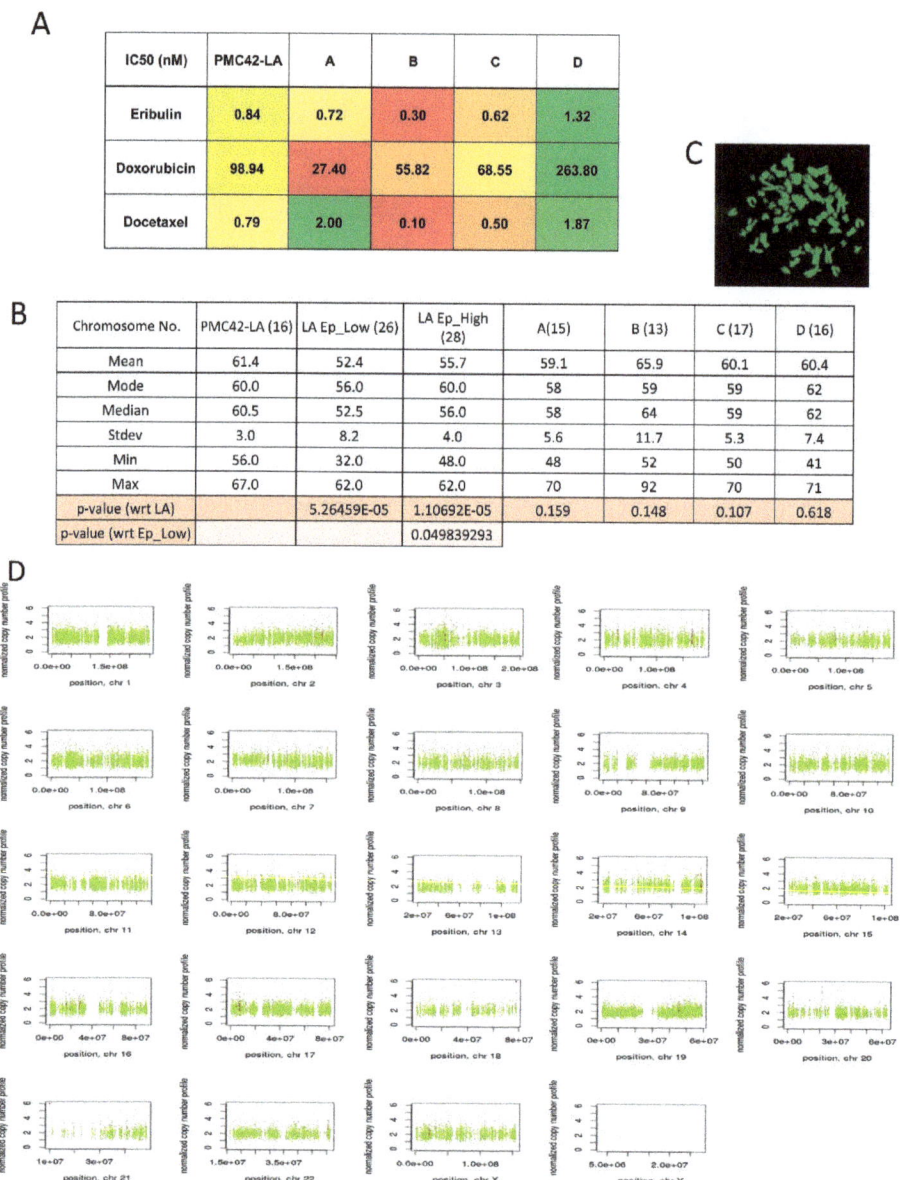

**Figure 8.** (**A**) Plot of heatmap on the basis of computed IC50 values of the drugs eribulin, doxorubicin, and docetaxel for PMC42-LA and the four selected clones. (**B**) Measurements of central tendency from distribution of chromosome number across PMC42 LA, EpCAM sorted subpopulations and four clones. Student *t*-test was applied to calculate *p*-value. (**C**) Metaphase spreads of PMC42-LA chromosomes stained with DAPI and imaged with confocal microscopy. (**D**) Visualization of Control-FREEC v6.0 output from PMC42-LA sorted EpCAM subpopulations whole exome sequencing data (Illumina HiSeq 2000). Copy number profiles for all chromosomes are shown for EpCAM[low] subpopulation in comparison to EpCAM[high]; normal copy number status is shown in green, copy number gains are represented in red, and copy number losses are represented in blue.

## 3.9. Chromosomal Instability (CIN) Reflected across EpCAM-Sorted Subpopulations

In order to determine the extent to which CIN may be associated with the intrinsic plasticity of PMC42-LA cells, we performed metaphase spreads and counted the abnormal chromosome numbers from parental PMC42-LA cells, EpCAM$^{Low}$ and $^{High}$ subpopulations, and the four single cell-derived clones from PMC42-LA. The EpCAM$^{Low}$ and EpCAM$^{High}$ subpopulations showed a significant deviation in their chromosome ploidy distribution, whereas numerical chromosomal aberrations per clone did not differ significantly from those of parental cell line PMC42-LA (Figure 8B,C).

In order to deeply examine the influence of chromosomal instability, whole exome sequencing (WES) of the sorted EpCAM$^{Low}$ and EpCAM$^{High}$ subpopulations and PMC42-LA cells was undertaken; however, comparing the copy number variation (CNV) data deciphered via WES for the EpCAM$^{Low}$ subpopulation to the EpCAM$^{High}$ subpopulation did not reveal any significant differences in the ploidy (Figure 8D). The data analyzed showed that the EpCAM$^{Low}$ and EpCAM$^{High}$ sorted subpopulations were not very different genetically.

## 4. Discussion

### 4.1. Dynamic EMT and MET Changes Observed in EpCAM-Profiled Subpopulations

Our findings established that epithelial and mesenchymal subpopulations, defined by their EpCAM expression, exist within the PMC42-LA breast cancer cell line, which maintains on average an EpCAM$^{+/High}$ epithelial and EpCAM$^{Low}$ mesenchymal population ratio of 80:20; whereas, the panel of other luminal cell lines (MCF7, T47D) and basal cell lines (MDA-MB-231, Sum159, HCC38), FACS profiled using EpCAM, displayed a uniform distribution of EpCAM high and EpCAM low states. Bidirectional transitions observed between the sorted epithelial and mesenchymal subpopulations in PMC42-LA suggest that intercellular regulation may exist to direct a phenotypic equilibrium inherent to the parental cell line. The time taken to achieve such a stable equilibrium from the purified mesenchymal subpopulation was longer than eight weeks and contrasts with studies with the SUM159 and SUM149 cell lines, where a phenotypically stable equilibrium was observed to occur rapidly after six days of growth [29]. CD44$^{low}$ non-CSC populations, isolated from five different basal breast cancer cell lines, also reported a return to CD44$^{high}$ state in vivo [66]. The dynamic EMT and MET was also observed in parental and HCC38 cells delineated by EpCAM profiling [26], in Zeb1 driving CD44$^{Low}$ to CD44$^{High}$ cellular plasticity [58] and in mammary carcinoma mouse MyPT models delineated by E-cadherin profiling [30]. Autocrine signaling is also speculated to play a significant role in EMP dynamics [67]. Recently, the exhibition of hysteretic patterns in TGF-β driven EMT also illustrated bi-stability of cellular states in tumor mammary epithelial cells, related to a higher propensity for metastatic colonization [68].

### 4.2. Inherent Phenotypic Plasticity and Differential Functional Attributes of the Single Cell-Derived Clones

The inherent plasticity was also evaluated in the sub-clones after isolating the single cells by their epithelial and mesenchymal traits as determined by their relative EpCAM high or low states. The proportion of epithelial and mesenchymal states varied across as well as within the sub-clones (Figures 3B and 5C) and also illustrates/renders the possibility of bi-directional phenotypic transitioning (interconversion between epithelial and mesenchymal states). None of the clones profiled for EpCAM displayed a similar distribution of EpCAM high and low states (80:20) as present in the parental PMC42-LA line, suggesting that stochastic fluctuations and inter-clonal cooperativity creates a special equilibrium [69,70], which can be of extreme relevance in mediating metastasis [71]. This plasticity across the EMP spectrum also elicits variable cellular behaviors, which may impact their tumorigenicity, therapy resistance, and proliferation.

The distinct clonal progenies derived from the parental line PMC42-LA displayed marked phenotypic heterogeneity. The presence of sub-clonal variants that exhibit phenotypic diversity across the epithelial-mesenchymal axis from populations of single cells in prostate and breast cancer, has also been verified recently, from in-vitro settings [42,46,72]. Observations based on assessing the four clonal populations in this study for their proliferation, transcriptional EMP status, migration, invasion, stemness, and chemoresistance demonstrated dynamics of intra-tumoral variability in the clones at a functional level. The presence of vimentin proved that the cells on the wound edge exhibited enhanced EMT consistent with cellular movement. However, the lower migratory phenotype in the mesenchymal Clone B led us to suspect that this context may require crosstalk as well as additional stimulation, or possess a defect in the way polarity proteins and extracellular proteins required for movement are trafficked [73,74]. The apparent differences observed in the expression and localization of various mesenchymal markers, such as marked increased in N-cadherin expression on the cell junctions in the Clone D also suggest multifactorial regulatory circuits, not only at the RNA or epigenetic level, but also at the protein level, that can impact intratumoral heterogeneity [75]. The level of CD24 was ~2-fold lower in the EpCAM$^{Low}$ population compared to the parental PMC42-LA cells, and was thus enriched for stem cell-like properties through enhancing their CD44(high)/CD24(low) ratio. Low CD24 expression also correlated positively with lower EpCAM expression in Basal B cell lines (Supplementary Figure S1C) [65]. The marked differences apparent in sub-clones for their proportion of CD44$^{High}$/CD24$^{Low}$ cells also highlight the additional clonal diversity at stemness level, and its relation to tumorigenic potential warrants further investigation. The differential expression of stemness markers was also consistent with the stochastic behavior of the sub-clones, in their response to next evaluated chemo-sensitivity.

Interestingly, in our PMC42-LA single cell-derived clones, the relatively slow proliferating clone with enriched mesenchymal traits (Clone B) did not possess high chemo-resistance against the panel of drugs tested, while counterintuitively, Clone D (with mixed phenotype states of 60 epithelial:40 mesenchymal) had more survival benefit as compared to the parental line and other clones. These results are in line with similar observations found in single cell-derived prostate cancer clones, where mesenchymal features (capable of undergoing EMT) did not necessarily enhance therapy resistance [72].

*4.3. Chromosomal Instability Doesn't Attribute to Intrinsic Phenotypic Plasticity*

We also observed that copy number variations from whole exome sequencing of EpCAM low versus high subpopulations did not correlate with significant differences seen at the chromosome level in ploidy analysis of metaphase spreads between the epithelial and mesenchymal subpopulation in comparison to PMC42-LA. Very few changes were seen at the somatic mutation or CNV level, and further validation from WES studies may be warranted. As presented in Supplementary Tables S4 and S5, several microRNAs (e.g., MIR-3648, MIR-3687) were highly amplified in copy number in the EpCAM$^{Low}$ subpopulation. These results indicate that intrinsic plasticity is contributed by factors other than CIN. Studies examining the contribution of genetic mutations to phenotypic plasticity within tumors and cell lines have resulted in inconsistent conclusions [76–79]. Determinants of metastatic competency investigated by sequencing of primary tumors and metastases from various cancers, such as colorectal cancer and ovarian cancer, have been unable to link specific genetic alterations with tumor dissemination per se [42,80]. Intra-tumoral heterogeneity beyond genetic determinants also had clinical implications in chemotherapy response [81–83]. Both intra-tumoral heterogeneity and intrinsic cellular plasticity warrant consideration as important non-genomic factors that may contribute to dynamic cellular behaviors. Various factors at the cellular or sub-cellular level, such as oscillations of gene expression by epigenetics, alternate splicing, or other unknown factors can also propagate cancer progression [84]. Most recently, the contribution of conformational dynamics of intrinsically disordered proteins, such as oncoproteins, reprogramming transcription factors (TFs) and EMT-TFs in cancer cells was also recognized [85–88]; these can also endow the cells with phenotypic diversity and robust survival potential during chemotherapy regimens. The computational models have also provided a rationale in decoding these intrinsic dynamics/the cell state transition of EMT based on epigenetic regulation and gene regulatory networks [89–92]. Further, the identification of tumor transition states occurring during EMT via phenotypic markers [25] and using a theoretical experimental framework approach to determine the plastic interplay of cell phenotypes [93] can herald a major refinement of our understanding of the intra-tumoral heterogeneity and plasticity within the tumor.

This work provides insight into the paradigm of the dynamic heterogeneity that exists within cancer cell populations and defines the contribution of intrinsic plasticity that endows the functional and phenotypic diversity to allow cancers to adapt within the tumor environment. It thus becomes imperative to develop approaches that allow us to estimate and model these dynamic processes that drive intra-tumoral heterogeneity and cellular plasticity. Tailored approaches need to be developed in such a way that therapy should not only reduce the tumor burden and prevent metastasis, but also address intra-tumoral heterogeneity to prevent adaptive responses.

**Supplementary Materials:** The following are available online at http://www.mdpi.com/2077-0383/8/6/893/s1, Figure S1: (A) FACS analysis of cell surface markers CD44 and CD24 in parental and EpCAM sorted low and high cells of PMC42-LA. (B) Percentages of the $CD44^+CD24^{Low}$ cells assessed through FACS in PMC42-LA and EpCAM sorted low and high subpopulations. (C) CD24 assessment in gene expression data of 50 breast cancer cell lines and 5 non-malignant breast cell lines, including three subtypes of luminal, basal A and basal B/mesenchymal. Data are from Array Express (accession no. E-MTAB-181) (Heiser et al., 2012) and are normalized log2-transformed values; * $P < 0.05$, ** $P < 0.01$ (one-way ANOVA, with Tukey's multiple comparisons). (D) Immunofluorescence microscopy analysis of EpCAM high and low sorted subpopulations of PMC42-LA cells using Cytell. Cells were stained with antibodies against E-cadherin, Vimentin, and EpCAM. (Scale bar, 100 µM), Figure S2: (A) Immunofluorescent staining for vimentin (green) reveals all cells in the vicinity of wound closure are vimentin positive for parental cell line and the clones. Scale bar: 100 µM. (B) Growth inhibitory effect of Eribulin, Doxorubicin, Docetaxel in PMC42-LA cell line after 72 h exposure. Table S1: List of Primers used in RT-qPCR annotated with their Gene Symbols and forward and reverse primer sequences information, Table S2: Antibodies used in this study along with their clone, supplier and catalog number information, Table S3: Fold change regulation of various EMT markers in PMC42-LA and single-cell derived clones after 10 ng/ml of EGF treatment for 3 days, Table S4: Copy Number Variations reflected in EPCAM_High vs. EpCAM_Low subpopulation of PMC42-LA cells, Table S5: SNVs identified in EpCAM_Low subpopulation wrt EpCAM_high subpopulation of PMC42-LA cells.

**Author Contributions:** S.B., T.B., C.P., and E.W.T. designed the experiments; S.B., J.M., and C.P. performed the experiments; C.P., T.B., and M.W. performed the work in mice; S.B., T.B., and E.W.T. analyzed the data; Genewiz personnel performed and analyzed the whole exome sequencing data; S.B., J.M., and E.W.T. wrote the manuscript; S.H.N. and E.W.T. supervised the study.

**Acknowledgments:** This work was supported in part by a National Breast Cancer Foundation grant (CG-10-04) to EWT. We would like to thank the FACS core facility, Microscopy core facility and Histology core facility teams based at TRI for their technical assistance. We also thank St Vincent's Experimental Medical and Surgical Unit as well as its BioResources Centre for the mouse-related work. The Translational Research Institute receives support from the Australian Government. During the course of the study, S.B. was supported by a QUTPRA scholarship.

**Conflicts of Interest:** The authors declare they have no competing financial interests in relation to the work described.

## References

1. Gerlinger, M.; Rowan, A.J.; Horswell, S.; Larkin, J.; Endesfelder, D.; Gronroos, E.; Martinez, P.; Matthews, N.; Stewart, A.; Tarpey, P.; et al. Intratumor Heterogeneity and Branched Evolution Revealed by Multiregion Sequencing. *N. Engl. J. Med.* **2012**, *366*, 883–892. [CrossRef] [PubMed]
2. Polyak, K.; Weinberg, R.A. Transitions between epithelial and mesenchymal states: acquisition of malignant and stem cell traits. *Nat. Rev. Cancer* **2009**, *9*, 265–273. [CrossRef] [PubMed]
3. Saunders, N.A.; Simpson, F.; Thompson, E.W.; Hill, M.M.; Endo-Munoz, L.; Leggatt, G.; Minchin, R.F.; Guminski, A. Role of intratumoural heterogeneity in cancer drug resistance: molecular and clinical perspectives. *EMBO Mol. Med.* **2012**, *4*, 675–684. [CrossRef] [PubMed]
4. Micalizzi, D.S.; Farabaugh, S.M.; Ford, H.L. Epithelial-mesenchymal transition in cancer: Parallels between normal development and tumor progression. *J. Mammary Gland Biol. Neoplasia* **2010**, *15*, 117–134. [CrossRef] [PubMed]
5. Chiou, S.H.; Yu, C.C.; Huang, C.Y.; Lin, S.C.; Liu, C.J.; Tsai, T.H.; Chou, S.H.; Chien, C.S.; Ku, H.H.; Lo, J.F. Positive correlations of Oct-4 and Nanog in oral cancer stem-like cells and high-grade oral squamous cell carcinoma. *Clin. Cancer Res. Off. J. Am. Assoc. Cancer Res.* **2008**, *14*, 4085–4095. [CrossRef] [PubMed]

6. Harris, M.A.; Yang, H.; Low, B.E.; Mukherjee, J.; Guha, A.; Bronson, R.T.; Shultz, L.D.; Israel, M.A.; Yun, K. Cancer stem cells are enriched in the side population cells in a mouse model of glioma. *Cancer Res.* **2008**, *68*, 10051–10059. [CrossRef] [PubMed]
7. Prat, A.; Parker, J.S.; Karginova, O.; Fan, C.; Livasy, C.; Herschkowitz, J.I.; He, X.; Perou, C.M. Phenotypic and molecular characterization of the claudin-low intrinsic subtype of breast cancer. *Breast Cancer Res.* **2010**, *12*, R68. [CrossRef]
8. Weigelt, B.; Horlings, H.M.; Kreike, B.; Hayes, M.M.; Hauptmann, M.; Wessels, L.F.; de Jong, D.; Van de Vijver, M.J.; Van't Veer, L.J.; Peterse, J.L. Refinement of breast cancer classification by molecular characterization of histological special types. *J. Pathol.* **2008**, *216*, 141–150. [CrossRef]
9. Caldarella, A.; Buzzoni, C.; Crocetti, E.; Bianchi, S.; Vezzosi, V.; Apicella, P.; Biancalani, M.; Giannini, A.; Urso, C.; Zolfanelli, F.; et al. Invasive breast cancer: A significant correlation between histological types and molecular subgroups. *J. Cancer Res. Clin. Oncol.* **2013**, *139*, 617–623. [CrossRef]
10. Joung, J.G.; Oh, B.Y.; Hong, H.K.; Al-Khalidi, H.; Al-Alem, F.; Lee, H.O.; Bae, J.S.; Kim, J.; Cha, H.U.; Alotaibi, M.; et al. Tumor Heterogeneity Predicts Metastatic Potential in Colorectal Cancer. *Clin. Cancer Res. Off. J. Am. Assoc. Cancer Res.* **2017**, *23*, 7209–7216. [CrossRef]
11. Lawson, D.A.; Kessenbrock, K.; Davis, R.T.; Pervolarakis, N.; Werb, Z. Tumour heterogeneity and metastasis at single-cell resolution. *Nat. Cell Biol.* **2018**, *20*, 1349–1360. [CrossRef] [PubMed]
12. Hallou, A.; Jennings, J.; Kabla, A.J. Tumour heterogeneity promotes collective invasion and cancer metastatic dissemination. *R. Soc. Open Sci.* **2017**, *4*, 161007. [CrossRef] [PubMed]
13. Neve, R.M.; Chin, K.; Fridlyand, J.; Yeh, J.; Baehner, F.L.; Fevr, T.; Clark, L.; Bayani, N.; Coppe, J.P.; Tong, F.; et al. A collection of breast cancer cell lines for the study of functionally distinct cancer subtypes. *Cancer Cell* **2006**, *10*, 515–527. [CrossRef] [PubMed]
14. Voduc, K.D.; Cheang, M.C.; Tyldesley, S.; Gelmon, K.; Nielsen, T.O.; Kennecke, H. Breast cancer subtypes and the risk of local and regional relapse. *J. Clin. Oncol. Off. J. Am. Soc. Clin. Oncol.* **2010**, *28*, 1684–1691. [CrossRef] [PubMed]
15. Perou, C.M.; Sorlie, T.; Eisen, M.B.; van de Rijn, M.; Jeffrey, S.S.; Rees, C.A.; Pollack, J.R.; Ross, D.T.; Johnsen, H.; Akslen, L.A.; et al. Molecular portraits of human breast tumours. *Nature* **2000**, *406*, 747–752. [CrossRef] [PubMed]
16. Sorlie, T.; Perou, C.M.; Tibshirani, R.; Aas, T.; Geisler, S.; Johnsen, H.; Hastie, T.; Eisen, M.B.; van de Rijn, M.; Jeffrey, S.S.; et al. Gene expression patterns of breast carcinomas distinguish tumor subclasses with clinical implications. *Proc. Natl. Acad. Sci. USA* **2001**, *98*, 10869–10874. [CrossRef] [PubMed]
17. Lehmann, B.D.; Bauer, J.A.; Chen, X.; Sanders, M.E.; Chakravarthy, A.B.; Shyr, Y.; Pietenpol, J.A. Identification of human triple-negative breast cancer subtypes and preclinical models for selection of targeted therapies. *J. Clin. Investig.* **2011**, *121*, 2750–2767. [CrossRef]
18. Du, T.; Zhu, L.; Levine, K.M.; Tasdemir, N.; Lee, A.V.; Vignali, D.A.A.; Houten, B.V.; Tseng, G.C.; Oesterreich, S. Invasive lobular and ductal breast carcinoma differ in immune response, protein translation efficiency and metabolism. *Sci. Rep.* **2018**, *8*, 7205. [CrossRef]
19. Tan, T.Z.; Miow, Q.H.; Huang, R.Y.J.; Wong, M.K.; Ye, J.; Lau, J.A.; Wu, M.C.; Bin Abdul Hadi, L.H.; Soong, R.; Choolani, M.; et al. Functional genomics identifies five distinct molecular subtypes with clinical relevance and pathways for growth control in epithelial ovarian cancer. *EMBO Mol. Med.* **2013**, *5*, 983–998. [CrossRef]
20. Tan, T.Z.; Miow, Q.H.; Miki, Y.; Noda, T.; Mori, S.; Huang, R.Y.; Thiery, J.P. Epithelial-mesenchymal transition spectrum quantification and its efficacy in deciphering survival and drug responses of cancer patients. *EMBO Mol. Med.* **2014**, *6*, 1279–1293. [CrossRef]
21. Tang, D.G. Understanding cancer stem cell heterogeneity and plasticity. *Cell Res.* **2012**, *22*, 457–472. [CrossRef] [PubMed]
22. Nieto, M.A.; Huang, R.Y.; Jackson, R.A.; Thiery, J.P. EMT: 2016. *Cell* **2016**, *166*, 21–45. [CrossRef] [PubMed]
23. Thompson, E.W.; Haviv, I. The social aspects of EMT-MET plasticity. *Nat. Med.* **2011**, *17*, 1048–1049. [CrossRef] [PubMed]
24. Jolly, M.K.; Tripathi, S.C.; Jia, D.; Mooney, S.M.; Celiktas, M.; Hanash, S.M.; Mani, S.A.; Pienta, K.J.; Ben-Jacob, E.; Levine, H. Stability of the hybrid epithelial/mesenchymal phenotype. *Oncotarget* **2016**, *7*, 27067–27084. [CrossRef] [PubMed]

25. Pastushenko, I.; Brisebarre, A.; Sifrim, A.; Fioramonti, M.; Revenco, T.; Boumahdi, S.; Van Keymeulen, A.; Brown, D.; Moers, V.; Lemaire, S.; et al. Identification of the tumour transition states occurring during EMT. *Nature* **2018**, *556*, 463–468. [CrossRef]
26. Yamamoto, M.; Sakane, K.; Tominaga, K.; Gotoh, N.; Niwa, T.; Kikuchi, Y.; Tada, K.; Goshima, N.; Semba, K.; Inoue, J.I. Intratumoral bidirectional transitions between epithelial and mesenchymal cells in triple-negative breast cancer. *Cancer Sci.* **2017**. [CrossRef]
27. Bierie, B.; Pierce, S.E.; Kroeger, C.; Stover, D.G.; Pattabiraman, D.R.; Thiru, P.; Liu Donaher, J.; Reinhardt, F.; Chaffer, C.L.; Keckesova, Z.; et al. Integrin-beta4 identifies cancer stem cell-enriched populations of partially mesenchymal carcinoma cells. *Proc. Natl. Acad. Sci. USA* **2017**, *114*, E2337–E2346. [CrossRef]
28. Chaffer, C.L.; Brueckmann, I.; Scheel, C.; Kaestli, A.J.; Wiggins, P.A.; Rodrigues, L.O.; Brooks, M.; Reinhardt, F.; Su, Y.; Polyak, K.; et al. Normal and neoplastic nonstem cells can spontaneously convert to a stem-like state. *Proc. Natl. Acad. Sci. USA* **2011**, *108*, 7950–7955. [CrossRef]
29. Gupta, P.B.; Fillmore, C.M.; Jiang, G.; Shapira, S.D.; Tao, K.; Kuperwasser, C.; Lander, E.S. Stochastic state transitions give rise to phenotypic equilibrium in populations of cancer cells. *Cell* **2011**, *146*, 633–644. [CrossRef]
30. Beerling, E.; Seinstra, D.; de Wit, E.; Kester, L.; van der Velden, D.; Maynard, C.; Schafer, R.; van Diest, P.; Voest, E.; van Oudenaarden, A.; et al. Plasticity between Epithelial and Mesenchymal States Unlinks EMT from Metastasis-Enhancing Stem Cell Capacity. *Cell Rep.* **2016**, *14*, 2281–2288. [CrossRef]
31. Marjanovic, N.D.; Weinberg, R.A.; Chaffer, C.L. Cell plasticity and heterogeneity in cancer. *Clin. Chem.* **2013**, *59*, 168–179. [CrossRef] [PubMed]
32. Biddle, A.; Liang, X.; Gammon, L.; Fazil, B.; Harper, L.J.; Emich, H.; Costea, D.E.; Mackenzie, I.C. Cancer stem cells in squamous cell carcinoma switch between two distinct phenotypes that are preferentially migratory or proliferative. *Cancer Res.* **2011**, *71*, 5317–5326. [CrossRef] [PubMed]
33. Bhatia, S.; Monkman, J.; Toh, A.K.L.; Nagaraj, S.H.; Thompson, E.W. Targeting epithelial-mesenchymal plasticity in cancer: clinical and preclinical advances in therapy and monitoring. *Biochem. J.* **2017**, *474*, 3269–3306. [CrossRef] [PubMed]
34. Arumugam, T.; Ramachandran, V.; Fournier, K.F.; Wang, H.; Marquis, L.; Abbruzzese, J.L.; Gallick, G.E.; Logsdon, C.D.; McConkey, D.J.; Choi, W. Epithelial to mesenchymal transition contributes to drug resistance in pancreatic cancer. *Cancer Res.* **2009**, *69*, 5820–5828. [CrossRef] [PubMed]
35. Zheng, X.; Carstens, J.L.; Kim, J.; Scheible, M.; Kaye, J.; Sugimoto, H.; Wu, C.-C.; LeBleu, V.S.; Kalluri, R. Epithelial-to-mesenchymal transition is dispensable for metastasis but induces chemoresistance in pancreatic cancer. *Nature* **2015**, *527*, 525–530. [CrossRef] [PubMed]
36. Fischer, K.R.; Durrans, A.; Lee, S.; Sheng, J.; Li, F.; Wong, S.T.C.; Choi, H.; El Rayes, T.; Ryu, S.; Troeger, J.; et al. Epithelial-to-mesenchymal transition is not required for lung metastasis but contributes to chemoresistance. *Nature* **2015**, *527*, 472–476. [CrossRef]
37. Eirew, P.; Steif, A.; Khattra, J.; Ha, G.; Yap, D.; Farahani, H.; Gelmon, K.; Chia, S.; Mar, C.; Wan, A.; et al. Dynamics of genomic clones in breast cancer patient xenografts at single-cell resolution. *Nature* **2015**, *518*, 422–426. [CrossRef] [PubMed]
38. Xu, X.; Hou, Y.; Yin, X.; Bao, L.; Tang, A.; Song, L.; Li, F.; Tsang, S.; Wu, K.; Wu, H.; et al. Single-cell exome sequencing reveals single-nucleotide mutation characteristics of a kidney tumor. *Cell* **2012**, *148*, 886–895. [CrossRef]
39. Hou, Y.; Guo, H.; Cao, C.; Li, X.; Hu, B.; Zhu, P.; Wu, X.; Wen, L.; Tang, F.; Huang, Y.; et al. Single-cell triple omics sequencing reveals genetic, epigenetic, and transcriptomic heterogeneity in hepatocellular carcinomas. *Cell Res.* **2016**, *26*, 304–319. [CrossRef]
40. Dalerba, P.; Kalisky, T.; Sahoo, D.; Rajendran, P.S.; Rothenberg, M.E.; Leyrat, A.A.; Sim, S.; Okamoto, J.; Johnston, D.M.; Qian, D.; et al. Single-cell dissection of transcriptional heterogeneity in human colon tumors. *Nat. Biotechnol.* **2011**, *29*, 1120–1127. [CrossRef]
41. Vermeulen, L.; Todaro, M.; de Sousa Mello, F.; Sprick, M.R.; Kemper, K.; Perez Alea, M.; Richel, D.J.; Stassi, G.; Medema, J.P. Single-cell cloning of colon cancer stem cells reveals a multi-lineage differentiation capacity. *Proc. Natl. Acad. Sci. USA* **2008**, *105*, 13427–13432. [CrossRef] [PubMed]
42. McPherson, A.; Roth, A.; Laks, E.; Masud, T.; Bashashati, A.; Zhang, A.W.; Ha, G.; Biele, J.; Yap, D.; Wan, A.; et al. Divergent modes of clonal spread and intraperitoneal mixing in high-grade serous ovarian cancer. *Nat. Genet.* **2016**, *48*, 758–767. [CrossRef] [PubMed]

43. Ting, D.T.; Wittner, B.S.; Ligorio, M.; Vincent Jordan, N.; Shah, A.M.; Miyamoto, D.T.; Aceto, N.; Bersani, F.; Brannigan, B.W.; Xega, K.; et al. Single-cell RNA sequencing identifies extracellular matrix gene expression by pancreatic circulating tumor cells. *Cell Rep.* **2014**, *8*, 1905–1918. [CrossRef] [PubMed]
44. Puram, S.V.; Parikh, A.S.; Tirosh, I. Single cell RNA-seq highlights a role for a partial EMT in head and neck cancer. *Mol. Cell. Oncol.* **2018**, *5*, e1448244. [CrossRef] [PubMed]
45. Puram, S.V.; Tirosh, I.; Parikh, A.S.; Patel, A.P.; Yizhak, K.; Gillespie, S.; Rodman, C.; Luo, C.L.; Mroz, E.A.; Emerick, K.S.; et al. Single-Cell Transcriptomic Analysis of Primary and Metastatic Tumor Ecosystems in Head and Neck Cancer. *Cell* **2017**, *171*, 1611–1624.e1624. [CrossRef] [PubMed]
46. Mathis, R.A.; Sokol, E.S.; Gupta, P.B. Cancer cells exhibit clonal diversity in phenotypic plasticity. *Open Biol.* **2017**, *7*, 160283. [CrossRef] [PubMed]
47. Patel, A.P.; Tirosh, I.; Trombetta, J.J.; Shalek, A.K.; Gillespie, S.M.; Wakimoto, H.; Cahill, D.P.; Nahed, B.V.; Curry, W.T.; Martuza, R.L.; et al. Single-cell RNA-seq highlights intratumoral heterogeneity in primary glioblastoma. *Science* **2014**, *344*, 1396–1401. [CrossRef]
48. Lee, M.C.; Lopez-Diaz, F.J.; Khan, S.Y.; Tariq, M.A.; Dayn, Y.; Vaske, C.J.; Radenbaugh, A.J.; Kim, H.J.; Emerson, B.M.; Pourmand, N. Single-cell analyses of transcriptional heterogeneity during drug tolerance transition in cancer cells by RNA sequencing. *Proc. Natl. Acad. Sci. USA* **2014**, *111*, E4726–E4735. [CrossRef]
49. Ackland, M.L.; Michalczyk, A.; Whitehead, R.H. PMC42, a novel model for the differentiated human breast. *Exp. Cell Res.* **2001**, *263*, 14–22. [CrossRef]
50. Ackland, M.L.; Newgreen, D.F.; Fridman, M.; Waltham, M.C.; Arvanitis, A.; Minichiello, J.; Price, J.T.; Thompson, E.W. Epidermal growth factor-induced epithelio-mesenchymal transition in human breast carcinoma cells. *Lab. Investig. J. Tech. Methods Pathol.* **2003**, *83*, 435–448. [CrossRef]
51. Hugo, H.J.; Kokkinos, M.I.; Blick, T.; Ackland, M.L.; Thompson, E.W.; Newgreen, D.F. Defining the E-cadherin repressor interactome in epithelial-mesenchymal transition: the PMC42 model as a case study. *Cells Tissues Organs* **2011**, *193*, 23–40. [CrossRef] [PubMed]
52. Lebret, S.C.; Newgreen, D.F.; Thompson, E.W.; Ackland, M.L. Induction of epithelial to mesenchymal transition in PMC42-LA human breast carcinoma cells by carcinoma-associated fibroblast secreted factors. *Breast Cancer Res.* **2007**, *9*, R19. [CrossRef] [PubMed]
53. Whitehead, R.H.; Bertoncello, I.; Webber, L.M.; Pedersen, J.S. A new human breast carcinoma cell line (PMC42) with stem cell characteristics. I. Morphologic characterization. *J. Natl. Cancer Inst.* **1983**, *70*, 649–661. [PubMed]
54. Whitehead, R.H.; Monaghan, P.; Webber, L.M.; Bertoncello, I.; Vitali, A.A. A new human breast carcinoma cell line (PMC42) with stem cell characteristics. II. Characterization of cells growing as organoids. *J. Natl. Cancer Inst.* **1983**, *71*, 1193–1203. [PubMed]
55. Whitehead, R.H.; Quirk, S.J.; Vitali, A.A.; Funder, J.W.; Sutherland, R.L.; Murphy, L.C. A new human breast carcinoma cell line (PMC42) with stem cell characteristics. III. Hormone receptor status and responsiveness. *J. Natl. Cancer Inst.* **1984**, *73*, 643–648. [PubMed]
56. Cursons, J.; Leuchowius, K.-J.; Waltham, M.; Tomaskovic-Crook, E.; Foroutan, M.; Bracken, C.P.; Redfern, A.; Crampin, E.J.; Street, I.; Davis, M.J.; et al. Stimulus-dependent differences in signalling regulate epithelial-mesenchymal plasticity and change the effects of drugs in breast cancer cell lines. *Cell Commun. Signal. CCS* **2015**, *13*, 26. [CrossRef] [PubMed]
57. Franken, N.A.; Rodermond, H.M.; Stap, J.; Haveman, J.; van Bree, C. Clonogenic assay of cells in vitro. *Nat. Protocols* **2006**, *1*, 2315–2319. [CrossRef] [PubMed]
58. Liu, H.; Patel, M.R.; Prescher, J.A.; Patsialou, A.; Qian, D.; Lin, J.; Wen, S.; Chang, Y.F.; Bachmann, M.H.; Shimono, Y.; et al. Cancer stem cells from human breast tumors are involved in spontaneous metastases in orthotopic mouse models. *Proc. Natl. Acad. Sci. USA* **2010**, *107*, 18115–18120. [CrossRef] [PubMed]
59. Li, H.; Durbin, R. Fast and accurate short read alignment with Burrows-Wheeler transform. *Bioinformatics* **2009**, *25*, 1754–1760. [CrossRef]
60. Li, H.; Handsaker, B.; Wysoker, A.; Fennell, T.; Ruan, J.; Homer, N.; Marth, G.; Abecasis, G.; Durbin, R. The Sequence Alignment/Map format and SAMtools. *Bioinformatics* **2009**, *25*, 2078–2079. [CrossRef]
61. McKenna, A.; Hanna, M.; Banks, E.; Sivachenko, A.; Cibulskis, K.; Kernytsky, A.; Garimella, K.; Altshuler, D.; Gabriel, S.; Daly, M.; et al. The Genome Analysis Toolkit: A MapReduce framework for analyzing next-generation DNA sequencing data. *Genome Res.* **2010**, *20*, 1297–1303. [CrossRef] [PubMed]

62. Wang, K.; Li, M.; Hakonarson, H. ANNOVAR: Functional annotation of genetic variants from high-throughput sequencing data. *Nucleic Acids Res.* **2010**, *38*, e164. [CrossRef] [PubMed]
63. Boeva, V.; Popova, T.; Bleakley, K.; Chiche, P.; Cappo, J.; Schleiermacher, G.; Janoueix-Lerosey, I.; Delattre, O.; Barillot, E. Control-FREEC: A tool for assessing copy number and allelic content using next-generation sequencing data. *Bioinformatics* **2012**, *28*, 423–425. [CrossRef] [PubMed]
64. Irigoyen, M.A.; Garcia, F.V.; Iturriagagoitia, A.C.; Beroiz, B.I.; Martinez, M.S.; Guillen Grima, F. [Molecular subtypes of breast cancer: Prognostic implications and clinical and immunohistochemical characteristics]. *Anales del Sistema Sanitario de Navarra* **2011**, *34*, 219–233. [PubMed]
65. Heiser, L.M.; Sadanandam, A.; Kuo, W.-L.; Benz, S.C.; Goldstein, T.C.; Ng, S.; Gibb, W.J.; Wang, N.J.; Ziyad, S.; Tong, F.; et al. Subtype and pathway specific responses to anticancer compounds in breast cancer. *Proce. Natl. Acad. Sci. USA* **2012**, *109*, 2724–2729. [CrossRef]
66. Chaffer, C.L.; Marjanovic, N.D.; Lee, T.; Bell, G.; Kleer, C.G.; Reinhardt, F.; D'Alessio, A.C.; Young, R.A.; Weinberg, R.A. Poised chromatin at the ZEB1 promoter enables breast cancer cell plasticity and enhances tumorigenicity. *Cell* **2013**, *154*, 61–74. [CrossRef] [PubMed]
67. Scheel, C.; Eaton, E.N.; Li, S.H.-J.; Chaffer, C.L.; Reinhardt, F.; Kah, K.-J.; Bell, G.; Guo, W.; Rubin, J.; Richardson, A.L.; et al. Paracrine and autocrine signals induce and maintain mesenchymal and stem cell states in the breast. *Cell* **2011**, *145*, 926–940. [CrossRef]
68. Celia-Terrassa, T.; Bastian, C.; Liu, D.D.; Ell, B.; Aiello, N.M.; Wei, Y.; Zamalloa, J.; Blanco, A.M.; Hang, X.; Kunisky, D.; et al. Hysteresis control of epithelial-mesenchymal transition dynamics conveys a distinct program with enhanced metastatic ability. *Nat. Commun.* **2018**, *9*, 5005. [CrossRef]
69. Neelakantan, D.; Drasin, D.J.; Ford, H.L. Intratumoral heterogeneity: Clonal cooperation in epithelial-to-mesenchymal transition and metastasis. *Cell Adhes. Migr.* **2014**, *9*, 265–276. [CrossRef]
70. Zhou, H.; Neelakantan, D.; Ford, H.L. Clonal cooperativity in heterogenous cancers. *Semin. Cell Dev. Biol.* **2017**, *64*, 79–89. [CrossRef]
71. Tsuji, T.; Ibaragi, S.; Shima, K.; Hu, M.G.; Katsurano, M.; Sasaki, A.; Hu, G.F. Epithelial-mesenchymal transition induced by growth suppressor p12CDK2-AP1 promotes tumor cell local invasion but suppresses distant colony growth. *Cancer Res.* **2008**, *68*, 10377–10386. [CrossRef] [PubMed]
72. Harner-Foreman, N.; Vadakekolathu, J.; Laversin, S.A.; Mathieu, M.G.; Reeder, S.; Pockley, A.G.; Rees, R.C.; Boocock, D.J. A novel spontaneous model of epithelial-mesenchymal transition (EMT) using a primary prostate cancer derived cell line demonstrating distinct stem-like characteristics. *Sci. Rep.* **2017**, *7*, 40633. [CrossRef] [PubMed]
73. Ozdamar, B.; Bose, R.; Barrios-Rodiles, M.; Wang, H.R.; Zhang, Y.; Wrana, J.L. Regulation of the polarity protein Par6 by TGFbeta receptors controls epithelial cell plasticity. *Science* **2005**, *307*, 1603–1609. [CrossRef] [PubMed]
74. Iden, S.; Collard, J.G. Crosstalk between small GTPases and polarity proteins in cell polarization. *Nat. Rev. Mol. Cell Biol.* **2008**, *9*, 846–859. [CrossRef] [PubMed]
75. Stefania, D.D.; Vergara, D. The Many-Faced Program of Epithelial–Mesenchymal Transition: A System Biology-Based View. *Front. Oncol.* **2017**, *7*, 274. [CrossRef] [PubMed]
76. Klevebring, D.; Rosin, G.; Ma, R.; Lindberg, J.; Czene, K.; Kere, J.; Fredriksson, I.; Bergh, J.; Hartman, J. Sequencing of breast cancer stem cell populations indicates a dynamic conversion between differentiation states in vivo. *Breast Cancer Res. BCR* **2014**, *16*, R72. [CrossRef] [PubMed]
77. Shipitsin, M.; Campbell, L.L.; Argani, P.; Weremowicz, S.; Bloushtain-Qimron, N.; Yao, J.; Nikolskaya, T.; Serebryiskaya, T.; Beroukhim, R.; Hu, M.; et al. Molecular definition of breast tumor heterogeneity. *Cancer Cell* **2007**, *11*, 259–273. [CrossRef] [PubMed]
78. Balic, M.; Schwarzenbacher, D.; Stanzer, S.; Heitzer, E.; Auer, M.; Geigl, J.B.; Cote, R.J.; Datar, R.H.; Dandachi, N. Genetic and epigenetic analysis of putative breast cancer stem cell models. *BMC Cancer* **2013**, *13*, 358. [CrossRef] [PubMed]
79. Park, S.Y.; Gonen, M.; Kim, H.J.; Michor, F.; Polyak, K. Cellular and genetic diversity in the progression of in situ human breast carcinomas to an invasive phenotype. *J. Clin. Investig.* **2010**, *120*, 636–644. [CrossRef]
80. Tauriello, D.V.; Calon, A.; Lonardo, E.; Batlle, E. Determinants of metastatic competency in colorectal cancer. *Mol. Oncol.* **2017**, *11*, 97–119. [CrossRef]

81. Kreso, A.; O'Brien, C.A.; van Galen, P.; Gan, O.I.; Notta, F.; Brown, A.M.; Ng, K.; Ma, J.; Wienholds, E.; Dunant, C.; et al. Variable clonal repopulation dynamics influence chemotherapy response in colorectal cancer. *Science* **2013**, *339*, 543–548. [CrossRef]
82. Boland, C.R.; Goel, A. Somatic evolution of cancer cells. *Semin. Cancer Biol.* **2005**, *15*, 436–450. [CrossRef] [PubMed]
83. Chapman, M.P.; Risom, T.; Aswani, A.J.; Langer, E.M.; Sears, R.C.; Tomlin, C.J. Modeling differentiation-state transitions linked to therapeutic escape in triple-negative breast cancer. *PLoS Comput. Biol.* **2019**, *15*, e1006840. [CrossRef] [PubMed]
84. Brock, A.; Chang, H.; Huang, S. Non-genetic heterogeneity—A mutation-independent driving force for the somatic evolution of tumours. *Nat. Rev. Genet.* **2009**, *10*, 336–342. [CrossRef] [PubMed]
85. Mooney, S.M.; Jolly, M.K.; Levine, H.; Kulkarni, P. Phenotypic plasticity in prostate cancer: Role of intrinsically disordered proteins. *Asian J. Androl.* **2016**, *18*, 704–710. [CrossRef] [PubMed]
86. Iakoucheva, L.M.; Brown, C.J.; Lawson, J.D.; Obradovic, Z.; Dunker, A.K. Intrinsic disorder in cell-signaling and cancer-associated proteins. *J. Mol. Biol.* **2002**, *323*, 573–584. [CrossRef]
87. Uversky, V.N.; Oldfield, C.J.; Dunker, A.K. Intrinsically disordered proteins in human diseases: Introducing the D2 concept. *Ann. Rev. Biophys.* **2008**, *37*, 215–246. [CrossRef]
88. Xue, B.; Oldfield, C.J.; Van, Y.Y.; Dunker, A.K.; Uversky, V.N. Protein intrinsic disorder and induced pluripotent stem cells. *Mol. BioSyst.* **2012**, *8*, 134–150. [CrossRef]
89. Joo, J.I.; Zhou, J.X.; Huang, S.; Cho, K.H. Determining Relative Dynamic Stability of Cell States Using Boolean Network Model. *Sci. Rep.* **2018**, *8*, 12077. [CrossRef]
90. Tripathi, S.; Levine, H.; Kumar Jolly, M. A Mechanism for Epithelial-Mesenchymal Heterogeneity in a Population of Cancer Cells. *bioRxiv* **2019**. [CrossRef]
91. Jia, W.; Deshmukh, A.; Mani, S.A.; Jolly, M.K.; Levine, H. A possible role for epigenetic feedback regulation in the dynamics of the Epithelial-Mesenchymal Transition (EMT). *bioRxiv* **2019**. [CrossRef]
92. Jolly, M.K.; Tripathi, S.C.; Somarelli, J.A.; Hanash, S.M.; Levine, H. Epithelial/mesenchymal plasticity: How have quantitative mathematical models helped improve our understanding? *Mol. Oncol.* **2017**, *11*, 739–754. [CrossRef] [PubMed]
93. Mandal, M.; Ghosh, B.; Anura, A.; Mitra, P.; Pathak, T.; Chatterjee, J. Modeling continuum of epithelial mesenchymal transition plasticity. *Integr. Biol. Quant. Biosci. Nano Macro* **2016**, *8*, 167–176. [CrossRef] [PubMed]

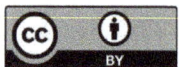

© 2019 by the authors. Licensee MDPI, Basel, Switzerland. This article is an open access article distributed under the terms and conditions of the Creative Commons Attribution (CC BY) license (http://creativecommons.org/licenses/by/4.0/).

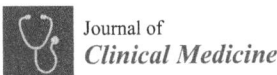 

*Article*

# Snail-Overexpression Induces Epithelial-mesenchymal Transition and Metabolic Reprogramming in Human Pancreatic Ductal Adenocarcinoma and Non-tumorigenic Ductal Cells

Menghan Liu [1,†], Sarah E. Hancock [1,†], Ghazal Sultani [1], Brendan P. Wilkins [1], Eileen Ding [1], Brenna Osborne [1], Lake-Ee Quek [1,2] and Nigel Turner [1,*]

1. Department of Pharmacology, School of Medical Sciences, University of New South Wales, Sydney, 2052 NSW, Australia; mliu6171@uni.sydney.unsw.edu.au (M.L.); sarah.hancock@unsw.edu.au (S.E.H.); ghazal.sultani@unsw.edu.au (G.S.); b.wilkins@victorchang.edu.au (B.P.W.); e.ding@unsw.edu.au (E.D.); b.osborne@unsw.edu.au (B.O.); lake-ee.quek@sydney.edu.au (L.-E.Q.)
2. Charles Perkins Centre, School of Mathematics and Statistics, The University of Sydney, Sydney, 2006 NSW, Australia
* Correspondence: n.turner@unsw.edu.au
† These authors contributed equally to this work.

Received: 5 April 2019; Accepted: 5 June 2019; Published: 8 June 2019

**Abstract:** The zinc finger transcription factor Snail is a known effector of epithelial-to-mesenchymal transition (EMT), a process that underlies the enhanced invasiveness and chemoresistance of common to cancerous cells. Induction of Snail-driven EMT has also been shown to drive a range of pro-survival metabolic adaptations in different cancers. In the present study, we sought to determine the specific role that Snail has in driving EMT and adaptive metabolic programming in pancreatic ductal adenocarcinoma (PDAC) by overexpressing Snail in a PDAC cell line, Panc1, and in immortalized, non-tumorigenic human pancreatic ductal epithelial (HPDE) cells. Snail overexpression was able to induce EMT in both pancreatic cell lines through suppression of epithelial markers and upregulation of mesenchymal markers alongside changes in cell morphology and enhanced migratory capacity. Snail-overexpressed pancreatic cells additionally displayed increased glucose uptake and lactate production with concomitant reduction in oxidative metabolism measurements. Snail overexpression reduced maximal respiration in both Panc1 and HPDE cells, with further reductions seen in ATP production, spare respiratory capacity and non-mitochondrial respiration in Snail overexpressing Panc1 cells. Accordingly, lower expression of mitochondrial electron transport chain proteins was observed with Snail overexpression, particularly within Panc1 cells. Modelling of $^{13}$C metabolite flux within both cell lines revealed decreased carbon flux from glucose in the TCA cycle in snai1-overexpressing Panc1 cells only. This work further highlights the role that Snail plays in EMT and demonstrates its specific effects on metabolic reprogramming of glucose metabolism in PDAC.

**Keywords:** SNA1; metabolomics; glucose metabolism; tumor metabolism; epithelial-mesenchymal transition; pancreatic adenocarcinoma

## 1. Introduction

Originating from the ductal cells of exocrine pancreas, pancreatic ductal adenocarcinoma (PDAC) is arguably the most lethal type of common cancer, and its dismal prognosis has remained relatively unchanged over the past three decades [1,2]. Decades of intensive research and clinical investigation have yielded a wealth of knowledge of pancreatic cancer pathophysiology, but effective treatment strategies are still in urgent demand to battle against the rise in pancreatic cancer-related mortalities [2]. The main causes of PDAC-related mortality are the frequent occurrence of metastatic spread and resistance to currently available therapeutic interventions, both of which are partially underlined by a complex process termed the epithelial-mesenchymal transition or EMT [3,4]. The cellular transition from epithelial to mesenchymal phenotype involves profound changes in gene expression patterns, which impart cells with a series of functional properties such as increased migratory potential, invasiveness, resistance to apoptotic stimuli and stemness [5]. In response to EMT-inducing signals commonly existing in the tumor micro-environment, a network of intracellular pathways is activated to convey the message to the EMT executioners for transcriptional regulation [6].

The zinc finger transcription factor Snail was the first identified and is the best characterized EMT effector, and it primarily controls EMT via repressing E-cadherin expression [7,8]. To orchestrate the EMT process, Snail is able to upregulate the mesenchymal genes N-cadherin, vimentin, fibronectin, the matrix metalloproteases (MMPs) and other EMT-inducing transcription factors including Twist1, Zeb1 and Zeb2 [7,9]. In PDAC, the functional significance of Snail-induced EMT has been exemplified by observations of clinical samples and experimental manipulations. Immunohistochemical staining of PDAC surgical specimens has revealed strong Snail expression in 35–80% of samples, which was tightly associated with lymph node invasion and distant metastasis [10,11]. Highly metastatic PDAC cell sublines have also been reported to possess EMT-like phenotype and Snail upregulation when compared with the bulk of tumor cells [12]. Such observations are confirmed by studies using cultured cells where Snail overexpression in Panc1, AsPC-1 and BxPC-3 cells led to overt EMT with alterations in morphology and gene expression and increased transwell invasion capacity [13–15]. Conversely, experimental knock-down of Snail in PDAC cell lines results in increased E-cadherin expression and translocation to the membrane and reduced tumorigenicity [16].

Over the past decade, metabolic reprogramming has been recognized as a hallmark in oncogenic transformation in PDAC and other cancers [17–19]. The well-known aerobic glycolysis or Warburg effect (upregulated glucose uptake and lactate production) has been shown to confer proliferative and survival advantages in multiple cancer types by supplying sufficient bioenergetic precursors and NADPH [20]. PDAC cells also display elevated glutaminolysis to maintain redox balance and scavenge extracellular fatty acids/amino acids to survive in a hostile microenvironment with limited fuel supply [18,21–23]. Heterogeneity exists between metabolic profiles of different cancer types and between different cancer cell populations within the same tumor, owing to the context-specific oncogenic signaling events and micro-environmental factors present [24,25]. The process of EMT involves major changes to the gene expression network and cellular phenotype. It is, therefore, likely to be accompanied by metabolic alterations to accommodate the shift in cell's priority from proliferation to invasion of neighboring tissues and to adapt to changes in the environment. Indeed, a wide range of metabolic alterations have been observed with induction of EMT status in breast, lung, ovarian, cervical and prostate cancers, although the nature of the metabolic reprogramming varies widely across the studies [26–40]. We have previously shown augmentations of glucose consumption and lactate output in Panc1 cells undergoing tumor necrosis factor-$\alpha$ (TNF$\alpha$)- and transformation growth factor-$\beta$ (TGF$\beta$)-induced EMT, with differential molecular changes observed in the two models [41].

Alongside changes to cell metabolism in our previous study [41], we also observed the induction of Snail expression concurrently with change in EMT status in Panc1 cell upon treatment with TGF$\beta$ or TGF$\beta$ combined TNF$\alpha$. In view of the importance of Snail-dependent EMT in underlying PDAC-related lethality, we sought to induce EMT in Panc1 and the non-tumorigenic human pancreatic ductal epithelial (HPDE) cells [42] via Snail overexpression to investigate the metabolic consequences. Specifically, we chose to compare the effects of Snail overexpression in a pancreatic cell line already on the EMT spectrum (Panc1) to that of a purely epithelial pancreatic cell line (HPDE) to study the specific consequences of Snail induction at different points across the EMT differentiation spectrum. Here we report that EMT in both cell lines is associated with elevated glucose uptake and lactate excretion, as well as downregulation of proteins in the mitochondrial electron transport chain (ETC).

## 2. Experimental Section

### 2.1. Antibodies and Reagents

Antibodies used are listed as follows: Snail (3879), Vimentin (5741), LDH-A (2012, Cell Signaling Technology, Danvers, MA, USA); E-cadherin (sc-21791), N-cadherin (sc-7939), Beta-actin (sc-47778, Santa Cruz, TX, USA); Hexokinase II (ab37593), Total OXPHOS Human WB Antibody Cocktail (ab110411, Abcam, Cambridge, UK). All other reagents were from Sigma-Aldrich (Sydney, NSW, Australia) unless stated otherwise.

### 2.2. Cell Culture

Panc1 cells from ATCC were cultured in Dulbecco's modified Eagle's medium (DMEM) containing 4.5 g/L glucose supplemented with 10% fetal bovine serum and penicillin-streptomycin. The human pancreatic ductal epithelial (HPDE) cell line [42] were a kind gift from Dr. Phoebe Phillips at Lowy Cancer Institute, UNSW Australia. HPDE cells were cultured in keratinocyte serum-free (KSF) media (ThermoFisher Scientific, Waltham, MA, USA) containing 1.6 g/L glucose supplemented with epidermal growth factor (5 ng/mL), bovine pituitary extract (50 ug/mL) and penicillin-streptomycin.

### 2.3. Overexpression of the SNAI1 Gene

Plasmid containing human SNAI1 (encoding Snail) cDNA (Addgene plasmid 23347) was a kind gift from Bob Weinberg [43]. Stable SNAI1-expressing Panc1 cell line was generated using retroviral-mediated pBabe-puro-Snail infection. Briefly, $8 \times 10^5$ Hek293-FT cells were seeded on 10 cm culture dishes and allowed to attach overnight before being transiently transfected with gag/pol and VSV-G packaging plasmids, along with the pBabe-puro-Snail plasmid or empty pBabe-puro vector. The culture media for Hek293-FT was refreshed 12 hours later and media containing viral particles were harvested 24 hours and 48 hours after media refreshment. The 24 hours and 48 hours media was combined and applied to target cells at 40% confluence with polybrene (8 µg/µL) for 24 hours. A pooled cell population was used for experiments following puromycin selection.

### 2.4. Cell Morphology

Pictures of cells were taken using a phase contrast microscope (Nikon Eclipse TS100, Nikon, Tokyo, Japan) attached to a camera (Nikon digital sight) under 40× or 100× magnification.

### 2.5. Western Blotting

Cells ($1 \times 10^6$) growing on 6-well plates were lysed in RIPA buffer containing protease inhibitors as described previously [44]. After denaturation, samples (20 ug protein) were resolved by 10% polyacrylamide gel electrophoresis (187 V, 1 h) and transferred to PVDF membranes (65 V, 65 min). For immunoblotting, membranes were blocked in 5% skim milk in tris-buffered saline containing Tween 20 (TBST), incubated with primary antibodies overnight at 4 °C, washed with TBST and incubated with secondary antibodies in 5% skim milk in TBST for an hour. After washing, membranes were developed with enhanced chemiluminescence reagents (Western Lighting Plus-ECL, Perkin Elmer, Waltham, MA, USA) and visualized under Las4000 imager (GE Healthcare, Chicage, IL, USA). Densitometry was performed using ImageJ software by obtaining the optical density of each band.

### 2.6. Quantitative PCR

Total RNA was extracted using the Roche High Pure RNA Extraction kit according to manufacturer's instructions (Roche, Basel, Switzerland). RNA (1 µg) was then reverse-transcribed using the Roche Transcriptor first strand cDNA synthesis kit. The resulting cDNA was mixed with primers (primer sequences sourced from Sigma KiCqstart or the Primer Bank [45]) and SYBR-Green (Roche, Basel, Switzerland) in 96-well plates. Quantitative PCR was performed using Roche 480

Light Cycler to obtain Ct values for each gene of interest and a housekeeper beta-actin. Analysis was conducted using the ΔΔCT method.

## 2.7. Wound Healing Assay

Cells were grown in 6-well plates and scratch wounds were created by scraping confluent cell monolayers with a sterile pipette tip on 3 sites on each well. The cells were then incubated under normal conditions with refreshed media under the Nikon Tie inverted time-lapse microscope for 24 hours. Migration at 24 hours was quantified by measuring the area closed between two moving borders of the cells from each scratch. Values from the 3 wounds on each of the triplicate wells were averaged and 3 independent experiments were carried out.

## 2.8. Measurement of Cell Proliferation

Cells were seeded in 6-well plates at a density of $1.5 \times 10^5$ per well. After 4 days, cells were rinsed with PBS and immersed in 0.5% crystal violet (w/v)/50% methanol (v/v) solution and left to fix for 20 min. After fixation, cells were gently rinsed to remove all the crystal violet solution and allowed to dry overnight. The next day, fixed cells were solubilized with 1% SDS at 37°C and 50 µL of the solution was taken for absorbance measurements at 570 nm using a plate reader as an indication of cell number of the well.

## 2.9. Glucose Uptake Assay

Glucose uptake was assessed using the glucose analogue 2-deoxyglucose (2-DG). Cytochalasin B (25 µM) was applied to control wells for 15 min before the assay and during the assay to give a measure of background glucose uptake.

After washing with PBS, cells in 6-well plates were incubated in Ringer solution (140 mM NaCl, 20 mM HEPES, 5 mM KCl, 2.5 mM MgSO4, 1.2 mM CaCl2, pH7.4) containing 10 µM 2-DG and 0.5 µCi/mL radio-labelled $^3$H-2-DG for exactly 8 min. Following incubation, cells were washed with cold PBS and lysed in 1 M NaOH. The amount of $^3$H radioactivity in lysates was counted using a beta-counter (Tri-Carb liquid scintillation counter, Perkin Elmer, Waltham, MA, USA) from which background was subtracted. Protein concentrations of lysates were measured using BCA assay (Pierce BCA protein assay kit, Thermo Fisher Scientific, Waltham, MA, USA) for normalization.

## 2.10. Lactate Assay

Lactate concentrations in cell culture media (72 hour after plating) were determined in a reaction mixture containing hydrazine hydrate (0.4 M, pH 9.0), EDTA (10 mM, pH 9.0) and NAD$^+$ (0.5 mM). Samples and standards were added into 96-well plates followed by lactate dehydrogenase (10 units/well) and the amount of lactate was assessed by measuring the amount of NADH formed at 340 nm after 2 hours of incubation at 37°C (a timepoint when lactate conversion is complete).

## 2.11. Bioenergetic Profiling of Oxygen Consumption and Extracellular Acidification in Snail Overexpressing and Control Cells

Cells were seeded at $2 \times 10^4$ per well on a XF96 seahorse cell plate (Agilent Technologies, Santa Clara, CA, USA) in their respective growth media. The next day, cells were washed with Seahorse assay media containing 25 mM glucose, 2 mM L-glutamine, 1 mM sodium pyruvate, pH 7.4 equilibrated in the same media at 37 °C for 30 min in a $CO_2$-free incubator. Bioenergetic profiling was performed by monitoring oxygen consumption and extracellular acidification rates at basal levels, followed by sequential injections of 1 µM oligomycin (an ATP synthase inhibitor), 0.5 µM Carbonyl cyanide-4-(trifluoromethoxy)-phenylhydrazone (FCCP) (a mitochondrial uncoupler) and 1 µM rotenone (a Complex I inhibitor) using the Seahorse XF96 Analyzer. The time-course of energetic profiles, as well as basal oxygen consumption, basal extracellular acidification rate and maximal oxygen consumption were calculated from the primary data.

## 2.12. Glucose Oxidation

Glucose oxidation was measured in cells seeded in 6-well plates ($1 \times 10^6$ cells per well). Briefly, cells were washed with PBS and incubated in DMEM containing 1 g/L D-glucose and 2 μCi/ml $^{14}$C-glucose for 1 hour at 37 °C. After incubation, the culture media was added to 1 M perchloric acid and the $CO_2$ released was absorbed in 1 M NaOH solution over 2 hours. The $CO_2$ produced was quantified by counting $^{14}$C content in the NaOH solution using a beta-counter (Tri-Carb liquid scintillation counter, Perkin Elmer, Waltham, MA, USA).

## 2.13. Measurement of Half-Maximal Inhibitory Concentration

The half-maximal inhibitory concentration ($IC_{50}$) was measured by crystal violet assay. Cells were seeded at $1 \times 10^4$ cells per well into a 96-well plate in triplicate and allowed to attach overnight. The next day cells were treated either with serial dilutions of gemcitabine or paclitaxel. The $IC_{50}$ was measured after 48 hours by crystal violet assay as described above ($n = 3$ biological replicates), with cell viability being expressed relative to vehicle control (phosphate buffered saline for gemcitabine, 0.1% ethanol for paclitaxel). The $IC_{50}$ was then calculated by non-linear regression by fitting the log-transformed drug concentration against relative cell viability.

For comparison under different glucose conditions, cells were allowed to adhere overnight in high glucose DMEM (i.e., 4.5 g/L glucose) before being treated with serial dilutions of gemcitabine spiked with an $IC_{75}$ dose of paclitaxel in media containing either high or no glucose.

## 2.14. $^{13}$C metabolic Tracer Experiment and Metabolomics

Triplicates of Panc1 and HPDE cells were cultured in 6-well plates in their respective glucose-free DMEM and KSF media as described earlier. Approximately 4.5 g/L and 2.9 g/L of uniformly labelled $^{13}C_6$-glucose was added to DMEM and KSF media respectively and cells were cultured for 5 hours. To measure the accumulation and $^{13}$C enrichment of extracellular pyruvate and lactate, 50 μL culture media was harvested hourly. The collected media were centrifuged ($300 \times g$, 4°C) for 5 min and the supernatant stored at −30 °C until analysis by gas chromatography mass spectrometry (GCMS) using an extraction and derivatization described previously [46]. To measure $^{13}$C enrichment of intracellular metabolites, cells were quenched at the end of the 5-hour culture, and metabolites were then extracted and derivatized for GCMS analysis [41]. GCMS of derivatized metabolites was conducted using g a HP-5ms capillary column (0.25 mm i.d. × 30 m × 0.25 μm; Agilent J&W, Agilent Technologies, Santa Clara, CA, USA) installed in an Agilent HP 6890-5973 gas chromatography/mass selective detector.

## 2.14. $^{13}$C Flux Analysis

Flux modelling was performed to explain the activity of catabolic pathways used by Panc1 and HPDE to metabolize glucose. Metabolic fluxes, which is a measure of metabolite flows, can be estimated by quantitatively fitting a metabolic model to the metabolite data [46]. A simple $^{13}$C metabolic flux analysis model was used, comprising of glycolysis, pentose-phosphate pathway and TCA cycle [47]. The metabolite data used for the fit included the isotopomer abundances of extracellular pyruvate and lactate, and the enrichment fractions of intracellular pyruvate, lactate, malate, 2-oxoglutarate, citrate, succinate, alanine and aspartate measured by GCMS [48]. Fluxes were then estimated by least-square optimization such that simulated results gave the best fit to the experimental data. Due to the lack of absolute abundance data for intracellular metabolites, metabolite data were simulated under the assumptions of both metabolic (i.e., constant fluxes) and isotopic steady-state (i.e., maximum intracellular $^{13}$C enrichment) [46]. Flux changes due to Snail overexpression was quantified by Monte-Carlo analysis [46]. In this bootstrapping approach, the dataset was repeatedly corrupted with Gaussian noise 200 times, and fluxes were re-estimated each time. The resulting flux distributions were then used to quantify flux changes. Full $^{13}$C flux analysis results are provided within the Supplementary Material, Table S1.

*2.15. Statistical Analysis*

Unless indicated otherwise, results comparing vector infected and Snail over-expressing Panc1 or HPDE cells were analyzed by student t-test and expressed as means ± standard error of the mean (SEM). Statistical significance was set at $p < 0.05$.

## 3. Results

*3.1. Comparison of Basal Levels of EMT Markers in Panc1 and HPDE Cells Establishes EMT Status in Panc1 Cells*

Prior to generation of Snail overexpressing Panc1 and HPDE cell lines, we first sought to determine their basal levels of EMT status. To achieve this, we performed immunoblotting on both Panc1 and HDPE cells cultured under normal conditions to look at basal markers of EMT status, including E-cadherin, N-cadherin, and vimentin (Figure 1). These preliminary immunoblotting experiments confirmed that Panc1 cells are natively somewhere along the EMT spectrum, displaying both markers of epithelial cell type (E-cadherin) as well as markers of mesenchymal status. Conversely, HPDE cells only displayed markers of epithelial status, indicating little to no induction of EMT.

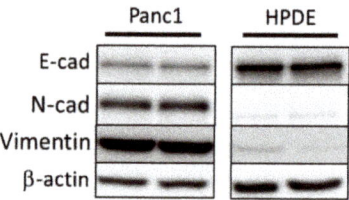

**Figure 1.** Immunoblotting of basal levels of EMT markers E-cadherin (E-cad), N-cadherin (N-cad), and vimentin in Panc1 and HPDE cells. β-actin was used as loading control.

*3.2. Snail Overexpression Induced EMT in Panc1 and HPDE Cells*

To study the metabolic changes associated pancreatic cells either already on the EMT spectrum or pancreatic cells with little EMT induction, we overexpressed the principal EMT-inducing transcription factor Snail in the PDAC cell line Panc1 and in non-tumorigenic HPDE cells respectively. Cells were infected with either the empty retroviral pBabe-puro vector (vector) or vector containing human SNAI1 (Snail). Two weeks after puromycin selection, surviving cells of the Snail clones in both cell lines displayed distinct morphology compared to the vector control in that they were more spindle like and dispersed, suggesting the dissociation of tight junctions (Figure 2A or Figure 2E). In Panc1, the increase in Snail (15-fold, $p < 0.01$) was coupled with marked reductions of E-cadherin levels ($p < 0.001$) in Snail-overexpressed cells, while levels of mesenchymal markers (N-cadherin and vimentin) presented little change (Figure 2B). In HPDE cells, N-cadherin and vimentin, as well as Snail, were only present at negligible levels in vector control but were remarkably induced upon Snail overexpression (80-fold increase, Figure 2F). The overexpression of Snail in HPDE also resulted in significant decreases in E-cadherin levels (Figure 2F).

To assess the functional effect of Snail overexpression in terms of migratory capacity, vector control and Snail-overexpressed cells were subjected to wound healing assays. Migration as indicated by the area of wound closure over 24 hours surprisingly did not differ between vector and Snail Panc1 cells (Figure 2C), while Snail resulted in increased percentage of wound closure over 24 hours in HPDE cells ($p < 0.05$, Figure 2G). The proliferation of cells over a 4-day period, measured by crystal violet assays, was slightly but significantly ($p < 0.01$) slowed down by Snail overexpression in Panc1 but not in HPDE cells (Figure 2D or Figure 2H).

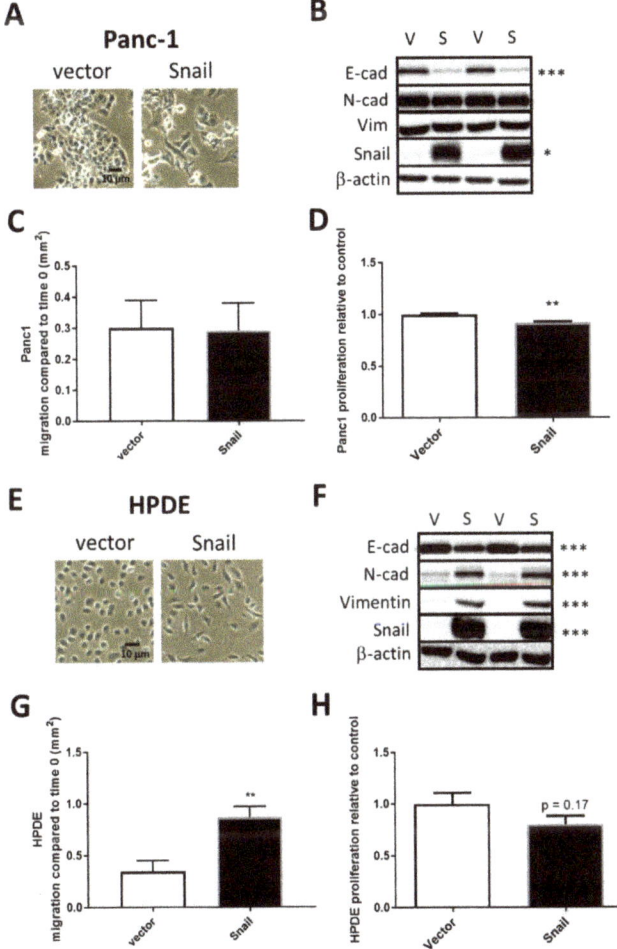

**Figure 2.** Snail overexpression induced EMT in Panc1 (**A–D**) and HPDE (**E–H**) cells. Vector control (V) and Snail-overexpressing (S) cells were generated in Panc1 via retroviral-mediated infections. (**A,E**) Representative cell images were taken under bright field microscopy. (**B,F**) Cell lysates were resolved by SDS-PAGE and immunoblotted with anti-E-cad, anti-N-cad, anti-vimentin, and anti-Snail antibodies with β-actin used as a loading control. (**C,G**) Cell migration as measured by wound healing assay. (**D,H**) Cell proliferation as measured by crystal violet assay. Results are shown as mean ± SEM with $n = 3$. * $p < 0.05$, ** $p < 0.01$, *** $p < 0.001$ for difference between vector control and Snail-overexpressing cells.

### 3.3. Snail Overexpression Resulted in Increased Glucose Uptake and Lactate Secretion in Panc1 Cells

The upregulation of aerobic glycolysis, or increased glycolysis and lactate production in the presence of sufficient oxygen, has been frequently observed during tumorigenesis and in some cancer cells undergoing EMT [26,27,32,34–36]. It was also one of the most pronounced changes seen with TGFβ-induced EMT in Panc1 cells, during which Snail was induced [41]. Here the overexpression of Snail in Panc1 cells also resulted in the upregulation of glucose uptake by nearly 2-fold ($p < 0.01$,

Figure 3A). There were no associated changes in SLC2A1 (encoding Glut1), SLC2A3 (encoding Glut3) or HK2, the enzyme converting glucose to glucose-6-phosphate (Figure 3D–F). Snail overexpression in Panc1 cells also caused a 2-fold increase in secreted lactate over a 3-day period ($p < 0.01$, Figure 3B). Using the Seahorse XF96 Analyzer system, lactate production was measured in a more acute setting as the basal extracellular acidification rate sampled over 20 min (Figure 3C). The basal extracellular acidification rate (ECAR; i.e., first 20 mins of assay) was slightly higher in Snail overexpressing Panc1 cells ($p < 0.05$, Figure 3C,D), while no difference was reported in maximal glycolysis after inhibition of mitochondrial ATP production by oligomycin. This lack of difference maximal glycolysis meant that Snail-overexpressing Panc1 cells had lower glycolytic capacity (i.e., the difference between maximal and basal glycolysis; $p < 0.05$; Figure 3C,D). Despite the changes in lactate production, no alterations were seen in LDH-A levels or LDH-B, MCT1 expressions whereas MCT4 expression was enhanced slightly ($p < 0.05$) (Figure 3F–I).

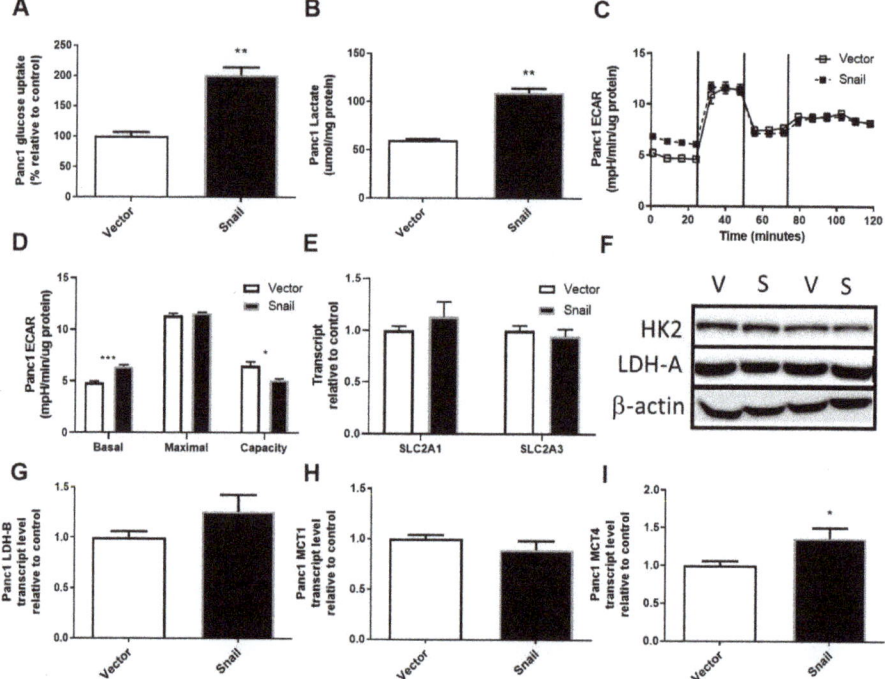

**Figure 3.** Effects of Snail overexpression on glucose uptake and lactate production in Panc1 cells. (**A**) Rate of glucose uptake measured using by $^3$H-2-Deoxy-Glucose uptake over an 8 min period. (**B**) Lactate assay performed on cell culture media after 72 hours of culture. (**C**) Extracellular acidification rate (ECAR) measured using the Seahorse XF96 Analyzer at basal levels for 30 min followed by sequential injections of 1 μM oligomycin, 0.5 μM Carbonyl cyanide-4-(trifluoromethoxy)-phenylhydrazone (FCCP) and 1 μM rotenone at 30 min intervals. (**D**) basal and maximal glycolytic activity and glycolytic capacity calculated from Seahorse data, (**E**) Fold-change in total RNA for SLC2A1 (encoding Glut1) and SLC2A3 (encoding Glut3) measured by qPCR using β-actin as housekeeper, (**F**) Immunoblotting results for hexokinase II (HK2) and lactate dehydrogenase A (LDH-A) with β-actin as loading control. (**G–I**) Fold change in total RNA detected for lactate dehydrogenase-B (LDH-B) and monocarboxylate transporter 1 (MCT1) and 4 (MCT4). Results are shown as mean ± SEM with $n = 3$. * $p < 0.05$, ** $p < 0.01$ for difference between vector control and Snail-overexpressing cells.

## 3.4. Snail Overexpression Resulted in Increased Glucose Uptake and Lactate Production in HPDE Cells

HPDE cells overexpressing Snail displayed elevated glucose uptake to a level comparable to Panc1 cells (2-fold, $p < 0.001$, Figure 4A). The augmentation of glucose uptake was accompanied by reduced SLC2A1 (Glut1) expression ($p < 0.001$, Figure 4D) and a 4-fold increase in SLC2A3 (Glut3) expression ($p < 0.01$, Figure 4E). The level of HK2 did not differ between vector and Snail clones (Figure 4F). Although levels of lactate production in vector control HPDE cells were higher than that observed for vector control Panc1 cells, Snail-overexpressing HPDE cells also showed an increase in lactate accumulation in the culture media (Figure 4B). This increase in lactate output was also apparent over the 30-minute period in which basal ECAR was measured using the Seahorse XF96 Analyzer (Figure 4C,D). Similar to Snail overexpressing Panc1 cells, there was no difference observed in maximal glycolysis rate leading to an overall decrease in glycolytic capacity in Snail overexpressing HPDE cells ($p < 0.05$). Among the lactate production (LDH-A and B) and secretion (MCT1 and 4) mRNA measured, only LDH-B transcript displayed a nearly 2-fold increase ($p < 0.001$) (Figure 4F–I).

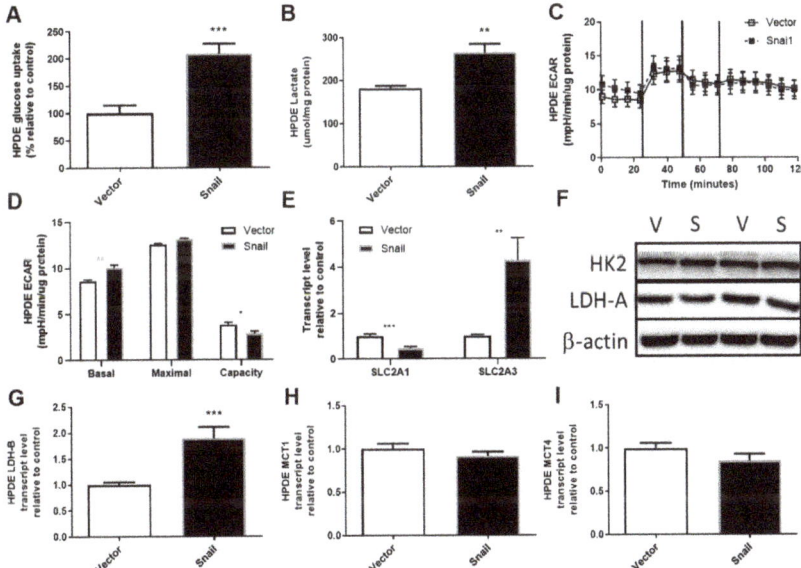

**Figure 4.** Effects of Snail overexpression on glucose uptake and lactate production in HPDE cells. (**A**) Rate of glucose uptake measured by $^3$H-2-Deoxy-Glucose tracer over an 8 min period. (**B**) Lactate assay performed on cell culture media collected after 72 hours of culturing. (**C**) Extracellular acidification rate (ECAR) measured using the Seahorse XF96 Analyzer at basal levels for 30 min followed by sequential injections of 1 µM oligomycin, 0.5 µM Carbonyl cyanide-4-(trifluoromethoxy)-phenylhydrazone (FCCP) and 1 µM rotenone at 30 min intervals. (**D**) basal and maximal glycolytic activity and glycolytic capacity calculated from Seahorse data. (**E**) Fold-change in total RNA for SLC2A1 (encoding Glut1) and SLC2A3 (encoding Glut3) measured by qPCR using β-actin as housekeeper. (**F**) Immunoblotting results for hexokinase II (HK2) and lactate dehydrogenase A (LDH-A) with β-actin as loading control. (**G–I**) Fold change in total RNA detected for lactate dehydrogenase-B (LDH-B) and monocarboxylate transporter 1 (MCT1) and 4 (MCT4). Results are shown as mean ± SEM with $n = 3$. ** $p < 0.01$, *** $p < 0.001$ for difference between vector control and Snail-overexpressing cells.

## 3.5. Snail Overexpression Impacted on Oxidative Metabolism in Both Panc1 and HPDE Cells

Following the observations of enhanced aerobic glycolysis, we next investigated the overall and glucose-specific oxidative metabolism in Panc1 and HPDE cells. Using the Seahorse XF96 Analyzer,

OCR at basal levels were not different in either the Panc1 or HPDE Snail overexpressing cells compared with their respective vector controls. Maximal OCR (after addition of the mitochondrial uncoupler FCCP that elicits maximal respiration) was significantly reduced upon Snail-overexpression-induced EMT in both Panc1 ($p < 0.001$) and HPDE ($p < 0.05$) cells (Figure 5B or Figure 5E). Notably, the maximally stimulated OCR in Snail-overexpressed Panc1 cells was nearly halved in comparison to vector control and was not higher than its basal level (Figure 5A). Alongside decreases in maximal respiration in Snail overexpressing Panc1 cells ($p < 0.001$), significant decreases were also observed in ATP production ($p < 0.05$), spare respiratory capacity ($p < 0.001$), and non-mitochondrial respiration ($p < 0.01$, Figure 5B). These observations were in line with significant ($p < 0.05$) decreases in the content of mitochondrial ETC subunits V, III, II and I in Snail-overexpressing Panc1 cells (Figure 5C). Glucose-specific oxidation measured using $^{14}$C-labelled glucose tracers was, however, not altered in Panc1 (Figure 5D).

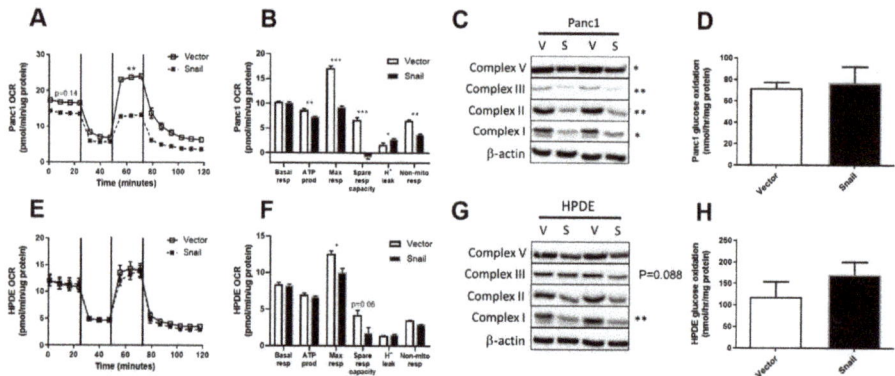

**Figure 5.** Effects of Snail overexpression on oxidative metabolism in Panc1 and HPDE cells. (**A,E**) Oxygen consumption rate (OCR) was measured using the Seahorse XF96 Analyzer at basal levels for 30 min followed by sequential injections of 1 µM oligomycin, 0.5 µM Carbonyl cyanide-4-(trifluoromethoxy)-phenylhydrazone (FCCP) and 1 µM rotenone at 30 min intervals. Basal and maximal (following FCCP injection) values of OCR from the time-course data were used for statistical analysis. (**B,F**) Basal respiration, ATP production, maximal respiration, spare respiratory capacity, proton leak and non-mitochondrial respiration calculated from Seahorse trace data for Panc1 and HPDE cells respectively. (**C,G**) Immunoblotting results for ETC complex I, II, III, V antibodies, with β-actin used as loading control. Densitometry on western blots was performed using image J. (**D,H**) Glucose oxidation was measured using the U-$^{14}$C-Glucose tracer over one-hour period. Results are shown as mean ± SEM with $n = 3$. * $p < 0.05$, ** $p < 0.01$ for difference between vector control and Snail-overexpressing cells.

In contrast to Panc1, the OCR at basal level and after addition of oligomycin, FCCP and rotenone remained unaffected by Snail overexpression in HPDE cells (Figure 5E). Snail overexpressing HPDE cells displayed a lower maximal respiration compared with vector control ($p < 0.05$), and a trend towards decreased spare respiratory capacity (Figure 5F). The decrease observed in maximal respiration observation was in line with reductions in the levels of ETC complexes in HPDE cells upon Snail-driven EMT ($p = 0.088$ for complex III; $p < 0.01$ for complex I), albeit to a lesser extent than Panc1 (Figure 5G). Glucose specific oxidative activity was unaltered in Snail overexpressed cells, as indicated by the $^{14}CO_2$ produced from $^{14}$C-glucose substrate (Figure 5H).

### 3.6. $^{13}$C Flux Analysis Validated Observed Changes in Aerobic Glycolysis and TCA Cycle Activity

A modelling approach was used to provide a coherent interpretation of metabolic fluxes using metabolite data obtained for Panc1 and HPDE cells with or without Snail overexpression (Figure 6A). Fluxes were estimated by fitting the metabolic model to the measured accumulation rate of extracellular lactate and pyruvate, and to the $^{13}$C enrichment pattern of intracellular metabolites (Figure 6B,C). Despite similarities in the enrichment fractions (Figure 6B), our analyses accounted for the fact that media used between the two cell lines (i.e., DMEM and KSF media) were different. In DMEM, glucose was 95% labelled and lactate was present, whereas in KSF media glucose was only 59% labelled and had no lactate (Figure 6A or Figure 6C). Similarly, only DMEM contained free alanine (results not shown), which explained the significant dilution of $^{13}$C-enriched intracellular alanine in Panc1 compared to HPDE (Figure 6B). The assimilation of unlabeled pyruvate was added ad-hoc to better fit metabolite data from HPDE cells.

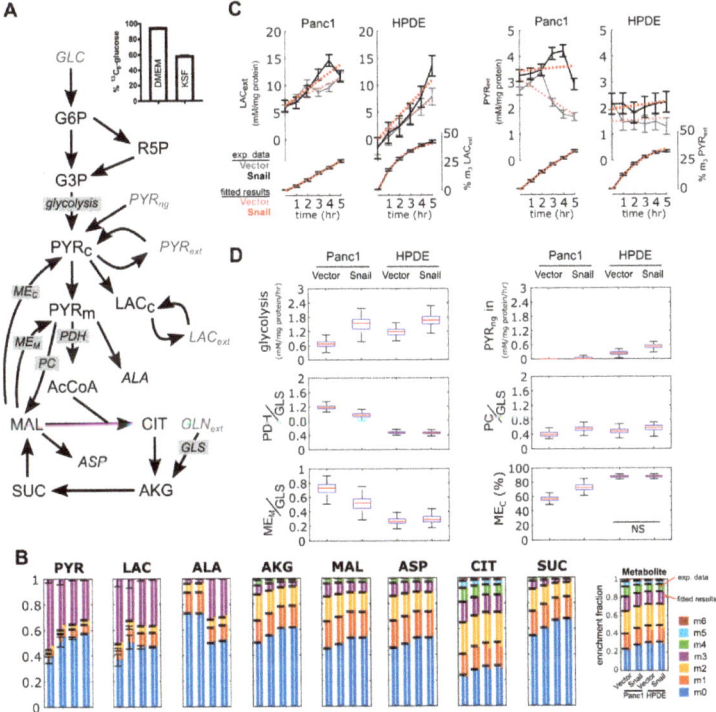

**Figure 6.** Metabolomics and flux analysis of the effects of Snail overexpression on glucose metabolism in Panc1 and HPDE cells. (**A**) 13C metabolic flux analysis model used to interpret metabolite data. Input substrates shown as gray. Average glucose $^{13}$C-enrichment in DMEM and KSF media shown to highlight differences in starting label. (**B**) $^{13}$C-enrichment of intracellular metabolites, showing measured fractional enrichments (left bars) and simulated results from the best fit (right bars). Data are shown with mean ± 1 SD with $n$ = 3. (**C**) Abundance and $^{13}$C-enrichment trajectories of extracellular lactate and pyruvate. "m3" represents fraction of lactate and pyruvate labelled at all three carbons. Results from the best fit are shown as red dotted lines. Error bars represent ± 1 SD. (**D**) Box-and-whiskers plots show estimated fluxes. PDH, PC and ME$_M$ fluxes normalized to glutamine uptake flux. ME$_C$ flux expressed as a fraction of total ME flux. All flux changes were significant, unless indicated otherwise. Enzyme: ME$_C$ (cytoplasmic malic enzyme), ME$_M$ (mitochondrial malic enzyme), PC (pyruvate carboxylase), GLS (glutaminase), glycolysis (pyruvate kinase), PDH (pyruvate dehydrogenase). Metabolites: PYR (pyruvate), LAC (lactate), ALA (alanine), AKG (2-oxoglutarate), MAL (malate), ASP (aspartate), CIT (citrate), SUC (succinate), R5P (ribose 5 phosphate), AcCoA (acetyl-CoA), GLN (glutamine). NS $p$ > 0.05.

Flux results confirmed that aerobic glycolysis increased in Snail overexpression, for both Panc1 and HPDE cells (Figure 6D). Basal lactate secretion rates were lower in Panc1 than HPDE cells; this is consistent with the results from the enzymatic lactate assay and ECAR (Figure 3B–D and Figure 4B–D). Likewise, the reduction of basal OCR in Panc1 but not HPDE (Figure 5A,E) was reproduced by the estimated pyruvate dehydrogenase fluxes (Figure 6D). Only Panc1 cells with Snail overexpression showed a net consumption of extracellular pyruvate (Figure 6C), although all cultures were secreting pyruvate from glucose.

Flux modelling revealed a few features not immediately observed from metabolite data. The overexpression of Snail in Panc1 cells reduced TCA cycle activity to a greater extent than HPDE cells. This was achieved by lowering both pyruvate dehydrogenase flux and complete oxidation of glutamine, with the latter indicated by a reduced mitochondrial malic enzyme activity and a concomitant shift towards cytoplasmic malic enzyme flux (Figure 6D). This metabolic configuration was required to reproduce the reduced enrichment of intracellular pyruvate and lactate, which could not be solely accomplished by the reversible exchange between the respective intracellular and extracellular pools. Overall, $^{13}$C flux analysis showed that Snail overexpression increased aerobic glycolysis and altered carbon flow in the TCA cycle, more so in Panc1 cells than in HPDE.

### 3.7. Snail Overexpression in Panc1 Cells Does Not Increase Resistance to Gemcitabine or Combination Gemcitabine-Paclitaxel Therapy

Given the known role of EMT in chemoresistance in PDAC [10], we sought to determine if Snail-overexpression and subsequent EMT induction in Panc1 cells could increase resistance to chemotherapies commonly used in PDAC treatment. To this end, we determined the half-maximal inhibitory concentration ($IC_{50}$) of gemcitabine, paclitaxel and gemcitabine combined with an $IC_{75}$ dose of paclitaxel (Table 1). Overexpression of Snail in Panc1 cells did not result in an increased resistance to gemcitabine alone or in combination with an $IC_{75}$ dose of paclitaxel, but Snail-overexpressing Panc1 cells were slightly more sensitive to paclitaxel monotherapy. We hypothesized that Snail overexpression may give PDAC cells enhanced chemoresistance under the low nutrient microenvironment conditions typically found in PDAC tumors as a result of the dense stromal/desmoplastic reaction [49], but no statistically significance differences were observed between the $IC_{50}$ of Snail-overexpressing and vector controls treated with combination therapy under limiting glucose conditions.

**Table 1.** The half-maximal inhibitory concentration ($IC_{50}$) of gemcitabine, paclitaxel and combination gemcitabine with an $IC_{75}$ dose of paclitaxel in vector control and Snail overexpressing Panc1 cells. Combination treatment was given under both high and no glucose media conditions.

| Panc1 | Gemcitabine | Paclitaxel * | Gemcitabine + $IC_{75}$ Paclitaxel | |
|---|---|---|---|---|
| | | | High Glucose | No Glucose |
| Vector | 1.8 (1.2–2.9) × 10$^{-7}$ | 3.3 (2.4–4.6) × 10$^{-9}$ | 1.3 (0.5–4.2) × 10$^{-7}$ | 1.3 (0.3–5.3) × 10$^{-7}$ |
| Snail | 1.4 (0.8–2.9) × 10$^{-7}$ | 2.0 (1.3–3.1) × 10$^{-9}$ | 3.0 (1.1–8.6) × 10$^{-7}$ | 6.3 (0.4–52.2) × 10$^{-7}$ |

$IC_{50}$ (M) with 95% confidence interval. Vector compared with Snail overexpression: * $p < 0.05$.

## 4. Discussion

The occurrence of EMT in response to micro-environmental factors partially underlines the malignant phenotype and chemoresistance of PDAC. High levels of Snail, a potent EMT-inducing transcription factor, closely correlate with lymph node invasion and distant metastasis in human PDAC samples [10–12,50–52]. Attenuation of Snail expression in PDAC cell lines resulted in the reversal of EMT, together with decreased sphere and colony formation capacity [16]. It has been shown in several studies that PDAC cells overexpressing Snail underwent EMT and exhibited EMT-associated invasive behaviors both in vitro and in vivo [10,13–15]. In the present study, stable overexpression of

Snail in the PDAC cell line Panc1 and non-tumorigenic HPDE cells resulted in pronounced EMT-like phenotypic change as evidenced by alterations in morphology, epithelial/mesenchymal markers and, in the case of HPDE, enhanced migratory capacity (Figure 2). There were also several adaptations in glucose and oxidative metabolism observed with snail overexpression in both cell lines. Despite these alterations to metabolism, Snail-overexpression in PDAC cells did not result in enhanced resistance to gemcitabine or combination gemcitabine/paclitaxel therapy when cultured under either high or limited glucose conditions (Table 1).

Over the past decade, metabolic reprogramming has been increasingly recognized as a hallmark of oncogenic transformation in PDAC and other cancers [17–19]. A small body of literature has also emerged in the last 5 years uncovering additional metabolic alterations related to EMT in breast, lung, ovarian, cervical and prostate cancers, but the actual changes vary considerably across different EMT models and cancer types [26–40]. The EMT events were mostly accompanied by elevated levels of more than one EMT-inducing transcription factors, with Snail being a principal player in the majority of cases [28–33,36]. In the context of PDAC, Snail was highly induced in Panc1 during TGFβ induced EMT, which was associated with upregulated aerobic glycolysis [41]. The induction of EMT by Snail overexpression in the current study was also accompanied by augmented glucose uptake, lactate production and increased levels of basal glycolytic activity, with changes in the expression of transporters and enzymes involved in these processes, namely increased MCT4 expression in Panc1 and higher GLUT3 as well as LDH-B expression in HPDE cells (Figures 3 and 4). In addition, marked downregulations of mitochondrial ETC subunits content and, particularly in the case of Panc1, impaired overall oxidative metabolism were evident.

A direct role of Snail in regulating the glycolytic process has been reported in several occasions. Dong et al. (2013) observed an inverse correlation between levels of Snail and the gluconeogenic enzyme FBP1 in breast cancers [27], hence favoring glucose flux through glycolysis rather than the reverse direction. In basal-like breast cancer, an aggressive subtype containing abundant EMT features, the Snail-G9a-Mnmt1 complex was shown to directly bind to the FBP1 promoter, leading to DNA methylation and transcriptional silencing of the gene [27]. The Snail-mediated suppression of FBP1 was thought to promote glucose uptake and lactate production via improving insulin sensitivity and decreasing PDH (the enzyme catalyzing the conversion of pyruvate to acetyl-CoA and therefore mitochondrial oxidation) activity [27]. In the same vein, Snail levels were high in the more aggressive and castration-resistant subtype of prostate cancer, in which Snail depletion reduced glucose consumption and lactate production [38]. Snail was found to regulate metabolism through miRNA-126-mediated RPS6KB1/HIF1α/PKM2 signaling [38]. In Madin Darby Canine Kidney (MDCK) cells, Snail overexpression resulted in increased activity of phosphofructokinase, a rate-limiting glycolytic enzyme promoting the opposite process to FBP1 [37]. Increased PDK1 expression and the consequent reduction of PDH activity also pointed to the diversion of glycolytic flux towards lactate synthesis [37]. The glycolytic switch was also observed in the breast cancer cell lines MCF-7 and MDA-MB-231 when Snail was induced by Wnt signaling or E-cadherin knock-down [39].

The augmentations of glucose uptake, lactate production, and basal glycolytic activity seen in both Panc1 and HPDE, despite differences in molecular changes, could contribute to EMT-related functional properties especially increased migratory and invasive potential. Enhanced aerobic glycolysis has been associated with invasive cancers and several glycolytic enzymes have been shown to stimulate migration via signaling effects [53–55]. The strongest argument in favor of the glycolytic dependency of migration came from observations that mesenchymal prostate and breast cancer cells exhibited higher aerobic glycolysis, cytoskeletal remodeling and faster migration than epithelial counterparts while no difference in mitochondrial ATP production was found [56]. Migration was attenuated only by inhibition of glycolysis but not mitochondrial respiration [56]. As cell migration is an energy-expensive process involving major remodeling of the cytoskeletal network [57,58], one benefit of the profound upregulation of the glycolytic pathway in PDAC EMT models is presumably to maintain a steady and rapid supply of ATP for cellular migration. The increased lactate secretion by tumor cells could result in an acidic peri-tumor microenvironment which induces MMP-9 expression and the release of other proteolytic enzymes to degrade components of the ECM [59,60]. This is of particular importance in PDAC, which exhibits a prominent desmoplastic reaction involving extensive proliferation of stromal cells and ECM deposition, constituting a physical barrier for tumor cell extravasation [49]. The flow of $H^+$ along its concentration gradient to adjacent normal tissues could also lead to toxic effects in normal cells such as stromal cells but not cancer cells that developed resistance to low pH environment during carcinogenesis [61]. In addition, lactate has been reported to directly enhance tumor cell motility and contribute to tumor immune escape by inhibiting monocyte migration and cytokine release [62]. However, overexpression of Snail within a metastatic subclone of PC-3 prostate cancer cells reduced both glucose and lactate consumption and increased oxidative metabolism, indicating that expression of EMT features may not always coincide with a higher glycolytic phenotype across all cancer types [63].

There was evidence of downregulation of ETC complex subunits in both cell lines with Snail overexpression. These changes were more pronounced in Panc1 cells compared to HPDE and translated into a functional deficit where both the maximal OCR and the flow of carbons into the TCA cycle decreased in Panc1 cells. The inhibition of oxidative phosphorylation by Snail was implicated in Dong et al. (2013) where Snail-mediated reduction in FBP1 resulted in the loss of mitochondrial transcription factor B1M (TFB1M), leading to defects of protein translation in ETC complex I components [27]. As complex I and III are the main sites of ROS production, the downregulation of complex I level caused by Snail was accompanied by ROS reduction [27]. Lee et al. (2012) showed the direct binding of Snail to promoters of three Cytochrome c oxidase (COX) subunits of ETC complex IV [39]. Complex IV activity and mitochondrial respiration were impaired as a result but no change in ATP status was seen, possibly owing to the compensatory increase in glycolytic ATP production [39]. Given that cell migration is an energy consuming process and the increased wound closure was only observed in HPDE cells overexpressing Snail that exhibit only a small change in maximal respiration (Figure 5F), one could speculate that the large decrease in maximal respiration and ATP production seen in Panc1-Snail cells limited their migratory capacity. This phenomenon was observed in other models of EMT induction where loss of oxidative metabolism impedes cell migration [64]. The dissociation of mitochondrial ETC content and basal/maximal OCR in HPDE cells with or without Snail might be attributed to decreased electron donation to the ETC complexes and increased energy consumption in other EMT-related processes. Alternatively, that fact that Panc1 cells are already on the EMT spectrum prior to Snail induction may limit any additional gain in migratory capacity (Figure 1).

There have been indications in the literature that the process of EMT promotes chemoresistance in various carcinomas including PDAC [65–68]. While the induction of several transcription factors and increased stemness were suggested as possible mechanisms, it is not clear if EMT-associated metabolic programming or increased glycolysis plays a role [66,67]. In the present study, Snail-induced EMT changes did not alter Panc1 sensitivity to gemcitabine or combination gemcitabine paclitaxel treatment despite marked enhancement of glycolysis and slight reduction on proliferation (Table 1 and Figure 1). Further work is required to probe the effects of EMT-related metabolic reprogramming on chemo-sensitivity in additional PDAC cell lines and with other first-line chemotherapeutic agents.

## 5. Conclusions

Collectively, Snail overexpression in the PDAC cell line Panc1 and in non-tumorigenic HPDE cells resulted in the induction of EMT and a range of accompanying metabolic changes. In both cell lines Snail overexpression resulted in increased glucose uptake and lactate production, as well as reductions in mitochondrial ETC protein content. Additionally, Snail overexpression caused decreased carbon flux from glucose in the TCA cycle in Panc1 cells only, with no change in Snail-overexpressing HPDE cells. Despite the induction of EMT status and detection of metabolic reprogramming of glucose metabolism in Panc1 cells Snail-overexpression did not result in enhanced resistance to gemcitabine or combination gemcitabine/paclitaxel therapy. This work highlights the role that Snail plays as an effector of EMT and its role in the induction of metabolic reprogramming in PDAC. Further research to uncover specific changes in metabolic enzymes, pathways and energetic profiles that are essential to EMT in PDAC is required to allow therapeutic interventions from a metabolic angle.

**Supplementary Materials:** The following are available online at http://www.mdpi.com/2077-0383/8/6/822/s1, Table S1: $^{13}$C metabolic flux analysis results.

**Author Contributions:** Conceptualization, M.L., L.-E.Q., N.T.; methodology, M.L., S.E.H., G.S., B.P.W., E.D., B.O., and L.-E.Q.; writing—original draft preparation, M.L., S.E.H. and L.-E.Q.; writing—review and editing, S.E.H. and N.T.; funding acquisition, L.-E.Q. and N.T.

**Funding:** This work was supported by an Australian Research Council Future Fellowship to N.T. M.L. was supported by an UNSW International Postgraduate Award, and L.-E.Q. by the Judith and Coffey Fund.

**Acknowledgments:** The authors wish to thank Phoebe Phillips for kind donation of the human pancreatic ductal epithelial cells. We also thank the staff at the Biomedical Imaging Facility at UNSW for their technical assistance. We gratefully acknowledge subsidized access to the Bioanalytical Mass Spectrometry Facility at UNSW, supported by the National Collaborative Research Infrastructure Scheme

**Conflicts of Interest:** The authors declare no conflict of interest.

## References

1. Falasca, M.; Kim, M.; Casari, I. Pancreatic cancer: Current research and future directions. *Biochim. Biophys. Acta* **2016**, *1865*, 123–132. [CrossRef] [PubMed]
2. Vincent, A.; Herman, J.; Schulick, R.; Hruban, R.H.; Goggins, M. Pancreatic cancer. *Lancet Lond. Engl.* **2011**, *378*, 607–620. [CrossRef]
3. Pan, J.-J.; Yang, M.-H. The role of epithelial-mesenchymal transition in pancreatic cancer. *J. Gastrointest. Oncol.* **2011**, *2*, 151–156. [PubMed]
4. Rhim, A.D.; Mirek, E.T.; Aiello, N.M.; Maitra, A.; Bailey, J.M.; McAllister, F.; Reichert, M.; Beatty, G.L.; Rustgi, A.K.; Vonderheide, R.H.; et al. EMT and Dissemination Precede Pancreatic Tumor Formation. *Cell* **2012**, *148*, 349–361. [CrossRef] [PubMed]
5. Lamouille, S.; Xu, J.; Derynck, R. Molecular mechanisms of epithelial–mesenchymal transition. *Nat. Rev. Mol. Cell Biol.* **2014**, *15*, 178–196. [CrossRef] [PubMed]
6. Craene, B.D.; Berx, G. Regulatory networks defining EMT during cancer initiation and progression. *Nat. Rev. Cancer* **2013**, *13*, 97–110. [CrossRef] [PubMed]
7. Cano, A.; Pérez-Moreno, M.A.; Rodrigo, I.; Locascio, A.; Blanco, M.J.; Del Barrio, M.G.; Portillo, F.; Nieto, M.A. The transcription factor Snail controls epithelial–mesenchymal transitions by repressing E-cadherin expression. *Nat. Cell Biol.* **2000**, *2*, 76–83. [CrossRef]
8. Batlle, E.; Sancho, E.; Francí, C.; Domínguez, D.; Monfar, M.; Baulida, J. Antonio García de Herreros the transcription factor Snail is a repressor of E-cadherin gene expression in epithelial tumour cells. *Nat. Cell Biol.* **2000**, *2*, 84–89. [CrossRef]
9. Peinado, H.; Olmeda, D.; Cano, A. Snail, Zeb and bHLH factors in tumour progression: An alliance against the epithelial phenotype? *Nat. Rev. Cancer* **2007**, *7*, 415–428. [CrossRef]
10. Yin, T.; Wang, C.; Liu, T.; Zhao, G.; Zha, Y.; Yang, M. Expression of Snail in Pancreatic Cancer Promotes Metastasis and Chemoresistance. *J. Surg. Res.* **2007**, *141*, 196–203. [CrossRef]
11. Hotz, B.; Arndt, M.; Dullat, S.; Bhargava, S.; Buhr, H.-J.; Hotz, H.G. Epithelial to Mesenchymal Transition: Expression of the Regulators Snail, Slug, and Twist in Pancreatic Cancer. *Clin. Cancer Res.* **2007**, *13*, 4769–4776. [CrossRef] [PubMed]
12. Von Burstin, J.; Eser, S.; Paul, M.C.; Seidler, B.; Brandl, M.; Messer, M.; Von Werder, A.; Schmidt, A.; Mages, J.; Pagel, P.; et al. E-cadherin regulates metastasis of pancreatic cancer in vivo and is suppressed by a SNAIL/HDAC1/HDAC2 repressor complex. *Gastroenterology* **2009**, *137*, 361–371.e5. [CrossRef] [PubMed]
13. Shields, M.A.; Dangi-Garimella, S.; Krantz, S.B.; Bentrem, D.J.; Munshi, H.G. Pancreatic Cancer Cells Respond to Type I Collagen by Inducing Snail Expression to Promote Membrane Type 1 Matrix Metalloproteinase-dependent Collagen Invasion. *J. Biol. Chem.* **2011**, *286*, 10495–10504. [CrossRef] [PubMed]

14. Nishioka, R.; Itoh, S.; Gui, T.; Gai, Z.; Oikawa, K.; Kawai, M.; Tani, M.; Yamaue, H.; Muragaki, Y. SNAIL induces epithelial-to-mesenchymal transition in a human pancreatic cancer cell line (BxPC3) and promotes distant metastasis and invasiveness in vivo. *Exp. Mol. Pathol.* **2010**, *89*, 149–157. [CrossRef]
15. Oyanagi, J.; Ogawa, T.; Sato, H.; Higashi, S.; Miyazaki, K. Epithelial-Mesenchymal Transition Stimulates Human Cancer Cells to Extend Microtubule-based Invasive Protrusions and Suppresses Cell Growth in Collagen Gel. *PLoS ONE* **2012**, *7*. [CrossRef] [PubMed]
16. Zhou, W.; Lv, R.; Qi, W.; Wu, D.; Xu, Y.; Liu, W.; Mou, Y.; Wang, L. Snail Contributes to the Maintenance of Stem Cell-Like Phenotype Cells in Human Pancreatic Cancer. *PLoS ONE* **2014**, *9*, e87409. [CrossRef] [PubMed]
17. Hanahan, D.; Weinberg, R.A. Hallmarks of Cancer: The Next Generation. *Cell* **2011**, *144*, 646–674. [CrossRef]
18. Blum, R.; Kloog, Y. Metabolism addiction in pancreatic cancer. *Cell Death Dis.* **2014**, *5*, e1065. [CrossRef]
19. Perera, R.M.; Bardeesy, N. Pancreatic Cancer Metabolism-Breaking it down to build it back up. *Cancer Discov.* **2015**, *5*, 1247–1261. [CrossRef]
20. Ward, P.S.; Thompson, C.B. Metabolic Reprogramming: A Cancer Hallmark Even Warburg Did Not Anticipate. *Cancer Cell* **2012**, *21*, 297–308. [CrossRef]
21. Son, J.; Lyssiotis, C.A.; Ying, H.; Wang, X.; Hua, S.; Ligorio, M.; Perera, R.M.; Ferrone, C.R.; Mullarky, E.; Shyh-Chang, N.; et al. Glutamine supports pancreatic cancer growth through a KRAS-regulated metabolic pathway. *Nature* **2013**, *496*, 101–105. [CrossRef] [PubMed]
22. Kamphorst, J.J.; Cross, J.R.; Fan, J.; De Stanchina, E.; Mathew, R.; White, E.P.; Thompson, C.B.; Rabinowitz, J.D. Hypoxic and Ras-transformed cells support growth by scavenging unsaturated fatty acids from lysophospholipids. *Proc. Natl. Acad. Sci. USA* **2013**, *110*, 8882–8887. [CrossRef] [PubMed]
23. Kamphorst, J.J.; Nofal, M.; Commisso, C.; Hackett, S.R.; Lu, W.; Grabocka, E.; Vander Heiden, M.G.; Miller, G.; Drebin, J.A.; Bar-Sagi, D.; et al. Human pancreatic cancer tumors are nutrient poor and tumor cells actively scavenge extracellular protein. *Cancer Res.* **2015**, *75*, 544–553. [CrossRef] [PubMed]
24. Al-Zhoughbi, W.; Huang, J.; Paramasivan, G.S.; Till, H.; Pichler, M.; Guertl-Lackner, B.; Hoefler, G. Tumor Macroenvironment and Metabolism. *Semin. Oncol.* **2014**, *41*, 281–295. [CrossRef] [PubMed]
25. Pavlova, N.N.; Thompson, C.B. The Emerging Hallmarks of Cancer Metabolism. *Cell Metab.* **2016**, *23*, 27–47. [CrossRef] [PubMed]
26. Li, W.; Wei, Z.; Liu, Y.; Li, H.; Ren, R.; Tang, Y. Increased 18F-FDG uptake and expression of Glut1 in the EMT transformed breast cancer cells induced by TGF-β. *Neoplasma* **2010**, *57*, 234–240. [CrossRef] [PubMed]
27. Dong, C.; Yuan, T.; Wu, Y.; Wang, Y.; Fan, T.W.M.; Miriyala, S.; Lin, Y.; Yao, J.; Shi, J.; Kang, T.; et al. Loss of FBP1 by Snail-mediated Repression Provides Metabolic Advantages in Basal-like Breast Cancer. *Cancer Cell* **2013**, *23*, 316–331. [CrossRef]
28. Aspuria, P.-J.P.; Lunt, S.Y.; Väremo, L.; Vergnes, L.; Gozo, M.; Beach, J.A.; Salumbides, B.; Reue, K.; Wiedemeyer, W.R.; Nielsen, J.; et al. Succinate dehydrogenase inhibition leads to epithelial-mesenchymal transition and reprogrammed carbon metabolism. *Cancer Metab.* **2014**, *2*, 21.
29. Sun, Y.; Daemen, A.; Hatzivassiliou, G.; Arnott, D.; Wilson, C.; Zhuang, G.; Gao, M.; Liu, P.; Boudreau, A.; Johnson, L.; et al. Metabolic and transcriptional profiling reveals pyruvate dehydrogenase kinase 4 as a mediator of epithelial-mesenchymal transition and drug resistance in tumor cells. *Cancer Metab.* **2014**, *2*, 20. [CrossRef]
30. Masin, M.; Vazquez, J.; Rossi, S.; Groeneveld, S.; Samson, N.; Schwalie, P.C.; Deplancke, B.; Frawley, L.E.; Gouttenoire, J.; Moradpour, D.; et al. GLUT3 is induced during epithelial-mesenchymal transition and promotes tumor cell proliferation in non-small cell lung cancer. *Cancer Metab.* **2014**, *2*, 11. [CrossRef]
31. Li, J.; Dong, L.; Wei, D.; Wang, X.; Zhang, S.; Li, H. Fatty Acid Synthase Mediates the Epithelial-Mesenchymal Transition of Breast Cancer Cells. *Int. J. Biol. Sci.* **2014**, *10*, 171–180. [CrossRef]
32. Kondaveeti, Y.; Guttilla Reed, I.K.; White, B.A. Epithelial-mesenchymal transition induces similar metabolic alterations in two independent breast cancer cell lines. *Cancer Lett.* **2015**, *364*, 44–58. [CrossRef] [PubMed]
33. Jiang, L.; Xiao, L.; Sugiura, H.; Huang, X.; Ali, A.; Kuro-o, M.; Deberardinis, R.J.; Boothman, D.A. Metabolic reprogramming during TGFβ1-induced epithelial-to-mesenchymal transition. *Oncogene* **2015**, *34*, 3908–3916. [CrossRef] [PubMed]
34. Lin, C.-C.; Cheng, T.-L.; Tsai, W.-H.; Tsai, H.-J.; Hu, K.-H.; Chang, H.-C.; Yeh, C.-W.; Chen, Y.-C.; Liao, C.-C.; Chang, W.-T. Loss of the respiratory enzyme citrate synthase directly links the Warburg effect to tumor malignancy. *Sci. Rep.* **2012**, *2*, 785. [CrossRef] [PubMed]

35. Fiaschi, T.; Marini, A.; Giannoni, E.; Taddei, M.L.; Gandellini, P.; Donatis, A.D.; Lanciotti, M.; Serni, S.; Cirri, P.; Chiarugi, P. Reciprocal Metabolic Reprogramming through Lactate Shuttle Coordinately Influences Tumor-Stroma Interplay. *Cancer Res.* **2012**, *72*, 5130–5140. [CrossRef] [PubMed]
36. Lucena, M.C.; Carvalho-Cruz, P.; Donadio, J.L.; Oliveira, I.A.; de Queiroz, R.M.; Marinho-Carvalho, M.M.; Sola-Penna, M.; de Paula, I.F.; Gondim, K.C.; McComb, M.E.; et al. Epithelial Mesenchymal Transition Induces Aberrant Glycosylation through Hexosamine Biosynthetic Pathway Activation. *J. Biol. Chem.* **2016**, *291*, 12917–12929. [CrossRef] [PubMed]
37. Haraguchi, M.; Indo, H.P.; Iwasaki, Y.; Iwashita, Y.; Fukushige, T.; Majima, H.J.; Izumo, K.; Horiuchi, M.; Kanekura, T.; Furukawa, T.; et al. Snail modulates cell metabolism in MDCK cells. *Biochem. Biophys. Res. Commun.* **2013**, *432*, 618–625. [CrossRef] [PubMed]
38. Tao, T.; Li, G.; Dong, Q.; Liu, D.; Liu, C.; Han, D.; Huang, Y.; Chen, S.; Xu, B.; Chen, M. Loss of SNAIL inhibits cellular growth and metabolism through the miR-128-mediated RPS6KB1/HIF-1α/PKM2 signaling pathway in prostate cancer cells. *Tumor Biol.* **2014**, *35*, 8543–8550. [CrossRef] [PubMed]
39. Lee, S.Y.; Jeon, H.M.; Ju, M.K.; Kim, C.H.; Yoon, G.; Han, S.I.; Park, H.G.; Kang, H.S. Wnt/Snail Signaling Regulates Cytochrome c Oxidase and Glucose Metabolism. *Cancer Res.* **2012**, *72*, 3607–3617. [CrossRef] [PubMed]
40. Shaul, Y.D.; Freinkman, E.; Comb, W.C.; Cantor, J.R.; Tam, W.L.; Thiru, P.; Kim, D.; Kanarek, N.; Pacold, M.E.; Chen, W.W.; et al. Dihydropyrimidine accumulation is required for the epithelial-mesenchymal transition. *Cell* **2014**, *158*, 1094–1109. [CrossRef]
41. Liu, M.; Quek, L.-E.; Sultani, G.; Turner, N. Epithelial-mesenchymal transition induction is associated with augmented glucose uptake and lactate production in pancreatic ductal adenocarcinoma. *Cancer Metab.* **2016**, *4*, 19. [CrossRef]
42. Ouyang, H.; Mou, L.; Luk, C.; Liu, N.; Karaskova, J.; Squire, J.; Tsao, M.-S. Immortal Human Pancreatic Duct Epithelial Cell Lines with Near Normal Genotype and Phenotype. *Am. J. Pathol.* **2000**, *157*, 1623–1631. [CrossRef]
43. Mani, S.A.; Yang, J.; Brooks, M.; Schwaninger, G.; Zhou, A.; Miura, N.; Kutok, J.L.; Hartwell, K.; Richardson, A.L.; Weinberg, R.A. Mesenchyme Forkhead 1 (FOXC2) plays a key role in metastasis and is associated with aggressive basal-like breast cancers. *Proc. Natl. Acad. Sci. USA* **2007**, *104*, 10069–10074. [CrossRef] [PubMed]
44. Turner, N.; Hariharan, K.; TidAng, J.; Frangioudakis, G.; Beale, S.M.; Wright, L.E.; Zeng, X.Y.; Leslie, S.J.; Li, J.-Y.; Kraegen, E.W.; et al. Enhancement of Muscle Mitochondrial Oxidative Capacity and Alterations in Insulin Action Are Lipid Species Dependent. *Diabetes* **2009**, *58*, 2547–2554. [CrossRef] [PubMed]
45. Spandidos, A.; Wang, X.; Wang, H.; Seed, B. PrimerBank: A resource of human and mouse PCR primer pairs for gene expression detection and quantification. *Nucleic Acids Res.* **2010**, *38*, D792–D799. [CrossRef] [PubMed]
46. Quek, L.-E.; Liu, M.; Joshi, S.; Turner, N. Fast exchange fluxes around the pyruvate node: A leaky cell model to explain the gain and loss of unlabelled and labelled metabolites in a tracer experiment. *Cancer Metab.* **2016**, *4*, 13. [CrossRef] [PubMed]
47. Quek, L.-E.; Nielsen, L.K. Customization of 13C-MFA Strategy According to Cell Culture System. *Metab. Flux Anal.* **2014**, *1191*, 81–90.
48. Quek, L.-E.; Wittmann, C.; Nielsen, L.K.; Krömer, J.O. OpenFLUX: Efficient modelling software for 13C-based metabolic flux analysis. *Microb. Cell Factories* **2009**, *8*, 25. [CrossRef]
49. Apte, M.V.; Xu, Z.; Pothula, S.; Goldstein, D.; Pirola, R.C.; Wilson, J.S. Pancreatic cancer: The microenvironment needs attention too! *Pancreatology* **2015**, *15*, S32–S38. [CrossRef]
50. Zhou, B.; Zhan, H.; Tin, L.; Liu, S.; Xu, J.; Dong, Y.; Li, X.; Wu, L.; Guo, W. TUFT1 regulates metastasis of pancreatic cancer through HIF1-Snail pathway induced epithelial-mesenchymal transition. *Cancer Lett.* **2016**, *382*, 11–20. [CrossRef]
51. Xu, Y.; Chang, R.; Peng, Z.; Wang, Y.; Ji, W.; Guo, J.; Song, L.; Dai, C.; Wei, W.; Wu, Y.; et al. Loss of polarity protein AF6 promotes pancreatic cancer metastasis by inducing Snail expression. *Nat. Commun.* **2015**, *6*, 7184. [CrossRef]
52. Guo, S.; Jing, W.; Hu, X.; Zhou, X.; Liu, L.; Zhu, M.; Yin, F.; Chen, R.; Zhao, J.; Guo, Y. Decreased TIP30 expression predicts poor prognosis in pancreatic cancer patients. *Int. J. Cancer* **2014**, *134*, 1369–1378. [CrossRef] [PubMed]

53. Gatenby, R.A.; Gillies, R.J. Why do cancers have high aerobic glycolysis? *Nat. Rev. Cancer* **2004**, *4*, 891–899. [CrossRef] [PubMed]
54. Han, T.; Kang, D.; Ji, D.; Wang, X.; Zhan, W.; Fu, M.; Xin, H.-B.; Wang, J.-B. How does cancer cell metabolism affect tumor migration and invasion? *Cell Adhes. Migr.* **2013**, *7*, 395–403. [CrossRef] [PubMed]
55. Shang, R.; Wang, J.; Sun, W.; Dai, B.; Ruan, B.; Zhang, Z.; Yang, X.; Gao, Y.; Qu, S.; Lv, X.; et al. RRAD inhibits aerobic glycolysis, invasion, and migration and is associated with poor prognosis in hepatocellular carcinoma. *Tumor Biol.* **2016**, *37*, 5097–5105. [CrossRef] [PubMed]
56. Shiraishi, T.; Verdone, J.E.; Huang, J.; Kahlert, U.D.; Hernandez, J.R.; Torga, G.; Zarif, J.C.; Epstein, T.; Gatenby, R.; McCartney, A.; et al. Glycolysis is the primary bioenergetic pathway for cell motility and cytoskeletal remodeling in human prostate and breast cancer cells. *Oncotarget* **2014**, *6*, 130–143. [CrossRef]
57. Fife, C.M.; McCarroll, J.A.; Kavallaris, M. Movers and shakers: Cell cytoskeleton in cancer metastasis. *Br. J. Pharmacol.* **2014**, *171*, 5507–5523. [CrossRef] [PubMed]
58. Cunniff, B.; McKenzie, A.J.; Heintz, N.H.; Howe, A.K. AMPK activity regulates trafficking of mitochondria to the leading edge during cell migration and matrix invasion. *Mol. Biol. Cell* **2016**, *27*, 2662–2674. [CrossRef]
59. Kato, Y.; Ozawa, S.; Tsukuda, M.; Kubota, E.; Miyazaki, K.; St-Pierre, Y.; Hata, R.-I. Acidic extracellular pH increases calcium influx-triggered phospholipase D activity along with acidic sphingomyelinase activation to induce matrix metalloproteinase-9 expression in mouse metastatic melanoma. *FEBS J.* **2007**, *274*, 3171–3183. [CrossRef]
60. Rothberg, J.M.; Bailey, K.M.; Wojtkowiak, J.W.; Ben-Nun, Y.; Bogyo, M.; Weber, E.; Moin, K.; Blum, G.; Mattingly, R.R.; Gillies, R.J.; et al. Acid-Mediated Tumor Proteolysis: Contribution of Cysteine Cathepsins. *Neoplasia* **2013**, *15*, 1125–1137. [CrossRef]
61. Gatenby, R.A.; Gawlinski, E.T.; Gmitro, A.F.; Kaylor, B.; Gillies, R.J. Acid-Mediated Tumor Invasion: A Multidisciplinary Study. *Cancer Res.* **2006**, *66*, 5216–5223. [CrossRef]
62. Goetze, K.; Walenta, S.; Ksiazkiewicz, M.; Kunz-Schughart, L.A.; Mueller-Klieser, W. Lactate enhances motility of tumor cells and inhibits monocyte migration and cytokine release. *Int. J. Oncol.* **2011**, *39*, 453–463. [CrossRef] [PubMed]
63. Aguilar, E.; de Mas, I.M.; Zodda, E.; Marin, S.; Morrish, F.; Selivanov, V.; Meca-Cortés, Ó.; Delowar, H.; Pons, M.; Izquierdo, I.; et al. Metabolic Reprogramming and Dependencies Associated with Epithelial Cancer Stem Cells Independent of the Epithelial-Mesenchymal Transition Program. *Stem Cells* **2016**, *34*, 1163–1176. [CrossRef] [PubMed]
64. LeBleu, V.S.; O'Connell, J.T.; Gonzalez Herrera, K.N.; Wikman, H.; Pantel, K.; Haigis, M.C.; de Carvalho, F.M.; Damascena, A.; Domingos Chinen, L.T.; Rocha, R.M.; et al. PGC-1α mediates mitochondrial biogenesis and oxidative phosphorylation in cancer cells to promote metastasis. *Nat. Cell Biol.* **2014**, *16*, 992–1003. [CrossRef] [PubMed]
65. Gaianigo, N.; Melisi, D.; Carbone, C. EMT and Treatment Resistance in Pancreatic Cancer. *Cancers* **2017**, *9*. [CrossRef] [PubMed]
66. Cho, E.S.; Kang, H.E.; Kim, N.H.; Yook, J.I. Therapeutic implications of cancer epithelial-mesenchymal transition (EMT). *Arch. Pharm. Res.* **2019**, *42*, 14–24. [CrossRef] [PubMed]
67. Izumiya, M.; Kabashima, A.; Higuchi, H.; Igarashi, T.; Sakai, G.; Iizuka, H.; Nakamura, S.; Adachi, M.; Hamamoto, Y.; Funakoshi, S.; et al. Chemoresistance Is Associated with Cancer Stem Cell-like Properties and Epithelial-to-Mesenchymal Transition in Pancreatic Cancer Cells. *Anticancer Res.* **2012**, *32*, 3847–3853. [PubMed]
68. Wang, R.; Cheng, L.; Xia, J.; Wang, Z.; Wu, Q.; Wang, Z. Gemcitabine resistance is associated with epithelial-mesenchymal transition and induction of HIF-1α in pancreatic cancer cells. *Curr. Cancer Drug Targets* **2014**, *14*, 407–417. [CrossRef] [PubMed]

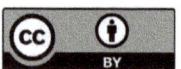

© 2019 by the authors. Licensee MDPI, Basel, Switzerland. This article is an open access article distributed under the terms and conditions of the Creative Commons Attribution (CC BY) license (http://creativecommons.org/licenses/by/4.0/).

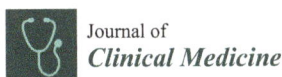

Article

# Phosphoproteomic Profiling Identifies Aberrant Activation of Integrin Signaling in Aggressive Non-Type Bladder Carcinoma

Barnali Deb [1,2], Vinuth N. Puttamallesh [1,3], Kirti Gondkar [1,3], Jean P. Thiery [4,5,6,*], Harsha Gowda [1,*] and Prashant Kumar [1,2,*]

1. Institute of Bioinformatics, International Technology Park, Bangalore 560066, India; barnali@ibioinformatics.org (B.D.); vinuth@ibioinformatics.org (V.N.P.); kirti@ibioinformatics.org (K.G.)
2. Manipal Academy of Higher Education, Madhav Nagar, Manipal 576104, India
3. School of Biotechnology, Amrita Vishwa Vidyapeetham, Kollam 690525, India
4. Cancer Science Institute of Singapore, National University of Singapore, Centre for Translational Medicine NUS Yong Loo Lin School of Medicine, Singapore 117597, Singapore
5. Comprehensive Cancer Center, Institut Gustave Roussy, 114 Rue Edouard Vaillant, 94800 Villejuif, France
6. CNRS UMR 7057, Matter and Complex Systems, Université Paris Diderot, 10 rue Alice Domon et Léonie Duquet Paris, 75205 Paris, France
* Correspondence: bchtjp@nus.edu.sg (J.P.T.); harsha@ibioinformatics.org (H.G.); prashant@ibioinformatics.org (P.K.); Tel.: +91-80-28416140 (P.K.); Fax: +91-80-28416132 (P.K.)

Received: 27 March 2019; Accepted: 23 April 2019; Published: 17 May 2019

**Abstract:** Bladder carcinoma is highly heterogeneous and its complex molecular landscape; thus, poses a significant challenge for resolving an effective treatment in metastatic tumors. We computed the epithelial-mesenchymal transition (EMT) scores of three bladder carcinoma subtypes—luminal, basal, and non-type. The EMT score of the non-type indicated a "mesenchymal-like" phenotype, which correlates with a relatively more aggressive form of carcinoma, typified by an increased migration and invasion. To identify the altered signaling pathways potentially regulating this EMT phenotype in bladder cancer cell lines, we utilized liquid chromatography-tandem mass spectrometry (LC-MS/MS)-based phosphoproteomic approach. Bioinformatics analyses were carried out to determine the activated pathways, networks, and functions in bladder carcinoma cell lines. A total of 3125 proteins were identified, with 289 signature proteins noted to be differentially phosphorylated ($p \leq 0.05$) in the non-type cell lines. The integrin pathway was significantly enriched and five major proteins (TLN1, CTTN, CRKL, ZYX and BCAR3) regulating cell motility and invasion were hyperphosphorylated. Our study reveals GSK3A/B and CDK1 as promising druggable targets for the non-type molecular subtype, which could improve the treatment outcomes for aggressive bladder carcinoma.

**Keywords:** urothelial cancer; phosphoproteomics; activated pathways; ingenuity pathway analysis; molecular subtypes

---

## 1. Introduction

Advanced cancer therapeutics demands a detailed understanding of the altered mechanisms operating in malignant disease. Notably, in bladder carcinoma, the current treatment regimens and interventions are mostly determined by the clinicopathological characteristics of the tumor. Bladder carcinoma is categorized into two clinicopathologically distinct subgroups: non-muscle-invasive bladder cancer (NMIBC) and muscle-invasive bladder cancer (MIBC). At diagnosis, 75% of bladder carcinoma is NMIBC, whereas 20% to 25% is MIBC. About 50% to 70% of NMIBC, including Ta- and T1-stage tumors, frequently recur [1], whereas 10% to 15% progress to MIBC (T2, T3, and T4 stages) [2]. Unlike most other carcinomas, carcinoma in situ (Tis) tumors, a superficial tumor, progress very rapidly to MIBC. Emerging evidence suggests that tumor heterogeneity alters treatment response and confers resistance, leading to recurrence. Thus, a detailed understanding of the clinicopathological subgroups and their molecular alterations is of paramount interest, especially for targeted therapy. Identification of distinct molecular subtypes of NMIBC and MIBC could highlight clinically relevant signaling pathways.

Clinical staging is still not precisely defined for bladder carcinoma because of its highly heterogeneous nature. The advent of whole-genomic and transcriptomic approaches has transformed our understanding of cancer heterogeneity. Whole-genome sequencing and expression profiling, have uncovered molecular subtypes that relate to distinct clinical entities in various cancers. For instance, several studies have identified intrinsic subtypes of MIBC that resemble the intrinsic subtypes of breast cancer [3–5]. Comprehensive studies have defined the molecular subtypes in bladder carcinoma, mainly by analyzing gene expression data, specific mutations, and copy-number changes with recent analyses suggesting that specific genetic alterations in fibroblast growth factor receptor 3 (*FGFR3*), tumor protein P53 (*TP53*), retinoblastoma 1 (*RB1*), Erb-B2 receptor tyrosine kinase 2 (*ERBB2*), nuclear-factor, erythroid 2 like 2 (*NFE2L2*), and lysine demethylase 6A (*KDM6A/UTX*) are enriched in different molecular subtypes and are clinically actionable [6–8].

So far, the intrinsic subtypes of bladder carcinoma have been categorized into two to seven classes by different groups. A broad stratification of high-grade bladder carcinoma was described by the University of North Carolina (UNC), where the subtypes (luminal and basal-like) reflected the hallmarks of breast cancer [4]. This study classified luminal and basal subtypes of bladder carcinoma using a 47-gene signature. Another similar molecular classification (MD Anderson) using gene expression profiling, restricted to MIBCs, found three subgroups: basal, luminal, and p53-like MIBCs [5]; the inclusion of the "p53-like" subtype was based on the mRNA expression of p53, which can predict MIBC chemoresistance. The Cancer Genome Atlas (TCGA) research network also categorized the intrinsic subtypes of bladder carcinoma into four clusters (Clusters I–IV) based on an integrated analysis of the mRNA, miRNA, and proteome expression profiling of 129 tumor samples. However, the most extensive classification by LUND University was conducted on gene expression profiling data for 308 tumor tissue samples, and resulted in five intrinsic types of carcinoma, designated Urobasal A, Genomically unstable, Urobasal B, Squamous cell carcinoma-like, and Infiltrated [9]. The LUND molecular subtypes were further characterized into seven gene signature (subdividing Urobasal A and Genomically instable subtypes into two groups each), based on the differential expression of genes associated with biological processes [10]. Using a 117-gene signature, Hedegaard et al. [11] classified only NMIBCs into three subclasses (Class I–III) with basal- and luminal-like characteristics as well as clinical features. A later meta-analysis on the molecular subtypes (established by UNC, MDA, TCGA and LUND) revealed some consensus patterning among the molecular subtyping strategies [10]. However, there remain inaccuracies in the current staging systems, and the clinicopathological features may also influence treatment selection [12]. Such inadequacies are to be expected due to the low sample size in these studies and a large, collaborative study is needed to identify the molecular signatures before assigning treatment with conventional chemotherapy.

In a study by Warrick et al., bladder carcinoma cell lines were used to study the molecular subtypes in a relevant in vitro model. A detailed analysis was carried out on the publicly available data for the 27 bladder carcinoma cell lines (CCLE database) [13] as per the TCGA study. The panel of bladder carcinoma cell lines was classified into three subtypes based on gene expression clusters: luminal, basal, and "non-type" [14]. The non-type subtype displayed low expression of both luminal and basal markers. We further included these three subtypes for our deeper understanding of the molecular events involved in bladder carcinoma.

We employed liquid chromatography tandem-mass spectrometry (LC-MS/MS)-based approach to identify differentially expressed proteins in all three distinct subtypes. We also sought to evaluate pathways enriched in luminal, basal, and non-type subtypes. We undertook an extensive quantitative phosphoproteomic analysis of six bladder carcinoma cell lines (RT112, SW780, VMCUB-1, T24, J82, and UMUC3) and compared the phosphoproteomic data of bladder carcinoma cell lines with a non-neoplastic bladder cell line (TERT-NHUC) [15]. The six cell lines were previously assigned to luminal (RT112 and SW780), basal (VMCUB-1), and non-type (UMUC3, J82 and T24) molecular subtypes [14]. To our knowledge, this is the first phosphoproteomic profiling of bladder carcinoma and it may provide a global platform to identify the complex kinase-driven signaling events in bladder carcinoma.

## 2. Experimental Section

### 2.1. Cell Culture

Bladder carcinoma cell lines, SW780, RT112, VMCUB-1, T24, J82, and UMUC3 were cultured in dulbecco's modified eagle's medium (DMEM; with high glucose, HIMEDIA), supplemented with 10% fetal bovine serum (FBS) and 1% penicillin/streptomycin. Cells were maintained in a humidified incubator at 37 °C and 5% $CO_2$. The non-neoplastic bladder cell line (TERT-NHUC) was cultured in KGM-Gold Media (Lonza Group, Allendale, NJ, USA) supplemented with hydrocortisone, transferrin, epinephrine, gentamicin, amphotericin B (GA-1000), bovine pituitary extract (BPE), recombinant human epidermal growth factor (rhEGF), and insulin in a humidified incubator at 37 °C and 5% $CO_2$.

TERT-NHUC cells were kindly provided by Prof. M.A. Knowles, University of Leeds, UK [15].

### 2.2. Cell Lysis, Protein Extraction, and Digestion

Cell lines were grown to 70% confluence, starved in serum-free medium for 12 h, and then lysed in cell lysis buffer (2% SDS, 5 mM sodium fluoride, 1 mM β-glycerophosphate, 1 mM sodium orthovanadate in 50 mM triethyl ammonium bicarbonate (TEABC)). Protein concentration was estimated using the BCA method (Pierce; Waltham, MA, USA). Equal amount of protein from each cell line was used for protein digestion. Cell lysates were reduced and alkylated using 5 mM dithiothreitol (DTT) and 20 mM iodoacetamide (IAA), respectively. Samples were then digested overnight at 37 °C using trypsin (1:20) (Promega; San Luis Obispo, CA, USA).

### 2.3. TMT Labeling

Before labeling, peptides were reconstituted in 50 mM TEABC (pH 8.0). Equal amounts of peptides from each condition were used for 10-plex Tandem Mass Tag (TMT) labeling (Thermo Fisher Scientific, Rockford, IL, USA). Labeling was carried out as per the manufacturer's protocol. TERT-NHUC was labeled with the channel 126, and SW780, RT112, VMCUB-1, T24, J82, and UMUC3 were labeled with 130N, 130C, 129C, 131, 128C, and 128N, respectively. The reaction was quenched by the addition of 8 μl of 5% hydroxylamine for 15 min at room temperature, and the samples were dried.

### 2.4. Basic pH RPLC (bRPLC) and $TiO_2$-Based Phosphopeptide Enrichment

TMT-labeled peptides were pooled and fractionated using an Agilent 1100 high-pH reverse-phase liquid chromatography (RPLC) system with a flow rate of 1 mL/min, as described earlier [16]. Briefly, labeled peptides, resuspended in 1 mL of bRPLC solvent (10 mM TEABC pH 8.4), were fractionated using high-pH, reverse-phase XBridge C18 columns (5 μm, 250 × 4.6 mm; Waters Corporation, Milford, MA, USA), with an increasing gradient of bRPLC solvent B (10 mM TEABC in 90% ACN, pH 8.4). A total of 96 fractions were collected in a 96-well plate containing 0.1% formic acid. The fractions were then concatenated into 12 pools, vacuum-dried, and subjected to $TiO_2$-based phosphopeptide enrichment [17]. The enriched phosphopeptides were eluted thrice into microfuge tubes with 40 μL of 2% ammonia solution containing 10 μL of 20% trifluoroacetic acid. The peptides were then dried, resuspended in 30 μL of 0.1% TFA, and desalted using C18 Stage Tips (Thermo Fisher Scientific). The eluted peptides were then subjected to LC-MS/MS analysis.

### 2.5. LC-MS/MS Analysis

Phosphoproteomic analyses were performed on an Orbitrap Fusion Tribrid mass spectrometer (Thermo Fisher Scientific) interfaced with an Easy-nLC II nanoflow liquid chromatography system

(Thermo Fisher Scientific), as described earlier [18]. Briefly, each fraction was reconstituted in Solvent A (0.1% Formic acid) and loaded on trap column (75 µm × 2 cm) packed with Magic C18 AQ (Michrom Bioresources, Inc., Auburn, CA, USA). Peptides were resolved on an analytical column (75 µm × 15 cm) at a flow rate of 350 nL/min using a linear gradient from 5% to 60% ACN in a 120 min run. MS data were acquired using scan range of 400–1,600 m/z at mass resolution of 120,000, and MS/MS data were acquired using resolution of 30,000 at m/z of 400. HCD fragmentation for MS/MS analysis was carried out with isolation width of 2 m/z and normalized collision energy of 34%. Data-dependent acquisition was carried out where the most intense precursor ions were detected.

### 2.6. Data Analysis

The MS-derived data were searched using Mascot and Sequest HT search engines with Proteome Discoverer 2.0 (Thermo Fisher Scientific). Phosphopeptide-enriched fractions from each replicate were searched against the RefSeq protein database (version 70), National Institutes of Health, USA with carbamidomethylation of cysteine residues as a fixed modification. Oxidation of methionine; the phosphorylations of serine, threonine, and tyrosine; and the deamidation of asparagine and glutamine were selected as dynamic modifications. Trypsin was set as the protease and a maximum of one missed cleavage was allowed. Precursor mass tolerance was set to 20 ppm, and a fragment mass tolerance of 0.05 Da was allowed. All peptide-spectrum matches (PSMs) were identified at a 1% false-discovery rate (FDR). Posterior error probability was calculated for individual PSMs using a percolator, providing statistical confidence for each spectral match. The probability of phosphorylation for each site was calculated by the phosphoRS node in Proteome Discoverer. Only phosphopeptides with >75% site localization probability were considered for further analysis. A 2-fold cut-off was used for dysregulated phosphopeptides compared to TERT-NHUC cell line.

### 2.7. Scratch Wound Assay

For each cell line, $3 \times 10^5$ cells were seeded into the wells of a 6-well plate. The experiment was conducted in triplicate. When the cells had reached 90% to 95% confluency, a scratch was made with a 20-µl pipette tip. Cells were washed gently with media, incubated with PBS, and then imaged. Cells were maintained in DMEM supplemented with 2% FBS. Cells were observed and imaged at 0 and 24 h. The rate of migration was calculated using ImageJ macros (v1.50i; National Institutes of Health, Maryland, USA). A $t$-test was used to calculate significance and the area covered by the migrating cells was plotted in a bar graph.

### 2.8. Invasion Assay

The transwell system was used to measure invasion, as reported earlier [19]. Briefly, 20,000 cells per 500µl of serum free media were seeded onto the Matrigel-coated PET membrane (BD Bio Coat Matrigel Invasion Chamber; BD Biosciences, CA, USA) in the upper compartment, while the lower compartment was filled with complete growth media. Plates were maintained at 37 °C for 48 h. After the incubation period, the upper membrane surface was wiped with a cotton-tip applicator to remove non-migratory cells. Cells that migrated to underside of membrane were fixed and stained using 4% methylene blue in 50% methanol. The number of cells that penetrated was counted for randomly selected viewing fields at 10× magnification using CX 41 Olympus Polarizing Trinocular microscope. The counting of cells was done using ImageJ multi-point cell counter (v1.50i; National Institutes of Health, Maryland, USA). The experiment was conducted in replicates.

### 2.9. Kinome Map

The kinome map was built using the KinMap tool (http://www.kinhub.org/kinmap/index.html). The list of identified kinases was searched and the relevant kinases are highlighted on the kinome map. Dysregulated kinases (hyper- or hypo-phosphorylated in any cell line) are also depicted.

*2.10. Clustering the Molecular Subtypes*

All quantified peptides (across all cell lines and in both replicates) were considered to identify differentially phosphorylated peptides. Fold-change was calculated by taking the intensity ratios with TERT-NHUC as the control. A *t*-test was used to determine the differentially phosphorylated peptides in the non-type subtype as compared with the luminal/basal subtype and the control cells. Differentially phosphorylated peptides ($p \leq 0.05$) were further considered for supervised clustering using Perseus data analysis tool v1.5.8.5, Martinsried, Germany (http://www.biochem.mpg.de/5111810/perseuss) [20].

*2.11. Ingenuity Pathway Analysis*

Pathway analysis was completed for significantly dysregulated phosphopeptides in the non-type subtype using the Ingenuity Pathway Analysis tool (IPA Build: 460209M; Version: 39480507; IPA, Qiagen, Redwood City, CA, USA). The Core Analysis module in the IPA Ingenuity Knowledge Base reference repository was used to predict relationships of differentially phosphorylated molecules in our dataset. IPA was used to overlay our input dataset with that of the knowledge base. Canonical pathway analyses identified the top canonical pathways significantly enriched in our datasets. The "integrin pathway" was enriched in the total quantified dataset across all tested cell lines and with a confident phosphosite assignment. Significantly enriched functions and networks were also obtained. The IPA analysis results were schematically replicated using Adobe Illustrator (vCS5.1; Adobe Systems, San Jose, CA, USA).

*2.12. Kinase-Substrate Enrichment Analysis*

Kinase-substrate enrichment analysis was done using the online KSEA tool (https://casecpb.shinyapps.io/ksea/) [21]. Proteins with differentially phosphorylated sites in the non-type subtype were used for the input file, and analyzed using PhosphoSitePlus and NetworKIN as the background datasets. The *p*-value cutoff (for plot) and number of substrates cutoff were set to 0.05 and 5, respectively.

*2.13. Motif Analysis*

Motifs enriched in the non-type subtype were analyzed using the motif-x algorithm v1.210.05.06 (http://motif-x.med.harvard.edu). The "phospho-window" (7 amino acid residues on either side of the phosphorylated residue) was extracted from the RefSeq database. Significance threshold was set to $p < 0.001$. The minimum occurrence of the motif was set to 20 for pSer peptides and 10 for pThr against an IPI (International Proteome Index) human proteome background with the central character as "s" and "t", respectively.

*2.14. Immunohistochemistry*

High-grade and low-grade bladder cancer FFPE tissue sections were obtained from Kidwai Institute of Molecular Oncology after informed patient consent. IHC was carried out on both the cases. Briefly, sections were deparaffinized and antigen retrieval was carried by incubating sections in antigen retrieval buffer (0.01 M Trisodium citrate buffer, pH 6) for 20 minutes. Endogenous peroxidases were quenched using (1:1) methanol: chloroform solution followed by washes with PBS plus 0.05% Tween-20. The sections were blocked using 5% goat serum to avoid non-specific binding of primary antibody for 30 minutes. Further sections were incubated with primary anti-Talin1 (S425) (Abcam, Cambridge, United Kingdom) antibody at 1:200 dilutions overnight at 4 °C in a humidified chamber. Next day, the sections were washed thrice with wash buffer and incubated with appropriate horseradish peroxidase conjugated rabbit secondary antibody for 30 minutes at room temperature. Excess secondary antibody was removed using wash buffer followed by addition of DAB substrate. The signal was developed using DAB chromogen (DAKO, Glostrup, Denmark) and counterstained by hematoxylin. The immunohistochemical labeling was assessed by an experienced pathologist. Images were taken at 10× on Olympus DP-21 microscope.

## 3. Results

### 3.1. EMT Scores of the Molecular Subtypes of Bladder Carcinoma Cell Lines

EMT (−1.0 to +1.0) scores were computed to estimate the EMT phenotype of the molecular subtypes of bladder carcinoma cell lines (Supplementary Table S1) [3]. To compute the EMT score in bladder carcinoma cell lines, we adopted a similar approach to that used in ssGSEA [22]. Empirical cumulative distribution function (ECDF) was estimated for Epithelial and Mesenchymal gene sets. The 2KS test was employed to compute the difference between the Mesenchymal ECDF ($ECDF_{Mes}$) and the epithelial ECDF ($ECDF_{Epi}$). The EMT signature specific to bladder was curated and applied to single sample gene set enrichment analysis (ssGSEA) to provide a gross assessment for the EMT phenotype for each cell line. The BinReg EMT signature was used to predict the EMT phenotype in the cell lines [3,23]. A cell line with a positive EMT score exhibits a more "mesenchymal-like" phenotype, whereas a negative EMT score reflected a more "epithelial-like" phenotype. EMT scores suggested that non-type cell lines were "mesenchymal-like", whereas the luminal and basal cell lines had an "epithelial-like" characteristic (Figure 1a).

### 3.2. Non-Type Bladder Carcinoma Has Increased Migration and Invasive Ability

We performed functional assays to determine and compare the tumorigenic properties of the non-type cell lines with the luminal/basal subtype. Using matrigel invasion assay, we estimated that the non-type were significantly more invasive as compared to the luminal ($p = 6.9 \times 10^{-14}$) and basal subtypes ($p = 0.03$) (Figure 1b,c). We found increased migration of non-type bladder carcinoma cell lines as compared to luminal ($p = 0.002$) and basal ($p = 0.007$) subtypes (Figure 1d,e).

### 3.3. Phosphoproteomic Analysis of Bladder Carcinoma Cell Lines

Phosphoproteomic profiling was conducted for six bladder carcinoma cell lines (RT112, SW780, VMCUB-1, J82, T24, and UMUC3) and the non-neoplastic bladder cell line (TERT-NHUC) using an established workflow for the enrichment of phosphopeptides (Figure 2). To increase the reliability of our phosphoproteomic analyses, we have included technical replicates in our study. The MS data were processed and searched against databases using SEQUEST-HT and MASCOT algorithms using the Proteome Discoverer 2.0 platform. Using an FDR cutoff of 1%, 10,979 phosphopeptides were identified, corresponding to 3125 proteins (Supplementary Table S2). The probability of Ser/Thr/Tyr phosphorylation sites on each peptide was calculated by the phosphoRS algorithm using a cut-off of >75%. We identified 4846 unique phosphopeptides corresponding to 2270 proteins (Supplementary Table S3), with a total of 4878 phosphosites identified: 4271 Ser residues, 574 Thr residues, and 33 Tyr residues (Figure 3a).

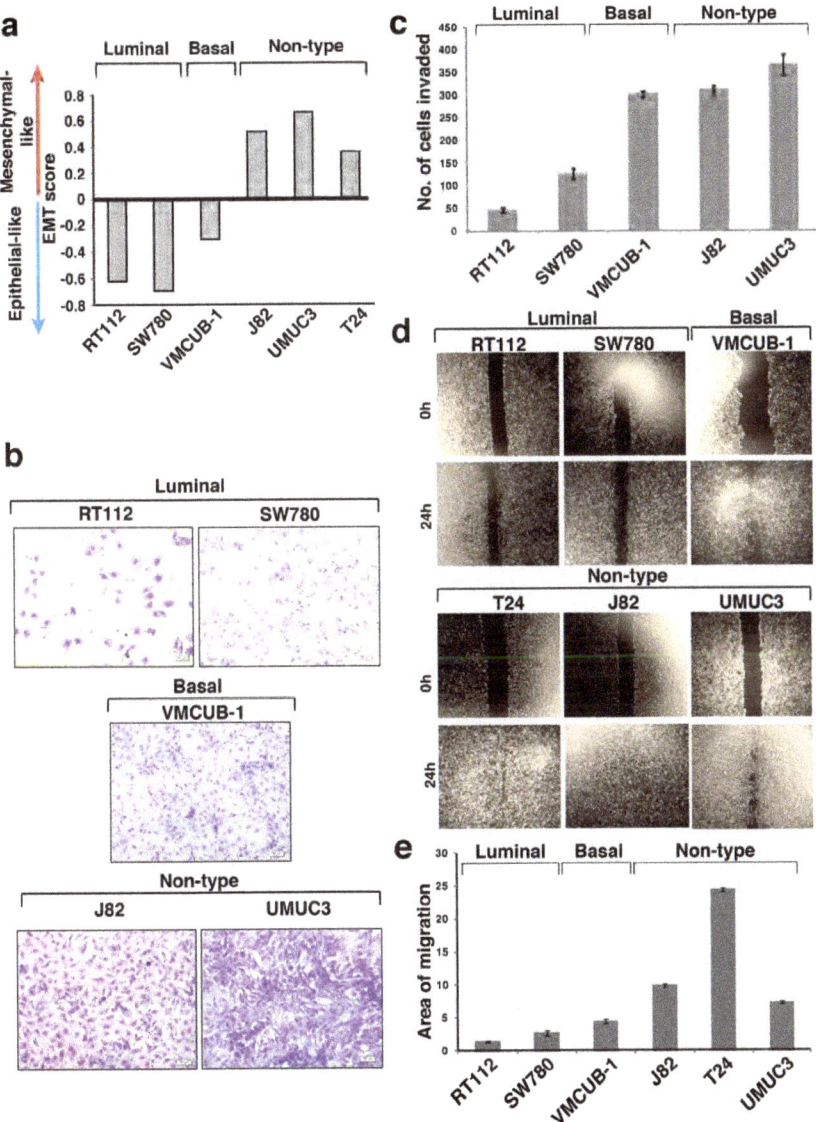

**Figure 1.** (**a**) Epithelial-mesenchymal transition score of the molecular subtypes of bladder carcinoma cell lines. (**b**) Invasion assay. Cells which invaded through the Matrigel were stained using methylene blue and imaged at 10× magnification. (**c**) Quantitative analysis of the number of cells which have invaded in each molecular subtype. (**d**) Scratch wound assay. Migration rate of the molecular subtypes of bladder carcinoma cell lines (magnification: 10×). (**e**) Quantitative analysis of scratch wound assay of the molecular subtype of bladder carcinoma.

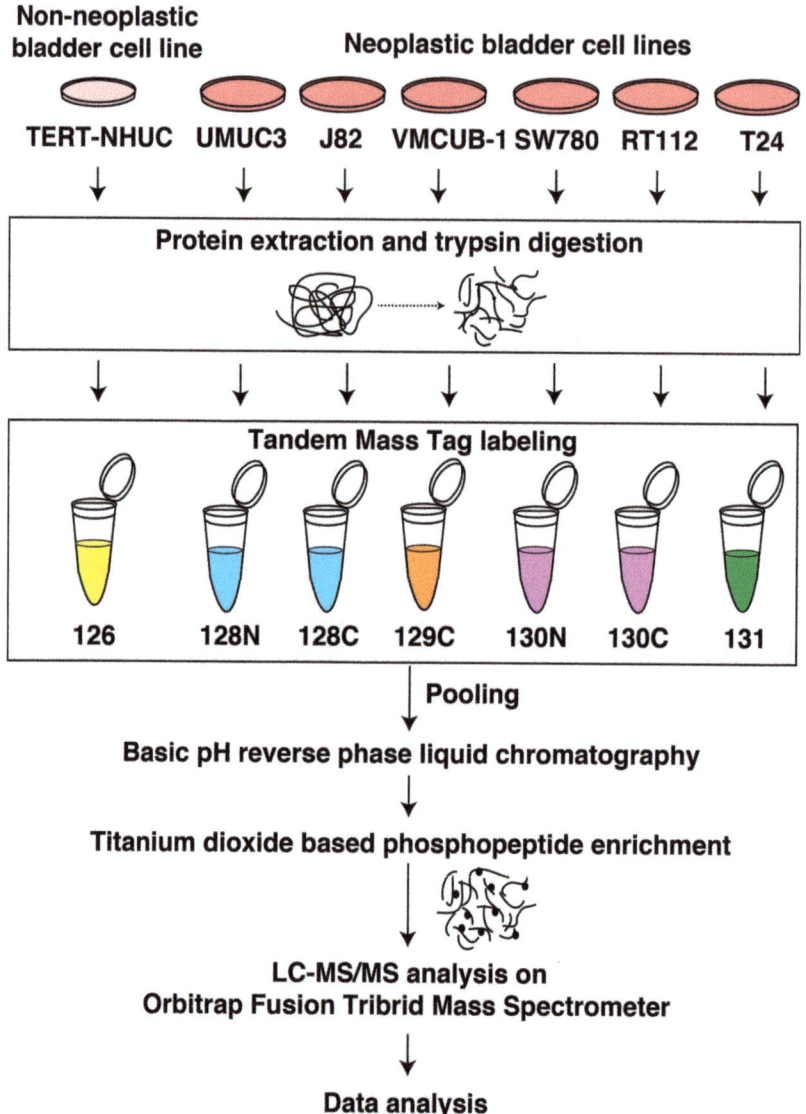

**Figure 2.** Workflow illustrating the quantitative phosphoproteomics analysis of bladder carcinoma cell lines. For sample processing, proteins were extracted from the bladder carcinoma and non-neoplastic cell lines and digested using trypsin. Each cell line was tagged using the tandem mass tags TMT labeling kit and lyophilized and enriched using the phosphopeptide enrichment protocol (titanium dioxide enrichment). The samples were run on Orbitrap Fusion Tribrid Mass Spectrometer and MS2-based quantitation was achieved. The files were searched against Mascot and Sequest HT search engines. PhosphoRS node was used for the phosphosite assignment. Data was acquired in technical replicates.

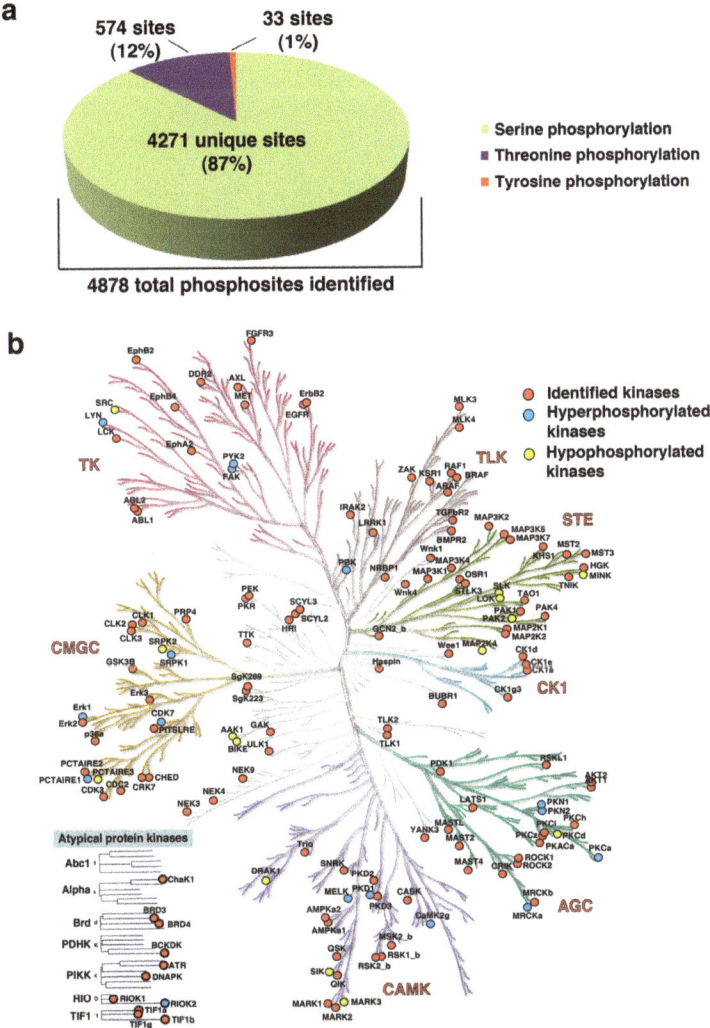

**Figure 3.** (a) Pie chart depicting the phosphosites identified in the study. Identification of the unique phosphosites (percentage of unique serine, threonine, and tyrosine sites identified in the study is mentioned). (b) Kinome map depicting the identified kinases in the dataset. Kinases are highlighted as in the inset legend. The map was built using the KinMap tool.

*3.4. Kinases Enriched in the Phosphoproteomics Dataset*

A total of 151 kinases were enriched in the phosphoproteomic analysis of the bladder carcinoma cell lines. Of these, 35 were CMGC (which refers to the CDK, MAPK, GSK3, and CLK set of families); 26 were of the homologs of yeast Sterile 7, Sterile 11, and Sterile 20 kinases (STE); 24 were from the protein kinase A, G, and C families (AGC); 20 were calmodulin/calcium regulated kinases (CAMK); 16 were tyrosine kinases (TK); 12 were tyrosine-like kinases (TLK); seven were casein kinases (CK1); and 11 were atypical kinases. In our dataset, 16 kinases were hyperphosphorylated and 14 were hypophosphorylated (in at least one cell line) (Figure 3b).

## 3.5. Unique Phosphorylation Signature Identified for the Non-Type Subtype of Bladder Carcinoma

In a recent detailed analysis, Warrick et al. used agglomerative methods (using the expression of a subtype-specific gene list from the TCGA study) to characterize molecular subtypes of bladder carcinoma cell lines [14]. Based on that report, we selected six bladder carcinoma cell lines to identify differential changes in the signaling pathways of the non-type molecular subtype (Table 1).

**Table 1.** General characterization and molecular subtypes of the bladder carcinoma cell lines.

| Cell Line | Source [a] | Molecular Subtype [b] | Derived from Male/Female | Grade |
|---|---|---|---|---|
| SW780 | UCC | Luminal | Female | Grade 1 |
| RT112 | UCC | Luminal | Female | Grade 2 |
| T24 | EC | Non-type | Female | Grade 3 |
| J82 | EC | Non-type | Male | Grade 3 |
| UMUC3 | UCC | Non-type | Male | - |
| VMCUB-1 | EC | Basal | Male | Grade 2 |

[a] UCC, urothelial cell carcinoma; EC, epithelial carcinoma; [b] Molecular subtypes are from Warrick et al., 2016 [14].

Unsupervised hierarchical clustering was employed to cluster quantified phosphopeptides across normal and malignant bladder cell lines (Supplementary Table S4). The luminal subtype showed distinct clusters (RT112 and SW780), whereas the non-type cell lines (J82, UMUC3 and T24) were clustered along with the basal type (VMCUB-1) (Supplementary Figure S1). Thus, we sought to use the phosphorylation pattern or signature in the non-type subtype to explain what drives the mesenchymal phenotype. 375 differentially phosphorylated peptides corresponding to 289 proteins were identified in the non-type cell lines as compared to the luminal/basal subtype ($p \leq 0.05$) (Supplementary Table S5). Supervised clustering of the 375 differentially phosphorylated peptides revealed distinct phosphopeptide signature. Two distinct clusters were observed: the non-type cell lines were clustered away from the luminal/basal cells (Figure 4).

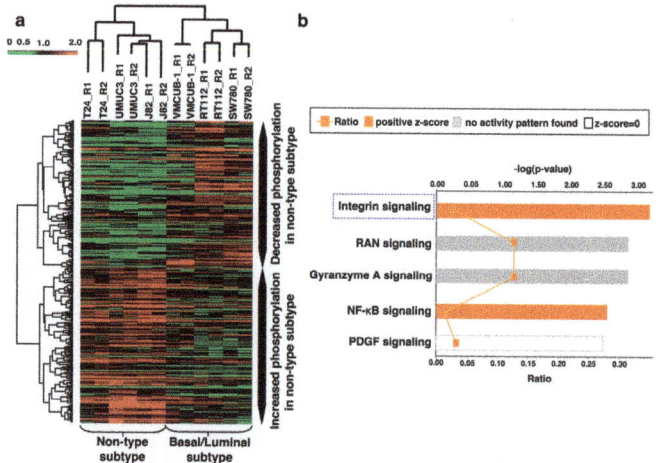

**Figure 4.** (**a**) Supervised clustering of the molecular subtypes of bladder carcinoma cell lines. A *t*-test conducted on the quantified data (across all cell lines) indicated that 375 peptides (corresponding to 289 proteins) were differentially phosphorylated in the non-type cell lines (T24, J82, and UMUC3) as compared with the luminal/basal subtype (SW780, RT112, and VMCUB-1) ($p \leq 0.05$). (**b**) Canonical pathways enriched in the non-type subtype of bladder carcinoma. IPA analysis identified the "integrin pathway" as the most significantly enriched pathway in the aggressive non-type bladder carcinoma subtype.

## 3.6. Ingenuity Pathway Analysis (IPA) Identifies Aberrant Activation of Pathways in the Molecular Subtypes of Bladder Carcinoma

IPA of 46 hyperphosphorylated peptides identified significant enrichment of "integrin pathway" components ($p$ = 6.29E-04; z-score = 2.00) (Figure 4b). Five proteins involved in cell motility had significantly increased phosphorylation in the non-type subtype as compared with the basal and luminal subtypes as well as the TERT-NHUC (control) cells (Supplementary Table S6). TLN1 was 3-fold hyperphosphorylated in the non-type and 2-fold in the basal. We further checked the hyperphosphorylation of TLN1 (S425) in bladder tumor sections. Immunohistochemical staining showed hyperphosphorylation of TLN1 (S425) in high-grade tumors as compared to low-grade tumors (Supplementary Figure S2). TLN1 is a major mediator of the integrin activation and crosstalk. It also stabilizes extracellular matrix-actin linkage [24]. CTTN and CRKL were 1.5-fold hyperphosphorylated in the non-type subtype. CTTN phosphorylation is reported to mediate and accompany integrin mediated cell adhesion to the extracellular matrix [25]. The translocation of CRKL to the focal adhesion activates integrin induced downstream signaling through Src family of kinases and further mediates cell migration [26]. ZYX and BCAR3 were 1.5-fold hyperphosphorylated in the non-type subtype whereas 0.5-fold hypophosphorylated in the luminal subtype. ZYX regulates cellular movement and binds strongly to the focal adhesions. Integrins bind its cytoplasmic tail to ZYX through alpha-actinin [27]. BCAR3 along with its binding partner BCAR1 leads to changes in cellular morphology, motility, and adhesion by the transduction of integrin signaling [28]. To check the global phosphorylation status in aggressive non-type we carried out a pathway analysis with the set of all the phosphopeptides quantified across all cell lines (2806 phosphopeptides). The analysis displayed integrin pathway enrichment which comprises global proposition of the other proteins (the other proteins which are identified/dysregulated in our study) ($p$ = 5.06E-04; z-score = 5.303) with the total inclusion of 49 proteins in the signaling network (Figure 5).

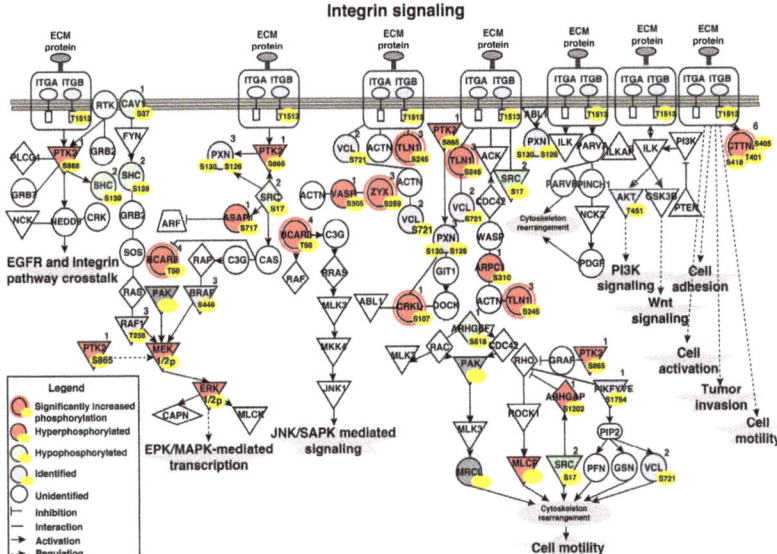

**Figure 5.** Schematic diagram of enriched integrin signaling pathway in non-type subtype of bladder carcinoma cell lines. Ingenuity pathway analysis lead to the identification of integrin signaling to be most enriched in the aggressive molecular subtype. The dysregulated proteins, the number of phosphopeptides, and the phosphosites identified are highlighted in the pathway.

For the luminal subtype, there was an enrichment of "phospholipase C signaling" components ($p = 6.29\text{E-}03$; z-score = 2.00), including four differentially phosphorylated proteins—Rho guanine nucleotide exchange factor 16 (AREGEF16), actin-related protein 2/3 complex subunit 1B (ARPC1B), cdc42 effector protein 1 (CDC42EP1), and stathmin1 (STMN1). The basal subtype showed enrichment of "signaling by Rho family GTPase" components ($p = 3.68\text{E-}03$; z-score = 2.00), and included the differential phosphorylation of neuroblast differentiation-associated protein (AHNAK), AREGEF16, myristoylated alanine-rich C-kinase substrate (MARCKS), and proto-oncogene tyrosine-protein kinase Src (SRC) (Supplementary Figure S3).

### 3.7. Regulatory Interaction Network Enriched in the Non-Type Subtype

Network analysis appeared to link key molecules not identified in our study which may be important regulators of the network along with the non-type subtype specific phosphoproteins. The most enriched network in the non-type subtype contained 25 proteins from our dataset (score = 46) (Supplementary Figure S4a). The primary hub proteins included protein kinase A catalytic subunit (PRKACA), Rac-alpha serine/threonine protein kinase (AKT) and nuclear factor NF-kappa-B (NFκB). PRKACA interacts with protein kinase A regulatory subunit 1A (PRKAR1A), ADP ribosylation factor guanine nucleotide exchange factor 2 (ARFGEF2) and A-kinase anchor protein (AKAP11). AKT interacts which TBC2 domain family 4 (TBC2D4) and interferon-induced, double-stranded RNA activated protein (EIF2AK2), desmoplakin (DSP), SRC, and integrin beta-4 (ITGB4). NFκB interacts with TGFβ-activated kinase 1 (TGFB1), MAP3K7-binding protein 2 (TAB2), TBC2D4, casein kinase II subunit beta (CSNK2B), EIF2AK2, CDC42, CDC42EP1, DNA polymerase alpha subunit B (PLOA2), sentrin-specific protease 1 (SENP1), PKA, and immunoglobulin G (IgG). Cell motility was the most enriched function determined by the IPA analysis. 21 proteins related to cell motility were enriched in the non-type subtype of bladder carcinoma (Supplementary Figure S4b).

### 3.8. CDK1 (Cyclin-Dependent Kinase 1) and GSK3A/GSK3B (Glycogen Synthase Kinase 3A and 3B) Are the Predicted Activated Kinases in Non-Type Subtype of Bladder Carcinoma Cell Lines

Eight kinases—GSK3A, GSK3B, CDK1, ribosomal protein S6 kinase alpha-1 (RPS6KA1), ribosomal protein S6 kinase alpha-1 (RPS6KB1), serine/threonine protein kinase Sgk 1 (SGK1), TGFβ receptor type-2 (TGFBR2), and 5′-AMP-activated protein kinase catalytic subunit alpha-2 (PRKAA2)—were predicted to be significantly enriched (Supplementary Table S7). GSK3A ($p = 0.003$; z-score = 2.7) and GSK3B ($p = 0.01$; z-score = 2.3) were predicted to be activated and responsible for the phosphorylation of four downstream proteins (tuberin (TSC2), AKAP11, MAP1B, and TBC1 domain family 4 (TBC1D4)). GSK3A was predicted to independently phosphorylate translocon-associated protein subunit alpha (SSR1), whereas GSK3B was predicted to be upstream of neurogenic locus notch homolog protein 2 (NOTCH2) and transcription factor RelB (RELB). CDK1 was also predicted as the upstream activated kinase ($p = 0.01$; z-score = 2.06) for 23 proteins at single, double, or triple phosphorylation sites (Supplementary Table S8). RPS6KA1, RPS6KB1, and SGK1 were predicted as the negatively regulated kinases ($p = 0.01$; z-score = $-2.10$) (Figure 6a–c).

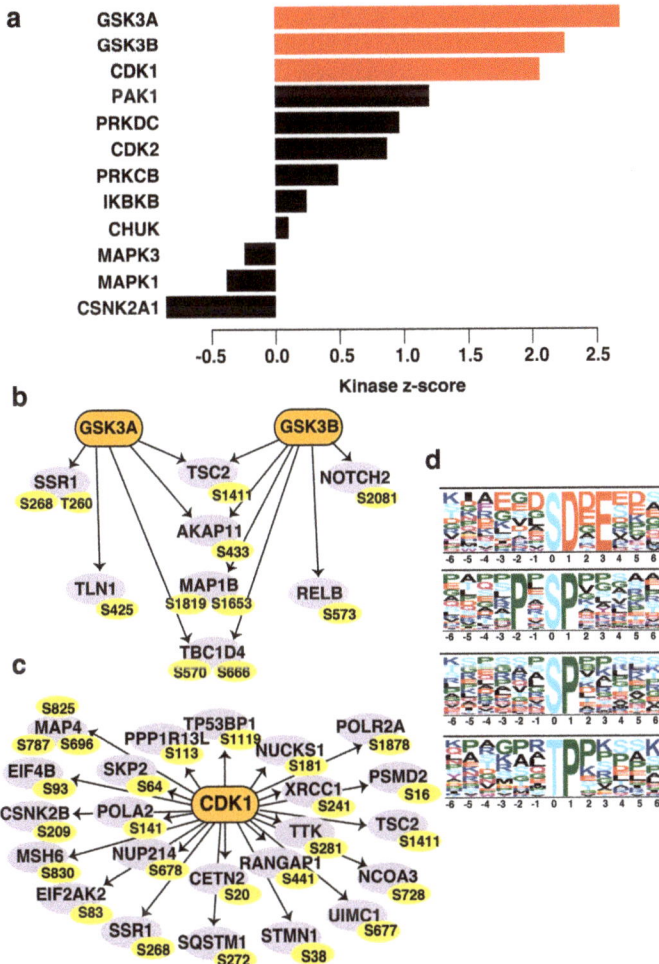

**Figure 6.** (a) Predicted upstream kinases enriched in the non-type subtype of bladder carcinoma cell lines. Graph showing the positively regulated upstream kinases (red bars) predicted to be activated in the non-type subtype. (b) Substrates of GSK3A/3B and (c) CDK1 enriched in non-type molecular subtype depicted by a schematic diagram. The respective phosphosites of the substrates identified are also highlighted. (d) Motif analysis of differentially phosphorylated peptides of non-type subtype bladder carcinoma. Serine and threonine motifs identified in the non-type subtype of bladder carcinoma.

*3.9. Active Proline-Directed Motifs Identified in the Non-Type Molecular Subtype*

In the non-type subtype, five serine and one threonine phosphorylated motifs were significantly differentially phosphorylated (among the 289 signature proteins). A maximum fold change of 36 was calculated for the pSDxE serine phosphorylated motif. The consensus motifs PxpSP and pSP motifs also showed a high fold change in phosphorylation of 7.5-fold. Supplementary Table S9 enlists the differentially phosphorylated protein sites matching to the consensus motifs. Only one motif for the threonine sites (pTP) was identified in the dataset (10-fold enriched among 24 phosphopeptides) (Figure 6d).

## 4. Discussion

A molecular subtype is an "intrinsic" feature that defines both clinical and biological stratification of a given tumor. The molecular subtypes of bladder carcinoma have not been extensively studied. In addition, switching between molecular subtypes and the multifocal characteristics of these tumors are two phenomena that preclude our understanding of the biological and clinical properties of these tumors. Most of the studies have defined the molecular subtypes by analyzing gene expression data based on the enrichment of specific genetic alterations and gene expression profiles. However, a comprehensive and quantitative phosphoproteomics study on bladder carcinoma has still not been reported. Here we provide compelling data that suggests the cellular signaling pathways that contribute to the mesenchymal phenotype in the non-type molecular subtype of bladder carcinoma. Our study identified 10,979 phosphopeptides corresponding to 3125 proteins from a panel of bladder carcinoma cell lines. This study offers new biological insight and identifies potential kinases that could be targeted in bladder carcinoma. We combined bioinformatics approaches with phosphoproteomic analyses of bladder carcinoma cell lines to generate highly enriched cellular signaling pathways. This provided the groundwork for defining the molecular subtypes in bladder carcinoma cell lines, which may help to identify and develop new therapeutic approaches within these model systems. Importantly, the study needs to be extended on large cohort of bladder tumor sections to validate a prognostic and predictive role of the subtype specific signature. This would aid in the clinical assessment of bladder carcinoma patients for appropriate treatment regimen based on the molecular subtypes. The computed EMT score suggests that the non-type molecular subtype is more "mesenchymal-like," whereas the luminal/basal subtypes are "epithelial-like." The non-type subtype cell lines show an increased migratory and invasive phenotype, reflecting typical characteristics of a mesenchymal-like phenotype. Non-type carcinomas may; thus, more readily invade the bladder wall, and this knowledge may provide the necessary evidence to spur a change in the field of muscle invasive bladder carcinoma, particularly in terms of their recurrent nature. Recently, existence of hybrid EMT state has also been reported by various groups [29,30]. A study by Jolly et al. showed that hybrid epithelial/mesenchymal cells adhere higher tumor-initiation capabilities and metastatic potential [31]. Another study by Yadavalli et al. computed the EMT score using transcriptomic datasets. The EMT scores distributed between −0.3 to +0.5, for cancer CTCs suggestive of intermediate phenotypes [32]. In our study, we observed the distribution of EMT scores in the aggressive non-type subtype were distributed between +0.35 to +0.65.

We identified the enrichment of the integrin signaling pathway in the non-type molecular subtype, with differential phosphorylation in five major proteins: TLN1, CTTN, BCAR3, CRKL, and ZYX. Integrins are a family of cell adhesion receptors that mediate cell–matrix and cell–cell interactions [33–35]. A major function of the integrins is to regulate the intracellular signaling cascades that lead to cell proliferation, survival, motility, and migration [36–38]. TLN1 is an adaptor protein critical to integrin signaling. In the non-type molecular subtype, TLN1 is significantly hyperphosphorylated at S425 in the head domain (band 4.1, ezrin, radixin, moesin homology domain) (Supplementary Figure S5), a site also known to be hyperphosphorylated in prostate cancer [39]. TLN1 S425 is phosphorylated by cyclin-dependent kinase 5 (CDK5), which controls the metastatic potential in prostate cancer [40]. S425 acts on integrin β with an "inside-out" mechanism; however, we did not identify a change in integrin β1. Cell migration is stimulated by TLN1 coupled to the integrin cytoplasmic domain: TLN1 connects ligand-bound integrins with the actin cytoskeleton, and this is needed for the catalysis of the focal adhesion-dependent pathways [41] to initiate cell movement. The phosphorylation of TLN1 at S425 limits focal-adhesion turnover, which, in turn, stabilizes the lamellipodia contributing to the sustained cell migration [42]. TLN1 overexpression is also correlated with advanced and aggressive oral squamous cell carcinoma [43]. In concordance with the reported studies, we also observed a hyperphosphorylation of TLN1 (S425) in high grade tumor sections. In our unpublished global proteomics data of bladder carcinoma cell lines, TLN1 is >1.5-fold overexpressed in the non-type cell lines; however, its role in bladder carcinoma and whether it contributes to the "mesenchymal-like" phenotype is unclear.

CTTN is an actin-binding protein significantly hyperphosphorylated at S418, S405, and T401 in the non-type molecular subtype. CTTN promotes cell migration by lengthening lamellipodia, increasing the number of filopodia, and increasing protrusion time [44]. CTTN is phosphorylated at S418 and S405 by the serine/threonine extracellular signal-regulated kinases (ERK1/2) [45], which, in turn, stimulates binding of the Arp2/3 complex to N-WASP via its SH3 domain [46]. CTTN phosphorylation is required for actin regulation and is responsible for lamellipodia formation and associated with enhanced cancer cell migration [47]. In bladder carcinoma, CTTN may be involved in the regulation of actin-based extravasation through invadopodia formation [48]. CRKL is another adaptor protein that is overexpressed in many cancers, including bladder carcinoma [49]. It regulates cyclin D1 and modulates ERK1/2 phosphorylation. In bladder carcinoma cell lines, CRKL is hyperphosphorylated at S107; however, the function of this phosphorylation is unclear. The two other differentially phosphorylated proteins identified in our study are ZYX and BCAR3. ZYX is a LIM domain protein with distinct actin polymerization activity. It also modulates cell adhesion and the expression of integrins, controlling cell motility in lung carcinoma. ZYX may also regulate EMT during lung cancer development and may regulate cell–cell adhesion, integrin α5β1 expression, and ECM adhesion [50]. ZYX is overexpressed in breast cancer and positively correlated with breast carcinoma metastasis [51]. Its depletion reduces cell proliferation, motility, and in vivo tumorigenic activity. BCAR3, on the other hand, binds to the C-terminal of its partner p130Cas (BCAR1) and co-ordinates the activation of SRC, a non-receptor tyrosine kinase [52]. The BCAR3–SRC activation axis is governed by PTPα, binding to its SH2 domain to recruit the BCAR3/Cas complex. T789 phosphorylation of PTPα is required for integrin induced-adhesion signaling [53]. The functional roles of ZYX (S259) and BCAR3 (T50) phosphorylation have not been studied in bladder carcinoma, but these proteins may contribute to invasion, as both proteins are involved in cell motility. However, EMT is regulated at several levels through transcriptional controls, epigenetic modifications, translational modifications, and alternative splicing [54–58].

Phospholipase C has a decisive role in skin cancer development [59], and its overexpression in gastric-mucosa cells perhaps offers an opportunity to differentiate gastric cancer and inflammatory lesions [60]. Thus, its overexpression in luminal bladder carcinoma is not unexpected, and may be the result of early pro-inflammatory signaling. Our pathway analysis also identified an enrichment of Rho signaling in the basal cell line. Activated Rho proteins can alter cell behavior as well as cell morphology. In breast cancer, Rho family GTPases regulates cell motility by cytoskeleton remodeling and altering focal adhesions [61]. High RhoA and RhoC expression is correlated with poor tumor differentiation, muscle invasion, and lymph node metastasis in bladder carcinoma [62]. The basal subtype of bladder carcinoma is relatively more aggressive than the luminal subtype, and activated Rho protein signaling may contribute to this aggressive clinical outcome [63].

In our IPA analysis, NFκB was highlighted as the regulatory hub molecule of the most enriched network in the non-type subtype. This transcriptional regulator largely affects the expression of cytokines, chemokines, adhesion molecules, and controls various mechanisms, including inflammation, proliferation, transformation, angiogenesis, invasion, and chemoresistance [64]. Interestingly, β1-integrin contains a unique NFκB-binding site in its promoter region, suggesting a potential regulatory role of NFκB in integrin signaling [65]. Thus, NFκB may regulate the expression of integrins and enhance signaling downstream, affecting cell proliferation and motility.

The non-type significantly enriched in golgi vesicle (0.09%), cytoskeleton (5.1%) and in nuclear compartment (75.2%). In addition, ubiquitin-specific proteases (4.9%), cytoskeleton protein binding (4.5%), and signal transducers (1.1%) were significantly active in non-type bladder carcinoma cell line (Supplementary Figure S6). Through our kinase-substrate enrichment analysis, we predicted that the two most activated kinases were GSK3A and GSK3B, two highly conserved serine/threonine protein kinases. The roles of these two kinases in cancer remain controversial, with little evidence in the literature to support their role in the disease. The Y216-phosphorylated active form of GSK3B is significantly decreased in squamous cell carcinoma [66] and in lung cancer, inhibiting GSK3B increases the expression of the transcriptional repressor Snail, which suppresses E-cadherin and promotes EMT [67]. A potent GSK3 inhibitor LY2090314 has been tested in clinical trials against metastatic pancreatic cancer (NCT0163230) and acute leukemia (NCT01214603) [68]. Others have reported that pharmacological inhibition of GSK3B can induce apoptosis by sorafenib in melanoma cell lines and leukemic cells [69,70]. Yet, in ovarian cancer, GSK3B activity was linked with cell proliferation, and overexpression of its active form can induce CDK1 expression and facilitate cell proliferation [71]. CDK1 is a major mitotic regulating kinase involved in the G2/M phase of the cell cycle, and is upregulated in several cancers and also associated with clinicopathological factors [72–74]. Various CDK inhibitors have been trialed for the treatment of breast cancer and chronic lymphocytic leukemia [75–77]. Nevertheless, the role of CDK1 in bladder carcinoma has yet to be elucidated. GSK3A/B and CDK1 could be potential druggable targets for the aggressive non-type bladder carcinoma. Intriguingly, we identified enrichment of proline-directed motifs (pSP/ pTP) in our dataset, which are known to be active mostly in proliferating cells and phosphorylated by CDK1 during mitosis [78]. We also identified the pSer and pThr motifs that recognize acidic casein kinase II in our dataset [79], yet the importance of these motifs in bladder carcinoma remains unclear.

## 5. Conclusions

We present the first comprehensive phosphoproteome of bladder carcinoma cells and offer a potential starting point for further mechanistic studies. Our phosphoproteomic data and bioinformatic analyses suggest two key activated kinases (GSK3A/B and CDK1) as potential druggable targets for the aggressive subtype of bladder carcinoma. We provide a glimpse of the dynamic process of phosphorylation in bladder carcinoma and also the differentially regulated phosphoproteins in this aggressive molecular non-type subtype.

**Supplementary Materials:** The following are available online at http://www.mdpi.com/2077-0383/8/5/703/s1, Figure S1: Unsupervised clustering of the bladder carcinoma cell lines of the quantified data across all the cell lines; Figure S2: Immunohistochemistry showing TLN1 (S425) hyperphosphorylation in high-grade tumors as compared to low-grade tumors; Figure S3: Top five canonical pathways enriched by IPA in (a) luminal and (b) basal subtypes of bladder carcinoma; Figure S4: (a) A global network interaction map of the differentially phosphorylated proteins in the non-type subtype. Most enriched network in the aggressive subtype with an enrichment score of 46 (IPA). (b) Cell motility is an intrinsic characteristic of the non-type subtype of bladder carcinoma. Phosphoproteins involved in cell motility, as depicted from the IPA analysis; Figure S5: Protein domain structure for TLN1. The domains of TLN1 and the significantly differentially phosphorylated sites (S425; head domain) in the non-type cell lines; Figure S6: Gene ontology enrichment of the differentially phosphorylated proteins in the non-type molecular subtype. Most of the proteins are nuclear proteins (75.2%). Proteins with kinase activity and signal transducer activity are also significantly enriched ($p \leq 0.05$). Data were analyzed using FunRich; Table S1: EMT score of bladder carcinoma cell lines molecular subtypes; Table S2: List of phosphopeptides identified in bladder carcinoma cell lines using SequestHT and Mascot search algorithms; Table S3: List of phosphopeptides identified in bladder carcinoma cell lines using SequestHT and Mascot search algorithms with a PhosphoRS probablity of $\geq 75\%$; Table S4: List of phosphopeptides identified in bladder carcinoma cell lines using SequestHT and Mascot search algorithms with a PhosphoRS probability of $\geq 75\%$ and quantified across all the cell lines; Table S5: A total of 375 differentially phosphorylated peptides in the non-type bladder carcinoma molecular subtype; Table S6: Proteins differentially phosphorylated in non-type subtype in integrin signaling (p-value $\leq 0.05$); Table S7: Kinase scores for the kinase-substrate enrichment analysis; Table S8: Kinase-substrate enrichment scores; and Table S9: Motifs identified by motif-x in the differentially phosphorylated peptides in non-type subtype.

**Author Contributions:** Conceptualization, P.K. and H.G.; methodology, B.D., V.N.P., and K.G.; software, B.D. and V.N.P.; validation, B.D. and K.G.; formal analysis, B.D., H.G., and P.K.; investigation, B.D., H.G., and P.K.; writing—original draft preparation, B.D. and P.K.; writing—review and editing, J.P.T., H.G., and P.K.; visualization, B.D., J.P.T., H.G., and P.K.; supervision, J.P.T., H.G., and P.K.; project administration, P.K.; funding acquisition, P.K. All authors have read and approved the final version of the manuscript.

**Funding:** This research was funded by Department of Science and Technology (DST), Ramanujan Fellowship, Government of India, grant number SB/S2/RJN-077/2015 and the APC was funded by SB/S2/RJN-077/2015, Department of Science and Technology (DST), Ramanujan Fellowship, Government of India.

**Acknowledgments:** We thank the Department of Biotechnology (DBT), Government of India for research support to the Institute of Bioinformatics, Bangalore. PK is a recipient of the Ramanujan Fellowship awarded by Department of Science and Technology (DST), Government of India. BD is a recipient of INSPIRE Fellowship from Department of Science and Technology (DST), Government of India. KG is a recipient of Senior Research Fellowship from

University Grants Commission (UGC), Government of India. We also thank Rebecca A. Jackson, Scientific Editor, for English editing.

**Conflicts of Interest:** The authors declare no conflicts of interest. The funders had no role in the design of the study; in the collection, analyses, or interpretation of data; in the writing of the manuscript, or in the decision to publish the results.

## References

1. Burger, M.; Oosterlinck, W.; Konety, B.; Chang, S.; Gudjonsson, S.; Pruthi, R.; Soloway, M.; Solsona, E.; Sved, P.; Babjuk, M.; et al. ICUD-EAU International Consultation on Bladder Cancer 2012: Non-muscle-invasive urothelial carcinoma of the bladder. *Eur. Urol.* **2013**, *63*, 36–44. [CrossRef] [PubMed]
2. Schrier, B.P.; Hollander, M.P.; van Rhijn, B.W.; Kiemeney, L.A.; Witjes, J.A. Prognosis of muscle-invasive bladder cancer: Difference between primary and progressive tumours and implications for therapy. *Eur. Urol.* **2004**, *45*, 292–296. [CrossRef]
3. Tan, T.Z.; Miow, Q.H.; Miki, Y.; Noda, T.; Mori, S.; Huang, R.Y.; Thiery, J.P. Epithelial-mesenchymal transition spectrum quantification and its efficacy in deciphering survival and drug responses of cancer patients. *EMBO Mol. Med.* **2014**, *6*, 1279–1293. [CrossRef]
4. Damrauer, J.S.; Hoadley, K.A.; Chism, D.D.; Fan, C.; Tiganelli, C.J.; Wobker, S.E.; Yeh, J.J.; Milowsky, M.I.; Iyer, G.; Parker, J.S.; et al. Intrinsic subtypes of high-grade bladder cancer reflect the hallmarks of breast cancer biology. *Proc. Natl. Acad. Sci. USA* **2014**, *111*, 3110–3115. [CrossRef] [PubMed]
5. Choi, W.; Porten, S.; Kim, S.; Willis, D.; Plimack, E.R.; Hoffman-Censits, J.; Roth, B.; Cheng, T.; Tran, M.; Lee, I.L.; et al. Identification of distinct basal and luminal subtypes of muscle-invasive bladder cancer with different sensitivities to frontline chemotherapy. *Cancer Cell* **2014**, *25*, 152–165. [CrossRef]
6. Fujimoto, K.; Yamada, Y.; Okajima, E.; Kakizoe, T.; Sasaki, H.; Sugimura, T.; Terada, M. Frequent association of p53 gene mutation in invasive bladder cancer. *Cancer Res.* **1992**, *52*, 1393–1398. [PubMed]
7. Van Rhijn, B.W.; Lurkin, I.; Radvanyi, F.; Kirkels, W.J.; van der Kwast, T.H.; Zwarthoff, E.C. The fibroblast growth factor receptor 3 (FGFR3) mutation is a strong indicator of superficial bladder cancer with low recurrence rate. *Cancer Res.* **2001**, *61*, 1265–1268. [PubMed]
8. Orlow, I.; Lacombe, L.; Hannon, G.J.; Serrano, M.; Pellicer, I.; Dalbagni, G.; Reuter, V.E.; Zhang, Z.F.; Beach, D.; Cordon-Cardo, C. Deletion of the p16 and p15 genes in human bladder tumors. *J. Natl. Cancer Inst.* **1995**, *87*, 1524–1529. [CrossRef]
9. Sjodahl, G.; Lauss, M.; Lovgren, K.; Chebil, G.; Gudjonsson, S.; Veerla, S.; Patschan, O.; Aine, M.; Ferno, M.; Ringner, M.; et al. A molecular taxonomy for urothelial carcinoma. *Clin. Cancer Res.* **2012**, *18*, 3377–3386. [CrossRef] [PubMed]
10. Aine, M.; Eriksson, P.; Liedberg, F.; Sjodahl, G.; Hoglund, M. Biological determinants of bladder cancer gene expression subtypes. *Sci. Rep.* **2015**, *5*, 10957. [CrossRef]
11. Hedegaard, J.; Lamy, P.; Nordentoft, I.; Algaba, F.; Hoyer, S.; Ulhoi, B.P.; Vang, S.; Reinert, T.; Hermann, G.G.; Mogensen, K.; et al. Comprehensive Transcriptional Analysis of Early-Stage Urothelial Carcinoma. *Cancer Cell* **2016**, *30*, 27–42. [CrossRef]
12. Svatek, R.S.; Shariat, S.F.; Novara, G.; Skinner, E.C.; Fradet, Y.; Bastian, P.J.; Kamat, A.M.; Kassouf, W.; Karakiewicz, P.I.; Fritsche, H.M.; et al. Discrepancy between clinical and pathological stage: External validation of the impact on prognosis in an international radical cystectomy cohort. *BJU Int.* **2011**, *107*, 898–904. [CrossRef]
13. Barretina, J.; Caponigro, G.; Stransky, N.; Venkatesan, K.; Margolin, A.A.; Kim, S.; Wilson, C.J.; Lehar, J.; Kryukov, G.V.; Sonkin, D.; et al. The Cancer Cell Line Encyclopedia enables predictive modelling of anticancer drug sensitivity. *Nature* **2012**, *483*, 603–607. [CrossRef]
14. Warrick, J.I.; Walter, V.; Yamashita, H.; Chung, E.; Shuman, L.; Amponsa, V.O.; Zheng, Z.; Chan, W.; Whitcomb, T.L.; Yue, F.; et al. FOXA1, GATA3 and PPAR Cooperate to Drive Luminal Subtype in Bladder Cancer: A Molecular Analysis of Established Human Cell Lines. *Sci. Rep.* **2016**, *6*, 38531. [CrossRef]
15. Chapman, E.J.; Hurst, C.D.; Pitt, E.; Chambers, P.; Aveyard, J.S.; Knowles, M.A. Expression of hTERT immortalises normal human urothelial cells without inactivation of the p16/Rb pathway. *Oncogene* **2006**, *25*, 5037–5045. [CrossRef]
16. Selvan, L.D.; Renuse, S.; Kaviyil, J.E.; Sharma, J.; Pinto, S.M.; Yelamanchi, S.D.; Puttamallesh, V.N.; Ravikumar, R.; Pandey, A.; Prasad, T.S.; et al. Phosphoproteome of Cryptococcus neoformans. *J. Proteomics* **2014**, *97*, 287–295. [CrossRef]

17. Pinto, S.M.; Nirujogi, R.S.; Rojas, P.L.; Patil, A.H.; Manda, S.S.; Subbannayya, Y.; Roa, J.C.; Chatterjee, A.; Prasad, T.S.; Pandey, A. Quantitative phosphoproteomic analysis of IL-33-mediated signaling. *Proteomics* **2015**, *15*, 532–544. [CrossRef]
18. Verma, R.; Pinto, S.M.; Patil, A.H.; Advani, J.; Subba, P.; Kumar, M.; Sharma, J.; Dey, G.; Ravikumar, R.; Buggi, S.; et al. Quantitative Proteomic and Phosphoproteomic Analysis of H37Ra and H37Rv Strains of Mycobacterium tuberculosis. *J. Proteome Res.* **2017**, *16*, 1632–1645. [CrossRef]
19. Subbannayya, Y.; Syed, N.; Barbhuiya, M.A.; Raja, R.; Marimuthu, A.; Sahasrabuddhe, N.; Pinto, S.M.; Manda, S.S.; Renuse, S.; Manju, H.C.; et al. Calcium calmodulin dependent kinase kinase 2-a novel therapeutic target for gastric adenocarcinoma. *Cancer Biol. Ther.* **2015**, *16*, 336–345. [CrossRef]
20. Tyanova, S.; Temu, T.; Sinitcyn, P.; Carlson, A.; Hein, M.Y.; Geiger, T.; Mann, M.; Cox, J. The Perseus computational platform for comprehensive analysis of (prote)omics data. *Nat. Methods* **2016**, *13*, 731–740. [CrossRef]
21. Wiredja, D.D.; Koyuturk, M.; Chance, M.R. The KSEA App: A web-based tool for kinase activity inference from quantitative phosphoproteomics. *Bioinformatics* **2017**. [CrossRef]
22. Verhaak, R.G.; Tamayo, P.; Yang, J.Y.; Hubbard, D.; Zhang, H.; Creighton, C.J.; Fereday, S.; Lawrence, M.; Carter, S.L.; Mermel, C.H.; et al. Prognostically relevant gene signatures of high-grade serous ovarian carcinoma. *J. Clin. Invest.* **2013**, *123*, 517–525. [CrossRef]
23. Gatza, M.L.; Lucas, J.E.; Barry, W.T.; Kim, J.W.; Wang, Q.; Crawford, M.D.; Datto, M.B.; Kelley, M.; Mathey-Prevot, B.; Potti, A.; et al. A pathway-based classification of human breast cancer. *Proc. Natl. Acad. Sci. USA* **2010**, *107*, 6994–6999. [CrossRef]
24. Das, M.; Ithychanda, S.; Qin, J.; Plow, E.F. Mechanisms of talin-dependent integrin signaling and crosstalk. *Biochim. Biophys. Acta* **2014**, *1838*, 579–588. [CrossRef]
25. Vuori, K.; Ruoslahti, E. Tyrosine phosphorylation of p130Cas and cortactin accompanies integrin-mediated cell adhesion to extracellular matrix. *J. Biol. Chem.* **1995**, *270*, 22259–22262. [CrossRef]
26. Li, L.; Guris, D.L.; Okura, M.; Imamoto, A. Translocation of CrkL to focal adhesions mediates integrin-induced migration downstream of Src family kinases. *Mol. Cell Biol.* **2003**, *23*, 2883–2892. [CrossRef]
27. Xu, C.; Yang, Y.; Yang, J.; Chen, X.; Wang, G. Analysis of the role of the integrin signaling pathway in hepatocytes during rat liver regeneration. *Cell Mol. Biol. Lett.* **2012**, *17*, 274–288. [CrossRef]
28. Green, Y.S.; Kwon, S.; Christian, J.L. Expression pattern of bcar3, a downstream target of Gata2, and its binding partner, bcar1, during Xenopus development. *Gene Expr. Patterns* **2016**, *20*, 55–62. [CrossRef]
29. Pastushenko, I.; Brisebarre, A.; Sifrim, A.; Fioramonti, M.; Revenco, T.; Boumahdi, S.; Van Keymeulen, A.; Brown, D.; Moers, V.; Lemaire, S.; et al. Identification of the tumour transition states occurring during EMT. *Nature* **2018**, *556*, 463–468. [CrossRef]
30. George, J.T.; Jolly, M.K.; Xu, S.; Somarelli, J.A.; Levine, H. Survival Outcomes in Cancer Patients Predicted by a Partial EMT Gene Expression Scoring Metric. *Cancer Res.* **2017**, *77*, 6415–6428. [CrossRef]
31. Jolly, M.K.; Somarelli, J.A.; Sheth, M.; Biddle, A.; Tripathi, S.C.; Armstrong, A.J.; Hanash, S.M.; Bapat, S.A.; Rangarajan, A.; Levine, H. Hybrid epithelial/mesenchymal phenotypes promote metastasis and therapy resistance across carcinomas. *Pharmacol. Ther.* **2019**, *194*, 161–184. [CrossRef]
32. Yadavalli, S.; Jayaram, S.; Manda, S.S.; Madugundu, A.K.; Nayakanti, D.S.; Tan, T.Z.; Bhat, R.; Rangarajan, A.; Chatterjee, A.; Gowda, H.; et al. Data-Driven Discovery of Extravasation Pathway in Circulating Tumor Cells. *Sci. Rep.* **2017**, *7*, 43710. [CrossRef]
33. Taherian, A.; Li, X.; Liu, Y.; Haas, T.A. Differences in integrin expression and signaling within human breast cancer cells. *BMC Cancer* **2011**, *11*, 293. [CrossRef]
34. Boudjadi, S.; Carrier, J.C.; Beaulieu, J.F. Integrin alpha1 subunit is up-regulated in colorectal cancer. *Biomark. Res.* **2013**, *1*, 16. [CrossRef]
35. Giancotti, F.G.; Ruoslahti, E. Integrin signaling. *Science* **1999**, *285*, 1028–1032. [CrossRef] [PubMed]
36. Hood, J.D.; Cheresh, D.A. Role of integrins in cell invasion and migration. *Nat. Rev. Cancer* **2002**, *2*, 91–100. [CrossRef]
37. Radeva, G.; Petrocelli, T.; Behrend, E.; Leung-Hagesteijn, C.; Filmus, J.; Slingerland, J.; Dedhar, S. Overexpression of the integrin-linked kinase promotes anchorage-independent cell cycle progression. *J. Biol. Chem.* **1997**, *272*, 13937–13944. [CrossRef]

38. Le Gall, M.; Grall, D.; Chambard, J.C.; Pouyssegur, J.; Van Obberghen-Schilling, E. An anchorage-dependent signal distinct from p42/44 MAP kinase activation is required for cell cycle progression. *Oncogene* **1998**, *17*, 1271–1277. [CrossRef] [PubMed]
39. Jin, J.K.; Tien, P.C.; Cheng, C.J.; Song, J.H.; Huang, C.; Lin, S.H.; Gallick, G.E. Talin1 phosphorylation activates beta1 integrins: A novel mechanism to promote prostate cancer bone metastasis. *Oncogene* **2015**, *34*, 1811–1821. [CrossRef] [PubMed]
40. Strock, C.J.; Park, J.I.; Nakakura, E.K.; Bova, G.S.; Isaacs, J.T.; Ball, D.W.; Nelkin, B.D. Cyclin-dependent kinase 5 activity controls cell motility and metastatic potential of prostate cancer cells. *Cancer Res.* **2006**, *66*, 7509–7515. [CrossRef]
41. Zhang, X.; Jiang, G.; Cai, Y.; Monkley, S.J.; Critchley, D.R.; Sheetz, M.P. Talin depletion reveals independence of initial cell spreading from integrin activation and traction. *Nat. Cell Biol.* **2008**, *10*, 1062–1068. [CrossRef]
42. Huang, C.; Rajfur, Z.; Yousefi, N.; Chen, Z.; Jacobson, K.; Ginsberg, M.H. Talin phosphorylation by Cdk5 regulates Smurf1-mediated talin head ubiquitylation and cell migration. *Nat. Cell Biol.* **2009**, *11*, 624–630. [CrossRef]
43. Lai, M.T.; Hua, C.H.; Tsai, M.H.; Wan, L.; Lin, Y.J.; Chen, C.M.; Chiu, I.W.; Chan, C.; Tsai, F.J.; Jinn-Chyuan Sheu, J. Talin-1 overexpression defines high risk for aggressive oral squamous cell carcinoma and promotes cancer metastasis. *J. Pathol.* **2011**, *224*, 367–376. [CrossRef]
44. He, Y.; Ren, Y.; Wu, B.; Decourt, B.; Lee, A.C.; Taylor, A.; Suter, D.M. Src and cortactin promote lamellipodia protrusion and filopodia formation and stability in growth cones. *Mol. Biol. Cell* **2015**, *26*, 3229–3244. [CrossRef]
45. Kruchten, A.E.; Krueger, E.W.; Wang, Y.; McNiven, M.A. Distinct phospho-forms of cortactin differentially regulate actin polymerization and focal adhesions. *Am. J. Physiol. Cell Physiol.* **2008**, *295*, C1113–C1122. [CrossRef]
46. Martinez-Quiles, N.; Ho, H.Y.; Kirschner, M.W.; Ramesh, N.; Geha, R.S. Erk/Src phosphorylation of cortactin acts as a switch on-switch off mechanism that controls its ability to activate N-WASP. *Mol. Cell Biol.* **2004**, *24*, 5269–5280. [CrossRef]
47. Kelley, L.C.; Hayes, K.E.; Ammer, A.G.; Martin, K.H.; Weed, S.A. Cortactin phosphorylated by ERK1/2 localizes to sites of dynamic actin regulation and is required for carcinoma lamellipodia persistence. *PLoS ONE* **2010**, *5*, e13847. [CrossRef]
48. Tokui, N.; Yoneyama, M.S.; Hatakeyama, S.; Yamamoto, H.; Koie, T.; Saitoh, H.; Yamaya, K.; Funyu, T.; Nakamura, T.; Ohyama, C.; et al. Extravasation during bladder cancer metastasis requires cortactinmediated invadopodia formation. *Mol. Med. Rep.* **2014**, *9*, 1142–1146. [CrossRef]
49. Han, B.; Luan, L.; Xu, Z.; Wu, B. Clinical significance and biological roles of CRKL in human bladder carcinoma. *Tumour. Biol.* **2014**, *35*, 4101–4106. [CrossRef]
50. Mise, N.; Savai, R.; Yu, H.; Schwarz, J.; Kaminski, N.; Eickelberg, O. Zyxin is a transforming growth factor-beta (TGF-beta)/Smad3 target gene that regulates lung cancer cell motility via integrin alpha5beta1. *J. Biol. Chem.* **2012**, *287*, 31393–31405. [CrossRef]
51. Ma, B.; Cheng, H.; Gao, R.; Mu, C.; Chen, L.; Wu, S.; Chen, Q.; Zhu, Y. Zyxin-Siah2-Lats2 axis mediates cooperation between Hippo and TGF-beta signalling pathways. *Nat. Commun.* **2016**, *7*, 11123. [CrossRef] [PubMed]
52. Riggins, R.B.; Quilliam, L.A.; Bouton, A.H. Synergistic promotion of c-Src activation and cell migration by Cas and AND-34/BCAR3. *J. Biol. Chem.* **2003**, *278*, 28264–28273. [CrossRef] [PubMed]
53. Sun, G.; Cheng, S.Y.; Chen, M.; Lim, C.J.; Pallen, C.J. Protein tyrosine phosphatase alpha phosphotyrosyl-789 binds BCAR3 to position Cas for activation at integrin-mediated focal adhesions. *Mol. Cell Biol.* **2012**, *32*, 3776–3789. [CrossRef]
54. Lu, M.; Jolly, M.K.; Levine, H.; Onuchic, J.N.; Ben-Jacob, E. MicroRNA-based regulation of epithelial-hybrid-mesenchymal fate determination. *Proc. Natl. Acad. Sci. USA* **2013**, *110*, 18144–18149. [CrossRef]
55. Roca, H.; Hernandez, J.; Weidner, S.; McEachin, R.C.; Fuller, D.; Sud, S.; Schumann, T.; Wilkinson, J.E.; Zaslavsky, A.; Li, H.; et al. Transcription factors OVOL1 and OVOL2 induce the mesenchymal to epithelial transition in human cancer. *PLoS ONE* **2013**, *8*, e76773. [CrossRef]

56. Feng, J.; Xu, G.; Liu, J.; Zhang, N.; Li, L.; Ji, J.; Zhang, J.; Zhang, L.; Wang, G.; Wang, X.; et al. Phosphorylation of LSD1 at Ser112 is crucial for its function in induction of EMT and metastasis in breast cancer. *Breast Cancer Res. Treat.* **2016**, *159*, 443–456. [CrossRef]
57. Sun, L.; Fang, J. Epigenetic regulation of epithelial-mesenchymal transition. *Cell Mol. Life Sci.* **2016**, *73*, 4493–4515. [CrossRef] [PubMed]
58. Warns, J.A.; Davie, J.R.; Dhasarathy, A. Connecting the dots: Chromatin and alternative splicing in EMT. *Biochem. Cell Biol.* **2016**, *94*, 12–25. [CrossRef]
59. Ikuta, S.; Edamatsu, H.; Li, M.; Hu, L.; Kataoka, T. Crucial role of phospholipase C epsilon in skin inflammation induced by tumor-promoting phorbol ester. *Cancer Res.* **2008**, *68*, 64–72. [CrossRef]
60. Chen, J.; Wang, W.; Zhang, T.; Ji, J.; Qian, Q.; Lu, L.; Fu, H.; Jin, W.; Cui, D. Differential expression of phospholipase C epsilon 1 is associated with chronic atrophic gastritis and gastric cancer. *PLoS ONE* **2012**, *7*, e47563. [CrossRef]
61. Burbelo, P.; Wellstein, A.; Pestell, R.G. Altered Rho GTPase signaling pathways in breast cancer cells. *Breast Cancer Res. Treat.* **2004**, *84*, 43–48. [CrossRef]
62. Kamai, T.; Tsujii, T.; Arai, K.; Takagi, K.; Asami, H.; Ito, Y.; Oshima, H. Significant association of Rho/ROCK pathway with invasion and metastasis of bladder cancer. *Clin. Cancer Res.* **2003**, *9*, 2632–2641.
63. Dadhania, V.; Zhang, M.; Zhang, L.; Bondaruk, J.; Majewski, T.; Siefker-Radtke, A.; Guo, C.C.; Dinney, C.; Cogdell, D.E.; Zhang, S.; et al. Meta-Analysis of the Luminal and Basal Subtypes of Bladder Cancer and the Identification of Signature Immunohistochemical Markers for Clinical Use. *EBioMedicine* **2016**, *12*, 105–117. [CrossRef]
64. Chaturvedi, M.M.; Sung, B.; Yadav, V.R.; Kannappan, R.; Aggarwal, B.B. NF-kappaB addiction and its role in cancer: 'One size does not fit all'. *Oncogene* **2011**, *30*, 1615–1630. [CrossRef]
65. Ahmed, K.M.; Zhang, H.; Park, C.C. NF-kappaB regulates radioresistance mediated by beta1-integrin in three-dimensional culture of breast cancer cells. *Cancer Res.* **2013**, *73*, 3737–3748. [CrossRef]
66. Leis, H.; Segrelles, C.; Ruiz, S.; Santos, M.; Paramio, J.M. Expression, localization, and activity of glycogen synthase kinase 3beta during mouse skin tumorigenesis. *Mol. Carcinog.* **2002**, *35*, 180–185. [CrossRef]
67. Caccavari, F.; Valdembri, D.; Sandri, C.; Bussolino, F.; Serini, G. Integrin signaling and lung cancer. *Cell Adh. Migr.* **2010**, *4*, 124–129. [CrossRef]
68. McCubrey, J.A.; Steelman, L.S.; Bertrand, F.E.; Davis, N.M.; Sokolosky, M.; Abrams, S.L.; Montalto, G.; D'Assoro, A.B.; Libra, M.; Nicoletti, F.; et al. GSK-3 as potential target for therapeutic intervention in cancer. *Oncotarget* **2014**, *5*, 2881–2911. [CrossRef]
69. Panka, D.J.; Cho, D.C.; Atkins, M.B.; Mier, J.W. GSK-3beta inhibition enhances sorafenib-induced apoptosis in melanoma cell lines. *J. Biol. Chem.* **2008**, *283*, 726–732. [CrossRef]
70. Mirlashari, M.R.; Randen, I.; Kjeldsen-Kragh, J. Glycogen synthase kinase-3 (GSK-3) inhibition induces apoptosis in leukemic cells through mitochondria-dependent pathway. *Leuk. Res.* **2012**, *36*, 499–508. [CrossRef]
71. Cao, Q.; Lu, X.; Feng, Y.J. Glycogen synthase kinase-3beta positively regulates the proliferation of human ovarian cancer cells. *Cell. Res.* **2006**, *16*, 671–677. [CrossRef]
72. Kang, J.; Sergio, C.M.; Sutherland, R.L.; Musgrove, E.A. Targeting cyclin-dependent kinase 1 (CDK1) but not CDK4/6 or CDK2 is selectively lethal to MYC-dependent human breast cancer cells. *BMC Cancer* **2014**, *14*, 32. [CrossRef] [PubMed]
73. Zeestraten, E.C.; Maak, M.; Shibayama, M.; Schuster, T.; Nitsche, U.; Matsushima, T.; Nakayama, S.; Gohda, K.; Friess, H.; van de Velde, C.J.; et al. Specific activity of cyclin-dependent kinase I is a new potential predictor of tumour recurrence in stage II colon cancer. *Br. J. Cancer* **2012**, *106*, 133–140. [CrossRef] [PubMed]
74. Chen, X.; Zhang, F.H.; Chen, Q.E.; Wang, Y.Y.; Wang, Y.L.; He, J.C.; Zhou, J. The clinical significance of CDK1 expression in oral squamous cell carcinoma. *Med. Oral Patol. Oral Cir. Bucal* **2015**, *20*, e7–e12. [CrossRef] [PubMed]
75. De Azevedo, W.F., Jr.; Mueller-Dieckmann, H.J.; Schulze-Gahmen, U.; Worland, P.J.; Sausville, E.; Kim, S.H. Structural basis for specificity and potency of a flavonoid inhibitor of human CDK2, a cell cycle kinase. *Proc. Natl. Acad. Sci. USA* **1996**, *93*, 2735–2740. [CrossRef] [PubMed]
76. Christian, B.A.; Grever, M.R.; Byrd, J.C.; Lin, T.S. Flavopiridol in the treatment of chronic lymphocytic leukemia. *Curr. Opin. Oncol.* **2007**, *19*, 573–578. [CrossRef]

77. Ghia, P.; Scarfo, L.; Perez, S.; Pathiraja, K.; Derosier, M.; Small, K.; McCrary Sisk, C.; Patton, N. Efficacy and safety of dinaciclib vs ofatumumab in patients with relapsed/refractory chronic lymphocytic leukemia. *Blood* **2017**, *129*, 1876–1878. [CrossRef] [PubMed]
78. Wu, C.F.; Wang, R.; Liang, Q.; Liang, J.; Li, W.; Jung, S.Y.; Qin, J.; Lin, S.H.; Kuang, J. Dissecting the M phase-specific phosphorylation of serine-proline or threonine-proline motifs. *Mol. Biol. Cell* **2010**, *21*, 1470–1481. [CrossRef]
79. Villen, J.; Beausoleil, S.A.; Gerber, S.A.; Gygi, S.P. Large-scale phosphorylation analysis of mouse liver. *Proc. Natl. Acad. Sci. USA* **2007**, *104*, 1488–1493. [CrossRef]

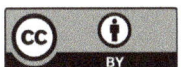

© 2019 by the authors. Licensee MDPI, Basel, Switzerland. This article is an open access article distributed under the terms and conditions of the Creative Commons Attribution (CC BY) license (http://creativecommons.org/licenses/by/4.0/).

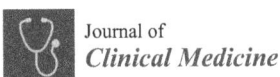 

Article

# Clinical Stratification of High-Grade Ovarian Serous Carcinoma Using a Panel of Six Biomarkers

Swapnil C. Kamble [1,2], Arijit Sen [3], Rahul D. Dhake [4], Aparna N. Joshi [5], Divya Midha [6] and Sharmila A. Bapat [1,*]

1. National Centre for Cell Science, Savitribai Phule Pune University, Ganeshkhind, Pune, Maharashtra 411007, India; sckamble@unipune.ac.in
2. Department of Technology, Savitribai Phule Pune University, Pune, Maharashtra 411007, India
3. Department of Pathology, Armed Forces Medical College, Pune, Maharashtra 411040, India; aseniaf@gmail.com
4. Department of Histopathology, Inlaks and Budrani Hospital, Morbai Naraindas Cancer Institute, Koregaon Park, Pune, Maharashtra 411001, India; drrahuldhake@gmail.com
5. Department of Pathology, KEM Hospital, Pune, Maharashtra 411011, India; draparnajoshi@gmail.com
6. Department of Oncopathology, Tata Medical Centre, Kolkata, West Bengal 700 156, India; divya.midha@tmckolkata.com
* Correspondence: sabapat@nccs.res.in; Tel.: +91-20-25708078

Received: 31 January 2019; Accepted: 21 February 2019; Published: 8 March 2019

**Abstract:** Molecular stratification of high-grade serous ovarian carcinoma (HGSC) for targeted therapy is a pertinent approach in improving prognosis of this highly heterogeneous disease. Enabling the same necessitates identification of class-specific biomarkers and their robust detection in the clinic. We have earlier resolved three discrete molecular HGSC classes associated with distinct functional behavior based on their gene expression patterns, biological networks, and pathways. An important difference revealed was that Class 1 is likely to exhibit cooperative cell migration (CCM), Class 2 undergoes epithelial to mesenchymal transition (EMT), while Class 3 is possibly capable of both modes of migration. In the present study, we define clinical stratification of HGSC tumors through the establishment of standard operating procedures for immunohistochemistry and histochemistry based detection of a panel of biomarkers including TCF21, E-cadherin, PARP1, Slug, AnnexinA2, and hyaluronan. Further development and application of scoring guidelines based on expression of this panel in cell line-derived xenografts, commercial tissue microarrays, and patient tumors led to definitive stratification of samples. Biomarker expression was observed to vary significantly between primary and metastatic tumors suggesting class switching during disease progression. Another interesting feature in the study was of enhanced CCM-marker expression in tumors following disease progression and chemotherapy. These stratification principles and the new information thus generated is the first step towards class-specific personalized therapies in the disease.

**Keywords:** high-grade serous ovarian carcinoma; epithelial-to-mesenchymal transition; molecular stratification; biomarkers; scoring system; immunohistochemistry

## 1. Introduction

Personalized therapeutic decisions in cancer necessitate the development of accurate stratification schemes based on mutations and/or association of tumor sub-groups with specific biomarkers and biological functions, besides well-elucidated principles for their detection [1]. Recent resolution of four gastric cancer molecular groups identified predictive amplifications for subtype-specific treatment [2], including *PDCD1LG2* locus for use of nivolumab and pembrolizumab in the Epstein-Barr virus-associated group, EGFR for cetuximab, panitumumab, nimotuzumab, or matuzumab treatment in the chromosome instability group and Aurora kinase A/B inhibitors for treatment of the genomically stable (GS) subgroup [3–6]. Immunohistochemical (IHC) has become a significant tool in clinical diagnostics and is frequently utilized to classify malignant cells [7]. In gastric cancer, a panel of six biomarkers was used in tumor stratification [8,9]. In a similar approach, cancers of the endometrium [10,11], lung [12], triple-negative breast [13], esophagogastric junction carcinomas [14] were stratified into discrete molecular classes using tumor-specific IHC-based biomarkers. Multiplexed IHC for the concurrent detection of a number of biomarkers in lung cancer is increasingly becoming point-of care in treatment [15]. Such translation of molecular information implies the feasibility of similar applications in other tumor types. High-grade serous ovarian cancer (HGSC) represents aggressive tumors characterized by swift metastatic progression and poor patient prognosis [16]. Despite radical surgery and initial response to platinum and taxane based chemotherapy, most patients relapse following median progression-free survival of ~18 months [17,18]. Clinical outcomes vary considerably emphasizing an imminent need to improve therapeutic options. Large-scale molecular analyses have recently identified diverse molecular pathways, mutations, gene expression, morphologies, cell(s) of origin, etc. leading to a systematic understanding of HGSC despite its heterogeneity [19–23]. Our earlier analyses of gene expression datasets also resolved three classes in HGSC that were associated with discrete mechanisms of metastases [24]. Development of targeted therapies now necessitates the establishment of a robust diagnostic pipeline for HGSC stratification. As a first step towards this aim, the present study evaluates the application of six markers using immunohistochemistry (IHC) and histochemistry (HC), the establishment of standard operating procedures (SOPs) and development of a reference human tissue library for these markers along with scoring guidelines for interpretation of marker expression. Further evaluation and application were performed in xenografts and commercial tissue microarrays (TMAs), along with the determination of thresholds for clinical classification in resected primary tumors and secondary metastases and/or cell blocks prepared from ascitic fluid of chemo-naïve and chemo-treated patients were also achieved (Supplementary Figure S1). These efforts define the establishment of diagnostic principles for application in clinical practice.

## 2. Materials and Methods

### 2.1. Sample Collection and Preparation

Formalin-fixed and paraffin-embedded (FFPE) tissue collection and processing using routine methods following surgery, after obtaining informed consent, were approved by the respective Institutional Review Board of NCCS with project identification code IEC/22/12/2014. All subjects gave their informed consent for inclusion before they participated in the study. The study was conducted in accordance with the Declaration of Helsinki, and the protocol was approved by the Ethics Committee of the National Centre for Cell Science IEC/22/12/2014. In all, retrospective 96 primary high-grade serous ovarian adenocarcinoma patient cases with information of name, age, grade, stage, and treatment status were selected, who had undergone surgery at the Armed Forces Medical College (Pune, India; 2008–2015), Tata Medical Centre (Kolkata, India; 2013–2014), Jehangir Hospital (Pune, India; 2003–2005), Command Hospital (Pune, India; 2010–2011) and Inlaks & Budhrani Hospital (Morbai Naraindas Budrani Cancer Institute, Pune, India; 2013–2015).

### 2.2. Animal Studies

Animal experimentation was in accordance with the rules and regulations of the National Centre for Cell Science (NCCS) Institutional Animal Ethics Committee. The study was approved with project number IAEC/2011/B-163. Xenografts were raised as described earlier [24]. In brief, $2.5 \times 10^6$ cells of cell lines OVCAR3, OV90, OVMZ6, A4, CP70, PEO14, and CAOV3 were injected subcutaneously in non-obese diabetic/severe combined immunodeficient (NOD/SCID) mice. Animals were maintained under pathogen-free conditions and assessed every 2 days until the tumor diameter was ~1 cm, whereupon animals were sacrificed and tumors harvested.

*2.3. Immunohistochemical (IHC) and Histochemical Staining (HC)*

IHC and HC were performed in 5 µm sections of FFPE blocks fixed by drying at 60 °C for at least 1 h in an oven using standard protocol, deparaffinized in xylene and hydrated in ethanol-distilled water gradient. Heat-induced epitope retrieval (HIER) was carried out for 30 min at pH = 9/pH = 6 (Himedia, India). For peroxidase inactivation, sections were incubated in 3% $H_2O_2$ for 30 min (Qualigens, MA, USA), followed by 1× Blocking Solution for 10 min (Biogenex, CA, USA) and overnight incubation in primary antibody (Abcam, MA, USA; E-cadherin ready-to-use, Biogenex, CA, USA; Santa Cruz Biotechnology Inc.Texas, USA; Abcam, MA, USA). Sections were washed and incubated with anti-rabbit HRP-conjugate (Jackson ImmunoResearch Laboratories, Inc., PA, USA) or anti-mouse HRP-conjugate (Jackson ImmunoResearch Laboratories, Inc., PA, USA) for 1 h, and color developed with DAB (Thermo Pierce, MA, USA); hematoxylin used as a counterstain. These sections were dehydrated and mounted in DPX (Qualigens, MA, USA). Negative controls were prepared in the absence of primary antibody. IHC methods were standardized for each marker as Standard Operating Procedures (SOPs; Supplementary Dataset 1). SOPs were developed considering the positive and negative expression tissue controls, and secondary antibody control for each batch of IHC run. For HC-based HA detection, test sections were exposed to freshly prepared hyaluronidase (1 mg/mL; Sigma-Aldrich, MA, USA); control slides were incubated in phosphate buffer for 1 h at 37 °C. Sections were washed in running water for 10 min and stained with Alcian blue for 30 min (pH = 2.5, Fluka, MA, USA), counterstained with Nuclear Fast Red Solution for 2 min (Sigma-Aldrich, MA, United States), and dehydrated and mounted in DPX (Qualigens, MA, USA). Positive experimental controls included testis (TCF21, PARP1), liver (E-cadherin), lymphocytes (Slug), gall bladder (ANXA2), and small intestine (hyaluronan); negative controls included heart (TCF21, E-cadherin, Slug, ANXA2) and mucosa of the small intestine (PARP1). Slides for human tissues, xenografts, and TMA were reviewed independently; a consensus was reached to establish tissues for reference score.

*2.4. Statistical Analysis*

Each observer scored the biomarkers for frequency, intensity, and localization. Computation of these scores led to the derivation of biomarker and class indices, which compared between groups by Pearson correlation using SPSS (version 20, SPSS Inc., Chicago, IL, USA) for Windows to delineate classes. Student's t-test and ANOVA were determined in Microsoft Excel 2016; $p < 0.05$ was considered significant.

## 3. Results

*3.1. Selection of Class-Specific Biomarkers, Development of SOPs for Detection, a Reference Human Tissue Library and Guidelines for Scoring*

A strong correlation of the transcription factors TCF21 and Slug with Class 1 (Cooperative Cell Migration/CCM-class) and Class 2 (Epithelial-to-Mesenchymal/EMT-class) tumors respectively [15] lent consideration to their inclusion in this study. E-cadherin was selected as a feature of cell-cell adhesion to substantiate CCM class-specific purported biological functions and PARP1 for defects in homologous recombination. Known associations of EMT with AnnexinA2 (ANXA2) and its interactions with Slug, and extra-cellular matrix components including hyaluronan (HA) and its synthesizing genes (*HAS1* and *HAS2*) suggested HA as a candidate marker (Supplementary Table S1, Supplementary Figure S2). Class 3 tumors lacked any unique biological features, hence no specific markers were assigned for their identification. An inability to correlate variations in Vimentin protein levels with either of the transcription factor present in these groups refrained its inclusion. The final screening biomarker panel thus comprised of TCF21, E-cadherin, PARP1, Slug, ANXA2, and HA (Figure 1A).

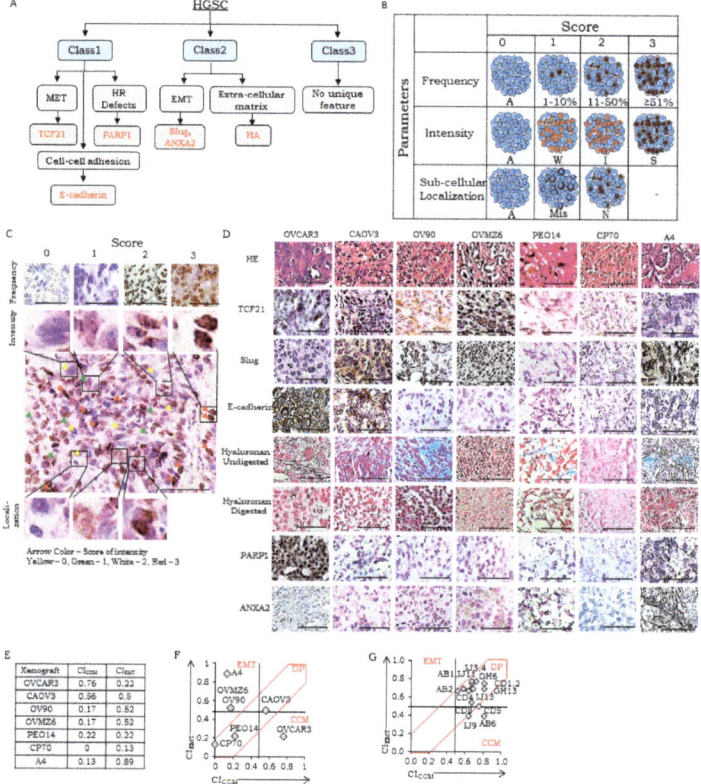

**Figure 1.** Class associations and marker scoring guidelines; (**A**) rationale for class-specific biological function based putative marker selection, MET: Mesenchymal-to-epithelial transition, HR: Homologous Recombination mediated DNA Damage Repair, EMT: Epithelial-to-mesenchymal transition; (**B**) schematic of scoring guidelines for IHC based staining of nuclear markers (TCF21, PARP1, Slug), A: Absent, W: Weak, I: Intermediate, S: Strong, Mis: Mislocalised, N: normal localization. A similar approach was used for scoring of membrane markers (E-cadherin, ANXA2) except that sub-cellular location was scored either 1 (cytoplasm) or 2 (cell membrane), while extracellular expression of hyaluronan fibers (evaluated as blue color developed by Alcian blue staining that is lost on hyaluronidase) was scored 1 in distant tumor stroma, and 2 in tumor epithelial cell nests. Scoring and analyses of marker expression in xenografts and TMAs; (**C**) Tissues and markers for Scoring of Frequency–0: A4 (TCF21), 1: OV90 (Slug), 2: OVCAR3 (PARP1), 3: A4 (Slug); scoring of intensity and localization-CAOV3 (TCF21), different regions representing scores of 0–3 (intensity) and 0–2 (localization), Scale bar is 50 µm; (**D**) Representative micrographs of HGSC xenografts for: Row 1-H&E (hematoxylin and eosin) stained section while Rows 2,3,4,7,8 represent IHC-based identification of TCF21, Slug, E-cadherin, PARP1, and ANXA2; Rows 5 and 6 represent HC-based identification of HA fibers in untreated and hyaluronidase digested xenograft sections respectively, scale bar is 50 µm; (**E**) class Indices of xenografts; (**F,G**) scatter plots of $CI_{CCM}$ vs. $CI_{EMT}$ in xenografts and high-grade serous ovarian carcinoma (HGSC) cases in TMA respectively. DP-double positive; CCM-cooperative cell migration.

Evaluation of any novel marker in tumor stratification necessitates the establishment of standard operating protocols (SOPs) to address pre-analytic (slide coating, tissue selection, fixation, processing), analytic (clone and antibody selection, buffers and instruments for antigen retrieval, antibody/enzyme concentration, duration of incubations at each step, etc.), and post-analytic parameters (interpretation, analyses and reporting of expression in the reference and control tissues). These were established for our panel (Supplementary Dataset 1), along with the development of a reference library based on the Human Protein Atlas (HPA) [25] using appropriate normal human tissues. Three specific metrics associated with IHC/HC detection viz. frequency, intensity, and localization were applied in developing universal guidelines for marker scoring (Figure 1B depicts a schematic for transcription factor marker scoring, while a reference score sheet is provided in Supplementary Figure S3). The subjectivity of analyses due to inter-personal observation variation was minimized by collecting independent scores from five observers followed by a comprehensive pathology review to arrive at a consensus in case of difference in opinions. Specific scoring guidelines for each marker that were thereby agreed on and corresponding healthy tissue included the following:

(i) Score for Marker Frequency ($S_{Freq}$)-percentage expression in total tumor cells of tissue section on a scale of 0–3 (0: absent, 1: 1–10%, 2: 11–50%, and 3: $\geq$51% marker-positive),

   a. TCF21: cardiac myocytes, ovarian stromal cells, and germinal cells of testis represented $S_{Freq}$ 0, 1, and 3 respectively; $S_{Freq}$ = 2 could not be identified in healthy tissues.
   b. E-cadherin: cardiac myocytes, liver hepatocytes, and prostate epithelial cells represented $S_{Freq}$ 0, 2, and 3 respectively; healthy tissues representing $S_{Freq}$ = 1 could not be identified.
   c. PARP1: mucosa of the small intestine, cardiac myocytes, germinal basal cells of testis represented $S_{Freq}$ as 0, 1, and 3 respectively; healthy tissues representing $S_{Freq}$ = 2 could not be identified.
   d. Slug: cardiac myocytes, smooth muscles of the appendix, lymphocytes of the small intestine represented $S_{Freq}$ 0, 1, and 2 respectively; healthy tissues representing $S_{Freq}$ = 3 could not be identified.
   e. HA: cartilage and sub-mucosa of the small intestine represented $S_{Freq}$ as 2 and 3 respectively; healthy tissues representing $S_{Freq}$ = 0 or 1 could not be identified.
   f. ANXA2: cardiac myocytes, the somatic muscle of the small intestine, epithelial cells of the gall bladder represented $S_{Freq}$ 0, 1, and 3 respectively; healthy tissues representing $S_{Freq}$ = 2 could not be identified.

(ii) Score for marker intensity ($S_{Int}$)-intensity of brown stain for IHC and blue for HC in positively stained tissue sections. A scale of 0–3 was established, 0: absent, 1: weak, 2: moderate, and 3: strong intensity of marker-positive cells,

   a. TCF21: cardiac myocytes, ovarian stromal cells, germinal basal cells of testis represented $S_{Int}$ 0, 1, and 2 respectively; $S_{Int}$ = 3 could not be identified in healthy tissues.
   b. E-cadherin: cardiac myocytes, epithelial cells of the small intestine, epithelial cells of prostate represented $S_{Int}$ 0, 2, and 3 respectively; healthy tissues representing $S_{Int}$ = 1 could not be identified.
   c. PARP1: mucosa of the small intestine, cardiac myocytes, and germinal basal cells of testis represented $S_{Int}$ 0, 1, and 2 respectively; healthy tissues representing $S_{Freq}$ = 3 could not be identified.
   d. Slug: cardiac myocytes, smooth muscle of the appendix, and lymphocytes of the small intestine represented $S_{Int}$ 0, 1, and 2 respectively; healthy tissues representing $S_{Int}$ = 3 could not be identified.
   e. HA: Intensity for hyaluronan was measured as blue color intensity developed by Alcian blue in comparison to hyaluronidase digested tissue section. Sub-mucosa of the small

intestine and cartilage tissues represented $S_{Int}$ 1 and 2 respectively; healthy tissues representing $S_{Int}$ = 0 or 3 could not be identified.

f. ANXA2: cardiac myocytes and epithelial cells of gall bladder represented $S_{Int}$ 0 and 2 respectively; healthy tissues representing $S_{Int}$ = 1 or 3 could not be identified.

(iii) Score for Marker Localization ($S_{Loc}$)-representing sub-cellular location of marker in the tissue section on a scale of 0–2, 0: Absent, 1: mislocalized (cellular localization does not correspond to known functionality, for example, cytoplasmic location for TCF21, PARP1, Slug, E-cadherin, ANXA2 or HA), 2: normal localization (for example, nuclear expression of TCF21, PARP1 or Slug, membrane for E-cadherin, membrane or cytoplasmic for ANXA2 and extracellular expression of HA.

a. TCF21: cardiac myocytes, liver hepatocytes, germinal basal cells of testis represented $S_{Loc}$ 0, 1, and 2 respectively.
b. E-cadherin: cardiac myocytes, prostate epithelial cells represented $S_{Loc}$ 0 and 2 respectively; healthy tissues representing $S_{Loc}$ = 1 could not be identified.
c. PARP1: mucosa of the small intestine, germinal basal cells of testis represented $S_{Loc}$ 0 and 2 respectively; healthy tissues representing $S_{Loc}$ = 1 could not be identified.
d. Slug: cardiac myocytes, the somatic muscle of the appendix, lymphocytes of the small intestine, represented $S_{Loc}$ 0, 1, and 2 respectively.
e. HA: cartilage represented $S_{Loc}$ of score 2; healthy tissues representing $S_{Loc}$ = 1 could not be identified. A further consensus was reached in the pathology review to consider extracellular staining in tumor nests that is eliminated following hyaluronidase treatment as a proper localization, while distant stroma-associated HA was considered as mislocalization.
f. ANXA2: cardiac myocytes, stromal cells of the gall bladder, epithelial cells of the gall bladder represented $S_{Loc}$ as 0, 1, and 2 respectively.

*3.2. Establishment of Scoring Guidelines for Stratification Using a Panel of Xenograft*

Initial validation of the biomarker expression and scoring scheme was achieved using HGSC cell line derived xenografts generated in NOD/SCID mice (Figure 1C,D). TCF21 localization in xenograft sections was either dominantly nuclear (CAOV3 and PEO14), cytoplasmic (OVMZ6, OV90, and OVCAR3), or negligible (CP70 and A4); similarly, Slug was nuclear (OVMZ6, OV90, and A4), cytoplasmic (CAOV3 and CP70), or absent (OVCAR3 and PEO14). Moderate intensity of E-cadherin at the cell membrane was observed in ~50% tumor cells in CAOV3 and OVCAR3 xenografts but was lower in OVMZ6, CP70, OV90, A4, and PEO14 xenografts. Significantly, high-intensity expression of nuclear PARP1 was evident only in OVCAR3 xenografts; while other xenografts had significantly lower expression. High frequency, moderate intensity of HA was observed in CAOV3, OV90, and A4 xenografts, while OVCAR3 and PEO14 expressed HA at low to moderate frequency with weak intensity. Significant expression of ANXA2 was evident only in OVMZ6 and A4 xenografts. Consensus marker scores consolidated by the pathologist panel for each marker and xenograft ($S_{Freq}$, $S_{Int}$, $S_{Loc}$; Table 1) were used to derive specific Biomarker Indices (BI; Equation (1)). Class-indices representing class-specific metrics of consolidated marker expression were derived from class-specific BI ($CI_{CCM}$ and $CI_{EMT}$; Equations (2) and (3) respectively; Table 1).

$$BI = \frac{1}{3}\left(\frac{observed\ S_{Freq}}{max\ S_{Freq}}\right) + \frac{1}{3}\left(\frac{observed\ S_{Int}}{max\ S_{Int}}\right) + \frac{1}{3}\left(\frac{observed\ S_{Loc}}{max\ S_{Loc}}\right) \quad (1)$$

$$CI_{CCM} = \frac{BI_{TCF21} + BI_{E-cadherin} + BI_{PARP1}}{3} \quad (2)$$

$$CI_{EMT} = \frac{BI_{Slug} + BI_{HA} + BI_{ANXA2}}{3} \tag{3}$$

Table 1. Scores, biomarker and class indices (BI and CI respectively) for cooperative cell migration (CCM) and epithelial-to-mesenchymal transition (EMT) markers in xenografts.

| Cell Line Derived Xenograft | CCM Markers | | | | | | | | | | | | $CI_{CCM}$ |
|---|---|---|---|---|---|---|---|---|---|---|---|---|---|
| | TCF21 | | | | E-cadherin | | | | PARP1 | | | | |
| | $S_{Freq}$ | $S_{Int}$ | $S_{Loc}$ | $BI_{TCF21}$ | $S_{Freq}$ | $S_{Int}$ | $S_{Loc}$ | $BI_{CDH1}$ | $S_{Freq}$ | $S_{Int}$ | $S_{Loc}$ | $BI_{PARP1}$ | |
| CAOV3 | 2 | 2 | 2 | 0.78 | 3 | 2 | 2 | 0.89 | 0 | 0 | 0 | 0 | 0.56 |
| OVMZ6 | 2 | 1 | 1 | 0.5 | 0 | 0 | 0 | 0 | 0 | 0 | 0 | 0 | 0.17 |
| CP70 | 0 | 0 | 0 | 0 | 0 | 0 | 0 | 0 | 0 | 0 | 0 | 0 | 0 |
| OV90 | 2 | 1 | 1 | 0.5 | 1 | 2 | 1 | 0.5 | 0 | 0 | 0 | 0 | 0.17 |
| A4 | 1 | 1 | 1 | 0.39 | 0 | 0 | 0 | 0 | 0 | 0 | 0 | 0 | 0.13 |
| OVCAR3 | 2 | 3 | 1 | 0.72 | 2 | 2 | 2 | 0.78 | 2 | 2 | 2 | 0.78 | 0.76 |
| PEO14 | 1 | 2 | 2 | 0.67 | 0 | 0 | 0 | 0 | 0 | 0 | 0 | 0 | 0.22 |

| Cell Line Derived Xenograft | EMT Markers | | | | | | | | | | | | $CI_{EMT}$ |
|---|---|---|---|---|---|---|---|---|---|---|---|---|---|
| | Slug | | | | HA | | | | ANXA2 | | | | |
| | $S_{Freq}$ | $S_{Int}$ | $S_{Loc}$ | $BI_{Slug}$ | $S_{Freq}$ | $S_{Int}$ | $S_{Loc}$ | $BI_{HA}$ | $S_{Freq}$ | $S_{Int}$ | $S_{Loc}$ | $BI_{AnxA2}$ | |
| CAOV3 | 3 | 1 | 1 | 0.61 | 3 | 2 | 2 | 0.89 | 0 | 0 | 0 | 0 | 0.5 |
| OVMZ6 | 2 | 1 | 2 | 0.67 | 0 | 0 | 0 | 0 | 3 | 2 | 2 | 0.89 | 0.52 |
| CP70 | 1 | 1 | 1 | 0.39 | 0 | 0 | 0 | 0 | 0 | 0 | 0 | 0 | 0.13 |
| OV90 | 1 | 1 | 2 | 0.56 | 3 | 3 | 2 | 1 | 0 | 0 | 0 | 0 | 0.52 |
| A4 | 3 | 3 | 2 | 1 | 3 | 2 | 2 | 0.89 | 3 | 1 | 2 | 0.78 | 0.89 |
| OVCAR3 | 0 | 0 | 0 | 0 | 2 | 1 | 2 | 0.67 | 0 | 0 | 0 | 0 | 0.22 |
| PEO14 | 0 | 0 | 0 | 0 | 2 | 1 | 2 | 0.67 | 0 | 0 | 0 | 0 | 0.22 |

Class indices represent class-specific metrics of consolidated markers expression; $CI_{CCM}$ and $CI_{EMT}$ computed for xenografts ranged from (0–0.76) and (0.22–0.89) respectively (Table 1; Figure 1D). The distribution of median $CI_{EMT}$ vs. $CI_{CCM}$ (±10%) values were further applied in class identification. Thus, OVCAR3 represents CCM-class; A4, OVMZ6, and OV90 the EMT-class; CAOV3, PEO14, and CP70 being double positive (DP; Figure 1E). Such inclusiveness of expression of the six markers quantifies molecular heterogeneity in mixed/unclassified tumors and assigns biological functions to the ambiguous Class 3 through relative marker expression.

### 3.3. Evaluation of Stratification Guidelines in TMAs

The above biomarker scoring and class identification guidelines were applied to commercial TMAs (duplicate cores per sample) which included two normal ovary and 13 HGSC tumor cases among other ovarian cancer subtypes. Availability of limited consecutive slides ($n$ = 5) led to screening of only four of the six biomarkers (TCF21, E-cadherin, Slug, and HA) and equations (ii) and (iii) were appropriately modified in consideration of a four marker-based class identification (Supplementary Figure S4; Supplementary Table S2). Biomarker score averages for clinical cases represented on TMAs were considered for computation of BI and CI values (of each core in duplicate showed a near-similar expression for all biomarkers). We observed that a majority of HGSC TMA-cores expressed high-intensity cytoplasmic TCF21, moderate nuclear expression of which was present in ~5–10% of tumor cells. Except in four cases, Slug expression was weak to moderate cytoplasmic and nuclear localization was evident in only 5–10% tumor cells. Moderate expression of E-cadherin at cell membranes was observed in nearly 50% of tumor cells, and extracellular HA fibers also stained at a moderate intensity in tumor cell nests. Consolidation of biomarker scores of each case, computation of BI and CI values followed by plotting the distribution of $CI_{CCM}$ vs. $CI_{EMT}$ values of TMA cores indicated three cases to represent CCM-Class while the remaining belonged to DP-Class; and EMT-Class remained unrepresented (Figure 1F).

### 3.4. Evaluation of Clinical Samples Associates CCM-Markers with Metastases and Chemotherapy

The variance in frequencies of class profiles between xenografts and TMAs emphasized the pertinence of screening larger numbers of clinical samples in validation. Towards assessing clinical representation, we obtained and stratified 160 tumor samples pathologically diagnosed as HGSC from 96 patients. These included primary (ovary (T), fallopian tube (FT)) and metastatic tumors (omentum (O), peritoneal ascites-derived cell blocks (A); Supplementary Table S3). BI and CI scores with $CI_{CCM}$ and $CI_{EMT}$ values for each tumor were computed from marker scores (Supplementary Tables S4–S8) followed by evaluation of CI distribution towards class assignment as performed for xenografts and TMA. Data analysis of this clinical cohort was conducted in tumor groups as given Table 2.

**Table 2.** Distribution of clinical cohort in tumor groups.

| Group | Analyses | Samples (n) |
|---|---|---|
| A | Between-group analyses of tumors in chemo-naïve tumors (T vs. FT vs. O) | 6 |
| B | Within the group of single tumors derived from either ovarian or FT sites, omental deposits or cell blocks from tumor ascites in chemo-naïve (CN) cases and chemo-treated (CT) cases | CN–51 (T), 8 (FT), 27 (O), 4 (A); CT–52 (T), 2 (FT), 17 (O), 2 (A) |
| C | Within groups of primary tumor & omental tumors pairs from either chemo-naïve (CN) or chemo-treated (CT) cases | CN–17; CT–16 |
| D | Between-group analyses of tumor samples of the same case before and after chemotherapy | 6 |

Examination of 'Group A' tumors representing different sites of metastases and stages of tumor progression in six chemo-naïve cases revealed consistent class-associations across different sites in two cases (B/2774/12 and B/3136/09), while suggesting class switching in the remaining four cases wherein marker expression was altered in following metastases (Figure 2A). One of the latter four cases expressed CCM-markers in ovarian tumors; FT and omental tumors were DP-Class (B/1627/13). The ovarian tumor of case B/825/10 expressed EMT-markers that switched to DP-Class in FT and omental tumors. Ovarian and omental tumors of the remaining two cases segregated into DP-Class, while FT tumors expressed either CCM (B/749/13) or EMT (B/1716/09) markers. Overall, the three tumor sites predominantly segregated into CCM or DP Class; only one case of ovarian and FT tumors was represented as EMT-Class (Figure 2B; Supplementary Tables S9 and S10).

CI-based class-assignment in 'Group B' tumors stratified chemo-naïve ovarian tumors into DP, CCM or EMT classes (33.3%, 29.4%, and 29.4% respectively; Figure 2C,E), while treated ovarian tumors exhibited dominant representation of CCM-Class with lower frequencies of EMT and DP classes (48.0%, 23.0%, and 19.2% respectively). Chemo-naïve FT tumors stratified into CCM, EMT or DP Class ($n = 2$, 1, and 8 respectively; Figure 2C,E), while those after treatment belonged to either CCM or DP Class. Omental tumor deposits were predominantly DP-Class, with a marginal increase in the frequency of CCM and EMT markers in treated samples (Figure 2D,E), while chemo-naïve as well as treated ascites cell blocks presented more frequently with the CCM-class (Figure 2D,E). Overall, 'Group B' patient tumors show predominantly CCM or DP expression (Supplementary Table S11) as compared with either xenografts (mostly EMT-class) or TMAs (CCM and DP class). These findings support metastasis/chemotherapy-induced HGSC tumor expression towards a CCM subtype.

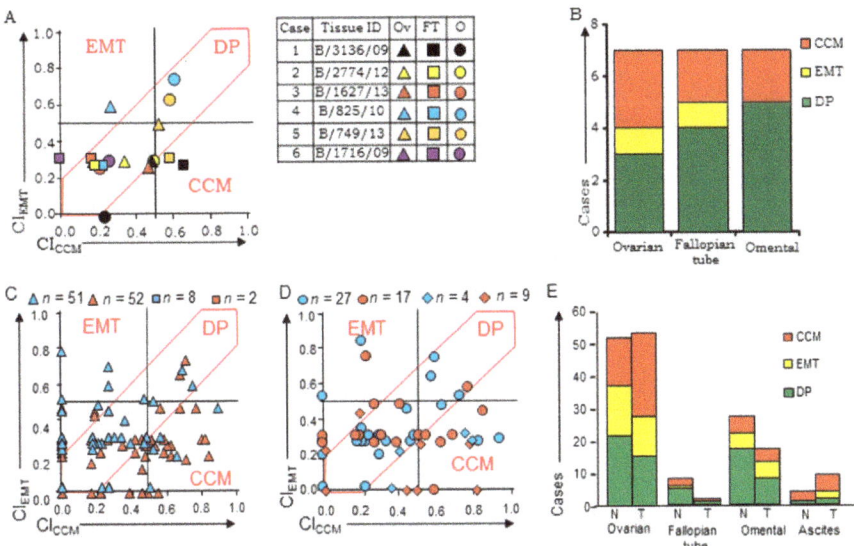

**Figure 2.** (**A**) Scatter plot of $CI_{CCM}$ vs. $CI_{EMT}$ distribution for chemo-naïve cases with tumors detected in ovary (Ov), fallopian tube (FT), and omentum (O) (left panel), and a reference case-chart (right panel), (**B**) graphical representation of class-specification of Group A tumors, (**C**) scatter plots of $CI_{CCM}$ vs. $CI_{EMT}$ distribution for single chemo-naïve or -treated (red and blue shapes respectively) tumors from-ovary △ & fallopian tube □, (**D**) omentum ○ and ascites cell blocks ◇, (**E**) graphical representation of Group B tumors (chemo-naïve-N; chemo-treated-T). EMT-epithelial to mesenchymal transition; DP-double positive; CCM-cooperative cell migration.

### 3.5. HGSC Tumors at Different Sites Exhibit Molecular Heterogeneity and Class-Switching

Class switching during tumor progression from ovarian to omental sites was further examined in 'Group C' samples that comprised of tumors from either chemo-naïve ($n = 17$) or -treated cases ($n = 16$). Almost half of the cases in both groups did indeed exhibit metastases associated class-switching (Figure 3(Ai,Aii); Supplementary Figure S5A), although lack of a specific direction to the switch possibly suggests the involvement of other factors in the determining marker expression.

The last analytical set of Group D tumors comprised of six ovarian, ascites, and/or omental tumor pairs before and after therapy (Figure 3B; Supplementary Figure S5B). Considering the limited cases that represent unique behavior, we have discussed them on a case to case basis. Cases 1 and 2 strongly conformed to CCM-class after disease progression as well as treatment, while the remaining four cases exhibited class-switching. Chemotherapy in Case 3 resulted in enhanced expression of CCM-markers over a DP-profile in untreated ovarian tumors, while Case 4 was associated with heterogeneity of marker expression following treatment. Case 5 was the most complex of all six and showed considerable marker heterogeneity between different tumor sites. Case 6 exhibited progression and therapy-associated class-shift towards the CCM class from a DP ovarian tumor. These findings further support the class-switching of HGSC tumors upon metastases and/or chemotherapy.

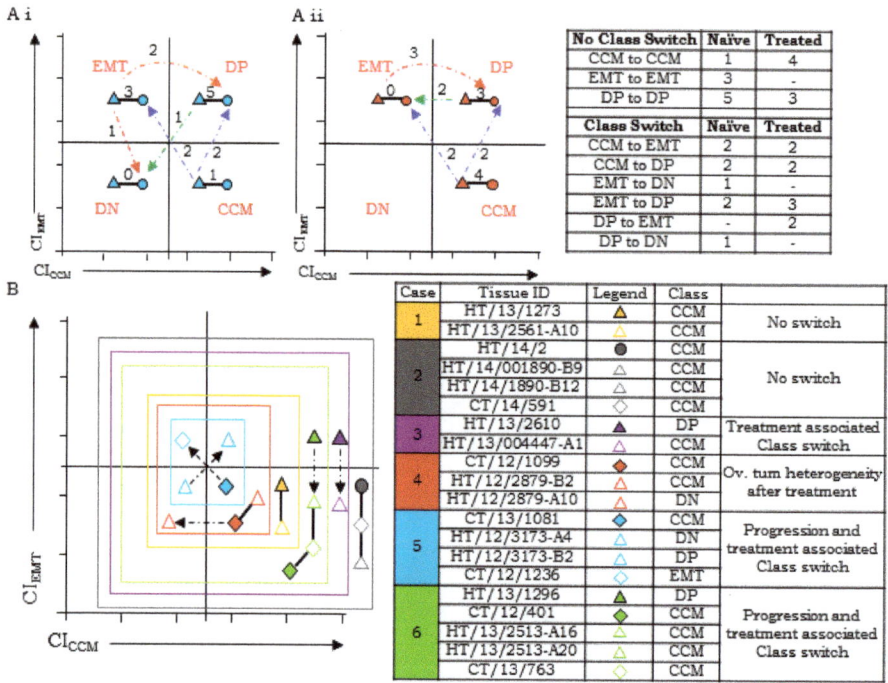

**Figure 3.** Class switching detected in cases with (**A**) ovarian and omental tumors tissues of (i) chemo-naïve (n = 17) and (ii) chemo-treated (n = 16) patient cohort; (**B**) class switching in tumors collected from patients (n = 6) prior to chemo-treatment (filled shapes) and post chemo-therapy (empty shapes) as determined through ascites (diamond), primary tumor (triangle), and omentum (circle). EMT-epithelial to mesenchymal transition; DP-double positive; DN-double negative; CCM-cooperative cell migration.

### 3.6. Disease Progression is Inclined Towards Enrichment of CCM-Markers

To evaluate the effects of therapy and disease progression vis-à-vis metastases and stage advancement on stratification, we further compared the means of $CI_{CCM}$ and $CI_{EMT}$ (M-$CI_{CCM}$ and M-$CI_{EMT}$ respectively) of ovarian, FT, and omental tumors from the same patient in chemo-naïve (CN) vs. chemo-treated (CT) groups. M-$CI_{CCM}$ of CN ovarian-omental (T-O) tumors (Group 'C') was lower than that of CN ovarian-FT-omental (T-F-O) tumors (Group 'A'), while M-$CI_{CCM}$ of CT T-O tumors was enhanced (Figure 4A, Supplementary Table S12). Interestingly, M-$CI_{EMT}$ of ovarian as well as omental tumors were similar between CN T-O vs. T-F-O tumors, and between CN T-O vs. CT T-O groups suggesting minimal effects of either disease progression or therapy on expression of EMT-markers. Towards elucidation of individual biomarker contribution likely to contribute to these differences, we analyzed their expression through means of BI (M-BI) during stage progression in CN HGSC cases represented on TMAs (T1 to T2) and in patient tumors. Nearly steady M-BI of TCF21, increased Slug, E-cadherin, and HA levels were revealed in the TMAs, with Slug expression being maximal at the T2 stage ($p < 0.007$; Figure 4B). Similar analyses of Group 'B' cases with available tumor stage information in CN (31-T, 1-FT, 17-O) and CT cases (35-T, 7-FT, and 9-O) were performed. CN T samples expressed comparable M-BI levels of TCF21 and HA, higher E-cadherin and PARP1 and lower Slug and ANXA2 at T3 over T1 stage; CT T samples had almost comparable M-BI profiles as CN tumors (Figure 4C, Supplementary Figure S6). Limited FT and O tumors at stages T1 and T2 restricted their analyses; CN- and CT-O tumors at stage T3 expressed comparable levels of markers. Group C CN O samples at stage T3 were associated with decreased TCF21 and E-cadherin concurrent with increased PARP1,

ANXA2, and HA M-BI profiles (Figure 4D). CT T tumors had low M-BI scores for TCF21, PARP1, and HA in comparison to O and similar levels of E-cadherin, Slug, and ANXA2. CT T samples in this group displayed steady levels of TCF21 and PARP1, lower E-cadherin, Slug, and ANXA2 and increased HA levels over CN tumors; while treatment was associated with higher BI levels of TCF21, PARP1, and HA and lower levels of E-cadherin, Slug, and ANXA2 in the O tumors. This suggests that selected biomarkers play a significant role during disease progression.

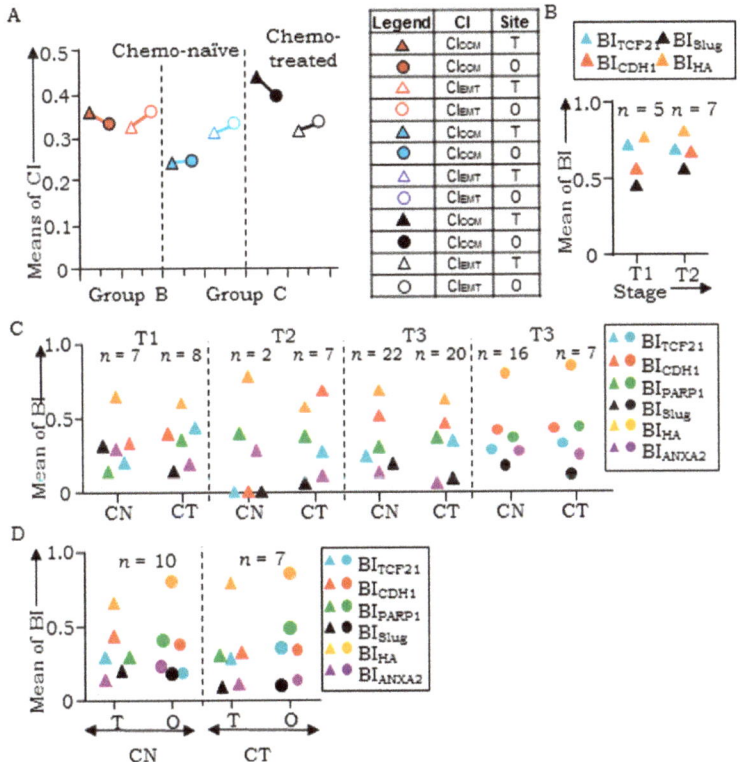

**Figure 4.** HGSC progression-associated marker expression. (**A**) Plot comparing $CI_{CCM}$ with $CI_{EMT}$ of tumors of Groups B and C respectively; (**B**) plot comparing biomarker (BI) scores for TCF21, E-cadherin, Slug, and HA in chemo-naïve ovarian tumors present in TMA for stages T1 and T2; (**C**) plot for chemo-naïve (left) and treated (right) paired ovarian (T)-omental (O) tumors; (**D**) plot for chemo-naïve (CN) and treated (CT) tumors at stages T1, T2, and T3 in ovarian △ and omental ○ tumors.

Class-switching in paired samples led us to examine similar effects of a chemotherapeutic challenge (paclitaxel) in the three classes representing cell lines derived xenografts viz. CCM-Class (OVCAR3), EMT-Class (A4, OVMZ6), and DP-Class (CAOV3, PEO14). Distribution of $CI_{CCM}$ and $CI_{EMT}$ values revealed a DP to CCM (CAOV3, PEO14) and EMT to DP (A4, OVMZ6) class switch. An outlier was the OVCAR3 xenograft (CCM class) that despite an increased CI score, provided no evidence of class switching (Figure 5A,B).

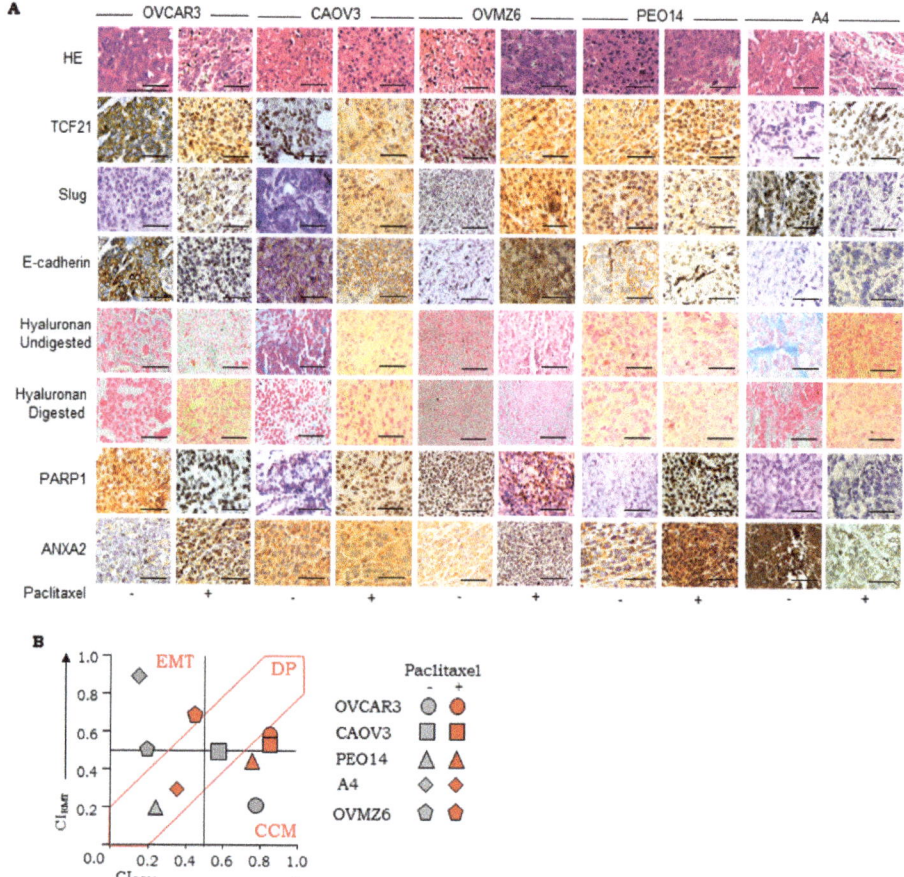

**Figure 5.** (**A**). Paclitaxel exposure alters scoring marker panel in HGSC cell line derived xenografts. Representative images of HGSC xenograft (control and paclitaxel treated) sections for Row 1-HE (hematoxylin and eosin), Rows 2,3,4,7,8 represent IHC-based detection of TCF21, Slug, E cadherin, PARP1, and ANXA2, Rows 5 and 6 represent HC-based identification of HA fibers in untreated and hyaluronidase digested sections respectively, scale bars-50 µm; (**B**) scatter plots of CI$_{CCM}$ vs. CI$_{EMT}$ derived from xenograft (control-grey and paclitaxel treated-red) scoring. EMT-epithelial to mesenchymal transition; DP-double positive; CCM-cooperative cell migration.

### 3.7. Correlation Between Transcript- and Protein-Based Stratification

Proteome-based profiling of TCGA samples has been reported earlier (Figure 6A) [26,27]. Comparison of tumor samples common to our earlier study and the five proteomic subtypes ($n = 61$; Refs. 24 vs. 26) indicated correlation between CCM and proliferative groups, while EMT tumors were dominantly mesenchymal, with a few being either immunoreactive or differentiated (Figure 6B); surprisingly, the stromal class had negligible associations. A similar comparison of tumor samples common to the transcript study and two proteomic subtypes ($n = 34$) [24,27] correlated the CCM-Class with TCGA-A/Epithelial cluster and EMT-Class with TCGA-B/mesenchymal cluster (Figure 6C). These observations indicate some degree of variation that could arise from differences between transcriptomic and protein abundances.

**A**

| Proteome sub-groups | | | | Transcript sub-groups | |
|---|---|---|---|---|---|
| Zhang et al. 2016 | Cases | Coscia et al. 2016 | Cases | Gardi et al. 2014 | Cases |
| Proliferative | 25 | TCGA-A | 51 | CCM-Class | 77 |
| Mesenchymal | 42 | TCGA-B | 33 | EMT-Class | 99 |
| Immuno-reactive | 32 | | | Class3 | 51 |
| Differentiated | 54 | | | | |
| Stromal | 16 | | | | |

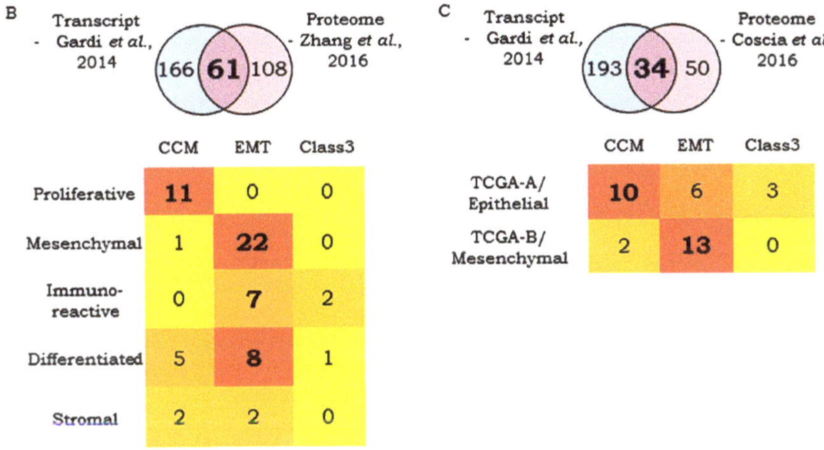

**B** Transcript - Gardi et al., 2014 (166 | 61 | 108) Proteome - Zhang et al., 2016

| | CCM | EMT | Class3 |
|---|---|---|---|
| Proliferative | 11 | 0 | 0 |
| Mesenchymal | 1 | 22 | 0 |
| Immuno-reactive | 0 | 7 | 2 |
| Differentiated | 5 | 8 | 1 |
| Stromal | 2 | 2 | 0 |

**C** Transcript - Gardi et al., 2014 (193 | 34 | 50) Proteome - Coscia et al., 2016

| | CCM | EMT | Class3 |
|---|---|---|---|
| TCGA-A/Epithelial | 10 | 6 | 3 |
| TCGA-B/Mesenchymal | 2 | 13 | 0 |

**Figure 6.** Comparison of HGSC stratification approaches. (**A**) Proteomics-based TCGA HGSC tumors stratification in 5 sub-groups by Zhang et al. 2016 (169 cases) and Coscia et al. 2016 (84 cases) and transcriptomics based HGSC stratification into three classes (Gardi et al. 2014); (**B**) comparison of Gardi et al. 2014 vs. Zhang et al., 2016; (**C**) comparison of Gardi et al. 2014 vs. Coscia et al. 2016.

## 4. Discussion

Molecular histology is a convenient tool in biomarker discovery, evaluation, and validation that could facilitate personalized therapeutic choices [28,29]. In the present study, we focused on evaluating our previous molecular stratification [24] through the establishment of reproducible SOPs and scoring guidelines for six biomarkers in xenografts (TCF21, E-cadherin, PARP1, Slug, ANXA2, and HA; Phase 0), and partial validation in TMAs (Phase I) and clinical samples (Phase II). In a routine pathology analysis, incorrect biomarker sub-cellular localization is usually ignored or considered an artifact. This is in contrast to several cells and macromolecular studies that attribute altered cellular functions to mislocalized proteins especially in the context of transformation that suggests different biological functions [30,31]. The inclusion of this parameter for biomarker evaluation was hence considered essential in the present study along with frequency and intensity. Results were interpreted based on individual scores and by deriving a relation between them. Individual biomarker scores were consolidated to derive CCM and EMT class specific indices that were applied for tumor stratification. The dominance of EMT-class in cell line-derived xenografts, DP-class in TMAs representing human cases and CCM-class in clinical tumor samples were observed. These differences might reflect on the purported cell culture driven mesenchymal phenotype [32,33] and expression of EMT markers in xenografts. The results suggest cross-talk between transcription factors TCF21 with Slug in regulating intrinsic cellular states and tumor subtypes. Importantly, we achieved tumor stratification through the incorporation of features of intermediate phenotypes that effectively accounts for tumor heterogeneity. Phenotypic transitions captured through different cell lines representing different phenotypes is a significant step towards understanding tumor heterogeneity. The existence of cellular plasticity has been attributed in cancers of the lung [34], ovary [35], pancreas [36], and prostate [37], that substantiates the presence of phenotypic heterogeneity in tumors. Likewise, restricted tissue sampling and representation of heterogeneity in TMAs could lead to incomplete tumor evaluation [38]. Therapy-influenced heterogeneity of molecular expression reported earlier in multi-drug resistant cancers [39–42] was noted as occasional class switching in the present study wherein tumors in the same patient stratified into different classes either during disease progression or following chemotherapy. We believe that these effects reflect the influences of a new/altered niche on molecular expression in the same tumor [43,44]. Analyses of a larger patient cohort could clarify the interplay of protein expression during treatment procedures.

Any improvement in the accuracy of current triaging using new biomarkers thereby is a likely value-addition in optimizing the selection of the right therapeutic drugs and regimens in patients. Our findings now set the stage for evaluation of class-specific inhibitors in this direction. Olaparib, Niraparib, Veliparib, and Rucaparib that are in different phases of research and clinical trials for cancers including HGSC may be evaluated in the CCM-Class for PARP1 as a potential therapeutic target [45,46] (ClinicalTrials.gov Identifier: NCT00535119, NCT00664781, and NCT00516373). In contrast, the PI3K-Akt signaling pathway driven EMT in ovarian cancer [47] suggests evaluation of PI3K inhibitors like BKM120 or BYL719 in patients presenting with this class of tumors; Phase I clinical trials for both these molecules is underway for recurrent TNBC and HGSC [ClinicalTrials.gov Identifier: NCT01623349]. While tumors segregating in Class 3 need further research for molecular target identification, the DP-class may be evaluated for efficacy of either PARP1 or PI3K inhibitors or a combination of both [48–51]. Thus, we hope that CCM-Class and EMT-Class tumors would respond specifically upon treatment with PARP1 inhibitors and PI3K-Akt inhibitors, respectively. However, this has to be substantiated by specific clinical studies. In conclusion, the current study establishes the diagnostic principles and possibilities for molecular stratification in HGSC to address a few missing steps in achieving a bench to bedside translation.

**Supplementary Materials:** The following are available online at http://www.mdpi.com/2077-0383/8/3/330/s1, Figure S1: Flowchart of the approach for molecular stratification of HGSC tumors, Table S1: Class-specific enrichment of extracellular matrix (ECM)-associated genes, Figure S2: Heatmap representing class distribution of ECM-genes in the 3 Classes of TCGA-HGSC samples, Dataset 1: Standard Operating Procedures for IHC Detection of TCF21, E-cadherin, PARP1, Slug, ANXA2, and Histochemical detection of Hyaluronic Acid, Figure S3: Reference tissue expression controls of scoring guidelines, Figure S4: Representative TMA case for CCM-Class and DP-Class, Table S2: Biomarker and Class Indices for normal and HGSC cases in TMA leads to Class identification, Table S3: Distribution of tumor tissues obtained from different sites in 96 clinical HGSC cases, Table S4: CI scores for chemo-naïve cases in unpaired ovarian tumors and omental tumors leading to Class assignment, Table S5: CI scores for chemo-naïve cases in ovarian tumors paired with omental tumor and fallopian tumor, and tumor collected with ascites leading to class assignment, Table S6: CI scores for chemo-treated cases in unpaired ovarian tumors or omental tumor or ascites cell block leading to Class assignment, Table S7: CI scores for chemo-treated cases in ovarian tumors paired with omental tumor or ascites, fallopian tumor and FT with ascites leading to Class assignment, Table S8: CI scores for chemo-naïve and chemo-treated pair cases, Table S9: Class comparison of tumors of ovary, fallopian tube, omentum, and ascites cell block, Table S10: CI scores for chemo-naïve ovarian tumors paired with tumors of fallopian tube and omentum, Table S11: Class comparison of tumors of ovary, fallopian tube, and omentum, Figure S5: Scatter plot for tumors of chemo-naïve and treated ovary, fallopian tube, and omentum and pre-post pairs, Table S12: Group analysis of tumors of Group 'B' and 'C' ovary, fallopian tube and omentum stratified into respective class for chemo-naïve and chemo-treated cases, Figure S6: Effect of marker expression with Stage of HGSC at presentation.

**Author Contributions:** S.C.K. designed methodology; S.A.B. conceived and designed methodology; S.C.K. performed experiments; S.C.K., A.S., A.N.J., R.D.D., D.M, and S.A.B. analyzed and interpreted data; S.C.K. and S.A.B. drafted, reviewed and edited the manuscript; all authors read and approved the final manuscript.

**Funding:** This research is funded through the following grants to SAB-(i) intra-mural funds from NCCS, (ii) extra-mural funds from the Department of Biotechnology, Government of India, New Delhi (BT/Indo-Aus/06/03/2011). SCK-research fellowship from the Council of Scientific and Industrial Research, New Delhi, India.

**Acknowledgments:** The authors acknowledge inputs in histological assessment and discussions with Avinash Pradhan, KEM, Pune and excellent technical support from Avinash Mali. Statistical analysis was performed by Aditi Deshpande, Amaze Stat, Pune.

**Conflicts of Interest:** The authors declare no conflict of interest.

**References**

1. Weigelt, B.; Reis-Filho, J.S.; Swanton, C. Genomic analyses to select patients for adjuvant chemotherapy: Trials and tribulations. *Ann. Oncol.* **2012**, *23*, 211–218. [CrossRef] [PubMed]
2. Bass, A.J.; Thorsson, V.; Shmulevich, I.; Reynolds, S.M.; Miller, M.; Bernard, B.; Hinoue, T.; Laird, P.W.; Curtis, C.; Shen, H.; et al. Comprehensive molecular characterization of gastric adenocarcinoma. *Nature* **2014**, *513*, 202–209. [CrossRef] [PubMed]
3. Gorgun, G.; Calabrese, E.; Hideshima, T.; Ecsedy, J.; Perrone, G.; Mani, M.; Ikeda, H.; Bianchi, G.; Hu, Y.; Cirstea, D.; et al. A novel aurora-A kinase inhibitor MLN8237 induces cytotoxicity and cell cycle arrest in multiple experimental multiple myeloma model. *Blood* **2010**, *115*, 5202–5213. [CrossRef] [PubMed]
4. Manfredi, M.G.; Ecsedy, J.A.; Chakravarty, A.; Silverman, L.; Zhang, M.; Hoar, K.M.; Stroud, S.G.; Chen, W.; Shinde, V.; Huck, J.J.; et al. Characterization of alisertib (MLN8237), an investigational small-molecule inhibitor of Aurora A kinase using novel in vivo pharmacodynamic assays. *Clin. Cancer Res.* **2011**, *17*, 7614–7624. [CrossRef] [PubMed]
5. Cidon, E.U.; Ellis, S.G.; Inam, Y.; Adeleke, S.; Zarif, S.; Geldart, T. Molecular targeted agents for gastric cancer: A step forward towards personalized therapy. *Cancers* **2013**, *5*, 64–91. [CrossRef] [PubMed]
6. Muro, K.; Chung, H.C.; Shankaran, V.; Geva, R.; Catenacci, D.; Gupta, S.; Eder, J.P.; Golan, T.; Le, D.T.; Burtness, B.; et al. Pembrolizumab for patients with PD-L1-positive advanced gastric cancer (KEYNOTE-012): A multicentre, open-label, phase 1b trial. *Lancet Oncol.* **2016**, *17*, 717–726. [CrossRef]
7. Magaki, S.; Hojat, S.A.; Wei, B.; So, A.; Yong, W.H. An Introduction to the Performance of Immunohistochemistry. In *Biobanking. Methods in Molecular Biology*; Humana Press: New York, NY, USA, 2019; pp. 289–298.
8. Cristescu, R.; Lee, J.; Nebozhyn, M.; Kim, K.-M.; Ting, J.C.; Wong, S.S.; Liu, J.; Yue, Y.G.; Wang, J.; Yu, K.; et al. Molecular analysis of gastric cancer identifies subtypes associated with distinct clinical outcomes. *Nat. Med* **2015**, *21*, 449–456. [CrossRef]
9. Díaz del Arco, C.; Estrada Muñoz, L.; Molina Roldán, E.; Cerón Nieto, M.Á.; Ortega Medina, L.; García Gómez de las Heras, S.; Fernández Aceñero, M.J. Immunohistochemical classification of gastric cancer based on new molecular biomarkers: A potential predictor of survival. *Virchows Arch.* **2018**, *473*, 687–695. [CrossRef]
10. Kim, J.; Kong, J.K.; Yang, W.; Cho, H.; Chay, D.B.; Lee, B.H.; Cho, S.J.; Hong, S.; Kim, J.-H. DNA Mismatch Repair Protein Immunohistochemistry and MLH1 Promotor Methylation Testing for Practical Molecular Classification and the Prediction of Prognosis in Endometrial Cancer. *Cancers* **2018**, *10*, 279. [CrossRef]
11. Karnezis, A.N.; Leung, S.; Magrill, J.; McConechy, M.K.; Yang, W.; Chow, C.; Kobel, M.; Lee, C.-H.; Huntsman, D.G.; Talhouk, A.; et al. Evaluation of endometrial carcinoma prognostic immunohistochemistry markers in the context of molecular classification. *J. Pathol. Clin. Res.* **2017**, *3*, 279–293. [CrossRef]
12. Ten Hoorn, S.; Trinh, A.; de Jong, J.; Koens, L.; Vermeulen, L. Classification of Colorectal Cancer in Molecular Subtypes by Immunohistochemistry. In *Methods in molecular biology (Clifton, N.J.)*; Beaulieu, J.-F., Ed.; Humana Press: New York, NY, USA, 2018.
13. Kim, S.; Moon, B.-I.; Lim, W.; Park, S.; Cho, M.S.; Sung, S.H. Feasibility of Classification of Triple Negative Breast Cancer by Immunohistochemical Surrogate Markers. *Clin. Breast Cancer* **2018**, *18*, e1123–e1132. [CrossRef] [PubMed]
14. Zou, L.; Wu, Y.; Ma, K.; Fan, Y.; Dong, D.; Geng, N.; Li, E. Molecular classification of esophagogastric junction carcinoma correlated with prognosis. *Onco. Targets. Ther.* **2017**, *10*, 4765–4772. [CrossRef] [PubMed]
15. Ilie, M.; Beaulande, M.; Hamila, M.; Erb, G.; Hofman, V.; Hofman, P. Automated chromogenic multiplexed immunohistochemistry assay for diagnosis and predictive biomarker testing in non-small cell lung cancer. *Lung Cancer* **2018**, *124*, 90–94. [CrossRef] [PubMed]
16. Siegel, R.L.; Miller, K.D.; Jemal, A. Cancer statistics, 2018. *CA. Cancer J. Clin.* **2018**, *68*, 7–30. [CrossRef] [PubMed]
17. Bast, R.C.; Hennessy, B.; Mills, G.B. The biology of ovarian cancer: New opportunities for translation. *Nat. Rev. Cancer* **2009**, *9*, 415–428. [CrossRef] [PubMed]
18. Yap, T.A.; Carden, C.P.; Kaye, S.B. Beyond chemotherapy: Targeted therapies in ovarian cancer. *Nat. Rev. Cancer* **2009**, *9*, 167–181. [CrossRef] [PubMed]

19. Tothill, R.W.; Tinker, A.V.; George, J.; Brown, R.; Fox, S.B.; Lade, S.; Johnson, D.S.; Trivett, M.K.; Etemadmoghadam, D.; Locandro, B.; et al. Novel Molecular Subtypes of Serous and Endometrioid Ovarian Cancer Linked to Clinical Outcome. *Clin. Cancer Res.* **2008**, *14*, 5198–5208. [CrossRef] [PubMed]
20. TCGA Network; Bell, D.; Berchuck, A.; Birrer, M.; Chien, J.; Cramer, D.W.; Dao, F.; Dhir, R.; DiSaia, P.; Gabra, H.; et al. Integrated genomic analyses of ovarian carcinoma. *Nature* **2011**, *474*, 609–615. [CrossRef]
21. Yang, D.; Sun, Y.; Hu, L.; Zheng, H.; Ji, P.; Pecot, C.V.; Zhao, Y.; Reynolds, S.; Cheng, H.; Rupaimoole, R.; et al. Integrated Analyses Identify a Master MicroRNA Regulatory Network for the Mesenchymal Subtype in Serous Ovarian Cancer. *Cancer Cell* **2013**, *23*, 186–199. [CrossRef]
22. Hoadley, K.A.; Yau, C.; Wolf, D.M.; Cherniack, A.D.; Tamborero, D.; Ng, S.; Leiserson, M.D.M.; Niu, B.; McLellan, M.D.; Uzunangelov, V.; et al. Multiplatform Analysis of 12 Cancer Types Reveals Molecular Classification within and across Tissues of Origin. *Cell* **2014**, *158*, 929–944. [CrossRef]
23. Kanchi, K.L.; Johnson, K.J.; Lu, C.; McLellan, M.D.; Leiserson, M.D.M.; Wendl, M.C.; Zhang, Q.; Koboldt, D.C.; Xie, M.; Kandoth, C.; et al. Integrated analysis of germline and somatic variants in ovarian cancer. *Nat. Commun.* **2014**, *5*, 3156. [CrossRef] [PubMed]
24. Gardi, N.L.; Deshpande, T.U.; Kamble, S.C.; Budhe, S.R.; Bapat, S.A. Discrete molecular classes of ovarian cancer suggestive of unique mechanisms of transformation and metastases. *Clin. Cancer Res.* **2014**, *20*, 87–99. [CrossRef] [PubMed]
25. Uhlen, M.; Fagerberg, L.; Hallstrom, B.M.; Lindskog, C.; Oksvold, P.; Mardinoglu, A.; Sivertsson, A.; Kampf, C.; Sjostedt, E.; Asplund, A.; et al. Tissue-based map of the human proteome. *Science* **2015**, *347*, 1260419. [CrossRef] [PubMed]
26. Zhang, H.; Liu, T.; Zhang, Z.; Chan, D.W.; Rodland, K.D.; Zhang, H.; Liu, T.; Zhang, Z.; Payne, S.H.; Zhang, B.; et al. Integrated Proteogenomic Characterization of Human High-Grade Serous Ovarian Cancer. *Cell* **2016**, *166*, 755–765. [CrossRef] [PubMed]
27. Coscia, F.; Watters, K.M.; Curtis, M.; Eckert, M.A.; Chiang, C.Y.; Tyanova, S.; Montag, A.; Lastra, R.R.; Lengyel, E.; Mann, M. Integrative proteomic profiling of ovarian cancer cell lines reveals precursor cell associated proteins and functional status. *Nat. Commun.* **2016**, *7*, 12645. [CrossRef] [PubMed]
28. Winget, M.D.; Baron, J.A.; Spitz, M.R.; Brenner, D.E.; Warzel, D.; Kincaid, H.; Thornquist, M.; Feng, Z. Development of common data elements: The experience of and recommendations from the early detection research network. *Int. J. Med. Inform.* **2003**, *70*, 41–48. [CrossRef]
29. Shariat, S.; Lotan, Y.; Vickers, A.; Karakiewicz, P.; Schmitz-Dräger, B.; Goebell, P.; Malats, N. Statistical consideration for clinical biomarker research in bladder cancer. *Urol. Oncol.* **2010**, *28*, 389–400. [CrossRef]
30. Kothe, S.; Muller, J.; Bohmer, S.-A.; Tschongov, T.; Fricke, M.; Koch, S.; Thiede, C.; Requardt, R.P.; Rubio, I.; Bohmer, F.D. Features of Ras activation by a mislocalized oncogenic tyrosine kinase: FLT3 ITD signals through K-Ras at the plasma membrane of acute myeloid leukemia cells. *J. Cell Sci.* **2013**, *126*, 4746–4755. [CrossRef]
31. Barham, W.; Chen, L.; Tikhomirov, O.; Onishko, H.; Gleaves, L.; Stricker, T.P.; Blackwell, T.S.; Yull, F.E. Aberrant activation of NF-κB signaling in mammary epithelium leads to abnormal growth and ductal carcinoma in situ. *BMC Cancer* **2015**, 1–17. [CrossRef]
32. Guttilla, I.K.; Phoenix, K.N.; Hong, X.; Tirnauer, J.S.; Claffey, K.P.; White, B.A. Prolonged mammosphere culture of MCF-7 cells induces an EMT and repression of the estrogen receptor by microRNAs. *Breast Cancer Res. Treat.* **2012**, *132*, 75–85. [CrossRef]
33. Sidney, L.E.; McIntosh, O.D.; Hopkinson, A. Phenotypic change and induction of cytokeratin expression during in vitro culture of corneal stromal cells. *Investig. Ophthalmol. Vis. Sci.* **2015**, *56*, 7225–7235. [CrossRef] [PubMed]
34. Jolly, M.K.; Tripathi, S.C.; Jia, D.; Mooney, S.M.; Celiktas, M.; Hanash, S.M.; Mani, S.A.; Pienta, K.J.; Ben-Jacob, E.; Levine, H. Stability of the hybrid epithelial/mesenchymal phenotype. *Oncotarget* **2016**, *7*, 27067–27084. [CrossRef] [PubMed]
35. Huang, R.Y.; Antony, J.; Tan, T.Z.; Tan, D.S. Targeting the AXL signaling pathway in ovarian cancer. *Mol. Cell Oncol.* **2016**, *4*, e1263716. [CrossRef] [PubMed]
36. Smigiel, J.M.; Parameswaran, N.; Jackson, M.W. Targeting Pancreatic Cancer Cell Plasticity: The Latest in Therapeutics. *Cancers* **2018**, *10*, 14. [CrossRef] [PubMed]

37. Banyard, J.; Chung, I.; Wilson, A.M.; Vetter, G.; Le Béchec, A.; Bielenberg, D.R.; Zetter, B.R. Regulation of epithelial plasticity by miR-424 and miR-200 in a new prostate cancer metastasis model. *Sci. Rep.* **2013**, *3*, 3151. [CrossRef] [PubMed]
38. Quagliata, L.; Schlageter, M.; Quintavalle, C.; Tornillo, L.; Terracciano, L. Identification of New Players in Hepatocarcinogenesis: Limits and Opportunities of Using Tissue Microarray (TMA). *Microarrays* **2014**, *3*, 91–102. [CrossRef] [PubMed]
39. Ku, M.; Kang, M.; Suh, J.; Yang, J. Effects for Sequential Treatment of siAkt and Paclitaxel on Gastric Cancer Cell Lines. *Int. J. Med. Sci.* **2016**, *13*, 708–716. [CrossRef]
40. Su, H.; Lin, F.; Deng, X.; Shen, L.; Fang, Y.; Fei, Z.; Zhao, L.; Zhang, X.; Pan, H.; Xie, D.; et al. Profiling and bioinformatics analyses reveal differential circular RNA expression in radioresistant esophageal cancer cells. *J. Transl. Med.* **2016**, *14*, 225. [CrossRef]
41. Litviakov, N.V.; Cherdyntseva, N.V.; Tsyganov, M.M.; Slonimskaya, E.M.; Ibragimova, M.K.; Kazantseva, P.V.; Kzhyshkowska, J.; Choinzonov, E.L. Deletions of multidrug resistance gene loci in breast cancer leads to the down-regulation of its expression and predict tumor response to neoadjuvant chemotherapy. *Oncotarget* **2016**, *5*, 7829–7841. [CrossRef]
42. Negrei, C.; Hudita, A.; Ginghina, O.; Galateanu, B.; Voicu, S.N.; Stan, M.; Costache, M.; Fenga, C.; Drakoulis, N.; Tsatsakis, A.M. Colon Cancer Cells Gene Expression Signature As Response to 5-Fluorouracil, Oxaliplatin, and Folinic Acid Treatment. *Front. Pharmacol.* **2016**, *7*, 172. [CrossRef]
43. Bjarnadottir, O.; Kimbung, S.; Johansson, I.; Veerla, S.; Jönsson, M.; Bendahl, P.-O.; Grabau, D.; Hedenfalk, I.; Borgquist, S. Global Transcriptional Changes Following Statin Treatment in Breast Cancer. *Clin. Cancer Res.* **2015**, *21*, 3402–3411. [CrossRef] [PubMed]
44. Chiu, J.W.; Hotte, S.J.; Kollmannsberger, C.K.; Renouf, D.J.; Cescon, D.W.; Hedley, D.; Chow, S.; Moscow, J.; Chen, Z.; Perry, M.; et al. A phase I trial of ANG1/2-Tie2 inhibitor trebaninib (AMG386) and temsirolimus in advanced solid tumors (PJC008/NCI#9041). *Invest. New Drugs* **2016**, *34*, 104–111. [PubMed]
45. Kim, G.; Ison, G.; McKee, A.E.; Zhang, H.; Tang, S.; Gwise, T.; Sridhara, R.; Lee, E.; Tzou, A.; Philip, R.; et al. FDA Approval Summary: Olaparib Monotherapy in Patients with Deleterious Germline BRCA-Mutated Advanced Ovarian Cancer Treated with Three or More Lines of Chemotherapy. *Clin. Cancer Res.* **2015**, *21*, 4257–4261. [CrossRef] [PubMed]
46. AlHilli, M.M.; Becker, M.A.; Weroha, S.J.; Flatten, K.S.; Hurley, R.M.; Harrell, M.I.; Oberg, A.L.; Maurer, M.J.; Hawthorne, K.M.; Hou, X.; et al. In vivo anti-tumor activity of the PARP inhibitor niraparib in homologous recombination deficient and proficient ovarian carcinoma. *Gynecol. Oncol.* **2016**, *143*, 379–388. [CrossRef] [PubMed]
47. Ke, Z.; Caiping, S.; Qing, Z.; Xiaojing, W. Sonic hedgehog-Gli1 signals promote epithelial-mesenchymal transition in ovarian cancer by mediating PI3K/AKT pathway. *Med. Oncol.* **2015**, *32*, 368. [CrossRef] [PubMed]
48. Ibrahim, Y.H.; García-García, C.; Serra, V.; He, L.; Torres-Lockhart, K.; Prat, A.; Anton, P.; Cozar, P.; Guzmán, M.; Grueso, J.; et al. PI3K inhibition impairs BRCA1/2 expression and sensitizes BRCA-proficient triple-negative breast cancer to PARP inhibition. *Cancer Discov.* **2012**, *2*, 1036–1047. [CrossRef] [PubMed]
49. Juvekar, A.; Burga, L.N.; Hu, H.; Lunsford, E.P.; Ibrahim, Y.H.; Balmañà, J.; Rajendran, A.; Papa, A.; Spencer, K.; Lyssiotis, C.A.; et al. Combining a PI3K inhibitor with a PARP inhibitor provides an effective therapy for BRCA1-related breast cancer. *Cancer Discov.* **2012**, *2*, 1048–1063. [CrossRef] [PubMed]
50. González-Billalabeitia, E.; Seitzer, N.; Song, S.J.; Song, M.S.; Patnaik, A.; Liu, X.-S.; Epping, M.T.; Papa, A.; Hobbs, R.M.; Chen, M.; et al. Vulnerabilities of PTEN-TP53-deficient prostate cancers to compound PARP-PI3K inhibition. *Cancer Discov.* **2014**, *4*, 896–904. [CrossRef] [PubMed]
51. Wang, D.; Li, C.; Zhang, Y.; Wang, M.; Jiang, N.; Xiang, L.; Li, T.; Roberts, T.M.; Zhao, J.J.; Cheng, H.; et al. Combined inhibition of PI3K and PARP is effective in the treatment of ovarian cancer cells with wild-type PIK3CA genes. *Gynecol. Oncol.* **2016**, *142*, 548–556. [CrossRef]

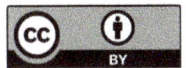

© 2019 by the authors. Licensee MDPI, Basel, Switzerland. This article is an open access article distributed under the terms and conditions of the Creative Commons Attribution (CC BY) license (http://creativecommons.org/licenses/by/4.0/).

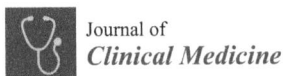

Article

# An Integrative Systems Biology and Experimental Approach Identifies Convergence of Epithelial Plasticity, Metabolism, and Autophagy to Promote Chemoresistance

Shengnan Xu [1], Kathryn E. Ware [1], Yuantong Ding [2], So Young Kim [3], Maya U. Sheth [1], Sneha Rao [4], Wesley Chan [1], Andrew J. Armstrong [1,5], William C. Eward [4], Mohit Kumar Jolly [6,7,*] and Jason A. Somarelli [1,*]

[1] Duke Cancer Institute and the Department of Medicine, Duke University Medical Center, Durham, NC 27710, USA; shengnan.xu@duke.edu (S.X.); kathryn.ware@duke.edu (K.E.W.); maya.sheth@duke.edu (M.U.S.); wesley.chan@duke.edu (W.C.); andrew.armstrong@duke.edu (A.J.A.)
[2] Department of Biology, Duke University Medical Center, Durham, NC 27710, USA; yuantong.ding@duke.edu
[3] Department of Molecular Genetics and Microbiology, Duke University Medical Center, Durham, NC 2 7710, USA; soyoung.kim@duke.edu
[4] Department of Orthopaedic Surgery, Duke University Medical Center, Durham, NC, 27710, USA; sneha.rao@duke.edu (S.R.); william.eward@duke.edu (W.C.E.)
[5] Solid Tumor Program and the Duke Prostate and Urologic Cancer Center, Duke University Medical Center, Durham, NC 27710, USA
[6] Center for Theoretical Biological Physics, Rice University, Houston, TX 77005-1827, USA
[7] Current address: Centre for BioSystems Science and Engineering, Indian Institute of Science, Bangalore 560012, India
* Correspondence: jason.somarelli@duke.edu (J.A.S.); mkjolly.15@gmail.com (M.K.J.)

Received: 7 January 2019; Accepted: 4 February 2019; Published: 7 February 2019

**Abstract:** The evolution of therapeutic resistance is a major cause of death for cancer patients. The development of therapy resistance is shaped by the ecological dynamics within the tumor microenvironment and the selective pressure of the host immune system. These selective forces often lead to evolutionary convergence on pathways or hallmarks that drive progression. Thus, a deeper understanding of the evolutionary convergences that occur could reveal vulnerabilities to treat therapy-resistant cancer. To this end, we combined phylogenetic clustering, systems biology analyses, and molecular experimentation to identify convergences in gene expression data onto common signaling pathways. We applied these methods to derive new insights about the networks at play during transforming growth factor-β (TGF-β)-mediated epithelial–mesenchymal transition in lung cancer. Phylogenetic analyses of gene expression data from TGF-β-treated cells revealed convergence of cells toward amine metabolic pathways and autophagy during TGF-β treatment. Knockdown of the autophagy regulatory, ATG16L1, re-sensitized lung cancer cells to cancer therapies following TGF-β-induced resistance, implicating autophagy as a TGF-β-mediated chemoresistance mechanism. In addition, high ATG16L expression was found to be a poor prognostic marker in multiple cancer types. These analyses reveal the usefulness of combining evolutionary and systems biology methods with experimental validation to illuminate new therapeutic vulnerabilities for cancer.

**Keywords:** evolution; systems biology; autophagy; lung cancer; epithelial–mesenchymal transition; tumor invasiveness; metabolism

## 1. Introduction

Mammalian cells respond to external stimuli through a coordinated system of signaling and gene expression circuitry. The inputs to this system are often the ligands for receptors, which initiate signaling cascades that ultimately lead to changes in gene expression. A cell can receive, process, and integrate multiple simultaneous inputs and respond to them with a coordinated phenotypic response [1,2].

Deregulation of the cellular signaling/response circuitry is a fundamental theme in cancer at both the tissue and single-cell levels. Indeed, deregulated intracellular signaling/gene expression circuitry is fundamental to many cancer hallmarks [3], including sustaining proliferation [4,5], evading growth suppression [5], inducing angiogenesis [5], tumor-promoting inflammation [5], invasion [6], and metastasis [7–9].

One well-studied signaling/expression circuit that is frequently dysregulated in cancer is the transforming growth factor β (TGF-β)/SMAD axis. The TGF-β/SMAD axis is a critical developmental pathway that controls differentiation and proliferation [10]. TGF-β/SMAD signaling is also important in wound healing and fibrosis (reviewed in [11,12]). One of the major phenotypic outputs of TGF-β/SMAD signaling is the phenotypic switch from an epithelial to a mesenchymal state, known traditionally as epithelial–mesenchymal transition (EMT) (reviewed in [13]). In the context of cancer, TGF-β-mediated EMT promotes downregulation of cell–cell adhesion and upregulation of migration and invasion [14,15]. This pro-invasive phenotype is usually activated at the expense of proliferation [15,16]: TGF-β induces potent cell cycle arrest through SMAD-mediated transcriptional activation of the cell cycle repressor, p21 [17]. TGF-β also reprograms cellular metabolism [18] and induces autophagy [19]—a process in which a cell self-digests its proteins and organelles. In addition to its cell autonomous role in promoting invasiveness, TGF-β also acts non-cell autonomously to create a tumor microenvironment more permissive to tumor growth [20,21]. These mechanisms can often drive resistance to chemotherapy and multiple targeted therapies [22,23].

However, the abovementioned effects of TGF-β/SMAD-induced EMT are typically studied in isolation with focus on a few nodes of the pathway, thereby neglecting the effects of crosstalk among multiple signaling pathways. Such crosstalk can often generate feedback loops with nonlinear dynamics, giving rise to emergent, complex, and non-intuitive behavior [24]. Hence, a systems biology approach, integrating computational and experimental components, can be essential to elucidating the dynamics of underlying interconnected cellular circuitry and identifying the fundamental organizational principles driving tumor progression [25]. Here, we used such an approach, incorporating multiple systems biology tools to analyze the dynamics of TGF-β-mediated EMT and to experimentally validate the computationally derived insights (Figure 1).

Cancer progression is an evolutionary process of selection over time [26,27]. Therefore, we postulated that tools developed for tracing evolutionary histories may provide new insights. One of the most commonly used methods of inferring ancestral relationships is phylogenetics. Phylogenetics uses a data matrix of character states to infer evolutionary relationships between groups [28]. Although phylogenetics was originally developed to reconstruct ancestral relationships between species, phylogenetic inference has also been applied to diverse datasets for which no underlying ancestral relationships exist, such as geography, linguistics, or astrophysics [28].

Given the flexibility of phylogenetics as a clustering tool for multiple data types and contexts, we hypothesized that analysis of time course gene expression data could provide crucial information about how circuits are integrated to lead to a given phenotype. We identified a convergence of gene expression data on amine metabolism pathways following TGF-β-induced EMT, and validated upregulation of ammonia production using wet bench experimentation. Interestingly, we also identified ATG16L1, a regulator of autophagy, as a central node in an ammonia production gene network, suggesting connections between elevated amine metabolism, EMT, and autophagy. ATG16L1 was also found to be upregulated during TGF-β-induced EMT. Finally, using high-throughput drug screens, we showed that siRNA-mediated inhibition of the autophagy regulator,

ATG16L1, rescued TGF-β-mediated chemoresistance. Together, this iterative combination of systems-based analyses and experimental validations suggests that TGF-β-mediated EMT converges on a gene expression network to induce autophagy and altered metabolism that can be targeted to overcome chemoresistance.

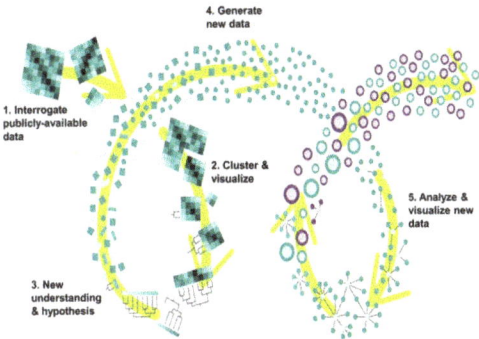

**Figure 1.** An integrated framework of iterative, systems-level analysis and experimental validation provides new insights. Large amounts of raw data, generated by new experimentation or re-analyzed from public databases (1), are analyzed by clustering approaches to easily visualize data topology (2). This visualization fosters a new, deeper understanding that informs a new hypothesis (3). Experimental validation of the new hypothesis generates new data (4), which is analyzed and visualized as a system (5).

## 2. Materials and Methods

### 2.1. Cell Culture

All cell lines were obtained from the Duke Cell Culture Facility. The Duke Cell Culture Facility routinely tests for mycoplasma and performs cell line authentication by short tandem repeat analysis. Cells were cultured in Dulbecco's Modified Eagle Medium (DMEM) with fetal bovine serum (FBS) and 1% penicillin–streptomycin in a standard 37 °C tissue culture incubator with 5% $CO_2$. Cell confluence during vehicle and TGF-β treatment was measured using the IncuCyte Zoom live cell analysis system (Sartorius, Goettingen, Germany).

### 2.2. RNA Extraction, Reverse Transcription, and RT-qPCR

RNA extraction, reverse transcription, and RT-qPCR were performed as previously described [29].

### 2.3. Western Blotting

Cells were prepared and lysed in 1× radioimmunoprecipitation assay (RIPA) buffer (Thermo, catalog number: 89900, Waltham, MA, USA) mixed with 1× protease and phosphatase inhibitor cocktail (Roche, San Jose, CA, USA). The composition of the RIPA buffer was 25 mM Tris·HCl pH 7.6, 150 mM NaCl, 1% Nonidet P-40 (NP-40), 1% sodium deoxycholate, and 0.1% sodium dodecyl sulfonate (SDS). Cell lysates were incubated at 4 °C for 20 min. and centrifuged at 14,000g for 5 min. Cleared lysates were mixed with 4× Laemmli loading buffer and incubated at 95 °C for 3 min. Lysates were separated in 4–12% NuPAGE Novex Bis-Tris gels (ThermoFisher, Waltham, MA, USA). Proteins were transferred to nitrocellulose membrane (GE Healthcare Life Sciences, Pittsburgh, PA, USA) in 1× NuPAGE Transfer Buffer (ThermoFisher, Waltham, MA, USA) for 2 h at 75 V at 4 °C in the cold room. Membranes were blocked at room temperature using Starting Block T20 TBS Blocking Buffer (ThermoFisher, Waltham, MA, USA). Primary antibodies were added to the blocking buffer and incubated at 4 °C overnight. Membranes were washed two times for 5 min. each with phosphate-buffered saline (PBS) and incubated with LI-COR goat anti-mouse or goat anti-rabbit secondary antibodies diluted 1:20,000 in Starting Block buffer. Membranes were visualized using the Odyssey Fc imager (27402864, LI-COR Biosciences, Lincoln, NE, USA). Primary antibodies used included glyceraldehyde-phosphate dehydrogenase (GAPDH) (C2415, Santa Cruz Biotechtology; 1:1000, Dallas, TX, USA), ATG16L1 (8089T, Cell Signaling; 1:1000, Danvers, MA, USA) and LC3 A/B (12741T, Cell Signaling; 1:1000, Danvers, MA, USA).

## 2.4. Ammonia Production Assay

A total of 200,000 cells were seeded in 6 cm dishes. At each time point, cells were washed with PBS, scraped, and lysed in Ammonia Assay Buffer provided in the Abcam ammonia assay kit (ab83360, Abcam, Cambridge, UK) after the end of each treatment time point. Ammonia production assays were performed after collecting all time points using the protocol recommended by the manufacturer.

## 2.5. Cytoscape Analysis

Gene networks were analyzed by importing all available human data on each gene in the Universal Interaction Database Client using Cytoscape version 3.5.1 (https://cytoscape.org/). All relevant networks of genes were merged to visualize interactions among genes.

## 2.6. Phylogenetic Reconstructions from Gene Expression Data

Distance-based dendograms were created by first constructing a distance matrix calculated based on the entire microarray dataset for each dataset to be analyzed, using the genes as the characters, the raw expression value for each gene as the set of character states, and the samples as the taxa. The Neighbor Joining method [30] was used for reconstructing phylogeny with distance matrices. To perform analysis based on maximum-likelihood (ML) and parsimony, the continuous gene expression data was converted into categorical variables. For example, for GSE23038, we used the passage 0 sample as an 'outgroup', and converted the gene expression data for all other samples into either upregulated, downregulated, or constant relative to passage 0. The reliability of the parsimony method is generally considered to increase with an increasing number of informative characters [31–33]. Therefore, cut-off thresholds of up- and downregulation were determined by calculating the maximum number of informative sites given different cut-offs, and a threshold was selected that provided the highest number of informative sites in each dataset. ML and parsimony analyses were then performed based on converted data. ML analysis after data conversion was performed online on a free phylogeny platform, PhyML 3.0 (14), whereas distance and parsimony tree constructions were performed using the APE [34] and Phangorn [35] packages implemented in R (15). Bootstrap tests of 100 pseudoreplicates were performed for all phylogenies to assess the branch support. Tree files were visualized in FigTree (Andrew Rambaut; http://tree.bio.ed.ac.uk/software/figtree/).

## 2.7. High-Throughput Screening

A549 cells were screened with the NCI Approved Oncology Drugs Set VI in the presence of vehicle (4 mM HCl and 2% bovine serum albumin (BSA)) or 4 ng/mL recombinant human TGF-β (R&D Systems, Minneapolis, MN, USA). Briefly, A549 cells were dispensed using liquid handling into 384 well plates with no drug, dimethyl sulfoxide (DMSO), or 1 µM drug at cell plating densities of 250 or 1000 cells/well. Plates were incubated at 37 °C, and cell viability was assayed by CellTiterGlo (Promega, Madison, WI, USA) after 72 h. Relative drug resistance or sensitivity was calculated as the fold change difference in CellTiterGlo value between vehicle-treated and TGF-β-treated wells. To perform the screen in the context of ATG16L1 knockdown, 20 nM siRNA targeting ATG16L1 was delivered to A549 cells by reverse transfection using RNAiMax and incubated at 37 °C for 24 h. After 24 h, the drug screen was performed −/+ TGF-β, as described above. All screens were performed in the Duke Functional Genomics Shared Resource. Raw data for the screens are provided in Supplementary Files 1 and 2.

*2.8. Correlation of ATG16L1 with Clinical Outcomes*

Kaplan–Meier curves were generated based on patients stratified by ATG16L1 expression level using R2: Genomics Analysis and Visualization Platform (https://hgserver1.amc.nl/cgi-bin/r2/main.cgi) and GEPIA (http://gepia.cancer-pku.cn/). The scan option was used to automatically select the cut-off values in the R2 platform, and default settings were used for GEPIA.

*2.9. Statistical Analyses*

All assays were performed in triplicate, and all experiments were repeated a minimum of two times. The real-time polymerase chain reaction (qRT-PCR) and ammonia production assays were analyzed using a one-way ANOVA with Tukey's post-hoc correction for multiple comparisons in JMP14.0 (SAS, Cary, NC, USA). Drug screen data was analyzed by linear regression and analysis of variance in JMP14.0. Pathway analyses were performed in FuncAssociate (http://llama.mshri.on.ca/funcassociate/) [36], which calculates an adjusted *p*-value as a fraction of 1000 simulations having attributes with the single hypothesis *p*-value. For Kaplan–Meier survival curves were analyzed by log-rank tests. All *p*-values <0.05 were considered statistically significant.

## 3. Results

*3.1. Phylogenetics Analyses Provide a Simple and Reliable Tool to Visualize Gene Expression Dynamics*

To test the feasibility and effectiveness of using phylogenetics as a clustering tool to analyze gene expression data, we tested if phylogenetic trees could recapitulate the temporal order of gene expression data collected at different time points. To do this, we constructed dendograms from publicly-available microarray data for immortalized prostate cells collected every 10 passages from 0 to 80 passages (GSE23038, [37]).

We first used distance-based trees to infer temporal relationships among the samples. Distance-based trees use a data matrix comprised of gene expression values as a continuous variable without the need for binning gene expression data into categorical variables of being upregulated, unchanged, and downregulated. Distance-based construction of a rooted tree with root at passage 0 produced a tree topology that, with the exception of passage 70, clustered samples according to their temporal order from passage 10 to 80 (Figure 2A).

We also analyzed GSE23038 [37] using maximum-likelihood and parsimony phylogenetics methods. The raw data matrix was converted into three character states based on a neutral evolution model, JC69, before being used as input for these two methods of tree construction. Importantly, for all three methods, trees constructed using gene expression data recapitulated the known temporal structure of the data with robust bootstrap support (Figure 2A–C, bootstrap values indicated above branches). A comparison of the three cladistical methods with clustering revealed that hierarchical clustering was unable to accurately reconstruct the temporal order of passages (Figure 2D,E).

Similarly, we performed phylogenetic clustering on additional datasets where samples had been analyzed longitudinally, including GSE17708 [38], microarray data from A549 lung adenocarcinoma cells treated with TGF-β over a period of 72 h, and GSE12548, microarray data from human ARPE-19 retinal pigment epithelium cells treated with TGF-β and TNF-α over 60 h [39]. For both of these datasets, phylogenetic clustering reconstructed the temporal order of treatments with strong bootstrap support (Figure 3A,B).

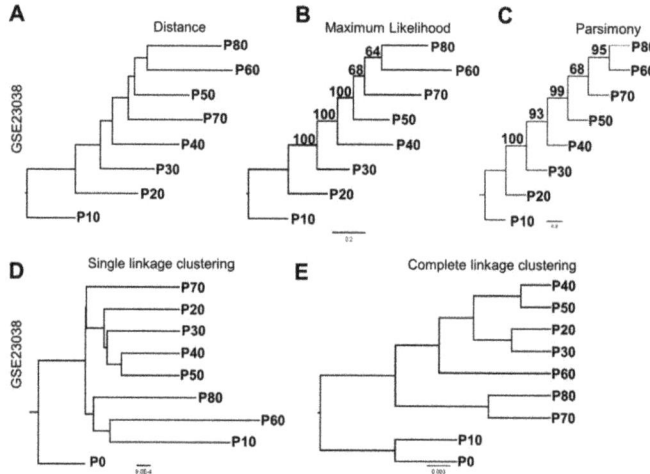

**Figure 2.** Phylogenetic reconstruction provides a simple visualization tool to view temporal changes in gene expression data. (**A**) Distance-based phylogeny of GSE23038; serial passage of normal prostate cells immortalized with hTERT using gene expression data as a continuous variable. (**B**) Maximum-likelihood and (**C**) maximum parsimony trees constructed based on gene expression data transformed to categorical variables. (**D**) Single and (**E**) complete linkage hierarchical clustering provides similar groupings of passage numbers, but lacks the temporal structure.

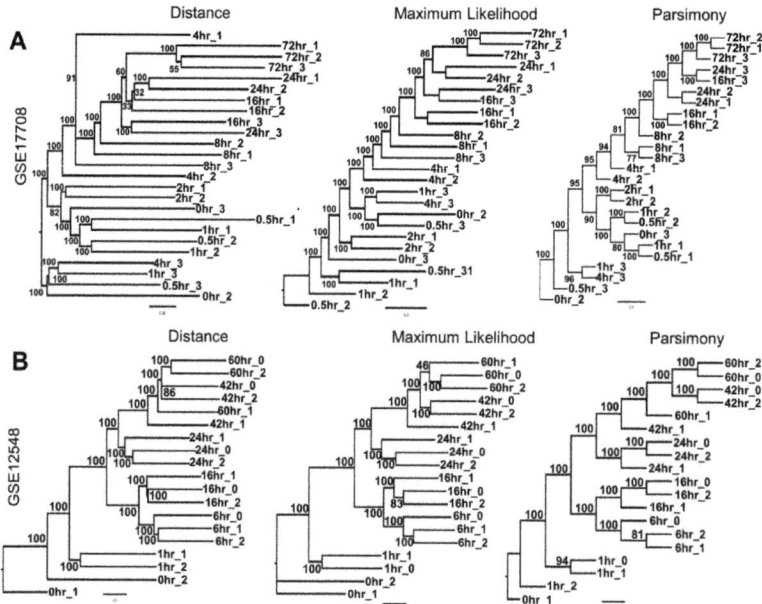

**Figure 3.** Phylogenetic clustering enables reconstruction of longitudinal data based on gene expression. (**A**) Distance, maximum parsimony, and maximum-likelihood dendograms of GSE17708; microarray analysis of A549 cells treated with TGF-β over 72 h. (**B**) Distance, maximum parsimony, and maximum-likelihood phylogeny construction of GSE12548; TGF-β and TNF-α treatment of human retinal pigment epithelium cells over 60 h.

## 3.2. Analyzing Dynamics of TGF-β Treatment through Visualization of Tree Structure Reveals Two Distinct Temporally-Resolved Clades

A major advantage of clustering is its ability to easily visualize relationships between large datasets and to derive novel insights. For example, re-analysis of microarray data from A549 cells treated with TGF-β over 72 h (GSE17708) revealed two distinctive patterns in the resulting phylogenies. First, early time points (0–8 h) were haphazardly organized in clades and subclades, where replicates of samples were admixed, indicating that phylogenetic analyses were not able to provide a clear signal based on the expression data that would predict timing of treatment (Figure 4A). Second, the later time points (≥8 h) were well resolved, suggesting the presence of a clear signal emerging in the gene expression data following long-term treatment with TGF-β (Figure 4A).

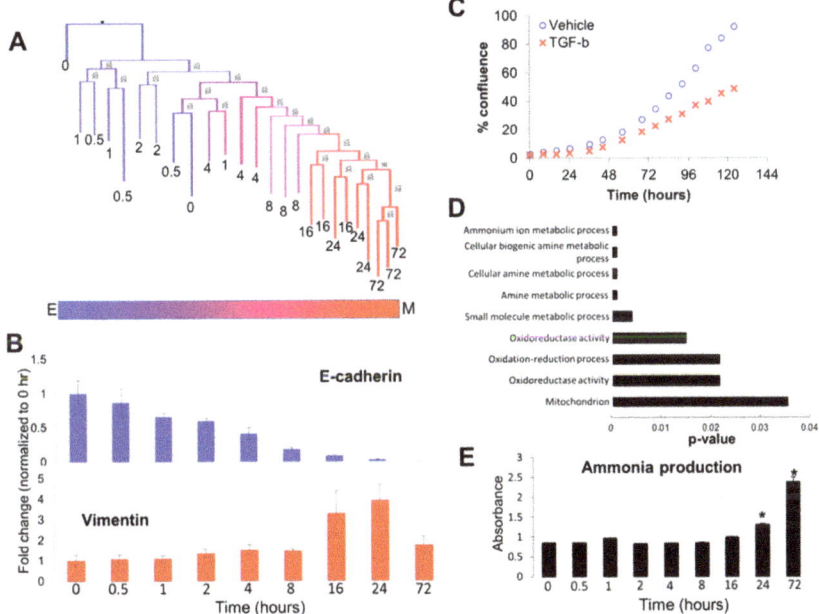

**Figure 4.** Visualization of tree topology reveals altered metabolism during epithelial–mesenchymal transition (EMT). (**A**) The topology of the maximum-likelihood reconstruction of GSE17708 showed an admixed clade at early time points in A549 cells with TGF-β treatment, with a clearly-resolved clade of later time points after eight hours as the phenotypic signal switched from epithelial to mesenchymal. (**B**) Consistent with the tree topology, changes in EMT biomarkers E-cadherin and vimentin were not apparent until after eight hours of treatment. * indicate $p < 0.05$ as compared to the 0 h time point (**C**) Growth curves of A549 cells treated with vehicle (blue circles) or TGF-β (red ×) analyzed by IncuCyte time-lapse imaging revealed TGF-β-induced growth inhibition at 48–72 h. (**D**) Pathway analysis of genes contributing to the bifurcation of early (<8 h) and late (≥8 h) time point clades revealed TGF-β-induced changes in amine metabolism pathways at the later time points as compared to the early time points. (**E**) Ammonia production assays validated the prediction that TGF-β induces upregulation of ammonia production.

Consistent with a convergence of signal at later time points, RT-qPCR analysis of the epithelial marker, E-cadherin, and the mesenchymal marker, vimentin, demonstrated that E-cadherin suppression and vimentin activation were not apparent until this bifurcation of early admixed time points vs. resolved late time points (Figure 4B). Likewise, our time-lapse imaging analysis of growth rate between vehicle-treated and TGF-β-treated A549 cells showed that differences in growth rate between the two conditions were not observed until approximately 72 h after the initiation of treatment (Figure 4C; Supplementary movies 1 and 2), consistent with reports demonstrating that EMT induces cell cycle arrest [40,41]. These experimental results suggest that the timing of both gene expression and phenotypic traits associated with EMT are consistent with the convergence of an emerging signal at later time points within the dendograms.

Next, we extracted genes that were differentially expressed across the two major clades of early and late treatment times. Pathway analysis of these genes showed that multiple amine metabolism pathways were significantly altered during TGF-β treatment (Figure 4D). To experimentally test if ammonia metabolism was altered during TGF-β treatment, we performed ammonia production assays on A549 cells from which the publicly available data were originally generated. Importantly, we found that ammonia production was altered significantly upon TGF-β treatment at later time points, with little change in ammonia production during earlier time points (Figure 4E). Together, these analyses demonstrated the utility of simple visualizations, such as phylogenetic trees and clustering dendograms, to yield new testable hypotheses.

### 3.3. Gene Expression Networks Couple Ammonia Production to Autophagy

Previous research has identified a connection between upregulation of ammonia production and induction of autophagy [42]. Based on this connection, we tested if TGF-β-induced EMT led to an increase in autophagy markers. In support of this hypothesis, TGF-β treatment led to upregulation of autophagy markers LC3A/B and ATG16L1 (Figure 5A,B). To better understand the connections between ammonia production and autophagy, we used Cytoscape to construct gene regulatory networks related to amine metabolism genes and autophagy regulators. We constructed gene networks that included the ammonia production genes identified by the pathway analysis, along with the autophagy markers LC3A/B and ATG16L1, that we identified in our western blots to be activated upon TGF-β treatment. Although we found few gene–gene interactions among amine metabolism genes alone (Figure 5C), when we added the autophagy regulator ATG16L1 to this network, it connected the entire set of previously-isolated amine metabolism subnetworks (Figure 5D). Our results suggest that TGF-β-mediated EMT is associated with increased amine production and upregulation of autophagy. It remains to be tested in this system if the ammonia production induces autophagy, as has been demonstrated previously in both yeast and mouse embryonic fibroblasts [42], or if TGF-β-induced autophagy upregulation leads to more ammonia. However, our results demonstrate a connection between TGF-β-mediated EMT, altered amine production, and upregulation of autophagy.

### 3.4. Autophagy Inhibition Re-sensitizes Cells to TGF-β-Induced Chemoresistance

Our data revealed that TGF-β-induced EMT leads to ammonia production and upregulation of autophagy. Interestingly, both EMT and autophagy are known to be involved in chemoresistance. EMT can drive chemoresistance in multiple cancers [43–46]. Likewise, autophagy is a pro-survival mechanism in response to cellular stresses, such as hypoxia and nutrient deprivation, and is increasingly implicated in resistance to cancer treatments [47,48]. Integrating our observations with these reports, we hypothesized that EMT-induced drug resistance is mediated, at least in part, by elevated levels of the autophagy regulator, ATG16L1.

To test this hypothesis, we used high-throughput drug screens of 119 FDA-approved small-molecule anticancer agents. To do this, we first tested if TGF-β-mediated EMT led to chemoresistance. We screened A549 cells treated with either vehicle or TGF-β and plated at both low and high density. After 72 h of incubation with each drug, the overall cell viability was analyzed with CellTiterGlo. We first performed quality control analyses of the screens. Linear regression of the empty and DMSO-treated wells showed virtually no relationship between the CellTiterGlo value and the position on the plate when comparing the same plate setup across multiple plates ($R^2 = 0.0862$), suggesting that the screen results did not suffer from plate effects (Figure S1). By contrast, the correlation coefficients in drug-containing wells were greater than 0.8 between high and low cell density for both vehicle- and TGF-β-treated conditions, suggesting high reproducibility across replicate plates when drug is present in the well (Figure S1).

Given the lack of apparent plate effects and strong reproducibility between replicate screens, we investigated whether TGF-β induced chemoresistance. Consistent with our hypothesis, TGF-β treatment increased resistance to 60% (71/119) of the compounds tested, as evaluated by an increase in CellTiterGlo absorbance as compared to vehicle-treated control wells (Figure 6A). Analysis of these compounds by pathway targets showed that TGF-β induced resistance to both broad spectrum chemotherapies, such as microtubule-targeting agents and topoisomerase inhibitors, as well as multiple targeted therapies, including those against HER2 and EGFR (Figure 6B).

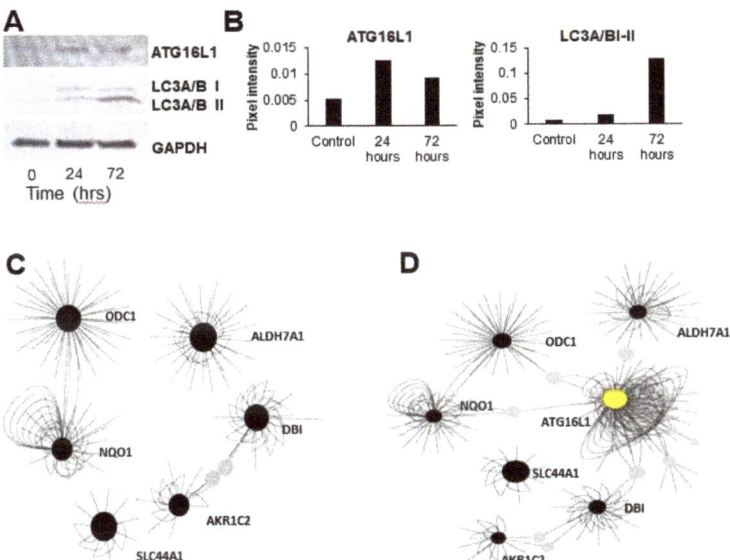

**Figure 5.** Epithelial-mesenchymal transition induces activation of autophagy and links to an amine production gene network. (**A**) TGF-β-induced epithelial-mesenchymal transition led to up-regulation of autophagy markers ATG16L1 and MAP1LC3A (LC3A/B). (**B**) Densitometric quantification of the western blotting data in A. (**C**) Cytoscape networks of amine production genes identified in Figure 4 showed few interactions between sub-networks. (**D**) Addition of the autophagy regulator, ATG16L1 (yellow circle), acted as a central hub to connect all amine metabolism sub-networks.

Next, to investigate the importance of autophagy in promoting TGF-β-induced therapy resistance, we performed siRNA-mediated knockdown of ATG16L1, the autophagy marker we identified as upregulated in TGF-β-treated cells. We first tested knockdown efficiency using four independent siRNAs and selected by Western blot analysis siRNA_1 for subsequent drug screens (Figure 6C). We then screened A549 with the same 119 drugs +/− TGF-β and treated with either a non-silencing siRNA or siRNA_1 targeting ATG16L1. Remarkably, ATG16L1 knockdown re-sensitized cells to 29/71 (41%) of drugs for which TGF-β treatment led to increased resistance (Figure 6D). Interestingly, these drugs included current standard-of-care therapies for small-cell lung cancer (SCLC), doxorubicin, and topotecan, as well as anti-VEGFR therapies, regorafenib, and axitinib, both of which have shown promising clinical benefits in early stage clinical trials against advanced non-small-cell lung cancer (NSCLC) [49,50], and cabozantinib, a tyrosine kinase inhibitor that has shown efficacy along with, or in combination with, erlotinib in the treatment of EGFR wild-type NSCLC patients [51]. Analysis by pathways showed that, on average, autophagy inhibition re-sensitized cells to multiple targeted therapies, including c-MET, c-RET, FLT3, TAM2, and dihydrofolate reductase (DHFR) (Figure 6E).

Together, our results support the hypothesis that TGF-β-mediated therapy resistance is driven, in part, by the autophagy regulator ATG16L1, suggesting the potential use of autophagy inhibitors as a concurrent or adjuvant therapy to counter resistance.

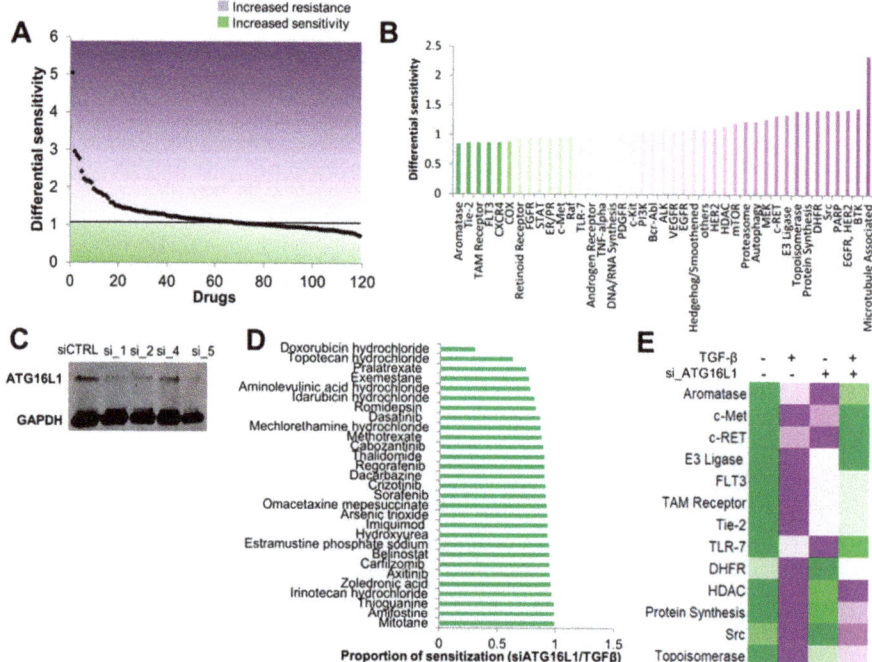

**Figure 6.** ATG16L1 knockdown rescues TGF-β-mediated chemoresistance. (**A**) A screen of 119 FDA-approved small molecule inhibitors demonstrated a broad increase in chemoresistance following TGF-β treatment. Each black dot represents one compound. Dots above the 1 were differentially resistant in TGF-β-treated cells as compared to vehicle-treated cells; dots below the 1 were more sensitive in the TGF-β-treated cells as compared to vehicle-treated cells. (**B**) Analysis of drug screen data by targets and pathways identified increased TGF-β-mediated resistance to several common chemotherapies, such as microtubule-associated and topoisomerase inhibitor therapies, and targeted therapies in lung cancer treatment, such as c-MET, VEGF, and EGFR (purple bars). (**C**) Knockdown of ATG16L1 by siRNAs was validated by western blotting. siCtrl = non-silencing siRNA; si_1, si_2, si_4, and si_5 are independent siRNAs targeting ATG16L1 (**D**) A549 lung adenocarcinoma cells −/+ TGF-β and −/+ siATG16_1 were screened against 119 FDA-approved compounds to identify drugs for which ATG16L1 rescued TGF-β-mediated therapy resistance. ATG16L1 knockdown re-sensitized cells to multiple therapeutic agents. (**E**) Pathway level analysis of compounds where TGF-β-mediated resistance was rescued by ATG16L1 knockdown.

To determine if ATG16L1 was related to clinical outcomes, we analyzed ATG16L1 expression in gene expression datasets from patient tumors. Analysis of Kaplan–Meier curves showed that low ATG16L1 expression is prognostic for improved overall survival in patients with lung and clear cell renal cancer (Figure 7A–C) and improved relapse-free survival in patients with colorectal cancer (Figure 7D). Together, these analyses indicate ATG16L1 as an important prognostic marker of clinical response and cancer cell aggression.

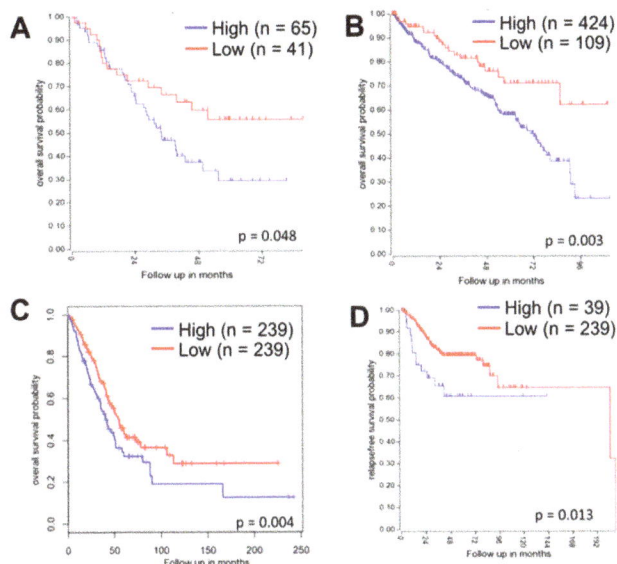

**Figure 7.** ATG16L1 is a prognostic biomarker of survival and progression in carcinoma patients. (**A**) Low ATG16L1 expression is prognostic for improved overall survival in lung adenocarcinoma patients. (**B**) Low ATG16L1 expression significantly predicts improved overall survival in kidney renal clear cell carcinoma patients. (**C**) Lower ATG16L1 expression in lung adenocarcinoma from The Cancer Genome Atlas dataset is prognostic for improved overall survival; data analyzed using GEPIA—http://gepia.cancer-pku.cn/. (**D**) Low ATG16L1 expression trends with better relapse-free survival in colorectal carcinoma patients.

## 4. Discussion

The progression of cancer from an indolent, slow-growing primary tumor to metastatic and therapy resistant disease is, at its foundation, an evolutionary process. Genetic and genomic dysregulation promotes heterogeneity in tumor cell populations [52], which provides raw materials for selection of the fittest cancer cells. During this process, mutations [53], epigenetic alterations [54], and gene expression changes [55] are selected that enable survival of individual cancer cells under the diverse environmental pressures not only within the tumor, but also during metastatic progression [56,57] and the emergence of therapy resistance [58].

Here, we combined methods rooted in evolutionary theory, such as phylogenetic inference, with pathway and network analyses, as well as experimental techniques, to yield new insights. By taking this novel approach to analyze a well-established system—TGF-β-induced EMT—we identified mechanisms of therapy resistance. Specifically, we found that EMT leads to increased production of intracellular ammonia. Ammonia is a by-product of protein breakdown and serves an important function in maintaining homeostasis in electrolyte concentration [59]. Recent evidence, however, also suggests that ammonia production is involved in regulating autophagy and pro-survival circuits that contribute to chemoresistance [42,60]. Importantly, autophagy can lead to increased aggressiveness in cancer, perhaps as an adaptive response to cellular stress. In our present study, downregulation of the autophagy regulator, ATG16L1, partially reversed EMT-induced therapy resistance, suggesting the potential benefits of concurrent uses of autophagy inhibitors with standard-of-care therapies.

TGF-β has also been reported to induce metabolic reprogramming of stromal cells, such as cancer-associated fibroblasts (CAFs), where CAFs overexpressing TGF-β ligands show increased autophagy and HIF-1α activation and concomitantly reduced oxidative phosphorylation [61].

The scaffolding/regulatory protein caveolin-1—a functional regulator of TGF-β signaling—can play a key role in coordinating these responses [62,63]. Thus, the nexus of TGF-β signaling, increased autophagy, and metabolic reprogramming may be a common design principle of multiple cell types.

Interestingly, inhibition of autophagy consistently led to re-sensitization to c-Met inhibitors during EMT. The c-Met oncogene is one of the two most highly-mutated tyrosine kinase receptors in NSCLC, and resistance to tyrosine kinase inhibitors (TKI) invariably follows after treatment [64]. Indeed, resistance to erlotinib is common in lung cancer, and ATG16L1 knockdown re-sensitized cells to increased EMT-induced erlotinib resistance. EMT has been shown as an important contributor to this resistance as TKI resistance NSCLC cell lines has a more mesenchymal phenotype, higher expression of mesenchymal markers, such as Zeb-1 and vimentin, and downregulation of E-cadherin [65]. Recent evidence has shown that c-Met promotes anoikis resistance and cell growth via activation of autophagy regulators, such as ATG5 and Beclin-1 [66]. These observations suggest that autophagy may be an important resistance mechanism and a combinatorial use of autophagy inhibitors with TKIs may increase therapeutic efficacy of TKIs and possibly prolong or reverse resistance.

## 5. Conclusions

By integrating systems biology and experimental methodologies we have revealed new connections between EMT, autophagy, ammonia production, and chemoresistance. These studies demonstrate the power of coupling tools from evolutionary biology with systems-level informatics analysis and experimental validation to yield novel insights. Future work is aimed at better understanding the mechanistic connections between autophagy, ammonia production, and EMT to design new therapies to treat chemo-resistant disease.

**Supplementary Materials:** The following are available online at http://www.mdpi.com/2077-0383/8/2/205/s1, Figure S1: Quality control analysis of high-throughput drug screen data, Video S1: A549vehicle; Video S2: A549vehicled.

**Author Contributions:** Conceptualization, S.X., K.E.W., M.K.J. and J.A.S.; Formal analysis, S.X., Y.D., W.C. and J.A.S.; Investigation, S.X., K.E.W. and S.Y.K.; Methodology, Y.D.; Supervision, K.E.W. and J.A.S.; Validation, S.Y.K.; Visualization, M.S. and S.R.; Writing—original draft, S.X. and J.A.S.; Writing—review & editing, S.X., K.E.W., Y.D., S.Y.K., M.S., S.R., W.C., W.C.E., A.J.A., K.E.W., M.K.J. and J.A.S.

**Acknowledgments:** J.A.S. wishes to acknowledge support from Meg and Bill Lindenberger, the Paul and Shirley Friedland Fund, the Triangle Center for Evolutionary Medicine, and funds raised in memory of Muriel E. Rudershausen (riding4research.org). The authors wish to thank Jeffrey Townsend and Herbert Levine for many helpful discussions in preparation of the manuscript. M.K.J. is supported by a training fellowship from the Gulf Coast Consortia on Computational Cancer Biology Training Program (CPRIT Grant No. RP170593).

**Conflicts of Interest:** The authors declare no conflict of interest.

## References

1. Chaiwanon, J.; Wang, W.; Zhu, J.Y.; Oh, E.; Wang, Z.Y. Information integration and communication in plant growth regulation. *Cell* **2016**, *164*, 1257–1268. [CrossRef]
2. Pawson, C.T.; Scott, J.D. Signal integration through blending, bolstering and bifurcating of intracellular information. *Nat. Struct. Mol. Biol.* **2010**, *17*, 653–658. [CrossRef]
3. Hanahan, D.; Weinberg, R.A. Hallmarks of cancer: The next generation. *Cell* **2011**, *144*, 646–674. [CrossRef]
4. Janda, E.; Litos, G.; Grunert, S.; Downward, J.; Beug, H. Oncogenic Ras/Her-2 mediate hyperproliferation of polarized epithelial cells in 3D cultures and rapid tumor growth via the PI3K pathway. *Oncogene* **2002**, *21*, 5148–5159. [CrossRef] [PubMed]
5. Sever, R.; Brugge, J.S. Signal transduction in cancer. *Cold Spring Harb Perspect. Med.* **2015**, *5*. [CrossRef] [PubMed]
6. Van Golen, K.L.; Bao, L.W.; Pan, Q.; Miller, F.R.; Wu, Z.F.; Merajver, S.D. Mitogen activated protein kinase pathway is involved in RhoC GTPase induced motility, invasion and angiogenesis in inflammatory breast cancer. *Clin. Exp. Metastasis* **2002**, *19*, 301–311. [CrossRef] [PubMed]

7. Iqbal, W.; Alkarim, S.; AlHejin, A.; Mukhtar, H.; Saini, K.S. Targeting signal transduction pathways of cancer stem cells for therapeutic opportunities of metastasis. *Oncotarget* **2016**, *7*, 76337–76353. [CrossRef]
8. Janda, E.; Lehmann, K.; Killisch, I.; Jechlinger, M.; Herzig, M.; Downward, J.; Beug, H.; Grunert, S. Ras and TGF-β cooperatively regulate epithelial cell plasticity and metastasis: Dissection of Ras signaling pathways. *J. Cell. Biol.* **2002**, *156*, 299–313. [CrossRef]
9. Brown, W.S.; Tan, L.; Smith, A.; Gray, N.S.; Wendt, M.K. Covalent targeting of fibroblast growth factor receptor inhibits metastatic breast cancer. *Mol. Cancer Ther.* **2016**, *15*, 2096–2106. [CrossRef]
10. Kitisin, K.; Saha, T.; Blake, T.; Golestaneh, N.; Deng, M.; Kim, C.; Tang, Y.; Shetty, K.; Mishra, B.; Mishra, L. TGF-β signaling in development. *Sci. STKE* **2007**, *2007*. [CrossRef]
11. Walton, K.L.; Johnson, K.E.; Harrison, C.A. Targeting TGF-β mediated SMAD signaling for the prevention of fibrosis. *Front. Pharmacol.* **2017**, *8*, 461. [CrossRef] [PubMed]
12. Carthy, J.M. TGF-β signaling and the control of myofibroblast differentiation: Implications for chronic inflammatory disorders. *J. Cell. Physiol.* **2018**, *233*, 98–106. [CrossRef]
13. Nawshad, A.; Lagamba, D.; Polad, A.; Hay, E.D. Transforming growth factor-beta signaling during epithelial-mesenchymal transformation: Implications for embryogenesis and tumor metastasis. *Cells Tissues Organs.* **2005**, *179*, 11–23. [CrossRef] [PubMed]
14. Papageorgis, P. TGF-β signaling in tumor initiation, epithelial-to-mesenchymal transition, and metastasis. *J. Oncol.* **2015**, *2015*, 587193. [CrossRef]
15. Fuxe, J.; Vincent, T.; Garcia de Herreros, A. Transcriptional crosstalk between TGF-β and stem cell pathways in tumor cell invasion: Role of EMT promoting SMAD complexes. *Cell Cycle* **2010**, *9*, 2363–2374. [CrossRef] [PubMed]
16. Huang, S.S.; Huang, J.S. TGF-β control of cell proliferation. *J. Cell. Biochem.* **2005**, *96*, 447–462. [CrossRef] [PubMed]
17. Moustakas, A.; Pardali, K.; Gaal, A.; Heldin, C.H. Mechanisms of TGF-β signaling in regulation of cell growth and differentiation. *Immunol. Lett.* **2002**, *82*, 85–91. [CrossRef]
18. Jiang, L.; Xiao, L.; Sugiura, H.; Huang, X.; Ali, A.; Kuro-o, M.; Deberardinis, R.J.; Boothman, D.A. Metabolic reprogramming during TGF-β-induced epithelial-to-mesenchymal transition. *Oncogene* **2015**, *34*, 3908–3916. [CrossRef]
19. Kiyono, K.; Suzuki, H.I.; Matsuyama, H.; Morishita, Y.; Komuro, A.; Kano, M.R.; Sugimoto, K.; Miyazono, K. Autophagy is activated by TGF-β and potentiates TGF-β-mediated growth inhibition in human hepatocellular carcinoma cells. *Cancer Res.* **2009**, *69*, 8844–8852. [CrossRef]
20. Hazelbag, S.; Gorter, A.; Kenter, G.G.; van den Broek, L.; Fleuren, G. Transforming growth factor-beta1 induces tumor stroma and reduces tumor infiltrate in cervical cancer. *Hum. Pathol.* **2002**, *33*, 1193–1199. [CrossRef]
21. Gigante, M.; Gesualdo, L.; Ranieri, E. TGF-β: A master switch in tumor immunity. *Curr. Pharm. Des.* **2012**, *18*, 4126–4134. [CrossRef] [PubMed]
22. Yao, Z.; Fenoglio, S.; Gao, D.C.; Camiolo, M.; Stiles, B.; Lindsted, T.; Schlederer, M.; Johns, C.; Altorki, N.; Mittal, V.; et al. TGF-β il-6 axis mediates selective and adaptive mechanisms of resistance to molecular targeted therapy in lung cancer. *Proc. Natl. Acad. Sci. USA* **2010**, *107*, 15535–15540. [CrossRef]
23. Brunen, D.; Willems, S.M.; Kellner, U.; Midgley, R.; Simon, I.; Bernards, R. TGF-β: An emerging player in drug resistance. *Cell Cycle* **2013**, *12*, 2960–2968. [CrossRef] [PubMed]
24. Magi, S.; Iwamoto, K.; Okada-Hatakeyama, M. Current status of mathematical modeling of cancer—From the viewpoint of cancer hallmarks. *Curr. Opin. Chem. Biol.* **2017**, *2*, 39–48.
25. Anderson, A.R.; Quaranta, V. Integrative mathematical oncology. *Nat. Rev. Cancer* **2008**, *8*, 227–234. [CrossRef]
26. Gerlinger, M.; McGranahan, N.; Dewhurst, S.M.; Burrell, R.A.; Tomlinson, I.; Swanton, C. Cancer: Evolution within a lifetime. *Annu. Rev. Genet.* **2014**, *48*, 215–236. [CrossRef] [PubMed]
27. Maley, C.C.; Aktipis, A.; Graham, T.A.; Sottoriva, A.; Boddy, A.M.; Janiszewska, M.; Silva, A.S.; Gerlinger, M.; Yuan, Y.; Pienta, K.J.; et al. Classifying the evolutionary and ecological features of neoplasms. *Nat. Rev. Cancer* **2017**, *17*, 605–619. [CrossRef]
28. Somarelli, J.A.; Ware, K.E.; Kostadinov, R.; Robinson, J.M.; Amri, H.; Abu-Asab, M.; Fourie, N.; Diogo, R.; Swofford, D.; Townsend, J.P. Phyloonocology: Understanding cancer through phylogenetic analysis. *Biochim. Biophys. Acta* **2017**, *1867*, 101–108. [CrossRef]

29. Somarelli, J.A.; Shetler, S.; Jolly, M.K.; Wang, X.; Bartholf Dewitt, S.; Hish, A.J.; Gilja, S.; Eward, W.C.; Ware, K.E.; Levine, H.; et al. Mesenchymal-epithelial transition in sarcomas is controlled by the combinatorial expression of MicroRNA 200s and GRHL2. *Mol. Cell. Biol.* **2016**, *36*, 2503–2513. [CrossRef]
30. Saitou, N.; Nei, M. The neighbor-joining method: A new method for reconstructing phylogenetic trees. *Mol. Biol. Evol.* **1987**, *4*, 406–425.
31. Hillis, D.M.; Bull, J.J. An empirical test of bootstrapping as a method for assessing confidence in phylogenetic analysis. *Syst. Biol.* **1993**, *42*, 182–192. [CrossRef]
32. Wiens, J.J. Polymorphic characters in phylogenetic systematics. *Syst. Biol.* **1995**, *44*, 482–500. [CrossRef]
33. Hillis, D.M.; Huelsenbeck, J.P.; Cunningham, C.W. Application and accuracy of molecular phylogenies. *Science* **1994**, *264*, 671–677. [CrossRef] [PubMed]
34. Paradis, E.; Claude, J.; Strimmer, K. Ape: Analyses of phylogenetics and evolution in R language. *Bioinformatics* **2004**, *20*, 289–290. [CrossRef]
35. Schliep, K.P. Phangorn: Phylogenetic analysis in R. *Bioinformatics* **2011**, *27*, 592–593. [CrossRef] [PubMed]
36. Berriz, G.F.; King, O.D.; Bryant, B.; Sander, C.; Roth, F.P. Characterizing gene sets with funcassociate. *Bioinformatics* **2003**, *19*, 2502–2504. [CrossRef] [PubMed]
37. Kogan-Sakin, I.; Tabach, Y.; Buganim, Y.; Molchadsky, A.; Solomon, H.; Madar, S.; Kamer, I.; Stambolsky, P.; Shelly, A.; Goldfinger, N.; et al. Mutant p53(R175H) upregulates Twist1 expression and promotes epithelial-mesenchymal transition in immortalized prostate cells. *Cell. Death Differ.* **2011**, *18*, 271–281. [CrossRef]
38. Sartor, M.A.; Mahavisno, V.; Keshamouni, V.G.; Cavalcoli, J.; Wright, Z.; Karnovsky, A.; Kuick, R.; Jagadish, H.V.; Mirel, B.; Weymouth, T.; et al. ConceptGen: A gene set enrichment and gene set relation mapping tool. *Bioinformatics* **2010**, *26*, 456–463. [CrossRef]
39. Takahashi, E.; Nagano, O.; Ishimoto, T.; Yae, T.; Suzuki, Y.; Shinoda, T.; Nakamura, S.; Niwa, S.; Ikeda, S.; Koga, H.; et al. Tumor necrosis factor-alpha regulates transforming growth factor-beta-dependent epithelial-mesenchymal transition by promoting hyaluronan-CD44-moesin interaction. *J. Biol. Chem.* **2010**, *285*, 4060–4073. [CrossRef]
40. Lovisa, S.; LeBleu, V.S.; Tampe, B.; Sugimoto, H.; Vadnagara, K.; Carstens, J.L.; Wu, C.C.; Hagos, Y.; Burckhardt, B.C.; Pentcheva-Hoang, T.; et al. Epithelial-to-mesenchymal transition induces cell cycle arrest and parenchymal damage in renal fibrosis. *Nat. Med.* **2015**, *21*, 998–1009. [CrossRef]
41. Vega, S.; Morales, A.V.; Ocana, O.H.; Valdes, F.; Fabregat, I.; Nieto, M.A. Snail blocks the cell cycle and confers resistance to cell death. *Genes Dev.* **2004**, *18*, 1131–1143. [CrossRef]
42. Cheong, H.; Lindsten, T.; Thompson, C.B. Autophagy and ammonia. *Autophagy* **2012**, *8*, 122–123. [CrossRef]
43. Du, B.; Shim, J.S. Targeting epithelial-mesenchymal transition (EMT) to overcome drug resistance in cancer. *Molecules* **2016**, *21*. [CrossRef] [PubMed]
44. Singh, A.; Settleman, J. Emt, cancer stem cells and drug resistance: An emerging axis of evil in the war on cancer. *Oncogene* **2010**, *29*, 4741–4751. [CrossRef]
45. Fischer, K.R.; Durrans, A.; Lee, S.; Sheng, J.; Li, F.; Wong, S.T.; Choi, H.; El Rayes, T.; Ryu, S.; Troeger, J.; et al. Epithelial-to-mesenchymal transition is not required for lung metastasis but contributes to chemoresistance. *Nature* **2015**, *527*, 472–476. [CrossRef] [PubMed]
46. Zheng, X.; Carstens, J.L.; Kim, J.; Scheible, M.; Kaye, J.; Sugimoto, H.; Wu, C.C.; Le Bleu, V.S.; Kalluri, R. Epithelial-to-mesenchymal transition is dispensable for metastasis but induces chemoresistance in pancreatic cancer. *Nature* **2015**, *527*, 525–530. [CrossRef] [PubMed]
47. Sui, X.; Chen, R.; Wang, Z.; Huang, Z.; Kong, N.; Zhang, M.; Han, W.; Lou, F.; Yang, J.; Zhang, Q.; et al. Autophagy and chemotherapy resistance: A promising therapeutic target for cancer treatment. *Cell. Death Dis* **2013**, *4*, e838. [CrossRef] [PubMed]
48. Yang, Z.J.; Chee, C.E.; Huang, S.; Sinicrope, F.A. The role of autophagy in cancer: Therapeutic implications. *Mol. Cancer Ther.* **2011**, *10*, 1533–1541. [CrossRef] [PubMed]
49. Schiller, J.H.; Larson, T.; Ou, S.H.; Limentani, S.; Sandler, A.; Vokes, E.; Kim, S.; Liau, K.; Bycott, P.; Olszanski, A.J.; et al. Efficacy and safety of axitinib in patients with advanced non-small-cell lung cancer: Results from a phase ii study. *J. Clin. Oncol.* **2009**, *27*, 3836–3841. [CrossRef] [PubMed]
50. Mross, K.; Frost, A.; Steinbild, S.; Hedbom, S.; Buchert, M.; Fasol, U.; Unger, C.; Kratzschmar, J.; Heinig, R.; Boix, O.; et al. A phase I dose-escalation study of regorafenib (BAY 73-4506), an inhibitor of oncogenic,

angiogenic, and stromal kinases, in patients with advanced solid tumors. *Clin. Cancer Res.* **2012**, *18*, 2658–2667. [CrossRef]
51. Neal, J.W.; Dahlberg, S.E.; Wakelee, H.A.; Aisner, S.C.; Bowden, M.; Huang, Y.; Carbone, D.P.; Gerstner, G.J.; Lerner, R.E.; Rubin, J.L.; et al. Erlotinib, cabozantinib, or erlotinib plus cabozantinib as second-line or third-line treatment of patients with EGFR wild-type advanced non-small-cell lung cancer (ECOG-ACRIN 1512): A randomised, controlled, open-label, multicentre, phase 2 trial. *Lancet Oncol.* **2016**, *17*, 1661–1671. [CrossRef]
52. Nowell, P.C. The clonal evolution of tumor cell populations. *Science* **1976**, *194*, 23–28. [CrossRef] [PubMed]
53. Lipinski, K.A.; Barber, L.J.; Davies, M.N.; Ashenden, M.; Sottoriva, A.; Gerlinger, M. Cancer evolution and the limits of predictability in precision cancer medicine. *Trends Cancer* **2016**, *2*, 49–63. [CrossRef] [PubMed]
54. Feinberg, A.P. Epigenetic stochasticity, nuclear structure and cancer: The implications for medicine. *J. Intern. Med.* **2014**, *276*, 5–11. [CrossRef]
55. Ostrow, S.L.; Barshir, R.; DeGregori, J.; Yeger-Lotem, E.; Hershberg, R. Cancer evolution is associated with pervasive positive selection on globally expressed genes. *PLoS Genet.* **2014**, *10*, e1004239. [CrossRef] [PubMed]
56. Casasent, A.K.; Edgerton, M.; Navin, N.E. Genome evolution in ductal carcinoma in situ: Invasion of the clones. *J. Pathol.* **2017**, *241*, 208–218. [CrossRef]
57. Seyfried, T.N.; Huysentruyt, L.C. On the origin of cancer metastasis. *Crit. Rev. Oncog.* **2013**, *18*, 43–73. [CrossRef]
58. Gatenby, R.; Brown, J. The evolution and ecology of resistance in cancer therapy. *Cold Spring Harb. Perspect. Med.* **2018**, *8*. [CrossRef]
59. Kurtz, I.; Dass, P.D.; Cramer, S. The importance of renal ammonia metabolism to whole body acid-base balance: A reanalysis of the pathophysiology of renal tubular acidosis. *Miner. Electrolyte Metab.* **1990**, *16*, 331–340.
60. Eng, C.H.; Yu, K.; Lucas, J.; White, E.; Abraham, R.T. Ammonia derived from glutaminolysis is a diffusible regulator of autophagy. *Sci. Signal.* **2010**, *3*. [CrossRef]
61. Guido, C.; Whitaker-Menezes, D.; Capparelli, C.; Balliet, R.; Lin, Z.; Pestell, R.G.; Howell, A.; Aquila, S.; Ando, S.; Martinez-Outschoorn, U.; et al. Metabolic reprogramming of cancer-associated fibroblasts by TGF-β drives tumor growth: Connecting TGF-β signaling with "warburg-like" cancer metabolism and l-lactate production. *Cell Cycle* **2012**, *11*, 3019–3035. [CrossRef] [PubMed]
62. Razani, B.; Zhang, X.L.; Bitzer, M.; von Gersdorff, G.; Bottinger, E.P.; Lisanti, M.P. Caveolin-1 regulates transforming growth factor TGF-β /SMAD signaling through an interaction with the TGF-β type I receptor. *J. Biol. Chem.* **2001**, *276*, 6727–6738. [CrossRef] [PubMed]
63. Shiroto, T.; Romero, N.; Sugiyama, T.; Sartoretto, J.L.; Kalwa, H.; Yan, Z.; Shimokawa, H.; Michel, T. Caveolin-1 is a critical determinant of autophagy, metabolic switching, and oxidative stress in vascular endothelium. *PLoS ONE* **2014**, *9*, e87871. [CrossRef]
64. Pasquini, G.; Giaccone, G. C-met inhibitors for advanced non-small cell lung cancer. *Expert Opin. Investig. Drugs* **2018**, *27*, 363–375. [CrossRef]
65. Rastogi, I.; Rajanna, S.; Webb, A.; Chhabra, G.; Foster, B.; Webb, B.; Puri, N. Mechanism of c-met and EGFR tyrosine kinase inhibitor resistance through epithelial mesenchymal transition in non-small cell lung cancer. *Biochem. Biophys. Res. Commun.* **2016**, *477*, 937–944. [CrossRef] [PubMed]
66. Barrow-McGee, R.; Kishi, N.; Joffre, C.; Menard, L.; Hervieu, A.; Bakhouche, B.A.; Noval, A.J.; Mai, A.; Guzman, C.; Robert-Masson, L.; et al. Beta 1-integrin-c-met cooperation reveals an inside-in survival signalling on autophagy-related endomembranes. *Nat. Commun.* **2016**, *7*, 11942. [CrossRef] [PubMed]

© 2019 by the authors. Licensee MDPI, Basel, Switzerland. This article is an open access article distributed under the terms and conditions of the Creative Commons Attribution (CC BY) license (http://creativecommons.org/licenses/by/4.0/).

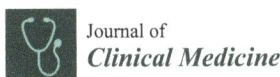 

Review

# Dynamics of Phenotypic Heterogeneity Associated with EMT and Stemness during Cancer Progression

Mohit Kumar Jolly [1],* and Toni Celià-Terrassa [2],*

[1] Centre for BioSystems Science and Engineering, Indian Institute of Science, Bangalore 560012, India
[2] Cancer Research Program, IMIM (Hospital del Mar Medical Research Institute), 08003 Barcelona, Spain
* Correspondence: mkjolly@iisc.ac.in (M.K.J.); acelia@imim.es (T.C.-T.)

Received: 30 July 2019; Accepted: 23 September 2019; Published: 25 September 2019

**Abstract:** Genetic and phenotypic heterogeneity contribute to the generation of diverse tumor cell populations, thus enhancing cancer aggressiveness and therapy resistance. Compared to genetic heterogeneity, a consequence of mutational events, phenotypic heterogeneity arises from dynamic, reversible cell state transitions in response to varying intracellular/extracellular signals. Such phenotypic plasticity enables rapid adaptive responses to various stressful conditions and can have a strong impact on cancer progression. Herein, we have reviewed relevant literature on mechanisms associated with dynamic phenotypic changes and cellular plasticity, such as epithelial–mesenchymal transition (EMT) and cancer stemness, which have been reported to facilitate cancer metastasis. We also discuss how non-cell-autonomous mechanisms such as cell–cell communication can lead to an emergent population-level response in tumors. The molecular mechanisms underlying the complexity of tumor systems are crucial for comprehending cancer progression, and may provide new avenues for designing therapeutic strategies.

**Keywords:** cellular dynamics; epithelial-to-mesenchymal transition; cell plasticity; cancer stem cells; mathematical modeling; population homeostasis

## 1. Introduction

Genetic and phenotypic tumor heterogeneity can act as a major bottleneck for the clinical management of cancers [1]. Genetic heterogeneity has been a long-standing focus in cancer progression research [2]. However, non-genetic factors such as phenotypic plasticity [3–5] and collective effects resulting from cell–cell communication [6–9] have gained recent attention for their proposed roles in tumor aggressiveness. Two major interconnected axes of phenotypic plasticity that have been extensively studied across multiple carcinomas are the epithelial–mesenchymal transition (EMT) and cancer stem cell (CSC) plasticity [10–14]. Initially, EMT was hypothesized to be an irreversible event similar to oncogenic transformation and was referred as "epithelial–mesenchymal transformation" [15]. However, during the last decade many studies have demonstrated beyond doubt its dynamic reversible nature in cancer. "Epithelial–mesenchymal plasticity" (EMP) has recently become commonly used terminology, encompassing bidirectional transitions among epithelial (E), mesenchymal (M), and one or more hybrid E/M phenotypes [16]. EMP is a "motor of cellular plasticity" [17], as it accompanies cell changes in immune response [18,19], tumor-initiation potential [8,20–22], metabolic reprogramming [23,24], senescence [25], cell proliferation [26,27], and drug resistance [14,28]. Similarly, the "cancer stem cell (CSC) model" initially portrayed CSCs as a small, fixed population which emerge from tissue-specific stem cells at the apex of hierarchical cellular differentiation in tumors. However, recent findings have demonstrated the transitionary nature of CSC populations and their different origins from differentiated cell types [29,30]. Thus, EMP and stemness can give rise to dynamic phenotypic heterogeneity in tumors by virtue of their reversibility and plasticity.

Various technological advancements and interdisciplinary cross-fertilization of ideas have led us through these paradigm shifts and emphasized the importance of unraveling the operating principles of cell state transitions along the axes of EMP and/or CSCs. Herein, we have reviewed how investigations at a single-cell level through reporter cell lines, real-time imaging, flow/mass cytometry, high-throughput dynamic measurements—integrated iteratively with mechanism-based mathematical modeling and data-based statistical modeling—have revealed unprecedented insights into the emergent dynamics of cancer progression, at both an intracellular and cell population level.

## 2. Dynamics of EMT

EMT is a nonlinear and reversible trans-differentiation process of an epithelial cell into a mesenchymal phenotype, encompassing changes in multiple phenotypic characteristics such as apico-basal polarity, cell–cell adhesion, cytoskeleton remodeling, cell–matrix adhesion, and cell migration and invasion [31,32]. EMT-inducing transcription factors include ZEB1/2, SNAI1/2, and TWIST, among others. The loss of epithelial molecules such as E-cadherin and the gain of mesenchymal markers such as vimentin and alpha smooth muscle actin ($\alpha$SMA) represent typical molecular features of EMT [16]. Furthermore, EMT is critical for embryonic development and wound healing, and is involved in pathological conditions such as cancer [16,33]. In cancer progression, EMT has been associated with metastasis, drug-resistance, immune evasion, and reduced patient survival/poor prognosis [14,17,34]. While the dynamics of EMT and its reverse mesenchymal-to-epithelial transition (MET) have been studied in developmental contexts for a long time [16,35], they have only recently received attention in the field of cancer [36–40].

EMT and MET have been canonically thought of as "all-or-none" responses, typically because only a few markers were used as a readout at the start and end points of the transition, with little attention to the dynamics and intermediate states. Recently, advanced live-cell imaging [41,42], transcriptomic profiling at multiple timepoints during EMT and/or MET [43,44], flow cytometry [45–47], high-throughput single-cell RNA-seq [48–50], morphological quantification [51,52], and mass cytometry analysis [53], coupled with mechanism-based mathematical modeling of EMT networks [54], have been used to reveal insights into the dynamics and intermediate states of EMT/MET. While these new sophisticated experimental tools and measurements allow the dynamics of EMT/MET to be tracked in multiple cells using a cohort of markers, mathematical models offer a framework in which to elucidate the mechanisms underlying these dynamics and generate hypotheses that can be experimentally tested. Thus, mathematical models can help to interpret experimental data, unveil complex dynamic patterns, predict cellular responses, and eventually contribute to the design of further expeirments [55]. Remarkably, mathematical models have decongested the understanding of EMT by predicting the existence of stable intermediate EMT or hybrid epithelial/mesenchymal (E/M) states [56–58]. Cells in these hybrid E/M phenotypes have been identified in cell lines in vitro and in vivo in primary tumors, circulating tumor cells, and metastases across multiple cancers [46,59–62]. These hybrid E/M phenotypes may be maintained by "phenotypic stability factors" such as NUMB, OVOL2, GRHL2, and NRF2 [57,63–65], a combination of EMT- and MET-inducing signals such as TGF-$\beta$ and all-trans retinoic acid (ATRA) [66,67], or via cell–cell communication through mechanisms such as Notch–Jagged signaling [68]. Strong evidence for the functional implications of these hybrid E/M phenotype(s) has been reported in both preclinical and clinical settings [46,69]. Examples include (a) their role in tumor formation in mice [20,60], (b) mediating collective cell migration and invasion through aggregates or clusters of circulating tumor cells (CTCs) [70], and (c) the correlation of hybrid E/M signatures with poor patient prognosis in many cancers [71].

Further, these mathematical models have also predicted the co-existence of multiple phenotypes in an otherwise genetically identical population [56]. Such non-genetic heterogeneity has been observed in multiple cell lines, wherein cells harboring both epithelial and mesenchymal signatures were found to co-exist alongside populations predominantly expressing either epithelial or mesenchymal markers [45,46,72]. The relative frequency of these phenotypes can vary depending on the genetic background and other factors, such as the micro-envrionmental milieu or markers used for identification [47,73–75]. Nonetheless, the co-existence of different cell subpopulations may enable cooperation among them during metastatic progression [8,9,76,77]. For instance, in vitro and in vivo mixing of more epithelial (PC-3/Mc) and more mesenchymal (PC-3/S) subpopulations of prostate cancer cells was reported to enhance local invasive potential and metastastic colonization of the former [8]. Other studies have documented the influence of paracrine signals from EMT-like cells on non-metastatic cell populations via activation of Hedgehog/GLI signaling to facilitate metastasis [9]. While the exact molecular mechanisms and emergent outcomes of such co-operation are yet to be experimentally determined, these processes are reminiscent of survival strategies observed in diverse ecological systems, such as quorum sensing in bacterial colonies, division of labor, and bet-hedging [78].

Intriguingly, the co-existence of these distinct phenotypes can be explained by the presence of multiple "attractors" or stable states in the multi-dimensional landscape of epithelial–mesenchymal plasticity. An attractor represents a stable cell phenotype which cells starting with varying levels of molecules can converge towards, depending on the crosstalk among different nodes of an interaction network. The concept of attractors is borrowed from a Waddington's landscape which depicts how a stem cell progresses from an undifferentiated state to a differentiated one [79]. In this framework, a stem cell—represented by a ball—rolls down the rugged landscape and eventually enters one of the valleys at the foot of the hill (Figure 1a). These valleys are the attaractors of a system [80]. Systems with more than one attractor are called "multistable" and have been experimentally observed in other biological contexts as well, such as during development, where one progenitor cell can give rise to two or more differentiated cell fates [81]. These attractors are governed by the complex, interlinked EMT regulatory networks operating at multiple levels—transcriptional, translational, post-translational, and epigenetic [80,82] (Figure 1a). The presence of these attractors raises the possibility that isogenic cells can respond differently to the same dose and duration of identical EMT-inducing stimuli. This cell-to-cell variability can arise due to multiple factors including cell cycle stage, stochasticity/fluctuations in biochemical reaction rates, concentrations of various molecular species, etc. [83]. Indeed, NMuMG mammary epithelial cells exposed to specific durations and concentrations of TGF-β were observed to respond largely in a bimodal manner—one subpopulation readily lost E-cadherin expression while the other remained epithelial; a similar trend was observed consistently across a larger panel of cell lines [47]. Notably, this bimodality existed only at intermediate concentrations or durations of TGF-β treatment; all cells maintained an E-cadherin$^{high}$ state at very low concentrations, and all of them switched to E-cadherin$^{low}$ at very high concentrations (Figure 1b). Such dose-/time-dependent bimodality indicates that isogenic cells can attain more than one phenotype under the same experimental conditions. The phenotype attained by an individual cell depends on its genetic and epigenetic background, which determines how "poised" a cell is to alter its biophysical and/or biochemical traits in response to varying extents of stimuli capable of eliciting an EMT response [32].

Multistability, or the presence of multiple attractors, can also drive non-genetic heterogeneity during chemotherapeutic responses and lead to resistance, a feature associated with EMT [28]. For instance, the treatment of a clonal cell population with apoptosis-inducing stimulus TRAIL (TNF-related apoptosis-inducing ligand) for the same duration and dose was shown to negatively affect viability only in a fraction of cells, while the rest survived [84]. This heterogeneity was attributed to a high variance in protein levels for a common set of apoptotic regulators. Such variability may contribute to treatment failure and provide a long-standing reservoir of cells that can gain drug resistance by virtue of newly acquired genetic alterations [85,86]. With this increased appreciation of the complexity associated with EMT/MET processes, we should practice caution in defining the exact parameters that should be referred to as EMT/MET (or various shades of these transitions) in vitro and in vivo to minimize further ambiguity.

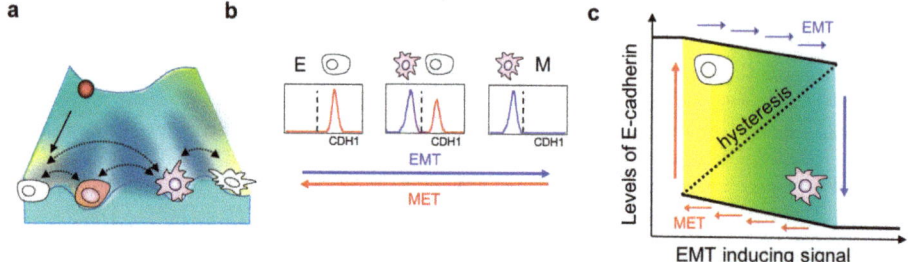

**Figure 1.** Non-genetic heterogeneity and hysteresis during epithelial–mesenchymal transition (EMT). (**a**) Representation of a Waddington's landscape with attractors of different EMT states. (**b**) Epithelial cells (left panel) from an isogenic population may respond differently to the same dose of EMT-inducing signals such as TGF-β (middle panel), while all of them may undergo a complete EMT at a higher dose of the signal (right panel). (**c**) Asymmetry in the "forward reaction" and "backward reaction", i.e., the concentration of the EMT-inducing signal at which all cells switch from being epithelial to mesenchymal (downward blue arrow) is not the same as the one at which all cells switch in the other direction (upward red arrow).

The presence of multiple attractors in a given system allows another interesting dynamic property: Cells exhibiting a particular phenotype (E, M, or hybrid E/M) can transition spontaneously to another phenotype under the influence of "intrinsic noise" or "extrinsic noise" in biological systems [87]. Such "spontaneous switching" between E and M states was recently demonstrated in mouse prostate cancer cells: The cell population was first sorted based on EpCAM and vimentin levels through fluorescence-activated cell sorting, and then cultured independently. Cells of each of the three sub-populations (EpCAM$^+$ Vim$^-$, EpCAM$^+$ Vim$^+$, and EpCAM$^-$ Vim$^+$), when cultured independently, were able to switch to the other two subpopulations [75]. Similar observations were made in a PMC42-LA breast cancer cell line where EpCAM levels were used to segregate cells as epithelial (EpCAM$^+$) or mesenchymal (EpCAM$^-$) [73]. These subpopulations underwent phenotypic transitions and reverted to the phenotypic distribution seen in the parental population. The authors demonstrated that these transitions were not driven by chromosomal instability, thus emphasizing a non-genetic mechanism underlying these phenotypic transitions. In vivo evidence for "spontaneous induction" of EMT was also reported recently in MMTV-PyMT mice [88]. However, the quantification of transition rates among different phenotypes has yet to be done rigorously. Mathematical models can play a crucial role in identifying the underlying context-dependent cues that can give rise to various EMT population distributions [89]. Future studies integrating experimental and theoretical approaches, similar to the attempts made for CSC dynamics, may pave the path to a holistic comprehension of these processes [12].

## 3. Hysteresis/Cellular Memory Effects during EMT Dynamics

Another hallmark of multistable systems is the possibility of cellular memory or hysteresis (Figure 1c). As discussed earlier, isogenic cells exposed to the same strength and duration of a signal may respond differently because they are placed in different attractors. Therefore, the response of a cell not only depends on the stimuli received in real time, but also on the history of input stimuli encountered previously that may have driven them to occupy specific attractors [90]. This property is typically described as "cellular memory". One of the first reports connecting multistability to cellular memory in mammalian systems exposed HL60 cells to increasing concentrations of DMSO for 7 days to differentiate them into neutrophils (forward reaction), and subsequently these fully differentiated neutrophils were resuspended in decreasing concentrations of DMSO for the same duration (backward reaction). Interestingly, the fraction of cells expressing CD11b—the surface marker for neutrophils—was different in the two trajectories for the same concentration of DMSO treatment.

This asymmetry in response was attributed to underlying multistability: Because every cell had multiple possible attractors—$CD11b^{hi}$ and $CD11b^{lo}$—their likelihood of acquiring one phenotype or the other depended not only on the DMSO received instantaneously, but also on all DMSO treatments received in the past [90]. Similar observations were recently made in cells undergoing EMT and their reverse MET [47,53]. HCC827 lung cancer cells treated with increasing concentrations of TGF-β to induce EMT (forward reaction) followed by progressively decreasing concentrations of TGF-β to induce MET (backward reaction) exhibited assymetric transition trajectories, as measured by 28 markers at a single-cell level. Furthermore, some cells did not revert to the epithelial phenotype even when TGF-β was completely withdrawn, indicating cellular memory [53]. The irreversibility of EMT has also been reported elsewhere [91–93], most likely due to "extreme" EMT induction. Nonetheless, the mechanisms of such irreversibility have yet to be identified comprehensively. However, preliminary evidence suggests that epigenetic treatments may help disrupt such irreversibility and permit the to reversion of cells to an epithelial phenotype [94,95], as many canonical epithelial genes such as E-cadherin can be epigenetically silenced during EMT progression [96,97].

Compared to EMT, molecular mechanisms mediating MET are relatively less characterized [98]. GRHL2—a transcription factor that activates CDH1 (E-cadherin) and CLDN4 (Claudin-4)—and OVOL1/2 can repress EMT-associated transcription factors and drive MET [99–101]. However, the overexpression of OVOL2, GRHL2, or E-cadherin may not always be sufficient to drive complete MET [95,102–104]. These observations reinforce the aspect that cells may navigate through different paths in the multi-dimensional landscape of EMP to undergo EMT or MET in a context-dependent manner; thus, the dynamics of EMT and MET need not be always symmetrical.

The bidirectional communication between computational and experimental approaches has been pivotal in gaining new insights into the dynamics of carcinoma EMT and MET. These insights have been suggestive of potential therapeutic strategies, particularly for reducing metastatic aggressiveness that exhibits a greater dependency on cellular plasticity than genetic mutations [105]. Firstly, driving tumor cells into a "locked" or "irreversible" mesenchymal state may compromise their ability to colonize distant organs, as observed in previous reports [8,20,46,106]. Secondly, mutually inhibitory feedback loops have been identified as regulators of multiple facets of cellular plasticity in cancer progression—EMT/MET [17,107], mesenchymal–amoeboid transition (MAT), and amoeboid–mesenchymal transition (AMT) [108], matrix-detached and matrix-attached states [109], and metabolic switching between oxidative phosphorylation and glycolysis [110]. Congruently, such feedback loops have also been observed to mediate various cell-fate decisions during embryonic development [111]. Disruption of such feedback loops may reduce cellular plasticity and curb metastatic potential in vivo [47]. Finally, the mechanisms responsible for maintaining the hybrid E/M phenotype(s)—considered more aggressive and metastatic in contrast to "extremely epithelial" or "extremely mesenchymal" ones [20,112]—can be targeted to reduce metastasis. These hybrid E/M cells exhibit higher tumor-initiating or cancer-stem-cell-like (CSC-like) properties than extremely epithelial or extremely mesenchymal populations [13,20], a notion supported by accumulating clinical evidence wherein co-expression of epithelial and mesenchymal markers tends to be associated with a poor patient survival across cancer types [71].

While an iterative interplay between mathematical models and experimental data has unraveled key design principles of the dynamics of cellular plasticity and heterogeneity during EMT/MET, many open questions remain. For instance, it remains to be identified how many hybrid E/M phenotypes exist and what the similarities and differences in their functional attributes are. While mathematical models of different regulatory networks have a common prediction that EMT/MET is not a binary process, different numbers of hybrid E/M states with varying molecular signatures have been predicted [113–115]. Which combination of molecular markers is most appropriate to experimentally identify these hybrid E/M phenotype(s) needs to be commonly agreed upon [71]. A robust identification of such markers could help affirm/falsify the predictions from these models, and fuel this interdisciplinary approach to classification of the '"common organizing principles" underlying the "myriad phenotypic complexities" [116] associated with various aspects of tumor progression, including metastasis.

## 4. Phenotypic Interconversions of Cancer Stem Cell Populations

Cancer stem cells (CSCs) are cells with self-renewal capacity that lead tumor initiation and give rise to the differentiated cells which constitute phenotypically heterogeneous tumors [29,117,118]. The notion of their existence has been around for over a century, but it gained more attention when the first CSC-specific markers were identified in hematological and solid tumors [119–121]. These populations have been reported to originate from normal stem cells, progenitor cells and differentiated cells that undergo a dedifferentiation process during malignant transformation (Figure 2a). Several markers have been described to define CSC populations in different cancer types; for instance, $CD24^{-/low}/CD44^{high}$ markers delineate a common CSC population for breast cancer, colorectal cancer, ovarian cancer, liver cancer, and others [122]. Interestingly, this population is characterized as the mesenchymal-like CSC population in breast cancer [123]. ALDH (aldehyde dehydrogenase) activity is another pan-CSC marker which can be employed for dissecting epithelial-like or E/M-hybrid-like CSCs [123], suggesting the existence of different CSC subsets within the same tumor depending on their EMT state. Indeed, CSCs can also exist in a quiescent or highly proliferative state, as has been reported since early seminal studies [124].

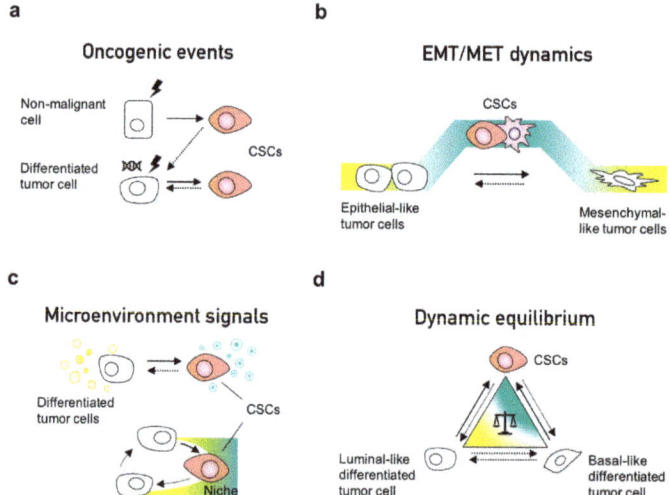

**Figure 2.** Origins and dynamics of cancer stem cells (CSCs). (**a**) CSCs can originate from normal cells during malignant transformation, induced by oncogenic events. Separately, additional genotoxic insults on malignant cells can lead to a dedifferentiation process of differentiated tumor cells into CSCs. Black and white cells are differentiated cells and colored cells are CSCs. (**b**) EMT/MET generates stem cell properties in cancer cells; however, extreme EMT can cause a loss of stemness potential. Therefore, cell plasticity and reversibility are important features in reversion to hybrid E/M states. (**c**) Microenvironmental signals can induce stemness in non-CSCs, e.g., cytokines such as IL-6 or TGF-β. In addition, tumor cells can hijack the niche of normal stem cells, inducing dedifferentiation and stemness in cancer cells. (**d**) Tumor cell populations tend to maintain their inherent proportion of CSCs. Differentiated phenotypes and lineages in tumours, either luminal and basal, can switch to CSCs when these are depleted or diminished due to experimental approaches or anticancer treatments.

The CSC phenotype is a dynamic state rather than a fixed population, as confirmed by lineage tracing in breast cancer models [125] and in human colorectal xenotransplants [30], wherein a continuous turnover of CSCs has been observed. Other in vitro models have also shown that CSCs can arise from non-CSCs [12,126,127]; for instance, cells undergoing EMT can convert from non-CSCs to CSCs [22] (Figure 2b). A recent study using lineage tracing and RNA-seq demonstrated that EMT occurs continuously during early tumorigenesis in individual clones [128], thus enabling CSC properties. EMT implies a transdifferentiation from an epithelial to a mesenchymal phenotype; therefore, it is not surprising that cells first dedifferentiate—increasing stemness—prior to their entry into the mesenchymal-like state. Thus, consistent with in silico predictions from mechanistic mathematical models [21], stemness has been observed to peak in the hybrid E/M state(s) rather than terminal epithelial or mesenchymal states [20,46]. Interestingly, in breast cancer, non-CSC to CSC conversions have been observed to occur more often in the basal-like subtype than in the luminal-like subtypes. This difference is due to the maintenance of bivalent or "poised" chromatin marks on the ZEB1promoter—an important EMT inducer—able to quickly respond to environmental signals [129]. Indeed, such poised marks have also been demonstrated for crucial cell-fate regulators in the differentiation of embryonic stem cells [130].

Dynamic reversible processes such as EMT can mediate interconversion among CSCs and non-CSCs. Besides EMT, cancer cells can also take alternate routes to acquire CSC properties, which include undergoing a dedifferentiation process by oncogenic transformation [127,131], acquisition of new mutations [132,133], reversible senescence [134], and in response to inflammatory signals from the microenvironment [11] (Figure 2a–c). In colorectal differentiated tumor cells, NF-κB signaling has been shown to activate the Wnt pathway to induce dedifferentiation, re-expression of Lgr5, gain of stem cell properties, and increased tumor initiation ability [135]. In addition, cancer cells can outcompete resident stem cells and occupy their supportive niches to acquire stem cell properties [11,136,137]. Interestingly, the depletion of Lgr5$^+$ cells ceases tumor growth of CRC, yet tumor growth is restored by the spontaneous reappearance of Lgr5$^+$ cells in a dedifferentiation event in the primary tumor but not in the metastatic liver site, suggesting the absence of a CSC-supportive niche in the liver [30,138]. Overall, these studies indicate that the CSC state is a dynamic and plastic condition coordinated by tumor intrinsic and extrinsic processes.

Phenotypic plasticity can explain the continuous appearance of CSCs reported in clonal evolution studies [125,139]. In fact, not all cancer types follow the hierarchical CSC model, as reported in melanoma and pancreatic studies by the lack of clonal expansion [139–142]. This observation can be a consequence of highly plastic tumors that continuously interconvert CSC states in equilibrium. In pancreatic cancer, CD133$^+$ tumor-initiating cells are transiently and continuouously generated, since their presence is required for tumor generation [139]. Therefore, the CSC phenotype—transient or sustained—seems to be crucial for tumor and metastasis initiation.

## 5. Dynamic Equilibrium within Cancer Cell Populations

Some studies have demonstrated a dynamic equilibrium between CSC and non-CSC populations (Figure 2d) [143,144]. Similarly to complex systems, tumors can maintain a phenotypic equilibrium for functional redundancy and feedback control [145]. A pioneering study demonstrated how a mixed population of CD44$^{high}$ and CD44$^{low}$ cells sorted from HME (normal human mammary epithelial cells) restored the parental stem-cell-like population. CD44$^{high}$ cells were observed to undergo differentiation while the CD44$^{low}$ population transitioned into the stem-cell-like CD44$^{high}$ phenotype, implying the existence of homeostatic control at population level. An alternate explanation could be different growth rates among stem-cell-like and differentiated cells; further investigation is required to deconvolute these different hypotheses [127]. Another landmark study combined the use of mathematical models and experimental approaches to characterize the equilibria of CSC and non-CSC populations [12]. Two breast cancer cell cell lines (SUM149 and SUM159) used in this study comprised different distributons in terms of luminal-like (L), basal-like (B), and stem cell-like (S) subpopulations. When these three subpopulations were segregated and cultured separately, all subpopulations returned to the original equilibrium of the parental cell line (SUM149 or SUM159, respectively), reminiscent of observations made in PMC42-LA systems [73]. Thus, de novo CSCs emerged independent of the starting point—L or B cells. These findings were later explained using a mathematical model proposing that phenotypic distributions in a given population (cell line) can be maintained due to stochastic cell-state transitions [12]. Another study using these cell lines showed how the aberrant regulation of cell fate determinants such as Slug can alter the balance of interconversion between luminal and basal cell populations [126]. Therefore, a perturbation in key regulatory genes can alter the relative stability of various possible attractors, and consequently generate different phenotypic distributions [146,147].

The population dynamics of cancer cells can also be influenced by extrinsic input fluctuations from microenvironmental signals. For instance, Zeb1 is epigenetically controlled, with bivalent histone marks allowing quick responses to TGF-β signals, impacting the dynamic equilibrium among $CD44^{low}$-non-CSCs and $CD44^{high}$-CSCs [129]. Thus, epigenetic marks can directly govern cell state transitions by affecting the transcriptional accesbility of genes involved in cellular plasticity [148]. TGF-β signaling also participates in maintenance of the equilibrium of non-CSC and $CD133^+$ CSCs, as reported in breast and colon cancer cells in vitro [144]. It is of note that TGF-β signaling also modulates the dynamic heterogeneity in embryonic stem cells by altering the balance of Nodal and BMP pathways [149]. In breast and prostate cancer, inflammatory cytokines such as IL-6, which are also involved in EMT [150], establish a dynamic balance of CSCs and non-CSCs. IL-6 secretion maintains the balance of newly generated CSCs and the CSC differentiation to non-CSCs [131]. In agreement with these studies, stochastic simulations estimated the rates of interconversion between epithelial-proliferative and mesenchymal-quiescence states in breast CSCs. Similarly, disrupting the inflammatory feedback loop signals of IL-6, Stat3, and NF-κB has been predicted to serve as a therapeutic intervention able to eliminate both types of CSCs [151]. This model prediction has yet to be experimentally tested.

## 6. Non-Cell Autonomous Effects of the EMT Process and CSC Identity

Tumors have been postulated to display collective behavior and can be viewed as a community of social cells [78,152]. Indeed, swarm-like behavior has been proposed to facilitate optimal utility of tissue space and induce motility beyond a threshold of tumor population density [153]. This collective behavior could be the result of the synchronized EMT evident in migrating individual mesenchymal cells documented in developmental and cancer models [35,88,154]. Synchronized EMT in cell populations can be observed in embryonic cells that ingress and form the mesoderm in the invagination and epiboly steps of gastrulation. The origins of this spatiotemporal synchrony are often assigned to the "organizer" group of cells, such as the Nieuwkoop center and Spemann organizer, which demarcate the onset of EMT in *Xenopus* embryos [155]. The signal gradients emanating from these node organizers, Wnt/β-catenin, and Nodal/TGF-β dictate the space and time of EMT during gastrulation [155,156]. In cancer, such structures have not yet been determined, as EMT is not likely to be restricted to a particular time or space; instead, it can occur spontaneously during different stages of disease progression and depending on microenvironmental changes.

The current observations of EMT in cancer have been mainly based on detecting morphologically visible invasive cells at tumor margins. Recent evidence suggests continuous EMT in the early stages of tumor development in different clones [128], even in preneoplastic stages [157]. Tumor marginal invasion has been captured by intravital microscopy (IVM), showing the occurrence of spontaneous EMT in individual cells of MMTV-PyMT breast tumors [88,158]. Another intravital imaging study implicated TGF-β in coordinating the local switch from attached groups of cells to cells displaying individual motility [159]. Overall, EMT might be synchronized at a population level in cancer.

Interestingly, E-cadherin has been reported to function as a sensor of cell population density, providing a mechanism by which cell populations may reach phenotypic equilibria through EMT in tissues. Mechanistically, E-cadherin can sense low cell densities and increase the availability of growth receptors, thus favoring downstream EGFR/ERK signaling and β-catenin stabilization to stimulate growth [160–162]. Computational studies have modeled "anti-social" behavior of E-cadherin-negative cells, typical of EMT-like cells, and predicted that their presence could disrupt existing population dynamics, depending on external environmental factors such as calcium levels [160]. This instance is a good example of "secrete-and-sense cells", by which an EMT event could alter homeostasis and influence the entire population.

## 7. Spatiotemporal Dynamics of EMT and CSCs

Cellular phenotypes displaying varying levels of EMT and/or CSCs have been witnessed in vitro and in vivo; one recent focus has been the identification of their spatial localizations within a tumor. One of the first reports on spatial heterogeneity in EMT proved a higher nuclear localization of β-catenin at the invasive edge of primary colorectal carcinomas, while a more cytoplasmic and membranous staining was evident in central tumor areas [163]. Concurrently, membranous E-cadherin was largely retained in central tumor areas but lost at the invasive edge [164,165]. More recently, subsets of CSCs ($CD44^+$/$CD24^-$ and $ALDH^+$) with varying EMT status (mesenchymal and hybrid E/M, respectively) have been described in breast cancers [123,166], with the mesenchymal subset located at the invasive edge and the hybrid E/M subset located in the tumor interior. This spatial distribution can be attributed to gradients of EMT-inducing signals and cell-to-cell communication in tumors [167]. In both aforementioned cases, the mesenchymal subpopulation at the invasive edge of primary tumors has been reported to be quiescent, while the central tumor subpopulation tends to be proliferative [123,163], consistent with the "go-or-grow" (i.e., migrating cells have low proliferation rates) paradigm, as witnessed in in vitro analysis of EMT and cell cycle regulators [26,168]. Single-cell transcriptomic analysis of primary head and neck tumors has further strengthened the finding of prominent mesenchymal features at the invasive edge [48]. Thus, a primary tumor may contain spatially distributed cells with varying extents of EMT [68,167].

Spatiotemporal patterns of EMT and non-EMT cells have been observed in vitro as well. EMT-like cells can induce EMT across the population by paracrine and/or juxtacrine signaling and generate an equilibrium of EMT-induced and non-EMT cells in tumor cell clusters [47,68]. The processes by which a cell population reaches these equilibria in a spatiotemporal manner require further investigation, and this is another example where mathematical modeling could reveal the underlying mechanisms.

This spectrum of heterogeneity has also been observed beyond the primary tumor in disseminated circulating tumor cells (CTCs) from patients across cancer types [59,69,169,170]. CTCs can migrate either as individual cells or in units of two or more cell clusters [169]. Various spatiotemporal patterns in EMT phenotypes may influence frequencies and size distributions of CTC clusters [171], which are considered the primary harbingers of metastasis [172]; thus, an understanding of their characteristics, such as size distribution, frequency, ability to traverse capillaries [173], and molecular profiles of their tumor and/or stromal cell populations [174], holds promise in highlighting new therapeutic vulnerabilities. Connecting these traits of CTC clusters to spatiotemporal dynamics of EMT in a primary tumor has yet to be undertaken comprehensively. Since these CTC clusters can contain various non-cancerous cells such as platelets and fibroblasts, their presence may have many functional consequences in accelerating metastasis; for instance, macrophages may facilitate transendothelial migration and neutrophils may drive cell cycle progression during circulation [175,176]. Thus, future efforts should focus on the mechanistic underpinnings of various modes of cell-to-cell communication, coordination, and cooperation among tumors and stromal cells during the various steps of the metastasis–invasion cascade.

## 8. Conclusions

Dynamic cell plasticity increases the phenotypic heterogeneity of tumors and thus tumor versatility at the population level. This phenomenon increases the complexity of the mechanisms underlying carcinogenesis, metastasis, and its treatment. The study of non-static systems is technically challenging, but the emergence of new techniques able to study single cell phenotypes and cell state transitions through reporter cell lines, real-time imaging in combination with mathematical modeling, and big data analysis sheds light on the existence of dynamic behaviors. Future studies need to focus on decoding the molecular mechanisms responsible for such emergent behaviors at cellular and population levels. An individual renegade cell has long been considered to be the unit of cancer progression. However, with accumulating evidence about collective phenomena at a tissue level, such as engineering of the primary tumor and/or metastatic niche [136,177], collective migration [175], and metabolic synergy [178], we must focus on non-cell autonomous mechanisms of cellular plasticity in the tumor microenvironment [179]. In addition, new studies should attempt to elucidate the nonlinear dynamics of cell-to-cell communication and co-operation in tumor progression. Such an integrative and dynamic understanding will steer us towards outsmarting cancer through innovative approaches such as blocking cellular plasticity bidirectionally and designing adaptive therapies that take into account the evolution of resistance [180].

**Author Contributions:** All authors made significant contributions to the article – conceptuliazation, M.K.J., T.C.-T.; writing – original draft preparation, M.K.J., T.C.-T.; writing—review and editing, M.K.J., T.C.-T.

**Funding:** The work was supported by Ramanujan Fellowship (SB/S2/RJN-049/2018) provided by SERB, Department of Science and Technology, Government of India to M.K.J.; and by the Instituto de Salud Carlos III-FSE (MS17/00037; PI18/00014) and the Cancer Research Institute CLIP grant to T.C.-T.

**Acknowledgments:** We thank the members of our laboratories for helpful discussions, and in particular, S. Varankar and M. von Locquenghiem for the critical reading. We apologize to the investigators whose important studies could not be cited here due to space limitations.

**Conflicts of Interest:** The authors declare no conflict of interest.

## References

1. Hinohara, K.; Polyak, K. Intratumoral Heterogeneity: More Than Just Mutations. *Trends Cell Biol.* **2019**, *29*, 569–579. [CrossRef] [PubMed]
2. Mcgranahan, N.; Swanton, C. Clonal Heterogeneity and Tumor Evolution: Past, Present, and the Future. *Cell* **2017**, *168*, 613–628. [CrossRef] [PubMed]
3. Gupta, P.B.; Pastushenko, I.; Skibinski, A.; Blanpain, C.; Kuperwasser, C. Phenotypic Plasticity: Driver of Cancer Initiation, Progression, and Therapy Resistance. *Cell Stem Cell* **2019**, *24*, 65–78. [CrossRef] [PubMed]
4. Bhatia, S.; Monkman, J.; Toh, A.K.L.; Nagaraj, S.H.; Thompson, E.W. Targeting epithelial–mesenchymal plasticity in cancer: Clinical and preclinical advances in therapy and monitoring. *Biochem. J.* **2017**, *474*, 3269–3306. [CrossRef] [PubMed]
5. Mooney, S.M.; Jolly, M.K.; Levine, H.; Kulkarni, P. Phenotypic plasticity in prostate cancer: Role of intrinsically disordered proteins. *Asian J. Androl.* **2016**, *18*, 704–710. [CrossRef] [PubMed]
6. Grosse-Wilde, A.; Kuestner, R.E.; Skelton, S.M.; MacIntosh, E.; Fouquier d'Herouei, A.; Ertaylan, G.; del Sol, A.; Skupin, A.; Huang, S. Loss of inter-cellular cooperation by complete epithelial-mesenchymal transition supports favorable outcomes in basal breast cancer patients. *Oncotarget* **2018**, *9*, 20018–20033. [CrossRef] [PubMed]
7. Chapman, A.; del Ama, L.F.; Ferguson, J.; Kamarashev, J.; Wellbrock, C.; Hurlstone, A. Heterogeneous tumor subpopulations cooperate to drive invasion. *Cell Rep.* **2014**, *8*, 688–695. [CrossRef] [PubMed]
8. Celià-Terrassa, T.; Meca-Cortés, Ó.; Mateo, F.; De Paz, A.M.; Rubio, N.; Arnal-Estapé, A.; Ell, B.J.; Bermudo, R.; Díaz, A.; Guerra-Rebollo, M.; et al. Epithelial-mesenchymal transition can suppress major attributes of human epithelial tumor-initiating cells. *J. Clin. Investig.* **2012**, *122*, 1849–1868. [CrossRef]
9. Neelakantan, D.; Zhou, H.; Oliphant, M.U.J.; Zhang, X.; Simon, L.M.; Henke, D.M.; Shaw, C.A.; Wu, M.F.; Hilsenbeck, S.G.; White, L.D.; et al. EMT cells increase breast cancer metastasis via paracrine GLI activation in neighbouring tumour cells. *Nat. Commun.* **2017**, *8*, 15773. [CrossRef]
10. Bocci, F.; Jolly, M.K.; George, J.T.; Levine, H.; Onuchic, J.N. A mechanism-based computational model to capture the interconnections among epithelial-mesenchymal transition, cancer stem cells and Notch-Jagged signaling. *Oncotarget* **2018**, *9*, 29906–29920. [CrossRef]
11. Varga, J.; Greten, F.R. Cell plasticity in epithelial homeostasis and tumorigenesis. *Nat. Cell Biol.* **2017**, *19*, 1133–1141. [CrossRef] [PubMed]

12. Gupta, P.B.; Fillmore, C.M.; Jiang, G.; Shapira, S.D.; Tao, K.; Kuperwasser, C.; Lander, E.S. Stochastic state transitions give rise to phenotypic equilibrium in populations of cancer cells. *Cell* **2011**, *146*, 633–644. [CrossRef] [PubMed]
13. Jolly, M.K.; Jia, D.; Boareto, M.; Mani, S.A.; Pienta, K.J.; Ben-Jacob, E.; Levine, H. Coupling the modules of EMT and stemness: A tunable 'stemness window' model. *Oncotarget* **2015**, *6*, 25161–25174. [CrossRef]
14. Singh, A.; Settleman, J. EMT, cancer stem cells and drug resistance: An emerging axis of evil in the war on cancer. *Oncogene* **2011**, *29*, 4741–4751. [CrossRef] [PubMed]
15. Hay, E.D. An overview of epithelio-mesenchymal transformation. *Acta Anat* **1995**, *154*, 8–20. [CrossRef]
16. Nieto, M.A.; Huang, R.Y.Y.J.; Jackson, R.A.A.; Thiery, J.P.P. Emt: 2016. *Cell* **2016**, *166*, 21–45. [CrossRef] [PubMed]
17. Brabletz, S.; Brabletz, T. The ZEB/miR-200 feedback loop—A motor of cellular plasticity in development and cancer? *EMBO Rep.* **2010**, *11*, 670–677. [CrossRef]
18. Tripathi, S.C.; Peters, H.L.; Taguchi, A.; Katayama, H.; Wang, H.; Momin, A.; Jolly, M.K.; Celiktas, M.; Rodriguez-Canales, J.; Liu, H.; et al. Immunoproteasome deficiency is a feature of non-small cell lung cancer with a mesenchymal phenotype and is associated with a poor outcome. *Proc. Natl. Acad. Sci. USA* **2016**, *113*, E1555–E1564. [CrossRef]
19. Chen, L.; Gibbons, D.L.; Goswami, S.; Cortez, M.A.; Ahn, Y.H.; Byers, L.A.; Zhang, X.; Yi, X.; Dwyer, D.; Lin, W.; et al. Metastasis is regulated via microRNA-200/ZEB1 axis control of tumour cell PD-L1 expression and intratumoral immunosuppression. *Nat. Commun.* **2014**, *5*, 1–12. [CrossRef]
20. Kröger, C.; Afeyan, A.; Mraz, J.; Eaton, E.N.; Reinhardt, F.; Khodor, Y.L.; Thiru, P.; Bierie, B.; Ye, X.; Burge, C.B.; et al. Acquisition of a hybrid E/M state is essential for tumorigenicity of basal breast cancer cells. *Proc. Natl. Acad. Sci. USA* **2019**, *116*, 7353–7362. [CrossRef]
21. Jolly, M.K.; Huang, B.; Lu, M.; Mani, S.A.; Levine, H.; Ben-jacob, E. Towards elucidating the connection between epithelial—Mesenchymal transitions and stemness. *J. R. Soc. Interface* **2014**, *11*, 20140962. [CrossRef] [PubMed]
22. Mani, S.A.; Guo, W.; Liao, M.-J.; Eaton, E.N.; Ayyanan, A.; Zhou, A.Y.; Brooks, M.; Reinhard, F.; Zhang, C.C.; Shipitsin, M.; et al. The epithelial-mesenchymal transition generates cells with properties of stem cells. *Cell* **2008**, *133*, 704–715. [CrossRef] [PubMed]
23. Liu, M.; Quek, L.-E.; Sultani, G.; Turner, N. Epithelial-mesenchymal transition induction is associated with augmented glucose uptake and lactate production in pancreatic ductal adenocarcinoma. *Cancer Metab.* **2016**, *4*, 19. [CrossRef] [PubMed]
24. Liu, M.; Hancock, S.E.; Sultani, G.; Wilkins, B.P.; Ding, E.; Osborne, B.; Quek, L.-E.; Turner, N. Snail-Overexpression Induces Epithelial-mesenchymal Transition and Metabolic Reprogramming in Human Pancreatic Ductal Adenocarcinoma and Non-tumorigenic Ductal Cells. *J. Clin. Med.* **2019**, *8*, 822. [CrossRef] [PubMed]
25. Smit, M.A.; Peeper, D.S. Epithelial-mesenchymal transition and senescence: Two cancer-related processes are crossing paths. *Aging* **2010**, *2*, 735–741. [CrossRef] [PubMed]
26. Vega, S.; Morales, A.V.; Ocaña, O.H.; Valdés, F.; Fabregat, I.; Nieto, M.A. Snail blocks the cell cycle and confers resistance to cell death. *Genes Dev.* **2004**, *18*, 1131–1143. [CrossRef] [PubMed]
27. Comaills, V.; Kabeche, L.; Morris, R.; Zou, L.; Daniel, A.; Yu, M.; Madden, M.W.; Licausi, J.A.; Boukhali, M.; Tajima, K.; et al. Genomic Instability Is Induced by Persistent Proliferation of Cells Undergoing Epithelial-to-Mesenchymal Transition. *Cell Rep.* **2016**, *17*, 2632–2647. [CrossRef]
28. Santamaria, P.G.; Moreno-Bueno, G.; Cano, A. Contribution of epithelial plasticity to therapy resistance. *J. Clin. Med.* **2019**, *8*, 676. [CrossRef]
29. Batlle, E.; Clevers, H. Cancer stem cells revisited. *Nat. Med.* **2017**, *23*, 1124–1134. [CrossRef]
30. Shimokawa, M.; Ohta, Y.; Nishikori, S.; Matano, M.; Takano, A.; Fujii, M.; Date, S.; Sugimoto, S.; Kanai, T.; Sato, T. Visualization and targeting of LGR5 + human colon cancer stem cells. *Nature* **2017**, *545*, 187–192. [CrossRef]
31. Savagner, P. Epithelial-mesenchymal transitions: From cell plasticity to concept elasticity. *Curr. Top. Dev. Biol.* **2015**, *112*, 273–300. [PubMed]
32. Jolly, M.K.; Ware, K.E.; Gilja, S.; Somarelli, J.A.; Levine, H. EMT and MET: Necessary or permissive for metastasis? *Mol. Oncol.* **2017**, *11*, 755–769. [CrossRef] [PubMed]

33. Jolly, M.; Boareto, M.; Huang, B.; Jia, D.; Lu, M.; Ben-Jacob, E.; Onuchic, J.N.; Levine, H. Implications of the hybrid epithelial/mesenchymal phenotype in metastasis. *Front. Oncol.* **2015**, *5*, 155. [CrossRef] [PubMed]
34. Dongre, A.; Rashidian, M.; Reinhardt, F.; Bagnato, A.; Keckesova, Z.; Ploegh, H.L.; Weinberg, R.A. Epithelial-to-mesenchymal transition contributes to immunosuppression in breast carcinomas. *Cancer Res.* **2017**, *77*, 3982–3989. [CrossRef] [PubMed]
35. Thiery, J.P.; Acloque, H.; Huang, R.Y.J.; Nieto, M.A. Epithelial-Mesenchymal Transitions in Development and Disease. *Cell* **2009**, *139*, 871–890. [CrossRef] [PubMed]
36. Nieto, M.A. Epithelial plasticity: A common theme in embryonic and cancer cells. *Science* **2013**, *342*, 1234850. [CrossRef] [PubMed]
37. Korpal, M.; Ell, B.J.; Buffa, F.M.; Ibrahim, T.; Blanco, M.A.; Celià-Terrassa, T.; Mercatali, L.; Khan, Z.; Goodarzi, H.; Hua, Y.; et al. Direct targeting of Sec23a by miR-200s influences cancer cell secretome and promotes metastatic colonization. *Nat. Med.* **2011**, *17*, 1101. [CrossRef] [PubMed]
38. Ocaña, O.H.; Córcoles, R.; Fabra, Á.; Moreno-Bueno, G.; Acloque, H.; Vega, S.; Barrallo-Gimeno, A.; Cano, A.; Nieto, M.A. Metastatic Colonization Requires the Repression of the Epithelial-Mesenchymal Transition Inducer Prrx1. *Cancer Cell* **2012**, *22*, 709–724. [CrossRef] [PubMed]
39. Pastushenko, I.; Blanpain, C. EMT Transition States during Tumor Progression and Metastasis. *Trends Cell Biol.* **2019**, *29*, 212–226. [CrossRef] [PubMed]
40. Tsai, J.H.; Donaher, J.L.; Murphy, D.A.; Chau, S.; Yang, J. Spatiotemporal Regulation of Epithelial-Mesenchymal Transition Is Essential for Squamous Cell Carcinoma Metastasis. *Cancer Cell* **2012**, *22*, 725–736. [CrossRef]
41. Toneff, M.J.; Sreekumar, A.; Tinnirello, A.; Hollander, P.D.; Habib, S.; Li, S.; Ellis, M.J.; Xin, L.; Mani, S.A.; Rosen, J.M. The Z-cad dual fluorescent sensor detects dynamic changes between the epithelial and mesenchymal cellular states. *BMC Biol.* **2016**, *14*, 47. [CrossRef] [PubMed]
42. Somarelli, J.A.; Schaeffer, D.; Marengo, M.S.; Bepler, T.; Rouse, D.; Ware, K.E.; Hish, A.J.; Zhao, Y.; Buckley, A.F.; Epstein, J.I.; et al. Distinct routes to metastasis: Plasticity-dependent and plasticity-independent pathways. *Oncogene* **2016**, *35*, 4302–4311. [CrossRef] [PubMed]
43. Stylianou, N.; Lehman, M.L.; Wang, C.; Fard, A.T.; Rockstroh, A.; Fazli, L.; Jovanovic, L.; Ward, M.; Sadowski, M.C.; Kashyap, A.S.; et al. A molecular portrait of epithelial–mesenchymal plasticity in prostate cancer associated with clinical outcome. *Oncogene* **2018**, *38*, 913–934. [CrossRef] [PubMed]
44. Xu, S.; Ware, K.E.; Ding, Y.; Kim, S.-Y.; Sheth, M.; Rao, S.; Chan, W.; Armstrong, A.J.; Eward, W.C.; Jolly, M.; et al. An integrative systems biology and experimental approach identifies convergence of epithelial plasticity, metabolism, and autophagy to promote chemoresistance. *J. Clin. Med.* **2019**, *8*, 205. [CrossRef] [PubMed]
45. George, J.T.; Jolly, M.K.; Xu, S.; Somarelli, J.A.; Levine, H. Survival outcomes in cancer patients predicted by a partial EMT gene expression scoring metric. *Cancer Res.* **2017**, *77*, 6415–6428. [CrossRef] [PubMed]
46. Grosse-Wilde, A.; Fouquier d' Herouei, A.; McIntosh, E.; Ertaylan, G.; Skupin, A.; Kuestner, R.E.; del Sol, A.; Walters, K.-A.; Huang, S. Stemness of the hybrid epithelial/mesenchymal state in breast cancer and its association with poor survival. *PLoS ONE* **2015**, *10*, e0126522. [CrossRef]
47. Celià-Terrassa, T.; Bastian, C.; Liu, D.; Ell, B.; Aiello, N.M.; Wei, Y.; Zamalloa, J.; Blanco, A.M.; Hang, X.; Kunisky, D.; et al. Hysteresis control of epithelial-mesenchymal transition dynamics conveys a distinct program with enhanced metastatic ability. *Nat. Commun.* **2018**, *9*, 5005. [CrossRef] [PubMed]
48. Puram, S.V.; Tirosh, I.; Parikh, A.S.; Patel, A.P.; Yizhak, K.; Gillespie, S.; Rodman, C.; Luo, C.L.; Mroz, E.A.; Emerick, K.S.; et al. Single-Cell Transcriptomic Analysis of Primary and Metastatic Tumor Ecosystems in Head and Neck Cancer. *Cell* **2017**, *171*, 1611–1624. [CrossRef]
49. McFaline-Figueroa, J.L.; Hill, A.J.; Qiu, X.; Jackson, D.; Shendure, J.; Trapnell, C. A pooled single-cell genetic screen identifies regulatory checkpoints in the continuum of the epithelial-to-mesenchymal transition. *Nat. Genet.* **2019**, *51*, 1389–1398. [CrossRef]
50. Cook, D.P.; Vanderhyden, B.C. Comparing transcriptional dynamics of the epithelial-mesenchymal transition. *bioRxiv* **2019**, 732412.
51. Devaraj, V.; Bose, B. Morphological State Transition Dynamics in EGF-Induced Epithelial to Mesenchymal Transition. *J. Clin. Med.* **2019**, *8*, 911. [CrossRef] [PubMed]
52. Leggett, S.E; Sim, J.Y.; Rubins, J.E.; Neronha, Z.J.; Williams, E.K.; Wong, I.Y. Morphological single cell profiling of the epithelial–mesenchymal transition. *Integr. Biol.* **2016**, *8*, 1133–1144. [CrossRef] [PubMed]

53. Karacosta, L.G.; Anchang, B.; Ignatiadis, N.; Kimmey, S.C.; Benson, J.A.; Shrager, J.B.; Tibshirani, R.; Bendall, S.C.; Plevritis, S.K. Mapping lung cancer epithelial-mesenchymal transition states and trajectories with single-cell resolution. *bioRxiv* **2019**, 570341.
54. Jolly, M.K.; Levine, H. Computational systems biology of epithelial-hybrid-mesenchymal transitions. *Curr. Opin. Syst. Biol.* **2017**, *3*, 1–6. [CrossRef]
55. Mobius, W.; Laan, L. Physical and Mathematical Modeling in Experimental Papers. *Cell* **2015**, *163*, 1577–1583. [CrossRef] [PubMed]
56. Lu, M.; Jolly, M.K.; Levine, H.; Onuchic, J.N.; Ben-Jacob, E. MicroRNA-based regulation of epithelial-hybrid-mesenchymal fate determination. *Proc. Natl. Acad. Sci. USA* **2013**, *110*, 18174–18179. [CrossRef]
57. Jolly, M.; Tripathi, S.C.; Jia, D.; Mooney, S.M.; Celiktas, M.; Hanash, S.M.; Mani, S.A.; Pienta, K.J.; Ben-Jacob, E.; Levine, H. Stability of the hybrid epithelial/mesenchymal phenotype. *Oncotarget* **2016**, *7*, 27067. [CrossRef] [PubMed]
58. Tian, X.-J.; Zhang, H.; Xing, J. Coupled Reversible and Irreversible Bistable Switches Underlying TGFβ-induced Epithelial to Mesenchymal Transition. *Biophys. J.* **2013**, *105*, 1079–1089. [CrossRef]
59. Yu, M.; Bardia, A.; Wittner, B.S.; Stott, S.L.; Smas, M.E.; Ting, D.T.; Isakoff, S.J.; Ciciliano, J.C.; Wells, M.N.; Shah, A.M.; et al. Circulating breast tumor cells exhibit dynamic changes in epithelial and mesenchymal composition. *Science* **2013**, *339*, 580–584. [CrossRef]
60. Pastushenko, I.; Brisebarre, A.; Sifrim, A.; Fioramonti, M.; Revenco, T.; Boumahdi, S.; Van Keymeulen, A.; Brown, D.; Moers, V.; Lemaire, S.; et al. Identification of the tumour transition states occurring during EMT. *Nature* **2018**, *556*, 463–468. [CrossRef]
61. Grigore, A.; Jolly, M.; Jia, D.; Farach-Carson, M.; Levine, H. Tumor Budding: The Name is EMT. Partial EMT. *J. Clin. Med.* **2016**, *5*, 51. [CrossRef] [PubMed]
62. Varankar, S.S.; Kamble, S.C.; Mali, A.M.; More, M.; Abraham, A.; Kumar, B.; Pansare, K.J.; Narayanan, N.J.; Sen, A.; Dhake, R.D.; et al. Functional Balance between TCF21-Slug defines phenotypic plasticity and sub-classes in high-grade serous ovarian cancer. *bioRxiv* **2018**, 307934.
63. Bocci, F.; Jolly, M.K.; Tripathi, S.C.; Aguilar, M.; Hanash, S.M.; Levine, H.; Onuchic, J.N. Numb prevents a complete epithelial-mesenchymal transition by modulating Notch signaling. *J. R. Soc. Interface* **2017**, *14*, 20170512. [CrossRef] [PubMed]
64. Hong, T.; Watanabe, K.; Ta, C.H.; Villarreal-Ponce, A.; Nie, Q.; Dai, X. An Ovol2-Zeb1 Mutual Inhibitory Circuit Governs Bidirectional and Multi-step Transition between Epithelial and Mesenchymal States. *PLoS Comput. Biol.* **2015**, *11*, e1004569. [CrossRef] [PubMed]
65. Bocci, F.; Tripathi, S.C.; Vilchez, M.S.A.; George, J.T.; Casabar, J.; Wong, P.; Hanash, S.; Levine, H.; Onuchic, J.; Jolly, M. NRF2 activates a partial Epithelial-Mesenchymal Transition and is maximally present in a hybrid Epithelial/Mesenchymal phenotype. *Integr. Biol.* **2019**, *11*, 251–263. [CrossRef] [PubMed]
66. Matsumura, Y.; Ito, Y.; Mezawa, Y.; Sulidan, K.; Daigo, Y.; Hiraga, T.; Mogushi, K.; Wali, N.; Suzuki, H.; Itoh, T.; et al. Stromal fibroblasts induce metastatic tumor cell clusters via epithelial–mesenchymal plasticity. *Life Sci. Alliance* **2019**, *2*, e201900425. [CrossRef]
67. Biddle, A.; Gammon, L.; Liang, X.; Costea, D.E.; Mackenzie, I.C. Phenotypic Plasticity Determines Cancer Stem Cell Therapeutic Resistance in Oral Squamous Cell Carcinoma. *EBioMedicine* **2016**, *4*, 138–145. [CrossRef]
68. Boareto, M.; Jolly, M.K.; Goldman, A.; Pietilä, M.; Mani, S.A.; Sengupta, S.; Ben-Jacob, E.; Levine, H.; Onuchic, J.N. Notch-Jagged signalling can give rise to clusters of cells exhibiting a hybrid epithelial/mesenchymal phenotype. *J. R. Soc. Interface* **2016**, *13*, 20151106. [CrossRef]
69. Armstrong, A.J.; Marengo, M.S.; Oltean, S.; Kemeny, G.; Bitting, R.L.; Turnbull, J.D.; Herold, C.I.; Marcom, P.K.; George, D.J.; Garcia-Blanco, M.A. Circulating tumor cells from patients with advanced prostate and breast cancer display both epithelial and mesenchymal markers. *Mol. Cancer Res.* **2011**, *9*, 997–1007. [CrossRef]
70. Pearson, G.W. Control of Invasion by Epithelial-to-Mesenchymal Transition Programs during Metastasis. *J. Clin. Med.* **2019**, *8*, 646. [CrossRef]
71. Jolly, M.K.; Somarelli, J.A.; Sheth, M.; Biddle, A.; Tripathi, S.C.; Armstrong, A.J.; Hanash, S.M.; Bapat, S.A.; Rangarajan, A.; Levine, H. Hybrid epithelial/mesenchymal phenotypes promote metastasis and therapy resistance across carcinomas. *Pharmacol. Ther.* **2019**, *194*, 161–184. [CrossRef] [PubMed]

72. Andriani, F.; Bertolini, G.; Facchinetti, F.; Baldoli, E.; Moro, M.; Casalini, P.; Caserini, R.; Milione, M.; Leone, G.; Pelosi, G.; et al. Conversion to stem-cell state in response to microenvironmental cues is regulated by balance between epithelial and mesenchymal features in lung cancer cells. *Mol. Oncol.* **2016**, *10*, 253–271. [CrossRef]
73. Bhatia, S.; Monkman, J.; Blick, T.; Pinto, C.; Waltham, A. Interrogation of phenotypic plasticity between epithelial and mesenchymal states in breast cancer. *J. Clin. Med.* **2019**, *8*, 893. [CrossRef] [PubMed]
74. Jia, D.; George, J.T.; Tripathi, S.C.; Kundnani, D.L.; Lu, M.; Hanash, S.M.; Onuchic, J.N.; Jolly, M.K.; Levine, H. Testing the gene expression classification of the EMT spectrum. *Phys. Biol.* **2019**, *16*, 025002. [CrossRef] [PubMed]
75. Ruscetti, M.; Dadashian, E.L.; Guo, W.; Quach, B.; Mulholland, D.J.; Park, J.W.; Tran, L.M.; Kobayashi, N.; Bianchi-Frias, D.; Xing, Y.; et al. HDAC inhibition impedes epithelial-mesenchymal plasticity and suppresses metastatic, castration-resistant prostate cancer. *Oncogene* **2016**, *35*, 3781–3795. [CrossRef]
76. Tsuji, T.; Ibaragi, S.; Shima, K.; Hu, M.G.; Katsurano, M.; Sasaki, A.; Hu, G.F. Epithelial-mesenchymal transition induced by growth suppressor p12 CDK2-AP1 promotes tumor cell local invasion but suppresses distant colony growth. *Cancer Res.* **2008**, *68*, 10377–10386. [CrossRef]
77. Westcott, J.M.; Prechtl, A.M.; Maine, E.A.; Dang, T.T.; Esparza, M.A.; Sun, H.; Zhou, Y.; Xie, Y.; Pearson, G.W. An epigenetically distinct breast cancer cell subpopulation promotes collective invasion. *J. Clin. Investig.* **2015**, *125*, 1927–1943. [CrossRef]
78. Ben-Jacob, E.; Coffey, D.S.; Levine, H. Bacterial survival strategies suggest rethinking cancer cooperativity. *Trends Microbiol.* **2012**, *20*, 403–410. [CrossRef]
79. Ferrell, J.E. Bistability, Bifurcations, and Waddington's Epigenetic Landscape. *Curr. Biol.* **2012**, *22*, R458–R466. [CrossRef]
80. Jia, D.; Jolly, M.K.; Kulkarni, P.; Levine, H. Phenotypic plasticity and cell fate decisions in cancer: Insights from dynamical systems theory. *Cancers* **2017**, *9*, 70. [CrossRef]
81. Ozbudak, E.M.; Thattai, M.; Lim, H.N.; Shraiman, B.I.; van Oudenaarden, A. Multistability in the lactose utilization network of *Escherichia coli*. *Nature* **2004**, *427*, 737–740. [CrossRef] [PubMed]
82. Aiello, N.M.; Kang, Y. Context-dependent EMT programs in cancer metastasis. *J. Exp. Med.* **2019**, *216*, 1016–1026. [CrossRef] [PubMed]
83. Balázsi, G.; van Oudenaarden, A.; Collins, J.J. Cellular Decision Making and Biological Noise: From Microbes to Mammals. *Cell* **2011**, *144*, 910–925. [CrossRef] [PubMed]
84. Spencer, S.L.; Gaudet, S.; Albeck, J.G.; Burke, J.M.; Sorger, P.K. Non-genetic origins of cell-to-cell variability in TRAIL-induced apoptosis. *Nature* **2009**, *459*, 428–432. [CrossRef] [PubMed]
85. Inde, Z.; Dixon, S.J. The impact of non-genetic heterogeneity on cancer cell death. *Crit. Rev. Biochem. Mol. Biol.* **2017**, *53*, 99–114. [CrossRef] [PubMed]
86. Jolly, M.K.; Kulkarni, P.; Weninger, K.; Orban, J.; Levine, H. Phenotypic plasticity, bet-hedging, and androgen independence in prostate cancer: Role of non-genetic heterogeneity. *Front. Oncol.* **2018**, *8*, 50. [CrossRef] [PubMed]
87. Elowitz, M.B.; Levine, A.J.; Siggia, E.D.; Swain, P.S. Stochastic gene expression in a single cell. *Science* **2002**, *297*, 1183–1186. [CrossRef] [PubMed]
88. Beerling, E.; Seinstra, D.; de Wit, E.; Kester, L.; van der Velden, D.; Maynard, C.; Schäfer, R.; van Diest, P.; Voest, E.; van Oudenaarden, A.; et al. Plasticity between Epithelial and Mesenchymal States Unlinks EMT from Metastasis-Enhancing Stem Cell Capacity. *Cell Rep.* **2016**, *14*, 2281–2288. [CrossRef] [PubMed]
89. Tripathi, S.; Levine, H.; Jolly, M.K. A Mechanism for Epithelial-Mesenchymal Heterogeneity in a Population of Cancer Cells. *bioRxiv* **2019**, 592691.
90. Chang, H.H.; Oh, P.Y.; Ingber, D.E.; Huang, S. Multistable and multistep dynamics in neutrophil differentiation. *BMC Cell Biol.* **2006**, *7*, 11. [CrossRef]
91. Gregory, P.A.; Bracken, C.P.; Smith, E.; Bert, A.G.; Wright, J.A.; Roslan, S.; Morris, M.; Wyatt, L.; Farshid, G.; Lim, Y.-Y.; et al. An autocrine TGF-beta/ZEB/miR-200 signaling network regulates establishment and maintenance of epithelial-mesenchymal transition. *Mol. Biol. Cell* **2011**, *22*, 1686–1698. [CrossRef] [PubMed]
92. Katsuno, Y.; Meyer, D.S.; Zhang, Z.; Shokat, K.M.; Akhurst, R.J.; Miyazono, K.; Derynck, R. Chronic TGF-β exposure drives stabilized EMT, tumor stemness, and cancer drug resistance with vulnerability to bitopic mTOR inhibition. *Sci. Signal.* **2019**, *12*, eaau8544. [CrossRef] [PubMed]

93. Zhang, J.; Tian, X.-J.; Zhang, H.; Teng, Y.; Li, R.; Bai, F.; Elankumaran, S.; Xing, J. TGF-β–induced epithelial-to-mesenchymal transition proceeds through stepwise activation of multiple feedback loops. *Sci. Signal.* **2014**, *7*, ra91. [CrossRef] [PubMed]
94. Jia, W.; Deshmukh, A.; Mani, S.A.; Jolly, M.K.; Levine, H. A possible role for epigenetic feedback regulation in the dynamics of the Epithelial-Mesenchymal Transition (EMT). *bioRxiv* **2019**, 651620. [CrossRef] [PubMed]
95. Somarelli, J.A.; Shetler, S.; Jolly, M.K.; Wang, X.; Dewitt, S.B.; Hish, A.J.; Gilja, S.; Eward, W.C.; Ware, K.E.; Levine, H.; et al. Mesenchymal-Epithelial Transition in Sarcomas Is Controlled by the Combinatorial Expression of MicroRNA 200s and GRHL2. *Mol. Cell. Biol.* **2016**, *36*, 2503–2513. [CrossRef] [PubMed]
96. Dumont, N.; Wilson, M.B.; Crawford, Y.G.; Reynolds, P.A.; Sigaroudinia, M.; Tlsty, T.D. Sustained induction of epithelial to mesenchymal transition activates DNA methylation of genes silenced in basal-like breast cancers. *Proc. Natl. Acad. Sci. USA* **2008**, *105*, 14867–14872. [CrossRef] [PubMed]
97. Peinado, H.; Ballestar, E.; Esteller, M.; Cano, A. Snail Mediates E-Cadherin Repression by the Recruitment of the Sin3A/Histone Deacetylase 1 (HDAC1)/HDAC2 Complex. *Mol. Cell. Biol.* **2004**, *24*, 306–319. [CrossRef] [PubMed]
98. Pei, D.; Shu, X.; Gassama-Diagne, A.; Thiery, J.P. Mesenchymal–epithelial transition in development and reprogramming. *Nat. Cell Biol.* **2019**, *21*, 44–53. [CrossRef] [PubMed]
99. Roca, H.; Hernandez, J.; Weidner, S.; McEachin, R.C.; Fuller, D.; Sud, S.; Schumann, T.; Wilkinson, J.E.; Zaslavsky, A.; Li, H.; et al. Transcription Factors OVOL1 and OVOL2 Induce the Mesenchymal to Epithelial Transition in Human Cancer. *PLoS ONE* **2013**, *8*, e76773. [CrossRef] [PubMed]
100. Frisch, S.M.; Farris, J.C.; Pifer, P.M. Roles of Grainyhead-like transcription factors in cancer. *Oncogene* **2017**, *36*, 6067–6073. [CrossRef]
101. Chung, V.Y.; Tan, T.Z.; Tan, M.; Wong, M.K.; Kuay, K.T.; Yang, Z.; Ye, J.; Muller, J.; Koh, C.M.; Guccione, E.; et al. GRHL2-miR-200-ZEB1 maintains the epithelial status of ovarian cancer through transcriptional regulation and histone modification. *Sci. Rep.* **2016**, *6*, 19943. [CrossRef] [PubMed]
102. Jolly, M.K.; Ware, K.E.; Xu, S.; Gilja, S.; Shetler, S.; Yang, Y.; Wang, X.; Austin, R.G.; Runyambo, D.; Hish, A.J.; et al. E-Cadherin Represses Anchorage-Independent Growth in Sarcomas through Both Signaling and Mechanical Mechanisms. *Mol. Cancer Res.* **2019**, *17*, 1391–1402. [CrossRef] [PubMed]
103. Chung, V.Y.; Tan, T.Z.; Ye, J.; Huang, R.-L.; Lai, H.-C.; Kappei, D.; Wollmann, H.; Guccione, E.; Huang, R.Y.-J. The role of GRHL2 and epigenetic remodeling in epithelial–mesenchymal plasticity in ovarian cancer cells. *Commun. Biol.* **2019**, *2*, 272. [CrossRef] [PubMed]
104. Qi, X.-K.; Han, H.-Q.; Zhang, H.-J.; Xu, M.; Li, L.; Chen, L.; Xiang, T.; Feng, Q.-S.; Kang, T.; Qian, C.-N.; et al. OVOL2 links stemness and metastasis via fine-tuning epithelial-mesenchymal transition in nasopharyngeal carcinoma. *Theranostics* **2018**, *8*, 2202–2216. [CrossRef] [PubMed]
105. Celià-Terrassa, T.; Kang, Y. Distinctive properties of metastasis- initiating cells. *Genes Dev.* **2016**, 892–908. [CrossRef] [PubMed]
106. Bierie, B.; Pierce, S.E.; Kroeger, C.; Stover, D.G.; Pattabiraman, D.R.; Thiru, P.; Liu Donaher, J.; Reinhardt, F.; Chaffer, C.L.; Keckesova, Z.; et al. Integrin-β4 identifies cancer stem cell-enriched populations of partially mesenchymal carcinoma cells. *Proc. Natl. Acad. Sci. USA* **2017**, *114*, E2337–E2346. [CrossRef] [PubMed]
107. Mooney, S.M.; Talebian, V.; Jolly, M.K.; Jia, D.; Gromala, M.; Levine, H.; McConkey, B.J. The GRHL2/ZEB Feedback Loop-A Key Axis in the Regulation of EMT in Breast Cancer. *J. Cell. Biochem.* **2017**, *118*, 2559–2570. [CrossRef] [PubMed]
108. Huang, B.; Lu, M.; Jolly, M.K.; Tsarfaty, I.; Onuchic, J.; Ben-Jacob, E. The three-way switch operation of Rac1/RhoA GTPase-based circuit controlling amoeboid-hybrid-mesenchymal transition. *Sci. Rep.* **2014**, *4*, 6449. [CrossRef] [PubMed]
109. Saha, M.; Kumar, S.; Bukhari, S.; Balaji, S.; Kumar, P.; Hindupur, S.; Rangarajan, A. AMPK-Akt Double-Negative Feedback Loop in Breast Cancer Cells Regulates Their Adaptation to Matrix Deprivation. *Cancer Res.* **2018**, *78*, 1497–1510. [CrossRef] [PubMed]
110. Yu, L.; Lu, M.; Jia, D.; Ma, J.; Ben-Jacob, E.; Levine, H.; Kaipparettu, B.A.; Onuchic, J.N. Modeling the Genetic Regulation of Cancer Metabolism: Interplay Between Glycolysis and Oxidative Phosphorylation. *Cancer Res.* **2017**, in press. [CrossRef] [PubMed]
111. Zhou, J.X.; Huang, S. Understanding gene circuits at cell-fate branch points for rational cell reprogramming. *Trends Genet.* **2011**, *27*, 55–62. [CrossRef] [PubMed]

112. Jolly, M.K.; Mani, S.A.; Levine, H. Hybrid epithelial/mesenchymal phenotype(s): The 'fittest' for metastasis? *Biochim. Biophys. Acta Rev. Cancer* **2018**, *1870*, 151–157. [CrossRef] [PubMed]
113. Jia, D.; Jolly, M.K.; Tripathi, S.C.; Den Hollander, P.; Huang, B.; Lu, M.; Celiktas, M.; Ramirez-Peña, E.; Ben-Jacob, E.; Onuchic, J.N.; et al. Distinguishing mechanisms underlying EMT tristability. *Cancer Converg.* **2017**, *1*, 2. [CrossRef] [PubMed]
114. Font-Clos, F.; Zapperi, S.; La Porta, C.A.M. Topography of epithelial–mesenchymal plasticity. *Proc. Natl. Acad. Sci. USA* **2018**, *115*, 5902–5907. [CrossRef]
115. Steinway, S.N.; Gomez Tejeda Zañudo, J.; Ding, W.; Rountree, C.B.; Feith, D.J.; Loughran, T.P.; Albert, R. Network modeling of TGFβ signaling in hepatocellular carcinoma epithelial-to-mesenchymal transition reveals joint Sonic hedgehog and Wnt pathway activation. *Cancer Res.* **2014**, *74*, 5963–5977. [CrossRef]
116. Hanahan, D.; Weinberg, R.A. Hallmarks of cancer: The next generation. *Cell* **2011**, *144*, 646–674. [CrossRef] [PubMed]
117. Reya, T.; Morrison, S.J.; Clarke, M.F.; Weissman, I.L. Stem cells, cancer, and cancer stem cells. *Nature* **2001**, *414*, 105. [CrossRef]
118. Visvader, J.E.; Lindeman, G.J. Cancer stem cells: Current status and evolving complexities. *Cell Stem Cell* **2012**, *10*, 717–728. [CrossRef] [PubMed]
119. Al-Hajj, M.; Wicha, M.S.; Benito-Hernandez, A.; Morrison, S.J.; Clarke, M.F. Prospective identification of tumorigenic breast cancer cells. *Proc. Natl. Acad. Sci. USA* **2003**, *100*, 3983–3988. [CrossRef] [PubMed]
120. Bonnet, D.; Dick, J.E. Human acute myeloid leukemia is organized as a hierarchy that originates from a primitive hematopoietic cell. *Nat. Med.* **1997**, *3*, 730. [CrossRef]
121. Lapidot, T.; Sirard, C.; Vormoor, J.; Murdoch, B.; Hoang, T.; Caceres-Cortes, J.; Minden, M.; Paterson, B.; Caligiuri, M.A.; Dick, J.E. A cell initiating human acute myeloid leukaemia after transplantation into SCID mice. *Nature* **1994**, *367*, 645. [CrossRef] [PubMed]
122. Medema, J.P. Cancer stem cells: The challenges ahead. *Nat. Cell Biol.* **2013**, *15*, 338. [CrossRef] [PubMed]
123. Liu, S.; Cong, Y.; Wang, D.; Sun, Y.; Deng, L.; Liu, Y.; Martin-Trevino, R.; Shang, L.; McDermott, S.P.; Landis, M.D.; et al. Breast cancer stem cells transition between epithelial and mesenchymal states reflective of their normal counterparts. *Stem Cell Rep.* **2014**, *2*, 78–91. [CrossRef] [PubMed]
124. Pierce, G.B.; Speers, W.C. Tumors as Caricatures of the Process of Tissue Renewal: Prospects for Therapy by Directing Differentiation. *Cancer Res.* **1988**, *48*, 1996–2004. [PubMed]
125. Zomer, A.; Ellenbroek, S.I.J.; Ritsma, L.; Beerling, E.; Vrisekoop, N.; Van Rheenen, J. Brief report: Intravital imaging of cancer stem cell plasticity in mammary tumors. *Stem Cells* **2013**, *31*, 602–606. [CrossRef] [PubMed]
126. Phillips, S.; Prat, A.; Sedic, M.; Proia, T.; Wronski, A.; Mazumdar, S.; Skibinski, A.; Shirley, S.H.; Perou, C.M.; Gill, G.; et al. Cell-state transitions regulated by SLUG are critical for tissue regeneration and tumor initiation. *Stem Cell Rep.* **2014**, *2*, 633–647. [CrossRef] [PubMed]
127. Chaffer, C.L.; Brueckmann, I.; Scheel, C.; Kaestli, A.J.; Wiggins, P.A.; Rodrigues, L.O.; Brooks, M.; Reinhardt, F.; Su, Y.; Polyak, K.; et al. Normal and neoplastic nonstem cells can spontaneously convert to a stem-like state. *Proc. Natl. Acad. Sci. USA* **2011**, *108*, 7950–7955. [CrossRef] [PubMed]
128. Rios, A.C.; Capaldo, B.D.; Vaillant, F.; Pal, B.; van Ineveld, R.; Dawson, C.A.; Chen, Y.; Nolan, E.; Fu, N.Y.; Jackling, F.C.; et al. Intraclonal Plasticity in Mammary Tumors Revealed through Large-Scale Single-Cell Resolution 3D Imaging. *Cancer Cell* **2019**, *35*, 618–632. [CrossRef] [PubMed]
129. Chaffer, C.L.; Marjanovic, N.D.; Lee, T.; Bell, G.; Kleer, C.G.; Reinhardt, F.; D'Alessio, A.C.; Young, R.A.; Weinberg, R.A. Poised chromatin at the ZEB1 promoter enables breast cancer cell plasticity and enhances tumorigenicity. *Cell* **2013**, *154*, 61–74. [CrossRef]
130. Bernstein, B.E.; Mikkelsen, T.S.; Xie, X.; Kamal, M.; Huebert, D.J.; Cuff, J.; Fry, B.; Meissner, A.; Wernig, M.; Plath, K.; et al. A Bivalent Chromatin Structure Marks Key Developmental Genes in Embryonic Stem Cells. *Cell* **2006**, *125*, 315–326. [CrossRef] [PubMed]
131. Iliopoulos, D.; Hirsch, H.A.; Wang, G.; Struhl, K. Inducible formation of breast cancer stem cells and their dynamic equilibrium with non-stem cancer cells via IL6 secretion. *Proc. Natl. Acad. Sci. USA* **2011**, *108*, 1397–1402. [CrossRef]
132. Blanpain, C.; Fuchs, E. Plasticity of epithelial stem cells in tissue regeneration. *Science* **2014**, *344*, 1242281. [CrossRef] [PubMed]

133. Koren, S.; Reavie, L.; Couto, J.P.; De Silva, D.; Stadler, M.B.; Roloff, T.; Britschgi, A.; Eichlisberger, T.; Kohler, H.; Aina, O.; et al. PIK3CAH1047R induces multipotency and multi-lineage mammary tumours. *Nature* **2015**, *525*, 114. [CrossRef] [PubMed]
134. Milanovic, M.; Fan, D.N.Y.; Belenki, D.; Däbritz, J.H.M.; Zhao, Z.; Yu, Y.; Dörr, J.R.; Dimitrova, L.; Lenze, D.; Monteiro Barbosa, I.A.; et al. Senescence-associated reprogramming promotes cancer stemness. *Nature* **2018**, *553*, 96. [CrossRef] [PubMed]
135. Schwitalla, S.; Fingerle, A.A.; Cammareri, P.; Nebelsiek, T.; Göktuna, S.I.; Ziegler, P.K.; Canli, O.; Heijmans, J.; Huels, D.J.; Moreaux, G.; et al. Intestinal tumorigenesis initiated by dedifferentiation and acquisition of stem-cell-like properties. *Cell* **2013**, *152*, 25–38. [CrossRef] [PubMed]
136. Celià-Terrassa, T.; Kang, Y. Metastatic niche functions and therapeutic opportunities. *Nat. Cell Biol.* **2018**, *20*, 868–877. [CrossRef] [PubMed]
137. Esposito, M.; Mondal, N.; Greco, T.M.; Wei, Y.; Spadazzi, C.; Lin, S.-C.; Zheng, H.; Cheung, C.; Magnani, J.L.; Lin, S.-H.; et al. Bone vascular niche E-selectin induces mesenchymal–epithelial transition and Wnt activation in cancer cells to promote bone metastasis. *Nat. Cell Biol.* **2019**, *21*, 627. [CrossRef]
138. De Sousa, E.; Melo, F.; Kurtova, A.V.; Harnoss, J.M.; Kljavin, N.; Hoeck, J.D.; Hung, J.; Anderson, J.E.; Storm, E.E.; Modrusan, Z.; et al. A distinct role for Lgr5 + stem cells in primary and metastatic colon cancer. *Nature* **2017**, *543*, 676–680. [CrossRef]
139. Ball, C.R.; Oppel, F.; Ehrenberg, K.R.; Dubash, T.D.; Dieter, S.M.; Hoffmann, C.M.; Abel, U.; Herbst, F.; Koch, M.; Werner, J.; et al. Succession of transiently active tumor-initiating cell clones in human pancreatic cancer xenografts. *EMBO Mol. Med.* **2017**, *9*, 918–932. [CrossRef]
140. Quintana, E.; Shackleton, M.; Foster, H.R.; Fullen, D.R.; Sabel, M.S.; Johnson, T.M.; Morrison, S.J. Phenotypic heterogeneity among tumorigenic melanoma cells from patients that is reversible and not hierarchically organized. *Cancer Cell* **2010**, *18*, 510–523. [CrossRef]
141. Quintana, E.; Shackleton, M.; Sabel, M.S.; Fullen, D.R.; Johnson, T.M.; Morrison, S.J. Efficient tumour formation by single human melanoma cells. *Nature* **2008**, *456*, 593. [CrossRef] [PubMed]
142. Kreso, A.; Dick, J.E. Evolution of the cancer stem cell model. *Cell Stem Cell* **2014**, *14*, 275–291. [CrossRef] [PubMed]
143. Wang, W.; Quan, Y.; Fu, Q.; Liu, Y.; Liang, Y.; Wu, J.; Yang, G.; Luo, C.; Ouyang, Q.; Wang, Y. Dynamics between cancer cell subpopulations reveals a model coordinating with both hierarchical and stochastic concepts. *PLoS ONE* **2014**, *9*, e84654. [CrossRef] [PubMed]
144. Yang, G.; Quan, Y.; Wang, W.; Fu, Q.; Wu, J.; Mei, T.; Li, J.; Tang, Y.; Luo, C.; Ouyang, Q.; et al. Dynamic equilibrium between cancer stem cells and non-stem cancer cells in human SW620 and MCF-7 cancer cell populations. *Br. J. Cancer* **2012**, *106*, 1512. [CrossRef] [PubMed]
145. Kitano, H. Cancer as a robust system: Implications for anticancer therapy. *Nat. Rev. Cancer* **2004**, *4*, 227–235. [CrossRef] [PubMed]
146. Jia, D.; Jolly, M.K.; Harrison, W.; Boareto, M.; Ben-Jacob, E.; Levine, H. Operating principles of tristable circuits regulating cellular differentiation. *Phys. Biol.* **2017**, *14*, 035007. [CrossRef] [PubMed]
147. Niu, Y.; Wang, Y.; Zhou, D. The phenotypic equilibrium of cancer cells: From average-level stability to path-wise convergence. *J. Theor. Biol.* **2015**, *386*, 7–17. [CrossRef]
148. Lotem, J.; Sachs, L. Epigenetics and the plasticity of differentiation in normal and cancer stem cells. *Oncogene* **2006**, *25*, 7663–7672. [CrossRef]
149. Galvin-Burgess, K.E.; Travis, E.D.; Pierson, K.E.; Vivian, J.L. TGF-β-superfamily signaling regulates embryonic stem cell heterogeneity: Self-renewal as a dynamic and regulated equilibrium. *Stem Cells* **2013**, *31*, 48–58. [CrossRef]
150. Xie, G.; Yao, Q.; Liu, Y.; Du, S.; Liu, A.; Guo, Z.; Sun, A.; Ruan, J.; Chen, L.; Ye, C.; et al. IL-6-induced epithelial-mesenchymal transition promotes the generation of breast cancer stem-like cells analogous to mammosphere cultures. *Int. J. Oncol.* **2012**, *40*, 1171–1179.
151. Sehl, M.E.; Shimada, M.; Landeros, A.; Lange, K.; Wicha, M.S. Modeling of cancer stem cell state transitions predicts therapeutic response. *PLoS ONE* **2015**, *10*, e0135797. [CrossRef]
152. Heppner, G.H. Cancer cell societies and tumor progression. *Stem Cells* **1993**, *11*, 199–203. [CrossRef] [PubMed]
153. Deisboeck, T.S.; Couzin, I.D. Collective behavior in cancer cell populations. *Bioessays* **2009**, *31*, 190–197. [CrossRef] [PubMed]

154. Campbell, K.; Casanova, J. A common framework for EMT and collective cell migration. *Development* **2016**, *143*, 4291–4300. [CrossRef]
155. Martinez Arias, A.; Steventon, B. On the nature and function of organizers. *Development* **2018**, *145*, dev159525. [CrossRef] [PubMed]
156. Micalizzi, D.S.; Farabaugh, S.M.; Ford, H.L. Epithelial-mesenchymal transition in cancer: Parallels between normal development and tumor progression. *J. Mammary Gland Biol. Neoplasia* **2010**, *15*, 117–134. [CrossRef]
157. Harper, K.L.; Sosa, M.S.; Entenberg, D.; Hosseini, H.; Cheung, J.F.; Nobre, R.; Avivar-Valderas, A.; Nagi, C.; Girnius, N.; Davis, R.J.; et al. Mechanism of early dissemination and metastasis in Her2+mammary cancer. *Nature* **2016**, *540*, 588–592. [CrossRef]
158. Zhao, Z.; Zhu, X.; Cui, K.; Mancuso, J.; Federley, R.; Fischer, K.; Teng, G.J.; Mittal, V.; Gao, D.; Zhao, H.; et al. In Vivo Visualization and Characterization of Epithelial-Mesenchymal Transition in Breast Tumors. *Cancer Res.* **2016**, *76*, 2094–2104. [CrossRef]
159. Giampieri, S.; Manning, C.; Hooper, S.; Jones, L.; Hill, C.S.; Sahai, E. Localized and reversible TGFβ signalling switches breast cancer cells from cohesive to single cell motility. *Nat. Cell Biol.* **2009**, *11*, 1287–1296. [CrossRef]
160. Walker, D.C.; Georgopoulos, N.T.; Southgate, J. Anti-social cells: Predicting the influence of E-cadherin loss on the growth of epithelial cell populations. *J. Theor. Biol.* **2010**, *262*, 425–440. [CrossRef]
161. Zhang, Z.; Bedder, M.; Smith, S.L.; Walker, D.; Shabir, S.; Southgate, J. Characterization and classification of adherent cells in monolayer culture using automated tracking and evolutionary algorithms. *Biosystems* **2016**, *146*, 110–121. [CrossRef] [PubMed]
162. Georgopoulos, N.T.; Kirkwood, L.A.; Southgate, J. A novel bidirectional positive-feedback loop between Wnt-β-catenin and EGFR-ERK plays a role in context-specific modulation of epithelial tissue regeneration. *J. Cell Sci.* **2014**, *127*, 2967–2982. [CrossRef] [PubMed]
163. Brabletz, T.; Jung, A.; Reu, S.; Porzner, M.; Hlubek, F.; Kunz-Schughart, L.A.; Knuechel, R.; Kirchner, T. Variable-catenin expression in colorectal cancers indicates tumor progression driven by the tumor environment. *Proc. Natl. Acad. Sci. USA* **2002**, *98*, 10356–10361. [CrossRef] [PubMed]
164. Schmalhofer, O.; Brabletz, S.; Brabletz, T. E-cadherin, beta-catenin, and ZEB1 in malignant progression of cancer. *Cancer Metastasis Rev.* **2009**, *28*, 151–166. [CrossRef] [PubMed]
165. Ramis-Conde, I.; Chaplain, M.A.J.; Anderson, A.R.A.; Drasdo, D. Multi-scale modelling of cancer cell intravasation: The role of cadherins in metastasis. *Phys. Biol.* **2009**, *6*, 016008. [CrossRef] [PubMed]
166. Colacino, J.A.; Azizi, E.; Brooks, M.D.; Harouaka, R.; Fouladdel, S.; McDermott, S.P.; Lee, M.; Hill, D.; Madden, J.; Boerner, J.; et al. Heterogeneity of Human Breast Stem and Progenitor Cells as Revealed by Transcriptional Profiling. *Stem Cell Rep.* **2018**, *10*, 1596–1609. [CrossRef]
167. Bocci, F.; Gearhart-Serna, L.; Boareto, M.; Ribeiro, M.; Ben-Jacob, E.; Devi, G.R.; Levine, H.; Onuchic, J.N.; Jolly, M.K. Toward understanding cancer stem cell heterogeneity in the tumor microenvironment. *Proc. Natl. Acad. Sci. USA* **2019**, *116*, 148–157. [CrossRef]
168. Lovisa, S.; LeBleu, V.S.; Tampe, B.; Sugimoto, H.; Vadnagara, K.; Carstens, J.L.; Wu, C.-C.; Hagos, Y.; Burckhardt, B.C.; Pentcheva-Hoang, T.; et al. Epithelial-to-mesenchymal transition induces cell cycle arrest and parenchymal damage in renal fibrosis. *Nat. Med.* **2015**, *21*, 998–1009. [CrossRef]
169. Jolly, M.K.; Boareto, M.; Debeb, B.G.; Aceto, N.; Farach-Carson, M.C.; Woodward, W.A.; Levine, H. Inflammatory Breast Cancer: A model for investigating cluster-based dissemination. *NPJ Breast Cancer* **2017**, *3*, 21. [CrossRef]
170. Sun, Y.; Wu, G.; Cheng, K.S.; Chen, A.; Neoh, K.H.; Chen, S.; Tang, Z.; Lee, P.F.; Dai, M.; Han, R.P.S. CTC phenotyping for a preoperative assessment of tumor metastasis and overall survival of pancreatic ductal adenocarcinoma patients. *EBioMedicine* **2019**, *46*, 133–149. [CrossRef]
171. Bocci, F.; Jolly, M.K.; Onuchic, J.N. A biophysical model of Epithelial-Mesenchymal Transition uncovers the frequency and size distribution of circulating tumor cell clusters across cancer types. *bioRxiv* **2019**, 563049.
172. Cheung, K.J.; Ewald, A.J. A collective route to metastasis: Seeding by tumor cell clusters. *Science* **2016**, *352*, 167–169. [CrossRef]
173. Au, S.H.; Storey, B.D.; Moore, J.C.; Tang, Q.; Chen, Y.-L.; Javaid, S.; Sarioglu, A.F.; Sullivan, R.; Madden, M.W.; O'Keefe, R.; et al. Clusters of circulating tumor cells traverse capillary-sized vessels. *Proc. Natl. Acad. Sci. USA* **2016**, *113*, 4947–4952. [CrossRef] [PubMed]

174. Gkountela, S.; Castro-Giner, F.; Szczerba, B.M.; Vetter, M.; Landin, J.; Scherrer, R.; Krol, I.; Scheidmann, M.C.; Beisel, C.; Stirnimann, C.U.; et al. Circulating Tumor Cell Clustering Shapes DNA Methylation to Enable Metastasis Seeding. *Cell* **2019**, *176*, 98–112. [CrossRef] [PubMed]
175. Giuliano, M.; Shaikh, A.; Lo, H.C.; Arpino, G.; De Placido, S.; Zhang, X.H.; Cristofanilli, M.; Schiff, R.; Trivedi, M.V. Perspective on Circulating Tumor Cell Clusters: Why It Takes a Village to Metastasize. *Cancer Res.* **2018**, *78*, 845–852. [CrossRef]
176. Szczerba, B.M.; Castro-Giner, F.; Vetter, M.; Krol, I.; Gkountela, S.; Landin, J.; Scheidmann, M.C.; Donato, C.; Scherrer, R.; Singer, J.; et al. Neutrophils escort circulating tumour cells to enable cell cycle progression. *Nature* **2019**, *566*, 553–557. [CrossRef]
177. Amend, S.R.; Roy, S.; Brown, J.S.; Pienta, K.J. Ecological paradigms to understand the dynamics of metastasis. *Cancer Lett.* **2016**, *380*, 237–242. [CrossRef]
178. Martinez-Outschoorn, U.; Sotgia, F.; Lisanti, M.P. Tumor microenvironment and metabolic synergy in breast cancers: Critical importance of mitochondrial fuels and function. *Semin. Oncol.* **2014**, *41*, 195–216. [CrossRef]
179. Li, X.; Jolly, M.K.; George, J.T.; Pienta, K.J.; Levine, H. Computational Modeling of the Crosstalk Between Macrophage Polarization and Tumor Cell Plasticity in the Tumor Microenvironment. *Front. Oncol.* **2019**, *9*, 1–12. [CrossRef]
180. Gallaher, J.A.; Enriquez-Navas, P.M.; Luddy, K.A.; Gatenby, R.A.; Anderson, A.R.A. Spatial heterogeneity and evolutionary dynamics modulate time to recurrence in continuous and adaptive cancer therapies. *Cancer Res.* **2018**, *78*, 2127–2139. [CrossRef]

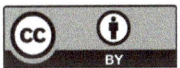

© 2019 by the authors. Licensee MDPI, Basel, Switzerland. This article is an open access article distributed under the terms and conditions of the Creative Commons Attribution (CC BY) license (http://creativecommons.org/licenses/by/4.0/).

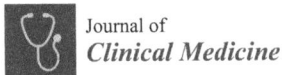

*Review*

# Markers of Cancer Cell Invasion: Are They Good Enough?

Tatiana S. Gerashchenko [1,*], Nikita M. Novikov [1,2], Nadezhda V. Krakhmal [3], Sofia Y. Zolotaryova [2], Marina V. Zavyalova [3,4], Nadezhda V. Cherdyntseva [1,5], Evgeny V. Denisov [1,6] and Vladimir M. Perelmuter [4]

1. Laboratory of Molecular Oncology and Immunology, Cancer Research Institute, Tomsk National Research Medical Center, 634009 Tomsk, Russia
2. Department of Cytology and Genetics, Tomsk State University, 634050 Tomsk, Russia
3. Department of Pathological Anatomy, Siberian State Medical University, 634050 Tomsk, Russia
4. Department of General and Molecular Pathology, Cancer Research Institute, Tomsk National Research Medical Center, 634009 Tomsk, Russia
5. Laboratory for Translational Cellular and Molecular Biomedicine, Tomsk State University, 634050 Tomsk, Russia
6. Department of Organic Chemistry, Tomsk State University, 634050 Tomsk, Russia
* Correspondence: t_gerashchenko@oncology.tomsk.ru

Received: 28 June 2019; Accepted: 22 July 2019; Published: 24 July 2019

**Abstract:** Invasion, or directed migration of tumor cells into adjacent tissues, is one of the hallmarks of cancer and the first step towards metastasis. Penetrating to adjacent tissues, tumor cells form the so-called invasive front/edge. The cellular plasticity afforded by different kinds of phenotypic transitions (epithelial–mesenchymal, collective–amoeboid, mesenchymal–amoeboid, and *vice versa*) significantly contributes to the diversity of cancer cell invasion patterns and mechanisms. Nevertheless, despite the advances in the understanding of invasion, it is problematic to identify tumor cells with the motile phenotype in cancer tissue specimens due to the absence of reliable and acceptable molecular markers. In this review, we summarize the current information about molecules such as extracellular matrix components, factors of epithelial–mesenchymal transition, proteases, cell adhesion, and actin cytoskeleton proteins involved in cell migration and invasion that could be used as invasive markers and discuss their advantages and limitations. Based on the reviewed data, we conclude that future studies focused on the identification of specific invasive markers should use new models one of which may be the intratumor morphological heterogeneity in breast cancer reflecting different patterns of cancer cell invasion.

**Keywords:** cancer; invasion; invasive front; epithelial–mesenchymal transition; heterogeneity

## 1. Introduction

Metastasis is a key feature of cancer and a "final chord" of the tumor progression [1]. The ability for metastasis enables tumor cells to leave the primary site and disseminate throughout the body, causing severe organ failure and leading to death. Understanding the mechanisms underlying metastasis is extremely important for the development of highly effective cancer therapies [2].

Metastasis is a complex process of stepwise events collectively termed the metastatic cascade and consisting of local invasion of tumor cells, intravasation to blood vessels, survival in the circulation, arrest at distant organs, extravasation into the parenchyma of distant tissues, micrometastasis formation, and metastatic colonization (macrometastasis) [1,2]. Invasion is the first step in the metastasis of tumor cells. From the morphological point of view, the invasion is a process during which malignant cells detach from the tumor mass, acquire the ability to actively move, and invade surrounding tissues through the adjacent basement membrane [3]. The interface of tumor and host tissue, in other words, the deepest rim of cancerous tissue grown in adjacent non-cancerous tissues, is called an "invasive front (edge)" [4]. Tumor cells constituting the invasive front are phenotypically different from cells in other tumor parts. Invasive front cells are believed to have a locomotor phenotype and demonstrate a variety of types and mechanisms of movement [5,6]. Tumor cells can move collectively or individually. The type of invasion depends on the molecular changes in tumor cells and the tumor microenvironment features [7–10]. The distinctive features of collective cell invasion include physical and functional relationships among tumor cells due to adhesion molecules as well as the presence of leader cells that are characterized by the mesenchymal phenotype and the ability to form lamellipodia, pull follower cells, and destroy the extracellular matrix (ECM) through production of proteases [11–13]. Interestingly, according some reports, invasive leaders do not express molecular features of epithelial–mesenchymal transition (EMT) [14], but exhibit a basal epithelial gene program, that is enriched in cytokeratin-14 and the transcription factor p63 [15,16].

Individual invasion can occur through mesenchymal and amoeboid cell migration mechanisms [17]. Sometimes, an intermediate amoeboid/mesenchymal (filopodial) cell migration mode is distinguished [18]. In mesenchymal movement, tumor cells exhibit a pronounced fibroblast-like phenotype, high expression of integrins, synthesis of proteolytic enzymes, and activity of small GTPases Rac1 and Cdc42 that are necessary to form lamellipodia and actomyosin contractions [7,12]. In amoeboid movement, cells are not capable of proteolysis and adhesion of the ECM but demonstrate the enhanced activity of the actomyosin machinery and the formation of cell membrane protrusions (blebs), which allow cells to squeeze through tight spaces in the surrounding matrix. Amoeboid movement directly depends on Rho/ROCK cell signaling and activity of type II myosin [13,17,19]. Tumor cells can transit from one cell migration phenotype to another via mesenchymal–amoeboid (MAT) and amoeboid–mesenchymal transition. The key role in these transitions is played by the balance of GTPases Rho and Rac, changes in expression of focal adhesion molecules and proteases, and ECM stiffness [13]. Importantly, the Rho/Rac feedback loop, particularly balanced relative high RhoA and Rac1, is also responsible for the hybrid amoeboid/mesenchymal phenotype in migrating cells [20].

EMT plays a key role in tumor dissemination. During EMT, tumor cells lose the epithelial phenotype and acquire the mesenchymal features and resistance to antitumor treatment; EMT also promotes immortalization and is involved in the prevention of apoptosis [21,22]. EMT is induced not only by molecular changes in tumor cells but also by cytokines and growth factors secreted by immune and stromal cells of the tumor microenvironment [23–26]. EMT may be incomplete (partial) when tumor cells still retain epithelial features but already acquire mesenchymal traits. During partial EMT, cells are described as a hybrid, with an intermediate epithelial/mesenchymal phenotype [27]. Partial EMT has been reported for both single tumor cells and tumor buds (groups of up to five cells) that are a variant of collective invasion [28]. The phenomenon "tumor budding" is regarded as a specific "signal" indicating the onset of cancer invasion and metastasis. The presence of tumor buds in the invasive front was found to be associated with increased metastasis and poor prognosis in various cancers [28–34].

Tumor cells can acquire the ability for migration not only through EMT but also through the so-called collective–amoeboid transition (CAT) when cells detach from the tumor mass and acquire an amoeboid phenotype rather than a mesenchymal phenotype. CAT is known to be regulated by the core regulatory circuits underlying EMT (miR-200/miR-34) and MAT (Rac1/RhoA) [35] and can be promoted by hypoxia-inducible factor 1 (HIF-1), which is accompanied by a decrease in E-cadherin expression [36]. However, CAT still remains a poorly understood phenomenon.

Active migration of tumor cells is not the only mechanism for invasive tumor growth. There is the so-called passive invasion when cells penetrate adjacent tissues under pressure from other tumor cells during proliferation (expansive growth) or due to an increase in the ECM density caused by the production of fibronectin and collagen by cancer-associated fibroblasts [37,38]. The fact that many circulating tumor cells are apoptotic [39,40], may be considered as indirect evidence of passive invasion, whereas active invasion is associated with viable cells [37].

Despite the fact that the mechanisms and types of cell migration and invasion have been described and studied quite well, there are currently no highly efficient and validated molecular markers for identification of migrating/invading tumor cells in tumors and, therefore, for assessment of their invasive potential. These markers could be used to identify patients at the high risk of distant metastasis and to prescribe therapy aimed at interrupting the metastatic process. In addition, these markers might represent targets for future therapeutics that block invasion and metastasis.

In this review, we systematized information about molecules that might be potential markers of tumor invasion and discussed the advantages and limitations of their use in clinical practice.

## 2. Potential Markers of Cancer Cell Invasion

The literature reports numerous studies describing various molecules that may act as markers of tumor cell invasion. Conventionally, they may be subdivided into several groups: ECM components, EMT, cell–cell and cell–ECM molecules, proteases, and actin cytoskeleton proteins (Table 1).

### 2.1. ECM Components

The first barrier to tumor cell invasion is the basement membrane that is a 100–300 nm thick ECM structure consisting of laminins, type IV collagen, and other non-cellular components, on which epithelial cells proliferate and differentiate [41–44]. Impaired integrity of the basement membrane is a histological marker indicating that carcinoma has acquired invasive properties [12,41,43]. A key component of the basement membrane, laminin-5, consists of α3, β3, and γ2 chains and plays a significant role in migration and invasion of tumor cells [43,45–48]. The interaction between laminin-5 and tumor cell integrins leads to the release of proteases and degradation of the basement membrane and ECM [43,47,49–51]. The laminin-5 γ2 chain monomer, which is considered as one of the most characteristic markers of invasion is found in the invasive front of different cancers [51,52]. For example, laminin γ2 expression combined with MMP-7 and EGFR expression in the invasive front is associated with gastric cancer aggressiveness [43]. In gastric cancer, cytoplasmic expression of laminin γ2 in tumor cells is related to lymph node metastasis and advanced stage [53]; in gallbladder cancer, stromal laminin γ2 expression is associated with a poor prognosis [54]. Laminin γ2 is also expressed in the invasive front of breast, pancreatic, colon, lung, and other cancers [46,51,52,55,56].

**Table 1.** Potential markers of cancer cell invasion.

| | Markers | Functions | Expression at the Invasive Front | Limitations |
|---|---|---|---|---|
| ECM components | Laminin-5, γ2 chain | ECM components, triggering MMP production through interaction with integrins | Breast, pancreatic, colon, lung, and other cancers [46,51,52,55,56] Oral and head and neck cancers [60,61] | Expression not only in the invasive front, but in other regions of the tumor [43,46,57–59] |
| | Fibronectin | | | |
| | Tenascin C | Modulation of cell adhesion | Melanoma, breast, lung, liver, and gallbladder cancers [57,62] | |
| EMT molecules | Snail, Twist, vimentin | EMT induction and regulation | Various cancers [63] | Snail and Twist: Unstable molecules [64,65], total expression in breast tumors [66]. Vimentin may not be expressed in invasive carcinomas [67] |
| Cell–cell and cell–ECM interaction molecules | Cadherin-catenin complex | Adherens junctions | Colorectal, oral, and basaloid carcinomas (loss of E-cadherin and nuclear localization of β-catenin) [68–71] | In some tumors, loss of E-cadherin is not indispensable for invasive growth [72] |
| | Integrins | Cell–ECM adhesion, involvement in MMP production | Melanoma (αvβ3), colon (αvβ6), head and neck (αvβ6), and lung (α6β4) cancers [73–76] | Involvement in other biological processes [77,78] |
| | Galectin 1 | Modulation of cell–cell and cell–ECM interactions | Oral and lung cancers, glioblastoma [47,79,80] | |
| | L1CAM | Cell adhesion | Colorectal and pancreatic cancers [81,82] | Dualistic role in cancer progression [83] |

Table 1. Cont.

| Markers | | Functions | Expression at the Invasive Front | Limitations |
|---|---|---|---|---|
| Serine proteases and MMPs | uPA | Proteolysis of plasminogen to plasmin | Oral and skin carcinomas [84,85] | Involvement in other biological processes [86,87] |
| | MMPs | ECM proteolysis | Melanoma (MMP-2), colorectal (MMP-7), gastric (MMP-7), endometrial (MMP-2, 9), ovarian (MMP-2, 9), and head and neck (MMP-2, 9) cancers [56,88–94] | |
| Actin cytoskeleton proteins | Ezrin | Actin polymerization, cytoskeletal dynamics | Lung cancer [95,96] | Involvement in other biological processes. Contradictory data on the role in cancer progression [96] |
| | WAVE2 | | Breast cancer [97] | - |
| | Cortactin | | Oral and laryngeal cancers [98,99] | - |
| | MENAinv | | Breast cancer [100] | - |
| | Fascin-1 | | Liver, colon, cervical, and endometrial cancers [101–104] | - |
| Other proteins | Ki-67 | Cell proliferation | Breast, oral, and endometrial cancers [6,105–107] | Contradictory data on the level of Ki-67 expression at the invasive front [56,69,108] |
| | FGFR2 | Cell division, growth and differentiation | Colorectal and cervical cancers [109,110] | Involvement in other biological processes [111] |

ECM, extracellular matrix; EMT, epithelial–mesenchymal transition; MMPs, matrix metalloproteinases.

After penetrating the basement membrane, invading cells enter the ECM. Fibronectin is the major ECM component that plays a key role in the stimulation of cell growth, adhesion, and cell migration. On the one hand, fibronectin forms a physical barrier for migrating cells; on the other hand, its interaction with tumor cell integrins, mainly with α5β1, triggers ECM proteolysis through secreting MMP-2 and MMP-9 [42,112]. Fibronectin was demonstrated to be involved in the regulation of cell invasion and migration in various cancers [113] and expressed at the invasive front of oral and head and neck squamous cell carcinomas [60,61].

The tenascin C protein also belongs to ECM glycoproteins; however, it is mainly active during embryogenesis. In the adult body, tenascin C is found only in some types of connective tissue (tendons, ligaments, etc.). Interestingly, tenascin C is often expressed in the invasive front of breast, lung, liver, and gallbladder cancers, as well as melanoma, and is associated with a poor prognosis particularly decreased recurrence-free and overall survival and a high rate of metastasis [57,62].

Despite the proven association of basement membrane and ECM components with invasiveness, their role as markers of tumor invasion is ambiguous. For example, laminin γ2 expression is not always observed in the invasive front. According to Sentani [43], cytoplasmic laminin γ2 expression in the invasive front of gastric cancer occurs only in 25% of cases, and stromal expression is observed in 8% of cases. According to García-Solano [58], laminin γ2 expression in tumor buds at the invasive front of colorectal adenocarcinoma is found only in 17–57% of cases. In addition to the invasive front, laminin γ2 is also found in the basement membrane and cytoplasm of tumor cells, outside the invasive front [46]. Fibronectin and tenascin C are also expressed not only in the invasive front [57,59].

## 2.2. EMT Factors

EMT is common to almost all cancers, but the transition is rarely implemented in full [67]. Partial EMT is mainly typical of tumor cell clusters. However, there is evidence that single migrating cells may be in partial EMT. During partial EMT, tumor cells show co-expression of molecules of epithelial (E-cadherin, EpCAM, cytokeratin 7, miR-200, miR-34, etc.) and mesenchymal (N-cadherin, vimentin, ZEB, SNAIL, etc.) phenotypes. Cells in a partial EMT are capable of both adhesion and migration [27,28,67].

Overexpression of EMT markers is often observed in the invasive front of various cancers [63]. Nevertheless, molecules involved or associated with EMT are characterized by a low diagnostic value in assessing the invasive potential of tumors. Snail and Twist transcription factors are unstable molecules and undergo rapid proteasomal degradation [64,65]. In contrast, according to our data, Snail and Twist are totally expressed in breast tumor, without any selectivity in the invasive front [66]. Vimentin, which is considered a marker of the final EMT stage, may not be expressed in invasive carcinomas at all [67]. Furthermore, EMT is not always necessary for invasion and metastasis. In Snail and Twist knockout mice, tumor dissemination and the number of metastases are comparable to those in control mice [114]. Therefore, the presence of EMT cannot always answer the question whether the tumor cell migrates at a given time.

However, it should be understood that EMT is a complex process in which each step is thought to be regulated by a distinct set of transcription factors and molecular circuits overlapping to each other and generating specific phenotypes [115,116]. The picture is complicated by the fact that EMT transcription factors control other cellular events, including apoptosis and stemness [116]. Moreover, induction of an EMT transcription factor is known to be sufficient to induce single-cell dissemination without orchestrating the molecular EMT program and with retaining epithelial identity [16,117]. Thus, further studies are needed to explore molecular mechanisms underlying each EMT module, namely cell motility, and to find markers that could be used to assess the invasive potential of tumor cells. In addition, it is necessary to consider the fact that cells are capable of amoeboid and hybrid amoeboid/mesenchymal movement. Therefore, a perfect method for determining the invasive phenotype in tumor cells is the simultaneous assessment of markers of mesenchymal and amoeboid migration.

### 2.3. Cell–Cell and Cell–ECM Interaction Molecules

Adhesion molecules, such as integrins and the cadherin-catenin complex, are the key components of tumor invasion. Changes in the activity of cadherins, which are proteins involved in the formation of cell–cell contacts, is a characteristic feature of invasive growth. E-cadherin, which forms adherens junctions in an epithelial cell layer, is repressed by Snail, Slug, and Twist transcription factors during EMT [64]. The loss of E-cadherin and the nuclear localization of β-catenin, involved in signaling to the actin cytoskeleton [118], were observed in tumor cells at the invasive front in various cancers [69]. Nuclear accumulation of β-catenin in tumor cells in the invasive front and in vessels was found to be a powerful predictor of liver metastasis in colorectal cancer [70,71]. However, the loss of E-cadherin expression is probably not an indispensable prerequisite for invasiveness of tumor cells [72] and, therefore, cannot be used as a marker for invasive growth, at least for some cancers. Moreover, in some tumors, a loss of E-cadherin has been shown to be detrimental to invasion and metastasis. For example, the presence of E-cadherin is a specific feature of a highly aggressive form of breast cancer, inflammatory carcinoma, and needed for successful invasion and metastatic colonization of bone by tumor cells [119]. In this regard, analysis of more effective markers is needed to assess the invasive tumor potential, along with markers of amoeboid movement, as mentioned above.

The key event initiating production of metalloproteinases is the interaction of integrins with ECM components. The main ligands for integrins are fibronectin ($α5β1$, $αvβ3$, and $α4β1$ integrins), collagens ($α1β1$, $α2β1$, and $α11β1$), and laminins ($α2β1$, $α3β1$, $α6β1$, and $α6β4$) [41,64,120–123]. For example, $α3β1$ integrin activates MMP-9 synthesis through interaction with laminins and triggers reorganization of the actin cytoskeleton [124]; $α6β1$ is involved in tumor invasion via activation of the urokinase plasminogen activator (uPA) receptor and MMP-2 [125]. Laminin-5 is the best-characterized ligand for $α3β1$ integrin. $α6β4$ integrin is involved in the regulation of tumor cell migration through activation of the Rho-A signaling cascade [121]. Binding of fibronectin to $α5β1$ integrin activates MMP-1 and stimulates migration through the ILK/Akt and GSK3β/Snail/E-cadherin signaling pathways [121,126]. Fibronectin-mediated migration is also associated with $αvβ3$ integrin. $αvβ3$ integrin is involved in activation of MMP-2 [127] and, under stress conditions, can trigger a ligand-independent signaling cascade leading to activation of NF-κB and Slug, acquisition of a stem phenotype, and promotion of migration [126].

Expression of integrins changes during tumor progression and is often elevated in the invasive front of tumors: $αvβ3$ in melanoma [75], $αvβ6$ in colon and head and neck cancers [73,76], and $α6β4$ in non-small cell lung cancer [74]. Furthermore, high expression of integrins in tumor cells may promote metastasis. For example, $α2β1$ enhances metastasis of rhabdomyosarcoma in nude mice after intravenous or subcutaneous injection [128], whereas α3β1 promotes lung metastasis through binding to laminin-5 in an exposed basement membrane in the pulmonary vasculature [50].

Signaling pathways activated by different integrins may lead to the same biological effects, while an individual contribution of each of the integrins is different. In neuroblastoma, tumor cell migration can be activated either via FAK-mediated α5β1 integrin signaling or via a FAK-independent pathway involving α4β1 integrin. Both signaling pathways lead to the induction of Src family protein kinases [129,130].

The use of integrins as markers of invasive growth is complicated by the fact that the same integrins can participate in both invasion and other biological processes [78]. For example, α6β1 integrin, apart from involvement in tumor invasion, also participates in $Ca^{2+}$ signaling [131] and platelet adhesion upon damage to the vascular wall [132].

There is evidence that changes in expression of other cell interaction proteins may be a marker of invasive tumor cells. Galectins, membrane glycoproteins, bound to integrins, laminins, and fibronectin, are used by cells to interact with each other and with the ECM [47,133]. Galectin-1 is involved in the regulation of cell adhesion and migration, on the one hand, through stimulation of MMP-2 and MMP-9 and, on the other hand, through activation of a small Rho GTPase Cdc42, which promotes the formation of actin filopodia. Increased expression of galectin-1 is associated with high invasiveness of lung adenocarcinoma and observed in the invasive front of oral squamous cell carcinoma and glioblastoma [47,79,80]. However, galectins have effects not only on tumor cells but also on immune cells promoting inflammation or dampening T cell-mediated immune responses [77]. The L1 cell adhesion molecule (L1CAM), which is involved in β-catenin/TCF signaling, is necessary for cell migration and invasion. Normally, L1CAM is present only in the nervous tissue, but its expression is induced in tumor cells. Increased expression of L1CAM was found in many cancers, including the invasive front of colorectal and pancreatic cancers [81,82]. Nevertheless, L1CAM can have a static function as a cell adhesion molecule and its expression is associated with good cancer prognosis [83,134].

*2.4. Serine Proteases and Matrix Metalloproteinases*

One of the main systems responsible for ECM proteolysis is the plasminogen activation system that triggers a powerful serine protease, plasmin. The central component of this system is the uPA and its receptor (uPAR), the interaction of which stimulates proteolysis of plasminogen to plasmin [135,136]. uPA is believed to play a significant role in tumor invasion and metastasis [135–137]. Experiments in model animals demonstrated that inhibition of uPA and/or the uPA/uPAR interaction slows down metastasis [135]. In contrast, expression of uPAR is associated with tumor invasion and is found in stromal and tumor cells in the invasive front of oral and skin squamous cell carcinomas [84,85].

Metalloproteinases are involved in proteolytic degradation of the basement membrane and ECM. MMP-7 activates MMP-2 and MMP-9 gelatinases exhibiting proteolytic activity against collagen IV, laminins, proteoglycans, and fibronectin [138]. Expression of MMPs is observed during cancer cell invasion [13,41]. MMP-7-positive tumor cells are predominantly found in the invasive front of gastric cancer, while their number is much higher in aggressive and late-stage tumors [90,91]. MMP-7 is also expressed in the invasive front of colon cancer and correlates with tumor stage [56,91,92]. Elevated MMP-2 and MMP-9 levels are observed in the invasive front of melanoma, endometrial cancer, and ovarian cancer [89,93]. High MMP-2 and MMP-9 expression is also observed in the invasive front of head and neck squamous cell carcinoma [88,94]. Assessment of MMP-2 and MMP-9 expression in the invasive tumor front may be helpful in the differentiation of verrucous carcinoma and squamous cell carcinoma of the oral cavity [139].

However, increased expression of uPA and MMPs is not a unique feature of invasive tumor cells and may be observed in other physiological processes. The components of the uPA system can be involved in the early stages of tumor formation and can increase cell proliferation, inhibit apoptosis, etc. [86]. MMPs are mediators between tumor cells and the microenvironment [87]. MMP-9 produced by inflammatory cells is involved in the proteolytic activation of anti-inflammatory cytokines

TGF-β2 and TGF-β3, and MMP-2 and MMP-14 participate in the activation of TGF-β1 [87,140,141]. MMP-2, MMP-9, and MMP-14 indirectly modulate TGF-β activity by cleaving an ECM component, the latent TGF-β binding protein 1 [87,142]. MMP-7 inhibits apoptosis and reduces the efficacy of chemotherapy by cleaving Fas ligands on the surface of cells exposed to doxorubicin [87,143]. MMP-2 and MMP-9 are also involved in the regulation of angiogenesis and lymphangiogenesis [87]. MMP-9 secreted by inflammatory cells modulates bioavailability of VEGF to the VEGFR2 receptor [87,144]. Experiments in mice demonstrated the role of MMP-9 in triggering the angiogenic switch and in vasculogenesis [87,145,146]. Therefore, the multifunctionality of MMPs reduces their significance as markers of invasive growth.

### 2.5. Actin Cytoskeleton Proteins

Proteins involved in actin cytoskeleton remodeling play an important role in the mechanisms of tumor cell migration and invasion [147]. The ezrin protein is a connecting link between actin filaments and membrane proteins involved in cell–cell adhesion and migration [148]. Ezrin was demonstrated to be localized together with the podoplanin in filopodia, stimulating cellular invasion [149], and expressed in the invasive front of lung cancer [95]. Many studies reported that upregulation of Ezrin is a negative prognostic factor in various cancers. However, there is an opposite data indicating the involvement of negative or reduced expression of Ezrin in cancer progression [96]. This contradiction can be explained by the fact that Ezrin is implicated in the regulation not only of cell motility but also of cell adhesion, ion channels, cell proliferation, etc. [150].

The WAVE2 protein is involved in actin filament reorganization and lamellipodia formation and was shown to colocalize with Arp2 at the invasive front of breast cancer [97,147].

Cortactin regulates cortical actin cytoskeleton dynamics by stabilizing F-actin networks and promoting actin polymerization via activating the Arp2/3 complex [47,151]. According to in vitro and in vivo experiments, cortactin promotes invasion of head and neck tumors [151], and its high expression is found in the invasive front of oral and laryngeal tumors [98,99].

The MENA protein regulates actin polymerization and cell migration. An elevated level of the MENA$^{inv}$ isoform, which is involved in the formation of invadopodia due to phosphorylation of cortactin and activation of the N-WASP/Arp2/3 complex, is found in invasive cells of human tumors and animal tumor models and is associated with a high risk of metastasis [100,152,153].

Fascin-1 is an actin-binding protein involved in filopodia formation. It is highly expressed in nervous tissue and is normally absent in epithelial cells. However, a high level of fascin-1 is found in many malignant neoplasms of the liver, gallbladder, stomach, intestines, lung, breast, etc., and is a marker of poor prognosis [154,155]. Increased expression of fascin-1 is found in the invasive front of liver, colon, cervical, and endometrial cancers and is associated with a high risk of metastasis [101–104].

### 2.6. Other Proteins

In the invasive front, there are highly proliferating tumor cells, which probably facilitate the more efficient dissemination of the tumor. Expression of Ki-67, a cell proliferation marker, was shown to be elevated in the invasive front of oral and endometrial cancers [6,105,106]. In breast cancer, nuclear expression of Ki-67 is two-fold higher in the invasive front than in other parts of the tumor and is associated with metastasis to bones and liver [107]. Increased proliferation of tumor cells in the invasive front is also indicated by elevated expression of FGFR2 that is involved in the induction of signaling pathways affecting division, growth, and differentiation of cells, as demonstrated in colorectal and cervical cancers [109,110]. However, there are also contradictory data on negative expression Ki-67 or the absence of differences in its level between the invasive front and the tumor center in oral and colorectal cancers [56,69,108]. Moreover, FGFR2 is a multifunctional protein that regulates different biological processes such as proliferation, differentiation, etc. [111].

At first glance, the prevalence of cell proliferation in the invasive front is in contradiction to the data that invading tumor cells are enriched in EMT markers [63] because EMT typically associates with cell cycle arrest [156]. However, in the invasive front, EMT-cell cycle connection can be broken. In other words, instead of "go-or-grow", tumor cells follow "go-and-grow" behavior [115,157].

The search for tumor invasion markers is an important issue aimed at assessing the risk of cancer metastasis. The role of the discussed molecules as invasive markers is controversial in most cases. Most of these molecules are involved not only in invasive growth but also in processes not related to cell migration. Nevertheless, some molecules such as WAVE2, cortactin, MENAinv, and fascin-1 are promising candidates for future studies of their roles as cancer cell invasion markers. In any case, the search for more specific markers of invasive growth is needed. In this regard, we think that the emphasis on intratumor morphological heterogeneity typical of many cancers may be very productive. In particular, investigation of the molecular make-up of various invasive tumor structures may enable identification of new molecules associated with invasion of tumor cells.

## 3. Intratumor Morphological Heterogeneity as a Model for Studying Cancer Cell Invasion

Based on more than 10-year morphological studies and detailed analysis of various structural features of invasive carcinoma of no special type of the breast (IC NST, previously classified as invasive ductal carcinoma), we have concluded that there are two types of tumors: Nonstructural and structural (Figure 1). Nonstructural breast carcinomas are characterized by a monomorphic pattern and are represented by large solid areas connected to each other, with thin layers of stromal elements (Figure 1).

Structural tumors are characterized by a polymorphic pattern and a pronounced phenotypic variety of the infiltrative (invasive) and stromal components (Figure 1). In other words, structural tumors demonstrate significant morphological heterogeneity. In initial attempts to determine the potential morphological IC NST features associated with cancer progression, we identified five main types of the invasive component in the tumor: Tubular, alveolar, solid, and trabecular structures, and discrete groups of tumor cells [158–161]. The tubular structures are tube-shaped and lumen-containing arrangements of single rows of rather monomorphic tumor cells with round monomorphic nuclei. The alveolar structures are clusters of round or slightly irregular tumor cells of different sizes, often with polymorphic nuclei. The number of cells in alveolar structures varies from 5–20. The solid structures are represented by large masses differing in size and shape, which consist of either small tumor cells with moderate cytoplasm and monomorphic nuclei or large cells with abundant cytoplasm and polymorphic nuclei. Although solid groups of tumor cells are a characteristic feature of nonstructural breast tumors, they are also observed in structural carcinomas. The trabecular structures are represented by either a single row of tumor cells (≥5 cells) or arrangements consisting of two rows of closely related monomorphic cells with moderate cytoplasm, which are parallel to each other. The discrete groups consist of small cell clusters (up to five cells) and single tumor cells (Figure 1). The size and shape of these cells and nuclei vary significantly [158–161].

Different morphological structures were shown to represent transcriptionally distinct tumor cell populations differing in the number of $CD44^+CD24^-$ cancer stem cells, epithelial and mesenchymal features, and enrichment of cancer invasion signaling pathways [160]. Tubular and alveolar structures are similar in gene expression and demonstrate co-expression of epithelial and mesenchymal markers. The solid structures retain the epithelial features but demonstrate an increase in the mesenchymal traits and collective cell migration hallmarks. Trabecular and discrete groups are enriched in mesenchymal genes and cancer invasion pathways. $CD44^+CD24^-$ cells are less common in the discrete groups and more abundant in the alveolar and solid structures [160]. Taken together, these data suggest that different morphological structures demonstrate varying degrees of EMT: From low in tubular, alveolar, and solid structures to advanced in trabecular and discrete groups of tumor cells [160].

The intratumor morphological heterogeneity of breast cancer is not an occasional phenomenon and is strongly associated with disease prognosis and therapy efficacy. Breast tumors with either alveolar or trabecular structures are characterized by a high rate of lymph node metastasis [161,162]. In neoadjuvant chemotherapy (NAC), tumors with alveolar or trabecular structures often demonstrate a poor response [162,163] and an increased risk of distant metastasis [162]. NAC-treated patients with alveolar or trabecular structures in breast tumors have decreased metastasis-free survival [162].

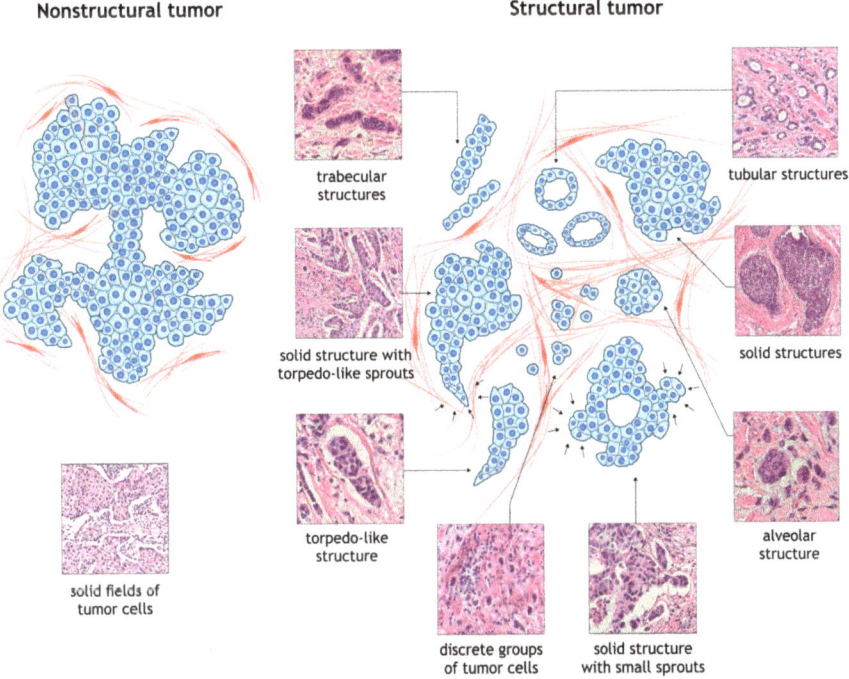

**Figure 1.** Two types of breast carcinomas based on a structural pattern. Nonstructural breast carcinomas are represented by large solid fields of cells connected to each other. Structural breast carcinomas are characterized by a phenotypic variety of the infiltrative (invasive) component, represented by certain types of morphological arrangements of tumor cells: Tubular structures, solid structures with small sprouts, solid structures with large torpedo-like sprouts, alveolar structures, torpedo-like structures, trabecular structures, and discrete groups of tumor cells. The images of hematoxylin and eosin-stained sections were obtained from the database of the Department of Pathological Anatomy, Siberian State Medical University, Tomsk, Russia.

In a longitudinal study of the morphological, molecular genetic and clinical features of breast cancer, we have clearly seen that the differences are present not only in the structural pattern of tumor tissue. It has become obvious that breast carcinoma is characterized by pronounced intratumor morphological heterogeneity when morphologically similar and almost identical structures can exhibit completely different expression profiles, and it may not be ruled out that this phenomenon may somehow affect the behavior of tumor [66]. This conclusion prompted us to differentiate in more detail the previously described morphological structures.

A morphological analysis of structural IC NSTs revealed significant diversity and variability in solid groups of tumor cells, among which we identified two different variants: Solid structures with large torpedo-like sprouts and solid structures with small bud-like sprouts (Figure 1). The first variant is represented by various differently-sized, merging solid areas of tightly packed tumor cells connected with each other. In these structures, there are elongated, mostly triangular sprouts consisting of two–three parallel cell rows. The base of torpedo-like sprouts is always pointed out to the body of solid structures, while the tip, consisting of one–three tumor cells, penetrates to different depths to the stroma. Importantly, torpedo-like sprouts can be presented as structures independent of solid groups of tumor cells (Figure 1). Another variant of solid structures is represented by the large masses of tumor cells. However, a distinctive feature is that any edge of a solid structure comprises rounded or spherical bud-like sprouts consisting of five–seven atypical cells penetrating to the stroma (Figure 1).

Thus, the structural diversity of the infiltrative component and the pronounced intratumor morphological heterogeneity in IC NST represent an attractive model for investigation of tumor cell invasion. The solid structures both with large torpedo-like and small bud-like sprouts, as well as trabecular structures, may be considered as a morphological manifestation of collective cell invasion. Discrete groups of tumor cells, mainly single tumor cells, are an example of individual cell invasion.

## 4. Conclusions

Invasion is a key event towards the acquisition of the metastatic phenotype by tumor cells and an attractive target for anticancer therapy aimed at the prevention of metastasis. In in vitro studies, EMT has been proved to play an important role in the appearance of migrating and invading tumor cells. However, the cell movement mechanisms working in vitro are frequently not related to the invasive growth in vivo. Molecules that have been identified in vitro to be involved in cancer cell invasion do not demonstrate selective expression at the invasive front or at the tips of invasive structures where tumor cells are rather motile. Moreover, the expression of these molecules does not often demonstrate clinical significance for the prediction of cancer metastasis risk. Thus, the question how to identify invading tumor cells in human cancer specimens remains unanswered. In this regard, new effective models should be developed to investigate the mechanisms of cancer cell invasion. In our opinion, one of these models, at least in case of breast cancer, can be intratumor morphological heterogeneity which is a manifestation of different patterns of tumor cell invasion. The investigation of the molecular make-up of invasive structures of tumor cells and their microenvironment may provide valuable information about new molecules involved in the invasive growth and may identify novel prognostic markers and therapeutic targets.

**Author Contributions:** Conceptualization, V.M.P. and M.V.Z.; writing—original draft preparation, T.S.G., N.M.N, N.V.K., and S.Y.Z.; writing—review and editing, E.V.D.; supervision, N.V.C.

**Funding:** The study was supported by the Russian Science Foundation (grant #19-75-30016).

**Conflicts of Interest:** The authors declare no conflict of interest.

## References

1. Hanahan, D.; Weinberg, R.A. Review Hallmarks of Cancer: The Next Generation. *Cell* **2011**, *144*, 646–674. [PubMed]
2. Jiang, W.G.; Sanders, A.J.; Katoh, M.; Ungefroren, H.; Gieseler, F.; Prince, M.; Thompson, S.K.; Zollo, M.; Spano, D.; Dhawan, P.; et al. Tissue invasion and metastasis: Molecular, biological and clinical perspectives. *Semin. Cancer Biol.* **2015**, *35*, 244–275.
3. Sahai, E. Mechanisms of cancer cell invasion. *Curr. Opin. Genet. Dev.* **2005**, *15*, 87–96. [PubMed]
4. Bànkfalvi, A.; Piffkò, J. Prognostic and predictive factors in oral cancer: The role of the invasive tumour front. *J. Oral Pathol. Med.* **2000**, *29*, 291–298. [PubMed]
5. Zlobec, I.; Lugli, A. Invasive front of colorectal cancer: Dynamic interface of pro-/anti-tumor factors. *World J. Gastroenterol.* **2009**, *15*, 5898–5906. [PubMed]
6. Rivera, C.; Venegas, B. Histological and molecular aspects of oral squamous cell carcinoma. *Oncol. Lett.* **2014**, *8*, 7–11. [PubMed]
7. Friedl, P.; Wolf, K. Tumour-cell invasion and migration: Diversity and escape mechanisms. *Nat. Rev. Cancer* **2003**, *3*, 362–374.
8. Wolf, K.; Friedl, P. Molecular mechanisms of cancer cell invasion and plasticity. *Br. J. Dermatol.* **2006**, *154*, 11–15.
9. Krakhmal, N.V.; Zavyalova, M.V.; Denisov, E.V.; Vtorushin, S.V.; Perelmuter, V.M. Cancer invasion: Patterns and mechanisms. *Acta Naturae* **2015**, *7*, 17–28.
10. Lintz, M.; Muñoz, A.; Reinhart-King, C.A. The Mechanics of Single Cell and Collective Migration of Tumor Cells. *J. Biomech. Eng.* **2017**, *139*, 021005.

11. Wang, X.; Enomoto, A.; Asai, N.; Kato, T.; Takahashi, M. Collective invasion of cancer: Perspectives from pathology and development. *Pathol. Int.* **2016**, *66*, 183–192. [PubMed]
12. Pandya, P.; Orgaz, J.L.; Sanz-Moreno, V. Modes of invasion during tumour dissemination. *Mol. Oncol.* **2017**, *11*, 5–27. [PubMed]
13. Friedl, P.; Alexander, S. Cancer invasion and the microenvironment: Plasticity and reciprocity. *Cell* **2011**, *147*, 992–1009. [PubMed]
14. Nguyen-Ngoc, K.-V.; Cheung, K.J.; Brenot, A.; Shamir, E.R.; Gray, R.S.; Hines, W.C.; Yaswen, P.; Werb, Z.; Ewald, A.J. ECM microenvironment regulates collective migration and local dissemination in normal and malignant mammary epithelium. *Proc. Natl. Acad. Sci.* **2012**, *109*, E2595–E2604. [PubMed]
15. Cheung, K.J.; Gabrielson, E.; Werb, Z.; Ewald, A.J. Collective invasion in breast cancer requires a conserved basal epithelial program. *Cell* **2013**, *155*, 1639–1651. [PubMed]
16. Cheung, K.J.; Ewald, A.J. Illuminating breast cancer invasion: Diverse roles for cell-cell interactions. *Curr. Opin. Cell Biol.* **2014**, *30*, 99–111. [PubMed]
17. Paňková, K.; Rösel, D.; Novotný, M.; Brábek, J. The molecular mechanisms of transition between mesenchymal and amoeboid invasiveness in tumor cells. *Cell. Mol. Life Sci.* **2010**, *67*, 63–71. [PubMed]
18. Chikina, A.S.; Alexandrova, A.Y. The cellular mechanisms and regulation of metastasis formation. *Mol. Biol.* **2014**, *48*, 165–180.
19. Paluch, E.K.; Raz, E. The role and regulation of blebs in cell migration. *Curr. Opin. Cell Biol.* **2013**, *25*, 582–590.
20. Huang, B.; Lu, M.; Jolly, M.K.; Tsarfaty, I.; Onuchic, J.; Ben-Jacob, E. The three-way switch operation of Rac1/RhoA GTPase-based circuit controlling amoeboid-hybrid-mesenchymal transition. *Sci. Rep.* **2014**, *4*, 1–11.
21. Kalluri, R.; Weinberg, R. The basics of epithelial-mesenchymal transition. *J. Clin. Invest.* **2009**, *119*, 1420–1428. [PubMed]
22. Lamouille, S.; Xu, J.; Derynck, R. Molecular mechanisms of epithelial–mesenchymal transition. *Nat. Rev. Mol. Cell Biol.* **2014**, *15*, 1–45.
23. Bonde, A.K.; Tischler, V.; Kumar, S.; Soltermann, A.; Schwendener, R.A. Intratumoral macrophages contribute to epithelial-mesenchymal transition in solid tumors. *BMC Cancer* **2012**, *12*, 35.
24. Nieto, M.A.; Huang, R.Y.Y.J.; Jackson, R.A.A.; Thiery, J.P.P. Emt: 2016. *Cell* **2016**, *166*, 21–45. [PubMed]
25. Lambert, A.W.; Pattabiraman, D.R.; Weinberg, R.A. Emerging Biological Principles of Metastasis. *Cell* **2017**, *168*, 670–691. [PubMed]
26. Gao, D.; Vahdat, L.T.; Wong, S.; Chang, J.C.; Mittal, V. Microenvironmental regulation of epithelial-mesenchymal transitions in cancer. *Cancer Res.* **2012**, *72*, 4883–4889. [PubMed]
27. Jolly, M.K.; Boareto, M.; Huang, B.; Jia, D.; Onuchic, J.N.; Levine, H. Implications of the hybrid epithelial/mesenchymal phenotype in metastasis. *Front Oncol.* **2015**, *5*, 1–19.
28. Grigore, A.D.; Jolly, M.K.; Jia, D. Tumor Budding: The Name is EMT. Partial EMT. *J. Clin. Med.* **2016**, *5*, 1–23.
29. Zhang, S.; Wang, X.; Gupta, A.; Fang, X.; Wang, L.; Zhang, C. Expression of IL-17 with tumor budding as a prognostic marker in oral squamous cell carcinoma. *Am. J. Transl. Res.* **2019**, *11*, 1876–1883.
30. Lorenzo Soriano, L.; Ordaz Jurado, G.; Pontones Moreno, J.L.; Villarroya Castillo, S.; Hernández Girón, S.; Sáez Moreno, I.; Ramos Soler, D. Tumor Budding: Prognostic Value in Muscle-Invasive Bladder Cancer. *Urology* **2019**.
31. Sirin, A.H.; Sokmen, S.; Unlu, S.M.; Ellidokuz, H.; Sarioglu, S. The prognostic value of tumor budding in patients who had surgery for rectal cancer with and without neoadjuvant therapy. *Tech. Coloproctol.* **2019**, *23*, 333–342. [PubMed]
32. Ekmekci, S.; Kucuk, U.; Kokkoz, S.; Cakir, E.; Gumussoy, M. Tumor budding in laryngeal carcinoma. *Indian J. Pathol. Microbiol.* **2019**, *62*, 7–10. [PubMed]
33. Agarwal, R.; Khurana, N.; Singh, T.; Agarwal, P.N. Tumor budding in infiltrating breast carcinoma: Correlation with known clinicopathological parameters and hormone receptor status. *Indian J. Pathol. Microbiol.* **2019**, *62*, 222–225. [PubMed]
34. Ogino, M.; Nakanishi, Y.; Mitsuhashi, T.; Hatanaka, Y.; Amano, T.; Marukawa, K.; Nitta, T.; Ueno, T.; Ono, M.; Kuwabara, S.; et al. Impact of Tumour Budding Grade in 310 Patients Who Underwent Surgical Resection for Extrahepatic Cholangiocarcinoma. *Histopathology* **2019**, *74*, 861–872. [PubMed]
35. Huang, B.; Jolly, M.K.; Lu, M.; Tsarfaty, I.; Ben-Jacob, E.; Onuchic, J.N. Modeling the Transitions between Collective and Solitary Migration Phenotypes in Cancer Metastasis. *Sci. Rep.* **2015**, *5*, 1–13.

36. Lehmann, S.; Boekhorst, V.; Odenthal, J.; Bianchi, R.; van Helvert, S.; Ikenberg, K.; Ilina, O.; Stoma, S.; Xandry, J.; Jiang, L.; et al. Hypoxia Induces a HIF-1-Dependent Transition from Collective-to-Amoeboid Dissemination in Epithelial Cancer Cells. *Curr. Biol.* **2017**, *27*, 392–400. [PubMed]
37. Bockhorn, M.; Jain, R.K.; Munn, L.L. Active versus passive mechanisms in metastasis: do cancer cells crawl into vessels, or are they pushed? *Lancet Oncol.* **2007**, *8*, 444–448.
38. Iguchi, T.; Aishima, S.; Taketomi, A.; Nishihara, Y.; Fujita, N.; Sanefuji, K.; Maehara, Y.; Tsuneyoshi, M. Extracapsular penetration is a new prognostic factor in human hepatocellular carcinoma. *Am. J. Surg. Pathol.* **2008**, *32*, 1675–1682. [PubMed]
39. Mehes, G.; Witt, A.; Kubista, E.; Ambros, P.F. Circulating Breast Cancer Cells Are Frequently Apoptotic. *Am. J. Pathol.* **2001**, *159*, 17–20. [PubMed]
40. Larson, C.J.; Moreno, J.G.; Pienta, K.J.; Gross, S.; Repollet, M.; O'Hara, S.M.; Russell, T.; Terstappen, L.W. Apoptosis of circulating tumor cells in prostate cancer patients. *Cytom. Part A* **2004**, *62*, 46–53.
41. Hood, J.D.; Cheresh, D.A. Role of integrins in cell invasion and migration. *Nat. Rev.* **2002**, *2*, 1–10.
42. Rowe, R.G.; Weiss, S.J. Navigating ECM Barriers at the Invasive Front: The Cancer Cell—Stroma Interface. *Annu. Rev. Cell Dev. Biol.* **2009**, *25*, 567–595. [PubMed]
43. Sentani, K.; Matsuda, M. Clinicopathological significance of MMP-7, laminin γ2 and EGFR expression at the invasive front of gastric carcinoma. *Gastric Cancer* **2014**, *17*, 412–422. [PubMed]
44. Halfter, W.; Oertle, P.; Monnier, C.A.; Camenzind, L.; Reyes-Lua, M.; Hu, H.; Candiello, J.; Labilloy, A.; Balasubramani, M.; Henrich, P.B.; et al. New concepts in basement membrane biology. *FEBS J.* **2015**, *282*, 4466–4479. [PubMed]
45. Hintermann, E.; Quaranta, V. Epithelial cell motility on laminin-5: Regulation by matrix assembly, proteolysis, integrins and erbB receptors. *Matrix Biol.* **2004**, *23*, 75–85. [PubMed]
46. Masuda, R.; Kijima, H.; Imamura, N.; Aruga, N.; Nakazato, K.; Oiwa, K.; Nakano, T.; Watanabe, H.; Ikoma, Y.; Tanaka, M.; et al. Laminin-5 gamma 2 chain expression is associated with tumor cell invasiveness and prognosis of lung squamous cell carcinoma. *Biomed. Res.* **2012**, *33*, 309–317. [PubMed]
47. Sharma, M.; Sah, P.; Sharma, S.S.; Radhakrishnan, R. Molecular changes in invasive front of oral cancer. *J. Oral Maxillofac. Pathol.* **2013**, *17*, 240–247. [PubMed]
48. Ramovs, V.; te Molder, L.; Sonnenberg, A. The opposing roles of laminin-binding integrins in cancer. *Matrix Biol.* **2017**, *57*, 213–243.
49. Ishikawa, T.; Wondimu, Z.; Oikawa, Y.; Gentilcore, G.; Kiessling, R.; Egyhazi Brage, S.; Hansson, J.; Patarroyo, M. Laminins 411 and 421 differentially promote tumor cell migration via α6β1 integrin and MCAM (CD146). *Matrix Biol.* **2014**, *38*, 69–83.
50. Wang, H.; Fu, W.; Im, J.H.; Zhou, Z.; Santoro, S.A.; Iyer, V.; DiPersio, C.M.; Yu, Q.C.; Quaranta, V.; Al-Mehdi, A.; et al. Tumor cell α3β1 integrin and vascular laminin-5 mediate pulmonary arrest and metastasis. *J. Cell Biol.* **2004**, *164*, 935–941.
51. Maltseva, D.V.; Rodin, S.A. Laminins in Metastatic Cancer. *Mol. Biol.* **2018**, *52*, 350–371.
52. Miyazaki, K. Laminin-5 (laminin-332): Unique biological activity and role in tumor growth and invasion. *Cancer Sci.* **2006**, *97*, 91–98. [PubMed]
53. Yamamoto, H.; Kitadai, Y.; Yamamoto, H.; Oue, N.; Ohdan, H.; Yasui, W.; Kikuchi, A. Laminin γ2 Mediates Wnt5a-Induced Invasion of Gastric Cancer Cells. *Gastroenterology* **2009**, *137*, 242–252. [PubMed]
54. Okada, K.-I.; Kijima, H.; Imaizumi, T.; Hirabayashi, K.; Matsuyama, M.; Yazawa, N.; Oida, Y.; Tobita, K.; Tanaka, M.; Dowaki, S.; et al. Stromal laminin-5γ2 chain expression is associated with the wall-invasion pattern of gallbladder adenocarcinoma. *Biomed. Res.* **2009**, *30*, 53–62. [PubMed]
55. Niki, T.; Kohno, T.; Iba, S.; Moriya, Y.; Takahashi, Y.; Saito, M.; Maeshima, A. Frequent Co-Localization of Cox-2 and Laminin-5 γ2 Chain at the Invasive Front of Early-Stage Lung Adenocarcinomas. *Am. J. Pathol.* **2002**, *160*, 1129–1141. [PubMed]
56. Karamitopoulou, E.; Zlobec, I.; Panayiotides, I.; Patsouris, E.S.; Peros, G.; Rallis, G.; Lapas, C.; Karakitsos, P.; Terracciano, L.M.; Lugli, A. Systematic analysis of proteins from different signaling pathways in the tumor center and the invasive front of colorectal cancer. *Hum. Pathol.* **2011**, *42*, 1888–1896. [PubMed]
57. Lowy, C.M.; Oskarsson, T.; Lowy, C.M.; Oskarsson, T. Tenascin C in metastasis: A view from the invasive front. *Cell Adh. Migr.* **2015**, *9*, 112–124.

58. García-Solano, J.; Conesa-Zamora, P.; Trujillo-Santos, J.; Torres-Moreno, D.; Mäkinen, M.J.; Pérez-Guillermo, M. Immunohistochemical expression profile of β-catenin, E-cadherin, P-cadherin, laminin-5γ2 chain, and SMAD4 in colorectal serrated adenocarcinoma. *Hum. Pathol.* **2012**, *43*, 1094–1102.
59. Bae, Y.K.; Kim, A.; Kim, M.K.; Choi, J.E.; Kang, S.H.; Lee, S.J. Fibronectin expression in carcinoma cells correlates with tumor aggressiveness and poor clinical outcome in patients with invasive breast cancer. *Hum. Pathol.* **2013**, *44*, 2028–2037.
60. Gopal, S.; Veracini, L.; Grall, D.; Butori, C.; Schaub, S.; Audebert, S.; Camoin, L.; Baudelet, E.; Adwanska, A.; Beghelli-De La Forest Divonne, S.; et al. Fibronectin-guided migration of carcinoma collectives. *Nat. Commun.* **2017**, *8*, 14105.
61. De Oliveira Ramos, G.; Bernardi, L.; Lauxen, I.; Filho, M.S.A.; Horwitz, A.R.; Lamers, M.L. Fibronectin modulates cell adhesion and signaling to promote single cell migration of highly invasive oral squamous cell carcinoma. *PLoS ONE* **2016**, *11*, 1–18.
62. Aishima, S.; Taguchi, K.; Terashi, T.; Matsuura, S.; Shimada, M.; Tsuneyoshi, M. Tenascin Expression at the Invasive Front Is Associated with Poor Prognosis in Intrahepatic Cholangiocarcinoma. *Mod. Pathol.* **2003**, *16*, 1019–1027. [PubMed]
63. Gurzu, S. Epithelial-mesenchymal, mesenchymal-epithelial, and endothelial-mesenchymal transitions in malignant tumors: An update. *World J. Clin. Cases* **2015**, *3*, 393–404. [PubMed]
64. Christofori, G. New signals from the invasive front. *Nature* **2006**, *441*, 444–450. [PubMed]
65. Zhong, J.; Ogura, K.; Wang, Z.; Inuzuka, H. Degradation of the Transcription Factor Twist, an Oncoprotein that Promotes Cancer Metastasis. *Discov Med.* **2013**, *15*, 7–15. [PubMed]
66. Krakhmal, N.V.; Zavyalova, M.V.; Perelmuter, V.M.; Vtorushin, S.V.; Slonimskaya, E.M.; Denisov, E.V. Heterogeneous expression of markers associated with invasive breast cancer (in Russ). *Sib. J. Oncol.* **2016**, *15*, 56–61.
67. Brabletz, T.; Kalluri, R.; Nieto, M.A.; Weinberg, R.A. EMT in cancer. *Nat. Rev. Cancer* **2018**, *18*, 128–134.
68. Brabletz, T.; Jung, A.; Reu, S.; Porzner, M.; Hlubek, F.; Kunz-Schughart, L.A.; Knuechel, R.; Kirchner, T. Variable β-catenin expression in colorectal cancers indicates tumor progression driven by the tumor environment. *Proc. Natl. Acad. Sci.* **2002**, *98*, 10356–10361.
69. Pereira, C.H.; Morais, M.O.; Martins, A.F.L.; Soares, M.Q.S.; de C.G. Alencar, R.; Batista, A.C.; Leles, C.R.; Mendonça, E.F. Expression of adhesion proteins (E-cadherin and β-catenin) and cell proliferation (Ki-67) at the invasive tumor front in conventional oral squamous cell and basaloid squamous cell carcinomas. *Arch. Oral Biol.* **2016**, *61*, 8–15.
70. Suzuki, H.; Masuda, N.; Shimura, T.; Araki, K.; Kobayashi, T.; Tsutsumi, S.; Asao, T.; Kuwano, H. Nuclear β-Catenin Expression at the Invasive Front and in the Vessels Predicts Liver Metastasis in Colorectal Carcinoma. *Anticancer Res.* **2008**, *28*, 1821–1830.
71. Wang, L.; Cheng, H.; Liu, Y.; Wang, L.; Yu, W.; Zhang, G.; Chen, B.; Yu, Z.; Hu, S. Prognostic value of nuclear β-catenin overexpression at invasive front in colorectal cancer for synchronous liver metastasis. *Ann. Surg. Oncol.* **2011**, *18*, 1553–1559. [PubMed]
72. Shamir, E.R.; Ewald, A.J. Adhesion in mammary development: Novel roles for E-cadherin in individual and collective cell migration. *Curr. Top. Dev. Biol.* **2015**, *112*, 353–382. [PubMed]
73. Yang, G.Y.; Guo, S.; Dong, C.Y.; Wang, X.Q.; Hu, B.Y.; Liu, Y.F.; Chen, Y.W.; Niu, J.; Dong, J.H. Integrin αvβ6 sustains and promotes tumor invasive growth in colon cancer progression. *World J. Gastroenterol.* **2015**, *21*, 7457–7467. [PubMed]
74. Stewart, R.L.; West, D.; Wang, C.; Weiss, H.L.; Gal, T.; Durbin, E.B.; O'Connor, W.; Chen, M.; O'Connor, K.L. Elevated integrin α6β4 expression is associated with venous invasion and decreased overall survival in non-small cell lung cancer. *Hum. Pathol.* **2016**, *54*, 174–183. [PubMed]
75. Albelda, S.M.; Mette, S.A.; Elder, D.E.; Stewart, R.M.; Damjanovich, L.; Herlyn, M.; Buck, C.A. Integrin Distribution in Malignant Melanoma: Association of the β3 Subunit with Tumor Progression. *Cancer Res.* **1990**, *50*, 6757–6764. [PubMed]
76. Koopman Van Aarsen, L.A.; Leone, D.R.; Ho, S.; Dolinski, B.M.; McCoon, P.E.; LePage, D.J.; Kelly, R.; Heaney, G.; Rayhorn, P.; Reid, C.; et al. Antibody-mediated blockade of integrin αvβ6 inhibits tumor progression in vivo by a transforming growth factor-β-regulated mechanism. *Cancer Res.* **2008**, *68*, 561–570.
77. Chou, F.C.; Chen, H.Y.; Kuo, C.C.; Sytwu, H.K. Role of galectins in tumors and in clinical immunotherapy. *Int. J. Mol. Sci.* **2018**, *19*, 430.

78. Richard, O. Hynes. Integrins: Bidirectional, Allosteric Signaling Machines. *Cell* **2002**, *110*, 673–687.
79. Wu, M.-H.; Hong, H.-C.; Cheng, H.-W.; Pan, S.-H.; Liang, Y.-R.; Hong, T.-M.; Chiang, W.-F.; Wong, T.-Y.; Shieh, D.-B.; Shiau, A.-L.; et al. Galectin-1-Mediated Tumor Invasion and Metastasis, Up-Regulated Matrix Metalloproteinase Expression, and Reorganized Actin Cytoskeletons. *Mol. Cancer Res.* **2009**, *7*, 311–318.
80. Toussaint, L.G.; Nilson, A.E.; Goble, J.M.; Ballman, K.V.; James, C.D.; Lefranc, F.; Kiss, R.; Uhm, J.H. Galectin-1, a gene preferentially expressed at the tumor margin, promotes glioblastoma cell invasion. *Mol. Cancer* **2012**, *11*, 32. [PubMed]
81. Gavert, N.; Conacci-sorrell, M.; Gast, D.; Schneider, A.; Altevogt, P.; Brabletz, T.; Ben-Ze'ev, A. L1, a novel target of β-catenin signaling, transforms cells and is expressed at the invasive front of colon cancers. *J. Cell Biol.* **2005**, *168*, 633–642. [PubMed]
82. Tsutsumi, S.; Morohashi, S.; Kudo, Y.; Akasaka, H.; Ogasawara, H.; Ono, M.; Takasugi, K.; Ishido, K.; Hakamada, K.; Kijima, H. L1 Cell adhesion molecule (L1CAM) expression at the cancer invasive front is a novel prognostic marker of pancreatic ductal adenocarcinoma. *J. Surg. Oncol.* **2011**, *103*, 669–673. [PubMed]
83. Altevogt, P.; Doberstein, K.; Fogel, M. L1CAM in human cancer. *Int. J. Cancer* **2016**, *138*, 1565–1576.
84. Shi, Z.; Stack, M.S. Urinary-type plasminogen activator (uPA) and its receptor (uPAR) in squamous cell carcinoma of the oral cavity. *Biochem. J.* **2007**, *407*, 153–159. [PubMed]
85. Rømer, J.; Pyke, C.; Lund, L.R.; Ralfkiær, E.; Danø, K. Cancer cell expression of urokinase-type plasminogen activator receptor mRNA in squamous cell carcinomas of the skin. *J. Invest. Dermatol.* **2001**, *116*, 353–358. [PubMed]
86. Mahmood, N.; Mihalcioiu, C.; Rabbani, S.A. Multifaceted Role of the Urokinase-Type Plasminogen Activator (uPA) and Its Receptor (uPAR): Diagnostic, Prognostic, and Therapeutic Applications. *Front. Oncol.* **2018**, *8*, 24. [PubMed]
87. Kessenbrock, K.; Plaks, V.; Werb, Z. Matrix Metalloproteinases: Regulators of the Tumor Microenvironment. *Cell* **2010**, *141*, 52–67. [PubMed]
88. Ondruschka, C.; Buhtz, P.; Motsch, C.; Freigang, B.; Schneider-Stock, R.; Roessner, A.; Boltze, C. Prognostic value of MMP-2, -9 and TIMP-1,-2 immunoreactive protein at the invasive front in advanced head and neck squamous cell carcinomas. *Pathol. Res. Pract.* **2002**, *198*, 509–515. [PubMed]
89. Ntayi, C.; Labrousse, A.L.; Debret, R.; Birembaut, P.; Bellon, G.; Antonicelli, F.; Hornebeck, W.; Bernard, P. Elastin-Derived Peptides Upregulate Matrix Metalloproteinase-2-ediated Melanoma Cell Invasion Through Elastin-Binding Protein. *J. Invest. Dermatol.* **2004**, *122*, 256–265.
90. Liu, X.P.; Kawauchi, S.; Oga, A.; Tsushimi, K.; Tsushimi, M. Prognostic significance of matrix metalloproteinase-7 (MMP-7) expression at the invasive front in gastric carcinoma. *Jpn. J. Cancer Res.* **2002**, *7*, 291–295.
91. Kitoh, T.; Yanai, H.; Saitoh, Y.; Nakamura, Y.; Matsubara, Y.; Kitoh, H.; Yoshida, T.; Okita, K. Increased expression of matrix metalloproteinase-7 in invasive early gastric cancer. *J. Gastroenterol.* **2004**, *39*, 434–440. [PubMed]
92. Adachi, Y.; Yamamoto, H.; Itoh, F.; Hinoda, Y.; Okada, Y.; Imai, K. Contribution of matrilysin (MMP-7) to the metastatic pathway of human colorectal cancers. *Gut* **1999**, *45*, 252–258. [PubMed]
93. Planagumà, J.; Liljeström, M.; Alameda, F.; Bützow, R.; Virtanen, I.; Reventós, J.; Hukkanen, M. Matrix metalloproteinase-2 and matrix metalloproteinase-9 codistribute with transcription factors RUNX1 / AML1 and ETV5 / ERM at the invasive front of endometrial and ovarian carcinoma. *Hum. Pathol.* **2011**, *42*, 57–67. [PubMed]
94. Sterz, C.M.; Kulle, C.; Dakic, B.; Makarova, G.; Böttcher, M.C.; Bette, M.; Werner, J.A.; Mandic, R. A basal-cell-like compartment in head and neck squamous cell carcinomas represents the invasive front of the tumor and is expressing MMP-9. *Oral Oncol.* **2010**, *46*, 116–122. [PubMed]
95. Li, Q.; Gao, H.; Xu, H.; Wang, X.; Pan, Y.; Hao, F.; Qiu, X.; Stoecker, M.; Wang, E.; Wang, E. Expression of ezrin correlates with malignant phenotype of lung cancer, and in vitro knockdown of ezrin reverses the aggressive biological behavior of lung cancer cells. *Tumour Biol.* **2012**, *33*, 1493–1504. [PubMed]
96. Li, J.; Wei, K.; Yu, H.; Jin, D.; Wang, G.; Yu, B. Prognostic Value of Ezrin in Various Cancers: A Systematic Review and Updated Meta-analysis. *Sci. Rep.* **2015**, *5*, 1–13.
97. Iwaya, K.; Norio, K.; Mukai, K. Coexpression of Arp2 and WAVE2 predicts poor outcome in invasive breast carcinoma. *Mod. Pathol.* **2007**, *20*, 339–343. [PubMed]

98. Ambrosio, P.E.; Rosa, E.F.; Aparecida, M.; Domingues, C.; André, R.; Villacis, R.; Coudry, R.D.A.; Tagliarini, J.V.; Soares, F.A. Cortactin is associated with perineural invasion in the deep invasive front area of laryngeal carcinomas. *Hum. Pathol.* **2011**, *42*, 1221–1229. [PubMed]
99. Yamada, S.I.; Yanamoto, S.; Kawasaki, G.; Mizuno, A.; Nemoto, T.K. Overexpression of cortactin increases invasion potential in oral squamous cell carcinoma. *Pathol. Oncol. Res.* **2010**, *16*, 523–531. [PubMed]
100. Toyoda, A.; Yokota, A.Y.A.; Saito, T.; Kawana, H. Overexpression of human ortholog of mammalian enabled (hMena) is associated with the expression of mutant p53 protein in human breast cancers. *Int. J. Oncol.* **2011**, *38*, 89–96.
101. Vignjevic, D.; Schoumacher, M.; Gavert, N.; Janssen, K.; Jih, G.; Lae, M.; Louvard, D.; Ben-ze, A.; Robine, S. Fascin, a Novel Target of β-Catenin-TCF Signaling, Is Expressed at the Invasive Front of Human Colon Cancer. *Cancer Res.* **2007**, *67*, 6844–6854. [PubMed]
102. Won, K.Y.; Kim, G.Y.; Lim, S.J.; Park, Y.K.; Kim, Y.W. Prognostic significance of fascin expression in extrahepatic bile duct carcinomas. *Pathol. Res. Pract.* **2009**, *205*, 742–748. [PubMed]
103. Stewart, C.J.R.; Crook, M.; Loi, S. Fascin expression in endocervical neoplasia: Correlation with tumour morphology and growth pattern. *J. Clin. Pathol.* **2012**, *65*, 213–217. [PubMed]
104. Stewart, C.J.R.; Crook, M.L. Fascin expression in undifferentiated and dedifferentiated endometrial carcinoma. *Hum. Pathol.* **2015**, *46*, 1514–1520. [PubMed]
105. Kurokawa, H.; Zhang, M.; Matsumoto, S.; Yamashita, Y.; Tanaka, T.; Tomoyose, T.; Takano, H.; Funaki, K.; Fukuyama, H.; Takahashi, T.; et al. The relationship of the histologic grade at the deep invasive front and the expression of Ki-67 antigen and p53 protein in oral squamous cell carcinoma. *J. Oral Pathol. Med.* **2005**, *34*, 602–607. [PubMed]
106. Horre, N.; Van Diest, P.J.; Sie-Go, D.M.; Heintz, A.P. The invasive front in endometrial carcinoma: higher proliferation and associated derailment of cell cycle regulators. *Hum. Pathol.* **2007**, *38*, 1232–1238.
107. Gong, P.; Wang, Y.; Liu, G.; Zhang, J.; Wang, Z. New Insight into Ki67 Expression at the Invasive Front in Breast Cancer. *PLoS ONE* **2013**, *8*, 1 5.
108. Rubio, C.A. Further studies on the arrest of cell proliferation in tumor cells at the invading front of colonic adenocarcinoma. *J. Gastroenterol. Hepatol.* **2007**, *22*, 1877–1881.
109. Matsuda, Y.; Ishiwata, T.; Yamahatsu, K.; Kawahara, K. Overexpressed fibroblast growth factor receptor 2 in the invasive front of colorectal cancer: A potential therapeutic target in colorectal cancer. *Cancer Lett.* **2011**, *309*, 209–219.
110. Kawase, R.; Ishiwata, T.; Matsuda, Y.; Onda, M.; Kudo, M.; Takeshita, T.; Naito, Z. Expression of fibroblast growth factor receptor 2 IIIc in human uterine cervical intraepithelial neoplasia and cervical cancer. *Int. J. Oncol.* **2010**, *38*, 257–266.
111. Turner, N.; Grose, R. Fibroblast growth factor signalling: From development to cancer. *Nat. Rev. Cancer* **2010**, *10*, 116–129. [PubMed]
112. Pal, S.; Ganguly, K.K.; Chatterjee, A. Extracellular matrix protein fibronectin induces matrix metalloproteinases in human prostate adenocarcinoma cells PC-3. *Cell Commun. Adhes.* **2013**, *20*, 105–114. [PubMed]
113. Wang, J.P.; Hielscher, A. Fibronectin: How its aberrant expression in tumors may improve therapeutic targeting. *J. Cancer* **2017**, *8*, 674–682. [PubMed]
114. Zheng, X.; Carstens, J.L.; Kim, J.; Scheible, M.; Kaye, J.; Sugimoto, H.; Wu, C.; Lebleu, V.S.; Kalluri, R.; Biology, C. EMT Program is Dispensable for Metastasis but Induces Chemoresistance in Pancreatic Cancer. *Nature* **2016**, *527*, 525–530.
115. Jolly, M.K.; Ware, K.E.; Gilja, S.; Somarelli, J.A.; Levine, H. EMT and MET: necessary or permissive for metastasis? *Mol. Oncol.* **2017**, *11*, 755–769. [PubMed]
116. Savagner, P. Epithelial-mesenchymal transitions: From cell plasticity to concept elasticity. *Curr. Top Dev. Biol.* **2015**, *112*, 273–300. [PubMed]
117. Shamir, E.R.; Pappalardo, E.; Jorgens, D.M.; Coutinho, K.; Tsai, W.T.; Aziz, K.; Auer, M.; Tran, P.T.; Bader, J.S.; Ewald, A.J. Twist1-induced dissemination preserves epithelial identity and requires E-cadherin. *J. Cell Biol.* **2014**, *204*, 839–856.
118. Isaeva, A.V.; Zima, A.P.; Shabalova, I.P.; Ryazantseva, N.V.; Vasil'eva, O.A.; Kasoayn, K.T.; Saprina, T.V.; Latypova, V.N.; Berezkina, I.S.; Novitskii, V.V. β-catenin: Structure, function and role in malignant transformation of epithelial cells (in Russ). *Vestn. Ross. Akad. Meditsinskikh Nauk* **2015**, *70*, 475–483.

119. Jolly, M.K.; Boareto, M.; Debeb, B.G.; Aceto, N.; Farach-Carson, M.C.; Woodward, W.A.; Levine, H. Inflammatory breast cancer: A model for investigating cluster-based dissemination. *NPJ Breast Cancer* **2017**, *3*, 1–7.
120. Friedl, P.; Gilmour, D. Collective cell migration in morphogenesis, regeneration and cancer. *Nat. Rev.* **2009**, *10*, 455–456.
121. Rathinam, R.; Alahari, S.K. Important role of integrins in the cancer biology. *Cancer Metastasis Rev.* **2010**, *29*, 223–237. [PubMed]
122. Huttenlocher, A.; Horwitz, A.R. Integrins in Cell Migration. *Cold Spring Harb. Perspect. Biol.* **2011**, 1–17.
123. Ganguly, K.K.; Pal, S.; Moulik, S.; Chatterjee, A. Integrins and metastasis. *Cell Adhes. Migr.* **2013**, *7*, 251–261.
124. Morini, M.; Marcella, M.; Nicoletta, F.; Federica, G.; Simonetta, B.; Roberta, M.; Douglas, M.N.; Pier Giorgio, N.; Adriana, A. The $\alpha 3\beta 1$ integrin is associated with mammary carcinoma cell metastasis, invasion, and gelatinase B (mmp-9) activity. *Int. J. Cancer* **2000**, *87*, 336–342. [PubMed]
125. He, Y.; Liu, X.D.; Chen, Z.Y.; Zhu, J.; Xiong, Y.; Li, K.; Dong, J.H.; Li, X. Interaction between cancer cells and stromal fibroblasts is required for activation of the uPAR-uPA-MMP-2 cascade in pancreatic cancer metastasis. *Clin. Cancer Res.* **2007**, *13*, 3115–3124. [PubMed]
126. Seguin, L.; Desgrosellier, J.S.; Weis, S.M.; Cheresh, D.A. Integrins and cancer: Regulators of cancer stemness, metastasis, and drug resistance. *Trends Cell Biol.* **2015**, *25*, 234–240.
127. Guo, W.; Giancotti, F.G. Integrin signalling during tumour progression. *Nat. Rev. Mol. Cell Biol.* **2004**, *5*, 816–826. [PubMed]
128. Chan, B.M.; Matsuura, N.; Takada, Y.; Zetter, B.R.; Hemler, M.E. In vitro and in vivo consequences of VLA-2 expression on rhabdomyosarcoma cells. *Science* **1991**, *251*, 1600–1602.
129. Desgrosellier, J.S.; Cheresh, D.A. Integrins in cancer: Biological implications and therapeutic opportunities. *Nat. Rev. Cancer* **2010**, *10*, 9–22.
130. Wu, L.; Bernard-Trifilo, J.A.; Lim, Y.; Lim, S.T.; Mitra, S.K.; Uryu, S.; Chen, M.; Pallen, C.J.; Cheung, N.K.V.; Mikolon, D.; et al. Distinct FAK-Src activation events promote $\alpha 5\beta 1$ and $\alpha 4\beta 1$ integrin-stimulated neuroblastoma cell motility. *Oncogene* **2008**, *27*, 1439–1448.
131. Schöttelndreier, H.; Potter, B.V.; Mayr, G.W.; Guse, A.H. Mechanisms involved in $\alpha 6\beta 1$-integrin-mediated Ca(2+) signalling. *Cell. Signal.* **2001**, *13*, 895–899. [PubMed]
132. Inoue, O.; Suzuki-Inoe, K.; McCarty, O.J.T.; Moroi, M.; Ruggeri, Z.M.; Kunicki, T.J. Laminin stimulates spreading of platelets through integrin $\alpha 6\beta 1$–dependent activation of GPVI. *Northwest Sci.* **2006**, *107*, 1405–1411.
133. Rapoport, E.M.; Kurmyshkina, O.V.; Bovin, N.V. Mammalian galectins: Structure, carbohydrate specificity, and functions. *Biochem.* **2008**, *73*, 393–405.
134. Kowitz, A.; Kadmon, G.; Verschueren, H.; Remels, L.; De Baetselier, P.; Hubbe, M.; Schachner, M.; Schirrmacher, V.; Altevogt, P. Expression of L1 cell adhesion molecule is associated with lymphoma growth and metastasis. *Clin. Exp. Metastasis* **1993**, *11*, 419–429. [PubMed]
135. Sidenius, N.; Blasi, F. The urokinase plasminogen activator system in cancer: Recent advances and implication for prognosis and therapy. *Cancer Metastasis Rev.* **2003**, *22*, 205–222. [PubMed]
136. Banys-Paluchowski, M.; Witzel, I.; Aktas, B.; Fasching, P.A.; Hartkopf, A.; Janni, W.; Kasimir-Bauer, S.; Pantel, K.; Schön, G.; Rack, B.; et al. The prognostic relevance of urokinase-type plasminogen activator (uPA) in the blood of patients with metastatic breast cancer. *Sci. Rep.* **2019**, *9*, 1–10.
137. Pavón, M.A.; Arroyo-Solera, I.; Céspedes, M.V.; Casanova, I.; León, X.; Mangues, R. uPA/uPAR and SERPINE1 in head and neck cancer: Role in tumor resistance, metastasis, prognosis and therapy. *Oncotarget* **2016**, *7*, 57351–57366.
138. Bozzuto, G.; Ruggieri, P.; Molinari, A. Molecular aspects of tumor cell migration and invasion. *Ann Ist Super Sanita* **2010**, *46*, 66–80.
139. Mohtasham, N.; Babakoohi, S.; Shiva, A.; Shadman, A.; Kamyab-Hesari, K.; Shakeri, M.-T.; Sharifi-Sistan, N. Immunohistochemical study of p53, Ki-67, MMP-2 and MMP-9 expression at invasive front of squamous cell and verrucous carcinoma in oral cavity. *Pathol. Res. Pract.* **2013**, *209*, 110–114.
140. Mu, D.; Cambier, S.; Fjellbirkeland, L.; Baron, J.L.; Munger, J.S.; Kawakatsu, H.; Sheppard, D.; Courtney Broaddus, V.; Nishimura, S.L. The integrin $\alpha v\beta 8$ mediates epithelial homeostasis through MT1-MMP-dependent activation of TGF-$\beta$1. *J. Cell Biol.* **2002**, *157*, 493–507.
141. Yu, Q.; Stamenkovic, I. Cell surface-localized matrix metalloproteinase-9 proteolytically activates TGF-$\beta$ and promotes tumor invasion and angiogenesis. *Genes Dev.* **2000**, *14*, 163–176. [PubMed]

142. Tatti, O.; Vehviläinen, P.; Lehti, K.; Keski-Oja, J. MT1-MMP releases latent TGF-β1 from endothelial cell extracellular matrix via proteolytic processing of LTBP-1. *Exp. Cell Res.* **2008**, *314*, 2501–2514. [PubMed]
143. Mitsiades, N.; Yu, W.H.; Poulaki, V.; Tsokos, M.; Stamenkovic, I. Matrix metalloproteinase-7-mediated cleavage of Fas ligand protects tumor cells from chemotherapeutic drug cytotoxicity. *Cancer Res.* **2001**, *61*, 577–581. [PubMed]
144. Bergers, G.; Brekken, R.; McMahon, G.; Vu, T.H.; Itoh, T.; Tamaki, K.; Tanzawa, K.; Thorpe, P.; Itohara, S.; Werb, Z.; et al. Matrix metalloproteinase-9 triggers the angiogenic switch during carcinogenesis. *Nat. Cell Biol.* **2000**, *2*, 737–744. [PubMed]
145. Ahn, G.O.; Brown, J.M. Matrix metalloproteinase-9 is required for tumor vasculogenesis but not for angiogenesis: role of bone marrow-derived myelomonocytic cells. *Cancer Cell* **2008**, *13*, 193–205. [PubMed]
146. Ardi, V.C.; Kupriyanova, T.A.; Deryugina, E.I.; Quigley, J.P. Human neutrophils uniquely release TIMP-free MMP-9 to provide a potent catalytic stimulator of angiogenesis. *Proc. Natl. Acad. Sci.* **2007**, *104*, 20262–20267. [PubMed]
147. Yamaguchi, H.; Condeelis, J. Regulation of the actin cytoskeleton in cancer cell migration and invasion. *Biochim. Biophys. Acta* **2007**, 642–652.
148. Clucas, J.; Valderrama, F. ERM proteins in cancer progression. *J. Cell Sci.* **2015**, *128*, 1253. [PubMed]
149. Martín-Villar, E.; Scholl, F.G.; Gamallo, C.; Yurrita, M.M.; Muñoz-Guerra, M.; Cruces, J.; Quintanilla, M. Characterization of human PA2.26 antigen (T1α-2, podoplanin), a small membrane mucin induced in oral squamous cell carcinomas. *Int. J. Cancer* **2005**, *113*, 899–910. [PubMed]
150. Fehon, R.G.; McClatchey, A.I.; Bretscher, A. Organizing the cell cortex: The role of ERM proteins. *Nat. Rev. Mol. Cell Biol.* **2010**, *11*, 276–287. [PubMed]
151. Clark, E.S.; Brown, B.; Whigham, A.S.; Kochaishvili, A.; Yarbrough, W.G.; Weaver, A.M. Aggressiveness of HNSCC tumors depends on expression levels of cortactin, a gene in the 11q13 amplicon. *Oncogene* **2009**, *28*, 431–444. [PubMed]
152. Roussos, E.T.; Balsamo, M.; Alford, S.K.; Wyckoff, J.B.; Gligorijevic, B.; Wang, Y.; Pozzuto, M.; Stobezki, R.; Goswami, S.; Segall, J.E.; et al. Mena invasive (MenaINV) promotes multicellular streaming motility and transendothelial migration in a mouse model of breast cancer. *J. Cell Sci.* **2011**, *124*, 2120–2131. [PubMed]
153. Weidmann, M.D.; Surve, C.R.; Eddy, R.J.; Chen, X.; Gertler, F.B.; Sharma, V.P.; Condeelis, J.S. MenaINV dysregulates cortactin phosphorylation to promote invadopodium maturation. *Sci. Rep.* **2016**, *6*, 1–18.
154. Machesky, L.M.; Li, A. Fascin. *Commun. Integr. Biol.* **2010**, *3*, 263–270. [PubMed]
155. Papaspyrou, K.; Brochhausen, C.; Schmidtmann, I.; Fruth, K.; Gouveris, H.; Kirckpatrick, J.; Mann, W.; Brieger, J. Fascin upregulation in primary head and neck squamous cell carcinoma is associated with lymphatic metastasis. *Oncol. Lett.* **2014**, *7*, 2041–2046. [PubMed]
156. Lovisa, S.; LeBleu, V.S.; Tampe, B.; Sugimoto, H.; Vadnagara, K.; Carstens, J.L.; Wu, C.C.; Hagos, Y.; Burckhardt, B.C.; Pentcheva-Hoang, T.; et al. Epithelial-to-mesenchymal transition induces cell cycle arrest and parenchymal damage in renal fibrosis. *Nat. Med.* **2015**, *21*, 998–1009. [PubMed]
157. Bauer, A.L.; Jackson, T.L.; Jiang, Y.; Rohlf, T. Receptor cross-talk in angiogenesis: Mapping environmental cues to cell phenotype using a stochastic, Boolean signaling network model. *J. Theor. Biol.* **2010**, *264*, 838–846. [PubMed]
158. Zavyalova, M.V.; Perelmuter, V.M.; Slonimskaya, E.M.; Vtorushin, S.V.; Garbukov, E.Y.; Gluschenko, S.A. Conjugation of lymphogenous metastatic spread and histologic pattern of infiltrative component of ductal breast cancer (in Russ). *Sib. J. Oncol.* **2006**, *1*, 32–35.
159. Perelmuter, V.M.; Zavyalova, M.V.; Slonimskaya, E.M.; Vtorushin, S.V.; Garbukov, E.Y. Hematogenous metastasis depending on histologic tumor pattern in breast cancer (In Russ). *Sib. J. Oncol.* **2006**, *3*, 29–33.
160. Denisov, E.V.; Skryabin, N.A.; Gerashchenko, T.S.; Tashireva, L.A.; Wilhelm, J.; Buldakov, M.A.; Sleptcov, A.A.; Lebedev, I.N.; Vtorushin, S.V.; Zavyalova, M.V.; et al. Clinically relevant morphological structures in breast cancer represent transcriptionally distinct tumor cell populations with varied degrees of epithelial-mesenchymal transition and CD44$^+$CD24$^-$ stemness. *Oncotarget* **2017**, *8*, 61163–61180.
161. Zavyalova, M.V.; Perelmuter, V.M.; Vtorushin, S.V.; Denisov, E.V.; Litvyakov, N.V.; Slonimskaya, E.M.; Cherdyntseva, N.V. The Presence of Alveolar Structures in Invasive Ductal NOS Breast Carcinoma is Associated with Lymph Node Metastasis. *Diagn. Cytopathol.* **2013**, *41*, 279–282. [PubMed]

162. Gerashchenko, T.S.; Zavyalova, M.V.; Denisov, E.V.; Krakhmal, N.V.; Pautova, D.N.; Litviakov, N.V.; Vtorushin, S.V.; Cherdyntseva, N.V.; Perelmuter, V.M. Intratumoral morphological heterogeneity of breast cancer as an indicator of the metastatic potential and tumor chemosensitivity. *Acta Naturae* **2017**, *9*, 56–67. [PubMed]
163. Denisov, E.V.; Litviakov, N.V.; Zavyalova, M.V.; Perelmuter, V.M.; Vtorushin, S.V.; Tsyganov, M.M.; Gerashchenko, T.S.; Garbukov, E.Y.; Slonimskaya, E.M.; Cherdyntseva, N.V. Intratumoral morphological heterogeneity of breast cancer: neoadjuvant chemotherapy efficiency and multidrug resistance gene expression. *Sci. Rep.* **2014**, *4*, 1–7.

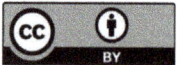 © 2019 by the authors. Licensee MDPI, Basel, Switzerland. This article is an open access article distributed under the terms and conditions of the Creative Commons Attribution (CC BY) license (http://creativecommons.org/licenses/by/4.0/).

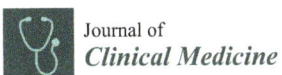 

*Review*

# Metabolic Plasticity and Epithelial-Mesenchymal Transition

Timothy M. Thomson [1,2,*], Cristina Balcells [3,4] and Marta Cascante [3,5]

1. Department of Cell Biology, Molecular Biology Institute of Barcelona, Science Research Council, 08028 Barcelona, Spain
2. Networked Center for Research in Liver and Digestive Diseases (CIBEREHD), Instituto de Salud Carlos III (ISCIII), 28029 Madrid, Spain
3. Department of Biochemistry and Molecular Biomedicine-Institute of Biomedicine (IBUB), University of Barcelona, 08028 Barcelona, Spain
4. Department of Materials Science and Physical Chemistry, University of Barcelona, 08028 Barcelona, Spain
5. Networked Center for Research in Liver and Digestive Diseases (CIBEREHD) and metabolomics node at INB-Bioinformatics Platform, Instituto de Salud Carlos III (ISCIII), 28029 Madrid, Spain
* Correspondence: titbmc@ibmb.csic.es

Received: 30 April 2019; Accepted: 28 June 2019; Published: 3 July 2019

**Abstract:** A major transcriptional and phenotypic reprogramming event during development is the establishment of the mesodermal layer from the ectoderm through epithelial-mesenchymal transition (EMT). EMT is employed in subsequent developmental events, and also in many physiological and pathological processes, such as the dissemination of cancer cells through metastasis, as a reversible transition between epithelial and mesenchymal states. The remarkable phenotypic remodeling accompanying these transitions is driven by characteristic transcription factors whose activities and/or activation depend upon signaling cues and co-factors, including intermediary metabolites. In this review, we summarize salient metabolic features that enable or instigate these transitions, as well as adaptations undergone by cells to meet the metabolic requirements of their new states, with an emphasis on the roles played by the metabolic regulation of epigenetic modifications, notably methylation and acetylation.

**Keywords:** epithelial-mesenchymal transition; metabolism; plasticity; epigenetics; drug resistance

---

## 1. Introduction

Cells undergoing switches from epithelial to mesenchymal states experience radical changes in motility, proliferation, morphology and interactions with their environment. Epithelial cells that undergo EMT lose cell-cell contacts, undergo extensive cytoskeletal remodeling and exponentially increase their motility and their ability to invade, through extracellular structures as individual cells [1]. At the same time, they adjust their rate of proliferation to the degree of motility, such that highly motile cells with strong acquired mesenchymal phenotypes may exhibit a diminished proliferative potential [2], while cells at "intermediate" states of EMT may retain or increase their proliferation rates relative to their initial epithelial states [3]. This suggests a balance between motility and proliferation [4,5], that may depend on the relative availability of common resources that can be spent on either motility or on proliferation. Indeed, cells can undergo EMT (or also mesenchymal–epithelial transition (MET)) to different extents [6], adopting a range of phenotypes. While "extreme" EMT can lead to stable mesenchymal phenotypes prone to enter pre-senescent states [5], "intermediate" forms of EMT endow cells with features shared with stem cells, including self-renewal or survival under stress and in non-adherent growth conditions [7,8].

Here we will review relevant interconnections between EMT and metabolism, with a particular emphasis on the modulation by metabolites of epigenetic readouts, including EMT.

## 2. Metabolic Reprogramming in EMT

As tumor cells proliferate, they require a constant availability of nutrients, and oxygen through cell metabolism for transformation into energy and the molecular components of progeny cells, which include nucleic acids, sugars, proteins, lipids and a myriad of small organic and inorganic molecules. On the other hand, highly motile disseminating tumor cells, or even tumor cells surviving in circulation, prioritize energetic yield over the production of building blocks, to ensure survival and fuel the cellular processes associated to cell motility [1].

While the generation of building blocks is most efficient through precursor, and reducing equivalent production by glycolysis and through precursor intake, the generation of energy in the form of adenosine triphosphate (ATP) is at its most efficient through mitochondrial oxidative phosphorylation (OXPHOS) [9]. However, when certain conditions, such as oncogenic signaling or hypoxia, force growth in spite of an absence of any optimal conditions for mitochondrial function (limited oxygen), cells resort to the activation of mechanisms that favor the derivation of glycolysis towards building block production at the expense of feeding mitochondrial functions (the Warburg effect).

The metabolic dichotomy established between highly proliferative and highly motile phenotypes is exemplified by a wide variety of observations. For instance, while epithelial cells display fragmented mitochondria dependent on the function of DRP1 mitochondrial fission protein, SNAI1 and TGF-β1-induced mesenchymal cells display mitochondria with predominant mitofusin-dependent fused/tubular morphologies in mammary stem cells [10]. Notably, mitochondrial fusion is associated with enhanced oxidation and tricarboxylic acid (TCA) cycle activity [11–13], and then the reversal of mitochondrial fusion leads to a decreased mitochondrial function and a reversal of EMT [10]. In line with this, TGF-β1 induces a shift from glycolysis to OXPHOS by its repression of PDK4, which counters the function of the pyruvate dehydrogenase (PDH) complex to introduce pyruvate into the mitochondria to feed the TCA cycle, as observed in lung cancer cells [14]. Other models of induced EMT, however, appear to favor a diversion of metabolic fluxes away from mitochondria. For example, in basal-like breast cancer, SNAI1 represses fructose-1,6-bisphophatase 1 (FBP1), promoting glucose uptake and the diversion of glycolytic carbons towards biosynthetic pathways, including the pentose phosphate pathway (PPP), and impairing the activity of the respiratory chain complex I [15]. Similarly, SNAI1 also represses phosphofructokinase platelet (PFKP) [16] and several subunits of cytochrome C oxidase (COX) [17] in breast cancer cells, further reinforcing a strongly glycolytic metabolic phenotype. Along the same lines, the silencing of aldolase A (ALDOA) or of glyceraldehyde-3-phosphate dehydrogenase (GAPDH) prevent EMT in various cancer cell models [18,19].

The first challenge that cancer cells face when undergoing the invasion-metastasis cascade resides in acquiring motile and invasive capacities in order to reach the bloodstream. The motile phenotype is driven in part by lipid rafts, cholesterol and sphingolipid-rich membranous structures that modulate cell adhesion by partnering with CD44, and are required for ECM degradation and invadopodia formation [20]. Sphingolipids themselves are also part of other oncogenic signaling cascades that lead to motile phenotypes [21]. Finally, different enzymes in fatty acid metabolism are also recruited for the metastatic process [22]. For example, ATP citrate lyase (ACLY) is required for low molecular weight cyclin E (LMW-E)-mediated transformation, migration, and invasion in breast cancer cells [23]. Similarly, fatty acid synthase (FASN) is also involved in invasion by promoting EMT in breast and ovarian cancer cells [24,25], and by interacting with wingless-related integration site (Wnt) signaling in metastatic colorectal cancer cells [26].

Upon detachment from an adherent layer, healthy non-hematopoietic cells are unable to uptake sufficient glucose, which subsequently leads to ATP shortage, a state that activates anoikis [27,28]. Circulating tumor cells (CTC) display metabolic adaptations specifically devoted to evade anoikis, and to favor anchorage-independent growth, a prerequisite state for metastatic dissemination [29].

Another possible trigger of anoikis is elevated levels of reactive oxygen species (ROS), which also contribute to inhibit ATP production [30]. Therefore, many of the adaptations displayed by CTCs may also be directed to scavenge or diminish the generation of ROS. One of these adaptations may be the reinforcement of a highly-glycolytic phenotype, since relying on glucose to generate ATP can decrease cellular ROS levels by two distinct mechanisms: First, diminished ROS-generating OXPHOS (Crabtree effect; [31]); and, second, increased NADPH production capacity through an enhanced flux through the PPP [32]. In contrast, invasive ovarian cancer cells grown under attachment-free conditions increase the pyruvate uptake for TCA cycle anaplerosis, which favors the adoption of a more oxidative metabolic state and a motile phenotype [33]. Similarly, the colorectal cancer cell line SW620, derived from a lymph node metastasis, exhibits an increase in EMT markers and invasiveness, and an enhanced mitochondrial metabolism to the detriment of aerobic glycolysis, when compared to its primary tumor counterpart, SW480 [34].

Not surprisingly, signaling cascades governing metabolic networks and EMT often display a remarkable level of overlapping. A prominent case is illustrated by glycogen synthase kinase-3 β (GSK3β), which targets the EMT transcription factor SNAI1, but is directly phosphorylated and inactivated by Akt. GSK3β phosphorylates SNAI1, targeting it for proteasomal degradation. Thus, Akt activation directly impacts SNAI1 levels through GSK3β, coupling the metabolic and the EMT phenotypes [35]. Importantly, this inhibition of GSK3 activates glycogen synthesis and glucose transport [36]. Thus, the induction of mesenchymal phenotypes by the inhibition of GSK3 and the subsequent SNAI1 (SNAIL) activation is associated with enhanced glucose transport and glycogen accumulation, which may represent a strategy to accumulate carbon and energy reservoirs to sustain cell motility.

## 3. Metabolism and the Epigenetic Control of Epithelial-Mesenchymal Plasticity

The transitions in EMT and MET are orchestrated by transcription factors, such as ZEB1/2, SNAI1/2, TWIST1/2, and microRNAs, including the miR-200 family and miR-205, whose expression is contingent upon epigenetic states determined by CpG island methylation and histone marks [37]. Enzymes that carry out epigenetic modifications commonly use key metabolites as either substrates or allosteric regulators [38] (Figure 1). Thus, cellular metabolic states can affect epigenetic regulatory proteins through metabolic signaling pathways. Intermediary metabolites involved in epigenetic regulation include acetyl-CoA, S-adenosyl methionine (SAM), α-ketoglutarate (α-KG), ATP, nicotinamide adenine dinucleotide (NAD+) and flavin adenine dinucleotide (FAD). Importantly, the cellular concentrations of many of these substrates can limit enzyme reaction rates [39]. As such, the availability and balance of metabolic resources can significantly modulate chromatin remodeling and transcription factor activities.

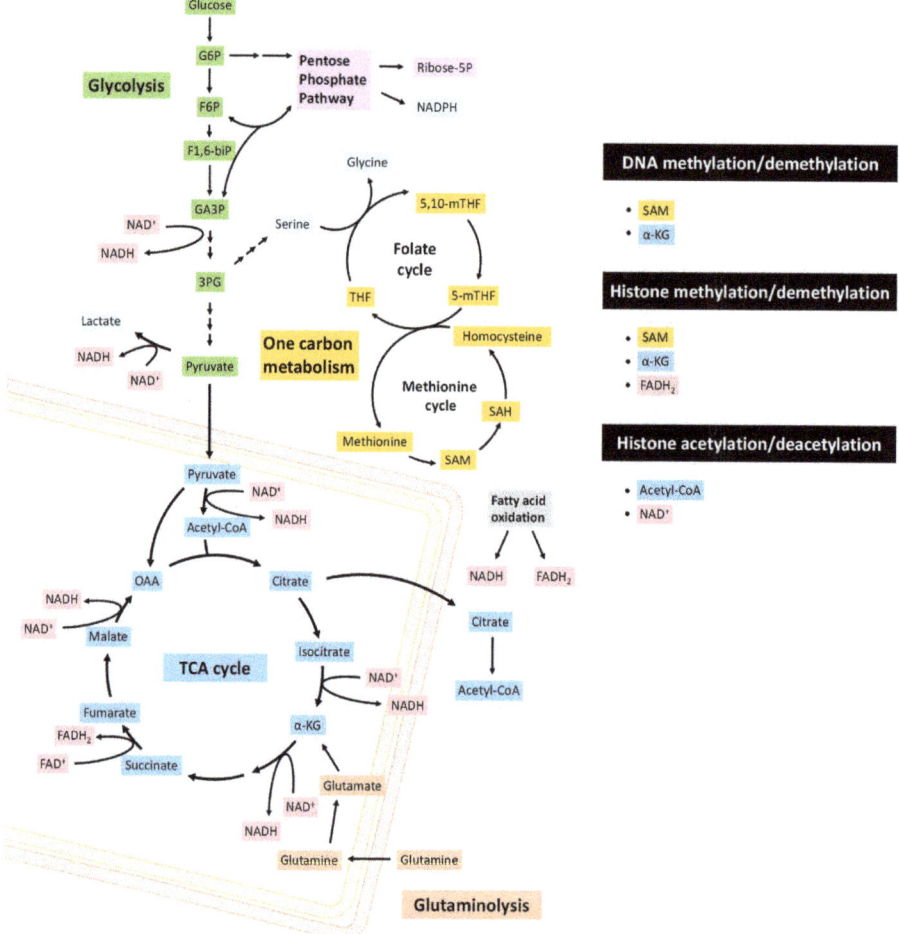

**Figure 1.** Metabolic requirements of protein and DNA methylation and protein acetylation. S-adenosyl-methionine (SAM) acts as a methyl donor for histone and DNA methylation. SAM is produced through one-carbon metabolism. Demethylation can require the tricarboxylic acid (TCA) cycle intermediate α-KG as a co-factor, and can be inhibited by other TCA cycle products: Succinate, fumarate or 2-hydroxyglutarate (2-HG). Histone demethylation by lysine-specific histone deacetylase 1 (LSD1) can also require the flavin adenine dinucleotide reduced form (FADH2), whose pools are dependent upon fatty acid oxidation and the TCA cycle. Histone acetylation requires acetyl-CoA, obtained from citrate or fatty acid oxidation in the TCA cycle. Histone deacetylation by sirtuin (SIRT) histone deacetylases is NAD+-dependent. NADH pools derive from multiple metabolic pathways, including glycolysis, pyruvate oxidation by pyruvate dehydrogenase (PDH), the TCA cycle, fatty acid oxidation, amino acid oxidation and OXPHOS. The metabolites involved in different pathways are shaded in different colors: Glycolysis (green), one carbon metabolism (yellow), pentose phosphate pathway (purple), TCA cycle (blue), NADH and FADH2 (pink) and glutaminolysis (orange).

### 3.1. Methylation

All methylation reactions require the one-carbon donor SAM, which is synthesized in the methionine cycle from methionine and ATP by methionine adenosyl-transferase (MAT). The transfer of the methyl group from SAM to the substrate produces S-adenosyl homocysteine (SAH), which in turn is converted to homocysteine, and finally regenerated to methionine after the donation of a methyl group from 5-methyl-tetrahydrofolate (5-MTHF) [40]. Methyl moieties are transferred from SAM to acceptor cytosine residues on DNA or lysine and arginine residues on histones in reactions catalyzed by DNA or histone methyltransferases, respectively (Figure 2). The availability of methionine determines the levels of histone and DNA methylation by modulating SAM and SAH [41]. These modifications are sensitive to the abundance of SAM or the [SAM]:[SAH] ratio, since SAH can act as an inhibitor of methyltransferases, and the Km and Ki for SAM and SAH, respectively, fall within physiological ranges [40]. The intracellular methionine concentration is also dependent on the expression of the cell surface amino acid transporter LAT1 (SLC7A5), which forms a heterodimer with SLC3A2 [42], and whose expression is regulated by MYC and the Akt-mTOR pathway [43–45].

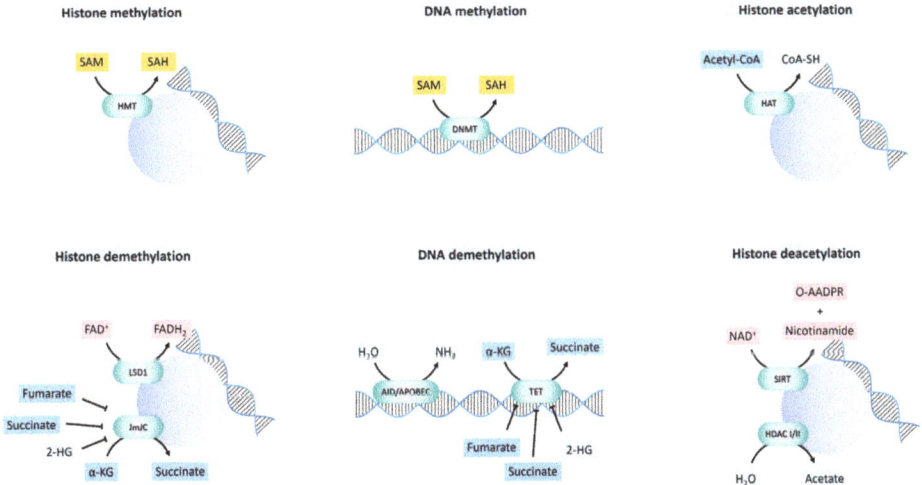

**Figure 2.** Mechanisms of histone and DNA methylation/demethylation and histone acetylation/deacetylation. S-adenosyl-methionine (SAM) acts as a methyl donor for histone and DNA methylation, yielding S-adenosyl homocysteine (SAH). DNA methylation is performed by DNA methyl transferases (DNMT), whereas histone methylation is performed by histone methyltransferases (HMT). Histone demethylation can be mediated by flavin adenine dinucleotide (FAD)-dependent lysine-specific demethylase 1 (LSD1); or by Jumonji C domain (JmjC) demethylases, that use α-ketoglutarate (α-KG) as a substrate, yielding succinate. JmjC demethylases can also be inhibited by other TCA cycle products: Succinate, fumarate or 2-hydroxyglutarate (2-HG). DNA demethylation can occur through the activation-induced deaminase/apolipoprotein B mRNA editing enzyme, catalytic (AID/APOBEC), or by ten-eleven translocation (TET) enzymes. TET dioxygenases use Fe(2+) and α-KG as co-factors, and their activity can also be inhibited by fumarate, succinate and 2-HG. Histone acetylation by histone acetyl-transferases (HAT) requires acetyl-CoA. Histone deacetylation can occur by class I and II histone deacetylases (HDAC I/II), and by class III histone deacetylases, also termed as sirtuins (SIRT). Sirtuins use nicotinamide adenine dinucleotide (NAD+), which is converted into nicotinamide and O-acetyl-ADP-ribose (O-AADPR).

SAM levels are also dependent on serine metabolism. Serine is a one-carbon donor to the folate cycle, and allows the regeneration of methionine for SAM synthesis. Serine conversion to glycine by serine hydroxymethyl transferase (SHMT) generates 5,10-methylene-THF, which is subsequently reduced by methylene tetrahydrofolate reductase (MTHFR) to 5-methyl-THF within the folate cycle [40]. Methionine is regenerated by the donation of a methyl group to homocysteine by 5-methyl-THF.

### 3.1.1. DNA Methylation and Demethylation

The m5C methyltransferases (C-5 cytosine-specific DNA methylases) catalyze the methylation of the C-5 carbon of cytosines in CpG islands to produce C5-methylcytosine [46]. Given the known switch in global DNA methylation associated with gene promoters and gene bodies that takes place during embryonic development, a relevant question is whether DNA methylation patterns are subjected to systematic changes during specific processes that determine cell-fate, including EMT. Although no changes in bulk DNA methylation are observed during EMT induced by TGF-β1 [47,48], differentially-methylated regions (DMR) were found to be induced in Madin-Darby Canine Kidney (MDCK) and human breast cancer cells [48]. In the latter study, unmethylated sequences tended to become methylated, and affected both intergenic and intragenic regions, as well as promoters and gene bodies. As expected, methylation in promoters is associated with transcript downregulation, mainly affecting cell adhesion, catabolism and protein transport and methylation, while methylation in gene bodies was associated with transcript upregulation, which affected signaling pathways, developmental processes, wound-healing and cell differentiation.

DNA can be indirectly demethylated through the deamination of 5mC by AID/APOBEC enzymes to give 5-hydroxymethyluracil [49], or through the oxidation of 5mC to 5-formylcytosine and 5-carboxylcytosine, catalyzed by ten-eleven translocation (TET) enzymes [50,51] (Figure 2). Activation-induced deaminase/apolipoprotein B mRNA editing enzymes, catalytic (AID/APOBEC) are zinc-dependent cytosine deaminases that function in antibody diversification and mRNA editing, with relatively weaker deamination-coupled demethylation activity on 5mC [49]. TET enzymes are dioxygenases that use $Fe(2+)$ and α-KG as co-factors. The deaminated or oxidized adducts are repaired by thymine DNA glycosylase (TDG) and base excision repair [52–54]. The carboxyl and formyl groups of 5-formylcytosine and 5-carboxylcytosine can be enzymatically removed without the excision of the base [53].

### 3.1.2. Histone Methylation and Demethylation

Histone methylation on lysine or arginine residues is catalyzed by lysine-specific (SET-domain or non-SET-domain) and arginine-specific histone methyltransferases (PRMTs) [55]. Histone methyl-ation at specific residues is associated with either the activation or the repression of transcription, depending on tethering "reader" proteins bearing domains that recognize specific histone modifications at specific lysines or arginines, which, in turn, recruit protein complexes that enable or repress transcription through chromatin remodeling [55]. Histone demethylation is catalyzed by two main classes of enzymes, flavin adenine dinucleotide (FAD)-dependent amine oxidases and $Fe(2+)$ and α-α-KG-dependent hydroxylases. Both operate by the hydroxylation of a methyl group, followed by the dissociation of formaldehyde [56].

#### 3.1.2.1. FAD-Dependent Demethylation

Lysine-specific histone demethylase 1A (LSD1), also known as lysine (K)-specific demethylase 1A (KDM1A) [56], catalyzes the FAD-dependent demethylation of mono- and dimethyl groups, but not trimethyl groups, at histone H3K4 and H3K9, generating formaldehyde and $H_2O_2$. FAD is derived from riboflavin (vitamin B2), and serves as a coenzyme in many oxidative reactions including mitochondrial fatty acid β-oxidation and in the respiratory chain (Figure 2). The catalytic activity of LSD1 may be directly connected to the cellular metabolic state via the fluctuation of the FAD/FADH2 ratio depending on the FAD oxidation processes, such as fatty acid β-oxidation and the TCA cycle. LSD1 is an integral component of the Mi-2/nucleosome remodeling and deacetylase (NuRD) complex [56], that can function as a co-repressor or a co-activator, but dependent on the interaction with specific chromatin regulatory complexes. When forming complexes with co-repressors, such as SNAI1, LSD1 demethylates H3K4me1/2 and represses transcription [57,58]. When associated with the androgen or estrogen nuclear receptors, LSD1 demethylates H3K9me1/2 [59,60], and activates the transcription of pro-invasive and ECM remodeling genes. In contrast, it has also been found that LSD1 inhibits the invasion of breast cancer cells in vitro, and suppresses breast cancer metastatic potential in vivo [61].

3.1.2.2. α-KG-Dependent Demethylation and Hydroxylation

The α-KG-dependent histone demethylases bear a Jumonji C domain (JmjC) [62]. Histone demethylation through the JmjC oxygenases occurs through a hydroxylation reaction, in which α-KG, oxygen, and Fe(2+) are used to produce succinate and $CO_2$ (Figure 2). The JmjC histone demethylases regulate chromatin states through the removal of mono-, di-, and tri-methylation marks upon specific lysine residues on histones. Different JmjC enzymes demethylate different methylated lysines on the histones, which imparts specific transcriptional outcomes (activation vs. repression) on each target gene [63].

Aside from JmjC demethylases, α-KG is a common substrate for several hydroxylases, including TET DNA hydroxylases [64] and prolyl hydroxylases, that regulate the stability of hypoxia-inducible factors (HIFs) [65]. Such hydroxylation reactions also require the co-factors Fe(2+) and vitamin C, as an electron donor that reduces ferric iron, Fe(3+), to ferrous iron, Fe(2+). This α-KG is an intermediary metabolite of the TCA cycle, produced by the isocitrate dehydrogenase (IDH)-catalyzed oxidative decarboxylation of isocitrate. This α-KG can also be produced in the reaction of glutamate and pyruvate, catalyzed by glutamate pyruvate transaminases (GPT1/2). Additionally, the reversible transfer of an amino group ($NH_3^+$) from glutamate to oxaloacetate, that has been catalyzed by glutamate oxaloacetate transaminases (GOT1/2) also results in the formation of α-KG and aspartate. Another non-TCA source of α-KG derives from glutaminolysis, in which glutamine transported into the cell is converted to glutamate and NH4+ in a deamination reaction catalyzed by glutaminases (GLS1/2). A second deamination reaction, catalyzed by mitochondrial glutamate dehydrogenase (GDH), reversibly converts glutamate to α-KG [66].

Importantly, succinate, fumarate, (D)-2-hydroxyglutarate (2-HG), and (L)-2-HG are α-KG structural analogs that competitively inhibit the hydroxylases which use α-KG as a substrate [65,67] (Figure 2). As a consequence, the relative concentrations of these metabolites are critical for histone and DNA methylation in the nucleus, and thus gene expression, as well as the regulation of HIF-1α levels. A compromise in SDH or FH activities leads to the accumulation of succinate or fumarate, respectively, causing the inhibition of DNA and histone demethylation [68,69]. Inactivating mutations in SDH are associated with pheochromocytomas and paragangliomas, sporadic renal cancer and gastrointestinal stromal tumors [69]. Accumulation of succinate causes epigenetic silencing of miR-200 and eventually EMT [70]. Similarly, loss-of-function FH mutations lead to hereditary leiomyomatosis and renal cell cancer (HLRCC), paragangliomas and pheochromocytomas [71–73]. Fumarate is accumulated in FH-deficient cells, inhibiting TET-dependent demethylation of miR200, which leads to its silencing and consequent EMT [68,70]. As a consequence of the competitive inhibition of α-KG by succinate and fumarate on proline hydroxylase activity, SDH or FH deficiencies promote the stabilization of HIF-1α in normoxic conditions, driving the expression of HIF target genes, including VEGF and GLUT1, that promote angiogenesis and glucose metabolism in renal and bile duct cancer cells [74].

IDH1 (cytosolic and peroxisomal) and IDH2 (mitochondrial) mutations occur frequently in a variety of human cancers, including malignant gliomas, AML, intrahepatic cholangiocarcinoma, chondrosarcoma, and thyroid carcinomas [75,76]. In addition, IDH2 mutations occur with high frequency in rare malignancies, such as angioimmunoblastic T cell lymphoma and solid papillary carcinoma with reverse polarity [77]. IDH-active site mutations confer a neomorphic activity that catalyzes the conversion of α-KG to D-2-hydroxyglutarate (D-2HG, or R-2HG) [76]. Under physiological conditions, cellular D-2HG accumulation is limited due to the actions of the endo-genous D-2HG dehydrogenase, which catalyzes the conversion of D-2HG to α-KG. Similar to high succinate or fumarate levels, high D-2HG levels competitively inhibit α-KG-dependent dioxygenases, causing the inhibition of JmjC and TET demethylases and histone and DNA hypermethylation, clinically associated with the increased methylation of patient tumor DNA in AML and gliomas, and in gliomas, a CpG island hypermethylator phenotype [76]. This is accompanied by an inhibition of normal differentiation processes and a promotion of tumorigenesis [78,79].

D-2HG levels have also been found elevated in breast cancer with wild-type IDH, driven by glutamine anaplerosis [80–82]. In colorectal cancer cells, D-2HG (but not its enantiomer L-2HG, produced from the reduction of α-KG by lactate dehydrogenase A, LDHA, or malate dehydrogenase, MDH) directly induces EMT in colorectal cancer cells by promoting H3K4me3 marks at the ZEB1 promoter and its transcription [83]. In this study, colorectal cancers with higher levels of D-2HG are associated with an increased frequency of distant metastasis, as well as an increased trend for a higher tumor stage. Further, hypoxia, independently of HIF, induces the LDH- and MDH-mediated production of the L-2HG enantiomer, which reinforces the hypoxic response, at least in part, through the stabilization of HIF-1α [84]. Accumulation of L-2HG, favored by acidic (low pH) conditions [85], slows glycolysis and mitochondrial respiration by reducing the rate of NAD+ regeneration [86], and promotes the same repressive chromatin marks that characterize the differentiation blockade of IDH-mutant malignancies. This provides a mechanistic link between hypoxic niches and stem-cell populations.

## 3.2. Acetylation

Protein acetylation is another major covalent modification directly linked to metabolite abundance that regulates gene programs as a result of histone acetylation and subsequent chromatin remodeling. The acetyl donor for acetylation reactions is acetyl-CoA, a central metabolic intermediate. The acetylation of histone lysines neutralizes the positive charges that govern the tight arrangement of nucleosomes and their interaction with DNA. As a result, chromatin becomes open to the access of bromodomain-containing proteins that dock at specific acetylated sites, and function as epigenetic readers or effectors, with critical roles in gene regulation.

### 3.2.1. Histone Acetylation and Deacetylation

The acetylation of the side-chain amino group of lysine residues on histones, and in some cases also other proteins, is mediated by histone acetyltransferases (HATs), or lysine acetyltransferases (KATs) [87]. HATs transfer the acetyl group from the acetyl-CoA cofactor to the ε nitrogen of a lysine side chain within the histones. In addition to charge neutralization and nucleosome remodeling, these histone modifications function as recognition sites for proteins bearing bromodomains (histone mark "readers") that further reinforce the chromatin remodeling initiated by acetylation [88], leading to outcomes such as ATP-dependent H2A/H2B dimer eviction or complete nucleosome disassembly, and consequent transcriptional regulation.

Histone acetylation is balanced by deacetylation catalyzed by HDACs, of which there are three major families in mammals: Class I, class IIa, class IIb and class III or sirtuins [87]. Unlike the constitutively nuclear class I HDACs, class IIa HDACs do not display an intrinsic HDAC activity, which is acquired only when in complex with class I HDACs, once they enter the nucleus [87]. The cytoplasmic-nuclear shuttling of class IIa HDACs is regulated by LKB1/AMPK-mediated phosphorylation, which results in the retention of phosphorylated forms in the cytoplasm, while dephosphorylated forms shuttle to the nucleus, where they act as scaffolds for the class I HDACs that then exert transcription regulatory activities [89]. Therefore, the function of these HDACs is sensitive to nutrient availability and cellular energy status. The unrelated class III HDACs, or sirtuins [90], are NAD+-dependent deacylases localized in the nucleus (SIRT1, 3, 6 and 7), cytoplasm (SIRT2 and SIRT1) and the mitochondria (SIRT 3, 4 and 5). SIRT4 and SIRT6 also have ADP-ribosyl transferase activity, and SIRT5 demalonylase and desuccinylase activity.

### 3.2.2. Regulation of Acetyl-CoA Pools

Global histone acetylation levels are sensitive to the availability of acetyl-CoA in the cell, which fluctuates in response to nutrient availability or metabolic reprogramming. In proliferating cells in culture, glucose fuels the majority of acetyl-CoA production used for acetylating histones. In mammalian cells, acetyl-CoA is produced within the mitochondria, the cytosol, and the nucleus [91]. Acetyl-CoA generated in mitochondria condenses with oxaloacetate to produce citrate, which is oxidized in the TCA cycle to provide ATP through OXPHOS. Citrate can be exported from mitochondria to the cytosol via the mitochondrial tricarboxylate transporter (SLC25A1), to regenerate acetyl-CoA and oxaloacetate by ATP-citrate lyase (ACLY). Because acetyl-CoA cannot be directly transported across mitochondrial membranes, citrate export and cleavage by ACLY is a major mechanism by which acetyl-CoA is generated outside of the mitochondria. Within the cytosol, acetyl-CoA is used in biosynthetic processes, including the synthesis of fatty acids and cholesterol. In addition to ACLY, another major source of acetyl-CoA outside of the mitochondria is ACSS2, which is localized to the cytosol and nucleus. ACSS2 is involved in the capture and use of exogenous acetate, as well as in the recycling of acetate produced by histone deacetylase (HDAC) reactions [92]. Additionally, the PDC can translocate to the nucleus under certain conditions, such as mitochondrial stress, where it contributes to provide acetyl-CoA for histone acetylation [93].

Since glucose is the preferred source of acetyl-CoA in proliferating cells, glucose limitation or glycolytic inhibition suppresses both acetyl-CoA and histone acetylation levels [94]. However, some cells can use carbon sources other than glucose to produce acetyl-CoA, such as exogenous acetate, in particular under metabolic stress conditions in hypoxia or fasting [95]. Acetate can be converted to acetyl-CoA by ACSS2, which is translocated to the nucleus in low oxygen and glucose conditions [96,97], thus mediating the recycling of the acetate produced by the HDAC reactions, instead of incorporating exogenous acetate. Therefore, nuclear ACSS2 may primarily rely on a locally-generated acetate pool for histone acetylation, while cytosolic ACSS2 promotes the use of exogenous acetate for lipid synthesis.

3.2.3. Regulation of NAD+/NADH Pools

NAD+ is a hydride-transfer acceptor, serving a wide variety of metabolic transformations, as it interconverts between its oxidized form (NAD+) and its reduced form (NADH) [98]. NAD+ directly participates in compartment-specific central metabolic pathways, such as glycolysis, PDH, the TCA cycle, fatty acid oxidation, amino acid oxidation and OXPHOS. In glycolysis, NAD+ is converted to NADH in the glyceraldehyde-3-phosphate dehydrogenase step. This process occurs in reverse for gluconeogenesis in the liver. NAD+ is also a precursor substrate for NADP+ and NADPH, which participate in biosynthesis and reactive oxygen detoxification. NADPH is a key reducing substrate to convert oxidized glutathione to reduced glutathione, a key protectant for cells to resist the toxicity of ROS.

In the nucleus, apart from its role in histone deacetylation, NAD+ is used by PARP, with essential functions in DNA damage repair, as well as by cyclic ADP-ribose synthases [99]. NAD+ is actively consumed during these enzymatic processes, serving as the donor of ADP-ribose in the reaction. The majority of PARP activity is distributed between PARP-1 and PARP-2. As the Km of PARP-1 for NAD+ is below its nuclear concentration, it is unlikely that the activity of PARP-1 is significantly affected by the fluctuations of NAD+. However, PARP-1 activity can reduce the effective concentration of the NAD+ available for other enzymes. As such, consumption of NAD+ by constitutive activation of PARP-1 hampers SIRT1 activity [99,100]. The PARP-2 dissociation constant for NAD+ is within the range of the physiological changes in NAD+ concentration (Km = 130 µM), and thus PARP-2 can directly compete with SIRT1 for NAD+ [101].

To summarize, the regulation of the expression of specific genes and entire gene programs by histone acetylation is orchestrated by metabolic inputs at multiple levels, including the availability of nuclear acetyl-CoA and the expression, activity and localization of HATs, bromodomain proteins and histone deacetylases, which in turn are also regulated by cellular metabolic states. Many of the genes thus regulated by metabolic inputs control the expression of proteins pertaining to the same or separate metabolic circuits, forming complex regulatory loops that enable a rapid fine-tuning of cell metabolic adaptations in response to a multiplicity of scenarios, from shifts in nutrient availability to environmental or oncogenic stress. Thus it is no surprise that changes in global or locus-specific histone acetylation have a significant impact on epithelial-mesenchymal plasticity, and conversely, these shifts utilize changes in histone acetylation.

In early embryonic development, mesoderm specification is accompanied by a downregulation of class I HDACs, and an induction of global histone acetylation by a treatment with the HDAC inhibitor trichostatin A (TSA) drives differentiation to the mesodermal lineage [102]. Consistently, treatment of epithelial tumor cells with TSA or other HDAC inhibitors, such as suberoylanilide hydroxamic acid (SAHA) or valproic acid (VPA), can induce EMT in certain cancer cells, with an upregulation of EMT factors such as ZEB1, ZEB2 or SLUG (SNAI2) [103–107]. This might explain the disappointing outcomes in the clinical trials of HDAC-targeting monotherapies for solid tumors [108]. However, HDACs are required to initiate or maintain EMT in other circumstances [109–114].

A possible explanation for these discrepant observations is the timing, dosing or the potency of HDAC inhibitor administration. As global histone acetylation generally enables open chromatin conformations associated with active transcription, the inhibition of HDACs or an abnormal accumulation of acetyl-CoA, as reported for hepatocellular carcinoma [115], would favor the expression of transcription factors necessary to initiate EMT in response to appropriate signals [116,117]. These factors tend to be transcriptional repressors for epithelial target genes, such as *CDH1*, for which function they recruit HDACs [118–123]. During EMT, the early repression of epithelial genes is later followed by a transcriptional activation of mesenchymal genes [124], which requires an open chromatin conformation enabled by the gain of histone acetylation. At least for *SNAI1*, the late wave of the transcriptional activation of mesenchymal genes is not associated with the binding of the EMT factor to their promoters [125]. These observations suggest that, in its early stages, EMT is established on cycles of transient histone acetylation and deacetylation at specific genes. The progressive stabilization of EMT is achieved through the deposition of any marks of stable chromatin repression [124] and, eventually, heritable DNA methylation of epithelial genes and regulators, such as the microRNA-200 family [125,126]. Cells that are in plastic, "intermediate" EMT states display bivalent marks associated with the promoters of EMT factors and effectors [124,127].

The effects of metabolism on the putative regulatory roles of the NAD+-dependent sirtuins on epithelial-mesenchymal plasticity is even less well understood than for class I and II HDACs [128]. Many reports generally provide evidences that one or more sirtuins favor EMT [129–133]. The ultimate mechanism of this function may be the recruitment of SIRT1 to the *CDH1* promoter by ZEB1 to the deacetylate histone H3 suppressing E-cadherin transcription [133–135], with the possible participation of other epigenetic regulators, such as MPP8, a methyl-H3K9 binding protein [136]. If this is the case, a depletion of NAD+, which occurs upon extensive DNA damage and an activation of PPAR with the consumption of NAD+, or during hypoxia, would be expected to blunt the activity of sirtuins and to impair EMT.

Figure 3 summarizes the descriptions provided in this section of some of the major directions that metabolic networks take to enable the epigenetic modifications necessary for the execution of the transcriptional programs orchestrating epithelial-mesenchymal plasticity.

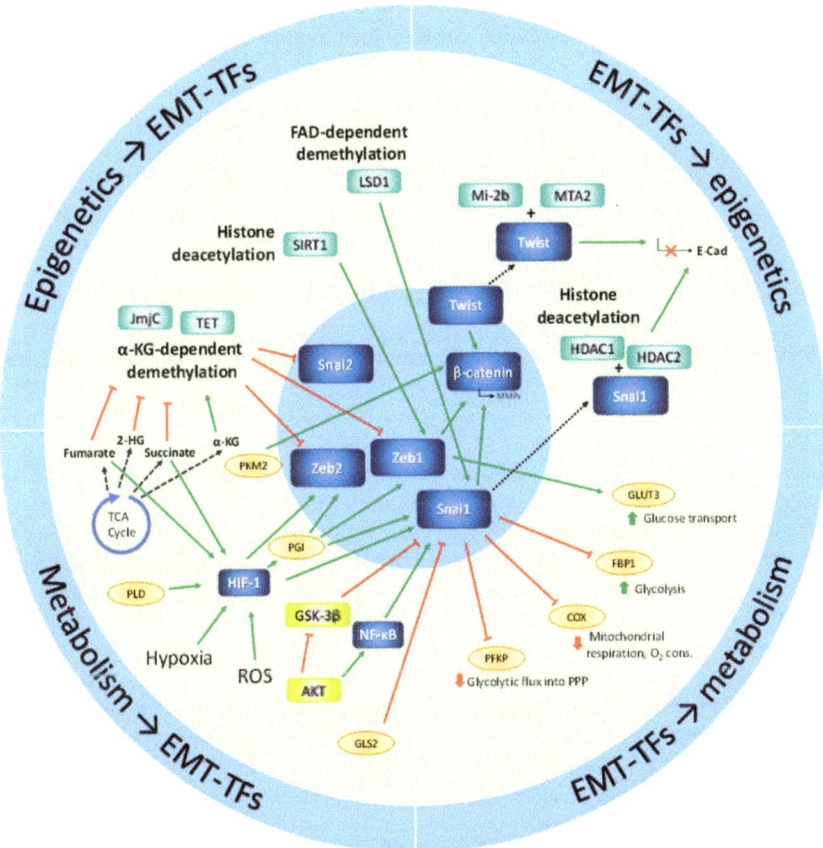

**Figure 3.** Relevant examples of crosstalk between metabolism, epithelial-mesenchymal plasticity and epigenetics. Epithelial-mesenchymal transition (EMT)-transcription factors (EMT-TFs) are regulated by histone and DNA methylation and by histone acetylation. These processes are, in turn, modulated by the intracellular levels of the metabolic products of the tricarboxylic acid (TCA) cycle. EMT-TFs also cooperate with histone deacetylases to repress the expression of cell adhesion molecules that modulate the EMT phenotype. Metabolic cues such as hypoxia, oxidative stress or nutrient availability can activate EMT-TFs through various signaling axes, such as HIF-1α, Akt, GSK-3β or NF-κB. Conversely, the expression of EMT-TFs can be directly modulated by metabolic enzymes, such as phosphoglucoisomerase (PGI) or pyruvate kinase isoform M2 (PKM2). In turn, EMT-TFs regulate central metabolic pathways, by activating or repressing the transcription of metabolic enzymes and metabolite transporters, such as phosphofructokinase platelet (PFKP), cytochrome c oxidase (COX), fructose-1,6-bisphophatase 1 (FBP1), or glucose transporter 3 (GLUT3).

## 4. EMT, Metabolism and Hypoxia

Hypoxia, nutrient starvation and lactate acidosis can each regulate gene expression at the transcriptional and posttranscriptional levels in vitro. Intratumoral hypoxia occurs when the partial pressure of $O_2$ is <5%, as tumor growth outpaces neoangiogenesis, generating heterogeneous $O_2$ gradients throughout the tumor. Tumor hypoxia promotes chemoresistance and radiation resistance [137]. Both the stabilization and activation of HIF-1α promote adaptation to hypoxic stress by modulating tumor cell metabolism, survival, angiogenesis, migration, invasion and metastasis.

High HIF-1α expression is associated with poor prognosis in many cancers [138]. Hypoxia induces ameboid motility [139] and invasive phenotypes, mediated by HIF-1α in multiple cancer types [140,141]. Interestingly, the enhanced motility and invasion elicited by hypoxia is not necessarily accompanied with an increased proliferation in ovarian cancer cells [142].

In normoxia, HIF-1α is a substrate of hydroxylation on specific prolines, catalyzed by oxygen-sensing prolyl hydroxylase domain (PHD) enzymes. Hydroxyprolyl-modified HIF-1α is recognized by the Cul2 subunit of the VHL E3 ubiquitin ligase, which mediates the polyubiquitylation and proteasome-mediated degradation of HIF-1α [143]. Low $O_2$ levels are accompanied with low PHD activity, and as a consequence, HIF-1α is stabilized during hypoxia. Loss-of-function mutations that affect the VHL ubiquitin ligase function, occurring in the von Hippel-Lindau disease [144], lead to an aberrant accumulation of HIF-1α. Since PHDs are αKG-dependent oxygenases [145], low levels of α-KG or high levels of its structural analogs and competitors succinate or fumarate (see Section 3.1.2.2) inhibit PHD enzymatic activity, causing the stabilization and accumulation of HIF-1α and leading to a state of pseudohypoxia.

As a transcription factor, HIF-1α activates the expression of the EMT factors *SNAI1* [146], *ZEB1/2* [147], *TCF3* [148,149] and *TWIST1* [150] to repress E-cadherin expression. It also elicits the expression of lysyl oxidase [151] and matrix metalloproteases for extracellular matrix remodeling, as well as angiogenic factors to promote the vascularization of the hypoxic areas and erythropoietin to boost red blood cell production in the bone marrow [138].

The major effects of HIF-1α activation on metabolism are to (1) stimulate glycolytic energy production by promoting the expression of the glucose transporter GLUT1 (SLC2A1) and glycolytic enzymes (such as hexokinase 1/2 (HK1/2), PFK1, PFKFB3 and aldolase); and (2) to downregulate mitochondrial OXPHOS by promoting the expression pyruvate dehydrogenase kinase 1 (PDK1) [152] and the MYC inhibitor MAX interactor 1 (MXI1) in renal cell carcinoma cells [153]. The combination of blunted mitochondrial function and high glycolytic activity associated with hypoxia and HIF-1α activity leads to the accumulation of cytoplasmic pyruvate and NADH. In order to dispose of these compounds, lactate dehydrogenase A (LDHA) is induced by HIF-1α and catalyzes the conversion of pyruvate and NADH to lactate and NAD+ [153], after which lactate is exported to the extracellular milieu through the HIF-inducible plasma membrane monocarboxylate transporter 4 (MCT4, SLC16A4) [154]. Thus, a collateral effect of these processes is the acidosis of the extracellular environment surrounding the tumor cells under hypoxia.

Acidosis is a characteristic feature of the tumor microenvironment that directly regulates tumor cell invasion by affecting immune cell function, clonal cell evolution and drug resistance [155]. Unlike normal cells, cancer cells can adapt to survive in low pH (acidic) environments through increased glycolytic activity and an expression of proton transporters that normalize intracellular pH [155]. Acidosis-driven adaptation also triggers the emergence of aggressive tumor cell subpopulations that exhibit increased invasion, proliferation and drug resistance [155]. Low extracellular pH induces increased histone deacetylation, thereby influencing the expression of stress-responsive genes and contributing to the normalization of intracellular pH through the enhanced release of acetate anions that are co-exported with protons through monocarboxylate transporters [156,157]. Low pH areas of these tumors are not necessarily restricted to hypoxic areas, and are enriched for cells that are invasive and proliferative. Acidic conditions induce a reversible transcriptomic rewiring, independent of lactate, involving RNA splicing and being enriched for the targets of RNA binding proteins with specificity for AU-rich motifs, including CD44 [158]. CD44 is a hyaluronan-binding receptor that mediates cell invasiveness and motility [159], expressed as two major isoforms associated with either epithelial or mesenchymal gene programs, and regulated by the alternative splicing factors ESRP1/2, that promote an epithelial program [160] or QKI and ROBFOX1/2, that promote a mesenchymal program [161–163].

## 5. EMT, Metabolism and Drug Resistance

Numerous experimental reports and studies with patient cohorts have found a significant association of EMT or mesenchymal traits of tumors with acquired resistance to chemotherapy, targeted drugs and immunotherapy [164–166]. No unifying theme has emerged that explains the specific mechanisms co-opted by EMT as a path to drug resistance. In one case, early adaptive resistance of lung cancer cells to the EGFR inhibitor erlotinib led to a metabolically quiescent state, albeit with increased glutamine addition and a survival attributed to an enhanced expression of BCL-2 and BCL-xL [167]. Resistance to the mitotic drug docetaxel was found to induce EMT in prostate cancer cells, accompanied with a more efficient respiratory phenotype, a utilization of glucose and glutamine and the production of lactate [168]. Short-term treatment of colorectal cancer cells with docetaxel induced an EMT phenotype in the surviving cells, which were more dependent on OXPHOS than sensitive cells [169]. Studies by our laboratory comparing the metabolic dependencies and vulnerabilities of clonal prostate cancer cell lines displaying either epithelial or marked mesenchymal phenotypes, indicated the establishment of a Warburg effect in epithelial cells with high lactate production and a strong reliance on glutaminolysis for the anaplerotic feeding of the TCA cycle. This rendered epithelial CSCs highly sensitive to glutaminase inhibitors, while mesenchymal cells more efficiently funneled glucose to the TCA cycle, displayed stronger OXPHOS dependency, and were more sensitive to mitochondrial complex I and III inhibitors [170].

When cells display a Warburg effect with an enhanced production of lactate, as observed in cells in intermediate EMT states concomitant with CSC features, the resulting acidic extracellular environment can promote drug resistance through several mechanisms, including the so-called "ion trapping" mechanism, by which molecules that are weak bases (e.g., anthracyclines, anthraquinones or vinca alkaloids) are protonated at an acidic pH, which impairs their diffusion through plasma membranes [171]. On the other hand, weak acids (e.g., chorambucil, cyclophosphamide, 5-FU) are not ionized at an acidic pH, and can more readily traverse membranes, reaching the slightly alkaline intracellular milieu, where they become negatively-charged, and accumulate for more efficacious cytotoxic effects [172]. Resistance to immunotherapy and immunosuppression is also tightly linked to tumor-generated metabolic microenvironments, including nutrient exhaustion (including glucose, glutamine or tryptophan) [173], hypoxia, or also enhanced acidosis by accumulation of lactate [174]. A more direct connection between EMT and tumor immune escape is provided by the demonstration that the immune checkpoint ligand PD-L1 is a target of miR-200 [175]. As such, ZEB1 expression downregulates miR-200 and enhances the expression of PD-L1 on tumor cells undergoing EMT. In turn, ligand-engaged PD-L1 can induce or reinforce EMT, as exemplified in renal cell carcinoma cells [176], thus establishing a positive feedback loop that potentiates acidic, inflammatory and immunosuppressive tumor microenvironments, that are also predicted to result in enhanced resistance to other drugs.

Therefore, differential glycolytic and mitochondrial efficiencies associated with epithelial or mesenchymal plasticity confer differential metabolic dependencies which can be exploited therapeutically in combinatorial schemes intended at overcoming drug resistance strategies adopted by cancer cells [177], including undergoing an EMT.

## 6. Concluding Remarks

From their earliest stages in development, multicellular organisms engage in asymmetric division followed by cell-cell communication in order to generate heterogeneity and specialization. Each stage in cell fate determination is exquisitely orchestrated by specific regulators that coordinate intricate transcriptional, signaling and metabolic networks that ultimately define cell identity and tissue and organ functions. Epithelial cells that enter a given differentiation lineage maintain degrees of plasticity before they acquire stable specialized features, and as such, they may exit or revert their committed paths, notably through EMT. In cancer, transformed cells endowed with phenotypic plasticity co-opt these same mechanisms as they evolve and adapt in response to environmental challenges, yielding intratumoral heterogeneity, which significantly impacts the biology and management of cancers.

Epithelial-mesenchymal plasticity is so deeply intertwined with metabolic reprogramming that the two processes may no longer be considered separately, in physiological or pathological scenarios. As such, signaling cues that drive EMT must concomitantly induce an appropriate reprogramming of metabolic networks in order to meet the requirements of the new cellular state, while conversely, endogenous or exogenous shifts in metabolic balances can drive EMT in their own right. This perspective opens the prospect that epithelial-mesenchymal plasticity may be modulated, in both clinical and experimental settings, through appropriate metabolic interventions. As discussed above, the inhibition of metabolic enzymes such as ALDOA, GAPDH or FASN can prevent or revert EMT in cell models, as can the neutralization of acidic tumor environments. The recent observations that mesenchymal properties require fused mitochondria endowed with efficient TCA and OXHPOS [10], while prostate CSCs rely on mitochondrial fission [178], afford the prediction that interventions directly aimed at mitochondrial function or dynamics will produce differential effects on cell plasticity, and thus are worth exploring as antineoplastic strategies.

Other metabolic interventions with the potential of impacting EMT and, consequently, tumor heterogeneity and drug resistance, include those that shift the intracellular balance of metabolites with direct effects on epigenetic marks and gene regulation. In this regard, an interesting recent study [179] has shown the feasibility of dietary methionine restriction as a strategy to target one-carbon metabolism, which modulated tumor growth and conferred tumor chemosensitivity to conventional drugs, thus opening the door to novel mechanistically-based dietary interventions designed at targeting specific metabolic pathways deranged in a given tumor type.

In summary, a deeper understanding of the multiple-level links between metabolism, epigenetics and epithelial-mesenchymal transition and their intimate interconnections should lead to the rational discovery of primary vulnerabilities as well as secondary vulnerabilities that emerge in response to first-line therapies, thus paving the way to propose combinatorial therapeutic strategies to combat advanced cancers and pharmacological or immunological resistance.

**Author Contributions:** Conceptualization, original draft preparation, review and edition, T.M.T., C.B. and M.C.

**Funding:** This work was funded by MINECO European Commission FEDER funds—"Una manera de hacer Europa" (SAF2015-66984-C2-1-R, SAF2017-89673-R and SAF2015-70270-REDT), Instituto de Salud Carlos III and Centro de Investigación Biomédica en Red de Enfermedades Hepáticas y Digestivas (CIBEREHD CB17/04/00023), Agència de Gestió d'Ajuts Universitaris i de Recerca (AGAUR)—Generalitat de Catalunya (2017SGR-1033). M.C. acknowledges the support received through the prize "ICREA Academia" for excellence in research, funded by ICREA foundation—Generalitat de Catalunya.

**Acknowledgments:** The authors are grateful to Míriam Tarrado (University of Barcelona and CIBER-EHD) for critical reading and suggestions to improve the manuscript.

**Conflicts of Interest:** The authors declare no conflicts of interest.

## References

1. Yilmaz, M.; Christofori, G. EMT, the cytoskeleton, and cancer cell invasion. *Cancer Metastasis Rev.* **2009**, *28*, 15–33. [CrossRef] [PubMed]
2. Vega, S.; Morales, A.V.; Ocaña, O.H.; Valdés, F.; Fabregat, I.; Nieto, M.A. Snail blocks the cell cycle and confers resistance to cell death. *Genes Dev.* **2004**, *18*, 1131–1143. [CrossRef] [PubMed]
3. Ye, X.; Weinberg, R.A. Epithelial-mesenchymal plasticity: A central regulator of cancer progression. *Trends Cell Biol.* **2015**, *25*, 675–686. [CrossRef] [PubMed]
4. Zheng, X.; Carstens, J.L.; Kim, J.; Scheible, M.; Kaye, J.; Sugimoto, H.; Wu, C.C.; LeBleu, V.S.; Kalluri, R. Epithelial-to-mesenchymal transition is dispensable for metastasis but induces chemoresistance in pancreatic cancer. *Nature* **2015**, *527*, 525–530. [CrossRef] [PubMed]

5. Celia-Terrassa, T.; Meca-Cortés, O.; Mateo, F.; Martínez de Paz, A.; Rubio, N.; Arnal-Estapé, A.; Ell, B.J.; Bermudo, R.; Díaz, A.; Guerra-Rebollo, M.; et al. Epithelial-mesenchymal transition can suppress major attributes of human epithelial tumor-initiating cells. *J. Clin. Investig.* **2012**, *122*, 1849–1868. [CrossRef] [PubMed]
6. Pastushenko, I.; Brisebarre, A.; Sifrim, A.; Fioramonti, M.; Revenco, T.; Boumahdi, S.; Van Keymeulen, A.; Brown, D.; Moers, V.; Lemaire, S.; et al. Identification of the tumour transition states occurring during EMT. *Nature* **2018**, *556*, 463–468. [CrossRef] [PubMed]
7. Kroger, C.; Afeyan, A.; Mraz, J.; Eaton, E.N.; Reinhardt, F.; Khodor, Y.L.; Thiru, P.; Bierie, B.; Ye, X.; Burge, C.B.; et al. Acquisition of a hybrid E/M state is essential for tumorigenicity of basal breast cancer cells. *Proc. Natl. Acad. Sci. USA* **2019**, *116*, 7353–7362. [CrossRef] [PubMed]
8. Dongre, A.; Weinberg, R.A. New insights into the mechanisms of epithelial-mesenchymal transition and implications for cancer. *Nat. Rev. Mol. Cell. Biol.* **2019**, *20*, 69–84. [CrossRef] [PubMed]
9. Porporato, P.E.; Payen, V.L.; Pérez-Escuredo, J.; De Saedeleer, C.J.; Danhier, P.; Copetti, T.; Dhup, S.; Tardy, M.; Vazeille, T.; Bouzin, C.; et al. A mitochondrial switch promotes tumor metastasis. *Cell Rep.* **2014**, *8*, 754–766. [CrossRef] [PubMed]
10. Wu, M.J.; Chen, Y.S.; Kim, M.R.; Chang, C.C.; Gampala, S.; Zhang, Y.; Wang, Y.; Chang, C.Y.; Yang, J.Y.; Chang, C.J. Epithelial-mesenchymal transition directs stem cell polarity via regulation of mitofusin. *Cell Metab.* **2019**, *29*, 993–1002. [CrossRef] [PubMed]
11. Gomes, L.C.; Di Benedetto, G.; Scorrano, L. During autophagy mitochondria elongate, are spared from degradation and sustain cell viability. *Nat. Cell Biol.* **2011**, *13*, 589–598. [CrossRef] [PubMed]
12. Rambold, A.S.; Kostelecky, B.; Elia, N.; Lippincott-Schwartz, J. Tubular network formation protects mitochondria from autophagosomal degradation during nutrient starvation. *Proc. Natl. Acad. Sci. USA* **2011**, *108*, 10190–10195. [CrossRef] [PubMed]
13. Mishra, P.; Chan, D.C. Metabolic regulation of mitochondrial dynamics. *J. Cell Biol.* **2016**, *212*, 379–387. [CrossRef] [PubMed]
14. Sun, Y.; Daemen, A.; Hatzivassiliou, G.; Arnott, D.; Wilson, C.; Zhuang, G.; Gao, M.; Liu, P.; Boudreau, A.; Johnson, L.; et al. Metabolic and transcriptional profiling reveals pyruvate dehydrogenase kinase 4 as a mediator of epithelial-mesenchymal transition and drug resistance in tumor cells. *Cancer Metab.* **2014**, *2*, 20. [CrossRef] [PubMed]
15. Dong, C.; Yuan, T.; Wu, Y.; Wang, Y.; Fan, T.W.; Miriyala, S.; Lin, Y.; Yao, J.; Shi, J.; Kang, T.; et al. Loss of FBP1 by Snail-mediated repression provides metabolic advantages in basal-like breast cancer. *Cancer Cell* **2013**, *23*, 316–331. [CrossRef] [PubMed]
16. Kim, N.H.; Cha, Y.H.; Lee, J.; Lee, S.H.; Yang, J.H.; Yun, J.S.; Cho, E.S.; Zhang, X.; Nam, M.; Kim, N.; et al. Snail reprograms glucose metabolism by repressing phosphofructokinase PFKP allowing cancer cell survival under metabolic stress. *Nat. Commun.* **2017**, *8*, 14374. [CrossRef]
17. Lee, S.Y.; Jeon, H.M.; Ju, M.K.; Kim, C.H.; Yoon, G.; Han, S.I.; Park, H.G.; Kang, H.S. Wnt/Snail signaling regulates cytochrome C oxidase and glucose metabolism. *Cancer Res.* **2012**, *72*, 3607–3617. [CrossRef] [PubMed]
18. Du, S.; Guan, Z.; Hao, L.; Song, Y.; Wang, L.; Gong, L.; Liu, L.; Qi, X.; Hou, Z.; Shao, S. Fructose-bisphosphate aldolase A is a potential metastasis-associated marker of lung squamous cell carcinoma and promotes lung cell tumorigenesis and migration. *PLoS ONE* **2014**, *9*, e85804. [CrossRef]
19. Liu, K.; Tang, Z.; Huang, A.; Chen, P.; Liu, P.; Yang, J.; Lu, W.; Liao, J.; Sun, Y.; Wen, S.; et al. Glyceraldehyde-3-phosphate dehydrogenase promotes cancer growth and metastasis through upregulation of SNAIL expression. *Int. J. Oncol.* **2017**, *50*, 252–262. [CrossRef]
20. Murai, T. The role of lipid rafts in cancer cell adhesion and migration. *Int. J. Cell Biol.* **2012**, *2012*, 763283. [CrossRef]
21. Ogretmen, B. Sphingolipid metabolism in cancer signalling and therapy. *Nat. Rev. Cancer* **2018**, *18*, 33–50. [CrossRef] [PubMed]
22. Luo, X.; Cheng, C.; Tan, Z.; Li, N.; Tang, M.; Yang, L.; Cao, Y. Emerging roles of lipid metabolism in cancer metastasis. *Mol. Cancer* **2017**, *16*, 76. [CrossRef] [PubMed]
23. Lucenay, K.S.; Doostan, I.; Karakas, C.; Bui, T.; Ding, Z.; Mills, G.; Hunt, K.K.; Keyomarsi, K. Cyclin E associates with the lipogenic enzyme ATP-citrate lyase to enable malignant growth of breast cancer cells. *Cancer Res.* **2016**, *76*, 2406–2418. [CrossRef] [PubMed]

24. Jiang, L.; Wang, H.; Li, J.; Fang, X.; Pan, H.; Yuan, X.; Zhang, P. Up-regulated FASN expression promotes transcoelomic metastasis of ovarian cancer cell through epithelial-mesenchymal transition. *Int. J. Mol. Sci.* **2014**, *15*, 11539–11554. [CrossRef] [PubMed]
25. Li, J.; Dong, L.; Wei, D.; Wang, X.; Zhang, S.; Li, H. Fatty acid synthase mediates the epithelial-mesenchymal transition of breast cancer cells. *Int. J. Biol. Sci.* **2014**, *10*, 171–180. [CrossRef] [PubMed]
26. Wang, H.; Xi, Q.; Wu, G. Fatty acid synthase regulates invasion and metastasis of colorectal cancer via Wnt signaling pathway. *Cancer Med.* **2016**, *5*, 1599–1606. [CrossRef] [PubMed]
27. Schafer, Z.T.; Grassian, A.R.; Song, L.; Jiang, Z.; Gerhart-Hines, Z.; Irie, H.Y.; Gao, S.; Puigserver, P.; Brugge, J.S. Antioxidant and oncogene rescue of metabolic defects caused by loss of matrix attachment. *Nature* **2009**, *461*, 109–113. [CrossRef] [PubMed]
28. Weber, G.F. Time and circumstances: Cancer cell metabolism at various stages of disease progression. *Front. Oncol.* **2016**, *6*, 257. [CrossRef] [PubMed]
29. Paoli, P.; Giannoni, E.; Chiarugi, P. Anoikis molecular pathways and its role in cancer progression. *Biochim. Biophys. Acta* **2013**, *1833*, 3481–3498. [CrossRef] [PubMed]
30. Buchheit, C.L.; Rayavarapu, R.R.; Schafer, Z.T. The regulation of cancer cell death and metabolism by extracellular matrix attachment. *Semin. Cell Dev. Biol.* **2012**, *23*, 402–411. [CrossRef] [PubMed]
31. Diaz-Ruiz, R.; Rigoulet, M.; Devin, A. The Warburg and Crabtree effects: On the origin of cancer cell energy metabolism and of yeast glucose repression. *Biochim. Biophys. Acta* **2011**, *1807*, 568–576. [CrossRef] [PubMed]
32. Patra, K.C.; Hay, N. The pentose phosphate pathway and cancer. *Trends Biochem. Sci.* **2014**, *39*, 347–354. [CrossRef] [PubMed]
33. Caneba, C.A.; Bellance, N.; Yang, L.; Pabst, L.; Nagrath, D. Pyruvate uptake is increased in highly invasive ovarian cancer cells under anoikis conditions for anaplerosis, mitochondrial function, and migration. *Am. J. Physiol. Endocrinol. Metab.* **2012**, *303*, E1036–E1052. [CrossRef] [PubMed]
34. Lin, C.S.; Liu, L.T.; Ou, L.H.; Pan, S.C.; Lin, C.I.; Wei, Y.H. Role of mitochondrial function in the invasiveness of human colon cancer cells. *Oncol. Rep.* **2018**, *39*, 316–330. [CrossRef] [PubMed]
35. Beurel, E.; Grieco, S.F.; Jope, R.S. Glycogen synthase kinase-3 (GSK3): Regulation, actions, and diseases. *Pharmacol. Ther.* **2015**, *148*, 114–131. [CrossRef] [PubMed]
36. Oreña, S.J.; Torchia, A.J.; Garofalo, R.S. Inhibition of glycogen-synthase kinase 3 stimulates glycogen synthase and glucose transport by distinct mechanisms in 3T3-L1 adipocytes. *J. Biol. Chem.* **2000**, *275*, 15765–15772. [CrossRef]
37. Nieto, M.A. The ins and outs of the epithelial to mesenchymal transition in health and disease. *Annu. Rev. Cell Dev. Biol.* **2011**, *27*, 347–376. [CrossRef]
38. Janke, R.; Dodson, A.E.; Rine, J. Metabolism and epigenetics. *Annu. Rev. Cell Dev. Biol.* **2015**, *31*, 473–496. [CrossRef]
39. Reid, M.A.; Dai, Z.; Locasale, J.W. The impact of cellular metabolism on chromatin dynamics and epigenetics. *Nat. Cell Biol.* **2017**, *19*, 1298–1306. [CrossRef]
40. Mentch, S.J.; Locasale, J.W. One-carbon metabolism and epigenetics: Understanding the specificity. *Ann. N. Y. Acad. Sci.* **2016**, *1363*, 91–98. [CrossRef]
41. Mentch, S.J.; Mehrmohamadi, M.; Huang, L.; Liu, X.; Gupta, D.; Mattocks, D.; Gómez Padilla, P.; Ables, G.; Bamman, M.M.; Thalacker-Mercer, A.E.; et al. Histone methylation dynamics and gene regulation occur through the sensing of one-carbon metabolism. *Cell Metab.* **2015**, *22*, 861–873. [CrossRef] [PubMed]
42. Napolitano, L.; Scalise, M.; Galluccio, M.; Pochini, L.; Albanese, L.M.; Indiveri, C. LAT1 is the transport competent unit of the LAT1/CD98 heterodimeric amino acid transporter. *Int. J. Biochem. Cell Biol.* **2015**, *67*, 25–33. [CrossRef] [PubMed]
43. Gao, P.; Tchernyshyov, I.; Chang, T.C.; Lee, Y.S.; Kita, K.; Ochi, T.; Zeller, K.I.; De Marzo, A.M.; Van Eyk, J.E.; Mendell, J.T.; et al. c-Myc suppression of miR-23a/b enhances mitochondrial glutaminase expression and glutamine metabolism. *Nature* **2009**, *458*, 762–765. [CrossRef] [PubMed]
44. Hayashi, K.; Jutabha, P.; Endou, H.; Anzai, N. c-Myc is crucial for the expression of LAT1 in MIA Paca-2 human pancreatic cancer cells. *Oncol. Rep.* **2012**, *28*, 862–866. [CrossRef] [PubMed]
45. Edinger, A.L.; Thompson, C.B. Akt maintains cell size and survival by increasing mTOR-dependent nutrient uptake. *Mol. Biol. Cell* **2002**, *13*, 2276–2288. [CrossRef] [PubMed]
46. Goll, M.G.; Bestor, T.H. Eukaryotic cytosine methyltransferases. *Annu. Rev. Biochem.* **2005**, *74*, 481–514. [CrossRef] [PubMed]

47. McDonald, O.G.; Wu, H.; Timp, W.; Doi, A.; Feinberg, A.P. Genome-scale epigenetic reprogramming during epithelial-to-mesenchymal transition. *Nat. Struct. Mol. Biol.* **2011**, *18*, 867–874. [CrossRef] [PubMed]
48. Carmona, F.J.; Davalos, V.; Vidal, E.; Gomez, A.; Heyn, H.; Hashimoto, Y.; Vizoso, M.; Martinez-Cardus, A.; Sayols, S.; Ferreira, H.J.; et al. A comprehensive DNA methylation profile of epithelial-to-mesenchymal transition. *Cancer Res.* **2014**, *74*, 5608–5619. [CrossRef] [PubMed]
49. Nabel, C.S.; Jia, H.; Ye, Y.; Shen, L.; Goldschmidt, H.L.; Stivers, J.T.; Zhang, Y.; Kohli, R.M. AID/APOBEC deaminases disfavor modified cytosines implicated in DNA demethylation. *Nat. Chem. Biol.* **2012**, *8*, 751–758. [CrossRef] [PubMed]
50. Guo, J.U.; Su, Y.; Zhong, C.; Ming, G.L.; Song, H. Hydroxylation of 5-methylcytosine by TET1 promotes active DNA demethylation in the adult brain. *Cell* **2011**, *145*, 423–434. [CrossRef]
51. Greer, E.L.; Shi, Y. Histone methylation: A dynamic mark in health, disease and inheritance. *Nat. Rev. Genet.* **2012**, *13*, 343–357. [CrossRef] [PubMed]
52. He, Y.F.; Li, B.Z.; Li, Z.; Liu, P.; Wang, Y.; Tang, Q.; Ding, J.; Jia, Y.; Chen, Z.; Li, L.; et al. Tet-mediated formation of 5-carboxylcytosine and its excision by TDG in mammalian DNA. *Science* **2011**, *333*, 1303–1307. [CrossRef] [PubMed]
53. Ito, S.; Shen, L.; Dai, Q.; Wu, S.C.; Collins, L.B.; Swenberg, J.A.; He, C.; Zhang, Y. Tet proteins can convert 5-methylcytosine to 5-formylcytosine and 5-carboxylcytosine. *Science* **2011**, *333*, 1300–1303. [CrossRef] [PubMed]
54. Maiti, A.; Drohat, A.C. Thymine DNA glycosylase can rapidly excise 5-formylcytosine and 5-carboxylcytosine: potential implications for active demethylation of CpG sites. *J. Biol. Chem.* **2011**, *286*, 35334–35338. [CrossRef] [PubMed]
55. Martin, C.; Zhang, Y. The diverse functions of histone lysine methylation. *Nat. Rev. Mol. Cell. Biol.* **2005**, *6*, 838–849. [CrossRef] [PubMed]
56. Hosseini, A.; Minucci, S. A comprehensive review of lysine-specific demethylase 1 and its roles in cancer. *Epigenomics* **2017**, *9*, 1123–1142. [CrossRef]
57. Lin, T.; Ponn, A.; Hu, X.; Law, B.; Lu, J. Requirement of the histone demethylase LSD1 in Snai1-mediated transcriptional repression during epithelial-mesenchymal transition. *Oncogene* **2010**, *29*, 4896–4904. [CrossRef]
58. Lin, Y.; Wu, Y.; Li, J.; Dong, C.; Ye, X.; Chi, Y.; Evers, B.M.; Zhou, B. The SNAG domain of Snail1 functions as a molecular hook for recruiting lysine-specific demethylase 1. *EMBO J.* **2010**, *29*, 1803–1816. [CrossRef]
59. Perillo, B.; Ombra, M.N.; Bertoni, A.; Cuozzo, C.; Sacchetti, S.; Sasso, A.; Chiariotti, L.; Malorni, A.; Abbondanza, C.; Avvedimento, E.V. DNA oxidation as triggered by H3K9me2 demethylation drives estrogen-induced gene expression. *Science* **2008**, *319*, 202–206. [CrossRef]
60. Carnesecchi, J.; Forcet, C.; Zhang, L.; Tribollet, V.; Barenton, B.; Boudra, R.; Cerutti, C.; Billas, I.M.; Sérandour, A.A.; Carroll, J.S.; et al. ERRalpha induces H3K9 demethylation by LSD1 to promote cell invasion. *Proc. Natl. Acad. Sci. USA* **2017**, *114*, 3909–3914. [CrossRef]
61. Hino, S.; Sakamoto, A.; Nagaoka, K.; Anan, K.; Wang, Y.; Mimasu, S.; Umehara, T.; Yokoyama, S.; Kosai, K.; Nakao, M. FAD-dependent lysine-specific demethylase-1 regulates cellular energy expenditure. *Nat. Commun.* **2012**, *3*, 758. [CrossRef] [PubMed]
62. Accari, S.L.; Fisher, P.R. Emerging roles of JmjC domain-containing proteins. *Int. Rev. Cell. Mol. Biol.* **2015**, *319*, 165–220. [PubMed]
63. Markolovic, S.; Leissing, T.M.; Chowdhury, R.; Wilkins, S.E.; Lu, X.; Schofield, C.J. Structure-function relationships of human JmjC oxygenases-demethylases versus hydroxylases. *Curr. Opin. Struct. Biol.* **2016**, *41*, 62–72. [CrossRef] [PubMed]
64. Wu, X.; Zhang, Y. TET-mediated active DNA demethylation: Mechanism, function and beyond. *Nat. Rev. Genet.* **2017**, *18*, 517–534. [CrossRef] [PubMed]
65. Nowicki, S.; Gottlieb, E. Oncometabolites: Tailoring our genes. *FEBS J.* **2015**, *282*, 2796–2805. [CrossRef] [PubMed]
66. Yang, L.; Venneti, S.; Nagrath, D. Glutaminolysis: A hallmark of cancer metabolism. *Annu. Rev. Biomed. Eng.* **2017**, *19*, 163–194. [CrossRef] [PubMed]
67. Xu, W.; Yang, H.; Liu, Y.; Yang, Y.; Wang, P.; Kim, S.H.; Ito, S.; Yang, C.; Wang, P.; Xiao, M.T.; et al. Oncometabolite 2-hydroxyglutarate is a competitive inhibitor of alpha-ketoglutarate-dependent dioxygenases. *Cancer Cell* **2011**, *19*, 17–30. [CrossRef]

68. Xiao, M.; Yang, H.; Xu, W.; Ma, S.; Lin, H.; Zhu, H.; Liu, L.; Liu, Y.; Yang, C.; Xu, Y.; et al. Inhibition of alpha-KG-dependent histone and DNA demethylases by fumarate and succinate that are accumulated in mutations of FH and SDH tumor suppressors. *Genes Dev.* **2012**, *26*, 1326–1338. [CrossRef]
69. Dalla Pozza, E.; Dando, I.; Pacchiana, R.; Liboi, E.; Scupoli, M.T.; Donadelli, M.; Palmieri, M. Regulation of succinate dehydrogenase and role of succinate in cancer. *Semin. Cell Dev. Biol.* **2019**. [CrossRef]
70. Sciacovelli, M.; Gonçalves, E.; Johnson, T.I.; Zecchini, V.R.; da Costa, A.S.; Gaude, E.; Drubbel, A.V.; Theobald, S.J.; Abbo, S.R.; Tran, M.G.; et al. Fumarate is an epigenetic modifier that elicits epithelial-to-mesenchymal transition. *Nature* **2016**, *537*, 544–547. [CrossRef]
71. Tomlinson, I.P.; Alam, N.A.; Rowan, A.J.; Barclay, E.; Jaeger, E.E.; Kelsell, D.; Leigh, I.; Gorman, P.; Lamlum, H.; Rahman, S.; et al. Germline mutations in FH predispose to dominantly inherited uterine fibroids, skin leiomyomata and papillary renal cell cancer. *Nat. Genet.* **2002**, *30*, 406–410. [PubMed]
72. Castro-Vega, L.J.; Buffet, A.; De Cubas, A.A.; Cascón, A.; Menara, M.; Khalifa, E.; Amar, L.; Azriel, S.; Bourdeau, I.; Chabre, O.; et al. Germline mutations in FH confer predisposition to malignant pheochromocytomas and paragangliomas. *Hum. Mol. Genet.* **2014**, *23*, 2440–2446. [CrossRef] [PubMed]
73. Clark, G.R.; Sciacovelli, M.; Gaude, E.; Walsh, D.; Kirby, G.; Simpson, M.A.; Trembath, R.C.; Berg, J.N.; Woodward, E.R.; Kinning, E.; et al. Germline FH mutations presenting with pheochromocytoma. *J. Clin. Endocrinol. Metab.* **2014**, *99*, E2046–E2050. [CrossRef] [PubMed]
74. Isaacs, J.S.; Jung, Y.J.; Mole, D.R.; Lee, S.; Torres-Cabala, C.; Chung, Y.L.; Merino, M.; Trepel, J.; Zbar, B.; Toro, J.; et al. HIF overexpression correlates with biallelic loss of fumarate hydratase in renal cancer: Novel role of fumarate in regulation of HIF stability. *Cancer Cell* **2005**, *8*, 143–153. [CrossRef] [PubMed]
75. Clark, O.; Yen, K.; Mellinghoff, I.K. Molecular pathways: Isocitrate dehydrogenase mutations in cancer. *Clin. Cancer Res.* **2016**, *22*, 1837–1842. [CrossRef] [PubMed]
76. Waitkus, M.S.; Diplas, B.H.; Yan, H. Biological role and therapeutic potential of IDH mutations in cancer. *Cancer Cell* **2018**, *34*, 186–195. [CrossRef] [PubMed]
77. Figueroa, M.E.; Abdel-Wahab, O.; Lu, C.; Ward, P.S.; Patel, J.; Shih, A.; Li, Y.; Bhagwat, N.; Vasanthakumar, A.; Fernandez, H.F.; et al. Leukemic IDH1 and IDH2 mutations result in a hypermethylation phenotype, disrupt TET2 function, and impair hematopoietic differentiation. *Cancer Cell* **2010**, *18*, 553–567. [CrossRef] [PubMed]
78. Lu, C.; Ward, P.S.; Kapoor, G.S.; Rohle, D.; Turcan, S.; Abdel-Wahab, O.; Edwards, C.R.; Khanin, R.; Figueroa, M.E.; Melnick, A.; et al. IDH mutation impairs histone demethylation and results in a block to cell differentiation. *Nature* **2012**, *483*, 474–478. [CrossRef] [PubMed]
79. Saha, S.K.; Parachoniak, C.A.; Ghanta, K.S.; Fitamant, J.; Ross, K.N.; Najem, M.S.; Gurumurthy, S.; Akbay, E.A.; Sia, D.; Cornella, H.; et al. Mutant IDH inhibits HNF-4alpha to block hepatocyte differentiation and promote biliary cancer. *Nature* **2014**, *513*, 110–114. [CrossRef]
80. Wise, D.R.; Ward, P.S.; Shay, J.E.; Cross, J.R.; Gruber, J.J.; Sachdeva, U.M.; Platt, J.M.; DeMatteo, R.G.; Simon, M.C.; Thompson, C.B. Hypoxia promotes isocitrate dehydrogenase-dependent carboxylation of alpha-ketoglutarate to citrate to support cell growth and viability. *Proc. Natl. Acad. Sci. USA* **2011**, *108*, 19611–19616. [CrossRef]
81. Mullen, A.R.; Hu, Z.; Shi, X.; Jiang, L.; Boroughs, L.K.; Kovacs, Z.; Boriack, R.; Rakheja, D.; Sullivan, L.B.; Linehan, W.M.; et al. Oxidation of alpha-ketoglutarate is required for reductive carboxylation in cancer cells with mitochondrial defects. *Cell Rep.* **2014**, *7*, 1679–1690. [CrossRef] [PubMed]
82. Terunuma, A.; Putluri, N.; Mishra, P.; Mathé, E.A.; Dorsey, T.H.; Yi, M.; Wallace, T.A.; Issaq, H.J.; Zhou, M.; Killian, J.K.; et al. MYC-driven accumulation of 2-hydroxyglutarate is associated with breast cancer prognosis. *J. Clin. Investig.* **2014**, *124*, 398–412. [CrossRef] [PubMed]
83. Colvin, H.; Nishida, N.; Konno, M.; Haraguchi, N.; Takahashi, H.; Nishimura, J.; Hata, T.; Kawamoto, K.; Asai, A.; Tsunekuni, K.; et al. Oncometabolite D-2-Hydroxyglurate directly induces epithelial-mesenchymal transition and is associated with distant metastasis in colorectal cancer. *Sci. Rep.* **2016**, *6*, 36289. [CrossRef] [PubMed]
84. Intlekofer, A.M.; Dematteo, R.; Venneti, S.; Finley, L.W.; Lu, C.; Judkins, A.R.; Rustenburg, A.S.; Grinaway, P.B.; Chodera, J.D.; Cross, J.R.; et al. Hypoxia induces production of L-2-Hydroxyglutarate. *Cell Metab.* **2015**, *22*, 304–311. [CrossRef] [PubMed]
85. Intlekofer, A.M.; Wang, B.; Liu, H.; Shah, H.; Carmona-Fontaine, C.; Rustenburg, A.S.; Salah, S.; Gunner, M.R.; Chodera, J.D.; Cross, J.R.; et al. L-2-Hydroxyglutarate production arises from noncanonical enzyme function at acidic pH. *Nat. Chem. Biol.* **2017**, *13*, 494–500. [CrossRef] [PubMed]

86. Oldham, W.M.; Clish, C.; Yang, Y.; Loscalzo, J. Hypoxia-mediated increases in L-2-hydroxyglutarate coordinate the metabolic response to reductive stress. *Cell Metab.* **2015**, *22*, 291–303. [CrossRef] [PubMed]
87. Haberland, M.; Montgomery, R.L.; Olson, E.N. The many roles of histone deacetylases in development and physiology: Implications for disease and therapy. *Nat. Rev. Genet.* **2009**, *10*, 32–42. [CrossRef]
88. Marmorstein, R.; Zhou, M.M. Writers and readers of histone acetylation: Structure, mechanism, and inhibition. *Cold Spring Harb. Perspect. Biol.* **2014**, *6*, a018762. [CrossRef]
89. Segre, C.V.; Chiocca, S. Regulating the regulators: The post-translational code of class I HDAC1 and HDAC2. *J. Biomed. Biotechnol.* **2011**, *2011*, 690848. [CrossRef]
90. Chang, H.C.; Guarente, L. SIRT1 and other sirtuins in metabolism. *Trends Endocrinol. Metab.* **2014**, *25*, 138–145. [CrossRef]
91. Sivanand, S.; Viney, I.; Wellen, K.E. Spatiotemporal control of acetyl-CoA metabolism in chromatin regulation. *Trends Biochem. Sci.* **2018**, *43*, 61–74. [CrossRef] [PubMed]
92. Bulusu, V.; Tumanov, S.; Michalopoulou, E.; van den Broek, N.J.; MacKay, G.; Nixon, C.; Dhayade, S.; Schug, Z.T.; Vande Voorde, J.; Blyth, K.; et al. Acetate recapturing by nuclear acetyl-CoA synthetase 2 prevents loss of histone acetylation during oxygen and serum limitation. *Cell Rep.* **2017**, *18*, 647–658. [CrossRef] [PubMed]
93. Sutendra, G.; Kinnaird, A.; Dromparis, P.; Paulin, R.; Stenson, T.H.; Haromy, A.; Hashimoto, K.; Zhang, N.; Flaim, E.; Michelakis, E.D. A nuclear pyruvate dehydrogenase complex is important for the generation of acetyl-CoA and histone acetylation. *Cell* **2014**, *158*, 84–97. [CrossRef] [PubMed]
94. Galdieri, L.; Vancura, A. Acetyl-CoA carboxylase regulates global histone acetylation. *J. Biol. Chem.* **2012**, *287*, 23865–23876. [CrossRef] [PubMed]
95. Kamphorst, J.J.; Chung, M.K.; Fan, J.; Rabinowitz, J.D. Quantitative analysis of acetyl-CoA production in hypoxic cancer cells reveals substantial contribution from acetate. *Cancer Metab.* **2014**, *2*, 23. [CrossRef] [PubMed]
96. Schug, Z.T.; Peck, B.; Jones, D.T.; Zhang, Q.; Grosskurth, S.; Alam, I.S.; Goodwin, L.M.; Smethurst, E.; Mason, S.; Blyth, K.; et al. Acetyl-CoA synthetase 2 promotes acetate utilization and maintains cancer cell growth under metabolic stress. *Cancer Cell* **2015**, *27*, 57–71. [CrossRef] [PubMed]
97. Li, X.; Yu, W.; Qian, X.; Xia, Y.; Zheng, Y.; Lee, J.H.; Li, W.; Lyu, J.; Rao, G.; Zhang, X.; et al. Nucleus-translocated ACSS2 promotes gene transcription for lysosomal biogenesis and autophagy. *Mol. Cell* **2017**, *66*, 684–697. [CrossRef] [PubMed]
98. Kirsch, M.; De Groot, H. NAD(P)H, a directly operating antioxidant? *FASEB J.* **2001**, *15*, 1569–1574. [CrossRef] [PubMed]
99. Choi, J.E.; Mostoslavsky, R. Sirtuins, metabolism, and DNA repair. *Curr. Opin. Genet. Dev.* **2014**, *26*, 24–32. [CrossRef] [PubMed]
100. Cantó, C.; Sauve, A.A.; Bai, P. Crosstalk between poly(ADP-ribose) polymerase and sirtuin enzymes. *Mol. Aspects Med.* **2013**, *34*. [CrossRef]
101. Zhang, N.; Sauve, A.A. Regulatory effects of NAD+ metabolic pathways on sirtuin activity. *Prog. Mol. Biol. Transl. Sci.* **2018**, *154*, 71–104. [PubMed]
102. Lv, W.; Guo, X.; Wang, G.; Xu, Y.; Kang, J. Histone deacetylase 1 and 3 regulate the mesodermal lineage commitment of mouse embryonic stem cells. *PLoS ONE* **2014**, *9*, e113262. [CrossRef] [PubMed]
103. Kong, D.; Ahmad, A.; Bao, B.; Li, Y.; Banerjee, S.; Sarkar, F.H. Histone deacetylase inhibitors induce epithelial-to-mesenchymal transition in prostate cancer cells. *PLoS ONE* **2012**, *7*, e45045. [CrossRef] [PubMed]
104. Giudice, F.S.; Pinto, D.S., Jr.; Nör, J.E.; Squarize, C.H.; Castilho, R.M. Inhibition of histone deacetylase impacts cancer stem cells and induces epithelial-mesenchyme transition of head and neck cancer. *PLoS ONE* **2013**, *8*, e58672. [CrossRef] [PubMed]
105. Feng, J.; Cen, J.; Li, J.; Zhao, R.; Zhu, C.; Wang, Z.; Xie, J.; Tang, W. Histone deacetylase inhibitor valproic acid (VPA) promotes the epithelial mesenchymal transition of colorectal cancer cells via up regulation of Snail. *Cell Adh. Migr.* **2015**, *9*, 495–501. [CrossRef] [PubMed]
106. Ji, M.; Lee, E.J.; Kim, K.B.; Kim, Y.; Sung, R.; Lee, S.J.; Kim, D.S.; Park, S.M. HDAC inhibitors induce epithelial-mesenchymal transition in colon carcinoma cells. *Oncol. Rep.* **2015**, *33*, 2299–2308. [CrossRef] [PubMed]

107. Koplev, S.; Lin, K.; Dohlman, A.B.; Ma'ayan, A. Integration of pan-cancer transcriptomics with RPPA proteomics reveals mechanisms of epithelial-mesenchymal transition. *PLoS Comput. Biol.* **2018**, *14*, e1005911. [CrossRef] [PubMed]
108. West, A.C.; Johnstone, R.W. New and emerging HDAC inhibitors for cancer treatment. *J. Clin. Investig.* **2014**, *124*, 30–39. [CrossRef]
109. Bruzzese, F.; Leone, A.; Rocco, M.; Carbone, C.; Piro, G.; Caraglia, M.; Di Gennaro, E.; Budillon, A. HDAC inhibitor vorinostat enhances the antitumor effect of gefitinib in squamous cell carcinoma of head and neck by modulating ErbB receptor expression and reverting EMT. *J. Cell Physiol.* **2011**, *226*, 2378–2390. [CrossRef]
110. Strobl-Mazzulla, P.H.; Bronner, M.E. A PHD12-Snail2 repressive complex epigenetically mediates neural crest epithelial-to-mesenchymal transition. *J. Cell Biol.* **2012**, *198*, 999–1010. [CrossRef]
111. Meidhof, S.; Brabletz, S.; Lehmann, W.; Preca, B.T.; Mock, K.; Ruh, M.; Schüler, J.; Berthold, M.; Weber, A.; Burk, U.; et al. ZEB1-associated drug resistance in cancer cells is reversed by the class I HDAC inhibitor mocetinostat. *EMBO Mol. Med.* **2015**, *7*, 831–847. [CrossRef] [PubMed]
112. Sakamoto, T.; Kobayashi, S.; Yamada, D.; Nagano, H.; Tomokuni, A.; Tomimaru, Y.; Noda, T.; Gotoh, K.; Asaoka, T.; Wada, H.; et al. A histone deacetylase inhibitor suppresses epithelial-mesenchymal transition and attenuates chemoresistance in biliary tract cancer. *PLoS ONE* **2016**, *11*, e0145985. [CrossRef] [PubMed]
113. Ruscetti, M.; Dadashian, E.L.; Guo, W.; Quach, B.; Mulholland, D.J.; Park, J.W.; Tran, L.M.; Kobayashi, N.; Bianchi-Frias, D.; Xing, Y.; et al. HDAC inhibition impedes epithelial-mesenchymal plasticity and suppresses metastatic, castration-resistant prostate cancer. *Oncogene* **2016**, *35*, 3781–3795. [CrossRef] [PubMed]
114. Mishra, V.K.; Wegwitz, F.; Kosinsky, R.L.; Sen, M.; Baumgartner, R.; Wulff, T.; Siveke, J.T.; Schildhaus, H.U.; Najafova, Z.; Kari, V.; et al. Histone deacetylase class-I inhibition promotes epithelial gene expression in pancreatic cancer cells in a BRD4- and MYC-dependent manner. *Nucleic Acids Res.* **2017**, *45*, 6334–6349. [CrossRef] [PubMed]
115. Lu, M.; Zhu, W.W.; Wang, X.; Tang, J.J.; Zhang, K.L.; Yu, G.Y.; Shao, W.Q.; Lin, Z.F.; Wang, S.H.; Lu, L.; et al. ACOT12-dependent alteration of acetyl-CoA drives hepatocellular carcinoma metastasis by epigenetic induction of epithelial-mesenchymal transition. *Cell Metab.* **2019**, *29*, 886–900.e5. [CrossRef] [PubMed]
116. Jiang, G.M.; Wang, H.S.; Zhang, F.; Zhang, K.S.; Liu, Z.; Fang, R.; Wang, H.; Cai, S.H.; Du, J. Histone deacetylase inhibitor induction of epithelial-mesenchymal transitions via up-regulation of Snail facilitates cancer progression. *Biochim. Biophys. Acta* **2013**, *1833*, 663–671. [CrossRef] [PubMed]
117. Mohd-Sarip, A.; Teeuwssen, M.; Bot, A.G.; De Herdt, M.J.; Willems, S.M.; Baatenburg de Jong, R.; Looijenga, L.J.; Zatreanu, D.; Bezstarosti, K.; van Riet, J.; et al. DOC1-dependent recruitment of NURD reveals antagonism with SWI/SNF during epithelial-mesenchymal transition in oral cancer cells. *Cell Rep.* **2017**, *20*, 61–75. [CrossRef] [PubMed]
118. Aghdassi, A.; Sendler, M.; Guenther, A.; Mayerle, J.; Behn, C.O.; Heidecke, C.D.; Friess, H.; Büchler, M.; Evert, M.; Lerch, M.M.; et al. Recruitment of histone deacetylases HDAC1 and HDAC2 by the transcriptional repressor ZEB1 downregulates E-cadherin expression in pancreatic cancer. *Gut* **2012**, *61*, 439–448. [CrossRef] [PubMed]
119. Cencioni, C.; Spallotta, F.; Savoia, M.; Kuenne, C.; Guenther, S.; Re, A.; Wingert, S.; Rehage, M.; Sürün, D.; Siragusa, M.; et al. Zeb1-Hdac2-eNOS circuitry identifies early cardiovascular precursors in naive mouse embryonic stem cells. *Nat. Commun.* **2018**, *9*, 1281. [CrossRef]
120. Fidalgo, M.; Faiola, F.; Pereira, C.F.; Ding, J.; Saunders, A.; Gingold, J.; Schaniel, C.; Lemischka, I.R.; Silva, J.C.; Wang, J. Zfp281 mediates Nanog autorepression through recruitment of the NuRD complex and inhibits somatic cell reprogramming. *Proc. Natl. Acad. Sci. USA* **2012**, *109*, 16202–16207. [CrossRef]
121. Peinado, H.; Ballestar, E.; Esteller, M.; Cano, A. Snail mediates E-cadherin repression by the recruitment of the Sin3A/histone deacetylase 1 (HDAC1)/HDAC2 complex. *Mol. Cell. Biol.* **2004**, *24*, 306–319. [CrossRef] [PubMed]
122. Qi, D.; Bergman, M.; Aihara, H.; Nibu, Y.; Mannervik, M. Drosophila Ebi mediates Snail-dependent transcriptional repression through HDAC3-induced histone deacetylation. *EMBO J.* **2008**, *27*, 898–909. [CrossRef] [PubMed]
123. Herranz, N.; Pasini, D.; Díaz, V.M.; Francí, C.; Gutierrez, A.; Dave, N.; Escrivà, M.; Hernandez-Muñoz, I.; Di Croce, L.; Helin, K.; et al. Polycomb complex 2 is required for E-cadherin repression by the Snail1 transcription factor. *Mol. Cell. Biol.* **2008**, *28*, 4772–4781. [CrossRef] [PubMed]

124. Javaid, S.; Zhang, J.; Anderssen, E.; Black, J.C.; Wittner, B.S.; Tajima, K.; Ting, D.T.; Smolen, G.A.; Zubrowski, M.; Desai, R.; et al. Dynamic chromatin modification sustains epithelial-mesenchymal transition following inducible expression of Snail-1. *Cell Rep.* **2013**, *5*, 1679–1689. [CrossRef] [PubMed]
125. Vrba, L.; Jensen, T.J.; Garbe, J.C.; Heimark, R.L.; Cress, A.E.; Dickinson, S.; Stampfer, M.R.; Futscher, B.W. Role for DNA methylation in the regulation of miR-200c and miR-141 expression in normal and cancer cells. *PLoS ONE* **2010**, *5*, e8697. [CrossRef] [PubMed]
126. Davalos, V.; Moutinho, C.; Villanueva, A.; Boque, R.; Silva, P.; Carneiro, F.; Esteller, M. Dynamic epigenetic regulation of the microRNA-200 family mediates epithelial and mesenchymal transitions in human tumorigenesis. *Oncogene* **2012**, *31*, 2062–2074. [CrossRef] [PubMed]
127. Chaffer, C.L.; Marjanovic, N.D.; Lee, T.; Bell, G.; Kleer, C.G.; Reinhardt, F.; D'Alessio, A.C.; Young, R.A.; Weinberg, R.A. Poised chromatin at the ZEB1 promoter enables breast cancer cell plasticity and enhances tumorigenicity. *Cell* **2013**, *154*, 61–74. [CrossRef] [PubMed]
128. Shi, L.; Tang, X.; Qian, M.; Liu, Z.; Meng, F.; Fu, L.; Wang, Z.; Zhu, W.G.; Huang, J.D.; Zhou, Z.; et al. A SIRT1-centered circuitry regulates breast cancer stemness and metastasis. *Oncogene* **2018**, *37*, 6299–6315. [CrossRef] [PubMed]
129. Jin, M.S.; Hyun, C.L.; Park, I.A.; Kim, J.Y.; Chung, Y.R.; Im, S.A.; Lee, K.H.; Moon, H.G.; Ryu, H.S. SIRT1 induces tumor invasion by targeting epithelial mesenchymal transition-related pathway and is a prognostic marker in triple negative breast cancer. *Tumour Biol.* **2016**, *37*, 4743–4753. [CrossRef]
130. Cheng, F.; Su, L.; Yao, C.; Liu, L.; Shen, J.; Liu, C.; Chen, X.; Luo, Y.; Jiang, L.; Shan, J.; et al. SIRT1 promotes epithelial-mesenchymal transition and metastasis in colorectal cancer by regulating Fra-1 expression. *Cancer Lett.* **2016**, *375*, 274–283. [CrossRef]
131. Feng, H.; Wang, J.; Xu, J.; Xie, C.; Gao, F.; Li, Z. The expression of SIRT1 regulates the metastatic plasticity of chondrosarcoma cells by inducing epithelial-mesenchymal transition. *Sci. Rep.* **2017**, *7*, 41203. [CrossRef] [PubMed]
132. Qiang, L.; Sample, A.; Liu, H.; Wu, X.; He, Y.Y. Epidermal SIRT1 regulates inflammation, cell migration, and wound healing. *Sci. Rep.* **2017**, *7*, 14110. [CrossRef] [PubMed]
133. Byles, V.; Zhu, L.; Lovaas, J.D.; Chmilewski, L.K.; Wang, J.; Faller, D.V.; Dai, Y. SIRT1 induces EMT by cooperating with EMT transcription factors and enhances prostate cancer cell migration and metastasis. *Oncogene* **2012**, *31*, 4619–4629. [CrossRef] [PubMed]
134. Chen, J.; Chan, A.W.; To, K.F.; Chen, W.; Zhang, Z.; Ren, J.; Song, C.; Cheung, Y.S.; Lai, P.B.; Cheng, S.H.; et al. SIRT2 overexpression in hepatocellular carcinoma mediates epithelial to mesenchymal transition by protein kinase B/glycogen synthase kinase-3beta/beta-catenin signaling. *Hepatology* **2013**, *57*, 2287–2298. [CrossRef] [PubMed]
135. Malik, S.; Villanova, L.; Tanaka, S.; Aonuma, M.; Roy, N.; Berber, E.; Pollack, J.R.; Michishita-Kioi, E.; Chua, K.F. SIRT7 inactivation reverses metastatic phenotypes in epithelial and mesenchymal tumors. *Sci. Rep.* **2015**, *5*, 9841. [CrossRef] [PubMed]
136. Sun, L.; Kokura, K.; Izumi, V.; Koomen, J.M.; Seto, E.; Chen, J.; Fang, J. MPP8 and SIRT1 crosstalk in E-cadherin gene silencing and epithelial-mesenchymal transition. *EMBO Rep.* **2015**, *16*, 689–699. [CrossRef] [PubMed]
137. Bertout, J.A.; Patel, S.A.; Simon, M.C. The impact of $O_2$ availability on human cancer. *Nat. Rev. Cancer* **2008**, *8*, 967–975. [CrossRef] [PubMed]
138. Schito, L.; Semenz, G.L. Hypoxia-inducible factors: Master regulators of cancer progression. *Trends Cancer* **2016**, *2*, 758–770. [CrossRef] [PubMed]
139. Lehmann, S.; Te Boekhorst, V.; Odenthal, J.; Bianchi, R.; van Helvert, S.; Ikenberg, K.; Ilina, O.; Stoma, S.; Xandry, J.; Jiang, L.; et al. Hypoxia induces a HIF-1-dependent transition from collective-to-amoeboid dissemination in epithelial cancer cells. *Curr. Biol.* **2017**, *27*, 392–400. [CrossRef] [PubMed]
140. Lewis, D.M.; Park, K.M.; Tang, V.; Xu, Y.; Pak, K.; Eisinger-Mathason, T.; Simon, M.C.; Gerecht, S. Intratumoral oxygen gradients mediate sarcoma cell invasion. *Proc. Natl. Acad. Sci. USA* **2016**, *113*, 9292–9297. [CrossRef] [PubMed]
141. Pennacchietti, S.; Michieli, P.; Galluzzo, M.; Mazzone, M.; Giordano, S.; Comoglio, P.M. Hypoxia promotes invasive growth by transcriptional activation of the met protooncogene. *Cancer Cell* **2003**, *3*, 347–361. [CrossRef]

142. Krtolica, A.; Ludlow, J.W. Hypoxia arrests ovarian carcinoma cell cycle progression, but invasion is unaffected. *Cancer Res.* **1996**, *56*, 1168–1173. [PubMed]
143. Maxwell, P.H.; Wiesener, M.S.; Chang, G.W.; Clifford, S.C.; Vaux, E.C.; Cockman, M.E.; Wykoff, C.C.; Pugh, C.W.; Maher, E.R.; Ratcliffe, P.J. The tumour suppressor protein VHL targets hypoxia-inducible factors for oxygen-dependent proteolysis. *Nature* **1999**, *399*, 271–275. [CrossRef] [PubMed]
144. Tarade, D.; Ohh, M. The HIF and other quandaries in VHL disease. *Oncogene* **2018**, *37*, 139–147. [CrossRef] [PubMed]
145. Markolovic, S.; Wilkins, S.E.; Schofield, C.J. Protein hydroxylation catalyzed by 2-oxoglutarate-dependent oxygenases. *J. Biol. Chem.* **2015**, *290*, 20712–20722. [CrossRef] [PubMed]
146. Yang, S.W.; Zhang, Z.G.; Hao, Y.X.; Zhao, Y.L.; Qian, F.; Shi, Y.; Li, P.A.; Liu, C.Y.; Yu, P.W. HIF-1alpha induces the epithelial-mesenchymal transition in gastric cancer stem cells through the Snail pathway. *Oncotarget* **2017**, *8*, 9535–9545. [PubMed]
147. Zhang, W.; Shi, X.; Peng, Y.; Wu, M.; Zhang, P.; Xie, R.; Wu, Y.; Yan, Q.; Liu, S.; Wang, J. HIF-1alpha promotes epithelial-mesenchymal transition and metastasis through direct regulation of ZEB1 in colorectal cancer. *PLoS ONE* **2015**, *10*, e0129603.
148. Krishnamachary, B.; Zagzag, D.; Nagasawa, H.; Rainey, K.; Okuyama, H.; Baek, J.H.; Semenza, G.L. Hypoxia-inducible factor-1-dependent repression of E-cadherin in von Hippel-Lindau tumor suppressor-null renal cell carcinoma mediated by TCF3, ZFHX1A, and ZFHX1B. *Cancer Res.* **2006**, *66*, 2725–2731. [CrossRef] [PubMed]
149. Kaidi, A.; Williams, B.V.; Paraskeva, C. Interaction between beta-catenin and HIF-1 promotes cellular adaptation to hypoxia. *Nat. Cell Biol.* **2007**, *9*, 210–217. [CrossRef]
150. Yang, M.H.; Wu, M.Z.; Chiou, S.H.; Chen, P.M.; Chang, S.Y.; Liu, C.J.; Teng, S.C.; Wu, K.J. Direct regulation of TWIST by HIF-1alpha promotes metastasis. *Nat. Cell Biol.* **2008**, *10*, 295–305. [CrossRef]
151. Erler, J.T.; Bennewith, K.L.; Cox, T.R.; Lang, G.; Bird, D.; Koong, A.; Le, Q.T.; Giaccia, A.J. Hypoxia-induced lysyl oxidase is a critical mediator of bone marrow cell recruitment to form the premetastatic niche. *Cancer Cell* **2009**, *15*, 35–44. [CrossRef] [PubMed]
152. Kim, J.W.; Tchernyshyov, I.; Semenza, G.L.; Dang, C.V. HIF-1-mediated expression of pyruvate dehydrogenase kinase: A metabolic switch required for cellular adaptation to hypoxia. *Cell Metab.* **2006**, *3*, 177–185. [CrossRef] [PubMed]
153. Zhang, H.; Gao, P.; Fukuda, R.; Kumar, G.; Krishnamachary, B.; Zeller, K.; Dang, C.V.; Semenza, G.L. HIF-1 inhibits mitochondrial biogenesis and cellular respiration in VHL-deficient renal cell carcinoma by repression of C-MYC activity. *Cancer Cell* **2007**, *11*, 407–420. [CrossRef] [PubMed]
154. Ullah, M.S.; Davies, A.J.; Halestrap, A.P. The plasma membrane lactate transporter MCT4, but not MCT1, is up-regulated by hypoxia through a HIF-1alpha-dependent mechanism. *J. Biol. Chem.* **2006**, *281*, 9030–9037. [CrossRef] [PubMed]
155. Estrella, V.; Chen, T.; Lloyd, M.; Wojtkowiak, J.; Cornnell, H.H.; Ibrahim-Hashim, A.; Bailey, K.; Balagurunathan, Y.; Rothberg, J.; Sloane, B.F.; et al. Acidity generated by the tumor microenvironment drives local invasion. *Cancer Res.* **2013**, *73*, 1524–1535. [CrossRef] [PubMed]
156. McBrian, M.A.; Behbahan, I.S.; Ferrari, R.; Su, T.; Huang, T.W.; Li, K.; Hong, C.S.; Christofk, H.R.; Vogelauer, M.; Seligson, D.B.; et al. Histone acetylation regulates intracellular pH. *Mol. Cell* **2013**, *49*, 310–321. [CrossRef] [PubMed]
157. Corbet, C.; Pinto, A.; Martherus, R.; Santiago de Jesus, J.P.; Polet, F.; Feron, O. Acidosis drives the reprogramming of fatty acid metabolism in cancer cells through changes in mitochondrial and histone acetylation. *Cell Metab.* **2016**, *24*, 311–323. [CrossRef]
158. Rohani, N.; Hao, L.; Alexis, M.S.; Joughin, B.A.; Krismer, K.; Moufarrej, M.N.; Soltis, A.R.; Lauffenburger, D.A.; Yaffe, M.B.; Burge, C.B.; et al. Acidification of tumor at stromal boundaries drives transcriptome alterations associated with aggressive phenotypes. *Cancer Res.* **2019**, *79*, 1952–1966. [CrossRef] [PubMed]
159. Brown, R.L.; Reinke, L.M.; Damerow, M.S.; Perez, D.; Chodosh, L.A.; Yang, J.; Cheng, C. CD44 splice isoform switching in human and mouse epithelium is essential for epithelial-mesenchymal transition and breast cancer progression. *J. Clin. Investig.* **2011**, *121*, 1064–1074. [CrossRef]
160. Warzecha, C.C.; Sato, T.K.; Nabet, B.; Hogenesch, J.B.; Carstens, R.P. ESRP1 and ESRP2 are epithelial cell-type-specific regulators of FGFR2 splicing. *Mol. Cell* **2009**, *33*, 591–601. [CrossRef]

161. Li, J.; Choi, P.S.; Chaffer, C.L.; Labella, K.; Hwang, J.H.; Giacomelli, A.O.; Kim, J.W.; Ilic, N.; Doench, J.G.; Ly, S.H.; et al. An alternative splicing switch in FLNB promotes the mesenchymal cell state in human breast cancer. *Elife* **2018**, *7*. [CrossRef] [PubMed]
162. Venables, J.P.; Brosseau, J.P.; Gadea, G.; Klinck, R.; Prinos, P.; Beaulieu, J.F.; Lapointe, E.; Durand, M.; Thibault, P.; Tremblay, K.; et al. RBFOX2 is an important regulator of mesenchymal tissue-specific splicing in both normal and cancer tissues. *Mol. Cell. Biol.* **2013**, *33*, 396–405. [CrossRef] [PubMed]
163. Yang, Y.; Park, J.W.; Bebee, T.W.; Warzecha, C.C.; Guo, Y.; Shang, X.; Xing, Y.; Carstens, R.P. Determination of a comprehensive alternative splicing regulatory network and combinatorial regulation by key factors during the epithelial-to-mesenchymal transition. *Mol. Cell. Biol.* **2016**, *36*, 1704–1719. [CrossRef] [PubMed]
164. Zhang, P.; Sun, Y.; Ma, L. ZEB1: At the crossroads of epithelial-mesenchymal transition, metastasis and therapy resistance. *Cell Cycle* **2015**, *14*, 481–487. [CrossRef] [PubMed]
165. Byers, L.A.; Diao, L.; Wang, J.; Saintigny, P.; Girard, L.; Peyton, M.; Shen, L.; Fan, Y.; Giri, U.; Tumula, P.K.; et al. An epithelial-mesenchymal transition gene signature predicts resistance to EGFR and PI3K inhibitors and identifies Axl as a therapeutic target for overcoming EGFR inhibitor resistance. *Clin. Cancer Res.* **2013**, *19*, 279–290. [CrossRef] [PubMed]
166. Emran, A.A.; Chatterjee, A.; Rodger, E.J.; Tiffen, J.C.; Gallagher, S.J.; Eccles, M.R.; Hersey, P. Targeting DNA methylation and EZH2 activity to overcome melanoma resistance to immunotherapy. *Trends Immunol.* **2019**, *40*, 328–344. [CrossRef] [PubMed]
167. Fan, W.; Tang, Z.; Yin, L.; Morrison, B.; Hafez-Khayyata, S.; Fu, P.; Huang, H.; Bagai, R.; Jiang, S.; Kresak, A.; et al. MET-independent lung cancer cells evading EGFR kinase inhibitors are therapeutically susceptible to BH3 mimetic agents. *Cancer Res.* **2011**, *71*, 4494–4505. [CrossRef] [PubMed]
168. Ippolito, L.; Marini, A.; Cavallini, L.; Morandi, A.; Pietrovito, L.; Pintus, G.; Giannoni, E.; Schrader, T.; Puhr, M.; Chiarugi, P.; et al. Metabolic shift toward oxidative phosphorylation in docetaxel resistant prostate cancer cells. *Oncotarget* **2016**, *7*, 61890–61904. [CrossRef]
169. Denise, C.; Paoli, P.; Calvani, M.; Taddei, M.L.; Giannoni, E.; Kopetz, S.; Kazmi, S.M.; Pia, M.M.; Pettazzoni, P.; Sacco, E.; et al. 5-fluorouracil resistant colon cancer cells are addicted to OXPHOS to survive and enhance stem-like traits. *Oncotarget* **2015**, *6*, 41706–41721. [CrossRef]
170. Aguilar, E.; Marin de Mas, I.; Zodda, E.; Marin, S.; Morrish, F.; Selivanov, V.; Meca-Cortés, Ó.; Delowar, H.; Pons, M.; Izquierdo, I.; et al. Metabolic reprogramming and dependencies associated with epithelial cancer stem cells independent of the epithelial-mesenchymal transition program. *Stem Cells* **2016**, *34*, 1163–1176. [CrossRef]
171. Taylor, S.; Spugnini, E.P.; Assaraf, Y.G.; Azzarito, T.; Rauch, C.; Fais, S. Microenvironment acidity as a major determinant of tumor chemoresistance: Proton pump inhibitors (PPIs) as a novel therapeutic approach. *Drug Resist. Update* **2015**, *23*, 69–78. [CrossRef] [PubMed]
172. Gerweck, L.E.; Seetharaman, K. Cellular pH gradient in tumor versus normal tissue: Potential exploitation for the treatment of cancer. *Cancer Res.* **1996**, *56*, 1194–1198. [PubMed]
173. Chang, C.H.; Qiu, J.; O'Sullivan, D.; Buck, M.D.; Noguchi, T.; Curtis, J.D.; Chen, Q.; Gindin, M.; Gubin, M.M.; van der Windt, G.J.; et al. Metabolic competition in the tumor microenvironment is a driver of cancer progression. *Cell* **2015**, *162*, 1229–1241. [CrossRef] [PubMed]
174. Angelin, A.; Gil-de-Gómez, L.; Dahiya, S.; Jiao, J.; Guo, L.; Levine, M.H.; Wang, Z.; Quinn, W.J., 3rd; Kopinski, P.K.; Wang, L.; et al. Foxp3 reprograms T cell metabolism to function in low-glucose, high-lactate environments. *Cell Metab.* **2017**, *25*, 1282–1293. [CrossRef] [PubMed]
175. Chen, L.; Gibbons, D.L.; Goswami, S.; Cortez, M.A.; Ahn, Y.H.; Byers, L.A.; Zhang, X.; Yi, X.; Dwyer, D.; Lin, W.; et al. Metastasis is regulated via microRNA-200/ZEB1 axis control of tumour cell PD-L1 expression and intratumoral immunosuppression. *Nat. Commun.* **2014**, *5*, 5241. [CrossRef] [PubMed]
176. Wang, Y.; Wang, H.; Zhao, Q.; Xia, Y.; Hu, X.; Guo, J. PD-L1 induces epithelial-to-mesenchymal transition via activating SREBP-1c in renal cell carcinoma. *Med. Oncol.* **2015**, *32*, 212. [CrossRef] [PubMed]
177. Elgendy, M.; Cirò, M.; Hosseini, A.; Weiszmann, J.; Mazzarella, L.; Ferrari, E.; Cazzoli, R.; Curigliano, G.; DeCensi, A.; Bonanni, B.; et al. Combination of hypoglycemia and metformin impairs tumor metabolic plasticity and growth by modulating the PP2A-GSK3β-MCL-1 axis. *Cancer Cell* **2019**, *35*, 1–18. [CrossRef]

178. Civenni, G.; Bosotti, R.; Timpanaro, A.; Vàzquez, R.; Merulla, J.; Pandit, S.; Rossi, S.; Albino, D.; Allegrini, S.; Mitra, A.; et al. Epigenetic control of mitochondrial fission enables self-renewal of stem-like tumor cells in human prostate cancer. *Cell Metab.* **2019**. [CrossRef]
179. Gao, X.; Sanderson, S.M.; Dai, S.; Reid, M.A.; Cooper, D.E.; Lu, M.; Richie, J.P., Jr.; Ciccarella, A.; Calcagnotto, A.; Mikhael, P.G.; et al. Dietary methionine restriction targets one carbon metabolism in humans and produces broad therapeutic responses in cancer. *bioRxiv* **2019**. [CrossRef]

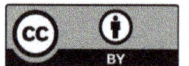

© 2019 by the authors. Licensee MDPI, Basel, Switzerland. This article is an open access article distributed under the terms and conditions of the Creative Commons Attribution (CC BY) license (http://creativecommons.org/licenses/by/4.0/).

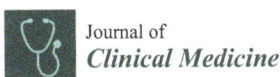

*Review*

# Uncoupling Traditional Functionalities of Metastasis: The Parting of Ways with Real-Time Assays

Sagar S. Varankar and Sharmila A. Bapat *

National Centre for Cell Science, Savitribai Phule Pune University, Ganeshkhind, Pune 411007, India
* Correspondence: sabapat@nccs.res.in; Tel.: +91-20-2570-8089

Received: 29 April 2019; Accepted: 4 June 2019; Published: 28 June 2019

**Abstract:** The experimental evaluation of metastasis overly focuses on the gain of migratory and invasive properties, while disregarding the contributions of cellular plasticity, extra-cellular matrix heterogeneity, niche interactions, and tissue architecture. Traditional cell-based assays often restrict the inclusion of these processes and warrant the implementation of approaches that provide an enhanced spatiotemporal resolution of the metastatic cascade. Time lapse imaging represents such an underutilized approach in cancer biology, especially in the context of disease progression. The inclusion of time lapse microscopy and microfluidic devices in routine assays has recently discerned several nuances of the metastatic cascade. Our review emphasizes that a complete comprehension of metastasis in view of evolving ideologies necessitates (i) the use of appropriate, context-specific assays and understanding their inherent limitations; (ii) cautious derivation of inferences to avoid erroneous/overestimated clinical extrapolations; (iii) corroboration between multiple assay outputs to gauge metastatic potential; and (iv) the development of protocols with improved in situ implications. We further believe that the adoption of improved quantitative approaches in these assays can generate predictive algorithms that may expedite therapeutic strategies targeting metastasis via the development of disease relevant model systems. Such approaches could potentiate the restructuring of the cancer metastasis paradigm through an emphasis on the development of next-generation real-time assays.

**Keywords:** metastasis; functional read-outs; metastatic modalities; live cell imaging; quantitative metrics

## 1. Introduction

Metastasis generates a systemic disease driven by the concerted alliance of tumor cell dissociation, physical translocation, and distant colonization. The dissociation of cells from the primary tumor initiates the metastatic cascade and generates distinct entities defined by severance dynamics of cell adhesion complexes. Further, acquisition of migratory/invasive properties by tumor cells facilitates their entry into circulation (or lymphatic system), wherein they evade host immune responses and endure extrinsic pressures followed by extravasation at secondary site(s). Tumor cell dormancy and secondary site remodeling then define the latency of colonization, which eventually establishes metastatic lesions [1–3]. An intricate interplay of molecular networks drives these programs and contributes to the efficacy of tumor progression [1–4]. Phenotypic switches induced by epithelial–mesenchymal transitions (EMT) are widely studied, and are deemed crucial for successful metastasis. Alternatively, recent studies highlight a collective mode of dissemination, wherein the retention of several epithelial properties is well documented [1–4]. These processes are further influenced by numerous physiological parameters, including the tissue stroma, architecture, and extra-cellular matrix (ECM) composition, in order to facilitate the successful establishment of a secondary disease [1–4]. Thus, collaboration amongst diverse functionalities outlines a complex blueprint of the process, wherein distinct modes of tumor cell dissemination can influence disease aggressiveness and therapeutic response.

Routine analyses in cancer metastasis studies inadvertently employ endpoint or "snapshot" assays that widely focus on the physical translocation of cancer cells. Functional read-outs tend to simplify various aspects of metastasis, and often neglect the role of tumor heterogeneity in disease progression. Furthermore, current notions extensively associate dissemination with a mesenchymal phenotype, and disregard the contributions of the alternate processes that are often unnoticed by existing experimental systems [3,5,6]. Detailed examination of the metastatic cascade thus necessitates the integration of the recent conceptual and technical advances for the development of informative assay protocols. In this article, we present a reassessment of the functional read-outs routinely employed in metastasis-associated studies, and accentuate the application of high-resolution imaging approaches to derive relevant patho-physiological conclusions.

## 2. Snapshot Assays for Metastasis Assessment

Reliance on snapshot assays in cancer research is accounted for by several advantages, including the ease of execution, reproducibility, and applicability in high throughput screens. In vitro functional read-outs provide a preliminary assessment of the metastatic capabilities, while the variables contributing to tumor heterogeneity viz., micro-environmental milieu, tissue specific metabolic gradients, and systemic architecture, are often assessed with in vivo models. While our review focusses on the widely employed functional assays corresponding to three distinct stages of metastasis, *viz.*, primary dissociation, physical translocation, and colonization, we briefly discuss the molecular approaches routinely used in cancer biology (Figure 1).

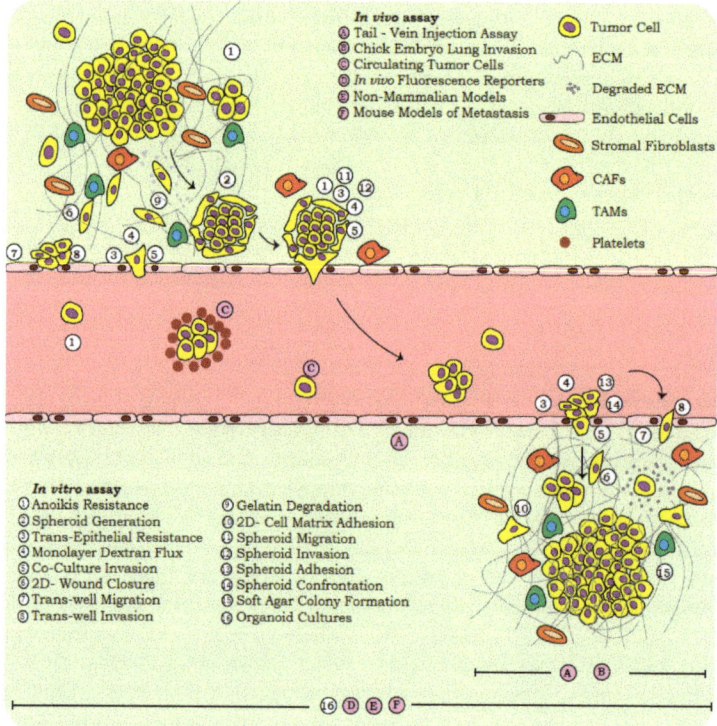

**Figure 1.** Functional assays for the metastatic cascade. Metastasis encompasses three distinct stages, *viz.* primary dissociation, physical translocation, and colonization. The interplay of complex processes severs cells from the primary tumor; these cells proliferate, migrate, and invade through the tissue matrix to initiate hematogenous or lymphatic dissemination.

Circulating tumor cells then overcome hydrostatic pressures and immune surveillance to extravasate and colonize distant tissues to seed micro-/macro-metastases. Diverse cellular functions activated during the metastatic cascade are evaluated experimentally by functional assays, and can be modified to accommodate multiple biological components (micro-environmental milieu, extra-cellular matrix–ECM, stromal cells, extrinsic physical pressures, immune cells, and so on). A list of the relevant assays employed across the metastatic cascade are listed and indicated in the schematic.

## 2.1. Molecular Assays

The functional assessment of metastasis is often correlated with the molecular signatures derived from tumor cells or cell line models. Primary profiling studies employ a wide range of markers identified across the metastatic cascade, which include cell junction and cytoskeletal components, transcription factors (TFs), secretory enzymes, and cell surface receptors [7]. Molecular profiles, averaged from a cell population, can often misrepresent disease heterogeneity, as affirmed by the reports on single cell characterization, besides over-emphasizing the role of EMT during metastasis [8–10]. Microscopy studies further associate the sub-cellular localization of several phenotype associated markers and TFs with distinct cellular functions [11,12]. Importantly, recent reports associating altered marker sub-cellular localization with pathological conditions necessitate the inclusion of this parameter in clinical assessments [13–15]. Furthermore, mechanistic studies on cell state maintenance employ fluorescence or enzyme (luciferase, β-galactosidase, and chloramphenicol acetyltransferase) assisted reporter systems for quantifying gene regulation [16,17]. Apart from the static molecular profiles, cytoskeletal, vesicular, and membrane dynamics, as captured by microscopy, offer deeper insight into the alterations of the cell shape and function [18–20].

Molecular assays, however, rely on markers that often exhibit extensive disparities across model systems, and are subject to cellular context-specific modulation [21–23]. E-cadherin expression and membrane localization, often gauged in clinical specimens by immuno-histochemical scoring, were exclusively associated with the lack of metastasis [24–26]; however, the detection of this adherens junction molecule in collectively metastasizing cells challenges its inverse correlation with dissemination [27,28]. Recently, E-cadherin negative cells have also been reported to exhibit collective migration by virtue of CD44 mediated cell-cell adhesion in invasive breast lobular carcinoma [29]. Such discrepancies arise from tissue-specific plasticity programs that are influenced by the local microenvironment. Similarly, the divergent contribution of regulatory TFs in metastasis has been reported; some examples include the stage specific roles of the EMT-mediating TFs Zeb1 and Zeb2 in pancreatic cancer and melanoma dissemination [30,31]; an EMT-TF circuitry switch in melanoma, wherein Slug–Zeb2 act as tumor suppressors in melanocytes, while Twist1–Zeb1 function towards neoplastic transformation [32]; the tissue-specific expression of the Prrx1 isoforms (Prrx1a and Prrx1b) that govern the distinct phenotypic states in pancreatic and breast cancer progression [33,34]; the co-operative role of Slug and Sox9 in the maintenance of breast epithelium homeostasis [35]; and so on. Thus, assigning relevance to metastases signatures requires an accompanying physiological comprehension of the cellular plasticity, and corroboration with tissue specific molecular profiles, mechanistic approaches, and imaging protocols.

## 2.2. Functional Assays

The examination of functionalities across the physiological and pathological states is robustly aided by cell-based assays. Routinely employed assays in cancer biology gauge the properties of anoikis resistance, stemness, migration, invasion, and colonization, so as to correlate with clinical observations (Table S1 and Figure 1).

2.2.1. In Vitro Assays

The loss of cell–cell and cell–matrix contacts initiates the anoikis cascade under physiological conditions, whereas resistance to this cell-death pathway in tumor cells permits effective disease progression [36]. The in vitro assessment of "anoikis" relies on the differential uptake of fluorescent dyes or the biochemical conversions of fluorophores by viable versus non-viable cells. Dissociated tumor cells exhibit a tendency to generate organized multi-cellular structures termed "spheroids", disorganized "cellular aggregates", or they exist as single cells [37]. Cell aggregates and spheroids exhibit stem-like and anoikis resistance properties, and are associated with disease aggressiveness [38,39].

The functional attributes of cell migration and invasion are also hijacked during tumor progression. Routine assessment of migratory capabilities by the "in vitro wound closure assays" is often enhanced by the fluorescent tagging of cells with reporter proteins or membrane labelling dyes [40,41]. The efficacy of tumor cell intra-/extra-vasation is recapitulated in vitro by trans-well inserts of pre-defined pore sizes. Such assays are employed widely to quantify "cell motility" in response to a chemotactic agent, while the layering of artificial matrix components (such as matrigel, carboxy methyl cellulose, and hydrogels) over these inserts gauge properties of "cell invasion" and "ECM remodeling" [38]. Recent trans-well systems employ micro-electrode coupled inserts that measure the impedance flux in response to cell migration/invasion, with enhanced precision [42]. Tumor cell invasion also entails the biochemical and mechanical modification of ECM components. "ECM degradation assays" measure the enzymatic activity of secreted matrix metalloproteinases (MMPs) by employing fluorescently labelled substrates and quantifying the signal intensity in the vicinity of invasive tumor cells [43]. Additional information pertaining to tumor cell invasion is gained from the "co-culture assays" that recapitulate the in-situ disruption of non-transformed tissue linings often encountered by metastasizing cancer cells [44]. The use of differentially labelled non-transformed and cancer cells improves the resolution of this assay, by enhancing the visualization and quantification of monolayer perturbance and invasion by tumor cells. Monolayer disruption by invading cancer cells is also quantified by the "trans-epithelial resistance (TER)" and "dextran flux assays" that gauge monolayer integrity and permeability, respectively [45,46]. Recent developments in advanced microfluidic and flow cytometry approaches have also facilitated the isolation of "circulating tumor cells (CTCs)", which are actual proof of an ongoing metastatic cascade [10,47]. Several recent reviews detail, at length, the role of CTCs in tumor biology and translational medicine, and associate them with stem-like properties, immune evasion signatures, and immense phenotypic plasticity [48–50]. CTCs also offer excellent diagnostic/prognostic value and specific targeting opportunities [51–53]. Hence, their detection, quantification, and analyses are being developed in view of clinical applications.

Cell-substrate adhesion, governed by tissue specific ECM components, represents a critical determinant of metastatic seeding [54–56]. The in vitro assessment of "adhesion" employs ECM pre-coated plates to identify the critical molecular players mediating cell–matrix interactions [57]. Separately, anchorage independent growth of tumor cells as gauged by the "soft agar assay" utilizes a three-dimensional (3D) matrix devoid of ECM components, and quantifies the tumor seeding capacity in vitro [58]. Apart from studies pertaining to single cell colonization, spheroids and cell aggregates are also functionally examined for their properties of adhesion, migration, and invasion, which can be extrapolated to the metastatic cascade [38]. Furthermore, the competitive interaction of these entities in suspension is assessed by "spheroid confrontation"; such an assay evaluates the differential invasive capabilities, as well as co-operation between these cell populations in view of metastases seeding [38].

Despite their obvious advantages, cell line models provide limited information on the in situ landscape of a disease, because of a lack of higher order organization conferred by the tissue architecture. "Organoid cultures" represent an in vitro 3D model system reminiscent of the in-situ organization, and provide improved clinical correlations [59]. The sustenance of genetic features from patient samples by organoids make them improved models for studying metastases as opposed to cell lines, which can often accumulate genetic aberrations over multiple passages [60]. Their amenability to in vitro functional assays further permits a high throughput assessment of pathological states. Studies with pancreatic and colorectal cancer organoids, established from clinical specimens, demonstrate the recapitulation of histological features reminiscent of the parental tissue, when injected into immunocompromised mice [61,62]. Interestingly, stage-specific organoids have also captured the evolving heterogeneity and molecular landscapes of tumors, and can improve the efficacy of therapeutic interventions in personalized medicine [63]. Similarly, organoids have been developed from CTCs that exhibit drug-resistance responses similar to the patients, and are amenable to high-throughput screening for the design of personalized therapeutic regimes [64]. Additional details on the advancements in organoid generation and utility in cancer biology are stated elsewhere [64–66].

2.2.2. In Vivo Systems

Despite the widespread applicability of in vitro systems, several aspects of metastasis that contribute to its complexity and heterogeneity are comprehended only when examined in vivo. Several non-mammalian systems have been extensively studied so as to comprehend the functionalities associated with the metastatic cascade. Examples include chemotactic migration observed in *Dictyostelium discoideum*, anchor cell invasion documented during vulva morphogenesis in *Caenorrhabditis elegans*, collective cell migration of ovarian border cells in *Drosophila melanogaster*, and the amoeboid migratory phenotype associated with primordial germ cells of *Danio rerio*. Extensive details on these non-mammalian models have been documented elsewhere [67]. Similarly, the developing chick embryo has been utilized for the assessment of its metastatic capabilities. The traditional chick "chorioallantoic membrane" assay quantifies tumor cell invasion across embryonic layers, and is assessed microscopically [68,69]. Recent "ex ovo embryo-xenograft models", however, serve as improved visual and quantitative systems for metastatic dissemination and intra-vital imaging [69]. Despite the evolutionary divergence, the conservation of distinct cellular functionalities in these animal models, along with their amenability to genetic screens and live cell imaging, permit the extrapolation of relevant observations to mammalian systems. However, the routine and widespread utility of mouse models in cancer biology as opposed to non-mammalian systems continues, because of emphasis on the clinically relevant settings that are more effectively mimicked by genetically engineered mice.

"Mouse models" recapitulate physiological variables contributing to disease progression, which are absent in vitro and allow for the derivation of clinically relevant outputs. We describe briefly a few mouse models and assays employed in tumor biology; interested readers may refer to other detailed articles [70–72]. The metastatic cascade is routinely captured by spontaneous models for metastasis that involves ectopic/orthotopic tumor cell transplantation in immunocompromised mice. Orthotopic models more effectively represent disease progression, as they expose tumor cells to the micro-environmental cues encountered in the tissue of origin. Alternatively, experimental models of metastasis include the inoculation of tumor cells into mice so as to assess the property of distant colonization. Intra-cardiac, intra-peritoneal, intra-splenic, the tail vein, and so on, are known routes of tumor cell injection, and have been documented to govern the tissue specificity of metastatic seeding [72]. Recent advances in bioluminescent imaging also permits the non-invasive detection of metastatic seeding by tagged tumor cells, thus ensuring real-time assessment [17,73]. These mouse models include cell-line generated allograft or xenograft systems that often lack the stromal/immune cell heterogeneity associated with the disease; the development of carcinogen-induced and genetically engineered mouse models has allowed cancer biologists to overcome this drawback. 7,12-Dimethylbenz[a]anthracene and azoxymethane-induced skin squamous cell and colorectal carcinoma mouse models, respectively, have been employed in deciphering the mechanisms of carcinogen mediated disease progression [74,75]. Cell lineage specific disease models, generated by Cre-lox approaches, have identified the molecular and cellular cascades contributing to metastasis and discerned disease associated patterns across stochastic cellular events [76,77]. For the improved recapitulation of breast cancer in mice, the mammary fat pad model system was developed so as to ensure the repopulation and manipulation of the mouse mammary gland with human-derived epithelia [78]. Similarly, patient-derived xenografts (PDXs) have been established, which can recapitulate metastatic and organ homing properties similar to the clinical specimen [79]. Fluorescent tagging of lineage-specific tumor cells and the establishment of confetti mouse models permits the tracing, isolation, and characterization of cell populations, thereby systematically dissecting the events involved in development and disease progression [80–83]. Reporter tags also facilitate CTC isolation and the detection of low frequency tumor cells at secondary sites during the colonization phase of metastasis [79]. Similarly, inducible reporter systems permit the fine tuning of specific molecular events, besides contributing to the spatiotemporal resolution of gene regulatory networks driving metastasis [75].

Functional assays and model systems thus simplify the comprehension of several mechanisms contributing to metastasis. However, the stromal and immune cell populations that facilitate metastasis are often under-represented in classical assays. These cellular interactions include platelet-coated CTCs, which exhibit enhanced survival and immune evasion; cancer associated fibroblasts (CAFs) or tumor associated macrophages (TAMs) in the primary and metastasizing tumor, which facilitate the generation of a supportive niche; and so on. [2,84,85]. Furthermore, the information provided by each assay exhibits cell-type and experimental-system associated context dependency [86]. Hence, an acknowledgement of the inherent shortcomings for each methodology is crucial, prior to the derivation of relevant conclusions, and may necessitate the development of improved protocols.

### 2.3. Scrutinizing Outcomes of Metastasis Assays

Most conventional in vitro assays associate metastasis with migratory and invasive capacities, while the processes of cell dissociation and colonization remain under-represented. Isolated read-outs can misrepresent the metastatic cascade and hinder effective translation of in vitro observations. Herein, we summarize the relevant biological limitations associated with in vitro read-outs (Table S2), and emphasize that a routine re-evaluation of assays is necessary for deriving appropriate clinical inferences.

The effective dissociation of cells from the primary tumor generates varied metastasizing entities (heterogeneous cell aggregates, single mesenchymal cells, and epithelial cell clusters) based on their modes of severance [37,87,88]. Differential molecular programs activated during cell dissociation from the primary tumor endow cells with functional signatures that can influence assay read-outs (Figure 2a). The acquisition of anoikis resistance by these entities is influenced by membrane dynamics, modified secretome, immune/stromal cell recruitment, and forces generated by primary tissue/interstitial fluids; parameters that are often neglected by in vitro assays [36,89,90]. Similar influences also distinguish cell aggregates from spheroids, and demand unambiguous identification approaches for these suspension entities [37]. The re-organization of tissue architecture during metastasis further employs processes that can degrade and/or realign specific ECM components in order to ensure optimal dissemination and colonization (Figure 2b.i) [91–93]. While ECM-based assays discern the molecular players of cell adhesion and degradation, there is limited comprehension of the influences from 3D-ECM rearrangement. For example, with minimal biochemical changes, collagens can undergo rearrangement with respect to fiber density and crosslinking, so as to alter cell–ECM interactions [94]. Similarly, degradation assays more commonly quantify the biochemical aspect of cell–ECM interaction, while the mechanical forces that can distort ECM arrangement are largely ignored (Figure 2b.ii) [43,95,96]. Existing assays also disregard the amoeboid mode of invasion, wherein cells exhibit a greater degree of deformability, which facilitates displacement across the ECM with minimal biochemical or mechanical alterations of the matrix [97,98].

In vitro migration and invasion assays present with similar shortcomings, wherein the heterogeneity and mechanics of these processes are excessively simplified and the modalities of translocation are overlooked. Wound closure assays widely imply cell migration, while disregarding the proliferative potential of the wound edge [99]. Similarly, experimental systems often employ scratch and gap closure assays interchangeably, with a complete disregard for the differential biological annotations represented by each method. While "gaps" (cell-free zones) are passively generated by artificial barriers positioned around proliferating cells, scratch assays involve the active disruption of cell monolayers. These differences can influence the activation of differential molecular networks and affect assay outputs [40,41]. Furthermore, trans-well assays restrict the movement of collectively invading cells, because of the pre-defined insert pore size that usually permits the passage of single cells. Similarly, co-culture systems often do not account for the paracrine effects of invading tumor cells on the epithelial/endothelial monolayers; these can activate the trans-differentiation and chemotaxis programs involved in the recruitment of CAFs, TAMs, and so on [84,85]. Most read-outs for migration and invasion also assume an onset of EMT, while the contributions of extra-tumoral cells recruited for their cooperative effects are often disregarded (Figure 2b.ii) [100]. Similarly, the plasticity of migratory/invasive modalities in response to differential ECM density, composition, and arrangement also requires critical scrutiny [101].

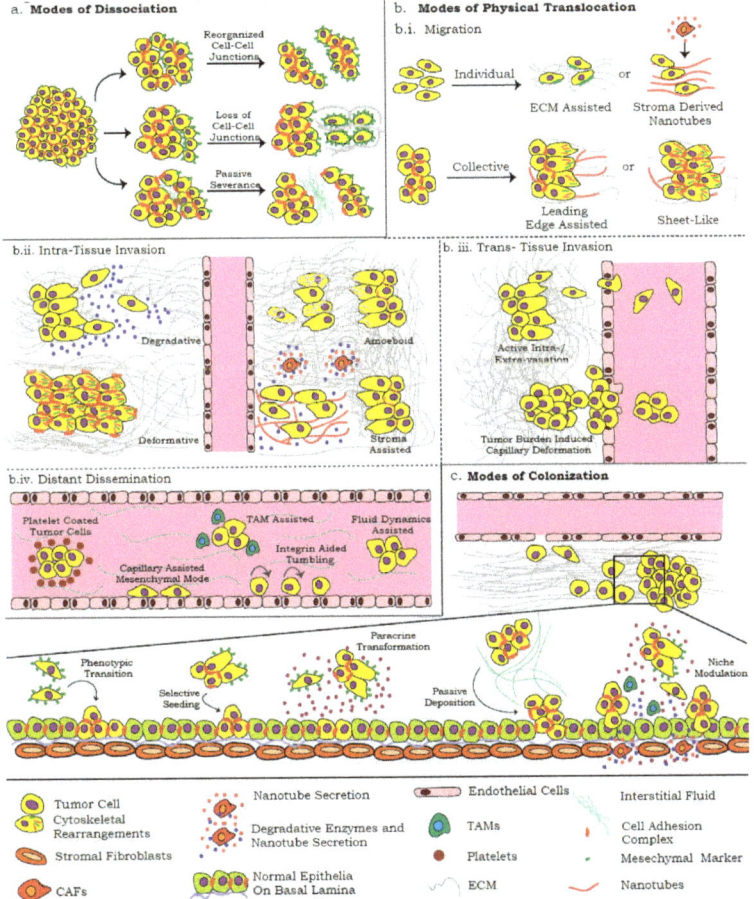

**Figure 2.** Modalities of metastasis. Metastasis is achieved by a step wise progression of tumor cell dissociation, physical translocation, and colonization. (**a.**) Cell dissociation entails a combination of cell–cell junctional complex rearrangements; phenotypic transitions, like EMT, that result in a loss of epithelial junctions; or the passive severance of cell clusters by virtue of forces exerted by the interstitial fluids. (**b.i.**)

Physical translocation involves a myriad of processes, amongst which cell migration is mediated by individual or collective clusters of cells. Individual cells migrate with the aid of ECM or stroma derived nanotubes, whereas collective migration is achieved by an active leading edge and/or by migration of cell sheets. (**b.ii.**) Migrating cells then undergo intra- and trans-tissue invasion by mediating distinct interactions with the ECM and non-transformed cell populations. Intra-tissue invasion involves the degradation and deformation of the ECM, either by the tumor or stromal cells. Alternatively, cells exhibit amoeboid invasion by altering their membrane fluidity so as to squeeze through the ECM with minimal disturbance to the surrounding architecture. (**b.iii.**) Trans-tissue invasion involves the disruption of endothelial linings by virtue of active intra-/extra-vasation or mechanical rupture because of an extensive tumor load. (**b.iv.**) Disseminating tumor cells in circulatory/lymphatic systems can exist either as platelet or tumor associated macrophage (TAMs) coated entities, mesenchymal cells along capillary linings, passively dispersed cell clusters, or exhibit an integrin mediated tumbling similar to cells of the immune system. (**c.**) The final stage of metastases establishment involves the colonization of tumor cells at distant sites mediated by phenotypic transitions, like mesenchymal to epithelial transition (MET), the selective seeding of epithelial cells from heterogeneous clusters, paracrine transformation of secondary site by the tumor cell secretome, passive deposition by interstitial fluids, and modulation of the secondary niche by activation of the tissue stromal compartment.

While several assays depict the properties associated with cell dissemination, the direct detection of metastatic seeding is not achieved in vitro. Metastasis-associated studies also disregard the stages of intra-/extra-vasation and the associated cellular plasticity that may govern efficacy of the metastatic cascade [102,103]. Importantly, routine in vivo models are usually limited by their inherent immunodeficiency that impacts the heterogeneity and efficiency of metastatic dissemination [104]. Similarly, the ectopic transplantation of tumor cells in mice and the infiltration of mouse stroma in these models make them less suitable for studying the role of tumor microenvironment on metastatic dissemination [104]. Thus, despite the existence of numerous elegant model systems, the complexity of metastasis necessitates regular improvements in assay resolution, and emphasizes the inclusion of recent ideologies when inferring from these outputs.

## 3. Uncoupling the Migration–Invasion–Metastasis Ideology

Tumors hijack several molecular programs associated with organogenesis; hence, concepts derived from developmental systems could elucidate the functional attributes observed during tumor progression and metastasis. Apart from tumor cells, the recruitment of tissue stroma/immune components vastly influences each stage of the metastatic cascade in a context dependent manner. The exclusion of several physiological parameters from experimental systems may stem from the limited familiarity and visualization of such processes, which can limit their collation with clinical observations. In this section, we aim to highlight the alternate physiological mechanisms adopted by tumors that uncouple the traditional migration–invasion–metastasis ideology, and warrant inclusion in routine assays (Figure 2).

The dissociation of cells from the primary tumor is widely attributed to active EMT as well as its molecular manifestations that affect cell adhesion and cytoskeletal complexes [105]; other studies highlight the realignment of adhesion complexes towards the generation of passively disseminating epithelial cell clusters [19]. Passive dissemination presents a challenge for experimental detection, although its contribution to metastasis is undeniable (Figure 2a) [106,107]. The degradative secretome that often accompanies EMT can further lead to the severance of single cells from the primary mass [96]. Tumors are also subject to hydrostatic pressures from organ-specific interstitial fluids that slough off weakly connected proliferative cell masses. Separately, the tumor edge can undergo cytoskeleton mediated delamination as epithelial sheets, a feature also noted during development [108].

Several existing studies associate metastatic efficacy with EMT facilitated migration and invasion [109–111]. However, recent reports highlight the differential migratory and invasive capabilities of tumor cells, significantly influenced by the microenvironment (Figure 2b.i). Passively dissociated cells can disperse and seed as proximal metastatic lesions in the absence of active migration/invasion programs [106,112]. Furthermore, efficient cell migration along chemo-/duro-tactic gradients relies on the sustained cellular contacts that underscore the existence of epithelial properties and fortify collective migration as a crucial process in disseminating tumor cells [112]. Recent studies also highlight the role of tumor/stroma cell derived membrane invaginations, termed "nanotubes" that can alter ECM arrangement and serve as directed migratory tracks for cancer cells [113].

The uncoupling of EMT from the metastatic cascade is also evident from reports highlighting the invasion of epithelial cell clusters by virtue of tensile forces exerted on the ECM (Figure 2b.ii) [114,115]. Invasion is also reported to be mediated by an amoeboid transition, which allows cells to squeeze through the ECM, without its biochemical or mechanical alteration [98]. Invasion modalities can be influenced by organ-specific architecture, which presents as an anatomical barrier for metastasis. For example, fenestrated bone marrow sinusoids offer a lower mechanical challenge for invasion, as opposed to the blood–brain barrier [116]. Distal metastasis is further ascertained by the density of lymphatic/blood vessels, and the ability of tumor cells to intra- and extra-vasate; invasive cell clusters capable of disrupting the basal lamina and entering circulation may stay lodged in the blood vessels and fail to extravasate (Figure 2b.iii) [117]. Tumor cells in capillaries or lymphatic vessels ensure survival in response to immune surveillance and hydrostatic pressures by existing as cell clusters or recruiting cells from the hematopoietic lineage [2]. Eventually, cells achieve distant dissemination under the influence of systemic circulatory flow, and can also exhibit migration along the capillary linings by virtue of mesenchymal motility or integrin mediated tumbling (Figure 2b.iv) [118,119].

Several of the above phenomena are reversed during the colonization stage of metastasis, wherein tumor cells re-establish cellular contacts and lodge into a supportive niche (Figure 2c). The reversal of certain mesenchymal properties is thus deemed crucial for colonization, as reports highlight the inability of rigid mesenchymal cells to metastasize, despite in vitro migratory and invasive capabilities [34,120]. Phenotypic plasticity plays a key role in enhancing the adaptability of cells to the altered niche, and may generate a heterogeneous disease at distinct sites in response to varying microenvironments [121,122]. The passive deposition and selective seeding of epithelial tumor cells from heterogeneous metastasizing clusters can dictate the efficacy of metastasis [106,107,112]. Sculpting of the secondary site is also undertaken by tumor cells, wherein paracrine signaling can result in a transformation of the secondary tissue or activate stromal cells, and generate a microenvironment conducive to metastases seeding [100]. Insights into the role of these extra-tumoral cellular components have been reviewed elsewhere [84,85]. Thus, a definitive comprehension of the metastatic cascade necessitates an approach wherein the aforementioned processes can be integrated into informative protocols.

## 4. Visualization of Metastatic Modalities with Real-Time Approaches

As discussed in previous sections, comprehending the biological heterogeneity of metastasis is often limited by the poor resolution of snapshot assays. Existing assays can provide an enhanced resolution of the cellular functionalities, when coupled with microfluidic approaches, real-time visualization, and intra-vital imaging. These methods can further reform traditional ideologies by including physiologically relevant variables and the development of quantitative parameters to delineate the metastatic cascade (Figure 3).

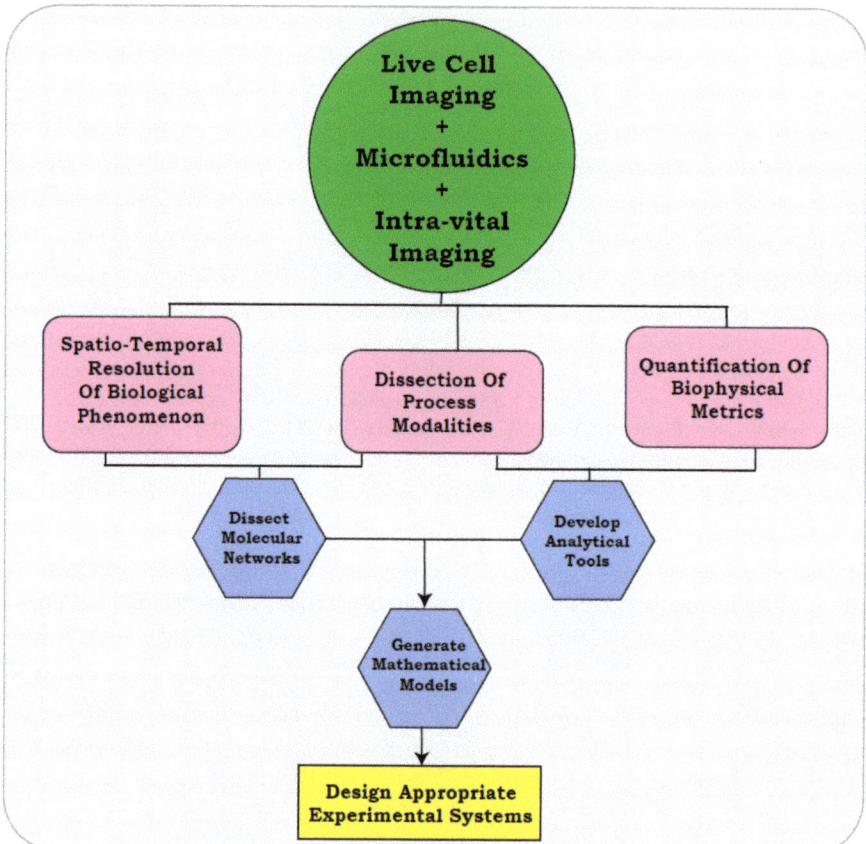

**Figure 3.** Era of real-time analysis. Routine implementation of real-time approaches in cancer biology can spatio-temporally resolve cellular processes and biological modalities by permitting the extraction of quantitative metrics associated with these states. Outputs from real-time studies can be collated to identify the regulatory networks governing the biological processes, and can be further applied to develop analytical tools/mathematical models for implementation in therapeutic/clinical screens. Such analyses support the design of relevant animal models, recapitulating the in situ patho-physiological parameters of the disease. Corroboration with microfluidic devices further enhances the outputs of these pipelines.

*4.1. Use of Microfluidics*

Microfluidic devices are recent advances in automation that have been applied in order to elucidate the distinct ECM components, widths of migratory paths, cell adhesion forces associated with collective migration, and the effect of extrinsic fluid pressures, amongst other metrics associated with metastasis [103,123–125]. In a recent study, an artificial circulatory system was generated on PDMS (polydimethylsiloxane) micro-capillaries lined with functional endothelial cells. This system was employed to model extra-/intra-vasation modalities under influences of extrinsic fluid pressure [102]. Label-free isolation and characterization of viable CTC clusters from blood samples has been achieved with Cluster-Chip, a microchip technology employing bifurcation traps. CTCs released from the microchip could be subjected to functional and molecular characterization in vitro, to comprehend their role in the metastatic cascade [126]. Similarly, an organ chip bioengineered to mimic the 3D microvascular networks has been effective in capturing and quantifying trans-endothelial migration, seeding, and micro-metastases formation [127]. Similar approaches have also used 3D bio-matrices to generate tissue models for studies pertaining to the interaction and infiltration of cancer cells [128–130]. Recently, the co-culture of breast cancer cells and CAFs on a microfluidic device successfully established a 3D-organotypic model to mimic stroma-driven tumor cell invasion. Live cell imaging coupled with transcriptome analysis of the co-cultured cells further discerned the novel molecular targets associated with invasion [131]. The recapitulation of spatio-temporal metabolic adaptations encountered by tumor cells was also achieved with a microfluidic organotypic breast cancer model, and employed to devise therapeutic strategies for targeting hypoxic cells [132].

*4.2. In Vitro Resolution of Metastatic Modalities with Live Cell Imaging*

Independent of microfluidic devices, live cell imaging has enabled the quantification of various functional properties by visually monitoring routine in vitro protocols. The spontaneous detachment of cells from 3D culture models of ovarian cancer was recently visualized with live cell imaging. These observations allowed for the development of in vivo lineage tracing methods, and discerned a collective dissociation of cells from the primary tumor, indicating the onset of metastasis [37]. A recent study from our group, coupling live cell imaging with the in vitro scratch assay, not only discerned the distinct migratory modalities in ovarian carcinoma (CCM versus EMT), but also resolved subtle variations within CCM; this defined CCM as being mediated either through proliferation (passive CCM) or sheet-like migration (active CCM). We quantified the altered migratory modalities in response to extrinsic and intrinsic stimuli, further establishing an improved prototype of the scratch assay [99]. In a separate study, CCM was assessed in the context of durotaxis, wherein live cell imaging successfully quantified the extent and pattern of migration in response to ECM variations [133]. Similar approaches were applied to invasion assays, so as to determine the morphological variations of patient derived spheroids invading into a carboxy–methyl cellulose matrix [134]. Separately, live cell imaging of the migrating cells in a confined micro-pillar array permitted the derivation of distinct quantitative parameters for distinguishing the individual and collective modes of migration [135].

Real-time studies can thus offer an improved comprehension of the bio-mechanical features associated with metastasis that are often overlooked by snapshot assays (Table S3). The corroboration of time-lapse microscopy with trans-well invasion assays could distinguish the degradative, deformative, and amoeboid modes of cell invasion [98,136]. Similar approaches with co-culture systems can delineate the proliferation driven disruption of endothelial linings from active events of intra-/extra-vasation, and in suspension cultures, distinguish the mechanical forces associated with spheroids versus cellular aggregates [38,115,137]. The assay resolution can be further enhanced by employing fluorescent dyes or protein tags that differentially label cell membranes, ECM fibers, cytoskeletal components, and so on. Importantly, the labelling methods adopted for real-time imaging studies must be permissive of the assay systems, and contribute minimal hindrance to the biological process under study [138,139]. Such real-time analysis can also be implemented in high-throughput screens, along with traditional assay outputs, so as to address the effects of growth additives and pharmacological compounds on diverse biological modalities.

*4.3. Intra-Vital Imaging Assisted Visualization of Cellular Properties*

As discussed previously, the limited in vitro recapitulation of the heterogeneity associated with metastasis has compelled cancer biologists to use animal models suitable for varied experimental approaches. The in vivo dynamics of migration and invasion have been previously noted in *C. elegans*, fruit fly, and zebrafish [67]. Recent advances in microscopy and fluorophore chemistry have also permitted the intra-vital single-cell resolution in vertebrate animal models. In a mouse model, intra-vital imaging assisted approaches elucidated the role of Rac1-dependent membrane protrusions in the maintenance of 3D spatial positions of mouse dermal fibroblasts during wound healing [140]. In yet another report, the transplantation of tumor cells into the mouse cerebellopontine angle region coupled with intra-vital imaging successfully developed a model to study the disease progression of vestibular schwannoma [141]. Separately, the intra-vital imaging of early breast carcinoma lesions identified a Her2 driven dissemination program that enables the dispersal of dormant cancer cells to distant organs, prior to the development of a primary tumor [142]. Intra-vital imaging also successfully discerned the significance of orthotopic, as opposed to subcutaneous, tumor models in prostate cancer wherein drastic differences in the overall vascularization and distant metastasis were duly noted [143]. Intra-vital imaging has been aided by confetti mouse models, which express a combination of fluorescent proteins in response to the Cre-recombinase, and permit the visualization of the in vivo heterogeneity inherent to tissue systems [144,145]. Confetti mice have been instrumental in comprehending squamous cell carcinoma progression, wherein the recruitment of the adjacent epithelium by monoclonal papillomas and intra-tumoural invasion by newly generated clones were effectively visualized [146]. Cell of origin studies in castration resistance prostate cancer, employing confetti mice, have previously assigned tumor formation to a population of $Bmi1^{+ve}$ luminal cells in the proximal prostate [83]. The in vivo fate and properties of transplanted corneal epithelium were also resolved with intra-vital imaging, which tracked the fluorescence signals from the confetti tagged donor cells [147].

Other advances in imaging technologies include improved tomography scans, fluorescence lifetime imaging microscopy (FLIM), coherent anti-Stokes Raman microscopy (CARS), and so on, and have been reviewed elsewhere in detail [148,149]. The routine application of such high-resolution approaches may be beneficial towards the development of more informative protocols, the quantification of key biomechanical features, and could overcome several limitations harbored by snapshot studies.

## 5. Quantitative Resolution of Biological Modalities

Examples of real-time assays discussed in previous sections not only emphasize their visual impact, but also highlight the derivation of varied quantitative metrics. The integration of live cell imaging into routine approaches can quantify diverse physiological parameters and enhance assay read-outs. We briefly familiarize readers with recent approaches developed for high-resolution real-time imaging, user-friendly analytical tools, and quantitative variables generated from imaging datasets (Table S3).

Continued technological advances and automation in the field of optics have provided high-resolution microscopes that facilitate the real-time visualization of dynamic biological processes, including the migration of metastatic cancer cells in vivo [150]. Similarly, atomic force microscopy (AFM) and protrusion force microscopy (PFM) have been employed to discern the mechanical forces involved in leukocyte–endothelial adhesion and invadosome–assisted extravasation, respectively [151]. CARS coupled with two-photon imaging has also emerged as a promising approach to describe multiple aspects of the tumor niche and disease progression, with minimal photo-damage to the specimen [73]. Interested readers may refer to several recent articles elaborating on the advances in microscope design, with significant implications in real-time cancer research [148,149].

Datasets generated by real-time imaging present a significant challenge for analysis, thus necessitating familiarity with relevant software and tools. While the adaptability of imaging tools across model systems is beneficial, optimal quantification can only be ensured when high-resolution/-contrast images are provided as inputs. The availability of user-friendly interfaces, improvements with recent plugins, and the development of codes for the customization of outputs enhance the applicability of imaging tools. Currently, a variety of programs facilitate time-lapse image analysis, and are available either commercially, viz., Metamorph (Olympus), Imaris (Bitplane), Zen (Zeiss), Elements (Nikon), Volocity (PerkinElmer), and so on, or as open source platforms, viz., Micro-manager, ImageJ, MotilityLab, and so on. Imaris is specifically useful for 4D data analysis, and can be substituted with the ImageJ post-installation of plugins that facilitate drift correction, volume measurement, free rotation, and so on [152]. COMBImage, a recent computational framework, has facilitated the automated analyses of cell morphology and confluence in cell viability assays [153]. The management and analysis of multi-dimensional imaging data have also been aided by support vector machines (SVM), which have been applied to group pixels for image segmentation, to detect cellular/sub-cellular phenotypes, or to categorize developmental stages at the level of entire organisms [154]. Similarly, mathematical approaches for migration track analysis have been developed [155]. A more comprehensive list of the currently available image processing software and tools is available elsewhere [156,157].

Analytical tools can yield extensive information from imaging datasets, and often confound untrained individuals. The extraction of relevant quantitative metrics must consider the biophysical properties of a system and examine the associative trends with the cellular processes under study. Examples highlighting the selection of quantitative metrics are summarized in Table S3, and include the micro-pillar array-based study, wherein six quantitative parameters extracted from individual cells generated a binary solidification model for describing the interconversion between collective versus individual modes of migration [135], fractal analysis that described the developing dermis as a lattice structure resulting from the dynamic stroma [158], derivation of migration modalities in ovarian cancer cell lines assisted by coupling live cell imaging with the in vitro scratch assay [99], and so on. Additional studies highlight the vast array of quantitative measures derived from real-time imaging datasets, and signify their contributions to an improved understanding of the biological processes [11,151,159–162].

## 6. The Era of Live Cell Imaging

The simple corroboration of time-lapse microscopy with endpoint assays can reveal the modalities of several biological processes, indicate differential routes of metastasis taken by tumors, and identify the associated molecular pathways (Figure 3). Collation of these datasets can generate multi-parametric simulations that define the biological thresholds associated with diverse cellular functions, and their modulation in response to various cues [163–165]. Such models or simulations could aid in the design of appropriate experimental systems that encompass heterogeneous processes contributing to metastasis. Similarly, analytical tools developed with real-time approaches can be integrated into drug development pipelines [166]. In accordance with our statements, a recent study employing intra-vital imaging discerned the crucial role of CD44 driven cell aggregation of CTCs in metastatic dissemination. The study established CD44–PAK2 interaction as a driving event of the process, thus providing clinically relevant information with the aid of visual outputs [167]. While snap-shot assays will continue to provide high-throughput readouts for cell systems, it is crucial that experimentalists acknowledge their limitations when deriving clinically relevant inferences. With the right amount of caution, real-time approaches could herald an "era of live cell imaging" in cancer biology.

Real-time approaches, in conjunction with lineage tracing, may initiate the next phase of resolving cancer heterogeneity, which continues to elude comprehension and is responsible for therapy resistance. In view of recent reports, real-time approaches may decipher functional nuances and provide insight into the concept of "metastability" predicted during phenotypic switches. Real-time dynamics of molecular turn-over can further identify the spatiotemporal alterations of markers over the course of disease progression, and improve clinical interventions. Moreover, intra-vital imaging approaches present an exciting opportunity to tackle a residual minimal disease, which often results in an aggressive relapse and overall poor prognosis. Similarly, extra-tumoral cell populations crucial for disease progression in vivo can be identified and probed in vitro with micro-fluidic and real-time studies. More importantly, the stages of primary dissociation and colonization during metastasis represent a "grey area" of information, which could be effectively resolved with the previously discussed approaches. The delineation of these diverse biophysical features essentially nurtures the model of personalized medicine. A careful combination of appropriate existing assays with live cell imaging can reveal several nuances of the metastatic cascade and reiterate the "seeing is believing" ideology.

## 7. Conclusions

Recent studies reveal a functional uncoupling of several physiological processes previously deemed crucial for successful metastasis. Our own observations associated with the evaluation of in vitro metastasis reflect on the shortcomings of routine assays. For the detection of distinct modalities associated across the metastatic cascade, we suggest the adoption of time lapse imaging in routine assays. This approach has the capability to (i) make a visual impact on biological processes, (ii) identify different routes undertaken by tumor cells towards achieving these functions, and (iii) provide metrics for quantifying these processes. The information obtained from these approaches can be applied towards establishing mathematical models and intuitive inferences that tackle the heterogeneity associated with disease progression. Inherent cellular plasticity that contributes to tissue homeostasis can also be deciphered in the context of pathological conditions, by developing novel assays that combine the ease of traditional approaches with the enhanced resolution of real-time imaging. We also emphasize on the routine re-evaluation of functional read-outs, so as to incorporate recent conceptual developments that improve the comprehension of biological systems. Together, these features are likely to be useful in elucidating the poorly understood areas of disease progression in cancer, and deriving clinically relevant conclusions over the current assays.

**Supplementary Materials:** The following are available online at http://www.mdpi.com/2077-0383/8/7/941/s1: Table S1. Metastasis associated functional read-outs. Details pertaining to the setup, quantification, and biological read-out associated with the in vitro and in vivo methods employed to study the metastatic cascade are enlisted. Table S2. Applications and limitations of metastasis associated functional read-outs. Details pertaining to the cellular functionality gauged, stage of metastasis represented, and inherent limitations of the in vitro and in vivo methods employed to study the metastatic cascade are enlisted. Table S3. The real-time approach. Details pertaining to the model systems, relevant instrumentation, quantitative tools and variables, and their biological relevance for recent real-time studies are enlisted. The table includes a summary of a limited number of studies, interested readers may refer to the available literature cited in the text for more information.

**Author Contributions:** Conceptualization, S.A.B. and S.S.V.; investigation, S.S.V.; writing (original draft preparation), S.A.B. and S.S.V.; funding acquisition, S.A.B.

**Funding:** This work was supported by funding to SAB from NCCS, Pune (Intramural), and the Department of Biotechnology, Government of India, New Delhi (Extramural grant, BT/Indo-Aus/06/03/2011). The research fellowship was availed by SSV from Council of Scientific and Industrial Research, New Delhi, India.

**Conflicts of Interest:** The authors declare no conflict of interest.

## References

1. Chaffer, C.L.; San Juan, B.P.; Lim, E.; Weinberg, R.A. EMT, cell plasticity and metastasis. *Cancer Metastasis Rev.* **2016**, *35*, 645–654. [CrossRef] [PubMed]
2. Nieto, M.A.; Huang, R.Y.Y.J.; Jackson, R.A.A.; Thiery, J.P.P. Emt: 2016. *Cell* **2016**, *166*, 21–45. [CrossRef] [PubMed]
3. Brabletz, T. To differentiate or not-routes towards metastasis. *Nat. Rev. Cancer* **2012**, *12*, 425–436. [CrossRef] [PubMed]
4. Campbell, K.; Casanova, J. A common framework for EMT and collective cell migration. *Development* **2016**, *143*, 4291–4300. [CrossRef] [PubMed]
5. Pastushenko, I.; Brisebarre, A.; Sifrim, A.; Fioramonti, M.; Revenco, T.; Boumahdi, S.; Van Keymeulen, A.; Brown, D.; Moers, V.; Lemaire, S.; et al. Identification of the tumour transition states occurring during EMT. *Nature* **2018**, *556*, 463–468. [CrossRef] [PubMed]
6. Jolly, M.K.; Mani, S.A.; Levine, H. Hybrid epithelial/mesenchymal phenotype(s): The 'fittest' for metastasis? *Biochim. Biophys. Acta Rev. Cancer* **2018**, *1870*, 151–157. [CrossRef] [PubMed]
7. Tsai, J.H.; Yang, J. Epithelial—Mesenchymal plasticity in carcinoma metastasis. *Genes Dev.* **2013**, *27*, 2192–2206. [CrossRef]
8. Chung, W.; Eum, H.H.; Lee, H.O.; Lee, K.M.; Lee, H.B.; Kim, K.T.; Ryu, H.S.; Kim, S.; Lee, J.E.; Park, Y.H.; et al. Single-cell RNA-seq enables comprehensive tumour and immune cell profiling in primary breast cancer. *Nat. Commun.* **2017**, *8*, 15081. [CrossRef]
9. MacLean, A.L.; Hong, T.; Nie, Q. Exploring intermediate cell states through the lens of single cells. *Curr. Opin. Syst. Biol.* **2018**, *9*, 32–41. [CrossRef]
10. Bednarz-Knoll, N.; Alix-Panabières, C.; Pantel, K. Plasticity of disseminating cancer cells in patients with epithelial malignancies. *Cancer Metastasis Rev.* **2012**, *31*, 673–687. [CrossRef]

11. Labernadie, A.; Kato, T.; Brugués, A.; Serra-Picamal, X.; Derzsi, S.; Arwert, E.; Weston, A.; González-Tarragó, V.; Elosegui-Artola, A.; Albertazzi, L.; et al. A mechanically active heterotypic E-cadherin/N-cadherin adhesion enables fibroblasts to drive cancer cell invasion. *Nat. Cell Biol.* **2017**, *19*, 224–237. [CrossRef] [PubMed]
12. Aman, A.; Piotrowski, T. Wnt/β-Catenin and Fgf Signaling Control Collective Cell Migration by Restricting Chemokine Receptor Expression. *Dev. Cell* **2008**, *15*, 749–761. [CrossRef] [PubMed]
13. Barham, W.; Chen, L.; Tikhomirov, O.; Onishko, H.; Gleaves, L.; Stricker, T.P.; Blackwell, T.S.; Yull, F.E. Aberrant activation of NF-κB signaling in mammary epithelium leads to abnormal growth and ductal carcinoma in situ. *BMC Cancer* **2015**, *15*, 647. [CrossRef] [PubMed]
14. Köthe, S.; Müller, J.P.; Böhmer, S.-A.; Tschongov, T.; Fricke, M.; Koch, S.; Thiede, C.; Requardt, R.P.; Rubio, I.; Böhmer, F.D. Features of Ras activation by a mislocalized oncogenic tyrosine kinase: FLT3 ITD signals through K-Ras at the plasma membrane of acute myeloid leukemia cells. *J. Cell Sci.* **2013**, *126*, 4746–4755. [CrossRef] [PubMed]
15. Celestini, V.; Tezil, T.; Russo, L.; Fasano, C.; Sanese, P.; Forte, G.; Peserico, A.; Lepore Signorile, M.; Longo, G.; De Rasmo, D.; et al. Uncoupling FoxO3A mitochondrial and nuclear functions in cancer cells undergoing metabolic stress and chemotherapy. *Cell Death Dis.* **2018**, *9*, 231. [CrossRef] [PubMed]
16. Hill, S.J.; Baker, J.G.; Rees, S. Reporter-gene systems for the study of G-protein-coupled receptors. *Curr. Opin. Pharmacol.* **2001**, *1*, 526–532. [CrossRef]
17. Fan, F.; Wood, K.V. Bioluminescent Assays for High-Throughput Screening. *Assay Drug Dev. Technol.* **2007**, *5*, 127–136. [CrossRef]
18. Hirata, E.; Park, D.; Sahai, E. Retrograde flow of cadherins in collective cell migration. *Nat. Cell Biol.* **2014**, *16*, 621–623. [CrossRef]
19. Peglion, F.; Llense, F.; Etienne-Manneville, S. Adherens junction treadmilling during collective migration. *Nat. Cell Biol.* **2014**, *16*, 639–651. [CrossRef]
20. Zhang, L.; Luo, J.; Wan, P.; Wu, J.; Laski, F.; Chen, J. Regulation of cofilin phosphorylation and asymmetry in collective cell migration during morphogenesis. *Development* **2011**, *138*, 455–464. [CrossRef]
21. Henkel, L.; Rauscher, B.; Boutros, M. Context-dependent genetic interactions in cancer. *Curr. Opin. Genet. Dev.* **2019**, *54*, 73–82. [CrossRef] [PubMed]
22. Kosztyu, P.; Slaninová, I.; Valčíková, B.; Verlande, A.; Müller, P.; Paleček, J.J.; Uldrijan, S. A Single Conserved Amino Acid Residue as a Critical Context-Specific Determinant of the Differential Ability of Mdm2 and MdmX RING Domains to Dimerize. *Front. Physiol.* **2019**, *10*, 390. [CrossRef] [PubMed]
23. Richelle, A.; Chiang, A.W.T.; Kuo, C.C.; Lewis, N.E. Increasing consensus of context-specific metabolic models by integrating data-inferred cell functions. *PLoS Comput. Biol.* **2019**, *15*, e1006867. [CrossRef] [PubMed]
24. Lin, D.; Wang, X.; Li, X.; Meng, L.; Xu, F.; Xu, Y.; Xie, X.; He, H.; Xu, D.; Wang, C.; et al. Apogossypolone acts as a metastasis inhibitor via up-regulation of E-cadherin dependent on the GSK-3/AKT complex. *Am. J. Transl. Res.* **2019**, *11*, 218–232. [PubMed]
25. Menezes, S.V.; Fouani, L.; Huang, M.L.; Geleta, B.; Maleki, S.; Richardson, A.; Richardson, D.R.; Kovacevic, Z. The metastasis suppressor, NDRG1, attenuates oncogenic TGF-β and NF-κB signaling to enhance membrane E-cadherin expression in pancreatic cancer cells. *Carcinogenesis* **2018**. [CrossRef]
26. Bendardaf, R.; Sharif-Askari, F.S.; Sharif-Askari, N.S.; Syrjänen, K.; Pyrhönen, S. Cytoplasmic E-Cadherin Expression Is Associated With Higher Tumour Level of VEGFA, Lower Response Rate to Irinotecan-based Treatment and Poorer Prognosis in Patients With Metastatic Colorectal Cancer. *Anticancer Res.* **2019**, *39*, 1953–1957. [CrossRef] [PubMed]
27. Aiello, N.M.; Maddipati, R.; Norgard, R.J.; Balli, D.; Li, J.; Yuan, S.; Yamazoe, T.; Black, T.; Sahmoud, A.; Furth, E.E.; et al. EMT Subtype Influences Epithelial Plasticity and Mode of Cell Migration. *Dev. Cell* **2018**, *45*, 681–695.e4. [CrossRef]
28. Reichert, M.; Bakir, B.; Moreira, L.; Pitarresi, J.R.; Feldmann, K.; Simon, L.; Suzuki, K.; Maddipati, R.; Rhim, A.D.; Schlitter, A.M.; et al. Regulation of Epithelial Plasticity Determines Metastatic Organotropism in Pancreatic Cancer. *Dev. Cell* **2018**, *45*, 696–711. [CrossRef]
29. Khalil, A.A.; Ilina, O.; Gritsenko, P.G.; Bult, P.; Span, P.N.; Friedl, P. Collective invasion in ductal and lobular breast cancer associates with distant metastasis. *Clin. Exp. Metastasis* **2017**, *34*, 421–429. [CrossRef]
30. Denecker, G.; Vandamme, N.; Akay, Ö.; Koludrovic, D.; Taminau, J.; Lemeire, K.; Gheldof, A.; De Craene, B.; Van Gele, M.; Brochez, L.; et al. Identification of a ZEB2-MITF-ZEB1 transcriptional network that controls melanogenesis and melanoma progression. *Cell Death Differ.* **2014**, *21*, 1250–1261. [CrossRef]

31. Krebs, A.M.; Mitschke, J.; Losada, M.L.; Schmalhofer, O.; Boerries, M.; Busch, H.; Boettcher, M.; Mougiakakos, Di.; Reichardt, W.; Bronsert, P.; et al. The EMT-activator Zeb1 is a key factor for cell plasticity and promotes metastasis in pancreatic cancer. *Nat. Cell Biol.* **2017**, *19*, 518–529. [CrossRef] [PubMed]
32. Caramel, J.; Papadogeorgakis, E.; Hill, L.; Browne, G.J.; Richard, G.; Wierinckx, A.; Saldanha, G.; Osborne, J.; Hutchinson, P.; Tse, G.; et al. A Switch in the Expression of Embryonic EMT-Inducers Drives the Development of Malignant Melanoma. *Cancer Cell* **2013**, *24*, 466–480. [CrossRef] [PubMed]
33. Takano, S.; Reichert, M.; Bakir, B.; Das, K.K.; Nishida, T.; Miyazaki, M.; Heeg, S.; Collins, M.A.; Marchand, B.; Hicks, P.D.; et al. Prrx1 isoform switching regulates pancreatic cancer invasion and metastatic colonization. *Genes Dev.* **2016**, *30*, 233–247. [CrossRef] [PubMed]
34. Ocaña, O.H.; Córcoles, R.; Fabra, Á.; Moreno-Bueno, G.; Acloque, H.; Vega, S.; Barrallo-Gimeno, A.; Cano, A.; Nieto, M.A. Metastatic Colonization Requires the Repression of the Epithelial-Mesenchymal Transition Inducer Prrx1. *Cancer Cell* **2012**, *22*, 709–724. [CrossRef]
35. Guo, W.; Keckesova, Z.; Donaher, J.L.; Shibue, T.; Tischler, V.; Reinhardt, F.; Itzkovitz, S.; Noske, A.; Zürrer-Härdi, U.; Bell, G.; et al. Slug and Sox9 cooperatively determine the mammary stem cell state. *Cell* **2012**, *148*, 1015–1028. [CrossRef] [PubMed]
36. Taddei, M.L.; Giannoni, E.; Fiaschi, T.; Chiarugi, P. Anoikis: An emerging hallmark in health and diseases. *J. Pathol.* **2012**, *226*, 380–393. [CrossRef] [PubMed]
37. Al Habyan, S.; Kalos, C.; Szymborski, J.; McCaffrey, L. Multicellular detachment generates metastatic spheroids during intra-abdominal dissemination in epithelial ovarian cancer. *Oncogene* **2018**, *37*, 5127–5135. [CrossRef] [PubMed]
38. Kramer, N.; Walzl, A.; Unger, C.; Rosner, M.; Krupitza, G.; Hengstschläger, M.; Dolznig, H. In vitro cell migration and invasion assays. *Mutat. Res. Rev. Mutat. Res.* **2013**, *752*, 10–24. [CrossRef]
39. Choi, M.; Yu, S.J.; Choi, Y.; Lee, H.R.; Lee, E.; Lee, E.; Lee, Y.; Song, J.; Son, J.G.; Lee, T.G.; et al. Polymer Thin Film-Induced Tumor Spheroids Acquire Cancer Stem Cell-like Properties. *Cancer Res.* **2018**, *78*, 6890–6902. [CrossRef]
40. Liang, C.C.; Park, A.Y.; Guan, J.L. In vitro scratch assay: A convenient and inexpensive method for analysis of cell migration in vitro. *Nat. Protoc.* **2007**, *2*, 329–333. [CrossRef]
41. Das, A.M.; Eggermont, A.M.M.; Ten Hagen, T.L.M. A ring barrier-based migration assay to assess cell migration in vitro. *Nat. Protoc.* **2015**, *10*, 904–915. [CrossRef] [PubMed]
42. Dowling, C.M.; Herranz Ors, C.; Kiely, P.A. Using real-time impedance-based assays to monitor the effects of fibroblast-derived media on the adhesion, proliferation, migration and invasion of colon cancer cells. *Biosci. Rep.* **2014**, *34*, 415–427. [CrossRef] [PubMed]
43. Anderl, J.; Ma, J.; Armstrong, L. Fluorescent Gelatin Degradation Assays for Investigating Invadopodia Formation. *Nat Methods* **2012**, *121007*, 1–6.
44. Dong, Y.; Stephens, C.; Walpole, C.; Swedberg, J.E.; Boyle, G.M.; Parsons, P.G.; McGuckin, M.A.; Harris, J.M.; Clements, J.A. Paclitaxel Resistance and Multicellular Spheroid Formation Are Induced by Kallikrein-Related Peptidase 4 in Serous Ovarian Cancer Cells in an Ascites Mimicking Microenvironment. *PLoS ONE* **2013**, *8*, e57056. [CrossRef] [PubMed]
45. Nakai, K.; Tanaka, T.; Murai, T.; Ohguro, N.; Tano, Y.; Miyasaka, M. Invasive human pancreatic carcinoma cells adhere to endothelial tri-cellular corners and increase endothelial permeability. *Cancer Sci.* **2005**, *96*, 766–773. [CrossRef] [PubMed]
46. Narai, A.; Arai, S.; Shimizu, M. Rapid decrease in transepithelial electrical resistance of human intestinal Caco-2 cell monolayers by cytotoxic membrane perturbents. *Toxicol. Vitr.* **1997**, *11*, 347–354. [CrossRef]
47. Francart, M.E.; Lambert, J.; Vanwynsberghe, A.M.; Thompson, E.W.; Bourcy, M.; Polette, M.; Gilles, C. Epithelial–mesenchymal plasticity and circulating tumor cells: Travel companions to metastases. *Dev. Dyn.* **2018**, *247*, 432–450. [CrossRef]
48. Bardelli, A.; Pantel, K. Liquid Biopsies, What We Do Not Know (Yet). *Cancer Cell* **2017**, *31*, 172–179. [CrossRef]
49. Dong, X.; Alpaugh, K.R.; Cristofanilli, M. Circulating tumor cells (CTCs) in breast cancer: A diagnostic tool for prognosis and molecular analysis. *Chin. J. Cancer Res.* **2012**, *24*, 388–398. [CrossRef]
50. Jolly, M.K. Implications of the Hybrid Epithelial/Mesenchymal Phenotype in Metastasis. *Front. Oncol.* **2015**, *5*, 155. [CrossRef]

51. Nel, I.; Gauler, T.C.; Bublitz, K.; Lazaridis, L.; Goergens, A.; Giebel, B.; Schuler, M.; Hoffmann, A.C. Circulating tumor cell composition in renal cell carcinoma. *PLoS ONE* **2016**, *11*, e0153018. [CrossRef] [PubMed]
52. McInnes, L.M.; Jacobson, N.; Redfern, A.; Dowling, A.; Thompson, E.W.; Saunders, C.M. Clinical Implications of Circulating Tumor Cells of Breast Cancer Patients: Role of Epithelial–Mesenchymal Plasticity. *Front. Oncol.* **2015**, *5*, 42. [CrossRef] [PubMed]
53. Alonso-Alconada, L.; Muinelo-Romay, L.; Madissoo, K.; Diaz-Lopez, A.; Krakstad, C.; Trovik, J.; Wik, E.; Hapangama, D.; Coenegrachts, L.; Cano, A.; et al. Molecular profiling of circulating tumor cells links plasticity to the metastatic process in endometrial cancer. *Mol. Cancer* **2014**, *13*, 223. [CrossRef]
54. Giussani, M.; Merlino, G.; Cappelletti, V.; Tagliabue, E.; Daidone, M.G. Tumor-extracellular matrix interactions: Identification of tools associated with breast cancer progression. *Semin. Cancer Biol.* **2015**, *35*, 3–10. [CrossRef] [PubMed]
55. Hoshino, A.; Costa-Silva, B.; Shen, T.L.; Rodrigues, G.; Hashimoto, A.; Tesic Mark, M.; Molina, H.; Kohsaka, S.; Di Giannatale, A.; Ceder, S.; et al. Tumour exosome integrins determine organotropic metastasis. *Nature* **2015**, *527*, 329–335. [CrossRef] [PubMed]
56. Peinado, H.; Zhang, H.; Matei, I.R.; Costa-Silva, B.; Hoshino, A.; Rodrigues, G.; Psaila, B.; Kaplan, R.N.; Bromberg, J.F.; Kang, Y.; et al. Pre-metastatic niches: Organ-specific homes for metastases. *Nat. Rev. Cancer* **2017**, *17*, 302–317. [CrossRef] [PubMed]
57. Khalili, A.A.; Ahmad, M.R. A Review of cell adhesion studies for biomedical and biological applications. *Int. J. Mol. Sci.* **2015**, *16*, 18149–18184. [CrossRef] [PubMed]
58. Borowicz, S.; Van Scoyk, M.; Avasarala, S.; Karuppusamy Rathinam, M.K.; Tauler, J.; Bikkavilli, R.K.; Winn, R.A. The Soft Agar Colony Formation Assay. *J. Vis. Exp.* **2014**, *92*, e51998. [CrossRef] [PubMed]
59. Weeber, F.; Ooft, S.N.; Dijkstra, K.K.; Voest, E.E. Tumor Organoids as a Pre-clinical Cancer Model for Drug Discovery. *Cell Chem. Biol.* **2017**, *24*, 1092–1100. [CrossRef] [PubMed]
60. Weeber, F.; van de Wetering, M.; Hoogstraat, M.; Dijkstra, K.K.; Krijgsman, O.; Kuilman, T.; Gadellaa-van Hooijdonk, C.G.M.; van der Velden, D.L.; Peeper, D.S.; Cuppen, E.P.J.G.; et al. Preserved genetic diversity in organoids cultured from biopsies of human colorectal cancer metastases. *Proc. Natl. Acad. Sci. USA* **2015**, *112*, 13308–13311. [CrossRef] [PubMed]
61. Patman, G. Pancreatic cancer: From normal to metastases-a whole gamut of pancreatic organoids. *Nat. Rev. Gastroenterol. Hepatol.* **2015**, *12*, 61. [CrossRef] [PubMed]
62. Buske, P.; Przybilla, J.; Loeffler, M.; Sachs, N.; Sato, T.; Clevers, H.; Galle, J. On the biomechanics of stem cell niche formation in the gut—Modelling growing organoids. *FEBS J.* **2012**, *279*, 3475–3487. [CrossRef] [PubMed]
63. Fujii, M.; Shimokawa, M.; Date, S.; Takano, A.; Matano, M.; Nanki, K.; Ohta, Y.; Toshimitsu, K.; Nakazato, Y.; Kawasaki, K.; et al. A Colorectal Tumor Organoid Library Demonstrates Progressive Loss of Niche Factor Requirements during Tumorigenesis. *Cell Stem Cell* **2016**, *18*, 827–838. [CrossRef] [PubMed]
64. Praharaj, P.P.; Bhutia, S.K.; Nagrath, S.; Bitting, R.L.; Deep, G. Circulating tumor cell-derived organoids: Current challenges and promises in medical research and precision medicine. *Biochim. Biophys. Acta Rev. Cancer* **2018**, *1869*, 117–127. [CrossRef] [PubMed]
65. Drost, J.; Clevers, H. Organoids in cancer research. *Nat. Rev. Cancer* **2018**, *18*, 407–418. [CrossRef]
66. Schumacher, L.J.; Kulesa, P.M.; McLennan, R.; Baker, R.E.; Maini, P.K. Multidisciplinary approaches to understanding collective cell migration in developmental biology. *Open Biol.* **2016**, *6*, 160056. [CrossRef]
67. Stuelten, C.H.; Parent, C.A.; Montell, D.J. Cell motility in cancer invasion and metastasis: Insights from simple model organisms. *Nat. Rev. Cancer* **2018**, *18*, 296–312. [CrossRef]
68. Lokman, N.A.; Elder, A.S.F.; Ricciardelli, C.; Oehler, M.K. Chick chorioallantoic membrane (CAM) assay as an in vivo model to study the effect of newly identified molecules on ovarian cancer invasion and metastasis. *Int. J. Mol. Sci.* **2012**, *13*, 9959–9970. [CrossRef]
69. Stoletov, K.; Willetts, L.; Paproski, R.J.; Bond, D.J.; Raha, S.; Jovel, J.; Adam, B.; Robertson, A.E.; Wong, F.; Woolner, E.; et al. Quantitative in vivo whole genome motility screen reveals novel therapeutic targets to block cancer metastasis. *Nat. Commun.* **2018**, *9*, 2343. [CrossRef]
70. Lengyel, E.; Burdette, J.E.; Kenny, H.A.; Matei, D.; Pilrose, J.; Haluska, P.; Nephew, K.P.; Hales, D.B.; Stack, M.S. Epithelial ovarian cancer experimental models. *Oncogene* **2014**, *33*, 3619–3633. [CrossRef]

71. Hou, W.; Ji, Z. Generation of autochthonous mouse models of clear cell renal cell carcinoma: Mouse models of renal cell carcinoma. *Exp. Mol. Med.* **2018**, *50*, 30. [CrossRef] [PubMed]
72. Gómez-Cuadrado, L.; Tracey, N.; Ma, R.; Qian, B.; Brunton, V.G. Mouse models of metastasis: Progress and prospects. *Dis. Model. Mech.* **2017**, *10*, 1061–1074. [CrossRef] [PubMed]
73. Lee, M.; Downes, A.; Chau, Y.; Serrels, B.; Hastie, N.; Elfick, A.; Brunton, V.; Frame, M.; Serrels, A. In vivo imaging of the tumor and its associated microenvironment using combined CARS/2-photon microscopy. *IntraVital* **2015**, *4*, e1055430. [CrossRef] [PubMed]
74. Romano, G.; Chagani, S.; Kwong, L.N. The path to metastatic mouse models of colorectal cancer. *Oncogene* **2018**, *37*, 2481–2489. [CrossRef] [PubMed]
75. Beck, B.; Lapouge, G.; Rorive, S.; Drogat, B.; Desaedelaere, K.; Delafaille, S.; Dubois, C.; Salmon, I.; Willekens, K.; Marine, J.C.; et al. Different levels of Twist1 regulate skin tumor initiation, stemness, and progression. *Cell Stem Cell* **2015**, *16*, 67–79. [CrossRef] [PubMed]
76. Sauer, B. Inducible gene targeting in mice using the Cre/lox system. *Methods* **1998**, *14*, 381–392. [CrossRef] [PubMed]
77. Barker, N.; Huch, M.; Kujala, P.; van de Wetering, M.; Snippert, H.J.; van Es, J.H.; Sato, T.; Stange, D.E.; Begthel, H.; van den Born, M.; et al. Lgr5+veStem Cells Drive Self-Renewal in the Stomach and Build Long-Lived Gastric Units In Vitro. *Cell Stem Cell* **2010**, *6*, 25–36. [CrossRef] [PubMed]
78. Proia, T.A.; Keller, P.J.; Gupta, P.B.; Klebba, I.; Jones, A.D.; Sedic, M.; Gilmore, H.; Tung, N.; Naber, S.P.; Schnitt, S.; et al. Genetic predisposition directs breast cancer phenotype by dictating progenitor cell fate. *Cell Stem Cell* **2011**, *8*, 149–163. [CrossRef]
79. Sikandar, S.S.; Kuo, A.H.; Kalisky, T.; Cai, S.; Zabala, M.; Hsieh, R.W.; Lobo, N.A.; Scheeren, F.A.; Sim, S.; Qian, D.; et al. Role of epithelial to mesenchymal transition associated genes in mammary gland regeneration and breast tumorigenesis. *Nat. Commun.* **2017**, *8*, 1669. [CrossRef]
80. Hsu, Y.-C. The Theory and Practice of Lineage Tracing. *Stem Cells* **2015**, *33*, 3197–3204. [CrossRef]
81. Tekeli, I.; Aujard, I.; Trepat, X.; Jullien, L.; Raya, A.; Zalvidea, D. Long-term in vivo single-cell lineage tracing of deep structures using three-photon activation. *Light Sci. Appl.* **2016**, *5*, e16084. [CrossRef] [PubMed]
82. Marx, V. Stem cells: Lineage tracing lets single cells talk about their past. *Nat. Methods* **2018**, *15*, 411–414. [CrossRef] [PubMed]
83. Yoo, Y.A.; Roh, M.; Naseem, A.F.; Lysy, B.; Desouki, M.M.; Unno, K.; Abdulkadir, S.A. Bmi1 marks distinct castration-resistant luminal progenitor cells competent for prostate regeneration and tumour initiation. *Nat. Commun.* **2016**, *7*, 12943. [CrossRef] [PubMed]
84. Yamauchi, M.; Barker, T.H.; Gibbons, D.L.; Kurie, J.M. The fibrotic tumor stroma. *J. Clin. Investig.* **2018**, *128*, 16–25. [CrossRef] [PubMed]
85. Williams, C.B.; Yeh, E.S.; Soloff, A.C. Tumor-associated macrophages: Unwitting accomplices in breast cancer malignancy. *NPJ Breast Cancer* **2016**, *2*, 15025. [CrossRef] [PubMed]
86. Brabletz, T.; Kalluri, R.; Nieto, M.A.; Weinberg, R.A. EMT in cancer. *Nat. Rev. Cancer* **2018**, *18*, 128–134. [CrossRef] [PubMed]
87. Jiang, W.G.; Sanders, A.J.; Katoh, M.; Ungefroren, H.; Gieseler, F.; Prince, M.; Thompson, S.K.; Zollo, M.; Spano, D.; Dhawan, P.; et al. Tissue invasion and metastasis: Molecular, biological and clinical perspectives. *Semin. Cancer Biol.* **2015**, *35*, S244–S275. [CrossRef] [PubMed]
88. Abu, M.; Muhamad, M.; Hassan, H.; Zakaria, Z.; Ali, S.A.M. Proximity coupled antenna with star geometry pattern amc ground plane. *ARPN J. Eng. Appl. Sci.* **2016**, *11*, 8822–8828.
89. Zhong, X.; Rescorla, F.J. Cell surface adhesion molecules and adhesion-initiated signaling: Understanding of anoikis resistance mechanisms and therapeutic opportunities. *Cell. Signal.* **2012**, *24*, 393–401. [CrossRef] [PubMed]
90. Cao, Z.; Livas, T.; Kyprianou, N. Anoikis and EMT: Lethal "Liaisons" during Cancer Progression. *Crit. Rev. Oncog.* **2016**, *21*, 155–168. [CrossRef] [PubMed]
91. Nasrollahi, S.; Walter, C.; Loza, A.J.; Schimizzi, G.V.; Longmore, G.D.; Pathak, A. Past matrix stiffness primes epithelial cells and regulates their future collective migration through a mechanical memory. *Biomaterials* **2017**, *146*, 146–155. [CrossRef] [PubMed]
92. Sharma, P.; Ng, C.; Jana, A.; Padhi, A.; Szymanski, P.; Lee, J.S.H.; Behkam, B.; Nain, A.S. Aligned fibers direct collective cell migration to engineer closing and nonclosing wound gaps. *Mol. Biol. Cell* **2017**, *28*, 2579–2588. [CrossRef]

93. Symowicz, J.; Adley, B.P.; Gleason, K.J.; Johnson, J.J.; Ghosh, S.; Fishman, D.A.; Hudson, L.G.; Stack, M.S. Engagement of collagen-binding integrins promotes matrix metalloproteinase-9-dependent E-cadherin ectodomain shedding in ovarian carcinoma cells. *Cancer Res.* **2007**, *67*, 2030–2039. [CrossRef] [PubMed]
94. Drifka, C.R.; Loeffler, A.G.; Mathewson, K.; Keikhosravi, A.; Eickhoff, J.C.; Liu, Y.; Weber, S.M.; Kao, W.J.; Eliceiri, K.W. Highly aligned stromal collagen is a negative prognostic factor following pancreatic ductal adenocarcinoma resection. *Oncotarget* **2016**, *7*, 76197–76213. [CrossRef] [PubMed]
95. Han, M.K.L.; de Rooij, J. Converging and Unique Mechanisms of Mechanotransduction at Adhesion Sites. *Trends Cell Biol.* **2016**, *26*, 612–623. [CrossRef]
96. Alaseem, A.; Alhazzani, K.; Dondapati, P.; Alobid, S.; Bishayee, A.; Rathinavelu, A. Matrix Metalloproteinases: A challenging paradigm of cancer management. *Semin. Cancer Biol.* **2017**, *56*, 100–115. [CrossRef] [PubMed]
97. Cantelli, G.; Orgaz, J.L.; Rodriguez-Hernandez, I.; Karagiannis, P.; Maiques, O.; Matias-Guiu, X.; Nestle, F.O.; Marti, R.M.; Karagiannis, S.N.; Sanz-Moreno, V. TGF-β-Induced Transcription Sustains Amoeboid Melanoma Migration and Dissemination. *Curr. Biol.* **2015**, *25*, 2899–2914. [CrossRef]
98. O'Neill, P.R.; Castillo-Badillo, J.A.; Meshik, X.; Kalyanaraman, V.; Melgarejo, K.; Gautam, N. Membrane Flow Drives an Adhesion-Independent Amoeboid Cell Migration Mode. *Dev. Cell* **2018**, *46*, 9–22. [CrossRef] [PubMed]
99. Varankar, S.S.; Bapat, S.A. Migratory Metrics of Wound Healing: A Quantification Approach for in vitro Scratch Assays. *Front. Oncol.* **2018**, *8*, 633. [CrossRef]
100. Celià-Terrassa, T.; Kang, Y. Metastatic niche functions and therapeutic opportunities. *Nat. Cell Biol.* **2018**, *20*, 868–877. [CrossRef]
101. Reid, S.E.; Kay, E.J.; Neilson, L.J.; Henze, A.; Serneels, J.; McGhee, E.J.; Dhayade, S.; Nixon, C.; Mackey, J.B.; Santi, A.; et al. Tumor matrix stiffness promotes metastatic cancer cell interaction with the endothelium. *EMBO J.* **2017**, *36*, 2373–2389. [CrossRef] [PubMed]
102. Wong, A.D.; Searson, P.C. Live-cell imaging of invasion and intravasation in an artificial microvessel platform. *Cancer Res.* **2014**, *74*, 4937–4945. [CrossRef] [PubMed]
103. Katt, M.E.; Placone, A.L.; Wong, A.D.; Xu, Z.S.; Searson, P.C. In Vitro Tumor Models: Advantages, Disadvantages, Variables, and Selecting the Right Platform. *Front. Bioeng. Biotechnol.* **2016**, *4*, 12. [CrossRef] [PubMed]
104. Kersten, K.; de Visser, K.E.; van Miltenburg, M.H.; Jonkers, J. Genetically engineered mouse models in oncology research and cancer medicine. *EMBO Mol. Med.* **2017**, *9*, 137–153. [CrossRef] [PubMed]
105. Savagner, P. The epithelial-mesenchymal transition (EMT) phenomenon. *Ann. Oncol.* **2010**, *21*, 89–92. [CrossRef] [PubMed]
106. Broggini, T.; Piffko, A.; Hoffmann, C.J.; Harms, C.; Vajkoczy, P.; Czabanka, M. Passive entrapment of tumor cells determines metastatic dissemination to spinal bone and other osseous tissues. *PLoS ONE* **2016**, *11*, e0162540. [CrossRef] [PubMed]
107. Yeung, T.-L.; Leung, C.S.; Yip, K.-P.; Au Yeung, C.L.; Wong, S.T.C.; Mok, S.C. Cellular and molecular processes in ovarian cancer metastasis. A Review in the Theme: Cell and Molecular Processes in Cancer Metastasis. *Am. J. Physiol. Cell Physiol.* **2015**, *309*, C444–C456. [CrossRef]
108. Blaue, C.; Kashef, J.; Franz, C.M. Cadherin-11 promotes neural crest cell spreading by reducing intracellular tension—Mapping adhesion and mechanics in neural crest explants by atomic force microscopy. *Semin. Cell Dev. Biol.* **2018**, *73*, 95–106. [CrossRef]
109. Alonso-Alconada, L.; Eritja, N.; Muinelo-Romay, L.; Barbazan, J.; Lopez-Lopez, R.; Matias-Guiu, X.; Gil-Moreno, A.; Dolcet, X.; Abal, M. ETV5 transcription program links BDNF and promotion of EMT at invasive front of endometrial carcinomas. *Carcinogenesis* **2014**, *35*, 2679–2686. [CrossRef]
110. Rhim, A.D.; Mirek, E.T.; Aiello, N.M.; Maitra, A.; Bailey, J.M.; McAllister, F.; Reichert, M.; Beatty, G.L.; Rustgi, A.K.; Vonderheide, R.H.; et al. EMT and dissemination precede pancreatic tumor formation. *Cell* **2012**, *148*, 349–361. [CrossRef]
111. Schlegel, N.C.; von Planta, A.; Widmer, D.S.; Dummer, R.; Christofori, G. PI3K signalling is required for a TGFβ-induced epithelial-mesenchymal-like transition (EMT-like) in human melanoma cells. *Exp. Dermatol.* **2015**, *24*, 22–28. [CrossRef] [PubMed]
112. Haeger, A.; Wolf, K.; Zegers, M.M.; Friedl, P. Collective cell migration: Guidance principles and hierarchies. *Trends Cell Biol.* **2015**, *25*, 556–566. [CrossRef] [PubMed]

113. Lou, E.; Gholami, S.; Romin, Y.; Thayanithy, V.; Fujisawa, S.; Desir, S.; Steer, C.J.; Subramanian, S.; Fong, Y.; Manova-Todorova, K.; et al. Imaging Tunneling Membrane Tubes Elucidates Cell Communication in Tumors. *Trends Cancer* **2017**, *3*, 678–685. [CrossRef] [PubMed]
114. Combedazou, A.; Choesmel-Cadamuro, V.; Gay, G.; Liu, J.; Dupré, L.; Ramel, D.; Wang, X. Myosin II governs collective cell migration behaviour downstream of guidance receptor signalling. *J. Cell Sci.* **2017**, *130*, 97–103. [CrossRef] [PubMed]
115. Iwanicki, M.P.; Davidowitz, R.A.; Ng, M.R.; Besser, A.; Muranen, T.; Merritt, M.; Danuser, G.; Ince, T.; Brugge, J.S. Ovarian cancer spheroids use myosin-generated force to clear the mesothelium. *Cancer Discov.* **2011**, *1*, 144–157. [CrossRef] [PubMed]
116. Jha, P.; Wang, X.; Auwerx, J. Analysis of Mitochondrial Respiratory Chain Supercomplexes Using Blue Native Polyacrylamide Gel Electrophoresis (BN-PAGE). *Curr. Protoc. Mouse Biol.* **2016**, *6*, 1–14. [PubMed]
117. Melzer, C.; von der Ohe, J.; Hass, R. Breast Carcinoma: From Initial Tumor Cell Detachment to Settlement at Secondary Sites. *BioMed Res. Int.* **2017**, *2017*, 8534371. [CrossRef]
118. Desgrosellier, J.; David, C. Integrins in cancer: Biological implications in therapeutic opportunities. *Cancer Nat. Rev.* **2015**, *10*, 9–22. [CrossRef]
119. Yilmaz, M.; Christofori, G. Mechanisms of Motility in Metastasizing Cells. *Mol. Cancer Res.* **2010**, *8*, 629–642. [CrossRef]
120. Yuzhalin, A.E.; Gordon-Weeks, A.N.; Tognoli, M.L.; Jones, K.; Markelc, B.; Konietzny, R.; Fischer, R.; Muth, A.; O'Neill, E.; Thompson, P.R.; et al. Colorectal cancer liver metastatic growth depends on PAD4-driven citrullination of the extracellular matrix. *Nat. Commun.* **2018**, *9*, 4783. [CrossRef]
121. Jia, D.; Jolly, M.K.; Kulkarni, P.; Levine, H. Phenotypic plasticity and cell fate decisions in cancer: Insights from dynamical systems theory. *Cancers* **2017**, *9*, 70. [CrossRef] [PubMed]
122. Jolly, M.K.; Kulkarni, P.; Weninger, K.; Orban, J.; Levine, H. Phenotypic Plasticity, Bet-Hedging, and Androgen Independence in Prostate Cancer: Role of Non-Genetic Heterogeneity. *Front. Oncol.* **2018**, *8*, 50. [CrossRef] [PubMed]
123. Ma, Y.-H.V.; Middleton, K.; You, L.; Sun, Y. A review of microfluidic approaches for investigating cancer extravasation during metastasis. *Microsyst. Nanoeng.* **2018**, *4*, 17104. [CrossRef]
124. Kocal, G.C.; Güven, S.; Foygel, K.; Goldman, A.; Chen, P.; Sengupta, S.; Paulmurugan, R.; Baskin, Y.; Demirci, U. Dynamic Microenvironment Induces Phenotypic Plasticity of Esophageal Cancer Cells under Flow. *Sci. Rep.* **2016**, *6*, 38221. [CrossRef] [PubMed]
125. Vedula, S.R.K.; Hirata, H.; Nai, M.H.; Brugués, A.; Toyama, Y.; Trepat, X.; Lim, C.T.; Ladoux, B. Epithelial bridges maintain tissue integrity during collective cell migration. *Nat. Mater.* **2014**, *13*, 87–96. [CrossRef] [PubMed]
126. Sarioglu, A.F.; Aceto, N.; Kojic, N.; Donaldson, M.C.; Zeinali, M.; Hamza, B.; Engstrom, A.; Zhu, H.; Sundaresan, T.K.; Miyamoto, D.T.; et al. A microfluidic device for label-free, physical capture of circulating tumor cell clusters. *Nat. Methods* **2015**, *12*, 685–691. [CrossRef] [PubMed]
127. Sandy, M.; Butler, A. Microbial iron acquisition: Marine and terrestrial siderophores. *Chem. Rev.* **2009**, *109*, 4580–4595. [CrossRef]
128. Tanner, K.; Gottesman, M.M. Beyond 3D culture models of cancer. *Sci. Transl. Med.* **2015**, *7*, 283ps9. [CrossRef]
129. Qiao, H.; Tang, T. Engineering 3D approaches to model the dynamic microenvironments of cancer bone metastasis. *Bone Res.* **2018**, *6*, 3. [CrossRef]
130. Shang, M.; Soon, R.H.; Lim, C.T.; Khoo, B.L.; Han, J. Microfluidic modelling of the tumor microenvironment for anti-cancer drug development. *Lab Chip* **2019**, *19*, 369–386. [CrossRef]
131. Truong, D.D.; Kratz, A.; Park, J.G.; Barrientos, E.S.; Saini, H.; Nguyen, T.; Pockaj, B.; Mouneimne, G.; LaBaer, J.; Nikkhah, M. A human organotypic microfluidic tumor model permits investigation of the interplay between patient-derived fibroblasts and breast cancer cells. *Cancer Res.* **2019**. [CrossRef] [PubMed]
132. Ayuso, J.M.; Gillette, A.; Lugo-cintrón, K.; Acevedo-acevedo, S.; Gomez, I.; Morgan, M.; Heaster, T.; Wisinski, K.B.; Palecek, S.P.; Skala, M.C.; et al. EBioMedicine Organotypic micro fl uidic breast cancer model reveals starvation-induced spatial-temporal metabolic adaptations. *EBioMedicine* **2018**, *37*, 144–157. [CrossRef] [PubMed]

133. Martinez, J.S.; Schlenoff, J.B.; Keller, T.C.S. Collective epithelial cell sheet adhesion and migration on polyelectrolyte multilayers with uniform and gradients of compliance. *Exp. Cell Res.* **2016**, *346*, 17–29. [CrossRef]
134. Zajac, O.; Raingeaud, J.; Libanje, F.; Lefebvre, C.; Sabino, D.; Martins, I.; Roy, P.; Benatar, C.; Canet-Jourdan, C.; Azorin, P.; et al. Tumour spheres with inverted polarity drive the formation of peritoneal metastases in patients with hypermethylated colorectal carcinomas. *Nat. Cell Biol.* **2018**, *20*, 296–306. [CrossRef] [PubMed]
135. Wong, I.Y.; Javaid, S.; Wong, E.A.; Perk, S.; Haber, D.A.; Toner, M.; Irimia, D. Collective and individual migration following the epithelial-mesenchymal transition. *Nat. Mater.* **2014**, *13*, 1063–1071. [CrossRef] [PubMed]
136. Mitchell, C.B.; ONeill, G.M. Cooperative cell invasion: Matrix metalloproteinase-mediated incorporation between cells. *Mol. Biol. Cell* **2016**, *27*, 3284–3292. [CrossRef]
137. Klymenko, Y.; Johnson, J.; Bos, B.; Lombard, R.; Campbell, L.; Loughran, E.; Stack, M.S. Heterogeneous Cadherin Expression and Multicellular Aggregate Dynamics in Ovarian Cancer Dissemination. *Neoplasia* **2017**, *19*, 549–563. [CrossRef]
138. Kilgore, J.A.; Dolman, N.J.; Davidson, M.W. A Review of Reagents for Fluorescence Microscopy of Cellular Compartments and Structures, Part II: Reagents for Non-Vesicular Organelles. In *Current Protocols in Cytometry*; John Wiley & Sons, Inc.: Hoboken, NJ, USA, 2013; pp. 12.31.1–12.31.24. ISBN 0471142956.
139. Kilgore, J.A.; Dolman, N.J.; Davidson, M.W. A Review of Reagents for Fluorescence Microscopy of Cellular Compartments and Structures, Part III: Reagents for Actin, Tubulin, Cellular Membranes, and Whole Cell and Cytoplasm. In *Current Protocols in Cytometry*; John Wiley & Sons, Inc.: Hoboken, NJ, USA, 2014; pp. 12.32.1–12.32.17. ISBN 0471142956.
140. Marsh, E.; Gonzalez, D.G.; Lathrop, E.A.; Boucher, J.; Marsh, E.; Gonzalez, D.G.; Lathrop, E.A.; Boucher, J.; Greco, V. Positional Stability and Membrane Occupancy Define Skin Fibroblast Homeostasis In Vivo Article Positional Stability and Membrane Occupancy Define Skin Fibroblast Homeostasis In Vivo. *Cell* **2018**, *175*, 1620–1633. [CrossRef]
141. Chen, J.; Landegger, L.D.; Sun, Y.; Ren, J.; Maimon, N.; Wu, L.; Ng, M.R.; Chen, J.W.; Zhang, N.; Zhao, Y.; et al. A cerebellopontine angle mouse model for the investigation of tumor biology, hearing, and neurological function in NF2-related vestibular schwannoma. *Nat. Protoc.* **2019**, *14*, 541–555. [CrossRef]
142. Harper, K.L.; Sosa, M.S.; Entenberg, D.; Hosseini, H.; Cheung, J.F.; Nobre, R.; Avivar-Valderas, A.; Nagi, C.; Girnius, N.; Davis, R.J.; et al. Mechanism of early dissemination and metastasis in Her2+ mammary cancer. *Nature* **2016**, *540*, 588–592. [CrossRef]
143. Yang, Z.; Hoffman, R.M.; Ma, H.; Toneri, M.; Goto, Y.; Zhang, Y.; Bouvet, M.; Seki, N. Real-Time GFP Intravital Imaging of the Differences in Cellular and Angiogenic Behavior of Subcutaneous and Orthotopic Nude-Mouse Models of Human PC-3 Prostate Cancer. *J. Cell. Biochem.* **2016**, *117*, 2546–2551.
144. Zomer, A.; Ellenbroek, S.I.J.; Ritsma, L.; Beerling, E.; Vrisekoop, N.; Van Rheenen, J. Brief report: Intravital imaging of cancer stem cell plasticity in mammary tumors. *Stem Cells* **2013**, *31*, 602–606. [CrossRef] [PubMed]
145. Ritsma, L.; Ellenbroek, S.I.J.; Zomer, A.; Snippert, H.J.; de Sauvage, F.J.; Simons, B.D.; Clevers, H.; van Rheenen, J. Intestinal crypt homeostasis revealed at single-stem-cell level by in vivo live imaging. *Nature* **2014**, *507*, 362–365. [CrossRef] [PubMed]
146. Reeves, M.Q.; Kandyba, E.; Harris, S.; Del Rosario, R.; Balmain, A. Multicolour lineage tracing reveals clonal dynamics of squamous carcinoma evolution from initiation to metastasis. *Nat. Cell Biol.* **2018**, *20*, 699–709. [CrossRef] [PubMed]
147. Richardson, A.; Park, M.; Watson, S.L.; Wakefield, D.; Di Girolamo, N. Visualizing the Fate of Transplanted K14-Confetti Corneal Epithelia in a Mouse Model of Limbal Stem Cell Deficiency. *Investig. Ophthalmol. Vis. Sci.* **2018**, *59*, 1630–1640. [CrossRef] [PubMed]
148. Nobis, M.; Warren, S.C.; Lucas, M.C.; Murphy, K.J.; Herrmann, D.; Timpson, P. Molecular mobility and activity in an intravital imaging setting—Implications for cancer progression and targeting. *J. Cell Sci.* **2018**, *131*, jcs206995. [CrossRef]
149. Chitty, J.L.; Filipe, E.C.; Lucas, M.C.; Herrmann, D.; Cox, T.R.; Timpson, P. Recent advances in understanding the complexities of metastasis. *F1000Research* **2018**, *7*, F1000. [CrossRef]
150. Liu, T.-L.; Upadhyayula, S.; Milkie, D.E.; Singh, V.; Wang, K.; Swinburne, I.A.; Mosaliganti, K.R.; Collins, Z.M.; Hiscock, T.W.; Shea, J.; et al. Observing the cell in its native state: Imaging subcellular dynamics in multicellular organisms. *Science* **2018**, *360*, eaaq1392. [CrossRef]

151. Labernadie, A.; Trepat, X. ScienceDirect Sticking, steering, squeezing and shearing: Cell movements driven by heterotypic mechanical forces. *Curr. Opin. Cell Biol.* **2018**, *54*, 57–65. [CrossRef]
152. Kelley, L.C.; Wang, Z.; Hagedorn, E.J.; Wang, L.; Shen, W.; Lei, S.; Johnson, S.A.; Sherwood, D.R. Live-cell confocal microscopy and quantitative 4D image analysis of anchor-cell invasion through the basement membrane in Caenorhabditis elegans. *Nat. Protoc.* **2017**, *12*, 2081–2096. [CrossRef]
153. Chantzi, E.; Jarvius, M.; Niklasson, M.; Segerman, A.; Gustafsson, M.G. COMBImage: A modular parallel processing framework for pairwise drug combination analysis that quantifies temporal changes in label-free video microscopy movies. *BMC Bioinform.* **2018**, *19*, 453. [CrossRef] [PubMed]
154. Wang, M.F.Z.; Fernandez-Gonzalez, R. (Machine-)Learning to analyze in vivo microscopy: Support vector machines. *Biochim. Biophys. Acta Proteins Proteom.* **2017**, *1865*, 1719–1727. [CrossRef] [PubMed]
155. Svensson, C.; Medyukhina, A.; Belyaev, I.; Al-Zaben, N.; Figge, M.T. Untangling cell tracks: Quantifying cell migration by time lapse image data analysis. *Cytom. Part A* **2018**, *93*, 357–370. [CrossRef] [PubMed]
156. Cohen, S.; Valm, A.M.; Lippincott-Schwartz, J. Multispectral Live-Cell Imaging. *Curr. Protoc. Cell Biol.* **2018**, *79*, e46. [CrossRef] [PubMed]
157. Piltti, K.M.; Cummings, B.J.; Carta, K.; Manughian-Peter, A.; Worne, C.L.; Singh, K.; Ong, D.; Maksymyuk, Y.; Khine, M.; Anderson, A.J. Live-cell time-lapse imaging and single-cell tracking of in vitro cultured neural stem cells—Tools for analyzing dynamics of cell cycle, migration, and lineage selection. *Methods* **2018**, *133*, 81–90. [CrossRef] [PubMed]
158. Jiang, D.; Correa-Gallegos, D.; Christ, S.; Stefanska, A.; Liu, J.; Ramesh, P.; Rajendran, V.; De Santis, M.M.; Wagner, D.E.; Rinkevich, Y. Two succeeding fibroblastic lineages drive dermal development and the transition from regeneration to scarring. *Nat. Cell Biol.* **2018**, *20*, 422–431. [CrossRef] [PubMed]
159. Huang, J.; Guo, P.; Moses, M.A. A time-lapse, label-free, quantitative phase imaging study of dormant and active human cancer cells. *J. Vis. Exp.* **2018**, *132*, e57035. [CrossRef] [PubMed]
160. Lee, R.M.; Stuelten, C.H.; Parent, C.A.; Losert, W. Collective cell migration over long time scales reveals distinct phenotypes. *Converg. Sci. Phys. Oncol.* **2016**, *2*, 025001. [CrossRef] [PubMed]
161. Chepizhko, O.; Giampietro, C.; Mastrapasqua, E.; Nourazar, M.; Ascagni, M.; Sugni, M.; Fascio, U.; Leggio, L.; Malinverno, C.; Scita, G.; et al. Bursts of activity in collective cell migration. *Proc. Natl. Acad. Sci. USA* **2016**, *113*, 11408–11413. [CrossRef] [PubMed]
162. Paul, C.D.; Mistriotis, P.; Konstantopoulos, K. Cancer cell motility: Lessons from migration in confined spaces. *Nat. Rev. Cancer* **2017**, *17*, 131–140. [CrossRef]
163. Rogers, S.; McCloy, R.A.; Parker, B.L.; Gallego-Ortega, D.; Law, A.M.K.; Chin, V.T.; Conway, J.R.W.; Fey, D.; Millar, E.K.A.; O'Toole, S.; et al. MASTL overexpression promotes chromosome instability and metastasis in breast cancer. *Oncogene* **2018**, *37*, 4518–4533. [CrossRef] [PubMed]
164. Hetmanski, J.H.R.; Zindy, E.; Schwartz, J.M.; Caswell, P.T. A MAPK-Driven Feedback Loop Suppresses Rac Activity to Promote RhoA-Driven Cancer Cell Invasion. *PLoS Comput. Biol.* **2016**, *12*, e1004909. [CrossRef] [PubMed]
165. Keller, S.; Kneissl, J.; Grabher-Meier, V.; Heindl, S.; Hasenauer, J.; Maier, D.; Mattes, J.; Winter, P.; Luber, B. Evaluation of epidermal growth factor receptor signaling effects in gastric cancer cell lines by detailed motility-focused phenotypic characterization linked with molecular analysis. *BMC Cancer* **2017**, *17*, 845. [CrossRef] [PubMed]
166. Shafqat-Abbasi, H.; Kowalewski, J.M.; Kiss, A.; Gong, X.; Hernandez-Varas, P.; Berge, U.; Jafari-Mamaghani, M.; Lock, J.G.; Strömblad, S. An analysis toolbox to explore mesenchymal migration heterogeneity reveals adaptive switching between distinct modes. *Elife* **2016**, *5*, e11384. [CrossRef] [PubMed]
167. Liu, X.; Taftaf, R.; Kawaguchi, M.; Chang, Y.F.; Chen, W.; Entenberg, D.; Zhang, Y.; Gerratana, L.; Huang, S.; Patel, D.B.; et al. Homophilic CD44 interactions mediate tumor cell aggregation and polyclonal metastasis in patient-derived breast cancer models. *Cancer Discov.* **2019**, *9*, 96–113. [CrossRef] [PubMed]

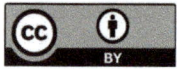

© 2019 by the authors. Licensee MDPI, Basel, Switzerland. This article is an open access article distributed under the terms and conditions of the Creative Commons Attribution (CC BY) license (http://creativecommons.org/licenses/by/4.0/).

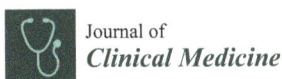 

Review

# Snail1: A Transcriptional Factor Controlled at Multiple Levels

Josep Baulida [1,*], Víctor M. Díaz [1,2,*] and Antonio García de Herreros [1,2,*]

[1] Programa de Recerca en Càncer, Institut Hospital del Mar d'Investigacions Mèdiques (IMIM), Unidad Asociada al CSIC, 08003 Barcelona, Spain
[2] Departament de Ciències Experimentals i de la Salut, Universitat Pompeu Fabra, 08003 Barcelona, Spain
* Correspondence: jbaulida@imim.es (J.B.); victor.diaz@upf.edu (V.M.D.); agarcia@imim.es (A.G.d.H.)

Received: 7 May 2019; Accepted: 23 May 2019; Published: 28 May 2019

**Abstract:** Snail1 transcriptional factor plays a key role in the control of epithelial to mesenchymal transition and fibroblast activation. As a consequence, Snail1 expression and function is regulated at multiple levels from gene transcription to protein modifications, affecting its interaction with specific cofactors. In this review, we describe the different elements that control Snail1 expression and its activity both as transcriptional repressor or activator.

**Keywords:** Snail1; transcriptional factor; Epithelial to mesenchymal transition (EMT); tumor invasion; drug resistance

## 1. Introduction

Epithelial to mesenchymal transition (EMT) is a progressive and reversible process that promotes epithelial cells to acquire a mesenchymal phenotype. During this transition, the cell-cell junction structures, including adherens junctions and desmosomes, are disassembled. Cells lose their cobblestone appearance and adopt a spindle-shaped morphology. EMT provides epithelial cells with different traits relevant for tumorigenesis since, upon EMT, cells become more motile and invasive, become more resistant to pro-apoptotic stimuli, reprogram their metabolism, and acquire characteristics of cancer stem cells. For these reasons, EMT has attracted the attention of many cancer biologists and has been extensively studied in recent years. Many excellent and recent reviews have addressed different insights in EMT and the acquisition of high-grade malignancy [1–3].

EMT is orchestrated by a set of EMT-activating transcriptional factors (EMT-TFs), whose core set includes Snail1 (Snail), Snail2 (Slug), Twist1, Zeb1, and Zeb2 [1]. Among these, a prominent role has been attributed to Snail1 since its expression is widely observed in EMT processes preceding the remaining EMT-TFs; moreover, ectopic Snail1 induces other EMT-TFs such as Zeb1/2 and Snail2 [4], and *Snail* depletion severely impacts mesoderm formation during embryogenesis [5]. For this reason, Snail1 has been extensively studied as key marker of EMT [6]. Besides this action in epithelial cells, Snail1 is also relevant for fibroblast activation [4], a process also driven in mesenchymal cells for conditions promoting EMT in epithelial cells. Fibroblast activation is required for the generation of cancer-associated fibroblasts (CAFs), a tumor stromal cell with a crucial role in tumor invasion or evasion from the immune system [7]. Without ignoring the contribution of other EMT-TFs to EMT and malignancy, our goal here has been to detail the different mechanisms that control Snail1 expression and function and therefore impact EMT and fibroblast activation.

## 2. Transcription

Snail1 expression was initially studied analyzing its mRNA. First, studies on the control of Snail1 were based on transcription and carried out with human and mouse proximal promoters that present less than 50% of homology. Accordingly, although many similarities are present, transcription factor binding elements described in one of these species cannot automatically be extrapolated to the other. In Table 1, we include a list of the transcriptional factors binding to the promoters of Snail1 genes both in mice and humans.

## 2.1. Murine Snai1 Transcription Regulation

TGFβ was the first factor reported to stimulate *Snai1* transcription and activity of a 900 pb fragment of the *Snai1* proximal promoter [8]. H-Ras transfection is as potent as TGFβ, and both MAPK and PI3K pathways are required for the H-Ras- and TGFβ1-mediated induction of the promoter activity [8]. The role of the canonical TGFβ pathway and Smads in activating *Snai1* promoter in mouse is controversial. The initial observations using a dominant negative form of Smad4 pointed to a Smad4-independent activation [8]; however, in lens epithelial cells, the proximal *Snai1* promoter was activated by TGFβ through the action of Smad2, -3, and -4 [9]. In addition, mice with a specific *Smad2* ablation in keratinocytes show an enhanced EMT during skin cancer formation and progression. In these animals, Smad4 binds to the *Snai1* promoter, and additional Smad3 or Smad4 knockdown abrogates Snai1 overexpression [10].

HMGA2 cooperates with the TGFβ/Smad pathway in the activation of *Snai1* gene expression concomitant to an increased binding of Smads to the proximal promoter. While HMGA2 binds to two A/T rich motifs at the −131/−92 region, Smad3 and -4, which physically interact with HMGA2, associate preferentially with the −230/−178 sequence [11]. Myc binding to the *Snai1* promoter is required for rapid *Snai1* activation upon TGFβ stimulation. Accordingly, knockdown of either c-Myc or Smad3/4 in epithelial cells eliminated Snail1 induction by TGFβ [12]. The hepatocyte growth factor (HGF) also activates *Snai1* promoter depending on Myc and Smad4 [12].

The mechanism regulating the expression of the *Snai1* gene has been studied in palatal shelves during the degradation of the midline epithelial seam. To activate expression of *Snai1* in palatal explants, TGFβ3 stimulates binding of Twist1/E47 dimers to the *Snai1* promoter; without E47, Twist1 represses *Snai1* expression [13]. Finally, in the mouse mammary epithelial cells, MMP-3 causes the binding of p65 and cRel NFκB subunits to the *Snai1* promoter, leading to its transcription [14].

## 2.2. Human SNAI1 Transcription Regulation

In humans, *SNAI1* transcription is also controlled by TGFβ and canonical Smads. In many cases, interference with this pathway decreases *SNAI1* mRNA; for instance, in A549 non-small lung cancer cells, the natural dietary flavonoid Kaempferol reverses TGFβ1-mediated *SNAI1* induction by weakening Smad3 binding to the promoter. This is dependent on the selective downregulation of the AKT1-dependent phosphorylation of Smad3 at T179 [15]. In HCCLM3 hepatocellular carcinoma cells, downregulation of AGO1 decreases Smad4 binding to *SNAI1* promoter and reduces its transcription [16]. Liver X receptor α (LXRα) also antagonizes TGFβ since the binding of LXRα to the *SNAI1* promoter prevents that of Smad3/4 [17].

NFκB is another potent stimulator of *SNAI1* transcription and promoter activity. Initial reporter assays with truncated promoters transfected in colon and pancreas cancer cells mapped the NFκB-responsive element to a sequence (−194/−78) located immediately upstream the minimal promoter (−78/+59) [18]. Erythropoietin also increases the binding of p50 and p65 NFκB subunits to the *SNAI1* promoter [19]. Overexpression of v-Akt increases *SNAI1* RNA and promoter activity [18,20]. This Akt effect involves several downstream factors since this protein kinase upregulates *SNAI1* RNA through the activation of NFκB [21] and Smad3 phosphorylation [15].

Another well documented factor that regulates *SNAI1* transcription is STAT3. Chromatin immunoprecipitation assays in cisplatin-resistant atypical teratoid/rhabdoid tumor cells indicated that STAT3 also binds to the *SNAI1* promoter, although in a more distant region than NFκB [22]. STAT3 was found to enhance *SNAI1* induction by TGF-β in cooperation with Ras [23]. In hepatoma cells, phosphorylated STAT3 was also found to bind to the *SNAI1* promoter; inhibition of STAT3 abrogated the hepatitis virus C core-induced Snail1 expression [24]. Additionally, in HCCLM3 hepatocellular carcinoma cells, the isoprenoid antibiotic ascochlorin increased the sensitivity to doxorubicin treatment by directly inhibiting binding of STAT3 to *SNAI1* promoter [25].

Factors downstream MAPK also bind and control *SNAI1* transcription; indeed, the minimal promoter fragment (−78/+59) is dependent on the ERK signaling pathway [18]. Ultraviolet (UV) irradiation transiently induces *SNAI1* expression in human skin and cultured human keratinocytes. Different MAPK pathways (ERK, p38, or JNK) participate in this *SNAI1* regulation, AP-1 sites present in human or mouse promoters and interacting with c-Jun are especially relevant for UV irradiation-increased *SNAI* promoter activity [26]. Osteoblast-derived CXCL5 increases Raf/MEK/ERK activation promoting MSK1 phosphorylation and binding to the *SNAI1* promoter [27]. In human gastric cancer cells, a pre-treatment with N-acetylcysteine attenuated the Helicobacter pylori-induced activation of ERK and *SNAI1* promoter activity [28].

HGF also stimulates Snail1 through MAPK stimulation and through Egr1 that binds to the *SNAI1* promoter [29]. Egr1 is also required for *SNAI1* expression in FGF2-activated cells [30]. Remarkably, Snail1 also binds the *EGR1* promoter and represses the expression of this transcriptional factor [29], demonstrating the existence of a self-inhibitory loop. Other similar loops have been described since Snail itself binds to the *SNAI1* promoter, limiting its own transcription [31]. As discussed in [32], such self-inhibition tends to prevent the aberrant activation of EMT by reducing noise in the system.

Table 1. Transcription factors binding to the *Snai1* or *SNAI1* promoter.

| Binding Factor | Cell Line or Tissue | References |
| --- | --- | --- |
| Smads | Lens epithelial cells, keratinocytes and lung and liver cancer cells | [9,10,15–17] |
| HMGA | Mammary and liver epithelial cells and fibroblasts | [11,12] |
| NFκB | Mammary epithelial cells and breast, colon, and pancreas tumor cells | [14,18,19] |
| STAT3 | Atypical teratoid/rhabdoid tumor cells, liver cancer, and pancreatic epithelial cells | [22–24] |
| Twist/E47 | Palatal shelves | [13] |
| AP1 | Skin keratinocytes | [26] |
| ELK1/MSK1 | Breast tumor cells | [27] |
| Egr1 | Stomach, esophagus, and liver cancer cells, kidney epithelial cells, and embryonic stem cells | [29,30] |
| Snail1 | Colon and pancreas cancer cells and fibroblasts | [31] |
| Forkhead box M1 | Lung adenocarcinoma cells and endothelial cells | [33,34] |
| PARP1 | Breast epithelial cells and prostate cancer cells | [35] |
| Polyomavirus-enhancer activator 3 | Lung and ovarian cancer cells | [36] |
| MUC1 | Renal carcinoma cells | [37] |
| P4R/EGFR | Liver cancer cells | [38] |
| COUP-TFII | Colon cancer cells | [39] |
| SP1 | Cholangiocarcinoma cell lines | [40] |
| HIF1α | Hepatocellular carcinoma | [41] |
| Estrogen receptor | Breast cancer cells | [42] |
| Wilms' tumor-1 | Epicardial cells | [43] |
| MTA3 | Breast cancer cells | [44] |
| Aryl Hydrocarbon receptor | Gastric carcinoma cells | [45] |
| CBX8 | Esophagus cancer cells | [46] |

Those commented in the text are in bold.

Besides these factors, other unrelated proteins, also presented in Table 1, bind and control *SNAI1* transcription [33–46]. Most proteins in this list stimulate *SNAI1* transcription; only metastasis-associated protein 3 (MTA3), aryl hydrocarbon receptor, and CBX8 repress *SNAI1* [44–46].

*2.3. Epigenetic Regulation of the SNAI1 Promoter*

*SNAI1* transcription is also regulated by epigenetic modifications at the promoter and enhancer regions. Initial epigenetic studies demonstrated that demethylation of the *Snai1* promoter accompanies its transcription in spindle or dedifferentiated cells and is associated with an increase in acetylated histone H4 [47]. After these studies, many others described methylation and acetylation marks with respect to the *SNAI1* promoter. For instance, in colon cancer cells, the *SNAI1* promoter is regulated by phosphorylated p68 RNA helicase, which induces the dissociation of the HDAC1 from the *SNAI1* promoter and activates its transcription [48]. In breast cancer cells, *SNAI1* is a direct target of JMJD5 and demethylated H3K36me2 [49]. HIV enhances the trimethylation of K4 in H3 at the *SNAI1* promoter site [50]. In nasopharyngeal carcinoma cells, HOPX mediates epigenetic silencing of *SNAI1* transcription through the enhancement of histone H3 K9 deacetylation. In one study, HOPX epigenetically suppressed SRF-dependent *SNAI1* transcription by recruiting histone deacetylase activity [51]. Other examples of epigenetic modifiers include DDX21, recruited to the *SNAI1* promoter together with EZH2 and SUZ12, which increased the trimethylation of H3 on K27 repressing *Snai1* transcription [52]; SETDB1 in MCF7 cells [53]; PDHE1α, which promoted H3K9 acetylation on the *Snai1* promoter to induce transcription and enhance cell motility [54]; MSK1, which enhanced histone H3 acetylation and phosphorylation (S10) at the *SNAI1* promoter [27]; and SATB2, which recruited HDAC1 to silence *SNAI1* transcription [55]. In general, with few exceptions, there is a gap of information on how epigenetic enzymes are activated by the transcription factors binding to the *SNAI1* gene.

Finally, a conserved 3′ region in the *SNAI1* gene acts as an enhancer. Contacting with the constitutively packaged promoter in a poised chromatin structure, this enhancer promotes the transcription associated with the enrichment of H3K4 dimethylation and H3 acetylation, at both the enhancer and the promoter [56]. *SNAI1* transcription is also controlled by a long noncoding RNA, lncRNA-a7, which acts in cis as an enhancer [56]. Accordingly, the deletion of lncRNA-a7 decreases the expression of *SNAI1* mRNA [57].

## 3. mRNA Stability

Many microRNAs (miRNAs) have been shown to negatively correlate with Snail1 levels in a variety of cellular contexts; however, only some of them directly bind and reduce *SNAI1* RNA levels. The earlier miRNA shown to bind to a highly conserved 3′ untranslated region (UTR) in *SNAI1* mRNA was the p53-dependent miR-34 in colon, breast and lung carcinomas. These results unveiled a link between p53, miR-34, and Snail1 in the regulation of cancer cell EMT programs [58]. Preventing miR-34a action by a long non-coding RNA, lncRNA-MUF, which acts as a competing endogenous RNA for miR-34a, leads to Snail1 upregulation and EMT activation [59]. In fact, double-negative feedback loops between the transcription factor Snail1 and the miR-34 family, and the transcription factor ZEB1 and the miR-200 control TGF-β1-induced EMT of MCF10A cells [60]. These loops explain the intermediate phenotypes observed during EMT ([61] and determine the hysteretic and bimodal responses in this transition [62].

The family of miR-30 is also involved in Snail1 repression. During differentiation of tracheal chondrocytes miR-125b and miR-30a/c keep Snail1 at low levels through their binding to the *Snai1* 3′ UTR [63]. In murine hepatocytes, the expression of miR-30 family members is significantly downregulated during TGF-β1-induced EMT, preventing their repressive actions on *Snai1* 3′UTR [64]. In liver fibrosis, miR-30c and miR-193 are a part of the TGF-β-dependent regulatory network controlling Snail1 and extracellular matrix genes [65]. miR-30c, in coordination with miR-26a, and miR-30e-3p also repress *SNAI1* mRNA in other cellular systems [66,67]. Accordingly, miR-30c protects against diabetic nephropathy by suppressing EMT in db/db mice [68].

Several experimental evidences also implicate miR-153 in controlling Snail1 and EMT. In hepatocellular carcinoma, miR-153 inhibits EMT by targeting *SNAI1* [69]. Indeed, the Krüppel-like factor 4 was found to suppress EMT in hepatocellular carcinoma cells in part by inducing miR-153 and repressing Snail1 [70]. Besides these, other reports have described additional miRNAs as also repressing *SNAI1* mRNA in other systems: miR-211-5p in renal cancer [71] and miR-122 in hepatocellular carcinoma [72].

## 4. Translation

Snail1 translation is also regulated both through cap-dependent and -independent mechanisms. Increased expression of Snail1 and a concomitant EMT is promoted by transfection of the Y-box binding protein-1 (YB-1), a protein that activates cap-independent translation of Snail1 mRNA [73]. This rise in Snail1 is antagonized by the cell fate determination factor Dachshund (DACH1) that binds and inactivates YB-1 [74]. Upregulated Snail1 translation caused by YB-1 is dependent on its binding to a putative IRES element contained in the 5′UTR *SNAI1* mRNA. Curiously, other transcriptional factors related to EMT (LEF-1, ZEB2, or HIF1α) are also translationally enriched upon enforced YB-1 expression [73] and contain IRES sequences in their 5′UTRs [75–77]. It remains to be established if these factors correspond to proteins activated during specific EMTs triggered by conditions that preclude cap-dependent translation, such as hypoxia.

Snail1 translation is also regulated through eIF4E- and cap-dependent translation. For instance, TGFβ-induced phosphorylation of eIF4E contributes to Snail1 expression during EMT [78]. Accordingly, a chemical antagonist of eIF4E blocks Snail1 mRNA recruitment to the polysomes and EMT [79]. Similar results have also being obtained by the expression of gain-of-function mutants of eIF4E-BP1, a repressor of eIF4E that downregulates Snail1 without affecting its transcription or protein stability [80]. Since eIF4E/eIF4BP1 interaction is disrupted by phosphorylation by TORC1, inhibitors of this modification decrease Snail1 expression. Remarkably, Snail1 also represses eIF4E-BP1 expression by direct binding to the promoter [81], demonstrating the existence of another loop of mutual repression, as has been shown above for Snail1 and miR-34. Accordingly, expression of eiF4E-BP1 and Snail1 is contrary in colorectal tumors [81].

Finally, Snail1 translation is also controlled by methylation of its mRNA. Methytransferase-like 3 (METTL3) modifies a GGAC motif present in the *Snai1* mRNA coding sequence, enhancing its presence in polysomes [82].

## 5. Protein Stability

Snail1 protein comprises two very well defined parts: the N-terminal or regulatory domain (amino acids 1–148) and the C-terminal or DNA-binding domain [83]. The regulatory domain contains a short sequence in the N-terminus, called the SNAG domain with a special relevance for the binding of co-repressors; other relevant regions are the Ser-rich subdomain (SRD) (amino acids 90–120) and the nuclear-export sequence (NES) (amino acids 138–146) [84] (Figure 1). The DNA-binding domain is composed of four zinc fingers (ZnF) of the C2H2 type although ZnF4 does not contain the consensus distance between these residues. A nuclear localization sequence (NLS) is also present in this domain [85].

Snail is a short-lived protein (with a half-life of about 25 min) since it is rapidly ubiquitinated and degraded by the 26S proteasome system [86]. Snail1 ubiquitination involves the participation of several E3 ubiquitin ligases of the multimeric SCF subtype (Skp1-Cullin1-F-box) [87]. From about 69 F-box proteins described, eight has been reported to participate in targeting Snail1: FBXW1, FBXW7, FBXL14, FBXL5, FBXO11, FBXO22, FBXO31, and FBXO45. This suggests a highly redundant mechanism of protein degradation to maintain Snail1 levels very low under non-pathological conditions. This seems to be common to other labile substrates with a central role in cancer, such as p53, β-catenin, or c-Myc.

Binding of Snail1 to the F-box module is often associated with Snail1 phosphorylation, although this is not always a prerequisite. The best example of a phosphorylation-dependent interaction is the one with FBXW1, commonly known as β-TrCP1 (β-transducin-repeat containing protein) [88]. SCF-FBXW1/β-TrCP1 recognizes the Snail1 phospho-degron sequence DpS96GxxpS100, a target sequence similarly found in β-catenin and other substrates, located in the SRD and phosphorylated by GSK-3β [89] (Figure 1). GSK-3β action requires the previous priming of Snail1 S92 by CK1ε or CK2β [90,91]. Other E3 ligases also require previous phosphorylation, such as SCF-FBXO11, which requires phosphorylation by the protein kinase D1 (PKD1) of Snail1-S11 in the SNAG domain [92]; however, according to other authors, it may also occur independently on phosphorylation [93]. Snail1 is degraded by the FBXW7 tumor suppressor [94,95]. Although FBXW7-mediated degradation will probably require Snail1 phosphorylation, as shown for ZEB2 [96] and many other substrates (cyclin E, Notch, c-Jun, c-Myc and mTOR) [97], this point has not been formally proven in the case of Snail1. Other F-box proteins have also been proposed as phosphorylation-dependent ubiquitin ligases for Snail1 such as SCF-FBXO22 and SCF-FBXO31 in mammary and gastric carcinomas, respectively [98,99].

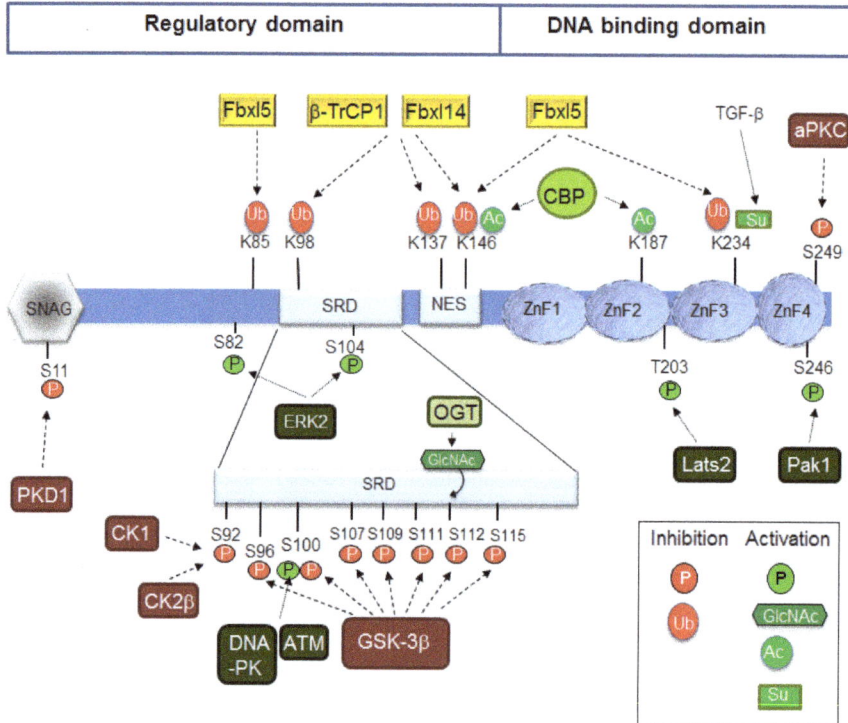

**Figure 1.** Post-translational modifications controlling Snail1 function. The figure shows a diagram of Snail1 protein with the N-terminal regulatory domain and the C-terminal DNA-binding domain. The SNAG, SRD, and NES elements are included in the N-terminal domain. The indicated covalent modifications of the amino acids are depicted in green or red if they activate or inhibit (respectively) Snail1 function. K48-mediated polyubiquitination is indicated by an oval (Ub); phosphorylation (P) and acetylation (Ac), by circles; glycosylation (NAcGlc), by a hexagon; sumoylation (Su), by a rectangle. The enzymes catalyzing these modifications are also shown when they have been described. Please notice that the phosphorylation of S100 can promote a positive or negative effect on Snail1 function depending on the protein kinase and the context. Only the F-box proteins acting on identified Lysine residues are shown.

The fact that in many cells Snail1 degradation is independent on GSK-3β suggested the participation of other E3s; accordingly, SCF-FBXL14 was identified as a potent, phosphorylation-independent Snail1 E3 ligase [100]. FBXL14 and β-TrCP1 redundantly modify the same group of Snail1 lysines (K98, K137, and K146) [100]. FBXL14 seems to have a central role in EMT since it also acts on other EMT-TFs and targets Snail2, Twist1, and Zeb2 [101]. SCF-FBXL14 is transcriptionally repressed during hypoxia, leading to Snail1 stabilization [100]. Importantly, hypoxia activates a full EMT program with the concomitant induction of Snail1, Twist1, and Zeb2 [102,103]. Recently, LKB1 protein has been shown to regulate FBXL14-Snail1 interaction by increasing their affinity [104].

An independent shRNA screening identified SCF-FBXL5 as a nuclear Snail1 E3 ubiquitin ligase binding to Snail1 C-terminal and targeting lysines 85, 146, and 234 [105]. Besides promoting degradation, Snail1-K234 ubiquitination by FBXL5 also decreases Snail1 interaction with the DNA. Curiously, FBXL5-mediated degradation is blocked after nuclear export inhibition, suggesting that the cytosolic relocation of ubiquitinated Snail1 is required in order to be efficiently degraded. FBXL5 protein stability requires iron and oxygen that bind to its N-terminal hemerythrin domain [106,107] and it is decreased by hypoxia [107] and by γ-irradiation (IR) [105]. FBXL5 suppresses invasion of gastric cancer cells by reducing the levels of Snail1 [108].

Finally, another E3 ligase acting on Snail1 is FBXO45 (F-box/SPRY domain–containing protein 1). Besides Snail1, this enzyme targets Snail2, Zeb1/2, and Twist1 [109]. In contrast to the other Snail1 E3 ligases, FBXO45 does not form an SCF complex [110].

It is remarkable that most FBX proteins controlling Snail1 stability are regulated by miRNAs: miR-17/20a controls FBXL14 [111], miR-27a targets FBXO45 [109], and FBXL5 mRNA levels are negatively regulated by miR-1306-3p; therefore, miR-1306-3p expression results in increased Snail1 protein stability [112].

As stated before, Snail1 degradation is intimately related with its phosphorylation status [86]. For this reason, Snail1 C-terminal domain dephosphorylation by small phosphatases promotes Snail1 stabilization [113,114]. Recently, the protein tyrosine phosphatase PTEN has been shown to change its tyrosine phosphatase activity after MEX3C-catalyzed K27-linked polyubiquitination triggered by high glucose, TGFβ or IL-6; K27-polyUb PTEN dephosphorylates the phosphoserine/threonine of several proteins involved in EMT, including S96 in Snail1, leading to its accumulation [115]. Snail1 stabilization is also triggered by TNF-α during inflammation and is mediated by the COP9 signalosome 2 protein (CSN2), which blocks the phosphorylation and ubiquitination of Snail1 by disrupting its binding to GSK-3β and β-TrCP1 [116]. However, phosphorylation is not always linked to degradation, and, intriguingly, some kinases may modify residues involved in protein instability to induce the contrary effect, Snail1 stabilization. This is the case for ATM that phosphorylates S100 increasing Snail1 half-life [117]; however this residue has also been related to GSK-3β-induced Snail1degradation [89]. This opposed regulation may be dependent on the different interaction of phosphorylated Snail1 with specific factors present in the nucleus or in the cytosol.

Other Snail1 stabilizing phosphorylations modify specific residues located in the C-terminal domain (Figure 1). This is the case for Lats2 kinase induced by TGFβ, which phosphorylates Snail1 on T203 [118] or the p21-activated kinase 1 (PAK1) that acts on S246 [119]. Curiously, whereas modification of this residue stabilizes Snail1, that of S249 by PAR-atypical protein kinase C (aPKC) leads to its degradation [120].

Interestingly, gamma-irradiation and DNA damage promote Snail1 expression and protein stabilization. This effect is mediated through the activation of PAK1 phosphorylating S246 [119] and by ATM and DNA-dependent protein kinase (DNA-PK) that modify S100 [117,121], suggesting the convergence of kinases regulated by cell stress. Other kinases inducing stabilization phosphorylate residues from the Snail1 N-terminal domain as ERK2, which acts on S82 and S104 after being activated by the collagen receptor known as Discoidin domain receptor 2 [122].

Ubiquitination can also promote an increase in Snail1 half-life when catalyzed by Pellino-1, which promotes Snail1 K63-mediated polyubiquitination [123], or by A20 that multi-monoubiquitinates Snail1 [124]. Other, less-studied post transcriptional modifications (PTMs), which also affect Snal1 stability, are polyADP-ribosylation (PARylation) [125] and glycosylation [126]. Snail1 modification by β-N-acetylglucosamine (O-GlcNAc) is triggered by high-glucose levels and has been mapped to S112, preventing phosphorylation by GSK-3β [126]. Snail1 is also modified by sumoylation of K234, a PTM enhanced by TGFβ that controlsSnail1 nuclear retention and cell invasion [127]. Finally, Snail1 is also acetylated by the CREB-binding protein (CBP) at lysines 146 and 187, a modification crucial for its transcriptional activity [128], as discussed below. It has been reported that Snail acetylation also enhances its stability by inhibiting phosphorylation and ubiquitination [129].

E3-dependent protein ubiquitination can be reverted by deubiquitinating enzymes (deubiquitinases, or DUBs), which play a decisive role in substrate stabilization [130]. Snail1 interacts and is deubiquitinated by DUB3 (also known as USP17L2) [131,132] and by USP27X [133]. These two DUBs are induced by cytokines: DUB3 by IL-6 [132] and USP27X by TGFβ [133]. Recently, other DUBs (OTUB1, PSMD14, USP11, USP26, and USP47) have been reported to promote Snail1 deubiquitination [134–138].

## 6. Subcellular Localization

Snail1 transcriptional action requires its accumulation in the nucleus, which seems to be the consequence of inhibited export. Besides being required for function, retention in the nucleus also indirectly controls Snail1 stability, since the most active Snail1 ligases (βTrCP1 and Fbxl14) are located in the cytosol [87]. Nuclear import is mediated by a C-terminus conserved NLS recognized by importins [85]. Nuclear export requires phosphorylation by GSK-3β on residues S104 and S107 to S119; this uncovers the NES (aa 132–143) that binds to Crm1 (Exportin-1) [84,89,139]. Alternatively, Snail1 ubiquitinylation by FBXL5, besides interfering with DNA-binding, facilitates nuclear export and Snail1 degradation in the cytosol [105].

Snail1 nuclear retention is triggered by GSK-3β inhibition. This is accomplished after Wnt stimulation that promotes the Axin2/GSK-3β nuclear export; therefore, phosphorylation-induced Snail1 traffic to the cytosol is blocked [140]. Akt phosphorylation of S9 in GSK-3β also inhibits this enzyme [89]; therefore, pathways activating Akt, such as TNFα, Wnt, and Notch, promote Snail1 nuclear retention [141]. Snail1 nuclear export is also prevented by dephosphorylation [113] or glycosylation, incompatible with the phosphorylation of S112 [126] (see Figure 1). Indirectly, inhibition of priming of GSK-3β phosphorylation also inhibits nuclear export [89,90,142,143]. Other protein kinases stabilizing Snail1 (Lats2, PAK1, or ERK2) also promote their effects enhancing Snail1 nuclear retention and preventing cytosolic degradation [118,119,122]. The mechanisms are not fully understood but may involve the participation of nuclear chaperones such as HSP90 or HSP27, which inhibit the binding of Snail1 to the Crm1 nuclear exporter [117,144]. Recently, the mitogen-activated sumoylation of nuclear Flotilin-1 has been reported to raise its interaction with Snail1 in this compartment and increase its stability [145].

## 7. Post-Translational Modifications Controlling Interaction with Co-Repressors and Co-Activators

Besides interacting with proteins involved in its stability or subcellular localization, Snail1 binds to other factors required for its transcriptional function. Although initially described as a repressor, several reports have determined that Snail1 also actively participates on gene transcription through its binding to mesenchymal promoters [128,146]. This different activity of Snail1 protein as transcriptional repressor or activator is controlled through its binding to different proteins, interactions that are also sensitive to post-translational modifications. We described here some of the cofactors required for these two Snail1 functions. A scheme of the binding of these different cofactors is presented in Figure 2A.

*7.1. Snail1 Binding to Co-Repressors*

The capability of Snail1 to inhibit gene transcription requires its interaction with specific E-boxes presenting a core sequence of 5'-CACCTG-3' (or inverse, 5'-CAGGTG-3'). This binding is mediated by the C-terminal Snail1 domain containing four zinc-fingers. Interestingly, the presence of a Smad-binding element closer to the E-box (about 100 bp) enhances Snail1 repression since Snail1 interacts with the Smad3/Smad4 complex [147]. This can indirectly potentiate the binding of Zeb1 and -2 proteins (also known as Tcf8 and Sip1, respectively) to adjacent E-boxes, since these two factors also associate with Smads [148,149], potentiating and temporally extending the Snail1 repression of epithelial genes.

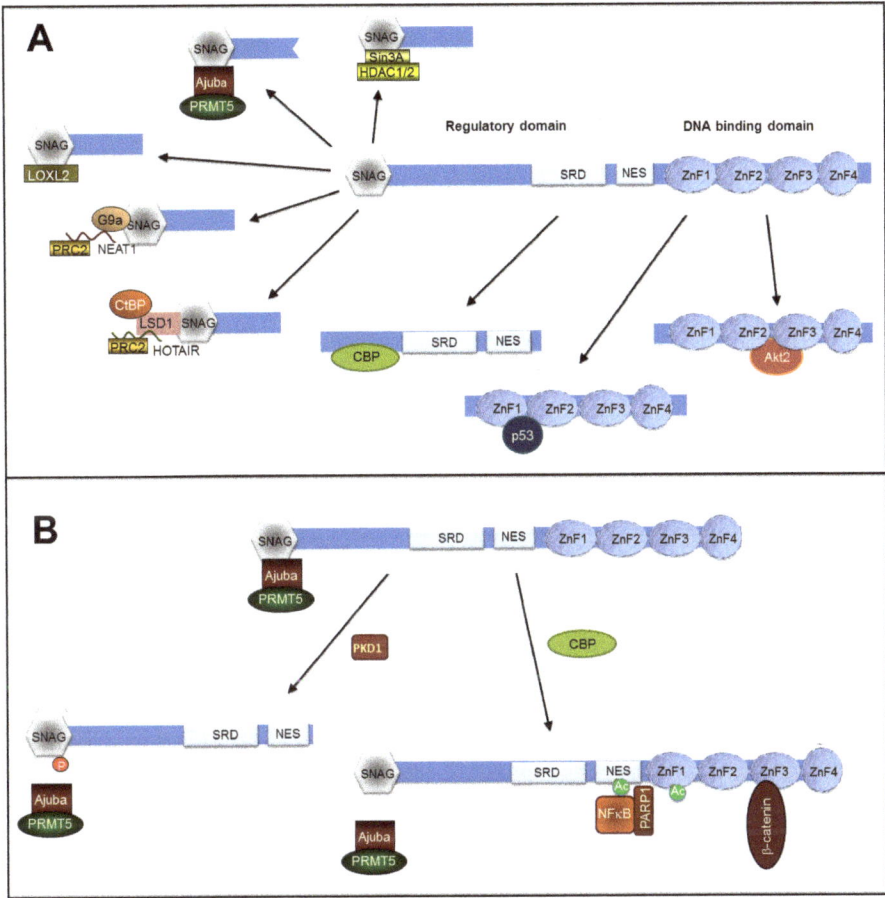

**Figure 2.** Transcriptional cofactors required for Snail1 function. The figure shows a diagram of Snail1 protein with the different corepressors interacting with the SNAG domain (**A**). The binding sites for CBP (required for Snail1-induced activation or mesenchymal genes), p53, and Akt2 are also shown. Other factors also interacting with Snail1 but with still uncharacterized sequences are not shown. In panel (**B**), the effect of PKD1-induced phosphorylation of S11 in the SNAG sequence on the interaction of Ajuba complex is presented. Moreover, this panel also illustrates the switch in Snail1 function promoted by the CBP-catalyzed phosphorylation of K146 and K187 that disrupts the association with Ajuba and facilitates binding to the p65/NFκB complex and presumably also to β-catenin. The Snail1 element interacting with NFκB has not been characterized; binding to β-catenin has been allocated to the C-terminal domain, likely to ZnF3 and -4 (see text).

In contrast to the Drosophila orthologue [150], Snail1 does not contain a binding site for the CtBP co-repressor. Instead, most of the cofactors involved in gene silencing interact with the short SNAG sequence (13 amino acids) placed in the very N-terminal end. For instance, Snail1 associates with the histone deacetylase (HDAC) complex Sin3a/HDAC1/HDAC2; this binding is dependent on the integrity of the SNAG domain [151]. It is unclear if this association is direct or mediated by LIM proteins, a family of proteins that mediate nuclear signaling events. Accordingly, the LIM proteins Ajuba and FHL2 interact with Snail1 and promote E-cadherin repression [152–154]. Besides HDACs, Ajuba also participates in the recruitment of protein arginine methyltransferase 5 (PMRT5), another histone modifier related to gene repression [155]. Snail1 phosphorylation in S11 by PKD1, besides promoting other negative effects on Snail1 function (see Section 5), prevents Snail1 repression by disrupting the interaction with Ajuba [142] (Figure 2B). It is remarkable that Ajuba, like β-catenin, is detected in cadherin-dependent junctions [156], representing an element of the cross-talk between cell–cell contacts, Snail1 function, and EMT (see also below).

Besides HDAC1/2 and PRMT5, other epigenetic regulators such as Polycomb repressive complex 2 (PRC2) are also necessary for Snail1-dependent E-cadherin repression [157]. PRC2 binding to Snail1 also requires the SNAG domain [157] and is associated with the formation of a complex also involving HDAC1 and -2 [158]. Since the PRC2 subunit EzH2 interacts with long non-coding RNAs (lncRNAs) [159], it has been proposed that the lncRNA HOTAIR mediates the interaction of Snail1 to EzH2 through the physical interaction of this lncRNA with both proteins [160]. However, it is possible that it is not Snail1 by itself that binds to HOTAIR but a Snail1-associated factor. A good candidate for this is the Lysine-specific methylase 1 (LSD1)/CoREST/REST complex since it interacts with HOTAIR [159] and to Snail1 through a mechanism in which the SNAG Snail1 domain mimics the histone tail and binds to the active site of LSD1 [161]. Moreover, since LSD1 also associates with CtBP1 [162], it provides the molecular connection between CtBP and the Snail1-repression complex, an association that in Drosophila Snail1 is accomplished by a direct Snail1-CtBP binding [150].

Another co-repressor binding to the Snail1 SNAG sequence is G9a, which forms part of the G9a histone methyltransferase/DNA methyltransferases complex [163]. This complex also interacts with another lncRNA, NEAT1, and is required for the NEAT1- and Snail1-dependent E-cadherin repression [164]; therefore, it is possible that G9a and NEAT1 might also participate in PRC2 recruitment to the Snail1 repressive complex.

Snail1 SNAG domain also binds to Lysyl oxidase-like 2 (LOXL2) [165]. Although it is still a matter of discussion, since for some authors the activity of this enzyme is not relevant in EMT [166], LOXL2 acts as an epigenetic modifier and participates in Snail1-induced gene repression by oxidizing and demethylating K4 in histone 3 [167] and TAF10, blocking TFIID-dependent gene transcription [168]. It is still unknown if, as is the case with Ajuba, binding of G9a, PRC2, and LOXL2 is also blocked by PKD1-dependent Snail1 phosphorylation in S11 or by acetylation (see below).

*7.2. Snail1 Binding to Transcriptional Activators*

Although Snail1 has been extensively studied as a transcriptional repressor, increasing evidence indicates that it also directly activates transcription. Binding of Snail1 to activated promoters of several genes has been reported [146,169–171]. In Drosophila, Snail positively modulates the transcriptional activation of target genes involved in the development through binding to active enhancers [172]. A kinetic study of Snail1 promoter binding during TGFβ-induced EMT has revealed that an initial phase of Snail1 association with repressed promoters, such as *CDH1* (E-cadherin), is followed by the later interaction with mesenchymal genes, such as *FN1* (fibronectin), concomitant with the transcriptional activation of these genes [146]. Whereas repression is dependent on canonical Snail1- binding 5'-CACCTG-3' boxes in the promoter, activation is not and is produced by a Snail1 association with an NFκB/PARP1 complex [146]. Snail1 also interacts with β-catenin stimulating β-catenin-mediated transcription [173]. In both cases, the association does not require the SNAG domain; the binding site in Snail1 has been characterized and corresponds to the C-terminal domain only for β-catenin [173]. Recently, a proposed Snail1-responsive motif, 5'-TCACA-3', has been identified in the promoters of ZEB1, MMP9, and p15INK4, genes activated by Snail1 in collaboration with EGR and SP1 [171]. This Snail1 switch from acting as a transcriptional repressor to an activator is dependent on its interaction with CBP, which acetylates K146 and K187 [128]. Accordingly, CBP and the co-repressors Ajuba and Sin3a are not present in the same Snail1 complexes and ectopic expression of CBP prevents the interaction of Snail1 and these co-repressors [128]. At present, it is not known how modification of these two Lysine residues might disrupt the association of repressors to the SNAG N-terminal sequence and facilitate the binding to co-activators (Figure 2B).

*7.3. Other*

As previously indicated (see Section 3), Snail1 and p53 are mutual antagonists, and p53 de-stabilizes *SNAI1* mRNA by activating miR-34 [58]. Snail1 also represses p53 function. The mechanism of this inhibition is still a matter of discussion: according to some authors, Snail1 and p53 interact [174]; as a consequence, p53 is secreted to the cellular medium and degraded [175]. Other authors have observed the presence of Snail1 and p53 in a complex with HDAC1, which promotes p53 deacetylation and further degradation by the proteasome [176]. However, in other cells, for instance in mesenchymal stem cells, p53 levels are not different in Snail1 KO or control cells [177]. It is unknown if the Snail1 interaction with p53, which requires the two first zinc-fingers in the C-terminal domain (aa 154–208) according to some authors [176] or the middle region (aa 91–112) according to others [174], is controlled by specific PTMs, which might explain the contradictory results observed in different cells.

Snail1 also binds to Akt2 [178], a protein kinase tightly associated with Snail1 function, since it is involved in Snail1 transcription and protein stabilization (see above) and is activated upon Snail1 expression [179,180]. Association with Snail1 enhances Akt activity on T45 in histone H3, a modification associated with transcription termination after DNA damage [181]. Since Snail1 is also upregulated by this insult [153] Snail1–Akt2 binding might contribute to the higher resistance to DNA damaging agents detected in Snail1-expressing cells.

## 8. Conclusions and Future Perspectives

Since Snail1 was characterized in 2000 as a transcriptional repressor of *CDH1* and an inducer of EMT and invasion in tumor cells [83,182], it has been the subject of study for many cancer biologists. Moreover, the implications of Snail1 and EMT in drug resistance, in the acquisition of cancer stem properties, and in other traits involved in tumor development have further fostered this interest. The analysis of Snail1 function has revealed a multilevel control that impinges on all the processes required for protein expression; moreover, multiple PTMs of this protein activate or inhibit Snail1 function. This multiple control has been frequently ignored, and the expression of Snail1 is usually determined only on the basis of its RNA levels, which do not necessarily correlate with protein or Snail1 function, as shown above. Moreover, several aspects of Snail1 action have yet to be clarified, especially those related to its role as a transcriptional activator of mesenchymal genes. It is likely that future research on Snail1 will clarify these issues and better explain Snail1 function in tumoral cells.

**Author Contributions:** Conceptualization: J.B., V.M.D., and A.G.d.H.; writing-original draft preparation: J.B., V.M.D., and A.G.d.H.; design of figures and tables: J.B., V.M.D., and A.G.d.H.; review and editing: J.B., V.M.D., and A.G.d.H.; funding acquisition: A.G.d.H.

**Funding:** Ministerio de Economía, Industria y Competitividad, Gobierno de España: SAF2016-76461-R.

**Acknowledgments:** Work in García de Herreros' laboratory was supported by the Ministerio de Economía y Competitividad (MINECO) co-funded by Fondo Europeo de Desarrollo Regional-FEDER-UE (SAF2016-76461-R).

**Conflicts of Interest:** The authors declare no conflict of interest.

## References

1. Stemmler, M.P.; Eccles, R.L.; Brabletz, S.; Brabletz, T. Non-redundant functions of EMT transcription factors. *Nat. Cell Biol.* **2019**, *21*, 102–112. [CrossRef] [PubMed]
2. Pastushenko, I.; Blanpain, C. EMT Transition States during Tumor Progression and Metastasis. *Trends Cell Biol.* **2019**, *29*, 212–226. [CrossRef] [PubMed]
3. Dongre, A.; Weinberg, R.A. New insights into the mechanisms of epithelial–mesenchymal transition and implications for cancer. *Nat. Rev. Mol. Cell Biol.* **2019**, *20*, 69–84. [CrossRef] [PubMed]
4. Baulida, J.; García de Herreros, A. Snail1-driven plasticity of epithelial and mesenchymal cells sustains cancer malignancy. *Biochim. Biophys. Acta* **2015**, *1856*, 55–61. [CrossRef] [PubMed]
5. Carver, E.A.; Jiang, R.; Lan, Y.; Oram, K.F.; Gridley, T. The mouse snail gene encodes a key regulator of the epithelial-mesenchymal transition. *Mol. Cell. Biol.* **2001**, *21*, 8184–8188. [CrossRef] [PubMed]

6. Nieto, M.A.; Huang, R.Y.; Jackson, R.A.; Thiery, J.P. Emt: 2016. *Cell* **2016**, *166*, 21–45. [CrossRef] [PubMed]
7. Kwa, M.Q.; Herum, K.M.; Brakebusch, C. Cancer-associated fibroblasts: How do they contribute to metastasis? *Clin. Exp. Metastasis* **2019**, *36*, 71–86. [CrossRef]
8. Peinado, H.; Quintanilla, M.; Cano, A. Transforming growth factor beta-1 induces snail transcription factor in epithelial cell lines: Mechanisms for epithelial mesenchymal transitions. *J. Biol. Chem.* **2003**, *278*, 21113–21123. [CrossRef]
9. Cho, H.J.; Baek, K.E.; Saika, S.; Jeong, M.-J.; Yoo, J. Snail is required for transforming growth factor-beta-induced epithelial-mesenchymal transition by activating PI3 kinase/Akt signal pathway. *Biochem. Biophys. Res. Commun.* **2007**, *353*, 337–343. [CrossRef]
10. Hoot, K.E.; Lighthall, J.; Han, G.; Lu, S.-L.L.; Li, A.; Ju, W.; Kulesz-Martin, M.; Bottinger, E.; Wang, X.-J.J. Keratinocyte-specific Smad2 ablation results in increased epithelial-mesenchymal transition during skin cancer formation and progression. *J. Clin. Investig.* **2008**, *118*, 2722–2732. [CrossRef]
11. Thuault, S.; Tan, E.-J.; Peinado, H.; Cano, A.; Heldin, C.-H.; Moustakas, A. HMGA2 and Smads co-regulate SNAIL1 expression during induction of epithelial-to-mesenchymal transition. *J. Biol. Chem.* **2008**, *283*, 33437–33446. [CrossRef] [PubMed]
12. Smith, A.P.; Verrecchia, A.; Faga, G.; Doni, M.; Perna, D.; Martinato, F.; Guccione, E.; Amati, B. A positive role for Myc in TGFbeta-induced Snail transcription and epithelial-to-mesenchymal transition. *Oncogene* **2009**, *28*, 422–430. [CrossRef] [PubMed]
13. Yu, W.; Zhang, Y.; Ruest, L.B.; Svoboda, K.K. Analysis of Snail1 function and regulation by Twist1 in palatal fusion. *Front. Physiol.* **2013**, *4*, 12. [CrossRef] [PubMed]
14. Cichon, M.A.; Radisky, D.C. ROS-induced epithelial-mesenchymal transition in mammary epithelial cells is mediated by NF-kB-dependent activation of Snail. *Oncotarget* **2014**, *5*, 2827–2838. [CrossRef] [PubMed]
15. Jo, E.; Park, S.J.; Choi, Y.S.; Jeon, W.-K.; Kim, B.-C. Kaempferol Suppresses Transforming Growth Factor-beta1-Induced Epithelial-to-Mesenchymal Transition and Migration of A549 Lung Cancer Cells by Inhibiting Akt1-Mediated Phosphorylation of Smad3 at Threonine-179. *Neoplasia* **2015**, *17*, 525–537. [CrossRef]
16. Wang, M.; Zhang, L.; Liu, Z.; Zhou, J.; Pan, Q.; Fan, J.; Zang, R.; Wang, L. AGO1 may influence the prognosis of hepatocellular carcinoma through TGF-beta pathway. *Cell Death Dis.* **2018**, *9*, 324. [CrossRef] [PubMed]
17. Bellomo, C.; Caja, L.; Fabregat, I.; Mikulits, W.; Kardassis, D.; Heldin, C.-H.; Moustakas, A. Snail mediates crosstalk between TGFbeta and LXRalpha in hepatocellular carcinoma. *Cell Death Differ.* **2018**, *25*, 885–903. [CrossRef] [PubMed]
18. Barberà, M.J.; Puig, I.; Domínguez, D.; Julien-Grille, S.; Guaita-Esteruelas, S.; Peiró, S.; Baulida, J.; Francí, C.; Dedhar, S.; Larue, L.; et al. Regulation of Snail transcription during epithelial to mesenchymal transition of tumor cells. *Oncogene* **2004**, *23*, 7345–7354. [CrossRef] [PubMed]
19. Ordoñez-Moreno, A.; Rodriguez-Monterrosas, C.; Cortes-Reynosa, P.; Perez-Carreon, J.I.; Perez Salazar, E. Erythropoietin Induces an Epithelial to Mesenchymal Transition-Like Process in Mammary Epithelial Cells MCF10A. *J. Cell. Biochem.* **2017**, *118*, 2983–2992. [CrossRef]
20. Grille, S.J.; Bellacosa, A.; Upson, J.; Klein-Szanto, A.J.; Van Roy, F.; Lee-Kwon, W.; Donowitz, M.; Tsichlis, P.N.; Larue, L. The protein kinase Akt induces epithelial mesenchymal transition and promotes enhanced motility and invasiveness of squamous cell carcinoma lines. *Cancer Res.* **2003**, *63*, 2172–2178.
21. Julien, S.; Puig, I.; Caretti, E.; Bonaventure, J.; Nelles, L.; Van Roy, F.; Dargemont, C.; García de Herreros, A.; Bellacosa, A.; Larue, L. Activation of NF-κB by Akt upregulates Snail expression and induces epithelium mesenchyme transition. *Oncogene* **2007**, *26*, 7445–7456. [CrossRef] [PubMed]
22. Liu, W.-H.; Chen, M.-T.; Wang, M.-L.; Lee, Y.-Y.; Chiou, G.-Y.; Chien, C.-S.; Huang, P.-I.; Chen, Y.-W.; Huang, M.-C.; Chiou, S.-H.; et al. Cisplatin-selected resistance is associated with increased motility and stem-like properties via activation of STAT3/Snail axis in atypical teratoid/rhabdoid tumor cells. *Oncotarget* **2015**, *6*, 1750–1768. [CrossRef] [PubMed]
23. Saitoh, M.; Endo, K.; Furuya, S.; Minami, M.; Fukasawa, A.; Imamura, T.; Miyazawa, K. STAT3 integrates cooperative Ras and TGF-beta signals that induce Snail expression. *Oncogene* **2016**, *35*, 1049–1057. [CrossRef] [PubMed]
24. Zhou, J.-J.; Meng, Z.; He, X.-Y.; Cheng, D.; Ye, H.-L.; Deng, X.-G.; Chen, R.-F. Hepatitis C virus core protein increases Snail expression and induces epithelial-mesenchymal transition through the signal transducer and activator of transcription 3 pathway in hepatoma cells. *Hepatol. Res.* **2017**, *47*, 574–583. [CrossRef] [PubMed]

25. Dai, X.; Ahn, K.S.; Wang, L.Z.; Kim, C.; Deivasigamni, A.; Arfuso, F.; Um, J.-Y.; Kumar, A.P.; Chang, Y.-C.; Kumar, D.; et al. Ascochlorin Enhances the Sensitivity of Doxorubicin Leading to the Reversal of Epithelial-to-Mesenchymal Transition in Hepatocellular Carcinoma. *Mol. Cancer Ther.* **2016**, *15*, 2966–2976. [CrossRef] [PubMed]
26. Li, Y.; Liu, Y.; Xu, Y.; Voorhees, J.J.; Fisher, G.J. UV irradiation induces Snail expression by AP-1 dependent mechanism in human skin keratinocytes. *J. Dermatol. Sci.* **2010**, *60*, 105–113. [CrossRef]
27. Hsu, Y.-L.; Hou, M.-F.; Kuo, P.-L.; Huang, Y.-F.; Tsai, E.-M. Breast tumor-associated osteoblast-derived CXCL5 increases cancer progression by ERK/MSK1/Elk-1/snail signaling pathway. *Oncogene* **2013**, *32*, 4436–4447. [CrossRef]
28. Ngo, H.-K.-C.; Lee, H.G.; Piao, J.-Y.; Zhong, X.; Lee, H.-N.; Han, H.-J.; Kim, W.; Kim, D.-H.; Cha, Y.-N.; Na, H.-K.; et al. Helicobacter pylori induces Snail expression through ROS-mediated activation of Erk and inactivation of GSK-3beta in human gastric cancer cells. *Mol. Carcinog.* **2016**, *55*, 2236–2246. [CrossRef]
29. Grotegut, S.; Von Schweinitz, D.; Christofori, G.; Lehembre, F. Hepatocyte growth factor induces cell scattering through MAPK/Egr-1-mediated upregulation of Snail. *EMBO J.* **2006**, *25*, 3534–3545. [CrossRef]
30. Kinehara, M.; Kawamura, S.; Mimura, S.; Suga, M.; Hamada, A.; Wakabayashi, M.; Nikawa, H.; Furue, M.K. Protein kinase C-induced early growth response protein-1 binding to SNAIL promoter in epithelial-mesenchymal transition of human embryonic stem cells. *Stem Cells Dev.* **2014**, *23*, 2180–2189. [CrossRef]
31. Peiró, S.; Escrivà, M.; Puig, I.; Barberà, M.J.; Dave, N.; Herranz, N.; Larriba, M.J.; Takkunen, M.; Francí, C.; Muñoz, A.; et al. Snail1 transcriptional repressor binds to its own promoter and controls its expression. *Nucleic Acids Res.* **2006**, *34*, 2077–2084. [CrossRef] [PubMed]
32. Lu, M.; Jolly, M.K.; Levine, H.; Onuchic, J.N.; Ben-Jacob, E. MicroRNA-based regulation of epithelial-hybrid-mesenchymal fate determination. *Proc. Natl. Acad. Sci. USA* **2013**, *110*, 18144–18149. [CrossRef]
33. Wei, P.; Zhang, N.; Wang, Y.; Li, D.; Wang, L.; Sun, X.; Shen, C.; Yang, Y.; Zhou, X.; Du, X. FOXM1 promotes lung adenocarcinoma invasion and metastasis by upregulating SNAIL. *Int. J. Biol. Sci.* **2015**, *11*, 186–198. [CrossRef]
34. Song, S.; Zhang, R.; Cao, W.; Fang, G.; Yu, Y.; Wan, Y.; Wang, C.; Li, Y.; Wang, Q. Foxm1 is a critical driver of TGF-beta-induced EndMT in endothelial cells through Smad2/3 and binds to the Snail promoter. *J. Cell. Physiol.* **2019**, *234*, 9052–9064. [CrossRef]
35. McPhee, T.R.; McDonald, P.C.; Oloumi, A.; Dedhar, S. Integrin-linked kinase regulates E-cadherin expression through PARP-1. *Dev. Dyn.* **2008**, *237*, 2737–2747. [CrossRef] [PubMed]
36. Yuen, H.-F.; Chan, Y.-K.; Grills, C.; McCrudden, C.M.; Gunasekharan, V.; Shi, Z.; Wong, A.S.-Y.; Lappin, T.R.; Chan, K.-W.; Fennell, D.A.; et al. Polyomavirus enhancer activator 3 protein promotes breast cancer metastatic progression through Snail-induced epithelial-mesenchymal transition. *J. Pathol.* **2011**, *224*, 78–89. [CrossRef] [PubMed]
37. Gnemmi, V.; Bouillez, A.; Gaudelot, K.; Hemon, B.; Ringot, B.; Pottier, N.; Glowacki, F.; Villers, A.; Vindrieux, D.; Cauffiez, C.; et al. MUC1 drives epithelial-mesenchymal transition in renal carcinoma through Wnt/beta-catenin pathway and interaction with SNAIL promoter. *Cancer Lett.* **2014**, *346*, 225–236. [CrossRef]
38. Zhang, M.; Zhang, H.; Cheng, S.; Zhang, D.; Xu, Y.; Bai, X.; Xia, S.; Zhang, L.; Ma, J.; Du, M.; et al. Prostaglandin E2 accelerates invasion by upregulating Snail in hepatocellular carcinoma cells. *Tumour Biol.* **2014**, *35*, 7135–7145. [CrossRef]
39. Bao, Y.; Gu, D.; Feng, W.; Sun, X.; Wang, X.; Zhang, X.; Shi, Q.; Cui, G.; Yu, H.; Tang, C.; et al. COUP-TFII regulates metastasis of colorectal adenocarcinoma cells by modulating Snail1. *Br. J. Cancer* **2014**, *111*, 933–943. [CrossRef]
40. Qian, Y.; Yao, W.; Yang, T.; Yang, Y.; Liu, Y.; Shen, Q.; Zhang, J.; Qi, W.; Wang, J. aPKC-iota/P-Sp1/Snail signaling induces epithelial-mesenchymal transition and immunosuppression in cholangiocarcinoma. *Hepatology* **2017**, *66*, 1165–1182. [CrossRef]
41. Zhang, L.; Huang, G.; Li, X.; Zhang, Y.; Jiang, Y.; Shen, J.; Liu, J.; Wang, Q.; Zhu, J.; Feng, X.; et al. Hypoxia induces epithelial-mesenchymal transition via activation of SNAI1 by hypoxia-inducible factor -1$\alpha$ in hepatocellular carcinoma. *BMC Cancer* **2013**, *13*, 108. [CrossRef] [PubMed]
42. Bossart, E.A.; Tasdemir, N.; Sikora, M.J.; Bahreini, A.; Levine, K.M.; Chen, J.; Basudan, A.; Jacobsen, B.M.; Burns, T.F.; Oesterreich, S. SNAIL is induced by tamoxifen and leads to growth inhibition in invasive lobular breast carcinoma. *Breast Cancer Res. Treat.* **2019**. [CrossRef] [PubMed]

43. Martínez-Estrada, O.M.; Lettice, L.A.; Essafi, A.; Guadix, J.A.; Slight, J.; Velecela, V.; Hall, E.; Reichmann, J.; Devenney, P.S.; Hohenstein, P.; et al. Wt1 is required for cardiovascular progenitor cell formation through transcriptional control of Snail and E-cadherin. *Nat. Genet.* **2010**, *42*, 89–93. [CrossRef] [PubMed]
44. Fujita, N.; Kajita, M.; Jaye, D.L.; Wade, P.A.; Geigerman, C.; Moreno, C.S. MTA3, a Mi-2/NuRD Complex Subunit, Regulates an Invasive Growth Pathway in Breast Cancer. *Cell* **2003**, *113*, 207–219. [CrossRef]
45. Lai, D.-W.; Liu, S.-H.; Karlsson, A.I.; Lee, W.-J.; Wang, K.-B.; Chen, Y.-C.; Shen, C.-C.; Wu, S.-M.; Liu, C.-Y.; Tien, H.-R.; et al. The novel Aryl hydrocarbon receptor inhibitor biseugenol inhibits gastric tumor growth and peritoneal dissemination. *Oncotarget* **2014**, *5*, 7788–7804. [CrossRef] [PubMed]
46. Wang, G.; Tang, J.; Zhan, W.; Zhang, R.; Zhang, M.; Liao, D.; Wang, X.; Wu, Y.; Kang, T. CBX8 Suppresses Tumor Metastasis via Repressing Snail in Esophageal Squamous Cell Carcinoma. *Theranostics* **2017**, *7*, 3478–3488. [CrossRef] [PubMed]
47. Fraga, M.F.; Herranz, M.; Espada, J.J.; Ballestar, E.; Paz, M.F.; Ropero, S.; Erkek, E.; Bozdogan, O.; Peinado, H.H.; Niveleau, A.; et al. A mouse skin multistage carcinogenesis model reflects the aberrant DNA methylation patterns of human tumors. *Cancer Res.* **2004**, *64*, 5527–5534. [CrossRef]
48. Carter, C.L.; Lin, C.; Liu, C.-Y.Y.; Yang, L.; Liu, Z.-R.R. Phosphorylated p68 RNA helicase activates snail1 transcription by promoting HDAC1 dissociation from the snail1 promoter. *Oncogene* **2010**, *29*, 5427–5436. [CrossRef]
49. Zhao, Z.; Sun, C.; Li, F.; Han, J.; Li, X.; Song, Z. Overexpression of histone demethylase JMJD5 promotes metastasis and indicates a poor prognosis in breast cancer. *Int. J. Clin. Exp. Pathol.* **2015**, *8*, 10325–10334.
50. Chandel, N.; Ayasolla, K.S.; Lan, X.; Sultana-Syed, M.; Chawla, A.; Lederman, R.; Vethantham, V.; Saleem, M.A.; Chander, P.N.; Malhotra, A.; et al. Epigenetic Modulation of Human Podocyte Vitamin D Receptor in HIV Milieu. *J. Mol. Biol.* **2015**, *427*, 3201–3215. [CrossRef]
51. Ren, X.; Yang, X.; Cheng, B.; Chen, X.; Zhang, T.; He, Q.; Li, B.; Li, Y.; Tang, X.; Wen, X.; et al. HOPX hypermethylation promotes metastasis via activating SNAIL transcription in nasopharyngeal carcinoma. *Nat. Commun.* **2017**, *8*, 14053. [CrossRef] [PubMed]
52. Zhang, H.; Zhang, Y.; Chen, C.; Zhu, X.; Zhang, C.; Xia, Y.; Zhao, Y.; Andrisani, O.M.; Kong, L. A double-negative feedback loop between DEAD-box protein DDX21 and Snail regulates epithelial-mesenchymal transition and metastasis in breast cancer. *Cancer Lett.* **2018**, *437*, 67–78. [CrossRef] [PubMed]
53. Yang, W.; Su, Y.; Hou, C.; Chen, L.; Zhou, D.; Ren, K.; Zhou, Z.; Zhang, R.; Liu, X. SETDB1 induces epithelialmesenchymal transition in breast carcinoma by directly binding with Snail promoter. *Oncol. Rep.* **2019**, *41*, 1284–1292. [PubMed]
54. Zhang, J.; Jia, L.; Liu, T.; Yip, Y.L.; Tang, W.C.; Lin, W.; Deng, W.; Lo, K.W.; You, C.; Lung, M.L.; et al. mTORC2-mediated PDHE1alpha nuclear translocation links EBV-LMP1 reprogrammed glucose metabolism to cancer metastasis in nasopharyngeal carcinoma. *Oncogene* **2019**. [CrossRef] [PubMed]
55. Wang, Y.-Q.; Jiang, D.-M.; Hu, S.-S.; Zhao, L.; Wang, L.; Yang, M.-H.; Ai, M.-L.; Jiang, H.-J.; Han, Y.; Ding, Y.-Q.; et al. SATB2-AS1 suppresses colorectal carcinoma aggressiveness by inhibiting SATB2-dependent Snail transcription and epithelial-mesenchymal transition. *Cancer Res.* **2019**. [CrossRef]
56. Palmer, M.B.; Majumder, P.; Green, M.R.; Wade, P.A.; Boss, J.M. A 3′ enhancer controls snail expression in melanoma cells. *Cancer Res.* **2007**, *67*, 6113–6120. [CrossRef] [PubMed]
57. Ørom, U.A.; Derrien, T.; Beringer, M.; Gumireddy, K.; Gardini, A.; Bussotti, G.; Lai, F.; Zytnicki, M.; Notredame, C.; Huang, Q.; et al. Long noncoding RNAs with enhancer-like function in human cells. *Cell* **2010**, *143*, 46–58. [CrossRef]
58. Kim, N.H.; Kim, H.S.; Li, X.-Y.; Lee, I.; Choi, H.-S.; Kang, S.E.; Cha, S.Y.; Ryu, J.K.; Yoon, D.; Fearon, E.R.; et al. A p53/miRNA-34 axis regulates Snail1-dependent cancer cell epithelial-mesenchymal transition. *J. Cell Biol.* **2011**, *195*, 417–433. [CrossRef]
59. Tang, Y.; Tang, Y.; Cheng, Y.-S. miR-34a inhibits pancreatic cancer progression through Snail1-mediated epithelial-mesenchymal transition and the Notch signaling pathway. *Sci. Rep.* **2017**, *7*, 38232. [CrossRef]
60. Zhang, J.; Tian, X.-J.; Zhang, H.; Teng, Y.; Li, R.; Bai, F.; Elankumaran, S.; Xing, J. TGF-beta-induced epithelial-to-mesenchymal transition proceeds through stepwise activation of multiple feedback loops. *Sci. Signal.* **2014**, *7*, ra91. [CrossRef]
61. Jolly, M.K.; Boareto, M.; Huang, B.; Jia, D.; Lu, M.; Ben-Jacob, E.; Onuchic, J.N.; Levine, H. Implications of the Hybrid Epithelial/Mesenchymal Phenotype in Metastasis. *Front. Oncol.* **2015**, *5*, 155. [CrossRef]

62. Celià-Terrassa, T.; Bastian, C.; Liu, D.D.; Ell, B.; Aiello, N.M.; Wei, Y.; Zamalloa, J.; Blanco, A.M.; Hang, X.; Kunisky, D.; et al. Hysteresis control of epithelial-mesenchymal transition dynamics conveys a distinct program with enhanced metastatic ability. *Nat. Commun.* **2018**, *9*, 5005. [CrossRef] [PubMed]
63. Gradus, B.; Alon, I.; Hornstein, E. miRNAs control tracheal chondrocyte differentiation. *Dev. Biol.* **2011**, *360*, 58–65. [CrossRef] [PubMed]
64. Zhang, J.; Zhang, H.; Liu, J.; Tu, X.; Zang, Y.; Zhu, J.; Chen, J.; Dong, L.; Zhang, J. miR-30 inhibits TGF-beta1-induced epithelial-to-mesenchymal transition in hepatocyte by targeting Snail1. *Biochem. Biophys. Res. Commun.* **2012**, *417*, 1100–1105. [CrossRef] [PubMed]
65. Roy, S.; Benz, F.; Vargas Cardenas, D.; Vucur, M.; Gautheron, J.; Schneider, A.; Hellerbrand, C.; Pottier, N.; Alder, J.; Tacke, F.; et al. miR-30c and miR-193 are a part of the TGF-beta-dependent regulatory network controlling extracellular matrix genes in liver fibrosis. *J. Dig. Dis.* **2015**, *16*, 513–524. [CrossRef] [PubMed]
66. Zheng, Z.; Guan, M.; Jia, Y.; Wang, D.; Pang, R.; Lv, F.; Xiao, Z.; Wang, L.; Zhang, H.; Xue, Y. The coordinated roles of miR-26a and miR-30c in regulating TGFbeta1-induced epithelial-to-mesenchymal transition in diabetic nephropathy. *Sci. Rep.* **2016**, *6*, 37492. [CrossRef]
67. Wang, D.; Zhu, C.; Zhang, Y.; Zheng, Y.; Ma, F.; Su, L.; Shao, G. MicroRNA-30e-3p inhibits cell invasion and migration in clear cell renal cell carcinoma by targeting Snail1. *Oncol. Lett.* **2017**, *13*, 2053–2058. [CrossRef]
68. Zhao, Y.; Yin, Z.; Li, H.; Fan, J.; Yang, S.; Chen, C.; Wang, D.W. MiR-30c protects diabetic nephropathy by suppressing epithelial-to-mesenchymal transition in db/db mice. *Aging Cell* **2017**, *16*, 387–400. [CrossRef]
69. Xia, W.; Ma, X.; Li, X.; Dong, H.; Yi, J.; Zeng, W.; Yang, Z. miR-153 inhibits epithelial-to-mesenchymal transition in hepatocellular carcinoma by targeting Snail. *Oncol. Rep.* **2015**, *34*, 655–662. [CrossRef]
70. Bracken, C.P.; Gregory, P.A.; Kolesnikoff, N.; Bert, A.G.; Wang, J.; Shannon, M.F.; Goodall, G.J. A double-negative feedback loop between ZEB1-SIP1 and the microRNA-200 family regulates epithelial-mesenchymal transition. *Cancer Res.* **2008**, *68*, 7846–7854. [CrossRef]
71. Wang, K.; Jin, W.; Jin, P.; Fei, X.; Wang, X.; Chen, X. miR-211-5p Suppresses Metastatic Behavior by Targeting SNAI1 in Renal Cancer. *Mol. Cancer Res.* **2017**, *15*, 448–456. [CrossRef]
72. Jin, Y.; Wang, J.; Han, J.; Luo, D.; Sun, Z. MiR-122 inhibits epithelial-mesenchymal transition in hepatocellular carcinoma by targeting Snail1 and Snail2 and suppressing WNT/beta-cadherin signaling pathway. *Exp. Cell Res.* **2017**, *360*, 210–217. [CrossRef] [PubMed]
73. Evdokimova, V.; Tognon, C.; Ng, T.; Ruzanov, P.; Melnyk, N.; Fink, D.; Sorokin, A.; Ovchinnikov, L.P.; Davicioni, E.; Triche, T.J.; et al. Translational Activation of Snail1 and Other Developmentally Regulated Transcription Factors by YB-1 Promotes an Epithelial-Mesenchymal Transition. *Cancer Cell* **2009**, *15*, 402–415. [CrossRef] [PubMed]
74. Wu, K.; Chen, K.; Wang, C.; Jiao, X.; Wang, L.; Zhou, J.; Wang, J.; Li, Z.; Addya, S.; Sorensen, P.H.; et al. Cell fate factor DACH1 represses YB-1-mediated oncogenic transcription and translation. *Cancer Res.* **2014**, *74*, 829–839. [CrossRef]
75. Jimenez, J.; Jang, G.M.; Semler, B.L.; Waterman, M.L. An internal ribosome entry site mediates translation of lymphoid enhancer factor-1. *RNA* **2005**, 1385–1399. [CrossRef] [PubMed]
76. Beltran, M.; Puig, I.; Peña, C.; García, J.M.; Álvarez, A.B.; Peña, R.; Bonilla, F.; García de Herreros, A. A natural antisense transcript regulates Zeb2/Sip1 gene expression during Snail1-induced epithelial-mesenchymal transition. *Genes Dev.* **2008**, *22*, 756–769. [CrossRef]
77. El-Naggar, A.M.; Veinotte, C.J.; Cheng, H.; Grunewald, T.G.P.; Negri, G.L.; Somasekharan, S.P.; Corkery, D.P.; Tirode, F.; Mathers, J.; Khan, D.; et al. Translational Activation of HIF1$\alpha$ by YB-1 Promotes Sarcoma Metastasis. *Cancer Cell* **2015**, *27*, 682–697. [CrossRef]
78. Robichaud, N.; Del Rincon, S.V.; Huor, B.; Alain, T.; Petruccelli, L.A.; Hearnden, J.; Goncalves, C.; Grotegut, S.; Spruck, C.H.; Furic, L.; et al. Phosphorylation of eIF4E promotes EMT and metastasis via translational control of SNAIL and MMP-3. *Oncogene* **2014**, *34*, 2032–2042. [CrossRef]
79. Smith, K.A.; Zhou, B.; Avdulov, S.; Benyumov, A.; Peterson, M.; Liu, Y.; Okon, A.; Hergert, P.; Braziunas, J.; Wagner, C.R.; et al. Transforming Growth Factor-$\beta$1 Induced Epithelial Mesenchymal Transition is blocked by a chemical antagonist of translation factor eIF4E. *Sci. Rep.* **2015**, *5*. [CrossRef]
80. Cai, W.; Ye, Q.; She, Q.-B. Loss of 4E-BP1 function induces EMT and promotes cancer cell migration and invasion via cap-dependent translational activation of snail. *Oncotarget* **2015**, *5*, 6015–6027. [CrossRef]

81. Wang, J.; Ye, Q.; Cao, Y.; Guo, Y.; Huang, X.; Mi, W.; Liu, S.; Wang, C.; Yang, H.S.; Zhou, B.P.; et al. Snail determines the therapeutic response to mTOR kinase inhibitors by transcriptional repression of 4E-BP1. *Nat. Commun.* **2017**, *8*, 2207. [CrossRef] [PubMed]
82. Lin, X.; Chai, G.; Wu, Y.; Li, J.; Chen, F.; Liu, J.; Luo, G.; Tauler, J.; Du, J.; Lin, S.; et al. RNA m6A methylation regulates the epithelial mesenchymal transition of cancer cells and translation of Snail1. *Nat. Commun.* **2019**, *10*, 2065. [CrossRef] [PubMed]
83. Batlle, E.; Sancho, E.; Francí, C.; Domínguez, D.; Monfar, M.; Baulida, J.; García de Herreros, A. The transcription factor snail is a repressor of E-cadherin gene expression in epithelial tumour cells. *Nat. Cell Biol.* **2000**, *2*, 84–89. [CrossRef] [PubMed]
84. Domínguez, D.; Montserrat-Sentís, B.; Virgós-Soler, A.; Guaita, S.; Grueso, J.; Porta, M.; Puig, I.; Baulida, J.; Francí, C.; García de Herreros, A. Phosphorylation regulates the subcellular location and activity of the snail transcriptional repressor. *Mol. Cell. Biol.* **2003**, *23*, 5078–5089. [CrossRef] [PubMed]
85. Mingot, J.-M.; Vega, S.; Maestro, B.; Sanz, J.M.; Nieto, M.A. Characterization of Snail nuclear import pathways as representatives of C2H2 zinc finger transcription factors. *J. Cell Sci.* **2009**, *122*, 1452–1460. [CrossRef] [PubMed]
86. Díaz, V.M.; Viñas-Castells, R.; García de Herreros, A. Regulation of the protein stability of EMT transcription factors. *Cell Adh. Migr.* **2014**, *8*, 418–428. [CrossRef] [PubMed]
87. Díaz, V.M.; García de Herreros, A. F-box proteins: Keeping the epithelial-to-mesenchymal transition (EMT) in check. *Semin. Cancer Biol.* **2016**, *36*, 71–79. [CrossRef]
88. Wu, G.; Xu, G.; Schulman, B.A.; Jeffrey, P.D.; Harper, J.W.; Pavletich, N.P. Structure of a β-TrCP1-Skp1-β-catenin complex: Destruction motif binding and lysine specificity of the SCFβ-TrCP1 ubiquitin ligase. *Mol. Cell* **2003**, *11*, 1445–1456. [CrossRef]
89. Zhou, B.P.; Deng, J.; Xia, W.; Xu, J.; Li, Y.M.; Gunduz, M.; Hung, M.-C. Dual regulation of Snail by GSK-3beta-mediated phosphorylation in control of epithelial-mesenchymal transition. *Nat. Cell Biol.* **2004**, *6*, 931–940. [CrossRef]
90. Xu, Y.; Lee, S.H.; Kim, H.S.; Kim, N.H.; Piao, S.; Park, S.H.; Jung, Y.S.; Yook, J.I.; Park, B.J.; Ha, N.C. Role of CK1 in GSK3B-mediated phosphorylation and degradation of Snail. *Oncogene* **2010**, *29*, 3124–3133. [CrossRef]
91. Deshiere, A.; Duchemin-Pelletier, E.; Spreux, E.; Ciais, D.; Combes, F.; Vandenbrouck, Y.; Couté, Y.; Mikaelian, I.; Giusiano, S.; Charpin, C.; et al. Unbalanced expression of CK2 kinase subunits is sufficient to drive epithelial-to-mesenchymal transition by Snail1 induction. *Oncogene* **2013**, *32*, 1373–1383. [CrossRef] [PubMed]
92. Zheng, H.; Shen, M.; Zha, Y.L.; Li, W.; Wei, Y.; Blanco, M.A.; Ren, G.; Zhou, T.; Storz, P.; Wang, H.Y.; et al. PKD1 Phosphorylation-Dependent Degradation of SNAIL by SCF-FBXO11 Regulates Epithelial-Mesenchymal Transition and Metastasis. *Cancer Cell* **2014**, *26*, 358–373. [CrossRef] [PubMed]
93. Jin, Y.; Shenoy, A.K.; Doernberg, S.; Chen, H.; Luo, H.; Shen, H.; Lin, T.; Tarrash, M.; Cai, Q.; Hu, X.; et al. FBXO11 promotes ubiquitination of the Snail family of transcription factors in cancer progression and epidermal development. *Cancer Lett.* **2015**, *362*, 70–82. [CrossRef] [PubMed]
94. Xiao, G.; Li, Y.; Wang, M.; Li, X.; Qin, S.; Sun, X.; Liang, R.; Zhang, B.; Du, N.; Xu, C.; et al. FBXW7 suppresses epithelial-mesenchymal transition and chemo-resistance of non-small-cell lung cancer cells by targeting snail for ubiquitin-dependent degradation. *Cell Prolif.* **2018**, *51*, e12473. [CrossRef] [PubMed]
95. Zhang, Y.; Zhang, X.; Ye, M.; Jing, P.; Xiong, J.; Han, Z.; Kong, J.; Li, M.; Lai, X.; Chang, N.; et al. FBW7 loss promotes epithelial-to-mesenchymal transition in non-small cell lung cancer through the stabilization of Snail protein. *Cancer Lett.* **2018**, *419*, 75–83. [CrossRef] [PubMed]
96. Li, N.; Babaei-Jadidi, R.; Lorenzi, F.; Spencer-Dene, B.; Clarke, P.; Domingo, E.; Tulchinsky, E.; Vries, R.G.J.; Kerr, D.; Pan, Y.; et al. An FBXW7-ZEB2 axis links EMT and tumour microenvironment to promote colorectal cancer stem cells and chemoresistance. *Oncogenesis* **2019**, *8*, 13. [CrossRef]
97. Cheng, Y.; Li, G. Role of the ubiquitin ligase Fbw7 in cancer progression. *Cancer Metastasis Rev.* **2012**, *31*, 75–87. [CrossRef]
98. Sun, R.; Xie, H.Y.; Qian, J.X.; Huang, Y.N.; Yang, F.; Zhang, F.L.; Shao, Z.M.; Li, D.Q. FBXO22 possesses both protumorigenic and antimetastatic roles in breast cancer progression. *Cancer Res.* **2018**, *78*, 5274–5286. [CrossRef]
99. Zou, S.; Ma, C.; Yang, F.; Xu, X.; Jia, J.; Liu, Z. FBXO31 Suppresses Gastric Cancer EMT by Targeting Snail1 for Proteasomal Degradation. *Mol. Cancer Res.* **2017**, *16*, 286–295. [CrossRef]

100. Viñas-Castells, R.; Beltran, M.; Valls, G.; Gómez, I.; García, J.M.; Montserrat-Sentís, B.; Baulida, J.; Bonilla, F.; García de Herreros, A.; Díaz, V.M. The hypoxia-controlled FBXL14 ubiquitin ligase targets SNAIL1 for proteasome degradation. *J. Biol. Chem.* **2010**, *285*, 3794–3805. [CrossRef]
101. Lander, R.; Nordin, K.; LaBonne, C. The F-box protein Ppa is a common regulator of core EMT factors Twist, Snail, Slug, and Sip1. *J. Cell Biol.* **2011**, *194*, 17–25. [CrossRef] [PubMed]
102. Yang, M.H.; Wu, M.Z.; Chiou, S.H.; Chen, P.M.; Chang, S.Y.; Liu, C.J.; Teng, S.C.; Wu, K.J. Direct regulation of TWIST by HIF-1α promotes metastasis. *Nat. Cell Biol.* **2008**, *10*, 295–305. [CrossRef] [PubMed]
103. Chen, J.; Imanaka, N.; Griffin, J.D. Hypoxia potentiates Notch signaling in breast cancer leading to decreased E-cadherin expression and increased cell migration and invasion. *Br. J. Cancer* **2009**, *102*, 351–360. [CrossRef] [PubMed]
104. Song, L.; Guo, J.; Chang, R.; Peng, X.; Li, J.; Xu, X.; Zhan, X.; Zhan, L. LKB1 obliterates Snail stability and inhibits pancreatic cancer metastasis in response to metformin treatment. *Cancer Sci.* **2018**, *109*, 1382–1392. [CrossRef] [PubMed]
105. Viñas-Castells, R.; Frías, Á.; Robles-Lanuza, E.; Zhang, K.; Longmore, G.D.; García de Herreros, A.; Díaz, V.M. Nuclear ubiquitination by FBXL5 modulates Snail1 DNA binding and stability. *Nucleic Acids Res.* **2014**, *42*, 1079–1094. [CrossRef] [PubMed]
106. Salahudeen, A.A.; Thompson, J.W.; Ruiz, J.C.; Ma, H.W.; Kinch, L.N.; Li, Q.; Grishin, N.V.; Bruick, R.K. An E3 ligase possessing an iron-responsive hemerythrin domain is a regulator of iron homeostasis. *Science* **2009**, *326*, 722–726. [CrossRef] [PubMed]
107. Vashisht, A.A.; Zumbrennen, K.B.; Huang, X.; Powers, D.N.; Durazo, A.; Sun, D.; Bhaskaran, N.; Persson, A.; Uhlen, M.; Sangfeit, O.; et al. Control of iron homeostasis by an iron-regulated ubiquitin ligase. *Science* **2009**, *326*, 718–721. [CrossRef] [PubMed]
108. Wu, W.; Ding, H.; Cao, J.; Zhang, W. FBXL5 inhibits metastasis of gastric cancer through suppressing Snail1. *Cell. Physiol. Biochem.* **2015**, *35*, 1764–1772. [CrossRef] [PubMed]
109. Xu, M.; Zhu, C.; Zhao, X.; Chen, C.; Zhang, H.; Yuan, H.; Deng, R.; Dou, J.; Wang, Y.; Huang, J.; et al. Atypical ubiquitin E3 ligase complex Skp1-Pam-Fbxo45 controls the core epithelial-to-mesenchymal transition-inducing transcription factors. *Oncotarget* **2015**, *6*, 979–994. [CrossRef] [PubMed]
110. Saiga, T.; Fukuda, T.; Matsumoto, M.; Tada, H.; Okano, H.J.; Okano, H.; Nakayama, K.I. Fbxo45 Forms a Novel Ubiquitin Ligase Complex and Is Required for Neuronal Development. *Mol. Cell. Biol.* **2009**, *29*, 3529–3543. [CrossRef] [PubMed]
111. Cui, Y.H.; Kim, H.; Lee, M.; Yi, J.M.; Kim, R.K.; Uddin, N.; Yoo, K.C.; Kang, J.H.; Choi, M.Y.; Cha, H.J.; et al. FBXL14 abolishes breast cancer progression by targeting CDCP1 for proteasomal degradation. *Oncogene* **2018**, *37*, 5794–5809. [CrossRef]
112. He, Z.J.; Li, W.; Chen, H.; Wen, J.; Gao, Y.F.; Liu, Y.J. miR-1306–3p targets FBXL5 to promote metastasis of hepatocellular carcinoma through suppressing snail degradation. *Biochem. Biophys. Res. Commun.* **2018**, *504*, 820–826. [CrossRef]
113. Wu, Y.; Mark Evers, B.; Zhou, B.P. Small C-terminal domain phosphatase enhances snail activity through dephosphorylation. *J. Biol. Chem.* **2009**, *284*, 640–648. [CrossRef]
114. Zhao, Y.; Liu, J.; Chen, F.; Feng, X.H. C-terminal domain small phosphatase-like 2 promotes epithelial-to-mesenchymal transition via Snail dephosphorylation and stabilization. *Open Biol.* **2018**, *8*, 170274. [CrossRef]
115. Hu, Q.; Li, C.; Wang, S.; Li, Y.; Wen, B.; Zhang, Y.; Liang, K.; Yao, J.; Ye, Y.; Hsiao, H.; et al. LncRNAs-directed PTEN enzymatic switch governs epithelial–mesenchymal transition. *Cell Res.* **2019**, *29*, 286–304. [CrossRef]
116. Wu, Y.; Deng, J.; Rychahou, P.G.; Qiu, S.; Evers, B.M.; Zhou, B.P. Stabilization of Snail by NF-κB Is Required for Inflammation-Induced Cell Migration and Invasion. *Cancer Cell* **2009**, *15*, 416–428. [CrossRef]
117. Sun, M.; Guo, X.; Qian, X.; Wang, H.; Yang, C.; Brinkman, K.L.; Serrano-Gonzalez, M.; Jope, R.S.; Zhou, B.; Engler, D.A.; et al. Activation of the ATM-Snail pathway promotes breast cancer metastasis. *J. Mol. Cell Biol.* **2012**, *4*, 304–315. [CrossRef]
118. Zhang, K.; Rodriguez-Aznar, E.; Yabuta, N.; Owen, R.J.; Mingot, J.M.; Nojima, H.; Nieto, M.A.; Longmore, G.D. Lats2 kinase potentiates Snail1 activity by promoting nuclear retention upon phosphorylation. *EMBO J.* **2012**, *31*, 29–43. [CrossRef]
119. Yang, Z.; Rayala, S.; Nguyen, D.; Vadlamudi, R.K.; Chen, S.; Kumar, R. Pak1 phosphorylation of Snail, a master regulator of epithelial-to- mesenchyme transition, modulates Snail's subcellular localization and functions. *Cancer Res.* **2005**, *65*, 3179–3184. [CrossRef]

120. Jung, H.Y.; Fattet, L.; Tsai, J.H.; Kajimoto, T.; Chang, Q.; Newton, A.C.; Yang, J. Apical–basal polarity inhibits epithelial–mesenchymal transition and tumour metastasis by PAR-complex-mediated SNAI1 degradation. *Nat. Cell Biol.* **2019**, *21*, 359–371. [CrossRef]
121. Pyun, B.J.; Seo, H.R.; Lee, H.J.; Jin, Y.B.; Kim, E.J.; Kim, N.H.; Kim, H.S.; Nam, H.W.; Yook, J.I.; Lee, Y.S. Mutual regulation between DNA-PKcs and snail1 leads to increased genomic instability and aggressive tumor characteristics. *Cell Death Dis.* **2013**, *4*, e517. [CrossRef]
122. Zhang, K.; Corsa, C.A.; Ponik, S.M.; Prior, J.L.; Piwnica-Worms, D.; Eliceiri, K.W.; Keely, P.J.; Longmore, G.D. The collagen receptor discoidin domain receptor 2 stabilizes SNAIL1 to facilitate breast cancer metastasis. *Nat. Cell Biol.* **2013**, *15*, 677–687. [CrossRef]
123. Jeon, Y.K.; Kim, C.K.; Hwang, K.R.; Park, H.Y.; Koh, J.; Chung, D.H.; Lee, C.W.; Ha, G.H. Pellino-1 promotes lung carcinogenesis via the stabilization of Slug and Snail through K63-mediated polyubiquitination. *Cell Death Differ.* **2017**, *24*, 469–480. [CrossRef]
124. Lee, J.H.; Jung, S.M.; Yang, K.M.; Bae, E.; Ahn, S.G.; Park, J.S.; Seo, D.; Kim, M.; Ha, J.; Lee, J.; et al. A20 promotes metastasis of aggressive basal-like breast cancers through multi-monoubiquitylation of Snail1. *Nat. Cell Biol.* **2017**, *19*, 1260–1273. [CrossRef]
125. Rodríguez, M.I.; González-Flores, A.; Dantzer, F.; Collard, J.; García de Herreros, A.; Oliver, F.J. Poly(ADP-ribose)-dependent regulation of Snail1 protein stability. *Oncogene* **2011**, *30*, 4365–4372. [CrossRef]
126. Park, S.Y.; Kim, H.S.; Kim, N.H.; Ji, S.; Cha, S.Y.; Kang, J.G.; Ota, I.; Shimada, K.; Konishi, N.; Nam, H.W.; et al. Snail1 is stabilized by O-GlcNAc modification in hyperglycaemic condition. *EMBO J.* **2010**, *29*, 3787–3796. [CrossRef]
127. Gudey, S.K.; Sundar, R.; Heldin, C.-H.; Bergh, A.; Landström, M. Pro-invasive properties of Snail1 are regulated by sumoylation in response to TGFβ stimulation in cancer. *Oncotarget* **2017**, *8*, 97703–97726. [CrossRef]
128. Hsu, D.S.-S.; Wang, H.-J.J.; Tai, S.-K.K.; Chou, C.-H.H.; Hsieh, C.-H.H.; Chiu, P.-H.H.; Chen, N.-J.J.; Yang, M.-H.H. Acetylation of snail modulates the cytokinome of cancer cells to enhance the recruitment of macrophages. *Cancer Cell* **2014**, *26*, 534–548. [CrossRef]
129. Xu, W.; Liu, H.; Liu, Z.G.; Wang, H.S.; Zhang, F.; Wang, H.; Zhang, J.; Chen, J.J.; Huang, H.J.; Tan, Y.; et al. Histone deacetylase inhibitors upregulate Snail via Smad2/3 phosphorylation and stabilization of Snail to promote metastasis of hepatoma cells. *Cancer Lett.* **2018**, *420*, 1–13. [CrossRef]
130. Komander, D.; Clague, M.J.; Urbé, S. Breaking the chains: Structure and function of the deubiquitinases. *Nat. Rev. Mol. Cell Biol.* **2009**, *10*, 550–563. [CrossRef]
131. Liu, T.; Yu, J.; Deng, M.; Yin, Y.; Zhang, H.; Luo, K.; Qin, B.; Li, Y.; Wu, C.; Ren, T.; et al. CDK4/6-dependent activation of DUB3 regulates cancer metastasis through SNAIL1. *Nat. Commun.* **2017**, *8*, 13923. [CrossRef]
132. Wu, Y.; Wang, Y.; Lin, Y.; Liu, Y.; Wang, Y.; Jia, J.; Singh, P.; Chi, Y.I.; Wang, C.; Dong, C.; et al. Dub3 inhibition suppresses breast cancer invasion and metastasis by promoting Snail1 degradation. *Nat. Commun.* **2017**, *8*, 14228. [CrossRef]
133. Lambies, G.; Miceli, M.; Martínez-Guillamon, C.; Olivera-Salguero, R.; Peña, R.; Frías, C.; Calderón, I.; Atanassov, B.; Dent, S.; Arribas, J.; et al. TGFβ-Activated USP27X Deubiquitinase Regulates Cell Migration and Chemoresistance via Stabilization of Snail1. *Cancer Res.* **2019**, *79*, 33–46. [CrossRef]
134. Li, L.; Zhou, H.; Zhu, R.; Liu, Z. USP26 promotes esophageal squamous cell carcinoma metastasis through stabilizing Snail. *Cancer Lett.* **2019**, *448*, 52–60.
135. Wang, W.; Wang, J.; Yan, H.; Zhang, K.; Liu, Y. Upregulation of USP11 promotes epithelial-to-mesenchymal transition by deubiquitinating Snail in ovarian cancer. *Oncol. Rep.* **2019**, *41*, 1739–1748. [CrossRef]
136. Zhou, H.; Liu, Y.; Zhu, R.; Ding, F.; Cao, X.; Lin, D.; Liu, Z. OTUB1 promotes esophageal squamous cell carcinoma metastasis through modulating Snail stability. *Oncogene* **2018**, *37*, 3356–3368. [CrossRef]
137. Zhu, R.; Liu, Y.; Zhou, H.; Li, L.; Li, Y.; Ding, F.; Cao, X.; Liu, Z. Deubiquitinating enzyme PSMD14 promotes tumor metastasis through stabilizing SNAIL in human esophageal squamous cell carcinoma. *Cancer Lett.* **2018**, *418*, 125–134. [CrossRef]
138. Choi, B.J.; Park, S.A.; Lee, S.Y.; Cha, Y.N.; Surh, Y.J. Hypoxia induces epithelial-mesenchymal transition in colorectal cancer cells through ubiquitin-specific protease 47-mediated stabilization of Snail: A potential role of Sox9. *Sci. Rep.* **2017**, *7*, 15918. [CrossRef]
139. Yook, J.I.; Li, X.Y.; Ota, I.; Fearon, E.R.; Weiss, S.J. Wnt-dependent regulation of the E-cadherin repressor snail. *J. Biol. Chem.* **2005**, *280*, 11740–11748. [CrossRef]

140. Yook, J.I.; Li, X.Y.; Ota, I.; Hu, C.; Kim, H.S.; Kim, N.H.; Cha, S.Y.; Ryu, J.K.; Choi, Y.J.; Kim, J.; et al. A Wnt-Axin2-GSK3beta cascade regulates Snail1 activity in breast cancer cells. *Nat. Cell Biol.* **2006**, *8*, 1398–1406. [CrossRef]
141. Frías, A.; Lambies, G.; Viñas-Castells, R.; Martínez-Guillamon, C.; Dave, N.; García de Herreros, A.; Díaz, V.M. A Switch in Akt Isoforms Is Required for Notch-Induced Snail1 Expression and Protection from Cell Death. *Mol. Cell. Biol.* **2015**, *36*, 923–940. [CrossRef]
142. Bastea, L.I.; Döppler, H.; Balogun, B.; Storz, P. Protein kinase D1 maintains the epithelial phenotype by inducing a DNA-bound, inactive SNAI1 transcriptional repressor complex. *PLoS ONE* **2012**, *7*, e30459. [CrossRef]
143. Mimoto, R.; Taira, N.; Takahashi, H.; Yamaguchi, T.; Okabe, M.; Uchida, K.; Miki, Y.; Yoshida, K. DYRK2 controls the epithelial-mesenchymal transition in breast cancer by degrading Snail. *Cancer Lett.* **2013**, *339*, 214–225. [CrossRef]
144. Wettstein, G.; Bellaye, P.S.; Kolb, M.; Hammann, A.; Crestani, B.; Soler, P.; Marchal-Somme, J.; Hazoume, A.; Gauldie, J.; Gunther, A.; et al. Inhibition of HSP27 blocks fibrosis development and EMT features by promoting snail degradation. *FASEB J.* **2013**, *27*, 1549–1560. [CrossRef]
145. Jang, D.; Kwon, H.; Choi, M.; Lee, J.; Pak, Y. Sumoylation of Flotillin-1 promotes EMT in metastatic prostate cancer by suppressing Snail degradation. *Oncogene* **2019**, *38*, 3248–3260. [CrossRef]
146. Stanisavljevic, J.; Porta-de-la-Riva, M.; Batlle, R.; García de Herreros, A.; Baulida, J. The p65 subunit of NF-κB and PARP1 assist Snail1 in activating fibronectin transcription. *J. Cell Sci.* **2011**, *124*, 4161–4171. [CrossRef]
147. Vincent, T.; Neve, E.P.A.; Johnson, J.R.; Kukalev, A.; Rojo, F.; Albanell, J.; Pietras, K.; Virtanen, I.; Philipson, L.; Leopold, P.L.; et al. A SNAIL1-SMAD3/4 transcriptional repressor complex promotes TGF-beta mediated epithelial-mesenchymal transition. *Nat. Cell Biol.* **2009**, *11*, 943–950. [CrossRef]
148. Verschueren, K.; Remacle, J.E.; Collart, C.; Kraft, H.; Baker, B.S.; Tylzanowski, P.; Nelles, L.; Su, M.; Bodmer, R.; Smith, C.; et al. SIP1, a Novel Zinc Finger / Homeodomain Repressor, Interacts with Smad Proteins Candidate Target Genes SIP1, a Novel Zinc Finger / Homeodomain Repressor, Interacts with Smad Proteins and Bin. *J. Biol. Chem.* **1999**, *274*, 20489–20498. [CrossRef]
149. Postigo, A.A. Opposing functions of ZEB proteins in the regulation of the TGFβ/BMP signaling pathway. *EMBO J.* **2003**, *22*, 2443–2452. [CrossRef]
150. Hemavathy, K.; Hu, X.; Ashraf, S.I.; Small, S.J.; Ip, Y.T. The repressor function of Snail is required for Drosophila gastrulation and is not replaceable by Escargot or Worniu. *Dev. Biol.* **2004**, *269*, 411–420. [CrossRef]
151. Peinado, H.; Ballestar, E.; Esteller, M.; Cano, A. Snail Mediates E-Cadherin Repression by the Recruitment of the Sin3A/Histone Deacetylase 1 (HDAC1)/HDAC2 Complex. *Mol. Cell. Biol.* **2004**, *24*, 306–319. [CrossRef]
152. Ayyanathan, K.; Peng, H.; Hou, Z.; Fredericks, W.J.; Goyal, R.K.; Langer, E.M.; Longmore, G.D.; Rauscher, F.J. The Ajuba LIM domain protein is a corepressor for SNAG domain mediated repression and participates in nucleocytoplasmic Shuttling. *Cancer Res.* **2007**, *67*, 9097–9106. [CrossRef]
153. Langer, E.M.; Feng, Y.; Zhaoyuan, H.; Rauscher, F.J.; Kroll, K.L.; Longmore, G.D. Ajuba LIM proteins are snail/slug corepressors required for neural crest development in Xenopus. *Dev. Cell* **2008**, *14*, 424–436. [CrossRef]
154. Zhang, W.; Wang, J.; Zou, B.; Sardet, C.; Li, J.; Lam, C.S.C.; Ng, L.; Pang, R.; Hung, I.F.N.; Tan, V.P.Y.; et al. Four and a half LIM protein 2 (FHL2) negatively regulates the transcription of E-cadherin through interaction with Snail1. *Eur. J. Cancer* **2011**, *47*, 121–130. [CrossRef]
155. Hou, Z.; Peng, H.; Ayyanathan, K.; Yan, K.-P.; Langer, E.M.; Longmore, G.D.; Rauscher, F.J. The LIM protein AJUBA recruits protein arginine methyltransferase 5 to mediate SNAIL-dependent transcriptional repression. *Mol. Cell. Biol.* **2008**, *28*, 3198–3207. [CrossRef]
156. Marie, H.; Pratt, S.J.; Betson, M.; Epple, H.; Kittler, J.T.; Meek, L.; Moss, S.J.; Troyanovsky, S.; Attwell, D.; Longmore, G.D.; et al. The LIM protein ajuba is recruited to cadherin-dependent cell junctions through an association with α-catenin. *J. Biol. Chem.* **2003**, *278*, 1220–1228. [CrossRef]
157. Herranz, N.; Pasini, D.; Díaz, V.M.; Francí, C.; Gutierrez, A.; Dave, N.; Escrivà, M.; Hernandez-Muñoz, I.; Di Croce, L.; Helin, K.; et al. Polycomb complex 2 is required for E-cadherin repression by the Snail1 transcription factor. *Mol. Cell. Biol.* **2008**, *28*, 4772–4781. [CrossRef]

158. Tong, Z.T.; Cai, M.Y.; Wang, X.G.; Kong, L.L.; Mai, S.J.; Liu, Y.H.; Zhang, H.B.; Liao, Y.J.; Zheng, F.; Zhu, W.; et al. EZH2 supports nasopharyngeal carcinoma cell aggressiveness by forming a co-repressor complex with HDAC1/HDAC2 and Snail to inhibit E-cadherin. *Oncogene* **2012**, *31*, 583–594. [CrossRef]
159. Tsai, M.C.; Manor, O.; Wan, Y.; Mosammaparast, N.; Wang, J.K.; Lan, F.; Shi, Y.; Segal, E.; Chang, H.Y. Long noncoding RNA as modular scaffold of histone modification complexes. *Science* **2010**, *329*, 689–693. [CrossRef]
160. Battistelli, C.; Cicchini, C.; Santangelo, L.; Tramontano, A.; Grassi, L.; Gonzalez, F.J.; De Nonno, V.; Grassi, G.; Amicone, L.; Tripodi, M. The Snail repressor recruits EZH2 to specific genomic sites through the enrollment of the lncRNA HOTAIR in epithelial-to-mesenchymal transition. *Oncogene* **2017**, *36*, 942–955. [CrossRef]
161. Lin, Y.; Wu, Y.; Li, J.; Dong, C.; Ye, X.; Chi, Y.-I.; Evers, B.M.; Zhou, B.P. The SNAG domain of Snail1 functions as a molecular hook for recruiting lysine-specific demethylase 1. *EMBO J.* **2010**, *29*, 1803–1816. [CrossRef]
162. Shi, Y.; Sawada, J.I.; Sui, G.; Affar, E.B.; Whetstine, J.R.; Lan, F.; Ogawa, H.; Luke, M.P.S.; Nakatani, Y.; Shi, Y. Coordinated histone modifications mediated by a CtBP co-repressor complex. *Nature* **2003**, *422*, 735–738. [CrossRef]
163. Dong, C.; Wu, Y.; Yao, J.; Wang, Y.; Yu, Y.; Rychahou, P.G.; Evers, B.M.; Zhou, B.P. G9a interacts with Snail and is critical for Snail-mediated E-cadherin repression in human breast cancer. *J. Clin. Investig.* **2012**, *122*, 1469–1486. [CrossRef]
164. Li, Y.; Cheng, C. Long noncoding RNA NEAT1 promotes the metastasis of osteosarcoma via interaction with the G9a-DNMT1-Snail complex. *Am. J. Cancer Res.* **2018**, *8*, 81–90.
165. Peinado, H.; Iglesias-de La Cruz, M.D.C.; Olmeda, D.; Csiszar, K.; Fong, K.S.K.; Vega, S.; Nieto, M.A.; Cano, A.; Portillo, F. A molecular role for lysyl oxidase-like 2 enzyme in Snail regulation and tumor progression. *EMBO J.* **2005**, *24*, 3446–3458. [CrossRef]
166. Cuevas, E.P.; Moreno-Bueno, G.; Canesin, G.; Santos, V.; Portillo, F.; Cano, A. LOXL2 catalytically inactive mutants mediate epithelial-to-mesenchymal transition. *Biol. Open* **2014**, *3*, 129–137. [CrossRef]
167. Herranz, N.; Dave, N.; Millanes-Romero, A.; Pascual-Reguant, L.; Morey, L.; Díaz, V.M.; Lórenz-Fonfría, V.; Gutierrez-Gallego, R.; Jerónimo, C.; Iturbide, A.; et al. Lysyl oxidase-like 2 (LOXL2) oxidizes trimethylated lysine 4 in histone H3. *FEBS J.* **2016**, *283*, 4263–4273. [CrossRef]
168. Iturbide, A.; Pascual-Reguant, L.; Fargas, L.; Cebrià, J.P.; Alsina, B.; García de Herreros, A.; Peiró, S. LOXL2 Oxidizes Methylated TAF10 and Controls TFIID-Dependent Genes during Neural Progenitor Differentiation. *Mol. Cell* **2015**, *58*, 755–766. [CrossRef]
169. Hu, C.T.; Chang, T.Y.; Cheng, C.C.; Liu, C.S.; Wu, J.R.; Li, M.C.; Wu, W.S. Snail associates with EGR-1 and SP-1 to upregulate transcriptional activation of p15INK4b. *FEBS J.* **2010**, *277*, 1202–1218. [CrossRef]
170. Hwang, W.; Yang, M.; Tsai, M.; Lan, H.; Su, S.; Chang, S.; Teng, H.; Yang, S.; Lan, Y.; Chiou, S.; et al. SNAIL regulates interleukin-8 expression, stem celllike activity, and tumorigenicity of human colorectal carcinoma cells. *Gastroenterology* **2011**, *141*, 279–291. [CrossRef]
171. Wu, W.S.; You, R.I.; Cheng, C.C.; Lee, M.C.; Lin, T.Y.; Hu, C.T. Snail collaborates with EGR-1 and SP-1 to directly activate transcription of MMP 9 and ZEB1. *Sci. Rep.* **2017**, *7*, 17753. [CrossRef]
172. Rembold, M.; Ciglar, L.; Omar Yáñez-Cuna, J.; Zinzen, R.P.; Girardot, C.; Jain, A.; Welte, M.A.; Stark, A.; Leptin, M.; Furlong, E.E.M. A conserved role for Snail as a potentiator of active transcription. *Genes Dev.* **2014**, *28*, 167–181. [CrossRef]
173. Stemmer, V.; De Craene, B.; Berx, G.; Behrens, J. Snail promotes Wnt target gene expression and interacts with β-catenin. *Oncogene* **2008**, *27*, 5075–5080. [CrossRef]
174. Lee, S.-H.; Lee, S.-J.; Jung, Y.S.; Xu, Y.; Kang, H.S.; Ha, N.-C.; Park, B.-J. Blocking of p53-Snail Binding, Promoted by Oncogenic K-Ras, Recovers p53 Expression and function. *Neoplasia* **2009**, *11*, 22–31. [CrossRef]
175. Lee, S.H.; Lee, S.J.; Chung, J.Y.; Jung, Y.S.; Choi, S.Y.; Hwang, S.H.; Choi, D.; Ha, N.C.; Park, B.J. P53, secreted by K-Ras-Snail pathway, is endocytosed by K-Ras-mutated cells; implication of target-specific drug delivery and early diagnostic marker. *Oncogene* **2009**, *28*, 2005–2014. [CrossRef]
176. Ni, T.; Li, X.-Y.; Lu, N.; An, T.; Liu, Z.-P.; Fu, R.; Lv, W.-C.; Zhang, Y.-W.; Xu, X.-J.; Grant Rowe, R.; et al. Snail1-dependent p53 repression regulates expansion and activity of tumour-initiating cells in breast cancer. *Nat. Cell Biol.* **2016**, *18*, 1221–1232. [CrossRef]
177. Alba-Castellón, L.; Batlle, R.; Francí, C.; Fernández-Aceñero, M.J.; Mazzolini, R.; Peña, R.; Loubat, J.; Alameda, F.; Rodríguez, R.; Curto, J.; et al. Snail1 expression is required for sarcomagenesis. *Neoplasia* **2014**, *16*, 413–421. [CrossRef]

178. Villagrasa, P.; Díaz, V.M.; Vīas-Castells, R.; Peiró, S.; Del Valle-Pérez, B.; Dave, N.; Rodríguez-Asiain, A.; Casal, J.I.; Lizcano, J.M.; Duñach, M.; et al. Akt2 interacts with Snail1 in the E-cadherin promoter. *Oncogene* **2012**, *31*, 4022–4033. [CrossRef]
179. Vega, S.; Morales, A.V.; Ocaña, O.H.; Valdés, F.; Fabregat, I.; Nieto, M.A. Snail blocks the cell cycle and confers resistance to cell death. *Genes Dev.* **2004**, *18*, 1131–1143. [CrossRef]
180. Escriva, M.; Peiro, S.; Herranz, N.; Villagrasa, P.; Dave, N.; Montserrat-Sentis, B.; Murray, S.A.; Franci, C.; Gridley, T.; Virtanen, I.; et al. Repression of PTEN Phosphatase by Snail1 Transcriptional Factor during Gamma Radiation-Induced Apoptosis. *Mol. Cell. Biol.* **2008**, *28*, 1528–1540. [CrossRef]
181. Lee, J.H.; Kang, B.H.; Jang, H.; Kim, T.W.; Choi, J.; Kwak, S.; Han, J.; Cho, E.J.; Youn, H.D. AKT phosphorylates H3-threonine 45 to facilitate termination of gene transcription in response to DNA damage. *Nucleic Acids Res.* **2015**, *43*, 4505–4516. [CrossRef]
182. Cano, A.; Pérez-Moreno, M.A.; Rodrigo, I.; Locascio, A.; Blanco, M.J.; del Barrio, M.G.; Portillo, F.; Nieto, M.A. The transcription factor snail controls epithelial-mesenchymal transitions by repressing E-cadherin expression. *Nat. Cell Biol.* **2000**, *2*, 76–83. [CrossRef]

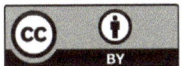

© 2019 by the authors. Licensee MDPI, Basel, Switzerland. This article is an open access article distributed under the terms and conditions of the Creative Commons Attribution (CC BY) license (http://creativecommons.org/licenses/by/4.0/).

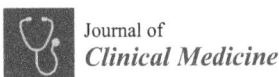 

Review

# Epithelial-Mesenchymal Plasticity in Organotropism Metastasis and Tumor Immune Escape

Xiang Nan [1,2,†], Jiang Wang [3,†], Haowen Nikola Liu [2], Stephen T.C. Wong [2,*] and Hong Zhao [2,*]

1. Center for Biomedical Engineering, University of Science and Technology of China, Hefei 230052, China; xnan2@houstonmethodist.org
2. Department of Systems Medicine and Bioengineering, Houston Methodist Cancer Center, Weill Cornell Medicine, Houston, TX 77030, USA; hnliu@houstonmethodist.org
3. Department of Orthopedics, Tongji Hospital, Wuhan 430050, China; wangjiangtjgk@163.com
* Correspondence: stwong@houstonmethodist.org (S.T.C.W.); hzhao@houstonmethodist.org (H.Z.)
† These authors contributed equally to this work.

Received: 25 March 2019; Accepted: 22 May 2019; Published: 25 May 2019

**Abstract:** Most cancer deaths are due to metastasis, and almost all cancers have their preferential metastatic organs, known as "organotropism metastasis". Epithelial-mesenchymal plasticity has been described as heterogeneous and dynamic cellular differentiation states, supported by emerging experimental evidence from both molecular and morphological levels. Many molecular factors regulating epithelial-mesenchymal plasticity have tissue-specific and non-redundant properties. Reciprocally, cellular epithelial-mesenchymal plasticity contributes to shaping organ-specific pre-metastatic niche (PMN) including distinct local immune landscapes, mainly through secreted bioactive molecular factors. Here, we summarize recent progress on the involvement of tumor epithelial-mesenchymal plasticity in driving organotropic metastasis and regulating the function of different immune cells in organ-specific metastasis.

**Keywords:** organotropism metastasis; EMT heterogeneity; tumor immune escape; cell–cell communication

## 1. Introduction

The mechanisms of organotropism metastasis is one of the most unanswered questions in the field of cancer research. From the original "seed and soil" theory to recent discoveries on pre-metastatic niches (PMNs), our current understanding of organotropic metastasis is that this process is regulated by multi-facet factors including intrinsic properties of cancer cells, characteristics of organ microenvironments, and cancer cell-organ interactions. Epithelial-mesenchymal transition (EMT) is recognized as an initial and critical event for the metastasis of carcinomas. Traditionally, tumor cells undergoing EMT lose their cell–cell adhesion and apico-basal polarity and gain the ability to migrate individually and invade basement membrane and blood vessels. Upon intravasation, these cells stay in the bloodstream as circulating tumor cells (CTCs) and evade immune attacks until extravasation at distant organs to seed micro-metastases. During seeding, they undergo the reverse EMT process, MET, to regain their epithelial characteristics and form secondary tumors or macro-metastases [1]. However, emerging studies identified the cellular plasticity of epithelial and mesenchymal state conversion of carcinoma cells during the metastasis process. Notably, tumor cells under partial EMT or hybrid EMT state, which means they keep both E and M properties, are likely to express or secret distinct bioactive factors and induce the formation of organ-specific PMNs; at seeding organs, the partial MET cells are more adaptive to the organ microenvironment and to forming colonization; these partial EMT and MET cells are more resistant to immune attacks by altering the function of different immune cells in systemic circulation and local organs. In this review, we focus on the heterogeneous EMT and

MET phenotypes in primary and metastatic tumors, the contribution of partial EMT and MET cells in organotropism metastasis, their regulation of the function of immune cells, and mostly, the secreted molecular factors regulating the cell–cell interactions in organ-specific tumor microenvironments.

### 1.1. Organotropic Metastasis

Metastasis is a fatal step in cancer progression, 90% of patient mortality is due to complications from metastatic diseases rather than from primary tumors [2]. Tumor metastases to different organs is not a random process but is known to have organ-specific preference or "organotropism". Organotropic metastasis remains the most intriguing but unanswered questions in cancer research. The "seed and soil" theory proposed by Steven first described site-specific metastasis [3]. Back to 1889, he proposed that metastatic tumor cells' ("seed") initiation of outgrowth in distant organs largely depends on crosstalk with the host microenvironment ("soil"). In the past several decades, extensive studies have enriched our understanding and indicate that organotropic metastasis is determined by multi-facet factors including cancer cells' intrinsic properties (cancer subtypes or cancer cell subpopulations), the distinct organ microenvironment, and cancer cells-organ interactions [4,5]. From the aspect of the intrinsic properties of cancer cells, for example, the hormone receptor positive (ER+/PR+) and human epidermal growth factor receptor 2 (HER2) positive (HER2+) breast cancer subtype has an especially high rate of bone metastases compared with other subtypes [6]. The triple-negative basal-like subtype is specifically associated with a low rate of bone and liver metastases but a high rate of brain metastasis [7]. At a genomics level, many exciting studies from Massagué's group identified altered gene expressions that mediate metastasis in breast cancer, lung adenocarcinoma, and renal cell carcinoma to sites including the bone, lung, and brain [8–13]. From the aspect of the host microenvironment, different anatomical and histological characteristics of the host organs determine the ease with which cancer cells can invade and outgrow. For example, in bone marrow and liver, fenestrated sinusoidal endothelia permits the high permeability of tumor cells [14], while in the brain the blood–brain barrier (BBB), formed by tight conjunct endothelia, astrocytes, and pericytes, restricts the entry of many molecules and cells [15]. In addition, the chemical compositions and mechanical forces presented by the extracellular matrix (ECM) [16] and local stromal cell populations [17] have been recognized to play critical roles in organotropic metastasis. Furthermore, immune cells in both the host organ microenvironment and systemic circulation have close interactions with tumor cells and regulate organotropic metastasis [18].

The recent discovery of organ-specific PMNs in both preclinical models and clinical samples is a new paradigm for metastasis initiation and explicitly organotropic metastasis [19–21]. Before tumor cells metastasize, the formation of PMNs at distant targeted organs are induced mainly by tumor cell-secreted factors and tumor-shed extracellular vesicles (EVs) that alter the organ's local milieu and create a tumor receptive microenvironment [19]. For example, PMNs consist of aberrant immune cells that are recruited from bone marrow [22–24]. Tumor cells seeding into PMNs get support to thrive and give rise to micro-metastasis; tumor cells seeding into non-PMN areas fail to form metastatic colonization. In contrast, specific niches, known as "sleepy niche" or dormant niches, also exist, in which disseminated tumor cells keep dormancy until the tissue homeostasis breaks and tumor cells awake to re-grow [19]. Because different sub-clones of tumor cells in one primary tumor can derive distinct and common secreted factors and Evs, and even one sub-clone of tumor cells can secret a variety of factors and Evs, multifocal PMNs in one organ and multiple PMNs in different organs can be formed, thus a primary tumor has the ability to metastasize to more than one organ and form polyclonal metastatic lesions within one organ. However, research in this field remains immature and there are many important questions that have not been elucidated, for example, studies on specific molecules expressed and/or shed by specific tumors to foster the formation of PMNs in specific organs are just emerging (see below section), thus this information is largely unknown; the dynamics of PMN formation has not been explored; and the contribution of other cellular components (such as adipocytes and sympathetic neurons) to PMN formation has not been explored [19]. Nonetheless, studying the molecular mechanisms of organotropism metastasis is critical, not only for biomarker-based prediction and prognosis, but also for the development of innovative therapeutic strategy, and the eventual prevention of cancer metastasis.

*1.2. Heterogeneous EMT Phenotypes and the Activation/Regulation Complexity*

Epithelial-mesenchymal plasticity is mostly referred to as the different cellular states when cells are undergoing EMT and its reverse program MET and intermediate states between these two, partial EMT or hybrid EMT. EMT is strictly defined as cell morphological changes from epithelioid to mesenchymal/fibroblastoid/spindle-shape and is accompanied by drastic and persistent molecular changes [25]. It has been accepted as a critical program allowing stationary epithelial cells to gain motility in order to migrate and invade during embryogenesis, organ development, tissue regeneration, and organ fibrosis. The activation of the EMT program has been implicated in cancer initiation, invasion, metastasis, and chemo-resistance as demonstrated by extensive studies in the past decade [26–29]. However, it is different from the context of wound healing and embryonic development where the intermediate states of EMT are distinct and well-studied, while in cancer, EMT and MET are not "all-or-none" processes. Cancer cells co-expressing both canonical epithelial and mesenchymal markers are stable over multiple passages and metastable [30]. Cancer EMT progression is a multi-dimensional nonlinear process and EMT and MET are not binary processes [30].

EMT primarily encompasses a cell morphological change. By performing intravital two-photon microscope imaging, our group was able to track and analyze individual EMT tumor cells in red (E)-to-green (M) fluorescent color switching mouse breast tumors [31]. Per the emergence of green (M) fluorescent cells in live mouse tumors, the cells' axial ratios and moving distances, we quantitatively identified the heterogeneous sub-populations of the EMT cells at different tumor stages, i.e., fibroblast-like EMT cells, migratory EMT cells, and quiescent EMT cells. For example, in the early-stage small tumors (~2 mm diameter), the fibroblast-like EMT cells constituted about 5% of all of the EMT cells. These cells were recognized by their spindle-like shape and long linear processes tightly attached to the ECM, but they do not have high migratory ability. About 50% of the EMT cells exhibited tropism movement and iterative elongation and contraction of the pseudopods toward one main direction; we defined them as migratory EMT cells. Another 20% of the green (M) cells kept an amoeboid appearance without pseudopods and were almost static without obvious shape changes during the 4–6 hours imaging period. These cells are mostly located in the surrounding of the migratory EMT cells, and we defined them as temporarily quiescent EMT cells [31]. The migratory EMT cells were characterized as losing cell polarity, acting like amoeba, and migrating towards stimuli, which may mainly contribute to metastasis [32]. The fibroblast-like EMT cells kept partial polarity and attached tightly to the ECM but without movement, which may develop into cancer associated fibroblasts [33]. In addition, a significant percentage (~20%) of EMT cells were of quiescent subtype, and we did not observe any changeovers between the quiescent and migratory EMT cells in the 4–6 hours imaging period. However, most of the migratory and quiescent EMT cells locate relatively closely (<50 um), but far apart from the clusters of fibroblast-like EMT cells (>100 um), which made us postulate that the migratory and quiescent EMT cells might have paracrine interplays or autocrine signals to maintain their equilibrium and give rise to metastasis [31]. Further characterization of the molecular composition of each subtype and delineation of their evolution or transformation is undergoing.

Aiello et al. also found the existence of divergent EMT programs in different cancer types [8]. In mouse pancreatic ductal adenocarcinoma (PDAC), the well-differentiated tumors are associated with a persistence of E-cadherin (ECAD) mRNA and a re-localization of ECAD protein inside the cells, which is termed as a partial EMT program (P-EMT). In contrast, the poorly-differentiated tumors tend to undergo a complete EMT (C-EMT) with losing ECAD mRNA and protein expression [34]. By cross-referencing the P-EMT and C-EMT gene signatures to the expression data from the Cancer Cell Line Encyclopedia (CCLE), several human pancreatic cancer cell lines were stratified as P-EMT or C-EMT. Similarly, basal-like breast cancer cells were characterized as C-EMT, but luminal A, B, or normal-like breast cancer cells were associated with P-EMT [34]. Puram et al. [35] profiled single cell transcriptome from matched pairs of primary tumors and lymph node metastases in head and neck cancer patients. They identified that cells expressing the P-EMT program spatially localized to the leading edge of primary tumors in proximity to cancer-associated fibroblasts (CAFs), and predict lymph node metastases.

Functionally, our studies and others found that many carcinoma cells may metastasize without completely losing the E (epithalial) and/or attaining the M (mesenchymal) traits [36,37]. Cells in the hybrid E/M phenotype keep both E and M traits, migrating collectively as commonly seen in the multicellular migration in ECM [31] and CTC clusters [38,39]. By examining the cell invasion and migration properties of the above mentioned histological-relevant EMT programs in PDAC, it was found that in the C-EMT tumorspheres, spindle-like protrusions of single cells at the edges of the primary cell mass were primarily observed. By contrast, in P-EMT spheres both budding cell clusters as a collective group and single cells escaped from the primary cell mass [34]. Furthermore, >95% of the CTCs in the C-EMT cell line-derived PDAC models were present as single cells, while >50% of CTCs existed as tumor cell clusters in the P-EMT cell line-derived models [34,40]. The single CTCs from the C-EMT tumors lacked staining of ECAD protein, and tumor cell clusters arising from P-EMT tumors retained ECAD staining only at the cell-cell contact points but not on the cluster surface [34]. The CTC cluster cells are resistant to anoikis, and they extravasate the vessels more efficiently and are 50 times more metastatic than individual CTCs [41,42]. Therefore, the P-EMT program poses a higher metastatic risk than the C-EMT program in cancer patients [43]. At the metastatic organs, heterogeneous MET phenotypes are also reported. Although metastatic carcinomas commonly express epithelial markers, mesenchymal markers are often examined in patients. For example, in the brain microenvironment, metastatic lung cancer cells showed increased expression of the epithelial marker ECAD as well as elevated levels of transcription factor ZEB1 and mesenchymal markers VIM [44,45], reflecting the partial EMT/MET phenotype. Recent studies revealed the existence of both MET-dependent and MET-independent metastasis, i.e., a MET-dependent metastasis in carcinosarcomas and a MET-independent metastasis in prostate cancer [46]. The traditional EMT "master" transcription factors (EMT-TFs) and miRNAs which maintain the epithelial phenotype mainly regulate the MET-dependent metastatic mechanisms [46].

In the complex process from primary tumor to metastasis, cancer cells adaptively change in the hostile environment by transitioning back-and-forth from differentiated to undifferentiated or partial EMT phenotypes [28,47]. The phenotypic plasticity of EMT subtypes is mainly regulated by functionally pleiotropic EMT-TFs and miRNAs [48,49]. Epithelial cell markers are transcriptionally repressed through the action of EMT-TFs. In parallel, mesenchymal markers are induced to express [50]. Furthermore, the EMT-TFs guide the recruitment of epigenetic machinery to the chromatin, thus allowing the proper regulation of gene expression [51,52]. For example, the E-cadherin promoter is regulated epigenetically via methylation in most intra-ductal breast carcinomas, thus E-cadherin expression is dynamically modulated by the microenvironment [53]. In addition, recent studies revealed post-transcriptional regulation of EMT activation. Studies on PDACs showed that C-EMT tumor cells lost both membranous and intracellular ECAD consistent with the loss of Ecad mRNA. By contrast, P-EMT cells store epithelial proteins (ECAD, β-catenin, Claudin-7 and EpCAM) intracellularly and re-locate them back to the cell surface through recycling endocytic vesicles [34]. Tumor microenvironment factors always activate EMT through multiple mechanisms. For example, under hypoxia the elevated hypoxia induced factor-1 (HIF-1) can bind to the promoter region of EMT-TFs and regulate their expressions [54]. In addition, inflammatory cells including neutrophils, lymphocytes, macrophages, and myeloid-derived suppressor cells (MDSCs), which secrete inflammatory cytokines stimulated by hypoxic stress, including tumor necrosis factor α, transforming growth factor β (TGF-β), interleukin 1 (IL-1), IL-6, and IL-8, all contribute to hypoxia-induced EMT [54–56]. For the P-EMT or E/M hybrid state, phenotypic stability factors (PSFs) including OVOL and GRHL2 have been characterized in stabilizing such EMT state [57], and OVOL by coupling with miR200/ZEB/LIN28/let-7 circuit has been examined to increase the stemness of the hybrid E/M phenotype [58,59].

## 2. Epithelial-Mesenchymal Plasticity and Cancer Organotropism Metastasis

A new mechanism revealed how epithelial/mesenchymal plasticity determines PDAC metastasizing to lung and liver [40,60]. The authors found that the expression of intact p120 Catenin (P120CTN), a protein that binds and stabilizes ECAD, appeared predominantly in liver metastasis of the PDAC mice; however, genetic abrogation of P120CTN significantly shifts the metastatic burden to the lungs [60]. This striking organotropism change is mediated by the differential epithelial status of tumor cells, i.e., invasive tumor cells in the primary tumor showed low E-cadherin expression but regained in liver metastatic lesions; in contrast, tumor cells in the lung metastases lacked expression of P120CTN or E-cadherin, suggesting the occurrence of MET in liver metastasis, but lung metastatic cells remained at the M state. This conclusion was further verified by an experiment that directly monitored the tumor cell colonization in liver and lung [60]. Cells with wild-type or single copy P120CTN, but not bi-allelic deletion, which kept the ability to stabilize ECAD and convert tumor cells to E state, are able to form liver metastases. However, PDAC cells with bi-allelic deletion of P120CTN lost the ability to stabilize ECAD and undergo MET, bypassed the liver, and preferentially went to the lung. The authors concluded that P120CTN modulated epithelial plasticity and liver or lung organotropic metastases in PDAC [60].

Although other mechanisms directly connecting EMT plasticity with organotropism metastasis are lacking, emerging evidence indicate that epithelial plasticity regulates cancer stemness [61], for which cancer stem cells (CSCs) are responsible for organotropism metastasis [62–64]. In certain studies inhibition of EMT has been reported to promote cancer stemness and is associated with tumor-initiating for metastatic colonization. However, activation of EMT was also shown to inhibit stem-like property [61]. MET has been noted to promote cancer stemness. For example, inhibitor of differentiation 1 (Id1) induces MET and stemness in breast cancer cells by antagonizing transcriptional factor Twist1 [65], and transient expression of Twist1 promotes the coexistence of both epithelial and mesenchymal features in the cells [66]. Existence of partial EMT/MET cells provides a reasonable explanation for this conflicting evidence, indicating that the 'intermediate state' of cancer cells may be more flexible in cell invasion and regulation of stem-like properties, especially when considering the temporal dynamics of the metastasis process in vivo. There are many observations to support this statement. For example, CTCs have been shown to express both epithelial and mesenchymal markers [67], and patients with advanced metastatic cancer have a high frequency of partial EMT/MET CTCs [39]. Furthermore, the partial EMT/MET cells in primary ovarian cancer and prostate cancer showed higher self-renewal and tumor-initiating ability [68,69]. Beerling et al. [70], tracked the ECAD$^{high}$ epithelial and ECAD$^{low}$ mesenchymal tumor cells in liver metastasis of PyMT-MMTV mouse breast tumors. They found that although intrinsically the epithelial and mesenchymal cells differ in stemness, this difference does not provide a significant metastatic outgrowth advantage because mesenchymal cells adapt an epithelial state after the first few cell divisions. This study further indicates the complex EMT plasticity in in vivo tumor metastasis. miRNAs were studied extensively in mediating the regulations of EMT/MET plasticity and stemness. miR-200 families were shown to promote MET, which also increases metastatic colonization in breast cancer [71]. miR-30 family members inhibited EMT through TWF1 and inhibited CSC-mediated lung metastasis [72]. miR-7 suppresses brain metastasis of breast cancer CSC by modulating KLF4 [73].

There are many more studies exploring miRNAs in cancer metastasis, and miRNAs in EMT regulation, thus we summarized here some speculations linking organ-specific EMT with metastasis initiation through miRNAs. For example, skeletons are the organ most affected by various metastatic cancer cells. Almost all important EMT regulators have been identified in the bone microenvironment facilitating bone metastasis formation, including hypoxia, various growth factors (TGF-β, epithelial growth factors, vascular endothelial growth factor, insulin-like growth factors, platelet-derived growth factor, and parathyroid hormone-related protein), cytokines (IL-1, 6, 8, 11), and other signaling molecules, including integrins, matrix metalloproteinases (MMPs), notch, Wnt, hedgehog signaling, and bone morphogenetic proteins (BMP) signaling pathways [74].

We speculate that miRNAs target host stroma in regulating organotropic metastasis by affecting tumor cell EMT. For example, breast cancer-secreted miR-122 promotes tumor metastasis to the brain and lungs by reprogramming glucose metabolism in the PMNs [75]. This process is likely accompanied by activated EMT in tumor cells [76]. Expression of miR-23b/27b/24 cluster promotes breast cancer lung metastasis by targeting metastasis-suppressive gene prosaposin [77]; these miRNAs also promote TGF-β1-induced EMT by directly targeting CDH1 and activating Wnt/β-catenin signaling [78,79]. Recently, Schirijver et al. compared global miRNAs expression in primary breast tumors and matched multiple distant metastases. miR-106b-5p was found to be an independent predictor of lung and gastrointestinal metastases, and miR-7-5p and miR-1273g-3p can predict skin and ovarian metastases, respectively [80]. These miRNAs have all been experimentally validated to regulate the EMT phenotypes of tumor cells [81–83].

Exosomes carrying specific miRNAs are recognized to not only function as vehicles to promote organ-specific metastasis but also mediate EMT regulation. Metastatic breast cancer cell-secreted miR-105 was shown to be transferred in exosome to endothelial cells and destroyed vascular endothelial barriers by targeting the tight junction protein Zonula occludens (ZO-1). This process was verified in experimental settings in promoting lung and brain metastasis [84]. Zhang et al. reported that brain astrocyte-derived exosomes promoted brain metastatic tumor growth from breast and lung cancer by transferring PTEN-targeting miR-19a to these cancer cells [85], and miR-19a has been well reported as an EMT promoting miRNA in lung cancer [86]. Tumor exosomes are shown to educate selected host tissues toward a prometastatic phenotype. In the rat pancreatic adenocarcinoma model ASML with preferential draining lymph nodes and lung metastasis, tumor exosomes and the exosomal mRNA and miRNA are taken up and recovered by lymph node stroma cells and lung fibroblasts after subcutaneous injection [87]. While the mRNAs' translation was barely detected in the target cells, the miRNAs profoundly affected the transcriptome of these cells. Remarkably, exosomal miR-494 and miR-542-3p suppressed the expression of cadherin-17, up-regulated the MMPs transcription, and prepared a pre-metastatic niche for the lymph node and lung metastasis [87]. Both miR-494 and miR-542-3p have been demonstrated as inhibitory factors for EMT in pancreatic cancer and other cancer types [88,89].

In addition to exosomal miRNAs, Lyden et al. demonstrated that the exosomes released from human lung-, liver- and brain-tropic tumor cells preferentially fuse with resident cells at their predicted destination, i.e., lung fibroblasts and epithelial cells, liver Kupffer cells, and brain endothelial cells [90]. These exosomes mediated tumor cell and organ cell interaction in the organotropic metastatic niche. The authors observed that treatment with exosomes from lung-tropic models redirected the metastasis of bone-tropic tumor cells to lung [90]. The distinct role of different exosomal integrins in the organotropic metastases was further elucidated, e.g., exosomal integrin αvβ5 in breast cancer cells specifically binds to Kupffer cells in facilitating liver metastasis, whereas exosomal integrins α6β4 and α6β1 bind lung fibroblasts and epithelial cells, facilitating lung metastasis [90]. Integrins comprise heterodimer ECM receptors that are essential in enabling tumor cells to interact with ECM remodeling in the initiation and progression of EMT [91]. Different integrins engage with different ECM components, i.e., collagen type IV (α1β1, α2β1), laminins (α3β1, α6β1), fibrillin (α5β1, αVβ3, αVβ6), perlecan, and versican (β1) [92]. Some are also associated with ECAD that are required for EMT progression by integrating the TGFβ and β-catenin signaling [91]. In addition, changes of the integrin repertoire during EMT correlate with the increased expression of proteases, such as MMP2 and MMP9, enhancing ECM protein degradation and enabling invasion [91].

## 3. Epithelial-Mesenchymal Plasticity and Tumor Immune Escape in Metastatic Organs

Clinical achievements of cancer immunotherapy are currently outpacing our scientific understanding of the immune-related mechanisms for organotropic metastasis. Different factors in regulating the sensitivity of organ-specific metastases versus primary tumors to immunomodulation remain understudied. However, the heterogeneity of tumor immune landscapes both locally and systemically [93] could be partly attributed to the tumor epithelial-mesenchymal plasticity in modulating antitumor immunity from tumor microenvironment components [94] (Figure 1).

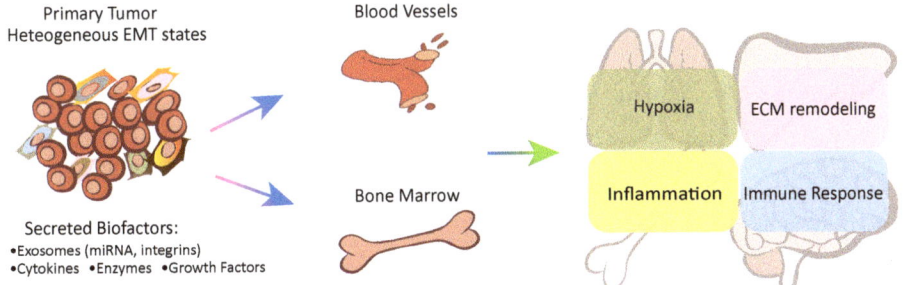

**Figure 1.** Epithelial-mesenchymal plasticity of carcinoma cells plays key roles in regulating organ microenvironment and local immune landscape in leading organotropism metastasis. Primary carcinoma cells under heterogeneous EMT states produce and secret a variety of bioactive factors, including exosomes carrying specific miRNAs, integrins, inflammatory cytokines, growth factors, and extracellular matrix enzymes to induce PMNs at distant organs. These bioactive factors mainly regulate microenvironmental hypoxia, inflammatory, ECM remodeling, and immune cell function.

Bone and the immune system are strictly linked to each other because all immune system cells are derived from hematopoietic stem cells that reside in bone, and many immunoregulatory cytokines influence the fate of bone cells. Moreover, many cytokines and secreted factors from immune and bone cells promote tumor growth in bone, contributing to the vicious cycle of bone metastasis [95]. As we mentioned before, almost all bone microenvironment factors are involved in regulating tumor EMT states [74]. The interactions between T cells and osteoclast precursors through reciprocal CD137/CD137L and RANK/RANKL regulate bone absorption in bone metastasis [96]; RANK/RANKL induces EMT in breast cancer [97]. Since MDSCs are progenitors of the osteoclast precursors, it is not surprising that they are largely increased in bone metastatic patients. MDSCs themselves could enhance tumor growth in bone through accumulating in secondary lymphoid organs and leading to a strong inhibition of the antitumor T cell response [95]. The accumulation of MDSCs in secondary lymphoid organs is mediated by the Wnt/β-catenin pathway [98], which is also an important EMT regulator. MDSCs have also been implicated in MET in lung metastasis. In the lung PMN of MMTV-PyMT breast tumor mice, accumulated MDSCs secrete versican, an extracellular matrix proteoglycan. Versican stimulated MET of metastatic tumor cells by attenuating phospho-Smad2 levels, which resulted in elevated cell proliferation and accelerated metastases [99]. As a primary tumor grows and becomes more hypoxic and inflammatory, tumor cells secret factors and extracellular vesicles [90,100] to attract MDSCs from bone marrow, initiating the pre-metastatic niche. The distant organ microenvironment is also adapted by these tumor secreted factors to accept the bone marrow derived cells and CTCs, thereby being shaped into a tumor-promoting metastatic niche characterized by increased angiogenesis and vascular permeability, ECM remodeling, chronic inflammation, and immunosuppression [21,101].

In brain metastasis, the STAT3-positive reactive astrocytes not only suppressed the activation of CD8+ T cells, but also promoted the expansion of CD74+ microglial/macrophages, which produces tumor growth promoting factors, thereby benefiting metastatic tumor growth in brain [102]. In patients, blocking STAT3 signaling in reactive astrocytes reduces experimental brain metastasis from different primary tumor sources, even at advanced stages of colonization [102]. STAT3 has long been recognized as a key stimulator of EMT in carcinoma [103], and recent studies revealed a EMT-like process in reactive astrocytes in primary brain tumors [104]. The increased expression of EMT-related factors in brain metastasis was found not only in tumor cells, but also in tumor-associated astrocytes [105].

Involvement of other immune cells in organ-specific metastasis have been explored in recent years as reviewed in [106], including metastasis-associated macrophages, neutrophils, natural killer (NK) cells, and T cells. Secreted factors from both tumor cells and stromal cells are the key factors controlling the functions of these immune cells, and again, many of them also regulate tumor epithelial-mesenchymal plasticity.

## 3.1. Metastasis-Associated Macrophages

Macrophages have been shown to promote lymph node, lung, and brain metastasis in breast cancer. Piao et al. reported that triple-negative breast cancer cell-derived exosomes induced M2 polarization of macrophages that created favorable conditions for lymph node metastasis, although the exact signaling factors in the exosomes were not characterized [107]. In the study by Linde et al. CD206$^{hi}$ intra-epithelial macrophages in the very early stage of mammary intra-epithelial neoplasia in mice, which is similar to ductal carcinoma in situ (DCIS) in humans, were shown to respond to tumor secreted chemokine ligand 2 (CCL-2), which in turn stimulates macrophages to produce Wnt-1, leading to disruption of E-cadherin junctions between early cancer cells and propelling lung dissemination. Transient depletion of macrophages in mice at the "DCIS" stage reduced lung metastatic burden later in mice life [108]. In addition, in breast cancer lung metastasis mouse models, CCL-2 secreted by both tumor cells and endothelial cells preferentially recruited C-C chemokine receptor type 2 (CCR2+) macrophages to lungs, resulting in increased metastatic seeding and tumor outgrowth [109]. Anti-CCL2 treatment in these mice showed good efficacy, and discontinuation of anti-CCL2 treatment increased lung metastasis and accelerates mice death [110]. CCL-2 also has also been shown to play a detrimental role in brain metastasis. Zhang et al. demonstrated that breast cancer cells secreted large amounts of CCL-2 in vivo when infiltrating the brain parenchyma, resulting in the recruitment of IBA1+ macrophages that reciprocally enhance the metastatic outgrowth [85]. EMT program has been reported to stimulate the production of proinflammatory factors by cancer cells including CCL-2 [111], and CCL-2 specifically has been demonstrated to induce EMT in cancer cells [112].

## 3.2. Metastasis-Associated Neutrophils

The role of neutrophils has been debated on both promoting and inhibiting metastasis [113]. Recent studies indicate that depletion of neutrophils inhibited lung metastasis, and the iron-transporting protein transferrin was identified as the major mitogen for tumor cells secreted by neutrophils [114]. Granulocyte-macrophage colony-stimulating factor (GM-CSF), which is produced primarily by tumor cells, is a selective inducer of de novo transferrin synthesis in neutrophils through the Jak/Stat5β pathway [114]. Interestingly, cancer cells that express the GM-CSF receptor may undergo EMT through the GM-CSF autocrine mechanism [115], and mesenchymal cells differentially secrete GM-CSF [116]. Neutrophils are the most abundant circulating immune cell population. They were shown to escort CTCs (form CTC-neutrophil clusters) and enable cell cycle progression in disseminated tumor cells [117]. Such CTC–neutrophil clusters represent the most efficient metastasis-forming cell subpopulation in breast cancer CTCs, and their presence in the patients' bloodstream is associated with a poor prognosis [117]. Vascular cell adhesion molecule 1 (VCAM1) was identified as the functional mediator for CTC-neutrophil interaction [117]. Although no difference on EMT-related genes was found between the CTCs with or without neutrophil escort, CTCs in general have been linked with C-EMT or P-EMT, as we discussed in the first section of this review. Intriguingly, VCAM-1 over-expression in normal breast epithelial cells controls the EMT program and has been associated with poor clinical prognosis in breast cancer patients [118].

## 3.3. Metastasis-Associated Natural Killer (NK) Cells

There is a general consensus that NK cells exert cytotoxicity against metastatic tumor cells. EMT activation in tumor cells during metastasis cascade is also accompanied by altered cell-surface ligands recognizable by NK cell-activating receptors, thus increasing susceptibility to NK cells [119,120].

A recent study by Chockley et al. reported that NK cells were activated to attack metastatic EMT tumor cells through the balance of activating and inhibitory receptors engaged by different ligands, and the EMT induced NK cell activity mediated immunosurveillance in lung metastasis [120]. Specifically, NK cells express killer lectin-like receptor G1 (KLRG1), which is an inhibitory receptor, and E-cad is an inhibitory ligand that engages KLRG1. The down-regulated E-cad during EMT released its inhibitory effect on KLRG1 and led to the activation of NK cells. Meanwhile, EMT also induced expression of cell adhesion molecule 1 (CADM1), which is an activating NK ligand and binds to the cytotoxic and regulatory T cell-associated molecule (CRTAM) receptor on NK cells. CADM1 is identified as a tumor suppressor and is frequently down-regulated in various types of tumors. Depletion of NK cells allowed spontaneous metastasis without affecting primary tumor growth in lung cancer [120].

*3.4. Metastasis-Associated T Cells*

T cell infiltration is crucial to tumor microenvironments and has been extensively studied in primary tumors [121]. However, T cell-dependent mechanisms involved in organ-specific metastasis remain underexplored. Mansfield et al. studied the T-cell clonal evolution in primary non-small cell lung tumors (NSCLC) and paired brain metastases [122]. They found significantly less numbers of unique T cell clones in brain metastases than those in primary tumors, and the clones were minimally overlapped, suggesting a divergent tumor immunogenicity following metastasis [122]. However, despite the contraction in the number of T cell clones, brain metastases harbored higher non-synonymous mutation burdens than primary lesions which may lead to the emergent expression of neoantigens [122]. Thereby, clinical response to anti-programmed cell death-1 (PD-1) monotherapy with pembrolizumab has shown intracranial response rates of 20–30% in patients with NSCLC or melanoma brain metastases [123]. The combination of nivolumab and ipilimumab (anti-PD-1 and anti-cytotoxic T-lymphocyte-associated protein 4 (CTLA-4)) showed an intracranial response rate of 55% in patients with melanoma brain metastases [124]. The emergence of neoantigens in brain metastatic tumors may be related to the very active neurogenesis, cellular differentiation and reprogramming state as evidenced by the co-expression of the epithelial marker with the mesenchymal marker and the high expression of stem cell markers [45].

## 4. Conclusions

In solid tumors, of which 90% are epithelial in nature, epithelial-mesenchymal plasticity is a fundamental factor in governing metastasis. As shown in Figure 2, emerging data have shown that certain types of tumors with heterogeneous EMT states or different degrees of EMT are prone to metastasize to different organs. Although the underlying mechanisms remain to be explored, the current studies indicate that cellular plasticity is linked with constant changes to produce various bioactive factors. The secreted bioactive factors not only contribute to shaping PMNs at specific organ sites, but also modify the local immune landscape, and in the meantime increase the plasticity of the niche cells. The niche cells reciprocally produce bioactive factors and interact with tumor cells and among themselves, leading to organotropism metastatic tumor growth. Thus, systematic studies of cell–cell communication on organ-specific tumor metastasis models will enable researchers to have a more precise picture of the co-evolution of metastatic tumor cells and their surrounding microenvironment, and offers new ways for therapeutic exploitation.

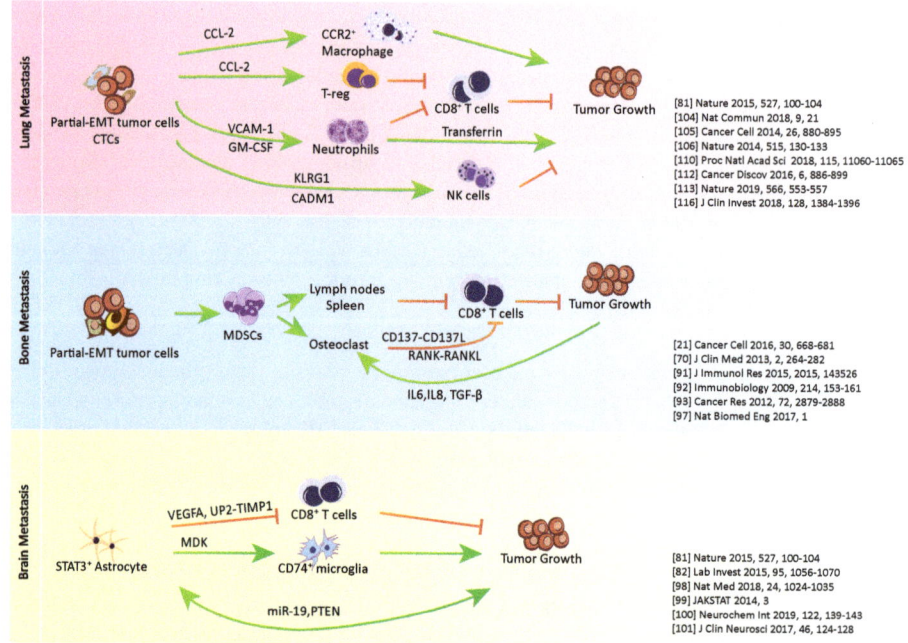

**Figure 2.** Crosstalk between cancer cells, immunosuppressive cells and immune effector cells in lung, bone, and brain metastasis.

**Author Contributions:** Writing—original draft preparation, X.N., J.W., H.N.L., and H.Z.; writing—review and editing, H.Z.; visualization, X.N.; supervision, H.Z., S.T.C.W.; funding acquisition, S.T.C.W.

**Funding:** This work was funded by NIH U54 CA149196, NIH U01CA188388, John S. Dunn Research Foundation, and TT and WF Chao Foundation to S.T.C.W., and China Scholarship Council to X.N.

**Acknowledgments:** The authors would like to thank Rebecca Danforth for proofreading the manuscript.

**Conflicts of Interest:** The authors declare no conflicts of interest.

## References

1. Chaffer, C.L.; Weinberg, R.A. A perspective on cancer cell metastasis. *Science* **2011**, *331*, 1559–1564. [CrossRef]
2. Turajlic, S.; Swanton, C. Metastasis as an evolutionary process. *Science* **2016**, *352*, 169–175. [CrossRef]
3. Paget, S. The distribution of secondary growths in cancer of the breast. 1889. *Cancer Metastasis Rev.* **1989**, *8*, 98–101.
4. Akhtar, M.; Haider, A.; Rashid, S.; Al-Nabet, A. Paget's "Seed and Soil" theory of cancer metastasis: An idea whose time has come. *Adv. Anat. Pathol.* **2019**, *26*, 69–74. [CrossRef] [PubMed]
5. Chen, W.; Hoffmann, A.D.; Liu, H.; Liu, X. Organotropism: New insights into molecular mechanisms of breast cancer metastasis. *NPJ Precis. Oncol.* **2018**, *2*, 4. [CrossRef] [PubMed]
6. Wu, Q.; Li, J.; Zhu, S.; Wu, J.; Chen, C.; Liu, Q.; Wei, W.; Zhang, Y.; Sun, S. Breast cancer subtypes predict the preferential site of distant metastases: A SEER based study. *Oncotarget* **2017**, *8*, 27990–27996. [CrossRef]
7. Kennecke, H.; Yerushalmi, R.; Woods, R.; Cheang, M.C.; Voduc, D.; Speers, C.H.; Nielsen, T.O.; Gelmon, K. Metastatic behavior of breast cancer subtypes. *J. Clin. Oncol.* **2010**, *28*, 3271–3277. [CrossRef]
8. Obenauf, A.C.; Massagué, J. Surviving at a distance: Organ specific metastasis. *Trends Cancer* **2015**, *1*, 76–91. [CrossRef] [PubMed]
9. Er, E.E.; Valiente, M.; Ganesh, K.; Zou, Y.; Agrawal, S.; Hu, J.; Griscom, B.; Rosenblum, M.; Boire, A.; Brogi, E.; et al. Pericyte-like spreading by disseminated cancer cells activates YAP and MRTF for metastatic colonization. *Nat. Cell Biol.* **2018**, *20*, 966–978. [CrossRef]

10. Valiente, M.; Obenauf, A.C.; Jin, X.; Chen, Q.; Zhang, X.H.; Lee, D.J.; Chaft, J.E.; Kris, M.G.; Huse, J.T.; Brogi, E.; et al. Serpins promote cancer cell survival and vascular co-option in brain metastasis. *Cell* **2014**, *156*, 1002–1016. [CrossRef] [PubMed]
11. Bos, P.D.; Zhang, X.H.; Nadal, C.; Shu, W.; Gomis, R.R.; Nguyen, D.X.; Minn, A.J.; van de Vijver, M.J.; Gerald, W.L.; Foekens, J.A.; et al. Genes that mediate breast cancer metastasis to the brain. *Nature* **2009**, *459*, 1005–1009. [CrossRef]
12. Minn, A.J.; Gupta, G.P.; Siegel, P.M.; Bos, P.D.; Shu, W.; Giri, D.D.; Viale, A.; Olshen, A.B.; Gerald, W.L.; Massague, J. Genes that mediate breast cancer metastasis to lung. *Nature* **2005**, *436*, 518–524. [CrossRef]
13. Kang, Y.; Siegel, P.M.; Shu, W.; Drobnjak, M.; Kakonen, S.M.; Cordon-Cardo, C.; Guise, T.A.; Massague, J. A multigenic program mediating breast cancer metastasis to bone. *Cancer Cell* **2003**, *3*, 537–549. [CrossRef]
14. Kan, C.; Vargas, G.; Pape, F.L.; Clezardin, P. Cancer cell colonisation in the bone microenvironment. *Int. J. Mol. Sci.* **2016**, *17*. [CrossRef]
15. Dong, X. Current strategies for brain drug delivery. *Theranostics* **2018**, *8*, 1481–1493. [CrossRef] [PubMed]
16. Walker, C.; Mojares, E.; Del Rio Hernandez, A. Role of extracellular matrix in development and cancer progression. *Int. J. Mol. Sci.* **2018**, *19*. [CrossRef] [PubMed]
17. Kaminska, K.; Szczylik, C.; Bielecka, Z.F.; Bartnik, E.; Porta, C.; Lian, F.; Czarnecka, A.M. The role of the cell–cell interactions in cancer progression. *J. Cell Mol. Med.* **2015**, *19*, 283–296. [CrossRef]
18. Blomberg, O.S.; Spagnuolo, L.; de Visser, K.E. Immune regulation of metastasis: Mechanistic insights and therapeutic opportunities. *Dis. Model Mech.* **2018**, *11*. [CrossRef]
19. Peinado, H.; Zhang, H.; Matei, I.R.; Costa-Silva, B.; Hoshino, A.; Rodrigues, G.; Psaila, B.; Kaplan, R.N.; Bromberg, J.F.; Kang, Y.; et al. Pre-metastatic niches: Organ-specific homes for metastases. *Nat. Rev. Cancer* **2017**, *17*, 302–317. [CrossRef]
20. Kaplan, R.N.; Riba, R.D.; Zacharoulis, S.; Bramley, A.H.; Vincent, L.; Costa, C.; MacDonald, D.D.; Jin, D.K.; Shido, K.; Kerns, S.A.; et al. VEGFR1-positive haematopoietic bone marrow progenitors initiate the pre-metastatic niche. *Nature* **2005**, *438*, 820–827. [CrossRef] [PubMed]
21. Liu, Y.; Cao, X. Characteristics and significance of the pre-metastatic niche. *Cancer Cell* **2016**, *30*, 668–681. [CrossRef]
22. Erler, J.T.; Bennewith, K.L.; Cox, T.R.; Lang, G.; Bird, D.; Koong, A.; Le, Q.T.; Giaccia, A.J. Hypoxia-induced lysyl oxidase is a critical mediator of bone marrow cell recruitment to form the premetastatic niche. *Cancer Cell* **2009**, *15*, 35–44. [CrossRef] [PubMed]
23. Giles, A.J.; Reid, C.M.; Evans, J.D.; Murgai, M.; Vicioso, Y.; Highfill, S.L.; Kasai, M.; Vahdat, L.; Mackall, C.L.; Lyden, D.; et al. Activation of hematopoietic stem/progenitor cells promotes immunosuppression within the pre-metastatic niche. *Cancer Res.* **2016**, *76*, 1335–1347. [CrossRef]
24. Sceneay, J.; Parker, B.S.; Smyth, M.J.; Moller, A. Hypoxia-driven immunosuppression contributes to the pre-metastatic niche. *Oncoimmunology* **2013**, *2*, e22355. [CrossRef]
25. Kalluri, R.; Weinberg, R.A. The basics of epithelial-mesenchymal transition. *J. Clin. Investig.* **2009**, *119*, 1420–1428. [CrossRef] [PubMed]
26. Yang, J.; Weinberg, R.A. Epithelial-mesenchymal transition: At the crossroads of development and tumor metastasis. *Dev. Cell* **2008**, *14*, 818–829. [CrossRef] [PubMed]
27. Roche, J. The epithelial-to-mesenchymal transition in cancer. *Cancers* **2018**, *10*. [CrossRef] [PubMed]
28. Brabletz, T.; Kalluri, R.; Nieto, M.A.; Weinberg, R.A. EMT in cancer. *Nat. Rev. Cancer* **2018**, *18*, 128–134. [CrossRef] [PubMed]
29. Chaffer, C.L.; San Juan, B.P.; Lim, E.; Weinberg, R.A. EMT, cell plasticity and metastasis. *Cancer Metastasis Rev.* **2016**, *35*, 645–654. [CrossRef]
30. Jolly, M.K.; Ware, K.E.; Gilja, S.; Somarelli, J.A.; Levine, H. EMT and MET: Necessary or permissive for metastasis? *Mol. Oncol.* **2017**, *11*, 755–769. [CrossRef]
31. Zhao, Z.; Zhu, X.; Cui, K.; Mancuso, J.; Federley, R.; Fischer, K.; Teng, G.; Mittal, V.; Gao, D.; Zhao, H.; et al. In vivo visualization and characterization of epithelial-mesenchymal transition in breast tumors. *Cancer Res.* **2016**, *76*, 2094–2104. [CrossRef] [PubMed]
32. Condeelis, J.; Segall, J.E. Intravital imaging of cell movement in tumours. *Nat. Rev. Cancer* **2003**, *3*, 921–930. [CrossRef]
33. Kalluri, R.; Zeisberg, M. Fibroblasts in cancer. *Nat. Rev. Cancer* **2006**, *6*, 392–401. [CrossRef] [PubMed]

34. Aiello, N.M.; Maddipati, R.; Norgard, R.J.; Balli, D.; Li, J.; Yuan, S.; Yamazoe, T.; Black, T.; Sahmoud, A.; Furth, E.E.; et al. EMT subtype influences epithelial plasticity and mode of cell migration. *Dev. Cell* **2018**, *45*, 681–695. [CrossRef]
35. Puram, S.V.; Tirosh, I.; Parikh, A.S.; Patel, A.P.; Yizhak, K.; Gillespie, S.; Rodman, C.; Luo, C.L.; Mroz, E.A.; Emerick, K.S.; et al. Single-cell transcriptomic analysis of primary and metastatic tumor ecosystems in head and neck cancer. *Cell* **2017**, *171*, 1611–1624. [CrossRef] [PubMed]
36. Christiansen, J.J.; Rajasekaran, A.K. Reassessing epithelial to mesenchymal transition as a prerequisite for carcinoma invasion and metastasis. *Cancer Res.* **2006**, *66*, 8319–8326. [CrossRef] [PubMed]
37. Fischer, K.R.; Durrans, A.; Lee, S.; Sheng, J.; Li, F.; Wong, S.T.; Choi, H.; El Rayes, T.; Ryu, S.; Troeger, J.; et al. Epithelial-to-mesenchymal transition is not required for lung metastasis but contributes to chemoresistance. *Nature* **2015**, *527*, 472–476. [CrossRef] [PubMed]
38. Lecharpentier, A.; Vielh, P.; Perez-Moreno, P.; Planchard, D.; Soria, J.C.; Farace, F. Detection of circulating tumour cells with a hybrid (epithelial/mesenchymal) phenotype in patients with metastatic non-small cell lung cancer. *Br. J. Cancer* **2011**, *105*, 1338–1341. [CrossRef] [PubMed]
39. Armstrong, A.J.; Marengo, M.S.; Oltean, S.; Kemeny, G.; Bitting, R.L.; Turnbull, J.D.; Herold, C.I.; Marcom, P.K.; George, D.J.; Garcia-Blanco, M.A. Circulating tumor cells from patients with advanced prostate and breast cancer display both epithelial and mesenchymal markers. *Mol. Cancer Res.* **2011**, *9*, 997–1007. [CrossRef]
40. Lo, H.C.; Zhang, X.H. EMT in metastasis: Finding the right balance. *Dev. Cell* **2018**, *45*, 663–665. [CrossRef]
41. Joosse, S.A.; Gorges, T.M.; Pantel, K. Biology, detection, and clinical implications of circulating tumor cells. *EMBO Mol. Med.* **2015**, *7*, 1–11. [CrossRef] [PubMed]
42. Aceto, N.; Bardia, A.; Miyamoto, D.T.; Donaldson, M.C.; Wittner, B.S.; Spencer, J.A.; Yu, M.; Pely, A.; Engstrom, A.; Zhu, H.; et al. Circulating tumor cell clusters are oligoclonal precursors of breast cancer metastasis. *Cell* **2014**, *158*, 1110–1122. [CrossRef]
43. Jolly, M.K.; Boareto, M.; Huang, B.; Jia, D.; Lu, M.; Ben-Jacob, E.; Onuchic, J.N.; Levine, H. Implications of the hybrid epithelial/mesenchymal phenotype in metastasis. *Front. Oncol.* **2015**, *5*, 155. [CrossRef]
44. Wingrove, E.; Liu, Z.Z.; Patel, K.D.; Arnal-Estape, A.; Cai, W.L.; Melnick, M.A.; Politi, K.; Monteiro, C.; Zhu, L.; Valiente, M.; et al. Transcriptomic hallmarks of tumor plasticity and stromal interactions in brain metastasis. *Cell Rep.* **2019**, *27*, 1277–1292. [CrossRef]
45. Jeevan, D.S.; Cooper, J.B.; Braun, A.; Murali, R.; Jhanwar-Uniyal, M. Molecular pathways mediating metastases to the brain via epithelial-to-mesenchymal transition: Genes, proteins, and functional analysis. *Anticancer Res.* **2016**, *36*, 523–532. [PubMed]
46. Somarelli, J.A.; Schaeffer, D.; Marengo, M.S.; Bepler, T.; Rouse, D.; Ware, K.E.; Hish, A.J.; Zhao, Y.; Buckley, A.F.; Epstein, J.I.; et al. Distinct routes to metastasis: Plasticity-dependent and plasticity-independent pathways. *Oncogene* **2016**, *35*, 4302–4311. [CrossRef] [PubMed]
47. Melzer, C.; von der Ohe, J.; Lehnert, H.; Ungefroren, H.; Hass, R. Cancer stem cell niche models and contribution by mesenchymal stroma/stem cells. *Mol. Cancer* **2017**, *16*, 28. [CrossRef] [PubMed]
48. Shibue, T.; Weinberg, R.A. EMT, CSCs, and drug resistance: The mechanistic link and clinical implications. *Nat. Rev. Clin. Oncol.* **2017**, *14*, 611–629. [CrossRef]
49. Puisieux, A.; Brabletz, T.; Caramel, J. Oncogenic roles of EMT-inducing transcription factors. *Nat. Cell Biol.* **2014**, *16*, 488–494. [CrossRef] [PubMed]
50. Nieto, M.A.; Huang, R.Y.; Jackson, R.A.; Thiery, J.P. EMT: 2016. *Cell* **2016**, *166*, 21–45. [CrossRef] [PubMed]
51. Battistelli, C.; Cicchini, C.; Santangelo, L.; Tramontano, A.; Grassi, L.; Gonzalez, F.J.; de Nonno, V.; Grassi, G.; Amicone, L.; Tripodi, M. The Snail repressor recruits EZH2 to specific genomic sites through the enrollment of the lncRNA HOTAIR in epithelial-to-mesenchymal transition. *Oncogene* **2017**, *36*, 942–955. [CrossRef] [PubMed]
52. Battistelli, C.; Tripodi, M.; Cicchini, C. Targeting of polycombs to DNA in EMT. *Oncotarget* **2017**, *8*, 57936–57937. [CrossRef] [PubMed]
53. Chao, Y.L.; Shepard, C.R.; Wells, A. Breast carcinoma cells re-express E-cadherin during mesenchymal to epithelial reverting transition. *Mol. Cancer* **2010**, *9*, 179. [CrossRef] [PubMed]
54. Jiang, J.; Tang, Y.L.; Liang, X.H. EMT: A new vision of hypoxia promoting cancer progression. *Cancer Biol. Ther.* **2011**, *11*, 714–723. [CrossRef] [PubMed]
55. Joseph, J.P.; Harishankar, M.K.; Pillai, A.A.; Devi, A. Hypoxia induced EMT: A review on the mechanism of tumor progression and metastasis in OSCC. *Oral Oncol.* **2018**, *80*, 23–32. [CrossRef] [PubMed]

56. Zhang, J.; Tian, X.J.; Xing, J. Signal transduction pathways of EMT induced by TGF-beta, SHH, and WNT and their crosstalks. *J. Clin. Med.* **2016**, *5*. [CrossRef] [PubMed]
57. Jolly, M.K.; Tripathi, S.C.; Jia, D.; Mooney, S.M.; Celiktas, M.; Hanash, S.M.; Mani, S.A.; Pienta, K.J.; Ben-Jacob, E.; Levine, H. Stability of the hybrid epithelial/mesenchymal phenotype. *Oncotarget* **2016**, *7*, 27067–27084. [CrossRef] [PubMed]
58. Jolly, M.K.; Jia, D.; Boareto, M.; Mani, S.A.; Pienta, K.J.; Ben-Jacob, E.; Levine, H. Coupling the modules of EMT and stemness: A tunable 'stemness window' model. *Oncotarget* **2015**, *6*, 25161–25174. [CrossRef]
59. Garg, M. Epithelial plasticity and cancer stem cells: Major mechanisms of cancer pathogenesis and therapy resistance. *World J. Stem Cells* **2017**, *9*, 118–126. [CrossRef] [PubMed]
60. Reichert, M.; Bakir, B.; Moreira, L.; Pitarresi, J.R.; Feldmann, K.; Simon, L.; Suzuki, K.; Maddipati, R.; Rhim, A.D.; Schlitter, A.M.; et al. Regulation of epithelial plasticity determines metastatic organotropism in pancreatic cancer. *Dev. Cell* **2018**, *45*, 696–711. [CrossRef] [PubMed]
61. Liao, T.T.; Yang, M.H. Revisiting epithelial-mesenchymal transition in cancer metastasis: The connection between epithelial plasticity and stemness. *Mol. Oncol.* **2017**, *11*, 792–804. [CrossRef] [PubMed]
62. Gao, W.; Chen, L.; Ma, Z.; Du, Z.; Zhao, Z.; Hu, Z.; Li, Q. Isolation and phenotypic characterization of colorectal cancer stem cells with organ-specific metastatic potential. *Gastroenterology* **2013**, *145*, 636–646. [CrossRef] [PubMed]
63. Yousefi, M.; Nosrati, R.; Salmaninejad, A.; Dehghani, S.; Shahryari, A.; Saberi, A. Organ-specific metastasis of breast cancer: Molecular and cellular mechanisms underlying lung metastasis. *Cell Oncol.* **2018**, *41*, 123–140. [CrossRef] [PubMed]
64. Ren, D.; Zhu, X.; Kong, R.; Zhao, Z.; Sheng, J.; Wang, J.; Xu, X.; Liu, J.; Cui, K.; Zhang, X.H.; et al. Targeting brain-adaptive cancer stem cells prohibits brain metastatic colonization of triple-negative breast cancer. *Cancer Res.* **2018**, *78*, 2052–2064. [CrossRef]
65. Stankic, M.; Pavlovic, S.; Chin, Y.; Brogi, E.; Padua, D.; Norton, L.; Massague, J.; Benezra, R. TGF-beta-Id1 signaling opposes Twist1 and promotes metastatic colonization via a mesenchymal-to-epithelial transition. *Cell Rep.* **2013**, *5*, 1228–1242. [CrossRef] [PubMed]
66. Schmidt, J.M.; Panzilius, E.; Bartsch, H.S.; Irmler, M.; Beckers, J.; Kari, V.; Linnemann, J.R.; Dragoi, D.; Hirschi, B.; Kloos, U.J.; et al. Stem-cell-like properties and epithelial plasticity arise as stable traits after transient Twist1 activation. *Cell Rep.* **2015**, *10*, 131–139. [CrossRef]
67. Yu, M.; Bardia, A.; Wittner, B.S.; Stott, S.L.; Smas, M.E.; Ting, D.T.; Isakoff, S.J.; Ciciliano, J.C.; Wells, M.N.; Shah, A.M.; et al. Circulating breast tumor cells exhibit dynamic changes in epithelial and mesenchymal composition. *Science* **2013**, *339*, 580–584. [CrossRef]
68. Ruscetti, M.; Quach, B.; Dadashian, E.L.; Mulholland, D.J.; Wu, H. Tracking and functional characterization of epithelial-mesenchymal transition and mesenchymal tumor cells during prostate cancer metastasis. *Cancer Res.* **2015**, *75*, 2749–2759. [CrossRef] [PubMed]
69. Strauss, R.; Li, Z.Y.; Liu, Y.; Beyer, I.; Persson, J.; Sova, P.; Moller, T.; Pesonen, S.; Hemminki, A.; Hamerlik, P.; et al. Analysis of epithelial and mesenchymal markers in ovarian cancer reveals phenotypic heterogeneity and plasticity. *PLoS ONE* **2011**, *6*, e16186. [CrossRef]
70. Beerling, E.; Seinstra, D.; de Wit, E.; Kester, L.; van der Velden, D.; Maynard, C.; Schafer, R.; van Diest, P.; Voest, E.; van Oudenaarden, A.; et al. Plasticity between epithelial and mesenchymal states unlinks EMT from metastasis-enhancing stem cell capacity. *Cell Rep.* **2016**, *14*, 2281–2288. [CrossRef]
71. Perdigao-Henriques, R.; Petrocca, F.; Altschuler, G.; Thomas, M.P.; Le, M.T.; Tan, S.M.; Hide, W.; Lieberman, J. miR-200 promotes the mesenchymal to epithelial transition by suppressing multiple members of the Zeb2 and Snail1 transcriptional repressor complexes. *Oncogene* **2016**, *35*, 158–172. [CrossRef]
72. Bockhorn, J.; Dalton, R.; Nwachukwu, C.; Huang, S.; Prat, A.; Yee, K.; Chang, Y.F.; Huo, D.; Wen, Y.; Swanson, K.E.; et al. MicroRNA-30c inhibits human breast tumour chemotherapy resistance by regulating TWF1 and IL-11. *Nat. Commun.* **2013**, *4*, 1393. [CrossRef] [PubMed]
73. Okuda, H.; Xing, F.; Pandey, P.R.; Sharma, S.; Watabe, M.; Pai, S.K.; Mo, Y.Y.; Iiizumi-Gairani, M.; Hirota, S.; Liu, Y.; et al. miR-7 suppresses brain metastasis of breast cancer stem-like cells by modulating KLF4. *Cancer Res.* **2013**, *73*, 1434–1444. [CrossRef] [PubMed]
74. Demirkan, B. The roles of epithelial-to-mesenchymal transition (EMT) and mesenchymal-to-epithelial transition (MET) in breast cancer bone metastasis: Potential targets for prevention and treatment. *J. Clin. Med.* **2013**, *2*, 264–282. [CrossRef]

75. Fong, M.Y.; Zhou, W.; Liu, L.; Alontaga, A.Y.; Chandra, M.; Ashby, J.; Chow, A.; O'Connor, S.T.; Li, S.; Chin, A.R.; et al. Breast-cancer-secreted miR-122 reprograms glucose metabolism in premetastatic niche to promote metastasis. *Nat. Cell Biol.* **2015**, *17*, 183–194. [CrossRef]
76. Sciacovelli, M.; Frezza, C. Metabolic reprogramming and epithelial-to-mesenchymal transition in cancer. *FEBS J.* **2017**, *284*, 3132–3144. [CrossRef] [PubMed]
77. Ell, B.; Qiu, Q.; Wei, Y.; Mercatali, L.; Ibrahim, T.; Amadori, D.; Kang, Y. The microRNA-23b/27b/24 cluster promotes breast cancer lung metastasis by targeting metastasis-suppressive gene prosaposin. *J. Biol. Chem.* **2014**, *289*, 21888–21895. [CrossRef]
78. Ma, F.; Li, W.; Liu, C.; Li, W.; Yu, H.; Lei, B.; Ren, Y.; Li, Z.; Pang, D.; Qian, C. MiR-23a promotes TGF-beta1-induced EMT and tumor metastasis in breast cancer cells by directly targeting CDH1 and activating Wnt/beta-catenin signaling. *Oncotarget* **2017**, *8*, 69538–69550.
79. Jiang, G.; Shi, W.; Fang, H.; Zhang, X. miR27a promotes human breast cancer cell migration by inducing EMT in a FBXW7dependent manner. *Mol. Med. Rep.* **2018**, *18*, 5417–5426.
80. Schrijver, W.A.; van Diest, P.J.; Dutch Distant Breast Cancer Metastases Consortium; Moelans, C.B. Unravelling site-specific breast cancer metastasis: A microRNA expression profiling study. *Oncotarget* **2017**, *8*, 3111–3123. [CrossRef]
81. Zhang, J.; Chen, D.; Liang, S.; Wang, J.; Liu, C.; Nie, C.; Shan, Z.; Wang, L.; Fan, Q.; Wang, F. miR-106b promotes cell invasion and metastasis via PTEN mediated EMT in ESCC. *Oncol. Lett.* **2018**, *15*, 4619–4626. [CrossRef] [PubMed]
82. Zhou, X.; Hu, Y.; Dai, L.; Wang, Y.; Zhou, J.; Wang, W.; Di, W.; Qiu, L. MicroRNA-7 inhibits tumor metastasis and reverses epithelial-mesenchymal transition through AKT/ERK1/2 inactivation by targeting EGFR in epithelial ovarian cancer. *PLoS ONE* **2014**, *9*, e96718. [CrossRef] [PubMed]
83. Mody, H.R.; Hung, S.W.; Pathak, R.K.; Griffin, J.; Cruz-Monserrate, Z.; Govindarajan, R. miR-202 diminishes TGFbeta receptors and attenuates TGFbeta1-induced EMT in pancreatic cancer. *Mol. Cancer Res.* **2017**, *15*, 1029–1039. [CrossRef]
84. Zhou, W.; Fong, M.Y.; Min, Y.; Somlo, G.; Liu, L.; Palomares, M.R.; Yu, Y.; Chow, A.; O'Connor, S.T.; Chin, A.R.; et al. Cancer-secreted miR-105 destroys vascular endothelial barriers to promote metastasis. *Cancer Cell* **2014**, *25*, 501–515. [CrossRef] [PubMed]
85. Zhang, L.; Zhang, S.; Yao, J.; Lowery, F.J.; Zhang, Q.; Huang, W.C.; Li, P.; Li, M.; Wang, X.; Zhang, C.; et al. Microenvironment-induced PTEN loss by exosomal microRNA primes brain metastasis outgrowth. *Nature* **2015**, *527*, 100–104. [CrossRef] [PubMed]
86. Li, J.; Yang, S.; Yan, W.; Yang, J.; Qin, Y.J.; Lin, X.L.; Xie, R.Y.; Wang, S.C.; Jin, W.; Gao, F.; et al. MicroRNA-19 triggers epithelial-mesenchymal transition of lung cancer cells accompanied by growth inhibition. *Lab. Investig.* **2015**, *95*, 1056–1070. [CrossRef]
87. Rana, S.; Malinowska, K.; Zoller, M. Exosomal tumor microRNA modulates premetastatic organ cells. *Neoplasia* **2013**, *15*, 281–295. [CrossRef] [PubMed]
88. Yang, Y.; Tao, X.; Li, C.B.; Wang, C.M. MicroRNA-494 acts as a tumor suppressor in pancreatic cancer, inhibiting epithelial-mesenchymal transition, migration and invasion by binding to SDC1. *Int. J. Oncol.* **2018**, *53*, 1204–1214. [CrossRef] [PubMed]
89. Tao, J.; Liu, Z.; Wang, Y.; Wang, L.; Yao, B.; Li, Q.; Wang, C.; Tu, K.; Liu, Q. MiR-542-3p inhibits metastasis and epithelial-mesenchymal transition of hepatocellular carcinoma by targeting UBE3C. *Biomed. Pharmacother.* **2017**, *93*, 420–428. [CrossRef] [PubMed]
90. Hoshino, A.; Costa-Silva, B.; Shen, T.L.; Rodrigues, G.; Hashimoto, A.; Tesic Mark, M.; Molina, H.; Kohsaka, S.; Di Giannatale, A.; Ceder, S.; et al. Tumour exosome integrins determine organotropic metastasis. *Nature* **2015**, *527*, 329–335. [CrossRef]
91. Lamouille, S.; Xu, J.; Derynck, R. Molecular mechanisms of epithelial-mesenchymal transition. *Nat. Rev. Mol. Cell Biol.* **2014**, *15*, 178–196. [CrossRef]
92. Friedl, P.; Alexander, S. Cancer invasion and the microenvironment: Plasticity and reciprocity. *Cell* **2011**, *147*, 992–1009. [CrossRef] [PubMed]
93. Gentles, A.J.; Newman, A.M.; Liu, C.L.; Bratman, S.V.; Feng, W.; Kim, D.; Nair, V.S.; Xu, Y.; Khuong, A.; Hoang, C.D.; et al. The prognostic landscape of genes and infiltrating immune cells across human cancers. *Nat. Med.* **2015**, *21*, 938–945. [CrossRef] [PubMed]

94. Terry, S.; Savagner, P.; Ortiz-Cuaran, S.; Mahjoubi, L.; Saintigny, P.; Thiery, J.P.; Chouaib, S. New insights into the role of EMT in tumor immune escape. *Mol. Oncol.* **2017**, *11*, 824–846. [CrossRef] [PubMed]
95. D'Amico, L.; Roato, I. The impact of immune system in regulating bone metastasis formation by osteotropic tumors. *J. Immunol. Res.* **2015**, *2015*, 143526. [CrossRef] [PubMed]
96. Senthilkumar, R.; Lee, H.W. CD137L- and RANKL-mediated reverse signals inhibit osteoclastogenesis and T lymphocyte proliferation. *Immunobiology* **2009**, *214*, 153–161. [CrossRef] [PubMed]
97. Palafox, M.; Ferrer, I.; Pellegrini, P.; Vila, S.; Hernandez-Ortega, S.; Urruticoechea, A.; Climent, F.; Soler, M.T.; Munoz, P.; Vinals, F.; et al. RANK induces epithelial-mesenchymal transition and stemness in human mammary epithelial cells and promotes tumorigenesis and metastasis. *Cancer Res.* **2012**, *72*, 2879–2888. [CrossRef]
98. Capietto, A.H.; Kim, S.; Sanford, D.E.; Linehan, D.C.; Hikida, M.; Kumosaki, T.; Novack, D.V.; Faccio, R. Down-regulation of PLCgamma2-beta-catenin pathway promotes activation and expansion of myeloid-derived suppressor cells in cancer. *J. Exp. Med.* **2013**, *210*, 2257–2271. [CrossRef]
99. Gao, D.; Joshi, N.; Choi, H.; Ryu, S.; Hahn, M.; Catena, R.; Sadik, H.; Argani, P.; Wagner, P.; Vahdat, L.T.; et al. Myeloid progenitor cells in the premetastatic lung promote metastases by inducing mesenchymal to epithelial transition. *Cancer Res.* **2012**, *72*, 1384–1394. [CrossRef]
100. Becker, A.; Thakur, B.K.; Weiss, J.M.; Kim, H.S.; Peinado, H.; Lyden, D. Extracellular vesicles in cancer: Cell-to-cell mediators of metastasis. *Cancer Cell* **2016**, *30*, 836–848. [CrossRef]
101. Aguado, B.A.; Bushnell, G.G.; Rao, S.S.; Jeruss, J.S.; Shea, L.D. Engineering the pre-metastatic niche. *Nat. Biomed. Eng.* **2017**, *1*. [CrossRef]
102. Priego, N.; Zhu, L.; Monteiro, C.; Mulders, M.; Wasilewski, D.; Bindeman, W.; Doglio, L.; Martinez, L.; Martinez-Saez, E.; Ramon, Y.C.S.; et al. STAT3 labels a subpopulation of reactive astrocytes required for brain metastasis. *Nat. Med.* **2018**, *24*, 1024–1035. [CrossRef] [PubMed]
103. Wendt, M.K.; Balanis, N.; Carlin, C.R.; Schiemann, W.P. STAT3 and epithelial-mesenchymal transitions in carcinomas. *JAKSTAT* **2014**, *3*, e28975. [CrossRef]
104. Iser, I.C.; Lenz, G.; Wink, M.R. EMT-like process in glioblastomas and reactive astrocytes. *Neurochem. Int.* **2019**, *122*, 139–143. [CrossRef] [PubMed]
105. Nagaishi, M.; Nakata, S.; Ono, Y.; Hirata, K.; Tanaka, Y.; Suzuki, K.; Yokoo, H.; Hyodo, A. Tumoral and stromal expression of Slug, ZEB1, and ZEB2 in brain metastasis. *J. Clin. Neurosci.* **2017**, *46*, 124–128. [CrossRef]
106. Gonzalez, H.; Robles, I.; Werb, Z. Innate and acquired immune surveillance in the postdissemination phase of metastasis. *FEBS J.* **2018**, *285*, 654–664. [CrossRef]
107. Piao, Y.J.; Kim, H.S.; Hwang, E.H.; Woo, J.; Zhang, M.; Moon, W.K. Breast cancer cell-derived exosomes and macrophage polarization are associated with lymph node metastasis. *Oncotarget* **2018**, *9*, 7398–7410. [CrossRef]
108. Linde, N.; Casanova-Acebes, M.; Sosa, M.S.; Mortha, A.; Rahman, A.; Farias, E.; Harper, K.; Tardio, E.; Reyes Torres, I.; Jones, J.; et al. Macrophages orchestrate breast cancer early dissemination and metastasis. *Nat. Commun.* **2018**, *9*, 21. [CrossRef]
109. Srivastava, K.; Hu, J.; Korn, C.; Savant, S.; Teichert, M.; Kapel, S.S.; Jugold, M.; Besemfelder, E.; Thomas, M.; Pasparakis, M.; et al. Postsurgical adjuvant tumor therapy by combining anti-angiopoietin-2 and metronomic chemotherapy limits metastatic growth. *Cancer Cell* **2014**, *26*, 880–895. [CrossRef] [PubMed]
110. Bonapace, L.; Coissieux, M.M.; Wyckoff, J.; Mertz, K.D.; Varga, Z.; Junt, T.; Bentires-Alj, M. Cessation of CCL2 inhibition accelerates breast cancer metastasis by promoting angiogenesis. *Nature* **2014**, *515*, 130–133. [CrossRef]
111. Suarez-Carmona, M.; Lesage, J.; Cataldo, D.; Gilles, C. EMT and inflammation: Inseparable actors of cancer progression. *Mol. Oncol.* **2017**, *11*, 805–823. [CrossRef] [PubMed]
112. Lin, W.J.; Izumi, K. Androgen receptor, CCL2, and epithelial-mesenchymal transition: A dangerous affair in the tumor microenvironment. *Oncoimmunology* **2014**, *3*, e27871. [CrossRef]
113. Tuting, T.; de Visser, K.E. How neutrophils promote metastasis. *Science* **2016**, *352*, 145–146. [CrossRef]
114. Liang, W.; Li, Q.; Ferrara, N. Metastatic growth instructed by neutrophil-derived transferrin. *Proc. Natl. Acad. Sci. USA* **2018**, *115*, 11060–11065. [CrossRef]
115. Chen, Y.; Zhao, Z.; Chen, Y.; Lv, Z.; Ding, X.; Wang, R.; Xiao, H.; Hou, C.; Shen, B.; Feng, J.; et al. An epithelial-to-mesenchymal transition-inducing potential of granulocyte macrophage colony-stimulating factor in colon cancer. *Sci. Rep.* **2017**, *7*, 8265. [CrossRef] [PubMed]

116. Waghray, M.; Yalamanchili, M.; Dziubinski, M.; Zeinali, M.; Erkkinen, M.; Yang, H.; Schradle, K.A.; Urs, S.; Pasca Di Magliano, M.; Welling, T.H.; et al. GM-CSF mediates mesenchymal-epithelial cross-talk in pancreatic cancer. *Cancer Discov.* **2016**, *6*, 886–899. [CrossRef] [PubMed]
117. Szczerba, B.M.; Castro-Giner, F.; Vetter, M.; Krol, I.; Gkountela, S.; Landin, J.; Scheidmann, M.C.; Donato, C.; Scherrer, R.; Singer, J.; et al. Neutrophils escort circulating tumour cells to enable cell cycle progression. *Nature* **2019**, *566*, 553–557. [CrossRef]
118. Wang, P.C.; Weng, C.C.; Hou, Y.S.; Jian, S.F.; Fang, K.T.; Hou, M.F.; Cheng, K.H. Activation of VCAM-1 and its associated molecule CD44 leads to increased malignant potential of breast cancer cells. *Int. J. Mol. Sci.* **2014**, *15*, 3560–3579. [CrossRef] [PubMed]
119. Lopez-Soto, A.; Gonzalez, S.; Smyth, M.J.; Galluzzi, L. Control of metastasis by NK cells. *Cancer Cell* **2017**, *32*, 135–154. [CrossRef]
120. Chockley, P.J.; Chen, J.; Chen, G.; Beer, D.G.; Standiford, T.J.; Keshamouni, V.G. Epithelial-mesenchymal transition leads to NK cell-mediated metastasis-specific immunosurveillance in lung cancer. *J. Clin. Investig.* **2018**, *128*, 1384–1396. [CrossRef]
121. Speiser, D.E.; Ho, P.C.; Verdeil, G. Regulatory circuits of T cell function in cancer. *Nat. Rev. Immunol.* **2016**, *16*, 599–611. [CrossRef] [PubMed]
122. Mansfield, A.S.; Ren, H.; Sutor, S.; Sarangi, V.; Nair, A.; Davila, J.; Elsbernd, L.R.; Udell, J.B.; Dronca, R.S.; Park, S.; et al. Contraction of T cell richness in lung cancer brain metastases. *Sci. Rep.* **2018**, *8*, 2171. [CrossRef] [PubMed]
123. Goldberg, S.B.; Gettinger, S.N.; Mahajan, A.; Chiang, A.C.; Herbst, R.S.; Sznol, M.; Tsiouris, A.J.; Cohen, J.; Vortmeyer, A.; Jilaveanu, L.; et al. Pembrolizumab for patients with melanoma or non-small-cell lung cancer and untreated brain metastases: Early analysis of a non-randomised, open-label, phase 2 trial. *Lancet Oncol.* **2016**, *17*, 976–983. [CrossRef]
124. Kamath, S.D.; Kumthekar, P.U. Immune checkpoint inhibitors for the treatment of central nervous system (CNS) metastatic disease. *Front. Oncol.* **2018**, *8*, 414. [CrossRef] [PubMed]

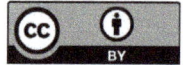

© 2019 by the authors. Licensee MDPI, Basel, Switzerland. This article is an open access article distributed under the terms and conditions of the Creative Commons Attribution (CC BY) license (http://creativecommons.org/licenses/by/4.0/).

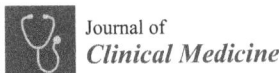 

*Review*

# Quantifying Cancer Epithelial-Mesenchymal Plasticity and its Association with Stemness and Immune Response

Dongya Jia [1], Xuefei Li [1], Federico Bocci [1,2], Shubham Tripathi [3], Youyuan Deng [1,4], Mohit Kumar Jolly [5,*], José N. Onuchic [1,2,6,7,*] and Herbert Levine [1,8,9,*]

1. Center for Theoretical Biological Physics, Rice University, Houston, TX 77005, USA; dj9@rice.edu (D.J.); Xuefei.Li@rice.edu (X.L.); fb20@rice.edu (F.B.); Youyuan.Deng@rice.edu (Y.D.)
2. Department of Chemistry, Rice University, Houston, TX 77005, USA
3. PhD Program in Systems, Synthetic, and Physical Biology, Rice University, Houston, TX 77005, USA; shubtri@rice.edu
4. Applied Physics Graduate Program, Rice University, Houston, TX 77005, USA
5. Centre for BioSystems Science and Engineering, Indian Institute of Science, Bangalore 560012, India
6. Department of Biosciences, Rice University, Houston, TX 77005, USA
7. Department of Physics and Astronomy, Rice University, Houston, TX 77005, USA
8. Department of Bioengineering, Northeastern University, Boston, MA 02115, USA
9. Department of Physics, Northeastern University, Boston, MA 02115, USA
* Correspondence: mkjolly@iisc.ac.in (M.K.J.); jonuchic@rice.edu (J.N.O.); h.levine@northeastern.edu (H.L.)

Received: 16 April 2019; Accepted: 20 May 2019; Published: 22 May 2019

**Abstract:** Cancer cells can acquire a spectrum of stable hybrid epithelial/mesenchymal (E/M) states during epithelial–mesenchymal transition (EMT). Cells in these hybrid E/M phenotypes often combine epithelial and mesenchymal features and tend to migrate collectively commonly as small clusters. Such collectively migrating cancer cells play a pivotal role in seeding metastases and their presence in cancer patients indicates an adverse prognostic factor. Moreover, cancer cells in hybrid E/M phenotypes tend to be more associated with stemness which endows them with tumor-initiation ability and therapy resistance. Most recently, cells undergoing EMT have been shown to promote immune suppression for better survival. A systematic understanding of the emergence of hybrid E/M phenotypes and the connection of EMT with stemness and immune suppression would contribute to more effective therapeutic strategies. In this review, we first discuss recent efforts combining theoretical and experimental approaches to elucidate mechanisms underlying EMT multi-stability (i.e., the existence of multiple stable phenotypes during EMT) and the properties of hybrid E/M phenotypes. Following we discuss non-cell-autonomous regulation of EMT by cell cooperation and extracellular matrix. Afterwards, we discuss various metrics that can be used to quantify EMT spectrum. We further describe possible mechanisms underlying the formation of clusters of circulating tumor cells. Last but not least, we summarize recent systems biology analysis of the role of EMT in the acquisition of stemness and immune suppression.

**Keywords:** epithelial–mesenchymal transition; EMT spectrum; hybrid epithelial/mesenchymal phenotypes; CTC clusters; stemness; immune suppression; EMT metrics; systems biology

## 1. Introduction

Metastasis remains the major cause of cancer-related deaths [1]. To enable successful metastasis, cancer cells often engage a trans-differentiation program referred to as epithelial–mesenchymal transition (EMT) [2]. During EMT, cells gradually lose epithelial features such as a cobblestone-like morphology, cell–cell adhesion, and apico-basal polarity and acquire mesenchymal features such as a spindle-like morphology, increased motility and invasiveness [2]. The concept of EMT was initially described during embryonic development. EMT was first observed in vitro by Greenberg and Hay showing that epithelial cells suspended in three-dimensional collagen gels lose their apical-basal polarity and acquire characteristics of migrating mesenchymal cells [3]. Later in vivo work by Nieto et al. argued that EMT is essential for the formation of mesoderm and the generation of the migratory neutral crest cells during chicken embryonic development [4]. EMT also plays a critical role during physiological wound repair and pathological fibrosis [5]. In the context of cancer metastasis, EMT has been proposed to be typically associated with enhanced metastatic potential of cancer cells [2] and the reverse process—mesenchymal–epithelial transition (MET)—has been considered to facilitate effective metastatic colonization by regaining epithelial and proliferative traits that are lost during EMT [6].

During metastasis of tumors, cells rarely undergo a complete EMT and enter a fully mesenchymal phenotype [7]. Instead, partial EMT leading to a hybrid epithelial/mesenchymal (E/M) phenotype has often been observed [8]. Thus, contrary to the prevailing dogma of EMT being a binary process, it is now accepted that there exists a spectrum of hybrid E/M phenotypes characterized by varying extents of epithelial and mesenchymal features and associated with metastatic potential and invasiveness [9,10]. Cancer cells in these hybrid E/M phenotypes tend to combine epithelial (e.g. cell–cell adhesion) and mesenchymal (e.g. increase motility) traits [11] and can thus migrate collectively, leading to formation of clusters of circulating tumor cells (CTCs). These clusters contribute much more than their proportional share to forming metastases relative to individual CTCs which are typically mesenchymal cells [12]. Moreover, the presence of CTC clusters in the peripheral blood has been shown to be a prognostic factor for poor patient survival across multiple types of cancer [13]. Therefore, a better understanding of the mechanisms underlying the emergence of hybrid E/M phenotypes and the formation of CTC clusters can lead to more effective therapeutic designs targeting metastasis.

Recently there have been ongoing debates regarding the necessity of EMT for metastasis [14]. Zheng et al. demonstrated that deletion of the EMT-inducing transcription factor (EMT-TF) SNAIL or TWIST in genetically engineered mouse models of pancreatic ductal adenocarcinoma (PDAC) did not cause any significant change in tumor progression and metastasis [15]. In addition, Fischer et al. suggested that EMT inhibition by over-expression of microRNA (miR)-200 led to no obvious change in lung metastasis development in spontaneous breast-to-lung metastasis mouse models [16]. From our perspective, these two studies assumed that EMT can be completely repressed by single factor manipulation, for example, deletion of SNAIL or TWIST in PDAC or over-expression of miR-200 in breast cancer. Following these studies, Krebs et al. used the same PDAC model [15] and showed that deletion of the EMT-TF ZEB1 significantly suppresses the colonization capacity of tumor cells and the formation of metastases [17], indicating a non-redundant role of EMT-TFs in regulating PDAC metastasis [18]. Moreover, another study by Cursons et al. showed that overexpression of miR-200c in the HMLE-derived mesenchymal cells established by exposing HMLE cells to TGF-β for 24 days can only drive a partial MET where the canonical epithelial marker E-cadherin increases but the mesenchymal maker vimentin remains [19]. One major contributing factor to these debates regarding the functional role of EMT in metastasis is the lack of consistency in defining EMT itself, owing to its highly nonlinear and multidimensional nature [20]. Thus, a rigorous quantification of the EMT status of tumor cells and a systematic analysis of the interacting EMT regulators such as interactions between miRNAs, EMT-TFs, and epigenetic factors is urgently needed.

Notably, various extracellular biochemical and biomechanical factors can induce and maintain a partial or complete EMT. For instance, neighboring cells can induce EMT through TGF-β [21] or Notch signaling [22], and also the alteration of stiffness of extracellular matrix (ECM) can trigger EMT [23]. In addition to the complexity of EMT itself, cancer cells undergoing EMT tend to acquire "stemness" characteristics, which are believed to be responsible for tumor-initiation ability and therapy resistance [24]. Moreover, cancer cells can interact with many other types of cells in the tumor microenvironment, such as fibroblasts, endothelial cells, and immune cells [25,26]. Specifically, the co-evolution of cancer and immune cells [27,28] has captured attention recently due to the promising effects of cancer immunotherapy [29,30]. Because of the typically enhanced metastatic potential and therapy resistance of cancer cells undergoing EMT, it is natural to analyze the correlation and causal relationship between EMT and immune response [31,32]. Furthermore, both EMT [1,2] and immune signatures [33–39] have been shown to be prognostic indicators for various types of cancer. A better understanding of their relationship can potentially contribute to more effective therapeutic designs.

In this review, we focus on how a combination of theoretical and experimental efforts has led to a better understanding of these aspects of EMT (Figure 1). We start with a discussion of mathematical modeling studies of EMT regulatory networks. Then we summarize recent in vitro and in vivo experimental studies that characterize EMT phenotypes. We then discuss non-cell-autonomous regulation of EMT. We further discuss metrics that have been developed to quantify EMT status. Finally, we extend our discussion to the coupling of EMT with stemness and immune response.

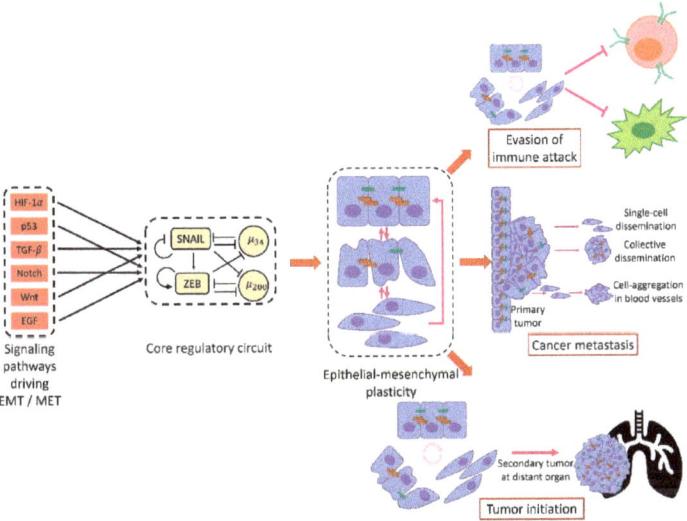

**Figure 1.** An overview of epithelial–mesenchymal plasticity causes and consequences. Multiple signaling pathways such as TGF-β, HIF-1α and Notch have been implicated in driving epithelial–mesenchymal transition (EMT). All these pathways tend to converge to a core regulatory circuit which includes two EMT-inducing transcription factors (EMT-TFs), SNAIL and ZEB, and two microRNAs, miR-34 and miR-200. The core regulatory circuit exhibits multi-stable dynamics: multiple stable steady states for the same level of EMT-inducing signal. These stable steady states contain different levels of SNAIL/ZEB/miR-34/miR-200 and thus corresponding to different EMT-associated phenotypes. The multi-stable dynamics of the core regulatory circuit allow for transitions among different stable states which leads to epithelial–mesenchymal plasticity. Cancer epithelial–mesenchymal plasticity typically enhances metastasis, allowing for disparate forms of migration and dissemination. In addition, epithelial–mesenchymal plasticity has been implicated in the acquisition of stem cell-like properties and immune evasion.

## 2. Emergence of Hybrid Epithelial/Mesenchymal Phenotypes

### 2.1. Hybrid E/M Phenotypes Are Predicted by Mathematical Modeling of EMT Regulation

EMT is governed by a complex gene regulatory network (GRN) including miRNAs, transcription factors (TFs), alternative spicing factors, epigenetic modifiers, growth factors, long non-coding RNAs, and others [7,40,41]. Several groups have proposed that two microRNA families miR-200 and miR-34 interacting with two EMT-TF families ZEB and SNAIL tend to form a core EMT regulatory network [40]. Many signaling pathways such as TGF-β, WNT, and Notch impinge upon this network to regulate

EMT. The miR-200 and miR-34 function as guardians of the epithelial phenotype and ZEB and SNAIL promote EMT. Mechanism-based mathematical modeling of this network that includes a detailed treatment of microRNA-mediated regulation suggests that it can give rise to three stable states: an epithelial phenotype characterized by miR-200$^{high}$/ZEB$^{low}$/miR-34$^{high}$/SNAIL$^{low}$; a mesenchymal phenotype characterized by miR-200$^{low}$/ZEB$^{high}$/miR-34$^{low}$/SNAIL$^{high}$; and a hybrid E/M phenotype characterized by co-expression of miR-200 and ZEB [42]. According to this model, the miR-200/ZEB circuit can function as a three-way decision-making switch governing the transitions between epithelial, mesenchymal, and hybrid E/M phenotypes and the miR-34/SNAIL circuit primarily functions as a noise-buffering integrator [42]. Alternatively, a different characterization of the hybrid E/M state has been proposed: starting from an epithelial state, miR-200$^{high}$/ZEB$^{low}$/miR-34$^{high}$/SNAIL$^{low}$, a hybrid state can be achieved when the miR-34/SNAIL circuit switches from miR-34$^{high}$/SNAIL$^{low}$ to miR-34$^{low}$/SNAIL$^{high}$, but the miR-200/ZEB circuit is maintained at miR-200$^{high}$/ZEB$^{low}$ [43]. Despite these differences [44], both of these mathematical models clearly indicate that EMT need not be a binary process and instead a stable hybrid E/M state expressing both epithelial and mesenchymal traits can be the end point of a transition.

The existence of hybrid E/M states has been further supported by other computational studies analyzing extended versions of the core EMT regulatory network [45–47]. Steinway et al. showed combinatorial intervention of TGF-β signal and SMAD suppression can lead to multiple hybrid E/M states using Boolean modeling [45]. Huang et al. and Font-Clos et al. showed that the hybrid E/M phenotypes are robust stable states emerging due to the topologies of EMT regulatory networks [46,48–50]. Mathematical modeling approaches have been further used to characterize phenotypic stability factors (PSFs) that can promote and stabilize hybrid E/M states. These PSFs include the transcription factors OVOL, GRHL2, NRF2, ΔNP63α, NUMB, and miR-145/OCT4 [50–54]. These PSFs can function in two related manners. First, coupling these PSFs with the decision-making circuit of EMT–miR-200/ZEB expands the parameter space and thereby the expected physiological conditions under which a hybrid E/M state can be attained [51–53]. In particular, PSF coupling can create a region of parameter space in which the only stable state is a hybrid one. Second, these PSFs increase the mean residence time of the hybrid E/M state, and thus its expected percentage in a cell population [50]. Experimental validation for these PSFs comes from observations that knocking them down destabilizes hybrid E/M phenotype and collective cell migration, instead promoting a complete EMT and individual cell migration. Other mechanisms through which a stable hybrid E/M phenotype can be acquired rely on combinatorial treatments with EMT-inducing and MET-inducing signals [54,55] or an increase in gene expression noise [56].

In summary, these mathematical modeling studies provide insights into the multi-stable nature of EMT, particularly the existence and characterization of hybrid E/M states. As we will now see, these modeling-predicted hybrid E/M states have been recently characterized experimentally both in vitro and in vivo.

*2.2. In vitro characterization of hybrid E/M phenotypes*

To map the EMT spectrum in ovarian carcinoma, Huang et al. analyzed the protein levels of epithelial markers, E-cadherin (E-Cad) and pan-cytokeratin (Pan-CK), and the mesenchymal marker, vimentin (Vim), of 42 ovarian carcinoma cell lines. Among these 42 cell lines, nine epithelial cell lines are characterized by E-Cad$^+$/Pan-CK$^+$/Vim$^-$, seven mesenchymal cell lines are characterized by E-Cad$^-$/Pan-CK$^-$/Vim$^+$, and 26 hybrid E/M cell lines are characterized by either E-Cad$^+$/Pan-CK$^+$/Vim$^+$ ($n = 18$, referred to as intermediate E) or E-Cad$^-$/Pan-CK$^+$/Vim$^-$ ($n = 8$, referred to as intermediate M) [57]. The intermediate E ovarian carcinoma cell lines exhibit significantly higher levels of SNAI1 mRNA and lower levels of ZEB1/2 mRNAs relative to the intermediate M ovarian carcinoma cell lines. The different expression patterns of SNAI1 and ZEB1/2 in intermediate E and intermediate M are reminiscent of the different characterizations of the hybrid E/M states by Lu et al. [42] and Zhang et al. [43]. Interestingly, the intermediate M ovarian carcinoma cell line SKOV3 exhibited significantly higher spheroidogenic efficiency, migratory and invasive potential relative to the ovarian carcinoma cell lines with other phenotypes. Further studies have revealed underlying feedback loops that can regulate such phenotypic plasticity in ovarian cancer [58].

Similarly, to characterize the EMT spectrum in lung adenocarcinoma, Schliekelman et al. analyzed the cell morphologies and the ratios of surface localized E-cadherin to vimentin of 38 non-small cell lung cancer (NSCLC) cell lines out of which nine were binned as epithelial, nine as mesenchymal, and 20 as hybrid E/M [59]. Notably, in these experiments the hybrid E/M cell lines are identified at a population level and therefore can contain purely individually hybrid E/M cells, or alternatively contain a mixture of epithelial and mesenchymal cells or both. Among these hybrid E/M NSCLC cell lines, almost all individual H1975 cells were shown to stably co-express E-cadherin and vimentin at least for two months over multiple passages, thus representing stable hybrid E/M cells [51]. In contrast, individual NSCLC H1944 or H2291 cells express either only E-cadherin or only vimentin, thus these cell lines are largely a mixture of epithelial and mesenchymal cells [60,61]. When knocking down the predicted PSFs—GRHL2, OVOL2, NUMB or NRF2—via siRNAs in H1975 cells, these hybrid E/M cells transition to a complete mesenchymal phenotype [51,53,62]. Another cell line that exhibits hybrid E/M phenotype characterized by co-expression of E-cadherin and ZEB1 at a single-cell level is human bladder cancer (HBC) RT4. Overexpression of the PSF NRF2 in RT4 cells increases the protein levels of both E-cadherin and ZEB1, supporting the predicted role of NRF2 in stabilizing a hybrid E/M phenotype.

In addition to cell lines containing either individual hybrid E/M cells or a mixture of E and M cells, there are cell lines that exhibit co-existence of hybrid E/M cells together with epithelial and/or mesenchymal cells. For example, the NSCLC HCC827 cells contain mostly epithelial cells and a subpopulation of individual hybrid E/M cells characterized by co-expression of epithelial markers including E-cadherin and miR-200a/b/c and mesenchymal markers including vimentin, ZEB1, and SNAI1 [63]. Treatment of the HCC827 cells with the epidermal growth factor receptor (EGFR) inhibitor erlotinib induces a stably erlotinib-resistant cell population among which the percentage of hybrid E/M cells is increased relative to their parental erlotinib-sensitive HCC827 cells [63], indicating a correlation of hybrid E/M phenotypes with therapy resistance. As expected, these HCC827-derived erlotinib-resistant cells exhibit collective migration and form more spheroids relative to their parental erlotinib-sensitive HCC827 cells [63]. Other NSCLC cell lines such as H920 and H2228 have been shown to be mixtures of hybrid E/M and epithelial cells with the hybrid E/M ones being dominant [60]. Aside from NSCLC cells, Grosse-Wilde et al. used flow cytometry analysis to isolate a subpopulation of breast cancer HMLER cells that are characterized by $CD24^+/CD44^+$. Most of these $CD24^+/CD44^+$ HMLER cells co-express epithelial genes such as CDH1 and EPCAM and mesenchymal genes such as VIM and ZEB2 and thus exist in a hybrid E/M phenotype [64]. These hybrid E/M HMLER cells demonstrate maximum mammosphere-forming ability relative to their epithelial and mesenchymal counterparts, highlighting that a hybrid E/M phenotype will often be more aggressive than a complete EMT phenotype, a theme which has also found emerging clinical support [65]. Later on, we will discuss how these additional properties of hybrid cells may arise due to a coupling of the EMT pathway and the network determining "stemness".

As already noted, hybrid E/M phenotypes can be acquired and maintained by combinatorial treatments of EMT- and MET-inducing signals. For example, Gould et al. showed that the epithelial colon carcinoma DLD1 cells can undergoing a partial EMT and acquire a hybrid E/M phenotype co-expressing E-cadherin and vimentin. Such hybrid E/M DLD1 cells are driven by simultaneous expression of the TFs, pSP1 and NFATc, in response to the combined treatment of VEGF-A and TGF-β1/2 [54]. Similarly, Biddle et al. showed that treatment of the oral squamous cell carcinoma (OSCC) CA1 and LM cells with TGF-β and retinoic acid simultaneously can stabilize a hybrid E/M subpopulation characterized by $CD44^{high}/EpCAM^{low/-}/CD24^+$ [55]. Additional experimental studies characterizing hybrid E/M phenotypes and their implications have been reviewed elsewhere [66,67].

In summary, hybrid E/M phenotypes have been observed in vitro at a single-cell level across multiple cancer types.

The co-existence of epithelial, mesenchymal, and hybrid E/M subpopulations in a single cell line indicates a population heterogeneity of EMT. Such heterogeneity can be generated and maintained via multiple mechanisms all of which can contribute to the acquisition and maintenance of hybrid E/M phenotypes (Figure 2). First, the EMT regulatory networks can be multi-stable [42,43,46,48]. Noise in the expression levels of the involved RNAs and proteins can thus cause transitions from one stable steady state to another [68]. Such noise may arise from the inherent stochasticity of the transcription process in cells [69] or from the random partitioning of parent cell RNAs and proteins among the daughter cells at the time of cell division (Figure 2A) [70–72]. Since both noise sources are cell-autonomous, individual epithelial cells may spontaneously undergo a phenotypic transition and acquire (or give rise to, in the second scenario) a hybrid E/M phenotype [73]. Thus, one must be careful when choosing a cell line for experiments: a cell line known to be epithelial may include substantial fractions of hybrid E/M and/or mesenchymal cells [55,73]. Second, the population heterogeneity of EMT can arise via cell–cell communication (Figure 2B). An example of such a communication channel is Notch-Delta-Jagged signaling. Some cells with high levels of Delta/Jagged expression act as senders, while other cells with high levels of Notch receptor expression act as receivers. This leads to a population that is inherently heterogeneous—a mix of sender and receiver cells. Notch-Delta-Jagged signaling-mediated heterogeneity is closely tied to the emergence of hybrid E/M phenotypes [74]. This will be discussed in more detail below. Third, population heterogeneity of EMT can arise due to different kinetic parameters controlling gene regulation in different cells (Figure 2C). Due to the multitude of peripheral factors involved in governing the behavior of a core regulatory circuit, the kinetics of the core circuit can vary from cell to cell leading to different responses to the same external cues in different cells [46]. This might be connected to the aforementioned random partitioning but might arise as well due to different long-lived fluctuations, perhaps related to chromatic structure heterogeneity.

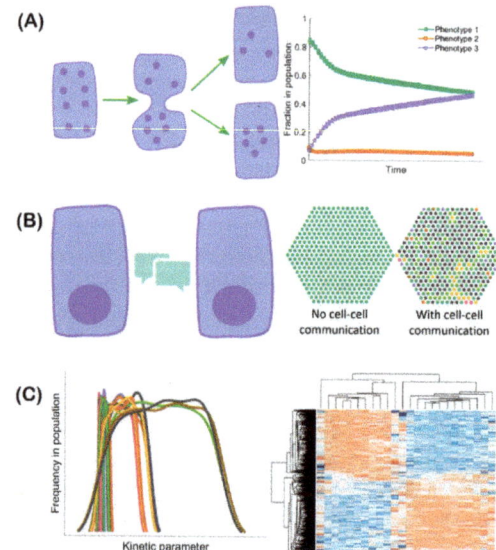

**Figure 2.** Multiple mechanisms can lead to EMT-associated population heterogeneity. (**A**) During cell division, noise can lead to asymmetric partitioning of molecules among daughter cells. This may lead to the daughter cell exhibiting a phenotype different from that of the parent cell. Consequently, the fractions of cells exhibiting different phenotypes can change over time. (**B**) Cell–cell communication

(left) mediated by, for example Notch-Delta-Jagged signaling, can lead to cells spontaneously acquiring "signal sender", "signal receiver", and "signal sender/receiver" phenotypes in a population (right: different colors correspond to different cell phenotypes). (**C**) The kinetics of gene regulation can vary in different cells due to stochasticity in kinetic parameters. Thus, each parameter can exhibit some variation in its value in a given isogenic population (left: each curve denotes the distribution of values of an individual parameter in a given population). This heterogeneity can lead to cells in the population acquiring different phenotypes in response to the same external cues (right: heatmap indicates the emergence of various phenotypes. Each row represents a cell and each column represents the expression level of one gene. Red color represents relatively high gene expression and blue color represents relatively low gene expression with white indicating intermediate expression levels).

### 2.3. In Vivo Characterization of Hybrid E/M Phenotypes

To identify whether cancer cells can acquire hybrid E/M phenotypes in vivo, Pastushenko et al. used fluorescence-activated cell sorting (FACS) to screen cell surface markers of skin squamous cell carcinoma (SCC) cells that can undergo spontaneous EMT and generate EpCAM$^+$ epithelial cells and EpCAM$^-$ mesenchymal-like cells in genetically engineered mouse models [10]. While the EpCAM$^+$ cells exhibit homogeneous expression of most of the markers, the EpCAM$^-$ cells exhibit heterogeneous expression of 17 cell surface markers among which the most heterogeneously expressed are CD61, CD51, and CD106. Consequently, the authors used combinatorial multicolor FACS analysis of these three markers to further classify the EpCAM$^-$ cells into six subpopulations among which the CD51$^-$CD61$^-$CD106$^-$, CD51$^+$, and CD106$^+$ subpopulations exhibit co-expression of the epithelial marker keratin 14 (K14) and the mesenchymal marker vimentin, and thus can be tentatively considered to be hybrid E/M phenotypes. The CD51$^+$CD61$^+$CD106$^+$ and CD51$^+$CD61$^+$ subpopulations, on the other hand, are vimentin positive and K14 negative and thus are mesenchymal-like. Intriguingly, the hybrid E/M CD51$^-$CD61$^-$CD106$^-$ and CD106$^+$ subpopulations generate significantly more metastases relative to other subpopulations, though all subpopulations here share similar tumor-propagating capacity. Similar results have also been observed in MMTV-PyMT mammary luminal tumors [10]. Another study performed by Aiello et al. that used a lineage-tracing mouse model of PDAC showed that the PDAC cells undergoing EMT can acquire a hybrid E/M phenotype via re-localization of epithelial proteins such as E-cadherin and claudin-7 from membrane to intracellular foci [75]. The emergence of these hybrid E/M PDAC cells indicates that besides transcriptional control, post-transcriptional regulation of localization can also be important to mediate the existence of hybrid E/M phenotypes. Finally, another study by Puram et al. showed that the head and neck squamous cell carcinoma (HNSCC) cells from patients exhibit a hybrid E/M phenotype characterized by co-expression of epithelial markers such as EPCAM and KRT17 and mesenchymal markers such as vimentin and TGF-β-induced (TGFBI) through single-cell transcriptomic analysis [76]. Intriguingly, these hybrid E/M HNSCC cells tend to localize at the leading edge of tumors close to surrounding stroma cells.

In summary, mathematical modeling together with both in vitro and in vivo experimental studies consistently demonstrate the existence of multiple hybrid E/M phenotypes characterized by varying extents of epithelial and mesenchymal features (Figure 3). It is worth noting that in addition to the characterization of the hybrid E/M phenotypes, mathematical modeling of EMT regulatory networks have generated many other interesting predictions that have been recently validated by experimental studies. First, modeling the core EMT regulatory network, miR-200/ZEB/miR-34/SNAIL, suggests a sequential response of the EMT-TFs SNAIL and ZEB to the EMT-inducing signal TGF-β [43,44]. When treated with different levels of TGF-β, SNAIL is predicted to precede ZEB and to be upregulated at relatively low TGF-β levels. The predicted different responses of SNAIL and ZEB has been verified in MCF10A cells [43]. Second, another prediction from modeling studies [42,43] is that EMT and MET are not necessarily symmetric processes and hysteresis is expected during EMT. The predicted hysteretic behavior of EMT has been recently demonstrated during TGF-β induced EMT of NMuMG and EpRAS cells, where the levels of E-cadherin exhibit a bimodal transition. Such hysteretic behavior of E-cadherin is regulated by the miR-200/ZEB1 circuit and blocking the inhibition of miR-200 by ZEB1 (referred to in this study as mutant cells) results in only a unimodal transition of E-cadherin, though these mutant cells can still undergo EMT with changes of EMT markers at a similar degree relative to the wild type [77]. Moreover, TGF-β induced EMT of mutant cells exhibits significantly decreased sphere-formation ability in vitro, decreased frequency of tumor-initiating cells and lung metastases in vivo relative to their wild types. These results also confirm a prominent role of the miR-200/ZEB circuit in regulating the aspects of EMT dynamics that result in a variety of functional consequences.

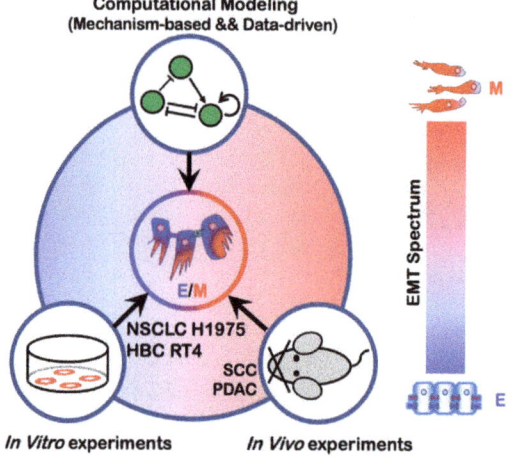

**Figure 3.** Emergence of hybrid E/M phenotypes demonstrated by a combination of theoretical and experimental efforts. The cell lines non-small cell lung cancer (NSCLC) H1975 and human bladder cancer (HBC) RT4 exhibit a hybrid E/M phenotype at a single-cell level. Hybrid E/M phenotypes have also been characterized in vivo using mouse models of squamous cell carcinoma (SCC) and pancreatic ductal adenocarcinoma (PDAC).

## 3. EMT Regulation by Cell Cooperation

### 3.1. Notch Signaling

Although EMT is fundamentally an individual cell phenomenon, it can also be regulated by cell cooperation such as Notch signaling. Notch signaling is a cell–cell communication mechanism and highly conserved across species. Originally characterized in Drosophila development, Notch signaling is a conserved and well-known regulator of multiple hallmarks of cancer, including angiogenesis and EMT [78–80].

The Notch signaling cascade is initiated by the binding of the Notch transmembrane receptor with a ligand belonging to a neighboring cell. This binding leads to the cleavage of the Notch intracellular domain (NICD), which is then released in the cytoplasm and transported to the cell nucleus, where it acts as a transcriptional cofactor [81]. Notch signaling is deeply coupled to the EMT regulatory networks discussed in previous sections. For example, on one hand, EMT-inhibiting miRNAs miR-34 and miR-200 reduce the levels of Notch receptor and ligands [82–84] by translational regulation [85]. On the other hand, NICD promotes the transcription of SNAIL and thus acts as an EMT inducer [86,87]. Therefore, cancer cells undergoing EMT can in turn induce EMT in their neighboring cells through the binding of their ligands to a neighbor's Notch receptors.

As often seen in the developmental context, Notch signaling can give rise to different spatial patterns of cell phenotypes due to feedback regulation between NICD and various alternate ligands. Specifically, NICD transcriptionally represses ligands of the Delta family but activates ligands of the Jagged family. Therefore, signaling through the Notch–Delta pathway typically promotes opposite cell fates in neighboring cells, or 'lateral inhibition'. This is accomplished by amplifying initial differences in the levels of receptors and ligands, ultimately leading to one cell with high levels of Notch receptor and low levels of Delta ligand (receiver cell) and a neighbor cell with low Notch and high Delta (sender cell) [88,89]. Conversely, Notch–Jagged signaling typically promotes a similar cell fate in neighboring cells, or 'lateral induction', because NICD upregulates Jagged ligands [90].

The cell patterning mediated by Notch ligands can modulate epithelial–mesenchymal plasticity in a tumor tissue due to the aforementioned coupling between Notch and the EMT regulatory circuits. Intracellular Notch signaling activated by either Delta or Jagged can activate EMT. However, mathematical modeling of the coupled regulatory networks regulating EMT and Notch signaling suggests that Notch–Delta and Notch–Jagged signaling have dramatically different outcomes at a multi-cellular level. While Notch–Delta signaling promotes a spatial arrangement where cells in a partial or complete EMT are surrounded by epithelial cells, Notch–Jagged signaling can give rise to clusters of hybrid epithelial/mesenchymal (E/M) cells [74] (Figure 4). Indeed, Jagged1 is one of the top differentially expressed genes in collectively migrating cells of breast cancer [12,91]. These observations suggest that Jagged1 can act as an intercellular PSF that stabilizes a hybrid E/M phenotype in a non-cell autonomous manner. Therefore, in addition to 'conventional' PSF proteins that promote a partial EMT through direct crosstalk with the EMT regulatory circuitry, such as OVOL, GRHL2, and NRF2 [51,52,62], other PSFs can facilitate a partial EMT and the formation of CTC clusters by activating Notch–Jagged signaling and/or inhibiting Notch–Delta signaling. For example, NUMB/NUMBL that forms a negative feedback loop with Notch [92–94] can prevent a complete EMT, and consistent with that identification, knockdown of NUMB/NUMBL results in a mesenchymal phenotype and enables individual migration of the hybrid E/M NSCLC H1975 cells that typically migrate collectively [53].

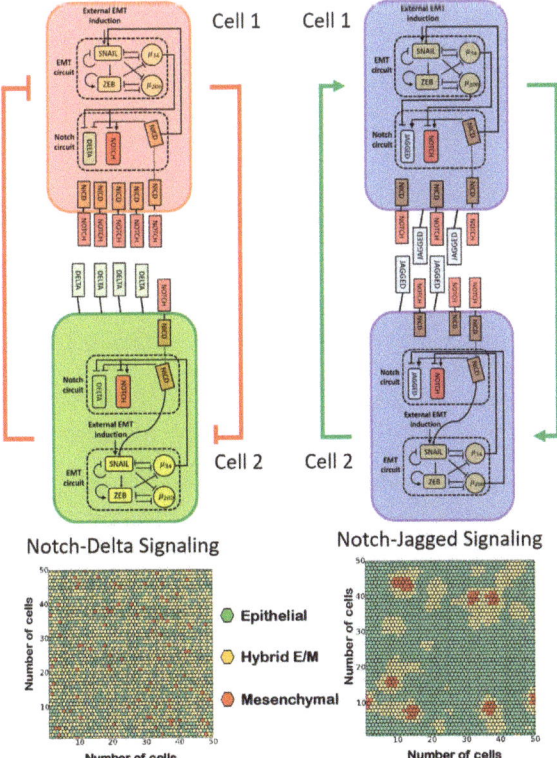

**Figure 4.** Notch–Delta and Notch–Jagged signaling give rise to opposite cell patterning of EMT.

(**A**) Coupling of Notch–Delta signaling with the core EMT regulatory circuit. The Notch intracellular domain NICD suppresses the endogenous expression of Delta ligands upon activation of Notch receptors by exogenous Delta ligands (top, red color represents the 'receiver phenotype' (high notch), green color represents 'sender phenotype' (high delta)). Cell patterning of EMT in presence of a strong Notch–Delta signaling (bottom). (**B**) Coupling of Notch–Jagged signaling with the core EMT regulatory circuit. NICD promotes the endogenous expression of Jagged ligands upon activation of Notch receptors by exogenous Jagged ligands (top, blue color represents a 'sender/receiver phenotype' (high Jagged)). Cell patterning of EMT in presence of a strong Notch–Jagged signaling (bottom). Hexagons with different colors depict epithelial (green), hybrid E/M (yellow), and mesenchymal (red) cells. Figures in the right panel are adapted from [53].

## 3.2. Interaction among Epithelial, Hybrid E/M, and Mesenchymal Cells

Similar to bidirectional interactions among epithelium and mesenchyme during organ development [95], there may be crosstalk and cooperation among cells exhibiting varying extents of EMT, which can accelerate tumor aggressiveness [96–98]. Hybrid E/M cells can facilitate such crosstalk, due to their plasticity that can generate and maintain epithelial–mesenchymal heterogeneity at a population level; such plasticity is limited for cells on either end of the EMT spectrum. Moreover, hybrid E/M cells can maintain cell–cell adhesion via E-cadherin, and thus potentially enabling formation of heterotypic clusters of CTCs with cells of varying EMT statuses [99]. Last but not least, a recent study highlighted that the hybrid E/M HMLER cells, but not a mixture of nonplastic 'extremely epithelial' (xE) cells and nonplastic 'extremely mesenchymal' (xM) cells, account for high tumorigenicity in vivo [100]. Notably, the nonplastic xE cells are created by ZEB1 knockdown and the nonplastic xM cells are created by constitutive ZEB1 expression, which supports the role of ZEB1 in mediating EMT [42,44].

Whether a mixture of E and M cells is sufficient to initiate the metastatic cascade and successfully form metastases remains to be resolved. Few molecular mechanisms enabling crosstalk between E and M cells have been elucidated recently. Tsuji et al. demonstrated that when EMT and non-EMT cells are inoculated subcutaneously in mice, they both establish primary tumors, but neither of them form lung metastases [96]; the ability to invade local tissues and enter circulation is demonstrated only by EMT cells. Further, when both cell types are injected intravenously, non-EMT cells form overt metastases, but the metastatic ability of EMT cells is compromised. Finally, when a mixture of EMT and non-EMT cells is subcutaneously injected, both cell types can intravasate but only non-EMT cells form lung metastases. Put together, these observations indicate a possible cooperation between EMT and non-EMT cells—while EMT cells can cleave the matrix to make way for both cell populations to intravasate, the non-EMT cells can colonize distant organs. This study did not identify any juxtacrine and/or paracrine signaling underlying this cooperation, but recent in vitro co-culture experiments of EMT and non-EMT cells have identified a few players that can mediate this crosstalk. HMLER cells overexpressing TWIST or SNAIL have been shown to impart migratory and invasive traits in vitro to control HMLER cells via paracrine Hedgehog signaling, but without explicitly inducing any morphological or molecular changes associated typically with EMT [97]. The authors also demonstrated that the EMT cells are able to increase the metastatic propensity of non-EMT cells in vivo, thus lending further credence to the notion that EMT cells can stimulate the migration of non-EMT cells. This idea is further strengthened by another in vitro analysis of sublines derived from prostate cancer PC-3 cells, where the relatively more epithelial PC-3/Mc cells, when co-cultured with post-EMT PC-3/S cells, have increased invasive potential which persisted for around seven days after the co-culture but eventually decline after being segregated from PC-3/S cells [101]. This increased invasive response is also observed upon co-culture of PC-3/Mc cells with NIH3T3 fibroblasts, suggesting that the invasiveness of non-EMT cells can be increased by both tumor and non-tumor mesenchymal cells [101]. In vivo experiments for individual or co-injection of PC-3/S and/or PC-3/Mc cells corroborate previous observations that the post-EMT cells had little, if any, contribution to distant organ colonization [101]. Put together, these findings are reminiscent of in vivo studies showing that a persistent EMT activation can reduce metastases formation [6,102], and clinical evidence that carcinoma metastases are largely epithelial [103].

Reversible transitions among epithelial and mesenchymal phenotypes of disseminating cells has been dogmatically considered as the driving engine of metastasis for a long time [1,104,105] (also referred to as the 'sequential metastasis' model) [98], but with the proposed key role of EMT and MET being relooked at more carefully [20], the possibility of a cooperative journey taken together by epithelial and mesenchymal cells where they necessarily do not change their phenotypes cannot be ruled out (also referred to as the 'cooperative metastasis model') [98]. Multiple possibilities may underlie this cooperation: (a) epithelial cells facilitate MET of mesenchymal cells; (b) mesenchymal cells facilitate the survival, persistence, and re-adhesion of epithelial cells during colonization; (c) epithelial and mesenchymal cells exchange survival signals; (d) a combination of the above. Nevertheless, collective transport of epithelial and mesenchymal cells is likely to be more effective for colonization as compared to that of one population alone. However, the role of hybrid E/M cells in this cooperative metastasis model remains to be explored.

What mechanisms may allow such collective migration of epithelial and mesenchymal cells? In developmental contexts, epithelial or mesenchymal cells have been seen to migrate collectively through respective cell–cell contacts mediated by E-cadherin or N-cadherin [106,107]. Recently, a N-cadherin/E-cadherin mechanically active heterophilic adhesion among the cancer-associated fibroblasts and cancer cells was reported to guide collective migration of tumor cells [108]. Given that the heterophilic E-cadherin/N-cadherin interaction has been proposed to be of similar affinity as that of homophilic E-cadherin interactions [109], collective cell migration can be expected to be observed among cells with varying levels of E-cadherin and N-cadherin. Another study reports a short-ranged interaction via EGF/CSF-1 paracrine axis to mediate macrophage-driven tumor cell migration [110,111]. CSF-1/CSF-1R axis has been recently proposed to associate with a hybrid E/M phenotype in inflammatory breast cancer [108]—a highly aggressive breast cancer subtype that metastasizes via clusters or emboli of circulating tumor cells [91]. These mechanisms may mediate, at least in part, a collective cooperative migration of cells in varying hues of EMT. Increased plasticity of hybrid E/M cells may be necessary and sufficient to maintain and propagate the non-genetic heterogeneity in terms of EMT status in a given isogenic cancer cell population.

## 4. Mechanical Control of EMT by ECM

In addition to chemical communication, the stiffness of ECM also plays a key role in regulating EMT. For example, cancer cells when cultured in stiffer substrates exhibit increased migratory and invasive ability and become more mesenchymal-like [112]. Alternation in ECM stiffness can trigger multiple signaling pathways to regulate EMT, such as TWIST1-G3BP2 [23], HA-CD44 [113], MRTF-A [114], PI3K/Akt [115], and YAP/TAZ [116]. Yet, the reversibility of ECM stiffness-induced EMT can be cell line-dependent. For example, the mammary epithelial cells that have undergone EMT in a stiff substrate partially revert to epithelial phenotype [117], while the colon carcinoma HCT-8 cells can retain their mesenchymal-like phenotype, after being re-cultured in the compliant substrate [118]. It is worth noting that cells undergoing EMT can in turn regulate ECM. For example, the LOX-family enzymes are upregulated in fibrosis and upregulation of LOX-family enzymes can directly increase connectivity of collagen fibers, stabilize and stiffen the collagen networks [119,120]. Given the importance of mechanical regulation of EMT, mathematical models that integrate mechanical with chemical signaling networks need to be developed to better understand EMT-ECM dynamics [121].

## 5. Quantification of the EMT Spectrum

Our discussion so far has hopefully made it clear that cells undergoing EMT can acquire a spectrum of hybrid E/M states both in vitro and in vivo. However, the lack of a rigorous quantification of the EMT spectrum, namely, the exact proportions of epithelial, mesenchymal, and hybrid E/M subpopulations of cell lines and clinical samples, can lead to potentially contradictory conclusions regarding the necessity and functional roles of EMT and MET in metastasis [15–17,102,122,123].

Cells undergoing EMT typically alter both their omics profiles and morphologies. Therefore, in principle, the EMT spectrum can be quantified via evaluating the change of cell morphology and/or their omics profiles. To classify epithelial and mesenchymal phenotype at a single-cell level, Leggett et al. developed a probabilistic classification scheme using Gaussian mixture model (GMM) focusing on four morphological features of single cells—maximum radius of the nucleus, vimentin area, cytoplasm form factor, and maximum feret diameter of cytoplasm [124]. The GMM is trained using the morphological features of DMSO-treated (epithelial) and 4-hydroxytamoxifen (OHT)-treated (mesenchymal) human mammary MCF-10A cells which are transfected with an inducible Snail construct, referred to as MCF-10A Snail cells. The probabilistic GMM model has revealed various EMT kinetics of MCF-10A Snail cells when induced by TGF-β1, plating density, and the microtubule inhibitor Taxol respectively. This GMM model also provides insight into the EMT status of individual cells which may be overlooked by population-average analysis. However, this method only focuses on a binary classification of EMT—epithelial or mesenchymal—and one missing piece of this model is the classification of hybrid E/M phenotypes.

To quantitatively measure the EMT status of cell lines with specific attention to a hybrid E/M phenotype, George et al. developed an EMT scoring metric to calculate the probability of a given sample to be hybrid E/M phenotype and assign a score between 0 and 2, with 0 being fully epithelial, 2 being fully mesenchymal, and 1 representing hybrid E/M [125]. Using the gene expression data of NCI-60 human tumor cell lines as the training set, the ratio of VIM to CDH1 together with CLDN7 expression are identified as the best-fit pair of predictors to classify EMT phenotypes. This EMT scoring metric has been used to characterize multiple hybrid E/M cancer cell lines including A549 and DU145. Furthermore, this EMT scoring metric has been extended to distinguish hybrid E/M cells from mixtures of epithelial and mesenchymal cells [60]. Another EMT scoring metric developed by Tan et al. assigns a score between -1 and 1 to a given sample with -1 being fully epithelial and 1 being fully mesenchymal [126]. Both George et al. and Tan et al. demonstrated that patient samples that are more mesenchymal-like do not necessarily correlate with worse overall and disease-free survival results and do not always show resistance to chemotherapy, indicating a subtype-dependent role of EMT in cancer progression and therapy resistance. In summary, these methods to quantify EMT status help address the multifaced roles of EMT in tumor progression and patient prognosis.

## 6. EMT and CTC Clusters

Cancer cells that acquire a hybrid E/M phenotype maintain both epithelial (e.g. cell–cell adhesion) and mesenchymal (e.g. migration) features thus can migrate collectively as a cluster. Such clusters of migrating tumor cells have been shown to be one of the primary instigators of metastases [12,127]. The experimental studies supporting this notion are discussed below.

Using multicolor lineage tracing, Cheung et al. showed by two sets of experiments that the CTC clusters are mainly formed by multi-cellular clusters from the primary tumors. In the first set of experiments, two differently colored populations—mTomato+ and CFP$^+$ MMTV-PyMT tumor organoids—were respectively transplanted into the right and left flanks of a nonfluorescent mouse. After six to eight weeks, only single-colored metastases were observed in lung. In the second set of experiments, mTomato$^+$ single cells isolated by FACS were transplanted into a nonfluorescent mouse via tail-vein injection and two days later FACS isolated CFP$^+$ single cells were injected into the same mouse. After two days, exclusively single-colored metastases were observed in lung. These two sets of experiments suggest that the polyclonal metastases in lung is more effectively generated by multicellular seeds and not by serial aggregation of single tumor cells [12]. The CTC clusters exhibit enriched expression of an epithelial cytoskeletal protein K14 that is required for the collective invasive behavior and distant metastasis. Another study supporting the idea that CTC clusters can arise as oligoclonal groups of cells detached from the primary tumors is Aceto et al. who identified plakoglobin as a key mediator for CTC cluster formation [128].

An alternative mechanism—that CTC clusters can be formed via aggregation of single CTCs in circulation—has been recently demonstrated by Liu et al. using intravital multiphoton microscopic imaging in both patient-derived xenograft (PDX) models of triple negative breast cancer (TNBC) and PyMT transgenic mouse models [127]. Liu et al. first showed that in chemoattractant-containing matrigel about 20% of invasion events of the tumor cells collected from the PDX models occur as multicellular aggregates, and in suspension culture individual CTCs derived from a breast cancer patient aggregate into clusters within one to two hours. These results indicate that single CTCs can aggregate in vitro. The authors further co-infused eGFP$^+$ and tdTomato$^+$ single MDA-MB-231 cells via the tail vein and observed that about 92% of lung metastasis are dual-color aggregates within 2 hours. The percentage of the dual-colored aggregates is affected by the timing of the eGFP$^+$ and tdTomato$^+$ entering blood vessels. Consequently, sequential infusion of the tdTomato$^+$ cells 5 minutes, 10 minutes, and 2 hours after the infusion of the eGFP$^+$ cells result in gradually decreased percentages (27%, 16% and 10%) of the dual-colored aggregates. The authors further showed that the CTC clusters exhibit notably enriched expression of CD44, and that the intercellular CD44 homophilic interaction is responsible for the aggregation of single CTCs.

One major difference in the studies by Cheung et al. and Liu et al. is the timing of the second-colored single cells entering the blood vessels. Cheung et al. injected the second-colored cells into the tail vein two days after the injection of the first-colored cells while Liu et al. waited for at most two hours to inject the second-colored cells. As discussed by Liu et al., the timing of the second-colored cells entering the blood vessel could have significant effect on the percentages of dual-colored lung metastases. From our perspective, the key issue in these two studies seems to be the lifetime and density of the injected single cancer cells. Since it is not clear how often the injected cells are expected to reach the bloodstream, it is hard to evaluate which protocol is a better match to reality. The experiments by Cheung et al., where two differently colored populations of tumor organoids are injected respectively into the right and left flanks of nonfluorescent mice, seems to be a better approach since the interaction of cells in the bloodstream is determined naturally rather than by the experimenters. Nonetheless, both studies showed that the CTC clusters significantly promote colony formation and lung polyclonal metastases in vivo. Liu et al. showed through CellSearch platform-based blood analysis that the breast cancer patients with CTC clusters exhibit significantly worse overall survival results relative to those with only single CTCs. And, CTC clusters in different contexts can be different. For example, though both invasive ductal carcinoma (IDC) and invasive lobular carcinoma (ILC) exhibit collective invasion patterns, the collective invasion in IDC lesions maintains intercellular E-cadherin while collective invasion in ILC lesions loses intercellular E-cadherin but retains CD44 for intercellular junctions [129]. The CTC clusters of SCC are regulated by the EMT-TF SNAIL [130]. All together, these studies suggest that CTC clusters can in principle be generated both by cohesive shedding from the primary tumors and/or serial aggregation of single cells in the circulation.

To model the migration of CTC clusters, Bocci et al. proposed a simple biophysical model where cancer cells can undergo a partial EMT that allows both single-cell and clustered-cell migration, or a complete EMT that only allows single-cell migration [131]. According to this reduced physical model, a tumor can undergo a transition from primarily single cell-based invasion to collective invasion. Strikingly, this theoretical framework reproduces multiple CTC cluster size distributions measured in patients and mouse models across cancer types, hence suggesting the existence of a unifying set of principles governing cancer cell migration [131].

Adding to the complexity of the problem, CTC clusters can associate with non-cancer cells including platelets and/or immune cells such as tumor-associated macrophages and neutrophils [132–134]. In particular, it is well recognized that interactions between macrophages and tumor cells are very important for tumor cell intravasation and extravasation, though the detailed mechanisms have not been elucidated [135,136]. In addition, the CTC-neutrophil clusters lead to more efficient metastasis relative to CTCs alone [132]. Future studies need to be performed to elucidate the cross-talk between CTC clusters and different types of immune cells.

## 7. EMT and Stemness in Tumor Microenvironment

We have already come across the fact that besides the migratory and invasive traits conferred by EMT, some cancer cells undergoing EMT can also acquire an enhanced ability to drive tumor initiation and an enhanced therapy resistance. These properties are associated with the notion of 'stemness', and such cells are sometimes referred to as cancer stem cells (CSCs). The connection between EMT and stemness was first proposed by Brabletz et al. [24] more than a decade ago based on the premise that EMT and stemness cannot explain the different steps of the metastatic cascade when considered as separate and independent processes [24]. Indeed, increasing experimental evidence suggests a strong association of EMT with stemness. For instance, human mammary epithelial cells (HMLEs) undergoing EMT can express stem cell markers and exhibit increased mammosphere formation [122]. Moreover, reversing EMT via knockdown of SNAIL represses stemness and tumor growth in ovarian cancer [137]. This and other evidence suggests that the activation of the EMT program leads to the acquisition of stemness [138]. This correlation, however, is not absolute, and several other experimental papers have claimed that stemness can occasionally correlate with an epithelial phenotype or suppression of EMT [101,102,139].

Revisiting the EMT-CSC connection through the lenses of epithelial–mesenchymal plasticity and hybrid E/M phenotypes, however, offers a more consistent picture. Mathematical modeling approaches have been applied to decode the connection of EMT with stemness via simulating the coupled decision-making regulatory networks of EMT and stemness. Specifically, EMT activation can downregulate let-7, a miRNA typically associated with repressing stemness [140]. Let-7 can bind to ZEB and promote its degradation. These two processes can settle at an intermediate level of let-7 and ZEB leading to hybrid E/M CSCs [141]. Indeed, characterization of CTCs in vivo revealed that circulating CSCs are typically associated with partial EMT [73,142]. This association, however, can vary depending on the coupling between the modules governing EMT and stemness, allowing for CSCs in an epithelial, mesenchymal, or hybrid E/M phenotype [141]. In addition, local perturbations in the tumor microenvironment such as TGF-β or Notch signaling also can modulate the association of CSCs with different EMT phenotypes [143,144]. All told, emerging evidence from theoretical and experimental studies tends to associate the hybrid epithelial/mesenchymal phenotypes with stemness [100,141,143,145–148].

Along these lines, the association of hybrid E/M phenotypes with stemness can be promoted by the PSFs—OVOL and Jagged1. Indeed, Jagged1 is typically overexpressed in CSC populations as compared with non-CSCs in multiple types of cancer including glioblastoma, pancreatic cancer, colon cancer, and breast cancer [22,149–151]. Through modeling the coupling of the regulatory networks governing EMT, stemness and Notch signaling, Bocci et al. proposed that Jagged1 facilitates a 'window of opportunity' that confers maximal invasion potential in terms of EMT and stemness [143,148]. A follow-up work showed that knockdown of Jagged1 impairs breast organoid formation in vitro, therefore highlighting a causal relationship between Jagged1 and stemness [144].

Subpopulations of CSCs with different EMT phenotypes can be representative of the spatial organization of a tumor tissue. In breast cancer, $CD24^-/CD44^+$ mesenchymal CSCs are typically located toward the invasive edge of the tumor by the tumor-stroma interface, while $ALDH1^+$ CSCs are found in the more interior region [152]. Interestingly, $ALDH1^+$ CSCs were originally considered as epithelial-like, but their RNA sequencing (RNA-Seq) data has later shown that these cells lean more toward a hybrid E/M phenotype and share several genes with TNBC signature [153]. Recently, Bocci et al. have argued that this spatial segregation can be qualitatively explained by the interplay of cancer cells with the tumor microenvironment [144]. Cytokines such as the EMT-inducer TGF-β are typically secreted at the tumor–stroma interface and give rise to a gradient of EMT-inducing signal throughout the tumor tissue. Therefore, CSCs at the invasive edge are highly exposed to TGF-β and tend to undergo a complete EMT leading to a fully mesenchymal phenotype, while CSCs in the interior maintain a hybrid E/M phenotype [144] (Figure 5). Consistently, in non-small cell lung CSCs, a subpopulation of mesenchymal CSCs exhibits high expression of TGF-β targets such as SNAI1 and ZEB1, as compared to a hybrid E/M CSC population [143].

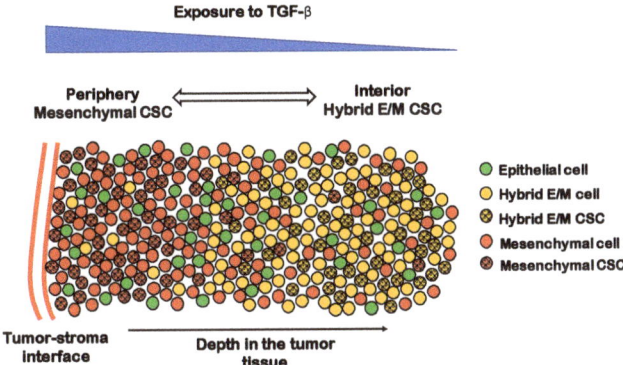

**Figure 5.** The spatial patterning of CSCs with different EMT phenotypes. Tumor-stroma interactions can give rise to a gradient of TGF- β (top, blue scale). In the periphery of the tumor, most cells are mesenchymal (red spheres), while the interior is mostly composed by hybrid E/M and epithelial cells (yellow and green spheres, respectively). CSCs are mostly mesenchymal in the periphery (black-dotted red spheres) and mostly hybrid E/M in the interior (black-dotted yellow spheres).

Besides a direct trigger of EMT through soluble inflammatory cytokines, the tumor microenvironment can induce EMT in cancer cells through hypoxia. The hypoxia inducible factor 1 alpha (HIF-1α) induces EMT through direct regulation of ZEB1 as shown in colorectal cancer [154]. Moreover, tumor hypoxia seems to regulate multiple aspects of tumor invasion. For instance, hypoxia correlates with EMT and CSC properties in pancreatic ductal adenocarcinoma (PDA) cells and gastric cancer cells [155,156].

In summary, EMT and CSC formation represent two essential axes of tumor progression, whose connection is modulated by factors in the tumor microenvironment such as signaling gradients and hypoxia, as well as cell–cell signaling [144,152,155–158]. The stem cell paradigm inherited from developmental biology implies a hierarchical lineage of cells that gradually but irreversibly differentiate [159,160]. In the context of cancer, however, stemness has proven to be a dynamical property that cells can gain and lose [161–163]. The complex interplay between EMT, stemness, and tumor microenvironment gives rise to tumor heterogeneity that still represents the major challenge hindering metastasis and therapy resistance [157].

## 8. EMT and Immune Suppression

In addition to cancer cells, a solid tumor harbors other types of cells which form the tumor microenvironment and strongly affects cancer outcome [26]. Specifically, many groups have investigated the roles of immune cells in cancer progression. Certain types of immune cells, such as macrophages and T cells, can comprise up to 50% of the cells in a solid tumor [27]. These immune cells usually polarize into phenotypes, such as M2-like macrophages and regulatory T helper cells (Tregs), that promote tumor progression via suppressing the activity or viability of anti-cancerous immune cells, e.g., M1-like macrophages and cancer-killing T effector cells [26,27,164]. Our goal here is to focus on the role of EMT in this tumor-immune interplay.

A series of mathematical models have been proposed to understand the roles of tumor-immune interactions in polarizing the cytokine-immune cell network into states dominated by either immune-promoting or immune-suppressing populations [165–170]. Such modeling frameworks can help to design effective perturbations to revert the immune microenvironment from an immune-suppressing to an immune-promoting one. Many of these models consider the fact that macrophages and cancer cells can directly interact with each other and regulate the behaviors of one another, as shown by many in vitro experiments [171–176]. The interactions between macrophages and cancer cells are formidably complex, and the emergent dynamics can be non-intuitive. A series of mathematical models capturing these interactions suggests that cancer cells in the epithelial-like state (less aggressive) and M1-like macrophages might form a stable ecosystem, whereas cancer cells in the mesenchymal-like state (more aggressive) and M2-like macrophages form another stable pair [177].

The question of establishing an immune-dominated versus immune-suppressed microenvironment should have an effect on the activity of cd8+ effector T-cells. There have been studies suggesting that T cells tend to be excluded from tumors enriched by mesenchymal-like cancer cells [178,179]; we will discuss this further below. Combining this data with the modeling results, one could argue that interactions between macrophages and cancer cells drive the macrophages to be M2-like and the cancer cells to be mesenchymal-like; and due to the effects of M2-like macrophages, T cells may be excluded from tumor areas enriched with mesenchymal-like cancer cells. Since both the infiltration of cancer-killing immune cells [33–39] and the epithelial–mesenchymal plasticity of cancer cells are important for the prognosis of cancer patients, it is clearly valuable to evaluate the association and ultimately the casual relationship between the two.

In the following, we will first describe in greater detail the corresponding in vitro and in vivo experiments as well as analyses of gene expression data from The Cancer Genome Atlas (TCGA) (Figure 6). Finally, we discuss the potential causal relationship between the EMT status of cancer cells and the infiltration of cancer-killing immune cells.

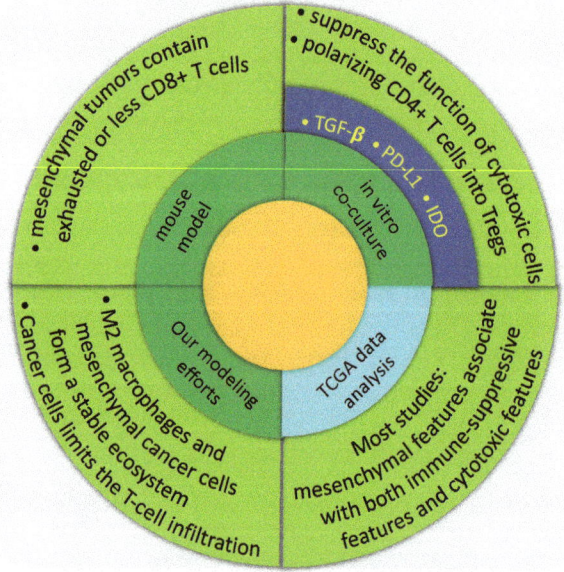

**Figure 6.** The relationship between EMT and immune response as shown by various approaches.

*8.1. In Vitro Characterization of the Immune-Suppressing Role of Mesenchymal-Like Cancer Cells*

For the interaction between mesenchymal-like cancer cells and immune cells, TGF-β signaling has been studied extensively. TGF-β is a well-known EMT inducer [21] and can be secreted by tumor-associated fibroblasts [180,181] and tumor-associated macrophages [182]. TGF-β signaling can impair maturation, differentiation, and/or activation of both innate and adaptive immune cells [31,183]. Specifically, TGF-β can inhibit the functions of cytotoxic T-cell functions [184,185]. In the co-culture experiments, Joffroy et al. showed that TGF-β secreted by cancer cells induces the differentiation of CD4$^+$ T cells into Treg (Foxp3$^+$) cells, which are immune-modulating cells [184]. Similar cancer-cell dependent expansion of CD4$^+$Foxp3$^+$ T cells is also shown by Kudo-Saito et al. when co-culturing SNAIL-enhanced mouse melanoma B16F10 cells with CD4$^+$ T cells [178]. For the innate immune cells, TGF-β secreted by cancer cells can help to polarize macrophages into M2-like ones, which potentially suppress the function of cytotoxic immune cells [186,187]. Furthermore, TGF-β can downregulate the MHC class I proteins as shown in prostate cancer [188] as well as NSCLC cell lines [189].

Aside from TGF-β, the PD-L1/PD-1 axis has also attracted attentions due to its implications in the immune-checkpoint blockade therapy. Presumably, PD-L1 expressed by cancer cells can bind to PD-1 expressed on the surface of cancer-killing immune cells, which will modulate their cytotoxic functions. It is shown that when driving EMT via downregulating miR-200 and overexpressing ZEB1, PD-L1 expression by cancer cells is upregulated [190]. Therefore, mesenchymal-like cancer cells could be more resistant to cancer-killing immune cells by upregulating PD-L1. Interestingly, expression levels of both TGF-β1 and PD-L1 by cancer cells can be induced under hypoxic conditions [191–193]. The hypoxia-induced EMT can promote immunosuppression via induced expression of indoleamine 2, 3-dioxygenase (IDO, another T-cell suppressing factor) in monocyte-derived macrophages [194].

EMT can also be induced when cancer cells are challenged by immune cells or inflammatory cytokines [195]. In addition, cancer cells can be equipped with immunomodulatory effects which interfere with proliferation, differentiation, and apoptosis of NK, T-cell, and B-cell populations [195]. As was the case for hypoxia, the IDO pathway is important for the immunomodulatory effects on T cells after inflammation-induced EMT [195]. These experimental results are potentially helpful for establishing a potential causal relationship between EMT of cancer cells and the infiltration of cytotoxic immune cells.

*8.2. In Vivo Characterization of the Immune-Suppressing Role of Mesenchymal-Like Cancer Cells*

Generally, in vivo experiments using mouse models show that tumors formed by mesenchymal-like cancer cells are less infiltrated with cancer-killing immune cells and/or more infiltrated by immune-suppressing immune cells. For example, Kudo-Saito et al. showed that in mice, compared with tumors formed by mock-transfected B16F10 cells, tumors derived from Snail-transduced B16F10 cells exhibit less tumor-infiltrating CD8$^+$ T cells, while more Tregs, and form more lung metastases [178]. In the same mouse model, the chemokine CCL2 can recruit immune-modulating populations such as MDSC and macrophages [196], which are responsible for creating the immune-suppressing microenvironment. In addition, in a mouse model of breast cancer [179], tumors formed by mesenchymal carcinoma cell lines contained more Tregs, M2 macrophages, and exhausted CD8$^+$ T cells, whereas tumors formed by more epithelial carcinoma cell lines contained CD8$^+$ T cells and M1 macrophages. Similarly, Suarez-Carmona et al. demonstrated that soluble factors regulated by EMT, such as IL-8, IL-6 and GM-CSF, mediate the recruitment of myeloid cells in xenograft mouse models [197,198]. Furthermore, using transgenic mouse models, Spranger et al. showed that an active β-catenin signaling in cancer cells contributes to a lack of T cell infiltration in tumor sites and resistance to anti-PD-L1 and/or anti-CTLA4 mAb therapy [199].

In summary, from the perspective of direct experiment in vitro or in preclinical models it is becoming clear that mesenchymal-like cancer cells can directly suppress the function of cancer-killing immune cells as well as promote the immune-suppressing microenvironment by recruiting or polarizing immune-suppressing immune cells. Following this logic, one would expect a lower presence of functional cancer-killing immune cells in the tumor area enriched with mesenchymal-like cancer cells.

*8.3. Gene Expression Data Analysis*

What about the results for patients? Unfortunately, the overall picture here as it emerges from TCGA data analyses tends to suggest that while mesenchymal tumors are generally enriched with immune-suppressing cells, they are often enriched with cancer-killing immune cells as well, as compared with epithelial tumors. For example, Mak et al. showed that the pan-cancer tumors samples with high EMT scores correlate with high expression of several immune checkpoints including PD-1, PD-L1, CTLA4, OX40L, and PD-L2 [200]. Lou et al. observed similar trend in lung cancer patients with early or advanced NSCLC adenocarcinomas [201]. Aside from the immune checkpoint markers, Lou et al. also found that the lung tumors that displayed an EMT phenotype also have a higher infiltration of Tregs. Interestingly, in their work, some immune costimulatory molecules such as CD80 and CD86 as well as IFN-$\gamma$ signals are more highly expressed in "mesenchymal" lung adenocarcinoma. Reports also suggest that, in the claudin-low subtype of breast and bladder cancer, which are mesenchymal-like, tumors are generally well-inflamed by immune-promoting immune cells but these cells are under active immunosuppression [202].

It should be noted that data in TCGA is rarely from tumor cells exclusively, thus the mesenchymal features seen there may be a consequence of higher infiltration of stromal cells. Conversely, analysis of epithelial markers [203] may not be biased by stromal cells. When investigating the epithelial marker ESRP1 for melanoma samples in TCGA dataset, Yao et al. found that a high infiltrating lymphocyte activity is enriched in ESRP1-low melanoma samples which have enhanced mesenchymal features [203]. The lymphocyte activity was evaluated by the gene expression of two cytotoxic agents—perforin (PRF1) and granzyme A (GZMA). Considering the use of an epithelial marker instead of mesenchymal markers, this work may be a strong piece of evidence, since the contamination by mesenchymal markers from non-cancer cells is supposed to be low. However, the immune infiltration still needs to be defined rigorously. It is possible that cytotoxic immune cells are constrained to lie in the tumor stroma instead of infiltrating into the tumor islets, though many of them infiltrate into the core of the tumor. For these tumors, the bulk tumor gene expression data will give a high infiltration score of cytotoxic immune cells. If these tumors happen to be ESRP1-low tumors, we are likely to conclude that a higher infiltration of cytotoxic immune cells is associated with more mesenchymal-like cancer cells.

Although the above-mentioned evidence tends to suggest that a higher infiltration of cytotoxic immune cells associates with the mesenchymal features of tumor samples, the jury is still out, and an opposite trend has been reported elsewhere. For example, Chae et al. reported that EMT is associated with significantly lower infiltration of CD4/CD8 T cells in squamous cell carcinoma [204]. In addition, high numbers of CD8$^+$ TILs have been shown to correlate with low SNAIL expression in extrahepatic cholangiocarcinoma [205]. Furthermore, in bladder cancers, patients with tumors characterized by an epithelial (luminal) phenotype have a better response rate when treated with anti-PD-L1 therapy compared to those harboring basal subtype [206], which are mesenchymal-like [207]. Since it has been suggested that patients who respond to anti-PD-L1 therapy usually have pre-existing CD8$^+$ T cells [208] which can be unleashed by the therapy, it is likely that in this particular study, epithelial-like tumors are better infiltrated by CD8$^+$ T cells than mesenchymal-like tumors. In addition, in muscle-invasive urothelial bladder cancer (MIUBC), activation of $\beta$-catenin pathway is found in the most common non-T cell-inflamed MIUBCs [209].

In summary, most of the gene expression analyses point towards a positive correlation between mesenchymal-like cancer cells and the higher infiltration of both immune-promoting and immune-suppressing immune cells, which seems the opposite of the trend revealed by in vitro co-culture experiments and in vivo mouse models. The inconsistency can be simply due to the fact that different analyses use varying standards of assessing the abundance of cancer-killing immune cells, for example, gene expression signatures of cancer-killing immune cells [199] or the percentage of cancer-killing immune cells among all (immune) cells [179]. In addition, the selected regions of interest (ROI) can also be inconsistent—core vs. margin—with varying immune-associated traits. Furthermore, the number of cancer cells in different ROI need to be evaluated for a fair comparison, i.e., a particular

ROI can be less inflamed. This confusion could be at least partially resolved if the infiltration could be quantified on the tumor islets level and the EMT status determined for single cancer cells instead of for the bulk population. For example, Seo et al. stained both EMT and CD8 markers for one breast cancer patient and found a positive correlation between the two [210]. However, the markers were not on the same section and there is still an issue of defining the immune infiltration. Therefore, it would be ideal to study the gene expression/protein abundance of the tumor islets or the sorted tumor cells in addition to the analysis of the corresponding images of the same tumor, so that we can have a better idea about whether there is any association between the EMT status of cancer cells and the infiltration of cancer-killing immune cells into the tumor islets.

*8.4. Causal Relationship between EMT and Infiltration of Cancer-Killing Immune Cells*

Even if we overcome the above-mentioned issues regarding the correlation between EMT and the infiltration of cancer-killing immune cells, there is still a hard problem to understand the causal relationship between the two. There is here an issue of the temporal coevolution of the tumor microenvironment which could play a role. Specifically, it is possible that apparently contradictory observations are in fact different snapshots of the co-evolution process of the two sets of cells. We can propose two potential scenarios on the causal relationship between the EMT status of cancer cells and the polarity of the immune microenvironment as well as the infiltration of cancer-killing immune cells.

The first scenario: tumor regions enriched with epithelial cancer cells first attract cancer-killing immune cells and then cancer cells are attacked by these immune cells. If one investigates the infiltration of immune cells at this stage, these epithelial tumors should be enriched by cancer-killing immune cells. The immune attack may convert epithelial-like cancer cells into mesenchymal-like ones [195]. Then the mesenchymal-like cancer cells can suppress the function of cancer-killing immune cells and start to promote the accumulation of immune-suppressing immune cells. Following this logic, at this stage, the mesenchymal-enriched tumors regions should have the infiltration of both cancer-killing and immune-suppressing immune cells. The TCGA data analysis results seem to support this hypothesis [200–202]. However, many in vivo experiments do not seem to support the late stage assumption of this scenario [178,199] even though experiments using epithelial-like cancer cell lines tend to support the early state aspects of this scenario at the early state [179].

The second scenario: before the engagement of immune systems, the cancer cells interact mainly with the cancer-associated fibroblasts (CAFs) or the tumor-associated macrophages (TAMs). The paracrine signaling between the two (cancer cells and CAFs, or cancer cells and TAMs) biases the cancer cells towards mesenchymal-like phenotypes [180–182]. Consequently, those mesenchymal-like cancer cells tend to exclude cancer-killing immune cells from the microenvironment. This exclusion may be also due to the accumulation of TAMs [196] or the absence of specific types of dendritic cells [199]. In addition, the mesenchymal-like cancer cells may also have their own ways to stop or exclude cancer-killing T cells [184,185,190]. In this scenario, epithelial tumors that do not undergo EMT (due to interactions with CAFs or TAMs) may be infiltrated by cancer-killing immune cells whereas mesenchymal tumors tend to exclude cancer-killing immune cells. Apparently, this scenario seems to be supported by the in vitro co-culture experiments as well as some in vivo studies but is not supported by most TCGA data analyses results.

In order to test different scenarios, it will be essential to monitor the trajectory of EMT of cancer cells as well as the evolution of the infiltration of cancer-killing immune cells in a single mouse. It has been shown that even in a single mouse model, some tumors can be "hot", and others can be "cold" [211]. The particular mouse model used in this recent study can be an ideal system to study the co-evolution of the EMT status of cancer cells as well as the infiltration pattern of cancer-killing immune cells to better understand the causal relationship between the two.

## 9. Hybrid E/M Phenotypes and Beyond

Our claim here has been that hybrid E/M phenotypes enable cancer cells metastatic plasticity to effectively metastasize. Notably, such stable hybrid phenotypes that combines features of two speciously exclusive phenotypes is not limited to EMT. For example, during pathological angiogenesis in cancer, a stable hybrid tip/stalk phenotype that results in poorly perfused and chaotic angiogenesis can be acquired due to the overexpressed Jagged [212]. The elevated production of Jagged in cancer can also promote the existence of a stable hybrid sender/receiver state where cells maintain intermediate levels of Jagged and Delta (ligands) and Notch (receptor) thus allowing cells the plasticity to both send and receive signals [90]. Another example of a hybrid phenotype in cancer appears to arise in cancer metabolic preprogramming. Some cancer cells can acquire a stable hybrid metabolic phenotype where both glycolysis and oxidative phosphorylation (OXPHOS) can be utilized [213–215]. Such hybrid metabolic phenotype enables cancer cell metabolic plasticity to grow and prosper in various hostile microenvironments. The hybrid metabolic phenotype has been observed in the human TNBC SUM159-PT and MDA-MB-231 and mouse breast cancer 4T1 cells at least at a population level. The emergence of the hybrid metabolic phenotype indicates that targeting both glycolysis and OXPHOS may be necessary to eliminate cancer metabolic plasticity. Notably, such a hybrid metabolic phenotype is not limited to cancer cells. For example, the naive pluripotent stem cells (PSCs) exhibit a hybrid glycolysis/OXPHOS phenotype relative to primed PSCs which primarily use glycolysis and somatic cells which primarily use OXPHOS [216]. As a result, activation of both OXPHOS and glycolysis, synergistically by the TFs Zic3 and Esrrb for example, is essential to reprogram somatic cells to acquire the naive pluripotency. In addition, regulatory T cells that utilize both glycolysis and fatty acid oxidation can be more effective in expansion than those that primarily use glycolysis [217]. In our final example, the T-helper (Th) cells can acquire a stable hybrid Th1/Th2 phenotype where cells co-express two mutually inhibiting TFs T-bet (stimulating Th1) and GATA3 (stimulating Th2) [218]. The hybrid Th1/Th2 phenotype combines the properties of Th1 and Th2 and can regulate effector T cell to function without excessive inflammation. In summary, it is reasonable to speculate that the hybrid phenotype is a common characteristic emerging from cellular plasticity.

## 10. Conclusions and Future Vision

Epithelial–mesenchymal plasticity has attracted much attention due to its critical roles in facilitating metastases, stemness, and immune repression. Emerging evidence suggests that cancer cells can acquire a spectrum of hybrid E/M phenotypes and cells can transition back and forth between different EMT phenotypes. Computational and experimental studies have been combined to deepen our understanding of EMT dynamics, the emergence of hybrid E/M phenotypes and the interplay of EMT with stemness and immune suppression. Notably, EMT is a multi-dimensional spatiotemporal program including alterations in mRNA and protein abundance, protein modification, and relocation which can mediate the changes in cell junction, morphology, and apico-basal polarity, resulting in adoption of cell migratory and invasive properties. Future computational studies need to integrate different facets of EMT to systemically elucidate EMT dynamics and quantify EMT status. The advance in experimental technologies such as simultaneous measurement of transcriptome and proteome at a single-cell level—CITE-seq [219] and REAP-seq [220]—intravital correlative microscopy [221] will contribute to high-resolution quantification of EMT in vivo. The combination of theoretical and experimental efforts will continue uncovering important mechanisms underlying epithelial–mesenchymal plasticity and its association with other hallmarks of cancer.

Thus, the emergence of hybrid phenotypes in cancer and the ability of cancer cells to switch back and forth between various phenotypes indicate that therapeutic strategies targeting cancer cell plasticity needs to be designed more carefully. Eliminating the notoriously aggressive hybrid phenotypes in cancer may serve as the first step towards conquering cancer.

**Acknowledgments:** This work is supported by the National Science Foundation (NSF) grant for the Center for Theoretical Biological Physics NSF PHY-1427654, by NSF grants PHY-1605817 and CHE-1614101 and by the John S. Dunn Foundation Collaborative Research Award. D.J. is supported by a training fellowship from the Gulf Coast Consortia, on the Computational Cancer Biology Training Program (CPRIT Grant No. RP170593). M.K.J. is supported by Ramanujan Fellowship awarded by SERB, DST, Government of India (SB/S2/RJN-049/2018). F.B. is supported by the Marjory Meyer Hasselmann Fellowship for academic excellence in chemistry.

**Conflicts of Interest:** The authors declare no conflict of interest.

## References

1. Chaffer, C.L.; Weinberg, R.A. A Perspective on Cancer Cell Metastasis. *Science* **2011**, *331*, 1559–1564. [CrossRef] [PubMed]
2. Ye, X.; Weinberg, R.A. Epithelial-Mesenchymal Plasticity: A Central Regulator of Cancer Progression. *Trends Cell Biol.* **2015**, *25*, 675–686. [CrossRef]
3. Greenburg, G.; Hay, E.D. Epithelia suspended in collagen gels can lose polarity and express characteristics of migrating mesenchymal cells. *J. Cell Biol.* **1982**, *95*, 333–339. [CrossRef] [PubMed]
4. Nieto, M.A.; Sargent, M.G.; Wilkinson, D.G.; Cooke, J. Control of cell behavior during vertebrate development by Slug, a zinc finger gene. *Science* **1994**, *264*, 835–839. [CrossRef]
5. Stone, R.C.; Pastar, I.; Ojeh, N.; Chen, V.; Liu, S.; Garzon, K.I.; Tomic-Canic, M. Epithelial-mesenchymal transition in tissue repair and fibrosis. *Cell Tissue Res.* **2016**, *365*, 495–506. [CrossRef] [PubMed]
6. Tsai, J.H.; Donaher, J.L.; Murphy, D.A.; Chau, S.; Yang, J. Spatiotemporal regulation of epithelial-mesenchymal transition is essential for squamous cell carcinoma metastasis. *Cancer Cell* **2012**, *22*, 725–736. [CrossRef]
7. Nieto, M.A.; Huang, R.Y.-J.; Jackson, R.A.; Thiery, J.P. EMT: 2016. *Cell* **2016**, *166*, 21–45. [CrossRef]
8. Bierie, B.; Pierce, S.E.; Kroeger, C.; Stover, D.G.; Pattabiraman, D.R.; Thiru, P.; Liu Donaher, J.; Reinhardt, F.; Chaffer, C.L.; Keckesova, Z.; et al. Integrin-β4 identifies cancer stem cell-enriched populations of partially mesenchymal carcinoma cells. *Proc. Natl. Acad. Sci. USA* **2017**, *114*, E2337–E2346. [CrossRef]
9. Jolly, M.K.; Ward, C.; Eapen, M.S.; Myers, S.; Hallgren, O.; Levine, H.; Sohal, S.S. Epithelial-mesenchymal transition, a spectrum of states: Role in lung development, homeostasis, and disease. *Dev. Dyn.* **2018**, *247*, 346–358. [CrossRef]
10. Pastushenko, I.; Brisebarre, A.; Sifrim, A.; Fioramonti, M.; Revenco, T.; Boumahdi, S.; Keymeulen, A.V.; Brown, D.; Moers, V.; Lemaire, S.; et al. Identification of the tumour transition states occurring during EMT. *Nature* **2018**, *556*, 463–468. [CrossRef]
11. Yu, M.; Bardia, A.; Wittner, B.S.; Stott, S.L.; Smas, M.E.; Ting, D.T.; Isakoff, S.J.; Ciciliano, J.C.; Wells, M.N.; Shah, A.M.; et al. Circulating Breast Tumor Cells Exhibit Dynamic Changes in Epithelial and Mesenchymal Composition. *Science* **2013**, *339*, 580–584. [CrossRef]
12. Cheung, K.J.; Padmanaban, V.; Silvestri, V.; Schipper, K.; Cohen, J.D.; Fairchild, A.N.; Gorin, M.A.; Verdone, J.E.; Pienta, K.J.; Bader, J.S.; et al. Polyclonal breast cancer metastases arise from collective dissemination of keratin 14-expressing tumor cell clusters. *Proc. Natl. Acad. Sci. USA* **2016**, *113*, E854–E863. [CrossRef] [PubMed]
13. Fabisiewicz, A.; Grzybowska, E. CTC clusters in cancer progression and metastasis. *Med. Oncol.* **2017**, *34*, 12. [CrossRef]
14. Brabletz, T.; Kalluri, R.; Nieto, M.A.; Weinberg, R.A. EMT in cancer. *Nat. Rev. Cancer* **2018**, *18*, 128–134. [CrossRef]
15. Zheng, X.; Carstens, J.L.; Kim, J.; Scheible, M.; Kaye, J.; Sugimoto, H.; Wu, C.-C.; LeBleu, V.S.; Kalluri, R. Epithelial-to-mesenchymal transition is dispensable for metastasis but induces chemoresistance in pancreatic cancer. *Nature* **2015**, *527*, 525–530. [CrossRef]
16. Fischer, K.R.; Durrans, A.; Lee, S.; Sheng, J.; Li, F.; Wong, S.T.C.; Choi, H.; El Rayes, T.; Ryu, S.; Troeger, J.; et al. Epithelial-to-mesenchymal transition is not required for lung metastasis but contributes to chemoresistance. *Nature* **2015**, *527*, 472–476. [CrossRef] [PubMed]
17. Krebs, A.M.; Mitschke, J.; Lasierra Losada, M.; Schmalhofer, O.; Boerries, M.; Busch, H.; Boettcher, M.; Mougiakakos, D.; Reichardt, W.; Bronsert, P.; et al. The EMT-activator Zeb1 is a key factor for cell plasticity and promotes metastasis in pancreatic cancer. *Nat. Cell Biol.* **2017**, *19*, 518–529. [CrossRef]
18. Stemmler, M.P.; Eccles, R.L.; Brabletz, S.; Brabletz, T. Non-redundant functions of EMT transcription factors. *Nat. Cell Biol.* **2019**, *21*, 102–112. [CrossRef]

19. Cursons, J.; Pillman, K.A.; Scheer, K.G.; Gregory, P.A.; Foroutan, M.; Hediyeh-Zadeh, S.; Toubia, J.; Crampin, E.J.; Goodall, G.J.; Bracken, C.P.; et al. Combinatorial targeting by microRNAs co-ordinates post-transcriptional control of EMT. *Cell Syst.* **2018**, *7*, 77.e7–91.e7. [CrossRef]
20. Jolly, M.K.; Ware, K.E.; Gilja, S.; Somarelli, J.A.; Levine, H. EMT and MET: Necessary or permissive for metastasis? *Mol. Oncol.* **2017**, *11*, 755–769. [CrossRef]
21. Xu, J.; Lamouille, S.; Derynck, R. TGF-beta-induced epithelial to mesenchymal transition. *Cell Res.* **2009**, *19*, 156–172. [CrossRef] [PubMed]
22. Wang, Z.; Li, Y.; Kong, D.; Banerjee, S.; Ahmad, A.; Azmi, A.S.; Ali, S.; Abbruzzese, J.L.; Gallick, G.E.; Sarkar, F.H. Acquisition of epithelial-mesenchymal transition phenotype of gemcitabine-resistant pancreatic cancer cells is linked with activation of the notch signaling pathway. *Cancer Res.* **2009**, *69*, 2400–2407. [CrossRef]
23. Wei, S.C.; Fattet, L.; Tsai, J.H.; Guo, Y.; Pai, V.H.; Majeski, H.E.; Chen, A.C.; Sah, R.L.; Taylor, S.S.; Engler, A.J.; et al. Matrix stiffness drives epithelial-mesenchymal transition and tumour metastasis through a TWIST1-G3BP2 mechanotransduction pathway. *Nat. Cell Biol.* **2015**, *17*, 678–688. [CrossRef] [PubMed]
24. Brabletz, T.; Jung, A.; Spaderna, S.; Hlubek, F.; Kirchner, T. Opinion: Migrating cancer stem cells—An integrated concept of malignant tumour progression. *Nat. Rev. Cancer* **2005**, *5*, 744–749. [CrossRef] [PubMed]
25. Hanahan, D.; Coussens, L.M. Accessories to the Crime: Functions of Cells Recruited to the Tumor Microenvironment. *Cancer Cell* **2012**, *21*, 309–322. [CrossRef] [PubMed]
26. Whiteside, T.L. The tumor microenvironment and its role in promoting tumor growth. *Oncogene* **2008**, *27*, 5904–5912. [CrossRef] [PubMed]
27. Gajewski, T.F.; Schreiber, H.; Fu, Y.-X. Innate and adaptive immune cells in the tumor microenvironment. *Nat. Immunol.* **2013**, *14*, 1014–1022. [CrossRef]
28. Schreiber, R.D.; Old, L.J.; Smyth, M.J. Cancer Immunoediting: Integrating Immunity's Roles in Cancer Suppression and Promotion. *Science* **2011**, *331*, 1565–1570. [CrossRef]
29. Rosenberg, S.A.; Restifo, N.P.; Yang, J.C.; Morgan, R.A.; Dudley, M.E. Adoptive cell transfer: A clinical path to effective cancer immunotherapy. *Nat. Rev. Cancer* **2008**, *8*, 299–308. [CrossRef]
30. Pardoll, D.M. The blockade of immune checkpoints in cancer immunotherapy. *Nat. Rev. Cancer* **2012**, *12*, 252–264. [CrossRef]
31. Terry, S.; Savagner, P.; Ortiz-Cuaran, S.; Mahjoubi, L.; Saintigny, P.; Thiery, J.-P.; Chouaib, S. New insights into the role of EMT in tumor immune escape. *Mol. Oncol.* **2017**, *11*, 824–846. [CrossRef] [PubMed]
32. Datar, I.; Schalper, K.A. Epithelial–Mesenchymal Transition and Immune Evasion during Lung Cancer Progression: The Chicken or the Egg? *Clin. Cancer Res.* **2016**, *22*, 3422–3424. [CrossRef] [PubMed]
33. Mahmoud, S.M.A.; Paish, E.C.; Powe, D.G.; Macmillan, R.D.; Grainge, M.J.; Lee, A.H.S.; Ellis, I.O.; Green, A.R. Tumor-infiltrating CD8+ lymphocytes predict clinical outcome in breast cancer. *J. Clin. Oncol.* **2011**, *29*, 1949–1955. [CrossRef]
34. Carstens, J.L.; Correa de Sampaio, P.; Yang, D.; Barua, S.; Wang, H.; Rao, A.; Allison, J.P.; LeBleu, V.S.; Kalluri, R. Spatial computation of intratumoral T cells correlates with survival of patients with pancreatic cancer. *Nat. Commun.* **2017**, *8*, 15095. [CrossRef] [PubMed]
35. Galon, J.; Costes, A.; Sanchez-Cabo, F.; Kirilovsky, A.; Mlecnik, B.; Lagorce-Pagès, C.; Tosolini, M.; Camus, M.; Berger, A.; Wind, P.; et al. Type, density, and location of immune cells within human colorectal tumors predict clinical outcome. *Science* **2006**, *313*, 1960–1964. [CrossRef] [PubMed]
36. Zhang, M.; He, Y.; Sun, X.; Li, Q.; Wang, W.; Zhao, A.; Di, W. A high M1/M2 ratio of tumor-associated macrophages is associated with extended survival in ovarian cancer patients. *J. Ovarian Res.* **2014**, *7*, 19. [CrossRef] [PubMed]
37. Edin, S.; Wikberg, M.L.; Dahlin, A.M.; Rutegård, J.; Öberg, Å.; Oldenborg, P.-A.; Palmqvist, R. The distribution of macrophages with a M1 or M2 phenotype in relation to prognosis and the molecular characteristics of colorectal cancer. *PLoS ONE* **2012**, *7*, e47045. [CrossRef]
38. Ma, J.; Liu, L.; Che, G.; Yu, N.; Dai, F.; You, Z. The M1 form of tumor-associated macrophages in non-small cell lung cancer is positively associated with survival time. *BMC Cancer* **2010**, *10*, 112. [CrossRef]
39. Ohri, C.M.; Shikotra, A.; Green, R.H.; Waller, D.A.; Bradding, P. Macrophages within NSCLC tumour islets are predominantly of a cytotoxic M1 phenotype associated with extended survival. *Eur. Respir. J.* **2009**, *33*, 118–126. [CrossRef]

40. De Craene, B.; Berx, G. Regulatory networks defining EMT during cancer initiation and progression. *Nat. Rev. Cancer* **2013**, *13*, 97–110. [CrossRef]
41. Grelet, S.; McShane, A.; Geslain, R.; Howe, P.H. Pleiotropic Roles of Non-Coding RNAs in TGF-β-Mediated Epithelial-Mesenchymal Transition and Their Functions in Tumor Progression. *Cancers* **2017**, *9*, 75. [CrossRef] [PubMed]
42. Lu, M.; Jolly, M.K.; Levine, H.; Onuchic, J.N.; Ben-Jacob, E. MicroRNA-based regulation of epithelial–hybrid–mesenchymal fate determination. *Proc. Natl. Acad. Sci. USA* **2013**, *110*, 18144–18149. [CrossRef] [PubMed]
43. Zhang, J.; Tian, X.-J.; Zhang, H.; Teng, Y.; Li, R.; Bai, F.; Elankumaran, S.; Xing, J. TGF-β–induced epithelial-to-mesenchymal transition proceeds through stepwise activation of multiple feedback loops. *Sci. Signal.* **2014**, *7*, ra91. [CrossRef]
44. Jia, D.; Jolly, M.K.; Tripathi, S.C.; Den Hollander, P.; Huang, B.; Lu, M.; Celiktas, M.; Ramirez-Peña, E.; Ben-Jacob, E.; Onuchic, J.N.; et al. Distinguishing mechanisms underlying EMT tristability. *Cancer Converg.* **2017**, *1*, 2. [CrossRef]
45. Steinway, S.N.; Zañudo, J.G.T.; Michel, P.J.; Feith, D.J.; Loughran, T.P.; Albert, R. Combinatorial interventions inhibit TGFβ-driven epithelial-to-mesenchymal transition and support hybrid cellular phenotypes. *NPJ Syst. Biol. Appl.* **2015**, *1*, 15014. [CrossRef]
46. Huang, B.; Lu, M.; Jia, D.; Ben-Jacob, E.; Levine, H.; Onuchic, J.N. Interrogating the topological robustness of gene regulatory circuits by randomization. *PLoS Comput. Biol.* **2017**, *13*, e1005456. [CrossRef]
47. Jolly, M.K.; Preca, B.-T.; Tripathi, S.C.; Jia, D.; George, J.T.; Hanash, S.M.; Brabletz, T.; Stemmler, M.P.; Maurer, J.; Levine, H. Interconnected feedback loops among ESRP1, HAS2, and CD44 regulate epithelial-mesenchymal plasticity in cancer. *APL Bioeng.* **2018**, *2*, 031908. [CrossRef]
48. Font-Clos, F.; Zapperi, S.; Porta, C.A.M.L. Topography of epithelial–mesenchymal plasticity. *Proc. Natl. Acad. Sci. USA* **2018**, *115*, 5902–5907. [CrossRef]
49. Li, C.; Hong, T.; Nie, Q. Quantifying the landscape and kinetic paths for epithelial–mesenchymal transition from a core circuit. *Phys. Chem. Chem. Phys.* **2016**, *18*, 17949–17956. [CrossRef]
50. Biswas, K.; Jolly, M.K.; Ghosh, A. Stability and mean residence times for hybrid epithelial/mesenchymal phenotype. *Phys. Biol.* **2019**, *16*, 025003. [CrossRef]
51. Jolly, M.K.; Tripathi, S.C.; Jia, D.; Mooney, S.M.; Celiktas, M.; Hanash, S.M.; Mani, S.A.; Pienta, K.J.; Ben-Jacob, E.; Levine, H. Stability of the hybrid epithelial/mesenchymal phenotype. *Oncotarget* **2016**, *7*, 27067–27084. [CrossRef]
52. Jia, D.; Jolly, M.K.; Boareto, M.; Parsana, P.; Mooney, S.M.; Pienta, K.J.; Levine, H.; Ben-Jacob, E. OVOL guides the epithelial-hybrid-mesenchymal transition. *Oncotarget* **2015**, *6*, 15436–15448. [CrossRef]
53. Bocci, F.; Jolly, M.K.; Tripathi, S.C.; Aguilar, M.; Hanash, S.M.; Levine, H.; Onuchic, J.N. Numb prevents a complete epithelial–mesenchymal transition by modulating Notch signalling. *J. R. Soc. Interface* **2017**, *14*. [CrossRef]
54. Gould, R.; Bassen, D.M.; Chakrabarti, A.; Varner, J.D.; Butcher, J. Population Heterogeneity in the Epithelial to Mesenchymal Transition Is Controlled by NFAT and Phosphorylated Sp1. *PLoS Comput. Biol.* **2016**, *12*, e1005251. [CrossRef]
55. Biddle, A.; Gammon, L.; Liang, X.; Costea, D.E.; Mackenzie, I.C. Phenotypic Plasticity Determines Cancer Stem Cell Therapeutic Resistance in Oral Squamous Cell Carcinoma. *EBioMedicine* **2016**, *4*, 138–145. [CrossRef]
56. Kohar, V.; Lu, M. Role of noise and parametric variation in the dynamics of gene regulatory circuits. *NPJ Syst. Biol. Appl.* **2018**, *4*, 40. [CrossRef]
57. Huang, R.Y.-J.; Wong, M.K.; Tan, T.Z.; Kuay, K.T.; Ng, A.H.C.; Chung, V.Y.; Chu, Y.-S.; Matsumura, N.; Lai, H.-C.; Lee, Y.F.; et al. An EMT spectrum defines an anoikis-resistant and spheroidogenic intermediate mesenchymal state that is sensitive to e-cadherin restoration by a src-kinase inhibitor, saracatinib (AZD0530). *Cell Death Dis.* **2013**, *4*, e915. [CrossRef]
58. Varankar, S.S.; Kamble, S.C.; Mali, A.M.; More, M.M.; Abraham, A.; Kumar, B.; Pansare, K.J.; Narayanan, N.J.; Sen, A.; Dhake, R.D.; et al. Functional Balance between TCF21-Slug defines phenotypic plasticity and sub-classes in high-grade serous ovarian cancer. *bioRxiv* **2018**, 307934.
59. Schliekelman, M.J.; Taguchi, A.; Zhu, J.; Dai, X.; Rodriguez, J.; Celiktas, M.; Zhang, Q.; Chin, A.; Wong, C.H.; Wang, H.; et al. Molecular portraits of epithelial, mesenchymal, and hybrid States in lung adenocarcinoma and their relevance to survival. *Cancer Res.* **2015**, *75*, 1789–1800. [CrossRef]

60. Jia, D.; George, J.T.; Tripathi, S.C.; Kundnani, D.L.; Lu, M.; Hanash, S.M.; Onuchic, J.N.; Jolly, M.K.; Levine, H. Testing the gene expression classification of the EMT spectrum. *Phys. Biol.* **2019**, *16*, 025002. [CrossRef]
61. Jolly, M.K.; Tripathi, S.C.; Somarelli, J.A.; Hanash, S.M.; Levine, H. Epithelial/mesenchymal plasticity: How have quantitative mathematical models helped improve our understanding? *Mol. Oncol.* **2017**, *11*, 739–754. [CrossRef]
62. Bocci, F.; Tripathi, S.C.; Mercedes, S.V.; George, J.T.; Casabar, J.; Wong, P.K.; Hanash, S.; Levine, H.; Onuchic, J.N.; Jolly, M.K. NRF2 activates a partial Epithelial-Mesenchymal Transition and is maximally present in a hybrid Epithelial/Mesenchymal phenotype. *bioRxiv* **2018**, 390237.
63. Fustaino, V.; Presutti, D.; Colombo, T.; Cardinali, B.; Papoff, G.; Brandi, R.; Bertolazzi, P.; Felici, G.; Ruberti, G. Characterization of epithelial-mesenchymal transition intermediate/hybrid phenotypes associated to resistance to EGFR inhibitors in non-small cell lung cancer cell lines. *Oncotarget* **2017**, *8*, 103340–103363. [CrossRef]
64. Grosse-Wilde, A.; d'Hérouël, A.F.; McIntosh, E.; Ertaylan, G.; Skupin, A.; Kuestner, R.E.; del Sol, A.; Walters, K.-A.; Huang, S. Stemness of the hybrid Epithelial/Mesenchymal State in Breast Cancer and Its Association with Poor Survival. *PLoS ONE* **2015**, *10*, e0126522. [CrossRef]
65. Grigore, A.D.; Jolly, M.K.; Jia, D.; Farach-Carson, M.C.; Levine, H. Tumor Budding: The Name is EMT. Partial EMT. *J. Clin. Med.* **2016**, *5*, 51. [CrossRef]
66. Jolly, M.K.; Somarelli, J.A.; Sheth, M.; Biddle, A.; Tripathi, S.C.; Armstrong, A.J.; Hanash, S.M.; Bapat, S.A.; Rangarajan, A.; Levine, H. Hybrid epithelial/mesenchymal phenotypes promote metastasis and therapy resistance across carcinomas. *Pharmacol. Ther.* **2019**, *194*, 161–184. [CrossRef]
67. Pastushenko, I.; Blanpain, C. EMT transition states during tumor progression and metastasis. *Trends Cell Biol.* **2019**, *29*, 212–226. [CrossRef]
68. Losick, R.; Desplan, C. Stochasticity and Cell Fate. *Science* **2008**, *320*, 65–68. [CrossRef]
69. Balaban, N.Q.; Merrin, J.; Chait, R.; Kowalik, L.; Leibler, S. Bacterial Persistence as a Phenotypic Switch. *Science* **2004**, *305*, 1622–1625. [CrossRef]
70. Huh, D.; Paulsson, J. Non-genetic heterogeneity from stochastic partitioning at cell division. *Nat. Genet.* **2011**, *43*, 95–100. [CrossRef]
71. Huh, D.; Paulsson, J. Random partitioning of molecules at cell division. *Proc. Natl. Acad. Sci. USA* **2011**, *108*, 15004–15009. [CrossRef]
72. Tripathi, S.; Levine, H.; Jolly, M.K. A Mechanism for Epithelial-Mesenchymal Heterogeneity in a Population of Cancer Cells. *bioRxiv* **2019**, 592691.
73. Ruscetti, M.; Quach, B.; Dadashian, E.L.; Mulholland, D.J.; Wu, H. Tracking and Functional Characterization of Epithelial-Mesenchymal Transition and Mesenchymal Tumor Cells During Prostate Cancer Metastasis. *Cancer Res.* **2015**, *75*, 2749–2759. [CrossRef]
74. Boareto, M.; Jolly, M.K.; Goldman, A.; Pietilä, M.; Mani, S.A.; Sengupta, S.; Ben-Jacob, E.; Levine, H.; Onuchic, J.N. Notch-Jagged signalling can give rise to clusters of cells exhibiting a hybrid epithelial/mesenchymal phenotype. *J. R. Soc. Interface* **2016**, *13*. [CrossRef]
75. Aiello, N.M.; Maddipati, R.; Norgard, R.J.; Balli, D.; Li, J.; Yuan, S.; Yamazoe, T.; Black, T.; Sahmoud, A.; Furth, E.E.; et al. EMT Subtype Influences Epithelial Plasticity and Mode of Cell Migration. *Dev. Cell* **2018**, *45*, 681.e4–695.e4. [CrossRef]
76. Puram, S.V.; Tirosh, I.; Parikh, A.S.; Patel, A.P.; Yizhak, K.; Gillespie, S.; Rodman, C.; Luo, C.L.; Mroz, E.A.; Emerick, K.S.; et al. Single-Cell Transcriptomic Analysis of Primary and Metastatic Tumor Ecosystems in Head and Neck Cancer. *Cell* **2017**, *171*, 1611.e24–1624.e24. [CrossRef]
77. Celià-Terrassa, T.; Bastian, C.; Liu, D.; Ell, B.; Aiello, N.M.; Wei, Y.; Zamalloa, J.; Blanco, A.M.; Hang, X.; Kunisky, D.; et al. Hysteresis control of epithelial-mesenchymal transition dynamics conveys a distinct program with enhanced metastatic ability. *Nat. Commun.* **2018**, *9*, 5005. [CrossRef]
78. Siebel, C.; Lendahl, U. Notch Signaling in Development, Tissue Homeostasis, and Disease. *Physiol. Rev.* **2017**, *97*, 1235–1294. [CrossRef]
79. Jolly, M.K.; Boareto, M.; Huang, B.; Jia, D.; Lu, M.; Ben-Jacob, E.; Onuchic, J.N.; Levine, H. Implications of the Hybrid Epithelial/Mesenchymal Phenotype in Metastasis. *Front. Oncol.* **2015**, *5*, 155. [CrossRef]
80. Li, D.; Masiero, M.; Banham, A.H.; Harris, A.L. The notch ligand JAGGED1 as a target for anti-tumor therapy. *Front. Oncol.* **2014**, *4*, 254. [CrossRef]
81. Bray, S.J. Notch signalling in context. *Nat. Rev. Mol. Cell Biol.* **2016**, *17*, 722–735. [CrossRef] [PubMed]

82. Brabletz, S.; Bajdak, K.; Meidhof, S.; Burk, U.; Niedermann, G.; Firat, E.; Wellner, U.; Dimmler, A.; Faller, G.; Schubert, J.; et al. The ZEB1/miR-200 feedback loop controls Notch signalling in cancer cells. *EMBO J.* **2011**, *30*, 770–782. [CrossRef] [PubMed]
83. de Antonellis, P.; Medaglia, C.; Cusanelli, E.; Andolfo, I.; Liguori, L.; Vita, G.D.; Carotenuto, M.; Bello, A.; Formiggini, F.; Galeone, A.; et al. MiR-34a Targeting of Notch Ligand Delta-Like 1 Impairs CD15+/CD133+ Tumor-Propagating Cells and Supports Neural Differentiation in Medulloblastoma. *PLoS ONE* **2011**, *6*, e24584. [CrossRef]
84. Bu, P.; Chen, K.-Y.; Chen, J.H.; Wang, L.; Walters, J.; Shin, Y.J.; Goerger, J.P.; Sun, J.; Witherspoon, M.; Rakhilin, N.; et al. A microRNA miR-34a-regulated bimodal switch targets Notch in colon cancer stem cells. *Cell Stem Cell* **2013**, *12*, 602–615. [CrossRef] [PubMed]
85. Bocci, F.; Jolly, M.K.; Levine, H.; Onuchic, J.N. Quantitative Characteristic of ncRNA Regulation in Gene Regulatory Networks. *Methods Mol. Biol.* **2019**, *1912*, 341–366.
86. Sahlgren, C.; Gustafsson, M.V.; Jin, S.; Poellinger, L.; Lendahl, U. Notch signaling mediates hypoxia-induced tumor cell migration and invasion. *Proc. Natl. Acad. Sci. USA* **2008**, *105*, 6392–6397. [CrossRef]
87. Niessen, K.; Fu, Y.; Chang, L.; Hoodless, P.A.; McFadden, D.; Karsan, A. Slug is a direct Notch target required for initiation of cardiac cushion cellularization. *J. Cell Biol.* **2008**, *182*, 315–325. [CrossRef] [PubMed]
88. Collier, J.R.; Monk, N.A.; Maini, P.K.; Lewis, J.H. Pattern formation by lateral inhibition with feedback: A mathematical model of delta-notch intercellular signalling. *J. Theor. Biol.* **1996**, *183*, 429–446. [CrossRef]
89. Shaya, O.; Sprinzak, D. From Notch signaling to fine-grained patterning: Modeling meets experiments. *Curr. Opin. Genet. Dev.* **2011**, *21*, 732–739. [CrossRef]
90. Boareto, M.; Jolly, M.K.; Lu, M.; Onuchic, J.N.; Clementi, C.; Ben-Jacob, E. Jagged–Delta asymmetry in Notch signaling can give rise to a Sender/Receiver hybrid phenotype. *Proc. Natl. Acad. Sci. USA* **2015**, *112*, E402–E409. [CrossRef]
91. Jolly, M.K.; Boareto, M.; Debeb, B.G.; Aceto, N.; Farach-Carson, M.C.; Woodward, W.A.; Levine, H. Inflammatory breast cancer: A model for investigating cluster-based dissemination. *NPJ Breast Cancer* **2017**, *3*, 21. [CrossRef]
92. Andersson, E.R.; Sandberg, R.; Lendahl, U. Notch signaling: Simplicity in design, versatility in function. *Development* **2011**, *138*, 3593–3612. [CrossRef]
93. Zhang, Y.; Li, F.; Song, Y.; Sheng, X.; Ren, F.; Xiong, K.; Chen, L.; Zhang, H.; Liu, D.; Lengner, C.J.; et al. Numb and Numbl act to determine mammary myoepithelial cell fate, maintain epithelial identity, and support lactogenesis. *FASEB J.* **2016**, *30*, 3474–3488. [CrossRef]
94. Flores, A.N.; McDermott, N.; Meunier, A.; Marignol, L. NUMB inhibition of NOTCH signalling as a therapeutic target in prostate cancer. *Nat. Rev. Urol.* **2014**, *11*, 499–507. [CrossRef]
95. Santosh, A.B.R.; Jones, T.J. The Epithelial-Mesenchymal Interactions: Insights into Physiological and Pathological Aspects of Oral Tissues. *Oncol. Rev.* **2014**, *8*, 239.
96. Tsuji, T.; Ibaragi, S.; Shima, K.; Hu, M.G.; Katsurano, M.; Sasaki, A.; Hu, G. Epithelial-mesenchymal transition induced by growth suppressor p12CDK2-AP1 promotes tumor cell local invasion but suppresses distant colony growth. *Cancer Res.* **2008**, *68*, 10377–10386. [CrossRef]
97. Neelakantan, D.; Zhou, H.; Oliphant, M.U.J.; Zhang, X.; Simon, L.M.; Henke, D.M.; Shaw, C.A.; Wu, M.-F.; Hilsenbeck, S.G.; White, L.D.; et al. EMT cells increase breast cancer metastasis via paracrine GLI activation in neighbouring tumour cells. *Nat. Commun.* **2017**, *8*, 15773. [CrossRef]
98. Grosse-Wilde, A.; Kuestner, R.E.; Skelton, S.M.; MacIntosh, E.; d'Hérouël, A.F.; Ertaylan, G.; Del Sol, A.; Skupin, A.; Huang, S. Loss of inter-cellular cooperation by complete epithelial-mesenchymal transition supports favorable outcomes in basal breast cancer patients. *Oncotarget* **2018**, *9*, 20018–20033. [CrossRef]
99. Campbell, K.; Casanova, J. A role for E-cadherin in ensuring cohesive migration of a heterogeneous population of non-epithelial cells. *Nat. Commun.* **2015**, *6*, 7998. [CrossRef]
100. Kröger, C.; Afeyan, A.; Mraz, J.; Eaton, E.N.; Reinhardt, F.; Khodor, Y.L.; Thiru, P.; Bierie, B.; Ye, X.; Burge, C.B.; et al. Acquisition of a hybrid E/M state is essential for tumorigenicity of basal breast cancer cells. *Proc. Natl. Acad. Sci. USA* **2019**, *116*, 7353–7362. [CrossRef]
101. Celià-Terrassa, T.; Meca-Cortés, O.; Mateo, F.; Martínez de Paz, A.; Rubio, N.; Arnal-Estapé, A.; Ell, B.J.; Bermudo, R.; Díaz, A.; Guerra-Rebollo, M.; et al. Epithelial-mesenchymal transition can suppress major attributes of human epithelial tumor-initiating cells. *J. Clin. Investig.* **2012**, *122*, 1849–1868. [CrossRef]

102. Ocaña, O.H.; Córcoles, R.; Fabra, A.; Moreno-Bueno, G.; Acloque, H.; Vega, S.; Barrallo-Gimeno, A.; Cano, A.; Nieto, M.A. Metastatic colonization requires the repression of the epithelial-mesenchymal transition inducer Prrx1. *Cancer Cell* **2012**, *22*, 709–724. [CrossRef]
103. Tarin, D.; Thompson, E.W.; Newgreen, D.F. The fallacy of epithelial mesenchymal transition in neoplasia. *Cancer Res.* **2005**, *65*, 5996–6000; discussion 6000–6001. [CrossRef]
104. Lee, J.M.; Dedhar, S.; Kalluri, R.; Thompson, E.W. The epithelial–mesenchymal transition: New insights in signaling, development, and disease. *J. Cell Biol.* **2006**, *172*, 973–981. [CrossRef]
105. Thiery, J.P. Epithelial-mesenchymal transitions in tumour progression. *Nat. Rev. Cancer* **2002**, *2*, 442–454. [CrossRef]
106. Ewald, A.J.; Brenot, A.; Duong, M.; Chan, B.S.; Werb, Z. Collective epithelial migration and cell rearrangements drive mammary branching morphogenesis. *Dev. Cell* **2008**, *14*, 570–581. [CrossRef]
107. Theveneau, E.; Mayor, R. Neural crest delamination and migration: From epithelium-to-mesenchyme transition to collective cell migration. *Dev. Biol.* **2012**, *366*, 34–54. [CrossRef]
108. Kai, K.; Iwamoto, T.; Zhang, D.; Shen, L.; Takahashi, Y.; Rao, A.; Thompson, A.; Sen, S.; Ueno, N.T. CSF-1/CSF-1R axis is associated with epithelial/mesenchymal hybrid phenotype in epithelial-like inflammatory breast cancer. *Sci. Rep.* **2018**, *8*, 9427. [CrossRef]
109. Tiwari, P.; Mrigwani, A.; Kaur, H.; Kaila, P.; Kumar, R.; Guptasarma, P. Structural-Mechanical and Biochemical Functions of Classical Cadherins at Cellular Junctions: A Review and Some Hypotheses. *Adv. Exp. Med. Biol.* **2018**, *1112*, 107–138.
110. Knútsdóttir, H.; Pálsson, E.; Edelstein-Keshet, L. Mathematical model of macrophage-facilitated breast cancer cells invasion. *J. Theor. Biol.* **2014**, *357*, 184–199. [CrossRef]
111. Wyckoff, J.; Wang, W.; Lin, E.Y.; Wang, Y.; Pixley, F.; Stanley, E.R.; Graf, T.; Pollard, J.W.; Segall, J.; Condeelis, J. A paracrine loop between tumor cells and macrophages is required for tumor cell migration in mammary tumors. *Cancer Res.* **2004**, *64*, 7022–7029. [CrossRef]
112. Matte, B.F.; Kumar, A.; Placone, J.K.; Zanella, V.G.; Martins, M.D.; Engler, A.J.; Lamers, M.L. Matrix stiffness mechanically conditions EMT and migratory behavior of oral squamous cell carcinoma. *J. Cell Sci.* **2019**, *132*, jcs224360. [CrossRef]
113. Razinia, Z.; Castagnino, P.; Xu, T.; Vázquez-Salgado, A.; Puré, E.; Assoian, R.K. Stiffness-dependent motility and proliferation uncoupled by deletion of CD44. *Sci. Rep.* **2017**, *7*, 16499. [CrossRef]
114. Gjorevski, N.; Boghaert, E.; Nelson, C.M. Regulation of Epithelial-Mesenchymal Transition by Transmission of Mechanical Stress through Epithelial Tissues. *Cancer Microenviron.* **2011**, *5*, 29–38. [CrossRef]
115. Leight, J.L.; Wozniak, M.A.; Chen, S.; Lynch, M.L.; Chen, C.S. Matrix rigidity regulates a switch between TGF-β1-induced apoptosis and epithelial-mesenchymal transition. *Mol. Biol. Cell* **2012**, *23*, 781–791. [CrossRef]
116. Dupont, S.; Morsut, L.; Aragona, M.; Enzo, E.; Giulitti, S.; Cordenonsi, M.; Zanconato, F.; Le Digabel, J.; Forcato, M.; Bicciato, S.; et al. Role of YAP/TAZ in mechanotransduction. *Nature* **2011**, *474*, 179–183. [CrossRef]
117. Ondeck, M.G.; Kumar, A.; Placone, J.K.; Plunkett, C.M.; Matte, B.F.; Wong, K.C.; Fattet, L.; Yang, J.; Engler, A.J. Dynamically stiffened matrix promotes malignant transformation of mammary epithelial cells via collective mechanical signaling. *Proc. Natl. Acad. Sci. USA* **2019**, *116*, 3502–3507. [CrossRef]
118. Tang, X.; Kuhlenschmidt, T.B.; Zhou, J.; Bell, P.; Wang, F.; Kuhlenschmidt, M.S.; Saif, T.A. Mechanical Force Affects Expression of an In Vitro Metastasis-Like Phenotype in HCT-8 Cells. *Biophys. J.* **2010**, *99*, 2460–2469. [CrossRef]
119. Cox, T.R.; Bird, D.; Baker, A.-M.; Barker, H.E.; Ho, M.W.-Y.; Lang, G.; Erler, J.T. LOX-Mediated Collagen Crosslinking Is Responsible for Fibrosis-Enhanced Metastasis. *Cancer Res.* **2013**, *73*, 1721–1732. [CrossRef]
120. Peng, D.H.; Ungewiss, C.; Tong, P.; Byers, L.A.; Wang, J.; Canales, J.R.; Villalobos, P.A.; Uraoka, N.; Mino, B.; Behrens, C.; et al. ZEB1 induces LOXL2-mediated collagen stabilization and deposition in the extracellular matrix to drive lung cancer invasion and metastasis. *Oncogene* **2017**, *36*, 1925–1938. [CrossRef]
121. Sun, M.; Spill, F.; Zaman, M.H. A Computational Model of YAP/TAZ Mechanosensing. *Biophys. J.* **2016**, *110*, 2540–2550. [CrossRef]
122. Mani, S.A.; Guo, W.; Liao, M.-J.; Eaton, E.N.; Ayyanan, A.; Zhou, A.Y.; Brooks, M.; Reinhard, F.; Zhang, C.C.; Shipitsin, M.; et al. The epithelial-mesenchymal transition generates cells with properties of stem cells. *Cell* **2008**, *133*, 704–715. [CrossRef]

123. Somarelli, J.A.; Schaeffer, D.; Marengo, M.S.; Bepler, T.; Rouse, D.; Ware, K.E.; Hish, A.J.; Zhao, Y.; Buckley, A.F.; Epstein, J.I.; et al. Distinct routes to metastasis: Plasticity-dependent and plasticity-independent pathways. *Oncogene* 2016, *35*, 4302–4311. [CrossRef]
124. Leggett, S.E.; Sim, J.Y.; Rubins, J.E.; Neronha, Z.J.; Williams, E.K.; Wong, I.Y. Morphological single cell profiling of the epithelial-mesenchymal transition. *Integr. Biol. (Camb.)* 2016, *8*, 1133–1144. [CrossRef]
125. George, J.T.; Jolly, M.K.; Xu, S.; Somarelli, J.A.; Levine, H. Survival Outcomes in Cancer Patients Predicted by a Partial EMT Gene Expression Scoring Metric. *Cancer Res.* 2017, *77*, 6415–6428. [CrossRef]
126. Tan, T.Z.; Miow, Q.H.; Miki, Y.; Noda, T.; Mori, S.; Huang, R.Y.-J.; Thiery, J.P. Epithelial-mesenchymal transition spectrum quantification and its efficacy in deciphering survival and drug responses of cancer patients. *EMBO Mol. Med.* 2014, *6*, 1279–1293. [CrossRef]
127. Liu, X.; Taftaf, R.; Kawaguchi, M.; Chang, Y.-F.; Chen, W.; Entenberg, D.; Zhang, Y.; Gerratana, L.; Huang, S.; Patel, D.B.; et al. Homophilic CD44 interactions mediate tumor cell aggregation and polyclonal metastasis in patient-derived breast cancer models. *Cancer Discov.* 2018, *9*, 96–113. [CrossRef]
128. Aceto, N.; Bardia, A.; Miyamoto, D.T.; Donaldson, M.C.; Wittner, B.S.; Spencer, J.A.; Yu, M.; Pely, A.; Engstrom, A.; Zhu, H.; et al. Circulating Tumor Cell Clusters Are Oligoclonal Precursors of Breast Cancer Metastasis. *Cell* 2014, *158*, 1110–1122. [CrossRef]
129. Khalil, A.A.; Ilina, O.; Gritsenko, P.G.; Bult, P.; Span, P.N.; Friedl, P. Collective invasion in ductal and lobular breast cancer associates with distant metastasis. *Clin. Exp. Metastasis* 2017, *34*, 421–429. [CrossRef]
130. Li, C.-F.; Chen, J.-Y.; Ho, Y.-H.; Hsu, W.-H.; Wu, L.-C.; Lan, H.-Y.; Hsu, D.S.-S.; Tai, S.-K.; Chang, Y.-C.; Yang, M.-H. Snail-induced claudin-11 prompts collective migration for tumour progression. *Nat. Cell Biol.* 2019, *21*, 251–262. [CrossRef]
131. Bocci, F.; Jolly, M.K.; Onuchic, J.N. A biophysical model uncovers the size distribution of migrating cell clusters across cancer types. *bioRxiv* 2019, 563049.
132. Szczerba, B.M.; Castro-Giner, F.; Vetter, M.; Krol, I.; Gkountela, S.; Landin, J.; Scheidmann, M.C.; Donato, C.; Scherrer, R.; Singer, J.; et al. Neutrophils escort circulating tumour cells to enable cell cycle progression. *Nature* 2019, *566*, 553–557. [CrossRef]
133. Sarioglu, A.F.; Aceto, N.; Kojic, N.; Donaldson, M.C.; Zeinali, M.; Hamza, B.; Engstrom, A.; Zhu, H.; Sundaresan, T.K.; Miyamoto, D.T.; et al. A microfluidic device for label-free, physical capture of circulating tumor cell clusters. *Nat. Methods* 2015, *12*, 685–691. [CrossRef]
134. Leone, K.; Poggiana, C.; Zamarchi, R. The Interplay between Circulating Tumor Cells and the Immune System: From Immune Escape to Cancer Immunotherapy. *Diagnostics (Basel)* 2018, *8*, 59. [CrossRef]
135. Mierke, C.T. *Physics of Cancer*; IOP Publishing: Bristol, UK, 2015; The Role of Macrophages during Cancer Cell Transendothelial Migration.
136. Nielsen, S.R.; Schmid, M.C. Macrophages as Key Drivers of Cancer Progression and Metastasis. *Mediators Inflamm.* 2017, *2017*, 9624760. [CrossRef]
137. Hojo, N.; Huisken, A.L.; Wang, H.; Chirshev, E.; Kim, N.S.; Nguyen, S.M.; Campos, H.; Glackin, C.A.; Ioffe, Y.J.; Unternaehrer, J.J. Snail knockdown reverses stemness and inhibits tumour growth in ovarian cancer. *Sci. Rep.* 2018, *8*, 8704. [CrossRef]
138. Tam, W.L.; Weinberg, R.A. The epigenetics of epithelial-mesenchymal plasticity in cancer. *Nat. Med.* 2013, *19*, 1438–1449. [CrossRef]
139. Patsialou, A.; Wang, Y.; Lin, J.; Whitney, K.; Goswami, S.; Kenny, P.A.; Condeelis, J.S. Selective gene-expression profiling of migratory tumor cells in vivo predicts clinical outcome in breast cancer patients. *Breast Cancer Res.* 2012, *14*, R139. [CrossRef]
140. Liao, T.-T.; Hsu, W.-H.; Ho, C.-H.; Hwang, W.-L.; Lan, H.-Y.; Lo, T.; Chang, C.-C.; Tai, S.-K.; Yang, M.-H. let-7 Modulates Chromatin Configuration and Target Gene Repression through Regulation of the ARID3B Complex. *Cell Rep.* 2016, *14*, 520–533. [CrossRef]
141. Jolly, M.K.; Jia, D.; Boareto, M.; Mani, S.A.; Pienta, K.J.; Ben-Jacob, E.; Levine, H. Coupling the modules of EMT and stemness: A tunable 'stemness window' model. *Oncotarget* 2015, *6*, 25161–25174. [CrossRef]
142. Strauss, R.; Li, Z.-Y.; Liu, Y.; Beyer, I.; Persson, J.; Sova, P.; Möller, T.; Pesonen, S.; Hemminki, A.; Hamerlik, P.; et al. Analysis of epithelial and mesenchymal markers in ovarian cancer reveals phenotypic heterogeneity and plasticity. *PLoS ONE* 2011, *6*, e16186. [CrossRef]

143. Bocci, F.; Jolly, M.K.; George, J.T.; Levine, H.; Onuchic, J.N. A mechanism-based computational model to capture the interconnections among epithelial-mesenchymal transition, cancer stem cells and Notch-Jagged signaling. *Oncotarget* **2018**, *9*, 29906–29920. [CrossRef]
144. Bocci, F.; Gearhart-Serna, L.; Boareto, M.; Ribeiro, M.; Ben-Jacob, E.; Devi, G.R.; Levine, H.; Onuchic, J.N.; Jolly, M.K. Toward understanding cancer stem cell heterogeneity in the tumor microenvironment. *Proc. Natl. Acad. Sci. USA* **2019**, *116*, 148–157. [CrossRef]
145. Shibue, T.; Weinberg, R.A. EMT, CSCs, and drug resistance: The mechanistic link and clinical implications. *Nat. Rev. Clin. Oncol.* **2017**, *14*, 611–629. [CrossRef]
146. Varga, J.; Greten, F.R. Cell plasticity in epithelial homeostasis and tumorigenesis. *Nat. Cell Biol.* **2017**, *19*, 1133–1141. [CrossRef]
147. Bocci, F.; Levine, H.; Onuchic, J.N.; Jolly, M.K. Deciphering the dynamics of Epithelial-Mesenchymal Transition and Cancer Stem Cells in tumor progression. *Curr. Stem Cell Rep.* **2019**, *5*, 11–21. [CrossRef]
148. Nie, Q. Stem cells: A window of opportunity in low-dimensional EMT space. *Oncotarget* **2018**, *9*, 31790–31791. [CrossRef]
149. Yamamoto, M.; Taguchi, Y.; Ito-Kureha, T.; Semba, K.; Yamaguchi, N.; Inoue, J. NF-κB non-cell-autonomously regulates cancer stem cell populations in the basal-like breast cancer subtype. *Nat. Commun.* **2013**, *4*, 2299. [CrossRef]
150. Sikandar, S.S.; Pate, K.T.; Anderson, S.; Dizon, D.; Edwards, R.A.; Waterman, M.L.; Lipkin, S.M. NOTCH Signaling Is Required for Formation and Self-Renewal of Tumor-Initiating Cells and for Repression of Secretory Cell Differentiation in Colon Cancer. *Cancer Res.* **2010**, *70*, 1469–1478. [CrossRef]
151. Zhu, T.S.; Costello, M.A.; Talsma, C.E.; Flack, C.G.; Crowley, J.G.; Hamm, L.L.; He, X.; Hervey-Jumper, S.L.; Heth, J.A.; Muraszko, K.M.; et al. Endothelial cells create a stem cell niche in glioblastoma by providing NOTCH ligands that nurture self-renewal of cancer stem-like cells. *Cancer Res.* **2011**, *71*, 6061–6072. [CrossRef]
152. Liu, S.; Cong, Y.; Wang, D.; Sun, Y.; Deng, L.; Liu, Y.; Martin-Trevino, R.; Shang, L.; McDermott, S.P.; Landis, M.D.; et al. Breast cancer stem cells transition between epithelial and mesenchymal states reflective of their normal counterparts. *Stem Cell Rep.* **2014**, *2*, 78–91. [CrossRef]
153. Colacino, J.A.; Azizi, E.; Brooks, M.D.; Harouaka, R.; Fouladdel, S.; McDermott, S.P.; Lee, M.; Hill, D.; Madden, J.; Boerner, J.; et al. Heterogeneity of Human Breast Stem and Progenitor Cells as Revealed by Transcriptional Profiling. *Stem Cell Rep.* **2018**, *10*, 1596–1609. [CrossRef]
154. Zhang, W.; Shi, X.; Peng, Y.; Wu, M.; Zhang, P.; Xie, R.; Wu, Y.; Yan, Q.; Liu, S.; Wang, J. HIF-1α Promotes Epithelial-Mesenchymal Transition and Metastasis through Direct Regulation of ZEB1 in Colorectal Cancer. *PLoS ONE* **2015**, *10*, e0129603. [CrossRef]
155. Guo, J.; Wang, B.; Fu, Z.; Wei, J.; Lu, W. Hypoxic Microenvironment Induces EMT and Upgrades Stem-Like Properties of Gastric Cancer Cells. *Technol. Cancer Res. Treat.* **2016**, *15*, 60–68. [CrossRef]
156. Salnikov, A.V.; Liu, L.; Platen, M.; Gladkich, J.; Salnikova, O.; Ryschich, E.; Mattern, J.; Moldenhauer, G.; Werner, J.; Schemmer, P.; et al. Hypoxia Induces EMT in Low and Highly Aggressive Pancreatic Tumor Cells but Only Cells with Cancer Stem Cell Characteristics Acquire Pronounced Migratory Potential. *PLoS ONE* **2012**, *7*, e46391. [CrossRef]
157. Jolly, M.K.; Kulkarni, P.; Weninger, K.; Orban, J.; Levine, H. Phenotypic Plasticity, Bet-Hedging, and Androgen Independence in Prostate Cancer: Role of Non-Genetic Heterogeneity. *Front. Oncol.* **2018**, *8*, 50. [CrossRef]
158. Goldman, A.; Majumder, B.; Dhawan, A.; Ravi, S.; Goldman, D.; Kohandel, M.; Majumder, P.K.; Sengupta, S. Temporally sequenced anticancer drugs overcome adaptive resistance by targeting a vulnerable chemotherapy-induced phenotypic transition. *Nat. Commun.* **2015**, *6*, 6139. [CrossRef]
159. Reya, T.; Morrison, S.J.; Clarke, M.F.; Weissman, I.L. Stem cells, cancer, and cancer stem cells. *Nature* **2001**, *414*, 105–111. [CrossRef]
160. Bjerkvig, R.; Tysnes, B.B.; Aboody, K.S.; Najbauer, J.; Terzis, A.J.A. Opinion: The origin of the cancer stem cell: Current controversies and new insights. *Nat. Rev. Cancer* **2005**, *5*, 899–904. [CrossRef]
161. Yang, G.; Quan, Y.; Wang, W.; Fu, Q.; Wu, J.; Mei, T.; Li, J.; Tang, Y.; Luo, C.; Ouyang, Q.; et al. Dynamic equilibrium between cancer stem cells and non-stem cancer cells in human SW620 and MCF-7 cancer cell populations. *Br. J. Cancer* **2012**, *106*, 1512–1519. [CrossRef]

162. Iliopoulos, D.; Hirsch, H.A.; Wang, G.; Struhl, K. Inducible formation of breast cancer stem cells and their dynamic equilibrium with non-stem cancer cells via IL6 secretion. *Proc. Natl. Acad. Sci. USA* **2011**, *108*, 1397–1402. [CrossRef]
163. Avgustinova, A.; Benitah, S.A. Epigenetic control of adult stem cell function. *Nat. Rev. Mol. Cell Biol.* **2016**, *17*, 643–658. [CrossRef]
164. Sica, A.; Mantovani, A. Macrophage plasticity and polarization: In vivo veritas. *J. Clin. Investig.* **2012**, *122*, 787–795. [CrossRef]
165. Norton, K.-A.; Jin, K.; Popel, A.S. Modeling triple-negative breast cancer heterogeneity: Effects of stromal macrophages, fibroblasts and tumor vasculature. *J. Theor. Biol.* **2018**, *452*, 56–68. [CrossRef]
166. Mahlbacher, G.E.; Reihmer, K.C.; Frieboes, H.B. Mathematical modeling of tumor-immune cell interactions. *J. Theor. Biol.* **2019**, *469*, 47–60. [CrossRef]
167. Mahlbacher, G.; Curtis, L.T.; Lowengrub, J.; Frieboes, H.B. Mathematical modeling of tumor-associated macrophage interactions with the cancer microenvironment. *J. ImmunoTher. Cancer* **2018**, *6*, 10. [CrossRef]
168. Robertson-Tessi, M.; El-Kareh, A.; Goriely, A. A mathematical model of tumor–immune interactions. *J. Theor. Biol.* **2012**, *294*, 56–73. [CrossRef]
169. Louzoun, Y.; Xue, C.; Lesinski, G.B.; Friedman, A. A mathematical model for pancreatic cancer growth and treatments. *J. Theor. Biol.* **2014**, *351*, 74–82. [CrossRef]
170. den Breems, N.Y.; Eftimie, R. The re-polarisation of M2 and M1 macrophages and its role on cancer outcomes. *J. Theor. Biol.* **2016**, *390*, 23–39. [CrossRef] [PubMed]
171. Yang, M.; Ma, B.; Shao, H.; Clark, A.M.; Wells, A. Macrophage phenotypic subtypes diametrically regulate epithelial-mesenchymal plasticity in breast cancer cells. *BMC Cancer* **2016**, *16*, 419. [CrossRef]
172. Sousa, S.; Brion, R.; Lintunen, M.; Kronqvist, P.; Sandholm, J.; Mönkkönen, J.; Kellokumpu-Lehtinen, P.-L.; Lauttia, S.; Tynninen, O.; Joensuu, H.; et al. Human breast cancer cells educate macrophages toward the M2 activation status. *Breast Cancer Res.* **2015**, *17*, 101. [CrossRef]
173. Weigert, A.; Tzieply, N.; von Knethen, A.; Johann, A.M.; Schmidt, H.; Geisslinger, G.; Brüne, B. Tumor Cell Apoptosis Polarizes Macrophages—Role of Sphingosine-1-Phosphate. *Mol. Biol. Cell* **2007**, *18*, 3810–3819. [CrossRef]
174. Yuan, A.; Hsiao, Y.-J.; Chen, H.-Y.; Chen, H.-W.; Ho, C.-C.; Chen, Y.-Y.; Liu, Y.-C.; Hong, T.-H.; Yu, S.-L.; Chen, J.J.W.; et al. Opposite Effects of M1 and M2 Macrophage Subtypes on Lung Cancer Progression. *Sci. Rep.* **2015**, *5*, 14273. [CrossRef] [PubMed]
175. Hollmén, M.; Roudnicky, F.; Karaman, S.; Detmar, M. Characterization of macrophage-cancer cell crosstalk in estrogen receptor positive and triple-negative breast cancer. *Sci. Rep.* **2015**, *5*, 9188. [CrossRef]
176. Su, S.; Liu, Q.; Chen, J.; Chen, J.; Chen, F.; He, C.; Huang, D.; Wu, W.; Lin, L.; Huang, W.; et al. A positive feedback loop between mesenchymal-like cancer cells and macrophages is essential to breast cancer metastasis. *Cancer Cell* **2014**, *25*, 605–620. [CrossRef]
177. Li, X.; Jolly, M.K.; George, J.T.; Pienta, K.J.; Levine, H. Computational Modeling of the Crosstalk Between Macrophage Polarization and Tumor Cell Plasticity in the Tumor Microenvironment. *Front. Oncol.* **2019**, *9*, 10. [CrossRef] [PubMed]
178. Kudo-Saito, C.; Shirako, H.; Takeuchi, T.; Kawakami, Y. Cancer metastasis is accelerated through immunosuppression during Snail-induced EMT of cancer cells. *Cancer Cell* **2009**, *15*, 195–206. [CrossRef] [PubMed]
179. Dongre, A.; Rashidian, M.; Reinhardt, F.; Bagnato, A.; Keckesova, Z.; Ploegh, H.L.; Weinberg, R.A. Epithelial-to-Mesenchymal Transition Contributes to Immunosuppression in Breast Carcinomas. *Cancer Res.* **2017**, *77*, 3982–3989. [CrossRef]
180. Ao, M.; Franco, O.E.; Park, D.; Raman, D.; Williams, K.; Hayward, S.W. Cross-talk between paracrine-acting cytokine and chemokine pathways promotes malignancy in benign human prostatic epithelium. *Cancer Res.* **2007**, *67*, 4244–4253. [CrossRef]
181. Yu, Y.; Xiao, C.-H.; Tan, L.-D.; Wang, Q.-S.; Li, X.-Q.; Feng, Y.-M. Cancer-associated fibroblasts induce epithelial-mesenchymal transition of breast cancer cells through paracrine TGF-β signalling. *Br. J. Cancer* **2014**, *110*, 724–732. [CrossRef]
182. Liu, Z.; Kuang, W.; Zhou, Q.; Zhang, Y. TGF-β1 secreted by M2 phenotype macrophages enhances the stemness and migration of glioma cells via the SMAD2/3 signalling pathway. *Int. J. Mol. Med.* **2018**, *42*, 3395–3403. [CrossRef]

183. Tu, E.; Chia, P.Z.C.; Chen, W. TGFβ in T cell biology and tumor immunity: Angel or devil? *Cytokine Growth Factor Rev.* **2014**, *25*, 423–435. [CrossRef] [PubMed]
184. Joffroy, C.M.; Buck, M.B.; Stope, M.B.; Popp, S.L.; Pfizenmaier, K.; Knabbe, C. Antiestrogens induce transforming growth factor beta-mediated immunosuppression in breast cancer. *Cancer Res.* **2010**, *70*, 1314–1322. [CrossRef] [PubMed]
185. Thomas, D.A.; Massagué, J. TGF-beta directly targets cytotoxic T cell functions during tumor evasion of immune surveillance. *Cancer Cell* **2005**, *8*, 369–380. [CrossRef]
186. Chockley, P.J.; Keshamouni, V.G. Immunological Consequences of Epithelial-Mesenchymal Transition in Tumor Progression. *J. Immunol.* **2016**, *197*, 691–698. [CrossRef] [PubMed]
187. Standiford, T.J.; Kuick, R.; Bhan, U.; Chen, J.; Newstead, M.; Keshamouni, V.G. TGF-β-induced IRAK-M expression in tumor-associated macrophages regulates lung tumor growth. *Oncogene* **2011**, *30*, 2475–2484. [CrossRef]
188. Chen, X.-H.; Liu, Z.-C.; Zhang, G.; Wei, W.; Wang, X.-X.; Wang, H.; Ke, H.-P.; Zhang, F.; Wang, H.-S.; Cai, S.-H.; et al. TGF-β and EGF induced HLA-I downregulation is associated with epithelial-mesenchymal transition (EMT) through upregulation of snail in prostate cancer cells. *Mol. Immunol.* **2015**, *65*, 34–42. [CrossRef]
189. Tripathi, S.C.; Peters, H.L.; Taguchi, A.; Katayama, H.; Wang, H.; Momin, A.; Jolly, M.K.; Celiktas, M.; Rodriguez-Canales, J.; Liu, H.; et al. Immunoproteasome deficiency is a feature of non-small cell lung cancer with a mesenchymal phenotype and is associated with a poor outcome. *Proc. Natl. Acad. Sci. USA* **2016**, *113*, E1555–E1564. [CrossRef]
190. Chen, L.; Gibbons, D.L.; Goswami, S.; Cortez, M.A.; Ahn, Y.-H.; Byers, L.A.; Zhang, X.; Yi, X.; Dwyer, D.; Lin, W.; et al. Metastasis is regulated via microRNA-200/ZEB1 axis control of tumour cell PD-L1 expression and intratumoral immunosuppression. *Nat. Commun.* **2014**, *5*, 5241. [CrossRef]
191. Hasmim, M.; Noman, M.Z.; Messai, Y.; Bordereaux, D.; Gros, G.; Baud, V.; Chouaib, S. Cutting Edge: Hypoxia-Induced Nanog Favors the Intratumoral Infiltration of Regulatory T Cells and Macrophages via Direct Regulation of TGF-β1. *J. Immunol.* **2013**, *191*, 5802–5806. [CrossRef]
192. Noman, M.Z.; Desantis, G.; Janji, B.; Hasmim, M.; Karray, S.; Dessen, P.; Bronte, V.; Chouaib, S. PD-L1 is a novel direct target of HIF-1α, and its blockade under hypoxia enhanced MDSC-mediated T cell activation. *J. Exp. Med.* **2014**, *211*, 781–790. [CrossRef]
193. Barsoum, I.B.; Smallwood, C.A.; Siemens, D.R.; Graham, C.H. A mechanism of hypoxia-mediated escape from adaptive immunity in cancer cells. *Cancer Res.* **2014**, *74*, 665–674. [CrossRef] [PubMed]
194. Ye, L.-Y.; Chen, W.; Bai, X.-L.; Xu, X.-Y.; Zhang, Q.; Xia, X.-F.; Sun, X.; Li, G.-G.; Hu, Q.-D.; Fu, Q.-H.; et al. Hypoxia-Induced Epithelial-to-Mesenchymal Transition in Hepatocellular Carcinoma Induces an Immunosuppressive Tumor Microenvironment to Promote Metastasis. *Cancer Res.* **2016**, *76*, 818–830. [CrossRef]
195. Ricciardi, M.; Zanotto, M.; Malpeli, G.; Bassi, G.; Perbellini, O.; Chilosi, M.; Bifari, F.; Krampera, M. Epithelial-to-mesenchymal transition (EMT) induced by inflammatory priming elicits mesenchymal stromal cell-like immune-modulatory properties in cancer cells. *Br. J. Cancer* **2015**, *112*, 1067–1075. [CrossRef] [PubMed]
196. Kudo-Saito, C.; Shirako, H.; Ohike, M.; Tsukamoto, N.; Kawakami, Y. CCL2 is critical for immunosuppression to promote cancer metastasis. *Clin. Exp. Metastasis* **2013**, *30*, 393–405. [CrossRef]
197. Suarez-Carmona, M.; Bourcy, M.; Lesage, J.; Leroi, N.; Syne, L.; Blacher, S.; Hubert, P.; Erpicum, C.; Foidart, J.-M.; Delvenne, P.; et al. Soluble factors regulated by epithelial-mesenchymal transition mediate tumour angiogenesis and myeloid cell recruitment. *J. Pathol.* **2015**, *236*, 491–504. [CrossRef]
198. Dominguez, C.; David, J.M.; Palena, C. Epithelial-mesenchymal transition and inflammation at the site of the primary tumor. *Semin. Cancer Biol.* **2017**, *47*, 177–184. [CrossRef]
199. Spranger, S.; Bao, R.; Gajewski, T.F. Melanoma-intrinsic β-catenin signalling prevents anti-tumour immunity. *Nature* **2015**, *523*, 231–235. [CrossRef]
200. Mak, M.P.; Tong, P.; Diao, L.; Cardnell, R.J.; Gibbons, D.L.; William, W.N.; Skoulidis, F.; Parra, E.R.; Rodriguez-Canales, J.; Wistuba, I.I.; et al. A Patient-Derived, Pan-Cancer EMT Signature Identifies Global Molecular Alterations and Immune Target Enrichment Following Epithelial-to-Mesenchymal Transition. *Clin. Cancer Res.* **2016**, *22*, 609–620. [CrossRef] [PubMed]

201. Lou, Y.; Diao, L.; Cuentas, E.R.P.; Denning, W.L.; Chen, L.; Fan, Y.H.; Byers, L.A.; Wang, J.; Papadimitrakopoulou, V.A.; Behrens, C.; et al. Epithelial–Mesenchymal Transition Is Associated with a Distinct Tumor Microenvironment Including Elevation of Inflammatory Signals and Multiple Immune Checkpoints in Lung Adenocarcinoma. *Clin. Cancer Res.* **2016**, *22*, 3630–3642. [CrossRef]
202. Kardos, J.; Chai, S.; Mose, L.E.; Selitsky, S.R.; Krishnan, B.; Saito, R.; Iglesia, M.D.; Milowsky, M.I.; Parker, J.S.; Kim, W.Y.; et al. Claudin-low bladder tumors are immune infiltrated and actively immune suppressed. *JCI Insight* **2016**, *1*, e85902. [CrossRef]
203. Yao, J.; Caballero, O.L.; Huang, Y.; Lin, C.; Rimoldi, D.; Behren, A.; Cebon, J.S.; Hung, M.-C.; Weinstein, J.N.; Strausberg, R.L.; et al. Altered Expression and Splicing of ESRP1 in Malignant Melanoma Correlates with Epithelial-Mesenchymal Status and Tumor-Associated Immune Cytolytic Activity. *Cancer Immunol. Res.* **2016**, *4*, 552–561. [CrossRef]
204. Chae, Y.K.; Chang, S.; Ko, T.; Anker, J.; Agte, S.; Iams, W.; Choi, W.M.; Lee, K.; Cruz, M. Epithelial-mesenchymal transition (EMT) signature is inversely associated with T-cell infiltration in non-small cell lung cancer (NSCLC). *Sci. Rep.* **2018**, *8*, 2918. [CrossRef]
205. Ueno, T.; Tsuchikawa, T.; Hatanaka, K.C.; Hatanaka, Y.; Mitsuhashi, T.; Nakanishi, Y.; Noji, T.; Nakamura, T.; Okamura, K.; Matsuno, Y.; et al. Prognostic impact of programmed cell death ligand 1 (PD-L1) expression and its association with epithelial-mesenchymal transition in extrahepatic cholangiocarcinoma. *Oncotarget* **2018**, *9*, 20034–20047. [CrossRef]
206. Rosenberg, J.E.; Hoffman-Censits, J.; Powles, T.; van der Heijden, M.S.; Balar, A.V.; Necchi, A.; Dawson, N.; O'Donnell, P.H.; Balmanoukian, A.; Loriot, Y.; et al. Atezolizumab in patients with locally advanced and metastatic urothelial carcinoma who have progressed following treatment with platinum-based chemotherapy: A single-arm, multicentre, phase 2 trial. *Lancet* **2016**, *387*, 1909–1920. [CrossRef]
207. Choi, W.; Porten, S.; Kim, S.; Willis, D.; Plimack, E.R.; Hoffman-Censits, J.; Roth, B.; Cheng, T.; Tran, M.; Lee, I.-L.; et al. Identification of distinct basal and luminal subtypes of muscle-invasive bladder cancer with different sensitivities to frontline chemotherapy. *Cancer Cell* **2014**, *25*, 152–165. [CrossRef]
208. Teng, M.W.L.; Ngiow, S.F.; Ribas, A.; Smyth, M.J. Classifying Cancers Based on T-cell Infiltration and PD-L1. *Cancer Res.* **2015**, *75*, 2139–2145. [CrossRef]
209. Sweis, R.F.; Spranger, S.; Bao, R.; Paner, G.P.; Stadler, W.M.; Steinberg, G.; Gajewski, T.F. Molecular Drivers of the Non-T-cell-Inflamed Tumor Microenvironment in Urothelial Bladder Cancer. *Cancer Immunol. Res.* **2016**, *4*, 563–568. [CrossRef]
210. Seo, A.N.; Lee, H.J.; Kim, E.J.; Kim, H.J.; Jang, M.H.; Lee, H.E.; Kim, Y.J.; Kim, J.H.; Park, S.Y. Tumour-infiltrating CD8+ lymphocytes as an independent predictive factor for pathological complete response to primary systemic therapy in breast cancer. *Br. J. Cancer* **2013**, *109*, 2705–2713. [CrossRef]
211. Li, J.; Byrne, K.T.; Yan, F.; Yamazoe, T.; Chen, Z.; Baslan, T.; Richman, L.P.; Lin, J.H.; Sun, Y.H.; Rech, A.J.; et al. Tumor Cell-Intrinsic Factors Underlie Heterogeneity of Immune Cell Infiltration and Response to Immunotherapy. *Immunity* **2018**, *49*, 178.e7–193.e7. [CrossRef]
212. Boareto, M.; Jolly, M.K.; Ben-Jacob, E.; Onuchic, J.N. Jagged mediates differences in normal and tumor angiogenesis by affecting tip-stalk fate decision. *Proc. Natl. Acad. Sci. USA* **2015**, *112*, E3836–E3844. [CrossRef]
213. Yu, L.; Lu, M.; Jia, D.; Ma, J.; Ben-Jacob, E.; Levine, H.; Kaipparettu, B.A.; Onuchic, J.N. Modeling the Genetic Regulation of Cancer Metabolism: Interplay between Glycolysis and Oxidative Phosphorylation. *Cancer Res.* **2017**, *77*, 1564–1574. [CrossRef]
214. Jia, D.; Lu, M.; Jung, K.H.; Park, J.H.; Yu, L.; Onuchic, J.N.; Kaipparettu, B.A.; Levine, H. Elucidating cancer metabolic plasticity by coupling gene regulation with metabolic pathways. *Proc. Natl. Acad. Sci. USA* **2019**, *116*, 3909–3918. [CrossRef] [PubMed]
215. Jia, D.; Park, J.; Jung, K.; Levine, H.; Kaipparettu, B. Elucidating the metabolic plasticity of cancer: Mitochondrial reprogramming and hybrid metabolic states. *Cells* **2018**, *7*, 21. [CrossRef]
216. Sone, M.; Morone, N.; Nakamura, T.; Tanaka, A.; Okita, K.; Woltjen, K.; Nakagawa, M.; Heuser, J.E.; Yamada, Y.; Yamanaka, S.; et al. Hybrid Cellular Metabolism Coordinated by Zic3 and Esrrb Synergistically Enhances Induction of Naive Pluripotency. *Cell Metab.* **2017**, *25*, 1103.e6–1117.e6. [CrossRef]
217. Pacella, I.; Procaccini, C.; Focaccetti, C.; Miacci, S.; Timperi, E.; Faicchia, D.; Severa, M.; Rizzo, F.; Coccia, E.M.; Bonacina, F.; et al. Fatty acid metabolism complements glycolysis in the selective regulatory T cell expansion during tumor growth. *Proc. Natl. Acad. Sci. USA* **2018**, *115*, E6546–E6555. [CrossRef]

218. Huang, S. Hybrid T-Helper Cells: Stabilizing the Moderate Center in a Polarized System. *PLoS Biol.* **2013**, *11*, e1001632. [CrossRef]
219. Stoeckius, M.; Hafemeister, C.; Stephenson, W.; Houck-Loomis, B.; Chattopadhyay, P.K.; Swerdlow, H.; Satija, R.; Smibert, P. Simultaneous epitope and transcriptome measurement in single cells. *Nat. Methods* **2017**, *14*, 865–868. [CrossRef]
220. Peterson, V.M.; Zhang, K.X.; Kumar, N.; Wong, J.; Li, L.; Wilson, D.C.; Moore, R.; McClanahan, T.K.; Sadekova, S.; Klappenbach, J.A. Multiplexed quantification of proteins and transcripts in single cells. *Nat. Biotechnol.* **2017**, *35*, 936–939. [CrossRef] [PubMed]
221. Karreman, M.A.; Hyenne, V.; Schwab, Y.; Goetz, J.G. Intravital correlative microscopy: Imaging life at the nanoscale. *Trends Cell Biol.* **2016**, *26*, 848–863. [CrossRef]

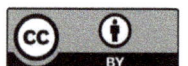

© 2019 by the authors. Licensee MDPI, Basel, Switzerland. This article is an open access article distributed under the terms and conditions of the Creative Commons Attribution (CC BY) license (http://creativecommons.org/licenses/by/4.0/).

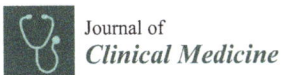 

*Review*

# Contribution of Epithelial Plasticity to Therapy Resistance

**Patricia G. Santamaría** [1,2,*], **Gema Moreno-Bueno** [1,2,3] **and Amparo Cano** [1,2,*]

1. Departamento de Bioquímica, Universidad Autónoma de Madrid (UAM), Instituto de Investigaciones Biomédicas 'Alberto Sols' (CSIC-UAM), IdiPAZ, c/ Arzobispo Morcillo 4, 28029 Madrid, Spain; gmoreno@iib.uam.es
2. Centro de Investigación Biomédica en Red de Cáncer (CIBERONC), c/ Monforte de Lemos 3-5, 28029 Madrid, Spain
3. Fundación MD Anderson Internacional, c/ Gómez Hemans 2, 28033 Madrid, Spain
* Correspondence: pgsantamaria@iib.uam.es (P.G.S.); acano@iib.uam.es (A.C.); Tel.: +34-91-497-2734 (P.G.S.); +34-91-497-5400 (A.C.)

Received: 15 April 2019; Accepted: 10 May 2019; Published: 14 May 2019

**Abstract:** Therapy resistance is responsible for tumour recurrence and represents one of the major challenges in present oncology. Significant advances have been made in the understanding of the mechanisms underlying resistance to conventional and targeted therapies improving the clinical management of relapsed patients. Unfortunately, in too many cases, resistance reappears leading to a fatal outcome. The recent introduction of immunotherapy regimes has provided an unprecedented success in the treatment of specific cancer types; however, a good percentage of patients do not respond to immune-based treatments or ultimately become resistant. Cellular plasticity, cancer cell stemness and tumour heterogeneity have emerged as important determinants of treatment resistance. Epithelial-to-mesenchymal transition (EMT) is associated with resistance in many different cellular and preclinical models, although little evidence derives directly from clinical samples. The recognition of the presence in tumours of intermediate hybrid epithelial/mesenchymal states as the most likely manifestation of epithelial plasticity and their potential link to stemness and tumour heterogeneity, provide new clues to understanding resistance and could be exploited in the search for anti-resistance strategies. Here, recent evidence linking EMT/epithelial plasticity to resistance against conventional, targeted and immune therapy are summarized. In addition, future perspectives for related clinical approaches are also discussed.

**Keywords:** epithelial–mesenchymal transition; hybrid E/M states; plasticity; tumour heterogeneity; treatment resistance; immunotherapy scape

---

## 1. Introduction

The emergence of therapy resistance is one of the main unsolved issues in present oncology and represents a major hurdle to defeating cancer.

Traditionally, two forms of tumour drug resistance, innate and acquired, have been considered responsible for tumour relapse either soon after initial treatment or even following several years of initial response and tumour shrinkage [1–3]. However, differences between both resistance definitions at mechanistic and molecular levels are somehow attenuated, especially after the accumulation of genomic and genetic data [2,4,5]. Accordingly, we will herein use the general term "treatment resistance" to refer to both types of resistance as well as to include resistance to diverse treatment regimens (radio, chemo or immune therapy, as well as targeted therapy).

A great effort has been made over the last two decades to unveil the molecular pathways responsible for therapy resistance. Such attempts have led to the identification of several molecular mechanisms involved in resistance to conventional (i.e., increased expression of anti-apoptotic or transporter proteins mediating multidrug resistance) and targeted therapies (like novel mutations bypassing specific inhibitors and/or activation of alternative signalling pathways) [6]. The introduction of next generation sequencing technology and the compilation of information regarding patients' responses to different therapies for distinct tumour types is providing powerful information towards personalized treatments as well as facilitating the prediction of recurrences [2,5]. Notwithstanding, we still have an insufficient knowledge of the mechanisms driving tumour resistance.

Three concepts that emerged over the last years have provided novel insights into our present understanding of tumour resistance: cancer stem cells (CSCs), epithelial-to-mesenchymal transition (EMT) and intra-tumour heterogeneity [7], all of them briefly discussed hereafter. The discovery of CSCs soon led to the exposure of their increased resistance to chemo- and radiotherapy compared to non-CSCs in the same tumour (reviewed in Reference [8]). This point has been confirmed in different experimental situations in which conventional therapies were able to eliminate non-CSCs while slowly proliferating CSCs were unaffected [9–12]. The subsequent link between EMT and cancer stem-cell properties [13–15] set the grounds to associate EMT with therapy resistance [16]. In fact, original studies in tumour cell lines revealed that cells undergoing EMT achieve resistance to genotoxic stress mediated by conventional radio- and chemotherapy [17–20]. This was later confirmed using different therapeutic drugs reinforcing the link between CSCs, EMT and resistance [8,16,21–23]. While this hypothesis is highly attractive, we have partial knowledge on how these two (clinically relevant) programs, cancer cell stemness and EMT are interrelated. Clinical evidence linking them to resistance is limited, mostly due to the lack of appropriate in vivo models and scarce patient samples to perform comprehensive studies.

A major problem to regard EMT as a relevant process in cancer progression has been the difficulty to unambiguously detect its occurrence in most human tumours. Nonetheless, the recognition that intermediate EMT or hybrid epithelial/mesenchymal (E/M) states represent a likely situation in tumours [24–27], has brought novel insights on the relationship between epithelial plasticity and treatment resistance [28,29]. The well-established intra-tumour heterogeneity (referred to from now as tumour heterogeneity), considered as a common feature of most solid tumours, has also powered the notion that heterogeneity might be key for treatment resistance [30,31]. The relationship among heterogeneity, phenotypic plasticity and tumour resistance is thus emerging as a forefront of research in oncology [28].

Several recent outstanding articles have reviewed the association between EMT and cancer stemness in tumour progression and/or treatment resistance [8,23–25,28,29,32] and this will not be considered here in extent. In the present review, we will thus summarize recent evidence linking EMT/epithelial plasticity to therapy resistance as well as to immune scape. Future perspectives for refining predictive resistance biomarkers and novel clinical approaches will be also discussed.

## 2. Tumour Heterogeneity and Epithelial Plasticity: Traits Conferring Tumour Aggressiveness and Resistance

### 2.1. Tumour Heterogeneity Links Phenotypic Plasticity and Therapy Resistance

Nowadays, increased evidence supports that heterogeneous cancer cell populations with distinct phenotypic features constitute the majority of tumours [2,7]. The heterogeneity of tumours represents new challenges in oncology with particular relevance for precision medicine. It is presently considered that the resistance to diverse treatments in many cancer patients relies on tumour heterogeneity [8,30,31], highlighting the importance of understanding cancer heterogeneity for prognosis and therapy choices. Despite the partial knowledge of the driving mechanisms leading to tumour heterogeneity, several common features are starting to emerge, summarized as: (a) tumour heterogeneity can arise from both genetic and epigenetic mechanisms; (b) tumour cells are able to shift among several phenotypic states during tumour evolution; and (c) discrete populations of cancer stem cells within the tumour mass can give rise to hierarchically organized phenotypically distinct subpopulations [5,7,8,25,28,30,33].

An additional consequence of tumour heterogeneity is phenotypic plasticity, a determinant factor for cancer progression and therapy resistance [34]. As extensively reviewed elsewhere, phenotypic plasticity is being recognized in several tumour types, including breast and lung cancer, involving the acquisition of different histological traits and/or differentiation states that, at least in some cases, are associated with therapy resistance [25,28,34].

*2.2. EMT and Epithelial Plasticity: A Short Story*

The EMT program, classically defined as a coordinated cell and molecular process by which epithelial tumour cells progressively lose cell junctions and apical–basal polarity while acquiring mesenchymal capacities [24,35–37], is likely one of the major manifestations of phenotypic epithelial plasticity in tumours. However, it is worth recalling here that EMT is an essential biological program for early development as well as for establishing key embryonic structures such as, but not limited to, derivatives from the neural crest or the cardiac cushions [35]. Importantly, developmental EMT is a highly dynamic and transient process acting at discrete spatio-temporal contexts, thus requiring its quick reversal through a mesenchymal-to-epithelial transition (MET) process. Moreover, several rounds of EMT and MET occur during development and morphogenesis of several embryonic tissues [35] reinforcing the dynamic nature of epithelial plasticity in physiological contexts.

Epithelial-to-mesenchymal transition was originally described in vitro in epithelial renal cells cultured under different substrates and characterized by the loss of intercellular adhesion and acquisition of migratory and mesenchymal-like traits [38], and later demonstrated to occur in vivo during chicken-embryo gastrulation [39]. Since the beginning of the present century, a myriad of articles have described the acquisition of EMT by normal and malignant epithelial cells under different stimulus in culture, starting from the original identification of Snail transcription factor as an E-cadherin repressor and EMT-inducer [40,41] followed by the identification of additional EMT-transcription factors (EMT-TFs), such as Slug, zinc finger E-box binding homeobox 1 and 2 (ZEB1, ZEB2), Twist or the basic-loop-helix transcription factor 3 E47/TCF3 (reviewed in References [37,42,43]), presently considered as classical or core EMT-TFs (Table 1). A plethora of extrinsic signalling pathways regulating EMT in non-malignant and tumour epithelial cells have been deciphered, as well as different intrinsic regulatory mechanisms acting at post-transcriptional, post-translational and epigenetic levels [23,24,35,42–44] that will not be further discussed here. However, it is important to remark that in tumours, most of the present data support that EMT is essential for metastasis, in particular for initial invasion, as well as for intra- and extravasation [8,24,25,37,45,46], while the reverse MET seems to be required for colonisation and macro-metastasis generation at distant sites [47–49].

**Table 1.** EMT-TFs and main characteristics associated with the EMT program.

| EMT State | Epithelial (E) | Hybrid E/M | Mesenchymal (M) |
|---|---|---|---|
| Morphology | Apical–basal polarity, cells attached to each other and to extracellular matrix (ECM) | Partial loss of cell–cell and cell–ECM attachment, epithelioid shape | Front–rear polarity, elongated shape, detached cells |
| Markers | E-cadherin, claudins, occludins, cytokeratins * | Co-expression of E and M markers: E-cadherin, cytokeratins *, vimentin | N-cadherin, vimentin, fibronectin, matrix metalloproteinases (MMPs), fibrillar collagens |
| Associated functional traits | Restrained motility, regulated proliferation | Motility, invasion, stemness, dissemination, metastasis, immune evasion, therapy resistance | |
| Core EMT-TFs: | Snail & Slug, ZEB1 & ZEB2, Twist, E47/TCF3 | | |

* Cytokeratins (Krts) such as Krt8/18 are commonly detected in E states whereas Krt5/14 in E/M states. EMT: epithelial-to-mesenchymal transition; EMT-TFs: EMT-transcription factors.

The relevance of the EMT program in cancer was strengthened by its connection to cancer cell stemness, initially described in normal and transformed human mammary cells in which EMT induction, by Snail or Twist expression, led to the acquisition of CSC markers, the ability to form mammospheres and tumour initiating capabilities [13,14]. Since then, the association of EMT and CSCs has been observed in several carcinoma types [8,13,15] supporting that the EMT program contributes to the self-renewing activity of CSCs in primary tumours and is potentially associated with therapeutic resistance [8,16,28]. Nevertheless, the association between EMT and CSCs during tumour progression and metastasis is not fully understood and, importantly, it might depend on particular tumour contexts [50], as exemplified by the non-classical EMT-TF paired related homeobox 1 (Prrx1) that represses CSC traits in triple-negative breast cancer (TNBC) cells while its silencing is required for metastatic colonization associated with the acquisition of stemness properties and an MET phenotype [47]. Further studies are undoubtedly needed to advance our knowledge on the EMT–CSCs link in connection to treatment resistance.

## 2.3. EMT In Vivo

In contrast to the overwhelming information on EMT in in vitro tumour cell models, the evidence for its occurrence in vivo is scarce. In fact, the relevance of EMT in human tumours has been widely questioned, in particular by pathologists, mainly because of the difficulty to detect full EMT inside tumours [51]. The generation of sophisticated genetically modified mouse models allowing EMT lineage tracing has provided convincing evidence for EMT occurrence in vivo (reviewed in References [26,27]). Some of these mouse cancer models combine the conditional deletion or activation of specific EMT-TFs and/or in vivo imaging. Information obtained from a genetic pancreatic mouse model showed that EMT cells (Zeb1$^+$) appear in precursor pancreatic intraepithelial neoplasia (PanIN) lesions and are able to generate heterogeneous tumours containing E-cadherin$^+$ and E-cadherin$^-$ cells [52]. Early disseminated tumour cells with partial EMT and high metastatic potential were also detected in the MMTV-Her2 breast cancer model [53]. Another elegant system designed to track endogenous E-cadherin in MMTV-PyMT breast cancer mouse model combined with high-resolution intravital imaging allowed the identification of a subpopulation of cells undergoing EMT with invasive and metastatic properties, exposing as well high the intrinsic plasticity of EMT cells at metastatic sites [54], similar to results obtained using a different breast cancer model [55]. Lineage tracing in a Notch-p53-based colorectal cancer (CRC) mouse model also provided evidence for invasive cells exhibiting a gradient of epithelial and mesenchymal phenotypes [56]. In addition, several mouse models based in the genetic manipulation of EMT-TFs have reported the implication of Snail or Twist1 in EMT induction in PyMT-breast cancer or skin squamous cell carcinomas (SCC), respectively [48,57]. Interestingly, these two studies demonstrated that both Snail and Twist1 are transiently expressed and needed for initial EMT-mediated invasion and dissemination, but their corresponding expression should be shut down for metastatic outgrowth in each tumour context.

Nonetheless, two recent studies using EMT lineage tracing and conditional deletion of specific EMT-TFs (Snail or Twist) in breast and pancreatic cancer mouse models, respectively, concluded that EMT is not required for metastasis but indeed contributes to chemoresistance [58,59]. As previously discussed by others [23,60,61], these unexpected and contradictory results can be explained either by the use of non-specific Cre-driver lines and/or by the redundant actions of specific EMT-TFs. In support of the later hypothesis, further analyses in the same pancreatic mouse cancer model by Zheng et al. [59] showed that the deletion of other EMT-TF such as Zeb1 strongly decreased lung metastasis, demonstrating that EMT is indeed required for distant metastasis [62]. Importantly, this particular study also contributed to establish that the role played by EMT-TFs can be redundant in a context-dependent fashion and that distinct EMT-TFs, or specific combinations of them also defined as "EMT-TF code", can be required to drive distant metastasis in different tumour settings [62–64].

*2.4. Intermediate EMT States in Tumours: Novel Insights on Epithelial Plasticity*

Present data suggest that EMT in vivo can be considered not as a binary process (epithelial versus mesenchymal states) but rather as a combination of several cellular states in which a spectrum of epithelial and mesenchymal traits can coexist [23,28,29] (Table 1). Hybrid E/M states can, theoretically, be associated with plasticity programs endowing tumour cells with a metastable state with the ability to rapidly respond to microenvironmental signals in either direction (i.e., towards an epithelial or a mesenchymal state) [24–26]. Accumulated data from cell lines and preclinical models are starting to provide evidence about the existence intermediate or hybrid E/M states in different tumour settings (see Reference [29] for a recent review). Computational and mathematical modelling analyses have been recently used to design hypothetical models of hybrid E/M states that are being tested to prove for tumour cell metastable or stable phenotypes as well as for their link to therapy resistance [65–68].

Initial insights for intermediate EMT states came from different studies showing the coexistence of epithelial and mesenchymal markers in tumour cell lines under various experimental conditions as well as in several tumour series (reviewed in Reference [27]). Of particular interest are the immunohistochemical analyses where the co-expression of epithelial (E-cadherin or keratins) and mesenchymal (N-cadherin or vimentin) markers was initially characterized in different breast tumour series [69,70]. Following studies characterized basal-like breast tumours as co-expressing vimentin and cytokeratins [71], and further identified an EMT immunohistochemical signature as specifically associated with basal-like breast tumours as well as the coexistence of epithelial and mesenchymal markers in the epithelial component of breast carcinosarcomas [72]. This later study represents one of the first hints pointing to the existence of a partial EMT in human tumours. However, until very recently, direct evidence for different intermediate E/M state occurrence in tumours was lacking. A recent study in a genetic mouse model of skin SCC has allowed to identify and isolate six intrinsic cell subpopulations with different combinations of epithelial and mesenchymal markers that define distinct EMT transition states in vivo [73]. This study shows that intermediate E/M populations are more metastatic than full M populations; in addition, intermediate E/M subpopulations exhibit a high degree of cell plasticity being able to switch into one another in secondary tumours [73]. Remarkably, and in agreement with those observations, depletion of the EMT-TF Zeb1 in pancreatic mouse tumours halts tumour cells in a stable epithelial state, losing their stemness and metastatic properties together with the ability to induce EMT upon transforming growth factor beta (TGFβ) signalling [62]. Overall, these recent studies support that epithelial plasticity conferred by intermediate E/M states is highly relevant for metastatic dissemination.

The influence of hybrid E/M states to treatment resistance is poorly understood, although several theoretical and experimental studies are starting to provide information of this relevant aspect, and they will be discussed below.

## 3. Evidence Linking EMT to Treatment Resistance

Work in cancer cellular models and patient samples, mostly analysing gene expression profiles that can be associated with therapy response, have allowed to establish a link between the gene expression associated with an EMT program and the development of therapeutic resistance [8]. The underlying mechanisms have been extensively reviewed [8,23,28] being essentially related to increased ability of EMT cells to avoid apoptosis induced by most standard anti-cancer drugs, implementation of mechanisms mediating drug detoxification and expression of immunosuppressive and immunoevasive molecules to avoid attack by the immune system. While the impact of hybrid E/M states to tumour aggressiveness is starting to be elucidated [29], several signalling pathways and molecular mechanisms are emerging as potential common traits of EMT and treatment resistance. For instance, a cellular signalling network consistently linked to EMT-mediated drug resistance across different cancer types is conveyed by the AXL tyrosine kinase receptor (known as AXL) that alters mitogen-activated protein kinase (MAPK)/ERK and phosphoinositide 3 kinase (PI3K)/Akt signalling pathways favouring proliferation, survival, migration and invasion [74]. Briefly, the AXL relationship to EMT (either as effector or inducer) has been explored in different tumour types, being associated with metastasis and drug resistance and, thus worse prognosis in patients (recently reviewed in Reference [74]). Additionally, AXL has been implicated in engaging other receptor tyrosine kinases (RTKs) and their downstream signalling in ovarian cancer [75] or epidermal growth factor receptor (EGFR) signalling in TNBC [76], which seem to be relevant in EMT cancer cells and associated resistance to RTK-targeted therapies.

In addition, a cellular adaptive mechanism known as the unfolded protein response (UPR) is activated to cope with the endoplasmic reticulum stress resulting from tumour progression (reviewed in References [77–79]). In cancer cells, UPR activation reduces the pro-apoptotic effects of several chemotherapeutic drugs and favours drug detoxifying mechanisms. Unfolded protein response activation has been suggested to uphold EMT, becoming both programs' allies in cancer initiation and progression (reviewed in another chapter in this special issue [80]) and contributing to cellular adaptive mechanisms responsible for chemotherapy resistance.

Tumour microenvironments can also have an important role in EMT and treatment resistance. Numerous studies have demonstrated that EMT programs in cancer cells are elicited by an array of signals originating from the different components of the tumour stroma [24,42,44]. Among them, cancer associated fibroblasts (CAFs), tumour associated macrophages (TAMs), infiltrating T-lymphocytes and myeloid-derived suppressor cells (MDSCs) can play prominent roles in the paracrine regulation of EMT induction, mainly mediated by TGFβ, tumor necrosis factor alpha (TNFα) or interleukin 6 (IL-6) secretion, among other cytokines and growth factors (reviewed in References [8,23]). The cytokine TGFβ is perhaps the most potent EMT-inducing signal in many different tumour contexts and indeed its secretion by CAFs and/or TAMs leads to EMT induction in breast cancer and hepatocarcinoma, among other tumour cells [81–84], while IL-6 secretion by CAFs has been associated to EMT-mediated resistance in non-small cell lung cancer (NSCLC) [85]. Interestingly, TGFβ has been proposed as a determinant of metastatic dissemination in CRC models [86] and poor prognosis CRC subtypes share a gene program driven by stromal TGFβ that seems to be associated with treatment resistance [87]. Recently, stromal TGFβ has been linked to immune evasion in CRC and urothelial tumours [88,89], although the potential connection to EMT induction has not been directly addressed. At present, the influence of the microenvironment in regulating intermediate E/M states and their association with therapeutic resistance is basically unknown, but it can be speculated that paracrine signals from CAFs, TAMs and other stromal components are relevant players in the dynamic regulation of epithelial plasticity in cancer progression.

*3.1. Studies on Tumour Cell Lines*

There are many examples in different cancer settings in which the expression of one or several core EMT-TFs is linked to increased resistance to radio- and chemotherapy as well as to targeted therapy [19,20,90–95]. Moreover, resistant tumour cells in culture frequently exhibit a mesenchymal phenotype [8] supporting the EMT involvement in therapy resistance. We will next discuss recent literature exemplifying such a link in several cellular cancer models.

3.1.1. Lung Cancer

In 2013, an EMT gene signature comprising 76 genes allowed to classify NSCLC cell lines as epithelial or mesenchymal, the latter expressing higher levels of ZEB1, *vimentin* or *AXL* [96]. This EMT signature also predicted the sensitivity of patient-derived NSCLC cell lines to different drugs, being the mesenchymal ones more resistant to the EGFR inhibitors (EGFRi) (erlotinib, gefitinib), as well as to PI3K inhibitors and common cytotoxic chemotherapies such as docetaxel or paclitaxel. However, the classification of a cell line as mesenchymal was not linked to widespread drug resistance since they were more sensitive to cisplatin or gemcitabine than the epithelial ones [96]. These studies and others have led to regard EMT as crucial for the generation of NSCLC resistance to EGFRi and the molecular mechanisms involved have been recently reviewed elsewhere [97]. In brief, cell stemness traits, anti-apoptotic signalling and chromatin remodelling imposed by EMT-TFs would cooperate to promote therapy resistance in NSCLC. As an example, the repression of the pro-apoptotic protein Bcl-2-like protein 11 (BIM) by ZEB1 seen in mesenchymal NSCLC cells is accountable for the increased resistance to EGFRi treatments [98].

Also, recent results link the presence of cells with hybrid E/M features in NSCLC cell lines to EGFRi resistance, increased sphere-forming ability and ZEB1 expression [99]. Other studies supporting the association of intermediate E/M phenotypes and resistance have described the expression of integrin beta4 (ITGB4), a proposed marker of the E/M state [100], in CSCs of NSCLC [101], although additional studies are required to sustain this connection.

In small cell lung cancer (SCLC) cells, the activation of the Met receptor with hepatocyte growth factor (HGF) induces a mesenchymal phenotype involving enhanced expression of EMT-TFs such as Snail together with increased invasion, tumorigenesis and chemoresistance to etoposide in xenograft assays [102]. Chemosensitivity could be restored in the presence of a Met inhibitor [102] further supporting the link between EMT and resistance in lung cancer.

3.1.2. Breast Cancer

Normal and transformed human mammary epithelial cells induced through an EMT by inhibition of E-cadherin expression or Twist overexpression are resistant to paclitaxel and doxorubicin, common chemotherapeutic drugs, whereas breast cancer cells with EMT traits show an increased sensitivity to paclitaxel [21,94]. A recent report has found links between EMT and endocrine therapy resistance in luminal breast cancer. Estrogen receptor alpha gene (*ESR1*) fusion proteins found in luminal tumours are responsible for endocrine therapy refractory disease [103]. In fact, when expressed in breast cancer cell lines, these functional fusion proteins (to the C-terminal sequence of the Hippo pathway coactivator yes-associated protein 1 (YAP1) or protocadherin 11X PCDH11X) promote an estrogen-independent activation of an EMT gene signature, Snail upregulation and E-cadherin downregulation resulting in increased migration in vitro and lung metastasis in xenograft models [103].

In basal-like breast cancer MDA-MB-231 cells, an early study showed that Snail confers resistance to the standard chemotherapeutic agents docetaxel and gemcitabine [20]. More recently, the ubiquitin editing enzyme A20 has been shown to ubiquitinate and stabilize Snail in basal-like breast cancer cells, favouring TGFβ-induced EMT and lung colonization of orthotopic tumours [104]. In vitro, A20 expression is associated with enhanced breast cancer cell viability upon doxorubicin and docetaxel treatment [104]. Another recent report has described that the deubiquitinase (DUB), USP27X, regulates Snail stability in MDA-MB-231 cells [105]. In the absence of USP27X, Snail is degraded, and the growth of xenograft tumours is delayed as well as Snail-mediated metastasis and resistance to cisplatin. The authors found a positive correlation of Snail and USP27X expression in TNBC patient-derived xenografts (PDX), although their status in relapsed patients requires further investigation. Besides USP27X, DUB3 has also been shown to stabilize Snail favouring EMT-related invasion, migration and metastasis of xenograft tumours whereas DUB3 levels in breast cancer patients are associated with metastatic progression and quicker relapse [106]. In addition, in basal-like breast cancer cells, DUB3 stabilizes Slug and Twist1 [107], suggesting that EMT-TF stabilization by preventing proteasome degradation is an important contributor to EMT and associated roles in tumour progression.

Recent studies also imply that hybrid E/M sates can more efficiently favour metastasis and therapy resistance than a complete mesenchymal state in breast cancer cells (reviewed in Reference [29]). The mechanistic pathways underlying chemotherapy resistance associated with E/M states in basal-like TNBC is being deciphered, as exemplified by ITGB4 expression regulated by ZEB1 and its downstream target Tap63a [100], but further studies are required.

3.1.3. Ovarian Cancer

In ovarian cancer, upregulation of Snail and Slug has been detected in cisplatin resistant cell lines [92]. Moreover, both EMT-TFs are associated with radio and chemoresistance by p53-dependent pro-survival signalling and regulation of stemness in this tumour context [108]. In response to cisplatin, doxorubicin or paclitaxel, ovarian cancer cells with CSCs traits are selected in vitro, characterized by a mesenchymal phenotype with downregulated transcript levels of *E-cadherin* and *occludin*, and higher transcript levels of *fibronectin*, *Snail*, *N-cadherin*, *TWIST*, *ZEB1* and *ZEB2* [109]. These cells, displaying chemokine receptor type 4 (CXCR4) surface markers, show enhanced migration, invasion and tumour-forming ability, and higher expression of ATP binding cassette subfamily B member 1 (ABCB1), a protein involved in acquiring multidrug resistance [109]. Besides, high-grade serous ovarian patients display higher levels of CXCR4 expression in their circulating tumour cells (CTCs), while targeting CXCR4 in preclinical models has been shown to decrease peritoneal dissemination in part by blocking EMT [110].

### 3.1.4. Prostate Cancer

Epithelial plasticity, noticed in some prostate cancer cell lines, was previously linked to cell stemness, tumour aggressiveness and metastatic potential [49,111,112], but few studies have so far analysed the relationship of EMT and hybrid E/M states to resistance in prostate cancer cells [29]. Recently, EMT has been involved in resistance to radiotherapy of prostate cancer cells. Lysyl oxidase-like 2 (LOXL2), a protein promoting EMT [113], is upregulated both in prostate cancer cell lines and radioresistant patient samples and seems to be responsible for radiotherapy resistance in prostate cancer cells and derived xenografts by implementing EMT [114]. Another study showed that chemoresistance to the taxane cabazitaxel was relieved by antiandrogen-mediated reversion of EMT towards MET in preclinical models such as PDX and genetic mouse models of advanced prostate cancer [115].

### 3.1.5. CRC

In CRC, a recent report depicts a novel mechanism involving EMT in progression and drug resistance [116]. While looking for substrates of the F-Box E3-ubiquitin ligase FBXW7 in intestinal stem cells, the authors find FBXW7 binds and ubiquitinates ZEB2 upon glycogen synthase kinase 3 beta (GSK3β) phosphorylation. In fact, in mouse and human CRC cell lines, ZEB2 induces EMT and is responsible for increased metastasis upon tail vein or orthotopic cell injection in nude mice. Also, ZEB2 is linked to the expression of stemness markers in colonospheres and organoids as well as increased drug resistance in CRC cell lines [116].

### 3.1.6. Melanoma

Malignant melanoma, an invasive tumour characterized by high genetic and phenotypic heterogeneity, commonly presents drug resistance. In melanoma, cell plasticity has been associated with resistance by means of ZEB1 reprogramming. Interestingly, low levels of *MITF*, a key melanocyte lineage TF, and high *ZEB1* levels are associated with B-Raf protein kinase inhibitor (BRAFi) resistance both in vitro and in tumour samples [117]. Using melanoma cellular models, Richard and co-authors [117] demonstrated that ZEB1 expression promotes the upregulation of stemness markers, increased tumorigenic potential and resistance to BRAFi. These observations are in agreement with the previous description that in vitro resistance to BRAFi is accompanied by loss of melanocyte inducing transcription factor (MITF), E-cadherin and *ZEB2* expression and upregulation of *ZEB1* and *TWIST*, linked as well to enhanced invasion [118]. Altogether, these data support the role of a mesenchymal phenotypic switching in melanoma related to dedifferentiation, invasiveness and drug resistance.

A recent report has linked microenvironmental cues such as nutrient starvation to translational reprogramming and therapeutic resistance in melanoma [119]. Upon glutamine starvation, melanoma cells downregulate MITF through UPR activation (eIF2α-ATF4), resulting in increased invasiveness linked to ZEB1, N-cadherin and fibronectin upregulation and Slug downregulation. Since ZEB1 and Slug have been previously involved in the phenotypic switch responsible for malignant melanoma [120], UPR activation is thus linked to the melanoma plasticity required for invasiveness. Indeed, ATF4 also correlates with higher AXL expression, a mediator of BRAF and MEK inhibitor (MAPKi) resistance in melanoma [121] also associated with anti-PD-1 therapy resistance [122]. These recent studies also indicate that MAPKi resistance in melanoma cells involves a mesenchymal signature, with decreased MITF and increased ZEB2 and Slug expression [121], suggestive of epigenetic regulatory mechanisms [122].

3.1.7. Glioblastoma

The EMT-TF ZEB1 has been involved in glioblastoma formation, invasion and chemoresistance in cellular models [123]. The proposed molecular mechanism involved EMT-induced cancer cell stemness and ZEB1-miR200 dependent upregulation of O-6-Methylguanine DNA methyltransferase (MGMT), responsible for resistance to the standard of care drug temozolomide (TMZ) [123]. Further studies to characterize ZEB1 involvement in glioblastoma by expression profiling and chromatin binding site analysis in CSCs have revealed that ZEB1 activates and represses distinct sets of target genes implementing a complex genetic program similar to EMT [124].

*3.2. Computational Modelling Analyses on Epithelial Plasticity and Tumour Resistance*

The presence of heterogeneous phenotypes within tumours before treatment and their plausible plastic transition across different E/M states might be useful to inform the outcome and, thus select therapies targeting particular phenotypes. To gain insight into phenotypic plasticity involvement in tumour heterogeneity and drug resistance, Gupta and co-workers [125] developed a method to mark the few cells within a breast cancer cell line that contain subpopulations of both epithelial and mesenchymal phenotypes. Expansion of this cell line originated clones composed of epithelial or mesenchymal cells or a mixture of both. In addition to concluding that phenotypic plasticity is inherited, these authors used these in vitro data gathered from these marked clones to perform computational simulations of the outcome of tumours containing mixed clones with different E/M phenotypes upon drug treatment. They modelled the effect of different chemotherapeutic drugs, selectively targeting epithelial or mesenchymal phenotypes, in different therapy regimens and concluded that the most efficient treatment is the combination therapy, repeated alternation of drugs targeting epithelial or mesenchymal phenotypes compared to monotherapy or sequential therapy [125].

Other computational modelling has provided an EMT metric to predict the extent of the EMT status, either epithelial, mesenchymal or hybrid E/M, of a given transcriptomic sample, aiming at being clinically informative [67]. Based on data from gene expression profiles, this EMT score has been validated in cancer cell lines with known EMT phenotypes and it provides valuable information regarding EMT score and survival as well as relapse upon treatment.

*3.3. Studies on Mouse Models*

At present, few reports have analysed EMT and treatment resistance in cancer mouse models, aside from analyses of xenografted tumour cell lines in immune-deficient mice.

A role for EMT in in vivo chemoresistance has been backed recently by two studies in mouse cancer models based on EMT downregulation [58,59]. Pancreatic mouse tumours generated after knocking down Snail or Twist were more sensitive to gemcitabine, the standard of care drug [59]. Additionally, in an EMT lineage tracing mouse model of breast cancer, EMT inhibition by miR-200 overexpression, which directly targeted *Zeb1* and *Zeb2*, the tumour resistance to the chemotherapy drug cyclophosphamide was abrogated [58]. Although the limitations of both studies regarding EMT contribution to metastasis have since been argued as already mentioned [46,60,61], they provided significant in vivo preclinical evidence of EMT involvement in chemoresistance.

## 4. Insights on EMT and Treatment Resistance in the Clinical Setting

The association of EMT and epithelial plasticity with resistance in the clinical context is not completely understood. As discussed above, EMT can provide tumour cells with the abilities to escape apoptosis, anoikis and senescence, among other traits and, thus confer treatment resistance in several preclinical models [8,28,29,126], but direct proof for this mechanistic link in tumours is still missing.

Nevertheless, different evidence supports the impact of EMT on treatment resistance in human tumours, such as the studies in which gene expression profiles from tumour samples are correlated to the clinical behaviour of treated patients. Some of these studies have resulted in the identification of several EMT-related gene expression signatures strongly associated with conventional and targeted therapy resistance, particularly in breast cancer and NSCLC [96,127,128].

## 4.1. EMT and Resistance to Conventional and Targeted Therapy

Epithelial plasticity and CSCs connection to treatment resistance is being recognised in particular tumour types [8,28,129,130] from where some common hints are emerging. In fact, it has been reported that in several tumour types, and particularly in pancreatic cancer, a minimal tumour fraction of resistant undifferentiated CSCs exhibit a spindle-shaped appearance typical of an EMT phenotype [8,29,126]. In this sense, both the expression of specific EMT-TFs and the acquisition of a mesenchymal or undifferentiated phenotype within tumours have been related to an adverse therapeutic outcome [28]. Nonetheless, few studies have so far focused on deciphering the clinical correlation between EMT and resistance (see Table 2 for examples) beyond lung cancer (see Reference [97] for a recent review).

**Table 2.** Examples of the contribution of epithelial plasticity to treatment resistance in cancer patients.

| Specific Therapy | Tumour Subtype | Status * | Phenotype # | Reference(s) |
|---|---|---|---|---|
| *Chemotherapy* | | | | |
| Platinum/etoposide | SCLC [1] | Clinical | Undifferentiated | [102] |
| Taxanes | NSCLC [1] | Clinical | Differentiated | [131] |
| Cisplatin | Ovarian | Clinical | Undifferentiated | [132] |
| Docetaxel/Cabazitaxel | Prostate | Clinical/preclinical | Differentiated | [115,133] |
| *Radiotherapy* | | | | |
| Radiotherapy | Prostate | Clinical | Differentiated | [114,134] |
| *Targeted therapy* | | | | |
| Temazolomide [2] | Glioblastoma MGMT-met | Clinical | Undifferentiated | [123] |
| Erlotinib [3]/temsirolimus [4] | HNSCC [1] | Clinical | Differentiated | [135] |
| Cobimetinib [3] | Melanoma | Preclinical | Undifferentiated | [117] |
| Vemurafenib [3] | Melanoma | Clinical/preclinical | Undifferentiated | [117] |
| Erlotinib/gefitinib [3] | NSCLC EGFR-mut | Preclinical | Undifferentiated | [96] |
| *Immunotherapy* | | | | |
| Nivulumab [5] | NSCLC (CTCs) [1] | Clinical | Undifferentiated | [136] |

* Clinical: study on patient tumour samples; Preclinical: study using preclinical models (like patient derived xenografts (PDXs)). # Estimated according to the tumour cell morphology. [1] SCLC: squamous cell lung cancer; HNSCC: head and neck squamous cell carcinoma; NSCLC: non-small cell lung cancer; CTCs: circulating tumour cells. [2] Alkylating cytotoxic prodrug. [3] Epidermal growth factor receptor/mitogen activated protein kinase/B-Raf protein kinase (EGFR/MAPK/BRAF) inhibitors. [4] mammalian target of rapamycin (mTOR) inhibitor. [5] monoclonal antibody against PD ligand 1 (mAb αPD-L1).

Regarding conventional chemotherapy, one example is seen in prostate cancer, in which resistance to docetaxel has been associated with EMT; presenting resistant tumours lower E-cadherin expression and decreased miR-200 levels [133]. In ovarian cancer patients, expression profiling analyses identified a molecular signature differentially expressed in chemoresistant and chemosensitive patients [132]. Importantly, *TWIST1* expression was significantly higher in ovarian cancer patients with poor therapeutic response upon platinum regimens (Table 2), and the authors proposed that chemoresistance was due to Twist1-mediated inhibition of apoptosis [132]. Moreover, biopsies from relapsed squamous cell lung carcinoma (SCLC) patients treated with platinum and etoposide showed enhanced levels of EMT-related mesenchymal proteins such as Snail, vimentin and the extracellular matrix protein SPARC and decreased expression of E-cadherin [102] (Table 2). Nonetheless, and in contrast to in vitro approaches, the association between EMT and resistance is not easy to characterize in the clinical context, probably because cancer patients normally receive complex therapeutic regimens, which would mask the relevance of cell plasticity to resistance against specific chemotherapeutic agents [137]. Despite this fact, the link between hybrid E/M states and chemoresistance has been established in a relevant study in human breast cancer, where the presence of CTCs, showing hybrid E/M traits, is associated with patients that exhibit increased resistance to combined chemotherapeutic and targeted agents [138].

On the other hand, the role of EMT in radioresistance has been studied in some tumour subtypes such as prostate cancer [134] (Table 2). Among different molecular mechanisms, including resistance to anoikis or PI3K/Akt pathway signalling activation, EMT induction has been observed in relapsed prostate cancer patients after radiotherapy. In this tumour context, radiation decreases E-cadherin expression by a mechanism dependent on Snail expression concomitant with N-cadherin and vimentin upregulation [139]. In addition, EMT-induced radioresistance is associated with a dramatic increase of the DNA repair gene poly (ADP-ribose) polymerase 1 (*PARP-1*) supporting that, in these radioresistant patients, treatment with PARP inhibitors might represent a new therapeutic approach worth being evaluated [139–141].

As already mentioned, the depiction of EMT in clinical samples has been linked to the lack of response to some particular targeted therapies, mostly by the association of specific EMT-TFs expression with resistance [28]. As examples, ZEB2 and Slug are overexpressed in MAPKi-resistant melanomas [121], while ZEB1 expression is linked to BRAFi resistance in melanoma patients [117], reduced response to the EGFRi erlotinib in NSCLC [96] and to TMZ in glioblastomas [123] (Table 2). Also, a correlation between Snail expression and resistance to erlotinib in head and neck squamous cell carcinoma (HNSCC) was described, at least in preclinical models [142]. Overall, these data gathered from clinical samples suggest that a dedifferentiation state (Table 2), modulated by the activation of an EMT program, appears as a key determinant for therapeutic resistance [28,29], although a thorough understanding of the mechanisms operating in cancer patients has not been achieved yet.

Despite numerous efforts to develop therapeutic strategies that directly or indirectly interfere with the EMT program (i.e., by blocking the secretion of EMT inducers, inhibiting EMT-TFs or targeting specific EMT-induced intracellular pathways [28]), none of them have so far benefitted patients in terms of resistance reversion. In fact, it was observed that these potential EMT-targeted therapies could trigger the activation of alternative pathways that behave as compensatory resistance mechanisms [143]. Likely, this could be related to the hybrid E/M phenotypes present in tumours as discussed above, even though EMT blockage remains nowadays a challenge in oncology and there are currently more than 30 clinical trials being conducted and focused on EMT reversion in many cancers, not only using chemo and/or targeted therapies (i.e., NCT01990196, NCT00769483 and NCT03509779) but also radiotherapy (i.e., NCT03660319 and NCT02913859) [144].

*4.2. EMT and Immunotherapy: A Further Link to Immune Evasion*

Immunotherapy approaches, including monoclonal antibodies, checkpoint inhibitors, therapeutic vaccines and adoptive cell transfer, have emerged as a promising therapeutic strategy for cancer treatment, particularly in melanoma, lung, bladder, NSCLC and HNSCC tumours. Immunotherapy, currently focused on immuno-inhibitors targeting the interaction of programmed cell death 1 (PD-1) with PD ligand 1 (PD-L1) or cytotoxic T-lymphocyte antigen 4 (CTLA-4) (reviewed in References [145,146]) provides clear benefit for some cancer patients. However, it is yet a challenge due to the high number of patients not profiting from immune-based treatments, some of them actually resistant to immunotherapy [147].

Tumour cells undergoing EMT have been shown to circumvent immune surveillance and become refractory to immune-based therapies [23,29,148]. Although not completely understood, recent evidence is providing some clues into the molecular bases of the link between EMT/epithelial plasticity and immune evasion [148]. The detected CTCs positive for PD-L1 show spindle-like morphology resembling intermediate EMT phenotypes [149]. Moreover, in NSCLC recurrent patients under treatment with the PD-L1 inhibitor nivulumab, the co-expression of some EMT markers (N-Cadherin and vimentin) and PD-L1 was detected in their CTCs [136] (Table 2) suggesting that the EMT phenotype of PD-L1 CTCs might identify those NSCLC patients not responding to immune therapy.

Furthermore, immunotherapy response deficiency, also known as tumour immune escape, has been partially associated with the upregulation of some EMT-TFs [148]. It has been recently noted that the suppression of anti-tumour immunity, affecting CD8+ T cells in the tumour microenvironment, could be due to the miR-200/ZEB1 axis, which directly regulates the expression of PD-L1 in lung cancer [150]. The association of EMT with an immunosuppressive phenotype has also been observed in melanoma, pancreatic and breast cancer patients [148]. Epithelial breast carcinoma cells expressing high levels of Snail showed significant susceptibility to CTL-mediated lysis reduction [151] and this has been related to the activation of pro-survival autophagy [152]. In colon cancer biopsies, PD-L1 expression has been detected in tumour buds, located at the invasive fronts of tumours and thought to be formed by cancer cells undergoing EMT [153]. In fact, PD-L1 expression in tumour buds positively correlates with ZEB1 and ZEB2 expression, suggesting that an EMT program might be linked to immune evasion by upregulating PD-L1 in CRC patients [153].

Besides, exome and transcriptome sequencing data obtained from melanoma samples, suggest that tumours unresponsive to anti-PD-L1 therapy display a gene signature related to mesenchymal phenotypes, also induced upon treatment with MAPKi and present in residual tumours treated with MAPKi, suggesting that common mesenchymal features are associated with resistance to targeted and immune therapies [122].

Furthermore, an EMT transcriptional score was measured in many tumour subtypes [128] and the immunotherapy response was better in those patients presenting tumours with luminal (epithelial) phenotype than in those patients with basal (undifferentiated or mesenchymal like) phenotype [154]. Furthermore, a high EMT score has been related to immune marker expression (i.e., PD-L1, PD-L2, and CTLA-4, among others) [155], and PD-L1 association with EMT was confirmed in lung adenocarcinomas [156] and HNSCC [157]. In NSCLC, the mesenchymal tumours showed an increase in tumour infiltrating lymphocytes (TILs) and regulatory T (Treg) cells [156]. A high EMT score in NSCLC tumours was also correlated with expression of the immune modulator CD276, regarded as a new prognostic marker for overall survival. Additionally, mesenchymal NSCLC tumour subclones, but not those with epithelial phenotype, presented increased ability to resist lysis-induced by natural killer (NK) cells [158]. Some studies also suggest that tumour cells undergoing EMT show a significant reduction in the MHC class I receptor [148], which participates in the activation of additional lytic cell death mediated by NK cells [148,159].

Further studies are required to precisely decipher the immune scape mechanisms occurring in cancer. Nevertheless, some hints point to an important contribution of EMT/epithelial plasticity to immune escape as well as a to the potential utility of EMT assessment in patients as a predictive biomarker for immune therapy selection.

## 5. Novel Perspectives for Targeting EMT-Mediated Resistance

Hitherto, the development of new therapeutic approaches to minimise EMT-induced treatment resistance in cancer is essential. The strategies for targeting EMT and resistance are particularly directed at the reversion of EMT and/or dedifferentiation programs. Various recent approaches will be briefly described in this section. With the objective to selectively kill cancer stem cells, several attempts have been implemented to find molecules targeting cells undergoing EMT [21,94,160]. In this sense, standard chemotherapy has been demonstrated to be unable of killing cells undergoing EMT in several carcinoma cellular models. Gupta and co-authors [21] exploited this fact in experimentally induced EMT in untransformed and transformed human mammary epithelial cells by downregulating E-cadherin and observed an increase in their resistance to several established chemotherapeutic drugs. In particular, treatment with paclitaxel selected resistant mesenchymal and migratory cells displaying markers associated with human mammary CSCs as well as showing increased tumour seeding and metastasis in xenografts [21]. This resistance model was used in a high-throughput screen of chemical compounds leading to the identification of salinomycin, a potassium ionophore, with cytotoxic activity on EMT cells [21]. Other high-throughput screening identified PKCα inhibitors able to eliminate human mammary cells that underwent EMT [161], further supporting that EMT can confer vulnerabilities in order to tackle tumour resistance.

Dedifferentiation compelled by EMT activation has also been linked to multidrug resistance in breast cancer cell lines [162]. In vitro, the overexpression of Twist increases resistance to chemotherapeutic drugs through enhanced ability to cope with oxidative stress by the activation of the UPR. Indeed, the inhibition of UPR prior to treatment with chemotherapeutic drugs leads to a delayed growth of basal breast xenografted tumours [162].

On the other hand, EMT-endowed plasticity can be exploited to favour drug-induced MET or transdifferentiation. With the aim of identify compounds inducing MET in mesenchymal breast cancer cells, a screening for drugs able to induce E-cadherin transcription uncovered two classical activators of PKA (cholera toxin and forskolin) as inducers of the epithelial state [163]. The epithelial-derived breast cancer cells upon treatment with PKA activators lose their stemness properties and develop increased sensitivity to conventional chemotherapy. Mechanistically, the phenotypic reversion depends on the PKA substrate H3K9 histone demethylase PHF2 that derepresses epithelial gene expression by epigenetic mechanisms [163]. This finding is also in agreement with the previous discovery that the HDAC inhibitor mocetinostat reverts ZEB1-associated resistance of cancer cells [164] lending further support to the potential use of epigenetic modulators to revert EMT-associated resistance [26].

In fact, transdifferentiation has been a long-standing goal in anti-cancer treatment. However, in the context of EMT/epithelial plasticity, reversion to a MET state can represent a double-edged strategy because of the association of MET with metastasis colonization at distant sites [47,48]. Therefore, complete eradication of EMT tumour cells, and particularly of those acquiring intermediate E/M states, can be envisioned as a steadier strategy against tumour metastasis and resistance. A recent elegant study has exploited the plasticity of intermediate E/M cancer cells to force their transdifferentiation into post-replicative adipocytes [165]. Murine breast cancer cells forced to undergo EMT were induced to irreversibly become adipocytes in vitro with a cocktail containing rosiglitazone, a peroxisome proliferator activated receptor gamma (PPARγ) agonist, and bone morphogenetic protein 2 (BMP2), being the cells in hybrid E/M states the most sensitive ones. During the cancer cell transdifferentiation, the expression of EMT-related and proliferation genes was reduced to become cell cycle arrested adipocytes. Indeed, Snail downregulation and ZEB1 upregulation were necessary, whereas MEK/ERK signalling had a negative effect towards adipogenesis of EMT cells. In vivo, the treatment with a MEKi (trametinib) and rosiglitazone, so-called adipogenesis therapy, reduced the growth and metastatic colonization of breast orthotopic tumours formed by injecting MDA-MD-231 LM basal-like breast cancer cells, similar to the results obtained in a TNBC-derived PDXs [165]. Interestingly, the analysis of the tumours upon adipogenesis therapy showed that the cancer-derived adipocytes were located at the tumour rims, where the expected EMT cells responsible for invasiveness and metastasis are located [166]. Furthermore, the tumours presented a rather differentiated phenotype with upregulation of E-cadherin expression. Since EMT cells were able to transdifferentiate into other mesenchymal cell types such as osteoblasts and chondrocytes depending on the differentiation protocol used [165], the therapeutic exploitation of the plasticity that EMT grants should be further explored in other solid tumours (Figure 1).

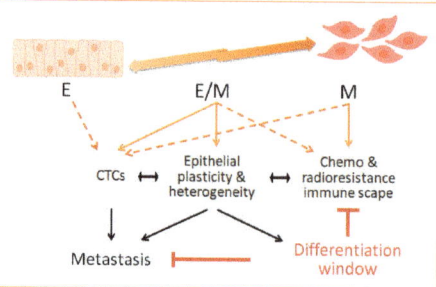

**Figure 1.** Tumours are formed by heterogeneous and phenotypically diverse cancer cell populations. During tumour progression, epithelial cells lose their apical–basal polarity and acquire mesenchymal traits through the Epithelial-to-mesenchymal transition (EMT) program. In vivo, EMT generates a wide spectrum of cellular phenotypes from epithelial (E) to mesenchymal (M) phenotypes, accompanied by gain of migratory and invasive abilities. Cells in hybrid E/M states give raise to heterogeneous populations, some endowed with stem cell-like features. These metastable E/M cells, able to rapidly adapt to changes in the tumour microenvironment, could ultimately be responsible for tumour resistance to anti-cancer therapy and immune scape. Indeed, hybrid E/M cells are associated with tumour progression, metastatic dissemination and tumour recurrence since they thrive in hostile situations due to their inherent plasticity. Circulating tumour cells (CTCs) isolated from patients display E/M traits and, in some tumour types, are considered crucial for metastatic colonization. Since treatment resistance and metastasis are the main consequences of cancer progression, drugs aimed at exploiting epithelial plasticity by promoting a cell irreversible differentiation state might constitute a successful anti-cancer strategy.

In melanoma, studies using single-cell sequencing showed that drug resistance is achieved through epigenetic reprogramming [167]. The authors found that rare cells within the bulk population expressed high levels of resistance markers (such as platelet-derived growth factor receptor (PDGFR) or AXL) in pre-treated cultures, giving then rise to a resistant population upon BRAFi treatment. They concluded that a transient pre-drug pre-resistant state allows tumour cells to readily acquire stable resistance when exposed to a drug and they suggest that this reprogramming is accompanied by phenotypic changes [167], which are reminiscent of EMT even if this point was not directly analysed. Interestingly as well, a recent study shows that minimal residual disease in melanoma is associated with cell and spatial heterogeneity and identifies transcriptional programs associated with neural crest cell stemness as key drivers of resistance to established targeted inhibitors [168]. Since a phenotypic switch associated with the change in expression of specific EMT-TF in melanoma progression has been previously identified [120], it is tempting to speculate that such phenotypic plasticity can also be exploited for epigenetic reprogramming associated with drug resistance in melanoma.

## 6. Conclusions

The EMT program and epithelial plasticity have been associated with resistance to chemo, radio and targeted therapies, as well as to novel immune-based treatments in different tumour contexts. Mechanistic insights behind such relationships are starting to emerge from experimental cellular and preclinical tumour models. Although evidence in clinical settings is still scarce, the recent appreciation that intermediate or hybrid E/M states might represent a more likely situation in tumours, together with their potential involvement in tumour heterogeneity and stemness, are providing new opportunities to expand our understanding of the contribution of epithelial plasticity to treatment resistance. As depicted in Figure 1, the attained knowledge will provide additional means to design therapeutic strategies aimed at reverting resistance by targeting epithelial plasticity and eliminating E/M cells similar to the induction of irreversible differentiated cell states.

**Author Contributions:** All authors made substantial contributions to the conception, design and writing of the article and approved the submitted version. (Conceptualization, P.G.S., G.M.-B. and A.C.; writing—original draft preparation, P.G.S., G.M.-B. and A.C.; design of Figures and Tables, P.G.S., G.M.-B.; review and editing, P.G.S., G.M.-B. and A.C.; funding acquisition, P.G.S., G.M.-B. and A.C.).

**Funding:** This work was supported by grants from the Spanish Ministerio de Economía y Competividad (SAF2013-44739-R, SAF2016-76504-R) and Instituto de Salud Carlos III (CIBERONC 16/12/00295; PI16/00134), all of them partly supported by EU-FEDER fund, FC AECC (Grupos Estables de Investigación 2018-AECC) and Worldwide Cancer Research UK (formerly AICR, 12-1057 and 16-0295).

**Acknowledgments:** We thank members of the A. Cano lab for their insightful discussions.

**Conflicts of Interest:** The authors declare no conflict of interest.

## References

1. Marusyk, A.; Polyak, K. Tumor heterogeneity: Causes and consequences. *Biochim. Biophys. Acta* **2010**, *1805*, 105–117. [CrossRef] [PubMed]
2. Davis, A.; Gao, R.; Navin, N. Tumor evolution: Linear, branching, neutral or punctuated? *Biochim Biophys. Acta Rev. Cancer* **2017**, *1867*, 151–161. [CrossRef] [PubMed]
3. Malek, R.; Wang, H.; Taparra, K.; Tran, P.T. Therapeutic Targeting of Epithelial Plasticity Programs: Focus on the Epithelial-Mesenchymal Transition. *Cells Tissues Organs* **2017**, *203*, 114–127. [CrossRef]
4. Almendro, V.; Cheng, Y.K.; Randles, A.; Itzkovitz, S.; Marusyk, A.; Ametller, E.; Gonzalez-Farre, X.; Munoz, M.; Russnes, H.G.; Helland, A.; et al. Inference of tumor evolution during chemotherapy by computational modeling and in situ analysis of genetic and phenotypic cellular diversity. *Cell Rep.* **2014**, *6*, 514–527. [CrossRef] [PubMed]
5. Burrell, R.A.; Swanton, C. Re-Evaluating Clonal Dominance in Cancer Evolution. *Trends Cancer* **2016**, *2*, 263–276. [CrossRef]
6. Gatenby, R.; Brown, J. The Evolution and Ecology of Resistance in Cancer Therapy. *Cold Spring Harb. Perspect. Med.* **2018**, *8*, a033415. [CrossRef]
7. McGranahan, N.; Swanton, C. Clonal Heterogeneity and Tumor Evolution: Past, Present, and the Future. *Cell* **2017**, *168*, 613–628. [CrossRef] [PubMed]
8. Shibue, T.; Weinberg, R.A. EMT, CSCs, and drug resistance: The mechanistic link and clinical implications. *Nat. Rev. Clin. Oncol.* **2017**, *14*, 611–629. [CrossRef]
9. Dean, M.; Fojo, T.; Bates, S. Tumour stem cells and drug resistance. *Nat. Rev. Cancer* **2005**, *5*, 275–284. [CrossRef]
10. Bao, S.; Wu, Q.; McLendon, R.E.; Hao, Y.; Shi, Q.; Hjelmeland, A.B.; Dewhirst, M.W.; Bigner, D.D.; Rich, J.N. Glioma stem cells promote radioresistance by preferential activation of the DNA damage response. *Nature* **2006**, *444*, 756–760. [CrossRef] [PubMed]
11. Eyler, C.E.; Rich, J.N. Survival of the fittest: Cancer stem cells in therapeutic resistance and angiogenesis. *J. Clin. Oncol.* **2008**, *26*, 2839–2845. [CrossRef] [PubMed]
12. Diehn, M.; Cho, R.W.; Lobo, N.A.; Kalisky, T.; Dorie, M.J.; Kulp, A.N.; Qian, D.; Lam, J.S.; Ailles, L.E.; Wong, M.; et al. Association of reactive oxygen species levels and radioresistance in cancer stem cells. *Nature* **2009**, *458*, 780–783. [CrossRef]
13. Mani, S.A.; Guo, W.; Liao, M.J.; Eaton, E.N.; Ayyanan, A.; Zhou, A.Y.; Brooks, M.; Reinhard, F.; Zhang, C.C.; Shipitsin, M.; et al. The epithelial-mesenchymal transition generates cells with properties of stem cells. *Cell* **2008**, *133*, 704–715. [CrossRef] [PubMed]
14. Morel, A.P.; Lievre, M.; Thomas, C.; Hinkal, G.; Ansieau, S.; Puisieux, A. Generation of breast cancer stem cells through epithelial-mesenchymal transition. *PLoS ONE* **2008**, *3*, e2888. [CrossRef]
15. Polyak, K.; Weinberg, R.A. Transitions between epithelial and mesenchymal states: Acquisition of malignant and stem cell traits. *Nat. Rev. Cancer* **2009**, *9*, 265–273. [CrossRef]
16. Singh, A.; Settleman, J. EMT, cancer stem cells and drug resistance: An emerging axis of evil in the war on cancer. *Oncogene* **2010**, *29*, 4741–4751. [CrossRef]
17. Inoue, A.; Seidel, M.G.; Wu, W.; Kamizono, S.; Ferrando, A.A.; Bronson, R.T.; Iwasaki, H.; Akashi, K.; Morimoto, A.; Hitzler, J.K.; et al. Slug, a highly conserved zinc finger transcriptional repressor, protects hematopoietic progenitor cells from radiation-induced apoptosis in vivo. *Cancer Cell* **2002**, *2*, 279–288. [CrossRef]

18. Perez-Losada, J.; Sanchez-Martin, M.; Perez-Caro, M.; Perez-Mancera, P.A.; Sanchez-Garcia, I. The radioresistance biological function of the SCF/kit signaling pathway is mediated by the zinc-finger transcription factor Slug. *Oncogene* **2003**, *22*, 4205–4211. [CrossRef] [PubMed]
19. Kajita, M.; McClinic, K.N.; Wade, P.A. Aberrant expression of the transcription factors snail and slug alters the response to genotoxic stress. *Mol. Cell. Biol.* **2004**, *24*, 7559–7566. [CrossRef]
20. Olmeda, D.; Moreno-Bueno, G.; Flores, J.M.; Fabra, A.; Portillo, F.; Cano, A. SNAI1 is required for tumor growth and lymph node metastasis of human breast carcinoma MDA-MB-231 cells. *Cancer Res.* **2007**, *67*, 11721–11731. [CrossRef] [PubMed]
21. Gupta, P.B.; Onder, T.T.; Jiang, G.; Tao, K.; Kuperwasser, C.; Weinberg, R.A.; Lander, E.S. Identification of selective inhibitors of cancer stem cells by high-throughput screening. *Cell* **2009**, *138*, 645–659. [CrossRef] [PubMed]
22. Holohan, C.; Van Schaeybroeck, S.; Longley, D.B.; Johnston, P.G. Cancer drug resistance: An evolving paradigm. *Nat. Rev. Cancer* **2013**, *13*, 714–726. [CrossRef] [PubMed]
23. Dongre, A.; Weinberg, R.A. New insights into the mechanisms of epithelial-mesenchymal transition and implications for cancer. *Nat. Rev. Mol. Cell Biol.* **2019**, *20*, 69–84. [CrossRef] [PubMed]
24. Nieto, M.A.; Huang, R.Y.; Jackson, R.A.; Thiery, J.P. Emt: 2016. *Cell* **2016**, *166*, 21–45. [CrossRef] [PubMed]
25. Chaffer, C.L.; San Juan, B.P.; Lim, E.; Weinberg, R.A. EMT, cell plasticity and metastasis. *Cancer Metastasis Rev.* **2016**, *35*, 645–654. [CrossRef] [PubMed]
26. Santamaria, P.G.; Moreno-Bueno, G.; Portillo, F.; Cano, A. EMT: Present and future in clinical oncology. *Mol. Oncol.* **2017**, *11*, 718–738. [CrossRef] [PubMed]
27. Pastushenko, I.; Blanpain, C. EMT Transition States during Tumor Progression and Metastasis. *Trends Cell Biol.* **2019**, *29*, 212–226. [CrossRef]
28. Gupta, P.B.; Pastushenko, I.; Skibinski, A.; Blanpain, C.; Kuperwasser, C. Phenotypic Plasticity: Driver of Cancer Initiation, Progression, and Therapy Resistance. *Cell Stem Cell* **2019**, *24*, 65–78. [CrossRef]
29. Jolly, M.K.; Somarelli, J.A.; Sheth, M.; Biddle, A.; Tripathi, S.C.; Armstrong, A.J.; Hanash, S.M.; Bapat, S.A.; Rangarajan, A.; Levine, H. Hybrid epithelial/mesenchymal phenotypes promote metastasis and therapy resistance across carcinomas. *Pharmacol. Ther.* **2019**, *194*, 161–184. [CrossRef] [PubMed]
30. Easwaran, H.; Tsai, H.C.; Baylin, S.B. Cancer epigenetics: Tumor heterogeneity, plasticity of stem-like states, and drug resistance. *Mol. Cell* **2014**, *54*, 716–727. [CrossRef] [PubMed]
31. Alizadeh, A.A.; Aranda, V.; Bardelli, A.; Blanpain, C.; Bock, C.; Borowski, C.; Caldas, C.; Califano, A.; Doherty, M.; Elsner, M.; et al. Toward understanding and exploiting tumor heterogeneity. *Nat. Med.* **2015**, *21*, 846–853. [CrossRef]
32. Da Silva-Diz, V.; Lorenzo-Sanz, L.; Bernat-Peguera, A.; Lopez-Cerda, M.; Munoz, P. Cancer cell plasticity: Impact on tumor progression and therapy response. *Semin. Cancer Biol.* **2018**, *53*, 48–58. [CrossRef] [PubMed]
33. Chaffer, C.L.; Brueckmann, I.; Scheel, C.; Kaestli, A.J.; Wiggins, P.A.; Rodrigues, L.O.; Brooks, M.; Reinhardt, F.; Su, Y.; Polyak, K.; et al. Normal and neoplastic nonstem cells can spontaneously convert to a stem-like state. *Proc. Natl. Acad. Sci. USA* **2011**, *108*, 7950–7955. [CrossRef] [PubMed]
34. Xue, Y.; Hou, S.; Ji, H.; Han, X. Evolution from genetics to phenotype: Reinterpretation of NSCLC plasticity, heterogeneity, and drug resistance. *Protein Cell* **2017**, *8*, 178–190. [CrossRef] [PubMed]
35. Thiery, J.P.; Acloque, H.; Huang, R.Y.; Nieto, M.A. Epithelial-mesenchymal transitions in development and disease. *Cell* **2009**, *139*, 871–890. [CrossRef] [PubMed]
36. Moreno-Bueno, G.; Peinado, H.; Molina, P.; Olmeda, D.; Cubillo, E.; Santos, V.; Palacios, J.; Portillo, F.; Cano, A. The morphological and molecular features of the epithelial-to-mesenchymal transition. *Nat. Protoc.* **2009**, *4*, 1591–1613. [CrossRef]
37. Nieto, M.A.; Cano, A. The epithelial-mesenchymal transition under control: Global programs to regulate epithelial plasticity. *Semin. Cancer Biol.* **2012**, *22*, 361–368. [CrossRef]
38. Greenburg, G.; Hay, E.D. Epithelia suspended in collagen gels can lose polarity and express characteristics of migrating mesenchymal cells. *J. Cell Biol.* **1982**, *95*, 333–339. [CrossRef]
39. Nieto, M.A.; Sargent, M.G.; Wilkinson, D.G.; Cooke, J. Control of cell behavior during vertebrate development by Slug, a zinc finger gene. *Science* **1994**, *264*, 835–839. [CrossRef]
40. Cano, A.; Perez-Moreno, M.A.; Rodrigo, I.; Locascio, A.; Blanco, M.J.; del Barrio, M.G.; Portillo, F.; Nieto, M.A. The transcription factor snail controls epithelial-mesenchymal transitions by repressing E-cadherin expression. *Nat. Cell Biol.* **2000**, *2*, 76–83. [CrossRef]

41. Batlle, E.; Sancho, E.; Franci, C.; Dominguez, D.; Monfar, M.; Baulida, J.; Garcia De Herreros, A. The transcription factor snail is a repressor of E-cadherin gene expression in epithelial tumour cells. *Nat. Cell Biol.* **2000**, *2*, 84–89. [CrossRef]
42. Peinado, H.; Olmeda, D.; Cano, A. Snail, Zeb and bHLH factors in tumour progression: An alliance against the epithelial phenotype? *Nat. Rev. Cancer* **2007**, *7*, 415–428. [CrossRef]
43. De Craene, B.; Berx, G. Regulatory networks defining EMT during cancer initiation and progression. *Nat. Rev. Cancer* **2013**, *13*, 97–110. [CrossRef] [PubMed]
44. Lamouille, S.; Xu, J.; Derynck, R. Molecular mechanisms of epithelial-mesenchymal transition. *Nat. Rev. Mol. Cell Biol.* **2014**, *15*, 178–196. [CrossRef]
45. Lambert, A.W.; Pattabiraman, D.R.; Weinberg, R.A. Emerging Biological Principles of Metastasis. *Cell* **2017**, *168*, 670–691. [CrossRef]
46. Brabletz, T.; Kalluri, R.; Nieto, M.A.; Weinberg, R.A. EMT in cancer. *Nat. Rev. Cancer* **2018**, *18*, 128–134. [CrossRef] [PubMed]
47. Ocaña, O.H.; Corcoles, R.; Fabra, A.; Moreno-Bueno, G.; Acloque, H.; Vega, S.; Barrallo-Gimeno, A.; Cano, A.; Nieto, M.A. Metastatic colonization requires the repression of the epithelial-mesenchymal transition inducer Prrx1. *Cancer Cell* **2012**, *22*, 709–724. [CrossRef] [PubMed]
48. Tsai, J.H.; Donaher, J.L.; Murphy, D.A.; Chau, S.; Yang, J. Spatiotemporal regulation of epithelial-mesenchymal transition is essential for squamous cell carcinoma metastasis. *Cancer Cell* **2012**, *22*, 725–736. [CrossRef]
49. Celia-Terrassa, T.; Meca-Cortes, O.; Mateo, F.; Martinez de Paz, A.; Rubio, N.; Arnal-Estape, A.; Ell, B.J.; Bermudo, R.; Diaz, A.; Guerra-Rebollo, M.; et al. Epithelial-mesenchymal transition can suppress major attributes of human epithelial tumor-initiating cells. *J. Clin. Investig.* **2012**, *122*, 1849–1868. [CrossRef]
50. Nieto, M.A. Epithelial plasticity: A common theme in embryonic and cancer cells. *Science* **2013**, *342*, 1234850. [CrossRef]
51. Tarin, D.; Thompson, E.W.; Newgreen, D.F. The fallacy of epithelial mesenchymal transition in neoplasia. *Cancer Res.* **2005**, *65*, 5996–6000. [CrossRef] [PubMed]
52. Rhim, A.D.; Mirek, E.T.; Aiello, N.M.; Maitra, A.; Bailey, J.M.; McAllister, F.; Reichert, M.; Beatty, G.L.; Rustgi, A.K.; Vonderheide, R.H.; et al. EMT and dissemination precede pancreatic tumor formation. *Cell* **2012**, *148*, 349–361. [CrossRef] [PubMed]
53. Harper, K.L.; Sosa, M.S.; Entenberg, D.; Hosseini, H.; Cheung, J.F.; Nobre, R.; Avivar-Valderas, A.; Nagi, C.; Girnius, N.; Davis, R.J.; et al. Mechanism of early dissemination and metastasis in Her2(+) mammary cancer. *Nature* **2016**, *540*, 588–592. [CrossRef] [PubMed]
54. Beerling, E.; Seinstra, D.; de Wit, E.; Kester, L.; van der Velden, D.; Maynard, C.; Schafer, R.; van Diest, P.; Voest, E.; van Oudenaarden, A.; et al. Plasticity between Epithelial and Mesenchymal States Unlinks EMT from Metastasis-Enhancing Stem Cell Capacity. *Cell Rep.* **2016**, *14*, 2281–2288. [CrossRef] [PubMed]
55. Zhao, Z.; Zhu, X.; Cui, K.; Mancuso, J.; Federley, R.; Fischer, K.; Teng, G.; Mittal, V.; Gao, D.; Zhao, H.; et al. In Vivo Visualization and Characterization of Epithelial-Mesenchymal Transition in Breast Tumors. *Cancer Res.* **2016**, *76*, 2094–2104. [CrossRef] [PubMed]
56. Chanrion, M.; Kuperstein, I.; Barriere, C.; El Marjou, F.; Cohen, D.; Vignjevic, D.; Stimmer, L.; Paul-Gilloteaux, P.; Bieche, I.; Tavares Sdos, R.; et al. Concomitant Notch activation and p53 deletion trigger epithelial-to-mesenchymal transition and metastasis in mouse gut. *Nat. Commun.* **2014**, *5*, 5005. [CrossRef]
57. Tran, H.D.; Luitel, K.; Kim, M.; Zhang, K.; Longmore, G.D.; Tran, D.D. Transient SNAIL1 expression is necessary for metastatic competence in breast cancer. *Cancer Res.* **2014**, *74*, 6330–6340. [CrossRef] [PubMed]
58. Fischer, K.R.; Durrans, A.; Lee, S.; Sheng, J.; Li, F.; Wong, S.T.; Choi, H.; El Rayes, T.; Ryu, S.; Troeger, J.; et al. Epithelial-to-mesenchymal transition is not required for lung metastasis but contributes to chemoresistance. *Nature* **2015**, *527*, 472–476. [CrossRef]
59. Zheng, X.; Carstens, J.L.; Kim, J.; Scheible, M.; Kaye, J.; Sugimoto, H.; Wu, C.C.; LeBleu, V.S.; Kalluri, R. Epithelial-to-mesenchymal transition is dispensable for metastasis but induces chemoresistance in pancreatic cancer. *Nature* **2015**, *527*, 525–530. [CrossRef]
60. Aiello, N.M.; Brabletz, T.; Kang, Y.; Nieto, M.A.; Weinberg, R.A.; Stanger, B.Z. Upholding a role for EMT in pancreatic cancer metastasis. *Nature* **2017**, *547*, E7–E8. [CrossRef] [PubMed]
61. Ye, X.; Brabletz, T.; Kang, Y.; Longmore, G.D.; Nieto, M.A.; Stanger, B.Z.; Yang, J.; Weinberg, R.A. Upholding a role for EMT in breast cancer metastasis. *Nature* **2017**, *547*, E1–E3. [CrossRef] [PubMed]

62. Krebs, A.M.; Mitschke, J.; Lasierra Losada, M.; Schmalhofer, O.; Boerries, M.; Busch, H.; Boettcher, M.; Mougiakakos, D.; Reichardt, W.; Bronsert, P.; et al. The EMT-activator Zeb1 is a key factor for cell plasticity and promotes metastasis in pancreatic cancer. *Nat. Cell Biol.* **2017**, *19*, 518–529. [CrossRef] [PubMed]
63. Nieto, M.A. Context-specific roles of EMT programmes in cancer cell dissemination. *Nat. Cell Biol.* **2017**, *19*, 416–418. [CrossRef] [PubMed]
64. Stemmler, M.P.; Eccles, R.L.; Brabletz, S.; Brabletz, T. Non-redundant functions of EMT transcription factors. *Nat. Cell Biol.* **2019**, *21*, 102–112. [CrossRef] [PubMed]
65. Jolly, M.K.; Tripathi, S.C.; Jia, D.; Mooney, S.M.; Celiktas, M.; Hanash, S.M.; Mani, S.A.; Pienta, K.J.; Ben-Jacob, E.; Levine, H. Stability of the hybrid epithelial/mesenchymal phenotype. *Oncotarget* **2016**, *7*, 27067–27084. [CrossRef] [PubMed]
66. Jia, D.; Jolly, M.K.; Kulkarni, P.; Levine, H. Phenotypic Plasticity and Cell Fate Decisions in Cancer: Insights from Dynamical Systems Theory. *Cancers* **2017**, *9*, 70. [CrossRef] [PubMed]
67. George, J.T.; Jolly, M.K.; Xu, S.; Somarelli, J.A.; Levine, H. Survival Outcomes in Cancer Patients Predicted by a Partial EMT Gene Expression Scoring Metric. *Cancer Res.* **2017**, *77*, 6415–6428. [CrossRef]
68. Bocci, F.; Jolly, M.K.; George, J.T.; Levine, H.; Onuchic, J.N. A mechanism-based computational model to capture the interconnections among epithelial-mesenchymal transition, cancer stem cells and Notch-Jagged signaling. *Oncotarget* **2018**, *9*, 29906–29920. [CrossRef]
69. Yagasaki, R.; Noguchi, M.; Minami, M.; Earashi, M. Clinical significance of E-cadherin and vimentin co-expression in breast cancer. *Int. J. Oncol.* **1996**, *9*, 755–761. [CrossRef] [PubMed]
70. Thomas, P.A.; Kirschmann, D.A.; Cerhan, J.R.; Folberg, R.; Seftor, E.A.; Sellers, T.A.; Hendrix, M.J. Association between keratin and vimentin expression, malignant phenotype, and survival in postmenopausal breast cancer patients. *Clin. Cancer Res.* **1999**, *5*, 2698–2703.
71. Livasy, C.A.; Karaca, G.; Nanda, R.; Tretiakova, M.S.; Olopade, O.I.; Moore, D.T.; Perou, C.M. Phenotypic evaluation of the basal-like subtype of invasive breast carcinoma. *Mod. Pathol.* **2006**, *19*, 264–271. [CrossRef] [PubMed]
72. Sarrio, D.; Rodriguez-Pinilla, S.M.; Hardisson, D.; Cano, A.; Moreno-Bueno, G.; Palacios, J. Epithelial-mesenchymal transition in breast cancer relates to the basal-like phenotype. *Cancer Res.* **2008**, *68*, 989–997. [CrossRef] [PubMed]
73. Pastushenko, I.; Brisebarre, A.; Sifrim, A.; Fioramonti, M.; Revenco, T.; Boumahdi, S.; Van Keymeulen, A.; Brown, D.; Moers, V.; Lemaire, S.; et al. Identification of the tumour transition states occurring during EMT. *Nature* **2018**, *556*, 463–468. [CrossRef] [PubMed]
74. Antony, J.; Huang, R.Y. AXL-Driven EMT State as a Targetable Conduit in Cancer. *Cancer Res.* **2017**, *77*, 3725–3732. [CrossRef] [PubMed]
75. Antony, J.; Tan, T.Z.; Kelly, Z.; Low, J.; Choolani, M.; Recchi, C.; Gabra, H.; Thiery, J.P.; Huang, R.Y. The GAS6-AXL signaling network is a mesenchymal (Mes) molecular subtype-specific therapeutic target for ovarian cancer. *Sci. Signal.* **2016**, *9*, ra97. [CrossRef] [PubMed]
76. Meyer, A.S.; Miller, M.A.; Gertler, F.B.; Lauffenburger, D.A. The receptor AXL diversifies EGFR signaling and limits the response to EGFR-targeted inhibitors in triple-negative breast cancer cells. *Sci. Signal.* **2013**, *6*, ra66. [CrossRef]
77. Wang, M.; Kaufman, R.J. The impact of the endoplasmic reticulum protein-folding environment on cancer development. *Nat. Rev. Cancer* **2014**, *14*, 581–597. [CrossRef]
78. Avril, T.; Vauleon, E.; Chevet, E. Endoplasmic reticulum stress signaling and chemotherapy resistance in solid cancers. *Oncogenesis* **2017**, *6*, e373. [CrossRef]
79. Papaioannou, A.; Chevet, E. Driving Cancer Tumorigenesis and Metastasis Through UPR Signaling. *Curr. Top. Microbiol. Immunol.* **2018**, *414*, 159–192. [PubMed]
80. Santamaría, P.G.; Mazón, M.J.; Eraso, P.; Portillo, F. UPR: An Upstream Signal to EMT Induction in Cancer. *J. Clin. Med.* **2019**, *8*, 624. [CrossRef]
81. Yu, Y.; Xiao, C.H.; Tan, L.D.; Wang, Q.S.; Li, X.Q.; Feng, Y.M. Cancer-associated fibroblasts induce epithelial-mesenchymal transition of breast cancer cells through paracrine TGF-beta signalling. *Br. J. Cancer* **2014**, *110*, 724–732. [CrossRef]
82. Soon, P.S.; Kim, E.; Pon, C.K.; Gill, A.J.; Moore, K.; Spillane, A.J.; Benn, D.E.; Baxter, R.C. Breast cancer-associated fibroblasts induce epithelial-to-mesenchymal transition in breast cancer cells. *Endocr. Relat. Cancer* **2013**, *20*, 1–12. [CrossRef]

83. Bonde, A.K.; Tischler, V.; Kumar, S.; Soltermann, A.; Schwendener, R.A. Intratumoral macrophages contribute to epithelial-mesenchymal transition in solid tumors. *BMC Cancer* **2012**, *12*, 35. [CrossRef] [PubMed]
84. Fan, Q.M.; Jing, Y.Y.; Yu, G.F.; Kou, X.R.; Ye, F.; Gao, L.; Li, R.; Zhao, Q.D.; Yang, Y.; Lu, Z.H.; et al. Tumor-associated macrophages promote cancer stem cell-like properties via transforming growth factor-beta1-induced epithelial-mesenchymal transition in hepatocellular carcinoma. *Cancer Lett.* **2014**, *352*, 160–168. [CrossRef] [PubMed]
85. Shintani, Y.; Fujiwara, A.; Kimura, T.; Kawamura, T.; Funaki, S.; Minami, M.; Okumura, M. IL-6 Secreted from Cancer-Associated Fibroblasts Mediates Chemoresistance in NSCLC by Increasing Epithelial-Mesenchymal Transition Signaling. *J. Thorac. Oncol.* **2016**, *11*, 1482–1492. [CrossRef] [PubMed]
86. Calon, A.; Espinet, E.; Palomo-Ponce, S.; Tauriello, D.V.; Iglesias, M.; Cespedes, M.V.; Sevillano, M.; Nadal, C.; Jung, P.; Zhang, X.H.; et al. Dependency of colorectal cancer on a TGF-beta-driven program in stromal cells for metastasis initiation. *Cancer Cell* **2012**, *22*, 571–584. [CrossRef] [PubMed]
87. Calon, A.; Lonardo, E.; Berenguer-Llergo, A.; Espinet, E.; Hernando-Momblona, X.; Iglesias, M.; Sevillano, M.; Palomo-Ponce, S.; Tauriello, D.V.; Byrom, D.; et al. Stromal gene expression defines poor-prognosis subtypes in colorectal cancer. *Nat. Genet.* **2015**, *47*, 320–329. [CrossRef] [PubMed]
88. Tauriello, D.V.F.; Palomo-Ponce, S.; Stork, D.; Berenguer-Llergo, A.; Badia-Ramentol, J.; Iglesias, M.; Sevillano, M.; Ibiza, S.; Canellas, A.; Hernando-Momblona, X.; et al. TGFbeta drives immune evasion in genetically reconstituted colon cancer metastasis. *Nature* **2018**, *554*, 538–543. [CrossRef]
89. Mariathasan, S.; Turley, S.J.; Nickles, D.; Castiglioni, A.; Yuen, K.; Wang, Y.; Kadel, E.E., III; Koeppen, H.; Astarita, J.L.; Cubas, R.; et al. TGFbeta attenuates tumour response to PD-L1 blockade by contributing to exclusion of T cells. *Nature* **2018**, *554*, 544–548. [CrossRef]
90. Yauch, R.L.; Januario, T.; Eberhard, D.A.; Cavet, G.; Zhu, W.; Fu, L.; Pham, T.Q.; Soriano, R.; Stinson, J.; Seshagiri, S.; et al. Epithelial versus mesenchymal phenotype determines in vitro sensitivity and predicts clinical activity of erlotinib in lung cancer patients. *Clin. Cancer Res.* **2005**, *11*, 8686–8698. [CrossRef] [PubMed]
91. Saxena, M.; Stephens, M.A.; Pathak, H.; Rangarajan, A. Transcription factors that mediate epithelial-mesenchymal transition lead to multidrug resistance by upregulating ABC transporters. *Cell Death Dis.* **2011**, *2*, e179. [CrossRef]
92. Haslehurst, A.M.; Koti, M.; Dharsee, M.; Nuin, P.; Evans, K.; Geraci, J.; Childs, T.; Chen, J.; Li, J.; Weberpals, J.; et al. EMT transcription factors snail and slug directly contribute to cisplatin resistance in ovarian cancer. *BMC Cancer* **2012**, *12*, 91. [CrossRef] [PubMed]
93. Mallini, P.; Lennard, T.; Kirby, J.; Meeson, A. Epithelial-to-mesenchymal transition: What is the impact on breast cancer stem cells and drug resistance. *Cancer Treat. Rev.* **2014**, *40*, 341–348. [CrossRef]
94. Feng, Y.X.; Sokol, E.S.; Del Vecchio, C.A.; Sanduja, S.; Claessen, J.H.; Proia, T.A.; Jin, D.X.; Reinhardt, F.; Ploegh, H.L.; Wang, Q.; et al. Epithelial-to-mesenchymal transition activates PERK-eIF2alpha and sensitizes cells to endoplasmic reticulum stress. *Cancer Discov.* **2014**, *4*, 702–715. [CrossRef]
95. Dong, J.; Zhai, B.; Sun, W.; Hu, F.; Cheng, H.; Xu, J. Activation of phosphatidylinositol 3-kinase/AKT/snail signaling pathway contributes to epithelial-mesenchymal transition-induced multi-drug resistance to sorafenib in hepatocellular carcinoma cells. *PLoS ONE* **2017**, *12*, e0185088. [CrossRef] [PubMed]
96. Byers, L.A.; Diao, L.; Wang, J.; Saintigny, P.; Girard, L.; Peyton, M.; Shen, L.; Fan, Y.; Giri, U.; Tumula, P.K.; et al. An epithelial-mesenchymal transition gene signature predicts resistance to EGFR and PI3K inhibitors and identifies Axl as a therapeutic target for overcoming EGFR inhibitor resistance. *Clin. Cancer Res.* **2013**, *19*, 279–290. [CrossRef] [PubMed]
97. Tulchinsky, E.; Demidov, O.; Kriajevska, M.; Barlev, N.A.; Imyanitov, E. EMT: A mechanism for escape from EGFR-targeted therapy in lung cancer. *Biochim. Biophys. Acta Rev. Cancer* **2019**, *1871*, 29–39. [CrossRef]
98. Song, K.A.; Niederst, M.J.; Lochmann, T.L.; Hata, A.N.; Kitai, H.; Ham, J.; Floros, K.V.; Hicks, M.A.; Hu, H.; Mulvey, H.E.; et al. Epithelial-to-Mesenchymal Transition Antagonizes Response to Targeted Therapies in Lung Cancer by Suppressing BIM. *Clin. Cancer Res.* **2018**, *24*, 197–208. [CrossRef]
99. Fustaino, V.; Presutti, D.; Colombo, T.; Cardinali, B.; Papoff, G.; Brandi, R.; Bertolazzi, P.; Felici, G.; Ruberti, G. Characterization of epithelial-mesenchymal transition intermediate/hybrid phenotypes associated to resistance to EGFR inhibitors in non-small cell lung cancer cell lines. *Oncotarget* **2017**, *8*, 103340–103363. [CrossRef]

100. Bierie, B.; Pierce, S.E.; Kroeger, C.; Stover, D.G.; Pattabiraman, D.R.; Thiru, P.; Liu Donaher, J.; Reinhardt, F.; Chaffer, C.L.; Keckesova, Z.; et al. Integrin-beta4 identifies cancer stem cell-enriched populations of partially mesenchymal carcinoma cells. *Proc. Natl. Acad. Sci. USA* **2017**, *114*, E2337–E2346. [CrossRef]
101. Zheng, Y.; de la Cruz, C.C.; Sayles, L.C.; Alleyne-Chin, C.; Vaka, D.; Knaak, T.D.; Bigos, M.; Xu, Y.; Hoang, C.D.; Shrager, J.B.; et al. A rare population of CD24(+)ITGB4(+)Notch(hi) cells drives tumor propagation in NSCLC and requires Notch3 for self-renewal. *Cancer Cell* **2013**, *24*, 59–74. [CrossRef] [PubMed]
102. Canadas, I.; Rojo, F.; Taus, A.; Arpi, O.; Arumi-Uria, M.; Pijuan, L.; Menendez, S.; Zazo, S.; Domine, M.; Salido, M.; et al. Targeting epithelial-to-mesenchymal transition with Met inhibitors reverts chemoresistance in small cell lung cancer. *Clin. Cancer Res.* **2014**, *20*, 938–950. [CrossRef]
103. Lei, J.T.; Shao, J.; Zhang, J.; Iglesia, M.; Chan, D.W.; Cao, J.; Anurag, M.; Singh, P.; He, X.; Kosaka, Y.; et al. Functional Annotation of ESR1 Gene Fusions in Estrogen Receptor-Positive Breast Cancer. *Cell Rep.* **2018**, *24*, 1434–1444.e7. [CrossRef]
104. Lee, J.H.; Jung, S.M.; Yang, K.M.; Bae, E.; Ahn, S.G.; Park, J.S.; Seo, D.; Kim, M.; Ha, J.; Lee, J.; et al. A20 promotes metastasis of aggressive basal-like breast cancers through multi-monoubiquitylation of Snail1. *Nat. Cell Biol.* **2017**, *19*, 1260–1273. [CrossRef] [PubMed]
105. Lambies, G.; Miceli, M.; Martinez-Guillamon, C.; Olivera-Salguero, R.; Pena, R.; Frias, C.P.; Calderon, I.; Atanassov, B.S.; Dent, S.Y.R.; Arribas, J.; et al. TGFbeta-Activated USP27X Deubiquitinase Regulates Cell Migration and Chemoresistance via Stabilization of Snail1. *Cancer Res.* **2019**, *79*, 33–46. [CrossRef]
106. Wu, Y.; Wang, Y.; Lin, Y.; Liu, Y.; Wang, Y.; Jia, J.; Singh, P.; Chi, Y.I.; Wang, C.; Dong, C.; et al. Dub3 inhibition suppresses breast cancer invasion and metastasis by promoting Snail1 degradation. *Nat. Commun.* **2017**, *8*, 14228. [CrossRef] [PubMed]
107. Lin, Y.; Wang, Y.; Shi, Q.; Yu, Q.; Liu, C.; Feng, J.; Deng, J.; Evers, B.M.; Zhou, B.P.; Wu, Y. Stabilization of the transcription factors slug and twist by the deubiquitinase dub3 is a key requirement for tumor metastasis. *Oncotarget* **2017**, *8*, 75127–75140. [CrossRef]
108. Kurrey, N.K.; Jalgaonkar, S.P.; Joglekar, A.V.; Ghanate, A.D.; Chaskar, P.D.; Doiphode, R.Y.; Bapat, S.A. Snail and slug mediate radioresistance and chemoresistance by antagonizing p53-mediated apoptosis and acquiring a stem-like phenotype in ovarian cancer cells. *Stem Cells* **2009**, *27*, 2059–2068. [CrossRef]
109. Lee, H.H.; Bellat, V.; Law, B. Chemotherapy induces adaptive drug resistance and metastatic potentials via phenotypic CXCR4-expressing cell state transition in ovarian cancer. *PLoS ONE* **2017**, *12*, e0171044. [CrossRef]
110. Figueras, A.; Alsina-Sanchis, E.; Lahiguera, A.; Abreu, M.; Muinelo-Romay, L.; Moreno-Bueno, G.; Casanovas, O.; Graupera, M.; Matias-Guiu, X.; Vidal, A.; et al. A Role for CXCR4 in Peritoneal and Hematogenous Ovarian Cancer Dissemination. *Mol. Cancer Ther.* **2018**, *17*, 532–543. [CrossRef]
111. Putzke, A.P.; Ventura, A.P.; Bailey, A.M.; Akture, C.; Opoku-Ansah, J.; Celiktas, M.; Hwang, M.S.; Darling, D.S.; Coleman, I.M.; Nelson, P.S.; et al. Metastatic progression of prostate cancer and e-cadherin regulation by zeb1 and SRC family kinases. *Am. J. Pathol.* **2011**, *179*, 400–410. [CrossRef] [PubMed]
112. Ruscetti, M.; Quach, B.; Dadashian, E.L.; Mulholland, D.J.; Wu, H. Tracking and Functional Characterization of Epithelial-Mesenchymal Transition and Mesenchymal Tumor Cells during Prostate Cancer Metastasis. *Cancer Res.* **2015**, *75*, 2749–2759. [CrossRef] [PubMed]
113. Cano, A.; Santamaria, P.G.; Moreno-Bueno, G. LOXL2 in epithelial cell plasticity and tumor progression. *Future Oncol.* **2012**, *8*, 1095–1108. [CrossRef] [PubMed]
114. Xie, P.; Yu, H.; Wang, F.; Yan, F.; He, X. Inhibition of LOXL2 Enhances the Radiosensitivity of Castration-Resistant Prostate Cancer Cells Associated with the Reversal of the EMT Process. *Biomed. Res. Int.* **2019**, *2019*, 4012590. [CrossRef] [PubMed]
115. Martin, S.K.; Pu, H.; Penticuff, J.C.; Cao, Z.; Horbinski, C.; Kyprianou, N. Multinucleation and Mesenchymal-to-Epithelial Transition Alleviate Resistance to Combined Cabazitaxel and Antiandrogen Therapy in Advanced Prostate Cancer. *Cancer Res.* **2016**, *76*, 912–926. [CrossRef] [PubMed]
116. Li, N.; Babaei-Jadidi, R.; Lorenzi, F.; Spencer-Dene, B.; Clarke, P.; Domingo, E.; Tulchinsky, E.; Vries, R.G.J.; Kerr, D.; Pan, Y.; et al. An FBXW7-ZEB2 axis links EMT and tumour microenvironment to promote colorectal cancer stem cells and chemoresistance. *Oncogenesis* **2019**, *8*, 13. [CrossRef]
117. Richard, G.; Dalle, S.; Monet, M.A.; Ligier, M.; Boespflug, A.; Pommier, R.M.; de la Fouchardiere, A.; Perier-Muzet, M.; Depaepe, L.; Barnault, R.; et al. ZEB1-mediated melanoma cell plasticity enhances resistance to MAPK inhibitors. *EMBO Mol. Med.* **2016**, *8*, 1143–1161. [CrossRef]

118. Muller, J.; Krijgsman, O.; Tsoi, J.; Robert, L.; Hugo, W.; Song, C.; Kong, X.; Possik, P.A.; Cornelissen-Steijger, P.D.; Geukes Foppen, M.H.; et al. Low MITF/AXL ratio predicts early resistance to multiple targeted drugs in melanoma. *Nat. Commun.* **2014**, *5*, 5712. [CrossRef]
119. Falletta, P.; Sanchez-Del-Campo, L.; Chauhan, J.; Effern, M.; Kenyon, A.; Kershaw, C.J.; Siddaway, R.; Lisle, R.; Freter, R.; Daniels, M.J.; et al. Translation reprogramming is an evolutionarily conserved driver of phenotypic plasticity and therapeutic resistance in melanoma. *Genes Dev.* **2017**, *31*, 18–33. [CrossRef]
120. Caramel, J.; Papadogeorgakis, E.; Hill, L.; Browne, G.J.; Richard, G.; Wierinckx, A.; Saldanha, G.; Osborne, J.; Hutchinson, P.; Tse, G.; et al. A switch in the expression of embryonic EMT-inducers drives the development of malignant melanoma. *Cancer Cell* **2013**, *24*, 466–480. [CrossRef]
121. Song, C.; Piva, M.; Sun, L.; Hong, A.; Moriceau, G.; Kong, X.; Zhang, H.; Lomeli, S.; Qian, J.; Yu, C.C.; et al. Recurrent Tumor Cell-Intrinsic and -Extrinsic Alterations during MAPKi-Induced Melanoma Regression and Early Adaptation. *Cancer Discov.* **2017**, *7*, 1248–1265. [CrossRef] [PubMed]
122. Hugo, W.; Zaretsky, J.M.; Sun, L.; Song, C.; Moreno, B.H.; Hu-Lieskovan, S.; Berent-Maoz, B.; Pang, J.; Chmielowski, B.; Cherry, G.; et al. Genomic and Transcriptomic Features of Response to Anti-PD-1 Therapy in Metastatic Melanoma. *Cell* **2016**, *165*, 35–44. [CrossRef]
123. Siebzehnrubl, F.A.; Silver, D.J.; Tugertimur, B.; Deleyrolle, L.P.; Siebzehnrubl, D.; Sarkisian, M.R.; Devers, K.G.; Yachnis, A.T.; Kupper, M.D.; Neal, D.; et al. The ZEB1 pathway links glioblastoma initiation, invasion and chemoresistance. *EMBO Mol. Med.* **2013**, *5*, 1196–1212. [CrossRef]
124. Rosmaninho, P.; Mukusch, S.; Piscopo, V.; Teixeira, V.; Raposo, A.A.; Warta, R.; Bennewitz, R.; Tang, Y.; Herold-Mende, C.; Stifani, S.; et al. Zeb1 potentiates genome-wide gene transcription with Lef1 to promote glioblastoma cell invasion. *EMBO J.* **2018**, *37*, e97115. [CrossRef]
125. Mathis, R.A.; Sokol, E.S.; Gupta, P.B. Cancer cells exhibit clonal diversity in phenotypic plasticity. *Open Biol.* **2017**, *7*, 160283. [CrossRef]
126. Mitra, A.; Mishra, L.; Li, S. EMT, CTCs and CSCs in tumor relapse and drug-resistance. *Oncotarget* **2015**, *6*, 10697–10711. [CrossRef]
127. Farmer, P.; Bonnefoi, H.; Anderle, P.; Cameron, D.; Wirapati, P.; Becette, V.; Andre, S.; Piccart, M.; Campone, M.; Brain, E.; et al. A stroma-related gene signature predicts resistance to neoadjuvant chemotherapy in breast cancer. *Nat. Med.* **2009**, *15*, 68–74. [CrossRef]
128. Tan, T.Z.; Miow, Q.H.; Miki, Y.; Noda, T.; Mori, S.; Huang, R.Y.; Thiery, J.P. Epithelial-mesenchymal transition spectrum quantification and its efficacy in deciphering survival and drug responses of cancer patients. *EMBO Mol. Med.* **2014**, *6*, 1279–1293. [CrossRef]
129. Findlay, V.J.; Wang, C.; Watson, D.K.; Camp, E.R. Epithelial-to-mesenchymal transition and the cancer stem cell phenotype: Insights from cancer biology with therapeutic implications for colorectal cancer. *Cancer Gene Ther.* **2014**, *21*, 181–187. [CrossRef] [PubMed]
130. Li, Y.; Kong, D.; Ahmad, A.; Bao, B.; Sarkar, F.H. Pancreatic cancer stem cells: Emerging target for designing novel therapy. *Cancer Lett.* **2013**, *338*, 94–100. [CrossRef]
131. Zhou, J.; Hu, Q.; Zhang, X.; Zheng, J.; Xie, B.; Xu, Z.; Zhang, W. Sensitivity to chemotherapeutics of NSCLC cells with acquired resistance to EGFR-TKIs is mediated by T790M mutation or epithelial-mesenchymal transition. *Oncol. Rep.* **2018**, *39*, 1783–1792. [CrossRef]
132. Wu, Y.H.; Huang, Y.F.; Chang, T.H.; Chou, C.Y. Activation of TWIST1 by COL11A1 promotes chemoresistance and inhibits apoptosis in ovarian cancer cells by modulating NF-kappaB-mediated IKKbeta expression. *Int. J. Cancer* **2017**, *141*, 2305–2317. [CrossRef]
133. Puhr, M.; Hoefer, J.; Schafer, G.; Erb, H.H.; Oh, S.J.; Klocker, H.; Heidegger, I.; Neuwirt, H.; Culig, Z. Epithelial-to-mesenchymal transition leads to docetaxel resistance in prostate cancer and is mediated by reduced expression of miR-200c and miR-205. *Am. J. Pathol.* **2012**, *181*, 2188–2201. [CrossRef] [PubMed]
134. Chang, L.; Graham, P.H.; Hao, J.; Bucci, J.; Cozzi, P.J.; Kearsley, J.H.; Li, Y. Emerging roles of radioresistance in prostate cancer metastasis and radiation therapy. *Cancer Metastasis Rev.* **2014**, *33*, 469–496. [CrossRef] [PubMed]
135. Bauman, J.E.; Arias-Pulido, H.; Lee, S.J.; Fekrazad, M.H.; Ozawa, H.; Fertig, E.; Howard, J.; Bishop, J.; Wang, H.; Olson, G.T.; et al. A phase II study of temsirolimus and erlotinib in patients with recurrent and/or metastatic, platinum-refractory head and neck squamous cell carcinoma. *Oral Oncol.* **2013**, *49*, 461–467. [CrossRef]

136. Raimondi, C.; Carpino, G.; Nicolazzo, C.; Gradilone, A.; Gianni, W.; Gelibter, A.; Gaudio, E.; Cortesi, E.; Gazzaniga, P. PD-L1 and epithelial-mesenchymal transition in circulating tumor cells from non-small cell lung cancer patients: A molecular shield to evade immune system? *Oncoimmunology* **2017**, *6*, e1315488. [CrossRef]
137. Akalay, I.; Tan, T.Z.; Kumar, P.; Janji, B.; Mami-Chouaib, F.; Charpy, C.; Vielh, P.; Larsen, A.K.; Thiery, J.P.; Sabbah, M.; et al. Targeting WNT1-inducible signaling pathway protein 2 alters human breast cancer cell susceptibility to specific lysis through regulation of KLF-4 and miR-7 expression. *Oncogene* **2015**, *34*, 2261–2271. [CrossRef]
138. Yu, M.; Bardia, A.; Wittner, B.S.; Stott, S.L.; Smas, M.E.; Ting, D.T.; Isakoff, S.J.; Ciciliano, J.C.; Wells, M.N.; Shah, A.M.; et al. Circulating breast tumor cells exhibit dynamic changes in epithelial and mesenchymal composition. *Science* **2013**, *339*, 580–584. [CrossRef] [PubMed]
139. Stark, T.W.; Hensley, P.J.; Spear, A.; Pu, H.; Strup, S.S.; Kyprianou, N. Predictive value of epithelial-mesenchymal-transition (EMT) signature and PARP-1 in prostate cancer radioresistance. *Prostate* **2017**, *77*, 1583–1591. [CrossRef] [PubMed]
140. Chatterjee, P.; Choudhary, G.S.; Sharma, A.; Singh, K.; Heston, W.D.; Ciezki, J.; Klein, E.A.; Almasan, A. PARP inhibition sensitizes to low dose-rate radiation TMPRSS2-ERG fusion gene-expressing and PTEN-deficient prostate cancer cells. *PLoS ONE* **2013**, *8*, e60408. [CrossRef]
141. Mateo, J.; Carreira, S.; Sandhu, S.; Miranda, S.; Mossop, H.; Perez-Lopez, R.; Nava Rodrigues, D.; Robinson, D.; Omlin, A.; Tunariu, N.; et al. DNA-Repair Defects and Olaparib in Metastatic Prostate Cancer. *N. Engl. J. Med.* **2015**, *373*, 1697–1708. [CrossRef]
142. St John, M.A. Inflammatory mediators drive metastasis and drug resistance in head and neck squamous cell carcinoma. *Laryngoscope* **2015**, *125* (Suppl. 3), S1–S11. [CrossRef]
143. Singh, M.; Yelle, N.; Venugopal, C.; Singh, S.K. EMT: Mechanisms and therapeutic implications. *Pharmacol. Ther.* **2018**, *182*, 80–94. [CrossRef] [PubMed]
144. ClinicalTrials.gov. Available online: https://clinicaltrials.gov (accessed on 13 May 2019).
145. Wei, S.C.; Duffy, C.R.; Allison, J.P. Fundamental Mechanisms of Immune Checkpoint Blockade Therapy. *Cancer Discov.* **2018**, *8*, 1069–1086. [CrossRef]
146. Havel, J.J.; Chowell, D.; Chan, T.A. The evolving landscape of biomarkers for checkpoint inhibitor immunotherapy. *Nat. Rev. Cancer* **2019**, *19*, 133–150. [CrossRef]
147. Sharma, P.; Hu-Lieskovan, S.; Wargo, J.A.; Ribas, A. Primary, Adaptive, and Acquired Resistance to Cancer Immunotherapy. *Cell* **2017**, *168*, 707–723. [CrossRef]
148. Terry, S.; Savagner, P.; Ortiz-Cuaran, S.; Mahjoubi, L.; Saintigny, P.; Thiery, J.P.; Chouaib, S. New insights into the role of EMT in tumor immune escape. *Mol. Oncol.* **2017**, *11*, 824–846. [CrossRef]
149. Satelli, A.; Batth, I.S.; Brownlee, Z.; Rojas, C.; Meng, Q.H.; Kopetz, S.; Li, S. Potential role of nuclear PD-L1 expression in cell-surface vimentin positive circulating tumor cells as a prognostic marker in cancer patients. *Sci. Rep.* **2016**, *6*, 28910. [CrossRef]
150. Chen, L.; Gibbons, D.L.; Goswami, S.; Cortez, M.A.; Ahn, Y.H.; Byers, L.A.; Zhang, X.; Yi, X.; Dwyer, D.; Lin, W.; et al. Metastasis is regulated via microRNA-200/ZEB1 axis control of tumour cell PD-L1 expression and intratumoral immunosuppression. *Nat. Commun.* **2014**, *5*, 5241. [CrossRef]
151. Akalay, I.; Janji, B.; Hasmim, M.; Noman, M.Z.; Andre, F.; De Cremoux, P.; Bertheau, P.; Badoual, C.; Vielh, P.; Larsen, A.K.; et al. Epithelial-to-mesenchymal transition and autophagy induction in breast carcinoma promote escape from T-cell-mediated lysis. *Cancer Res.* **2013**, *73*, 2418–2427. [CrossRef] [PubMed]
152. Akalay, I.; Janji, B.; Hasmim, M.; Noman, M.Z.; Thiery, J.P.; Mami-Chouaib, F.; Chouaib, S. EMT impairs breast carcinoma cell susceptibility to CTL-mediated lysis through autophagy induction. *Autophagy* **2013**, *9*, 1104–1106. [CrossRef]
153. Martinez-Ciarpaglini, C.; Oltra, S.; Rosello, S.; Roda, D.; Mongort, C.; Carrasco, F.; Gonzalez, J.; Santonja, F.; Tarazona, N.; Huerta, M.; et al. Low miR200c expression in tumor budding of invasive front predicts worse survival in patients with localized colon cancer and is related to PD-L1 overexpression. *Mod. Pathol.* **2019**, *32*, 306–313. [CrossRef]
154. Choi, W.; Porten, S.; Kim, S.; Willis, D.; Plimack, E.R.; Hoffman-Censits, J.; Roth, B.; Cheng, T.; Tran, M.; Lee, I.L.; et al. Identification of distinct basal and luminal subtypes of muscle-invasive bladder cancer with different sensitivities to frontline chemotherapy. *Cancer Cell* **2014**, *25*, 152–165. [CrossRef] [PubMed]

155. Mak, M.P.; Tong, P.; Diao, L.; Cardnell, R.J.; Gibbons, D.L.; William, W.N.; Skoulidis, F.; Parra, E.R.; Rodriguez-Canales, J.; Wistuba, I.I.; et al. A Patient-Derived, Pan-Cancer EMT Signature Identifies Global Molecular Alterations and Immune Target Enrichment Following Epithelial-to-Mesenchymal Transition. *Clin. Cancer Res.* **2016**, *22*, 609–620. [CrossRef] [PubMed]
156. Lou, Y.; Diao, L.; Cuentas, E.R.; Denning, W.L.; Chen, L.; Fan, Y.H.; Byers, L.A.; Wang, J.; Papadimitrakopoulou, V.A.; Behrens, C.; et al. Epithelial-Mesenchymal Transition Is Associated with a Distinct Tumor Microenvironment Including Elevation of Inflammatory Signals and Multiple Immune Checkpoints in Lung Adenocarcinoma. *Clin. Cancer Res.* **2016**, *22*, 3630–3642. [CrossRef] [PubMed]
157. Ock, C.Y.; Kim, S.; Keam, B.; Kim, M.; Kim, T.M.; Kim, J.H.; Jeon, Y.K.; Lee, J.S.; Kwon, S.K.; Hah, J.H.; et al. PD-L1 expression is associated with epithelial-mesenchymal transition in head and neck squamous cell carcinoma. *Oncotarget* **2016**, *7*, 15901–15914. [CrossRef]
158. Terry, S.; Buart, S.; Tan, T.Z.; Gros, G.; Noman, M.Z.; Lorens, J.B.; Mami-Chouaib, F.; Thiery, J.P.; Chouaib, S. Acquisition of tumor cell phenotypic diversity along the EMT spectrum under hypoxic pressure: Consequences on susceptibility to cell-mediated cytotoxicity. *Oncoimmunology* **2017**, *6*, e1271858. [CrossRef]
159. Vivier, E.; Tomasello, E.; Baratin, M.; Walzer, T.; Ugolini, S. Functions of natural killer cells. *Nat. Immunol.* **2008**, *9*, 503–510. [CrossRef]
160. Vijay, G.V.; Zhao, N.; Den Hollander, P.; Toneff, M.J.; Joseph, R.; Pietila, M.; Taube, J.H.; Sarkar, T.R.; Ramirez-Pena, E.; Werden, S.J.; et al. GSK3beta regulates epithelial-mesenchymal transition and cancer stem cell properties in triple-negative breast cancer. *Breast Cancer Res.* **2019**, *21*, 37. [CrossRef] [PubMed]
161. Tam, W.L.; Lu, H.; Buikhuisen, J.; Soh, B.S.; Lim, E.; Reinhardt, F.; Wu, Z.J.; Krall, J.A.; Bierie, B.; Guo, W.; et al. Protein kinase C alpha is a central signaling node and therapeutic target for breast cancer stem cells. *Cancer Cell* **2013**, *24*, 347–364. [CrossRef] [PubMed]
162. Del Vecchio, C.A.; Feng, Y.; Sokol, E.S.; Tillman, E.J.; Sanduja, S.; Reinhardt, F.; Gupta, P.B. De-differentiation confers multidrug resistance via noncanonical PERK-Nrf2 signaling. *PLoS Biol.* **2014**, *12*, e1001945. [CrossRef] [PubMed]
163. Pattabiraman, D.R.; Bierie, B.; Kober, K.I.; Thiru, P.; Krall, J.A.; Zill, C.; Reinhardt, F.; Tam, W.L.; Weinberg, R.A. Activation of PKA leads to mesenchymal-to-epithelial transition and loss of tumor-initiating ability. *Science* **2016**, *351*, aad3680. [CrossRef]
164. Meidhof, S.; Brabletz, S.; Lehmann, W.; Preca, B.T.; Mock, K.; Ruh, M.; Schuler, J.; Berthold, M.; Weber, A.; Burk, U.; et al. ZEB1-associated drug resistance in cancer cells is reversed by the class I HDAC inhibitor mocetinostat. *EMBO Mol. Med.* **2015**, *7*, 831–847. [CrossRef] [PubMed]
165. Ishay-Ronen, D.; Diepenbruck, M.; Kalathur, R.K.R.; Sugiyama, N.; Tiede, S.; Ivanek, R.; Bantug, G.; Morini, M.F.; Wang, J.; Hess, C.; et al. Gain Fat-Lose Metastasis: Converting Invasive Breast Cancer Cells into Adipocytes Inhibits Cancer Metastasis. *Cancer Cell* **2019**, *35*, 17–32.e6. [CrossRef] [PubMed]
166. Kalluri, R.; Weinberg, R.A. The basics of epithelial-mesenchymal transition. *J. Clin. Investig.* **2009**, *119*, 1420–1428. [CrossRef]
167. Shaffer, S.M.; Dunagin, M.C.; Torborg, S.R.; Torre, E.A.; Emert, B.; Krepler, C.; Beqiri, M.; Sproesser, K.; Brafford, P.A.; Xiao, M.; et al. Rare cell variability and drug-induced reprogramming as a mode of cancer drug resistance. *Nature* **2017**, *546*, 431–435. [CrossRef] [PubMed]
168. Rambow, F.; Rogiers, A.; Marin-Bejar, O.; Aibar, S.; Femel, J.; Dewaele, M.; Karras, P.; Brown, D.; Chang, Y.H.; Debiec-Rychter, M.; et al. Toward Minimal Residual Disease-Directed Therapy in Melanoma. *Cell* **2018**, *174*, 843–855.e19. [CrossRef] [PubMed]

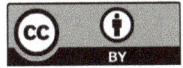

© 2019 by the authors. Licensee MDPI, Basel, Switzerland. This article is an open access article distributed under the terms and conditions of the Creative Commons Attribution (CC BY) license (http://creativecommons.org/licenses/by/4.0/).

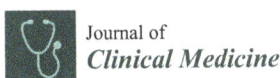 

*Review*

# Control of Invasion by Epithelial-to-Mesenchymal Transition Programs during Metastasis

Gray W. Pearson

Lombardi Comprehensive Cancer Center and Department of Oncology, Georgetown University, Washington, DC 20057, USA; gp507@georgetown.edu; Tel.: +1-202-687-0807

Received: 16 April 2019; Accepted: 8 May 2019; Published: 10 May 2019

**Abstract:** Epithelial-to-mesenchymal transition (EMT) programs contribute to the acquisition of invasive properties that are essential for metastasis. It is well established that EMT programs alter cell state and promote invasive behavior. This review discusses how rather than following one specific program, EMT states are diverse in their regulation and invasive properties. Analysis across a spectrum of models using a combination of approaches has revealed how unique features of distinct EMT programs dictate whether tumor cells invade as single cells or collectively as cohesive groups of cells. It has also been shown that the mode of collective invasion is determined by the nature of the EMT, with cells in a trailblazer-type EMT state being capable of initiating collective invasion, whereas cells that have undergone an opportunist-type EMT are dependent on extrinsic factors to invade. In addition to altering cell intrinsic properties, EMT programs can influence invasion through non-cell autonomous mechanisms. Analysis of tumor subpopulations has demonstrated how EMT-induced cells can drive the invasion of sibling epithelial populations through paracrine signaling and remodeling of the microenvironment. Importantly, the variation in invasive properties controlled by EMT programs influences the kinetics and location of metastasis.

**Keywords:** metastasis; epithelial-to-mesenchymal transition; collective invasion; heterogeneity; hybrid

## 1. Introduction

The acquisition of invasive ability (Figure 1) is an essential first step towards the development of metastatic cancer [1]. After invading into the connective tissue, tumor cells can intravasate into blood vessels and disseminate to new tissues [2]. Early attempts to define the properties of invasive tumor cells revealed that tumor cell cohesion is reduced relative to the tissue of origin [3], and that tumor cells could migrate as solitary cells or as multicellular groups in culture [4]. Notably, it was recognized that the duration of the tumor growth and the number of tumor cells entering the blood stream correlated with the extent of metastasis [5]. These collective findings have suggested that alterations to cell features that promote dissemination contribute to metastasis.

The acquisition of invasive traits by tumor cells mirrors the phenotypic changes of epithelial-to-mesenchymal transitions (EMTs) that take place during embryogenesis and wound healing [6]. The EMT process involves a loss of polarity, a disruption of cell–cell adhesion, and the acquisition of migratory ability [7]. These changes in cell state are coordinated by a combination of secondary modifications to existing proteins and alterations to cell signaling pathways through transcriptional and post-transcriptional changes that alter the pattern of gene expression [8]. Given that the properties of developmental EMT programs mirror essential features of invasive tumor cells, processes that regulate EMTs have been investigated in the context of neoplastic cell behavior [9]. Importantly, advances made in unravelling the regulation of EMTs that contribute to tissue development and inflammatory responses have established a signaling framework that has been used to reveal that EMTs contribute to tumor invasion and metastasis [10].

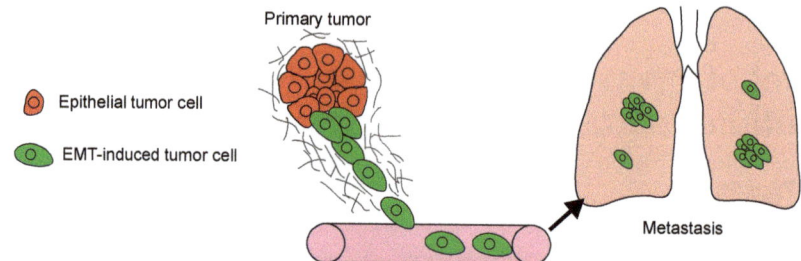

**Figure 1.** The model summarizes the steps involved in the development of metastasis. Epithelial-to-mesenchymal transition (EMT) program activation in tumor cells (green) promotes local invasion. The invasive cells intravasate into blood vessels and disseminate to new tissues, in this case the lungs. Disseminated tumor cells then initiate colonizing metastatic growth in the new organ.

## 2. EMT Program Regulation and Function

Epithelial tissue is comprised of adherent polarized sheets of cells that, depending on tissue type, are sculpted into ducts and lobules [11]. Tumors initially proliferate within luminal spaces and are separated from the stromal compartment containing conduits of metastasis [12]. The durable cell–cell attachments formed by normal and tumor cells within these lesions prevent spontaneous movement and invasion [13]. As is observed during embryogenesis and tissue morphogenesis, EMTs in tumor populations promote invasion by triggering a loss of polarity and cellular cohesion, while also conferring migratory properties and the ability to reorganize the extracellular matrix (ECM) [14].

### 2.1. Mechanism EMT Program Activation

EMT programs are normally initiated by ligands that bind to transmembrane receptors capable of activating intracellular signaling pathways. Examples include members of the TGFβ family, growth factors that bind to receptor tyrosine kinases (RTKs), and WNT ligands [15]. These signaling cues are expressed in the tumor microenvironment by recruited fibroblasts and leukocytes, which create niches where tumor cells undergo EMTs [16]. Genetic abnormalities also contribute to tumor cell EMTs, as evidenced by the ability of tumor cells to sustain mesenchymal features in the absence of extrinsic signaling cues from non-tumor populations [17]. The signaling pathways coordinated by these various receptors share the general feature of activating transcription factors that induce the expression of the core EMT transcription factors (EMT-TFs), Snail, Slug, Twist, Zeb1, and Zeb2. These EMT-TFs then directly repress epithelial cell–cell adhesion and polarity genes, while also inducing mesenchymal factors that alter the organization of the cytoskeleton, contribute to protrusion formation, and modulate the rate of cell migration. The induction of EMT programs is influenced by cell lineage-associated microRNAs (miRNAs), including miR200a, miR203, and miR205, which directly target EMT-TFs to restrict expression [18]. Additional layers of regulation include differential splicing and post-translational modifications that enhance EMT-TF stability, and epigenetic modifications that control chromatin accessibility [19]. Biomechanical feedback also influences EMT program transcription through control of EMT-TF subcellular localization [20].

## 2.2. Suppression of Epithelial Traits

The most established mechanism by which EMT programs promote cell migration is the suppression of the cell–cell adhesion protein E-cadherin. Reduced E-cadherin expression correlates with poor patient outcome [21–24] and is associated with enhanced invasive traits and metastatic capability [25]. Snail, Slug, Zeb1, and Zeb2 directly bind E-Box recognition sites in the E-cadherin promoter [26] and recruit histone methyltransferases, demethylases, and deacetylases to create a repressed chromatin architecture that drastically reduces or eliminates E-cadherin expression [27]. The loss of E-cadherin in transformed mammary epithelial cells is sufficient to promote the further induction of an EMT, invasion, and metastasis [28], highlighting the critical function of E-cadherin in sustaining epithelial fidelity. However, the loss of E-cadherin alone is not able to induce an EMT in all contexts [29], as it is typically a downstream signaling event coordinated by a more elaborate EMT program. As an alternative to transcriptional silencing, E-cadherin can be subjected to an increased rate of recycling by endocytosis [30,31], with the net effect of allowing transient adhesion formation that permits migration while retaining cell–cell cohesion [32]. In addition, cell cohesion is reduced by EMT-TF mediated suppression of proteins that contribute to tight junction, gap junction and desmosome formation [33]. The destabilization of cell–cell junctional integrity induced by EMTs also causes a disruption in the establishment of adhesion-associated PAR and the Crumbs polarity complexes [34]. Loss of apical-basal polarity is further reinforced by the suppression of polarity protein expression [35].

## 2.3. Induction of Mesenchymal Features

The loss of epithelial features alone is not sufficient to promote migration and invasion. EMT-TFs also induce mesenchymal genes that promote alterations in cell morphology, enhance migratory properties, and influence the ability to remodel the ECM [7]. EMTs also confer cells with the capacity to form protrusive structures and acquire a bipolar morphology [36] through the induction and alternative splicing of genes that regulate localization and duration of actin polymerization [37,38]. The induction of the intermediate filament protein vimentin is a canonical feature of EMT programs that is frequently used as a marker of cells that have undergone an EMT [39]. Tissue-specific keratin expression is also suppressed as cells progress to a more fully mesenchymal state [39]. One of the consequences of this change in intermediate filament composition is a perturbation in protein trafficking and interactions with motor proteins [27]. Cell substrate adhesion proteins and receptor composition are also altered to change the stability and duration of adhesive structures and how cells respond to new ECM niches [40]. These changes in cell morphology allow EMT-induced cells to respond to chemotactic signals and migrate through existing tracks in the ECM created by non-tumor populations in the microenvironment [41]. EMT programs also endow tumor cells with the ability to remodel the ECM themselves. The induction of matrix metalloproteinases, which cleave basement membrane proteins and collagens, facilitates the initial invasion from ductal structures, migration through stromal tissue, and intravasation into blood vessels [42]. The composition and adhesive properties of the ECM can be further altered through secretion of proteins such as fibronectin and Tenascin-C [43,44].

## 3. EMT Program Heterogeneity Confers Distinct Invasive Phenotypes

There is heterogeneity in the composition and functions of EMT programs. The elements of epithelial suppression and mesenchymal induction just described are not a part of a single EMT program through which cells progress over time. Thus, it should not be assumed that a feature of one EMT program is a trait of all EMT programs. There are a range of unique EMT states, reflecting distinct activating signals and intrinsic cell-lineage features, that determine the extent of epithelial gene suppression and mesenchymal gene induction that occurs as part of an EMT program. This heterogeneity in EMT programs contributes to the significant phenotypic variability observed in the modes of tumor cells invasion [45] (Figure 2).

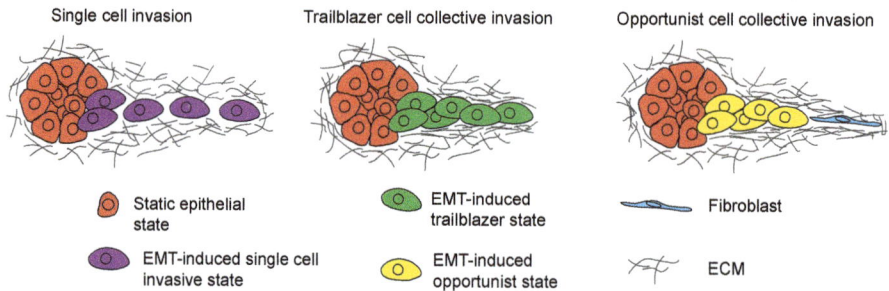

**Figure 2.** Model shows the different modes of invasion induced by EMT programs. Tumor cells can engage in single cell invasion (purple), trailblazer type collective invasion (green) or opportunistic collective invasion (yellow) depending on the nature of the EMT program that is activated.

## 3.1. Regulation of Single-Cell Invasion

Tumor cell invasion is frequently conceptualized as a process undertaken by solitary cells that detach from a multicellular tumor mass and migrate into the ECM. There are distinct modes of single-cell invasion [46]. Cells can engage in a mesenchymal mode that is dependent on the activity of proteases, such as matrix metalloproteinases, that degrade ECM proteins [47]. Tumor cells can also migrate using force-dependent cytoplasmic blebbing to push through gaps in the ECM, independent of protease activity [48,49]. A more fully mesenchymal state characterized by E-cadherin suppression and vimentin induction is associated with the ability of tumor cells to dissociate and invade as individual cells [17,50,51]. However, it should be noted that there is evidence suggesting that the retention of epithelial traits, such as E-cadherin expression, does not preclude the induction of single-cell invasion and may be promoted by a hybrid EMT state [52–54]. Single-cell invasion can be induced by a range of signals, including TGFβ [55], CXCL family chemokines, RTK ligands, and hypoxia [56]. Single-cell invasion is a relatively rare event in primary tumors and is most frequently detected proximal to blood vessels [51]. Intravital imaging has revealed that single cells can move rapidly along pre-existing aligned ECM fibers that act as paths towards blood vessels [57]. Evidence of both mesenchymal and rounded or ameboid modes of single-cell invasion is detected in EMT-induced cells [51]. In addition, EMT-induced tumor cells can convert between mesenchymal and ameboid modes of migration spontaneously, or in response to changes in ECM composition or experimental intervention [45]. The extent to which EMT programs directly control a switch between modes of single-cell invasion is not known.

## 3.2. Collective Invasion Is the Predominant Mode of Tumor Cell Invasion

Tumor cells frequently engage in a process called collective invasion, in which cells migrate through the ECM in groups of cells that retain cellular cohesion [58]. During collective invasion a leading tumor cell extends protrusions that establish traction and exert force on the ECM [59]. These protrusions also secrete proteases to further promote ECM degradation [60]. Additional cells track along the paths created by the first leading cell [61], widening the path in the ECM, and allowing the parallel invasion of cells [62]. Importantly, collective invasion is the principal mode of tumor invasion, as determined by the reconstruction of the primary tumor organization [63], evaluation of tumor explants [64,65], and intravital imaging [54,66]. There is variability in the mode of collective invasion induced by EMT programs. One class of EMT programs confers a trailblazer phenotype that is characterized by an enhanced ability to initiate collective invasion [67–69]. A second class of EMT programs induces an opportunistic state in which cells are motile, but are dependent on extrinsic factors, such as the recruitment of fibroblasts, to collectively invade [70,71].

## 3.3. Trailblazer-Type Collective Invasion

The trailblazer EMT program is distinguished by the induction of genes that are specifically required to form cellular protrusions that provide traction and reorganize collagen into parallel fibrils [68,72]. These trailblazer-specific proteins include DOCK10, a guanine nucleotide exchange factor that activates Cdc42 [73], integrin α11, a collagen 1 specific integrin [74], DAB2, which contributes to integrin endocytosis [75], and PDFGRA, which activates signaling pathways necessary for ECM degradation [76]. These proteins coordinate distinct pathways that are integrated together to promote this highly invasive phenotype [68]. Cells with trailblazer features also secrete fibronectin and express higher levels of vimentin [69]. Trailblazer cells investigated to date lack E-cadherin expression, yet retain cellular cohesion [68,69]. A switch from E-cadherin to N-cadherin expression is a feature of some EMT programs [77], and thus potentially provide a mechanism for trailblazer cells to retain cell–cell attachments. In squamous carcinoma models, the cohesion of trailblazer-type cells is sustained by Snail-dependent expression of the tight junction protein Claudin 11 [78]. Genes required for trailblazer cell collective invasion are also necessary for metastasis [68], suggesting that the intrinsic ability of cells to initiate collective invasion influences dissemination.

## 3.4. Opportunistic-Type Collective Invasion

Opportunistic EMT states can be induced by hybrid programs that confer mesenchymal features while allowing cells to retain epithelial character. Hybrid states are a general property of carcinomas [79] and collectively invading hybrid tumor cells are detected in breast, lung, and pancreatic patient tumors [63]. Live-imaging of 3-dimensional culture systems has revealed that cells in a hybrid state are motile within spheroids, yet are unable to initiate invasion into the ECM [70,80,81]. The opportunistic nature of hybrid EMT migration can also be inferred by contrasting the ability of these cells to collectively migrate in wound closure assays with their inability to degrade and reorganize the ECM [82]. Motile opportunist cells are able to collectively invade when the ECM is organized into tracks by fibroblasts, or enriched in collagen I, which promotes protrusion formation in both normal and mammary tumor cells [65]. Notably, activation of these hybrid EMT programs is essential for opportunist invasion [70,83,84].

## 3.5. Regulation of Hybrid EMT States That Promote Opportunistic Collective Invasion

The precise nature of hybrid EMT programs that confer an opportunist phenotype have begun to become unraveled. ΔNp63 is necessary for opportunistic invasion in multiple breast cancer models [83,84] and confers a hybrid EMT by directly inducing the expression of Slug and Axl [84,85]. Other EMT-TFs are not induced by ΔNp63 and E-cadherin expression is retained, possibly due to the parallel ΔNp63-mediated induction of miR205 [85]. This ΔNp63-induced hybrid EMT state is also activated in lung squamous cancer cells [84]. In models of breast ductal carcinoma in situ, ΔNp63 is activated in collectively invading cells by the recruitment of fibroblasts [85]. ΔNp63 induction is also necessary for luminal-type mammary tumor cells to invade in a genetically engineered mouse model of breast cancer [83]. These results indicate that the nature of the EMT activating signal can dictate the mode of collective invasion by being unable to induce further progression to a complete mesenchymal state. A hybrid state can also be conferred by cell lineage-specific transcription factors that restrict responses to EMT initiating signals. In this regulatory framework, loss of the restriction mechanism permits further progression towards a mesenchymal phenotype. For instance, the transcription factors GRHL2 and OVOL2 suppress Zeb1 to restrict EMT progression in lung cancer cells and promote a collective form of migration [86]. MicroRNA expression patterns also restrict EMT progression by targeting EMT-TFs and downstream mesenchymal genes that are necessary for inducing a mesenchymal state [87]. One of these mechanisms may be responsible for sustaining a hybrid state in a model of Luminal B-type breast cancer in which Snail is activated in collectively invading cells that sustain E-cadherin expression [83,88].

In addition to the underlying transcription regulation conferring an opportunistic hybrid state, properties of hybrid EMT cells that directly promote collective invasion have begun to be investigated. In pancreatic cancer models, a hybrid EMT state correlates with an increased storage of E-cadherin in recycling endosomes, potentially due to the increased expression of Rab11 [32]. This mechanism for promoting hybrid EMT collective invasion may be a property of breast and colon cancer cells as well [32]. Indeed, activation of ERK1/2 MAP kinases and ΔNp63 promote intracellular localization of E-cadherin in motile hybrid EMT cells, possibly through the expression of FAT2 [81,84]. KRT14 is necessary for invasion of Snail-expressing hybrid cells [83] and Axl is necessary for ΔNp63-induced invasion [85], although the specific function for these genes in this context is not known. Features of EMT programs that are necessary for single-cell invasion likely contribute to opportunist invasion if they are activated as part of a specific hybrid EMT program. However, the assigning of specific functions for these traits requires experimental confirmation.

## 4. EMT-Induced Cells Can Influence the Invasive Properties of Siblings

### 4.1. Subpopulation Interactions That Promote Single-Cell Invasion

EMT induction occurs in a fraction of cells in primary tumors [39,51,63,88,89]. In addition to conferring these cells with new invasive properties, EMT-induced cells can influence the invasive character of sibling epithelial subpopulations (Figure 3). In prostate cancer models, cells that have acquired a stable mesenchymal phenotype promote the invasion of a sibling epithelial subpopulation [90]. In this interaction, undefined secreted factors from the mesenchymal population promoted the conversion of epithelial cells into a more invasive state. This induction of single-cell invasion correlated with the activation of an EMT program in the epithelial cells, as indicated by the expression of fibronectin. The conversion of epithelial cells to a more invasive state was sustained for seven days after interacting with the mesenchymal subpopulation [90]. Consistent with this finding, cells that have undergone TGFβ-induced EMT are capable of propagating EMT induction in untreated sibling cells, which was detected by the silencing of E-cadherin [91]. Undefined paracrine signals from EMT-induced cells can also promote the invasion of neuroendocrine subpopulations in a small-cell lung cancer (SCLC) model [92]. In addition, EMT-induced cells can confer invasive properties through mechanisms that allow siblings to sustain epithelial character. Cells that have undergone an EMT in response to exogenous Twist, Snail, or Six1 expression are capable of activating a Gli1-dependent signaling pathway in epithelial cells that promotes their migration and invasion [93].

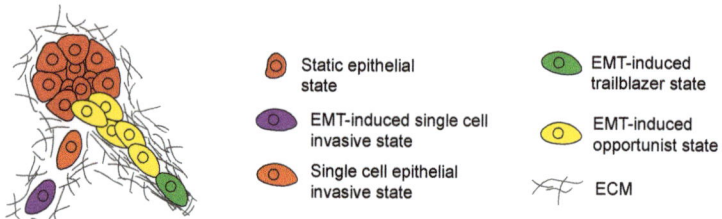

**Figure 3.** Model shows how a subpopulation of EMT induced cells can promote the invasion of siblings that lack intrinsic invasive properties. EMT induced cells (purple) can promote single cell invasion of sibling epithelial tumor cells (orange) through paracrine signaling. Cells in a trailblazer EMT state (green) can create paths in the ECM then promote the collective invasion of siblings in an opportunist EMT state (yellow).

### 4.2. Subpopulation Interactions That Promote Collective Invasion

Trailblazer cells can promote sibling opportunist-cell invasion through a paracrine signaling independent mechanism. In this mode of interaction, paths in the ECM created by trailblazer cells promote the collective invasion of motile opportunist sibling tumor cells or normal mammary epithelial cells that lack the intrinsic capacity to initiate invasion [68]. Interestingly, paracrine signaling is not sufficient for trailblazer cells to induce the opportunist subpopulation invasion [68]. Importantly, opportunist cells are also not conferred with a trailblazer phenotype in this mode of interaction [68]. A similar type of trailblazer cell-induced invasion through path generation has been detected in lung cancer cell lines [69]. Trailblazer and opportunist cells from both breast and lung cancer populations have EMT program activation, indicating that they are in distinct EMT states [68,69]. Breast cancer trailblazer and opportunist cells express high-levels of canonical EMT-TF and vimentin, in addition to having low E-cadherin expression. Lung cancer trailblazer and opportunist populations also lack E-cadherin expression [69].

Genes that are specifically required for trailblazer cell invasion that were described earlier, including, DOCK10, integrin α11, DAB2, and PDGFRA, are expressed at least four-fold higher in trailblazer cells, relative to opportunist siblings [68,85]. In lung cancer populations, trailblazer cells express higher levels of VEGFA and fibronectin, both of which are required for invasion [69]. Whether these functional requirements for trailblazer-induced invasion of sibling cells are conserved across tumor types is not known. Breast cancer trailblazer and opportunist subpopulations are epigenetically distinct and the phenotypes are semi-stable, with spontaneous conversion events detected over time [68]. However, the epigenetic control mechanism itself has not been established and processes that directly control the changes in gene expression that confer the trailblazer phenotype have not been established in breast or lung cancer populations. In addition, whether signals from the microenvironment, such as TGFβ, promote a trailblazer-opportunist relationship has not been analyzed. Thus, further investigation is needed to determine the details of the mechanisms underlying these interactions and the relative contribution of the EMT-induced cells and epithelial siblings towards metastasis and treatment response.

## 5. EMT Invasion Programs Determine Metastatic Traits

### 5.1. EMT Activation Promotes Early Dissemination

Analysis of mouse models of breast and pancreatic cancer suggest that an EMT is induced in a subpopulation of cells prior to detectable primary tumor formation [94–97]. These EMT-induced cells disseminate to distant tissues [95,96] and can form up to 80% of detected metastases [97]. In a HER2/Neu amplification model, this migratory program is inactivated during tumor progression as part of a pro-growth signaling program [97]. This suggests the intriguing possibility that normal mammary tissue is more permissive to EMT induction than highly proliferative cells in primary tumors. Early tumor cell dissemination is also detected in patients with pancreatic cysts [98], although the clinical contribution of early dissemination remains largely undefined. Also, the neoplastic perturbations driving tumor growth in these genetically engineered mouse models are present throughout the epithelium, creating a greater number of potential cells that can undergo EMT. In addition, widespread oncogene may create interactions with the microenvironment that are not normally present until later in tumor development, when these genetic abnormalities are frequently acquired. Thus, the precise role of early versus late dissemination requires further evaluation.

### 5.2. There Is EMT Program Heterogeneity in Primary Tumors

It is well-established that EMT programs are activated in invasive primary tumor cells [39,63]. In principle, EMT induction can promote the initial induction of invasion into the ECM. Consistent with this possibility, EMT program activation is sufficient to promote invasion, which triggers a transition from in situ to invasive growth in an orthotopic tumor model [85]. Moreover, trailblazer cells can induce the collective invasion of epithelial siblings in a model of ductal carcinoma in situ through a non-cell autonomous mechanism [68]. Consistent with this interaction between populations, distinct clones invade together during the initial induction of invasion in breast cancer patient tumors [99]. However, the precise point when EMT programs are activated in patient tumors remains unresolved [1]. This is, in part, due to the technical challenges of determining the timing of EMT activation with respect to occurring before or after invasion, which is impossible with current technology. Immunostaining and genetic reporters indicate that there is topographical variation with respect to EMT induction in invasive primary tumors [39,51,55,89]. The extent and nature of EMT program activation is also heterogeneous, yielding an assortment of EMT states with distinct invasive and metastatic properties [32,39,55]. This heterogeneity is influenced by clonal variability and the diversity of the tumor microenvironment [39,89]. The existence of distinct EMT states influences how and where tumor cells metastasize. In pancreatic cancer models, both hybrid and complete EMT programs are active in the same tumor. Hybrid EMT-induced cells collectively invade and disseminate as clusters of cells that specifically colonize the liver, whereas cells that have undergone a complete EMT engage in single-cell invasion and colonize the lungs [100]. In an orthotopic breast cancer model, collectively invading cells metastasize to lymph nodes while single invasive cells disseminate to the lungs [55]. Polyclonal tumor cell clusters seed lung metastases in a different set of breast cancer models [101,102], indicating that yet to be defined features of primary tumors dictate how the mode of invasion influences organotropism.

### 5.3. EMT Program Traits Influence Colonization Ability

The nature of the EMT program influences the ability of tumor cells to engage in colonizing metastatic growth. Stable and complete induction of EMTs promotes dissemination to new tissues [55,103]. However, sustained EMT induction can cause a loss of proliferative capacity and render cells dormant [55,104,105]. A mesenchymal-to-epithelial (MET) conversion after dissemination, either due to the removal of an EMT activation signal or to the induction of a reversion program, can re-initiate growth and promote colonization [103,106]. There are potential alternatives to the EMT-MET reversion mechanism for metastasis. Hybrid EMT states confer invasive properties while allowing cells to retain intrinsic metastatic growth potential [39,107,108]. In addition, cells that have acquired a mesenchymal phenotype can promote metastasis of a second population that lacked stable EMT features at the time of injection into the mouse in breast, prostate, and SCLC tumor models [90,92,93]. Notably, the cells that had undergone a stable EMT did not form metastases, highlighting the potential importance of non-cell autonomous mechanisms in promoting dissemination and colonization [90,92,93].

### 6. Conclusions

Extensive investigation using an array of tumor models supported by patient tumor analysis has demonstrated that EMT programs contribute to tumor invasion and metastasis. The basic features of EMT programs that control invasion have been established. More recently, the diversity of EMT programs and the phenotypes they induce during tumorigenesis have been recognized. Building upon these discoveries, there are a number of challenges that must be addressed to understand the regulation and function of EMTs with the goal of improving cancer patient diagnosis and treatment. It is critical to determine at which point EMTs are induced during tumor progression to define precisely how EMTs influence metastasis. The contributions of EMTs towards metastasis has largely relied on models in which tumor cells have progressed to a near fully mesenchymal state. However, hybrid states are frequently detected in primary tumors and may be the predominant type of EMT [109]. Yet the processes that confer hybrid EMTs and the functional requirements for hybrid cells to metastasize are unknown. How variability in EMT states present in a tumor contribute to metastasis has begun to be appreciated and requires further investigation. In particular, whether a specific subset of EMT states influences metastasis and if distinct EMT states create synergistic relationships that contribute to metastasis should be determined. Notably, certain transcription factors or EMT state-specific components may not be involved in metastatic events, but may be necessary for other features, such as acquired resistance to chemotherapy [110–113]. Thus, it is essential to define the composition of EMT signaling networks that are active in vivo and to determine their precise functions in promoting metastasis. Finally, any new analysis of EMTs should consider cell autonomous and non-cell autonomous functions, which have begun to be recognized, however lack a detailed mechanistic understanding.

**Funding:** This research was funded by the National Institute of Health, grant number R01CA218670, and Georgetown Women and Wine.

**Conflicts of Interest:** The author declares no conflict of interest. The funders had no role in the design of the study; in the collection, analyses, or interpretation of data; in the writing of the manuscript, or in the decision to publish the results.

## References

1. Lambert, A.W.; Pattabiraman, D.R.; Weinberg, R.A. Emerging biological principles of metastasis. *Cell* **2017**, *168*, 670–691. [CrossRef] [PubMed]
2. Fidler, I.J. Tumor heterogeneity and the biology of cancer invasion and metastasis. *Cancer Res.* **1978**, *38*, 2651–2660. [CrossRef] [PubMed]
3. Mc, C.M.; Coman, D.R.; Moore, F.B. Studies on invasiveness of cancer; adhesiveness of malignant cells in various human adenocarcinomas. *Cancer* **1948**, *1*, 460–467.
4. Enterline, H.T.; Coman, D.R. The ameboid motility of human and animal neoplastic cells. *Cancer* **1950**, *3*, 1033–1038. [CrossRef]
5. Zeidman, I.; Mc, C.M.; Coman, D.R. Factors affecting the number of tumor metastases; experiments with a transplantable mouse tumor. *Cancer Res.* **1950**, *10*, 357–359. [PubMed]
6. Nieto, M.A.; Cano, A. The epithelial-mesenchymal transition under control: Global programs to regulate epithelial plasticity. *Semin. Cancer Biol.* **2012**, *22*, 361–368. [CrossRef] [PubMed]
7. Thiery, J.P.; Acloque, H.; Huang, R.Y.; Nieto, M.A. Epithelial-mesenchymal transitions in development and disease. *Cell* **2009**, *139*, 871–890. [CrossRef] [PubMed]
8. Nieto, M.A. The ins and outs of the epithelial to mesenchymal transition in health and disease. *Annu. Rev. Cell Dev. Biol.* **2011**, *27*, 347–376. [CrossRef] [PubMed]
9. Thiery, J.P. Epithelial-mesenchymal transitions in tumour progression. *Nat. Rev. Cancer* **2002**, *2*, 442–454. [CrossRef] [PubMed]
10. Chaffer, C.L.; San Juan, B.P.; Lim, E.; Weinberg, R.A. EMT, cell plasticity and metastasis. *Cancer Metastasis Rev.* **2016**, *35*, 645–654. [CrossRef]
11. Debnath, J.; Brugge, J.S. Modelling glandular epithelial cancers in three-dimensional cultures. *Nat. Rev. Cancer* **2005**, *5*, 675–688. [CrossRef]
12. Jacks, T.; Weinberg, R.A. Taking the study of cancer cell survival to a new dimension. *Cell* **2002**, *111*, 923–925. [CrossRef]
13. Rorth, P. Collective cell migration. *Annu. Rev. Cell Dev. Biol.* **2009**, *25*, 407–429. [CrossRef] [PubMed]
14. Grunert, S.; Jechlinger, M.; Beug, H. Diverse cellular and molecular mechanisms contribute to epithelial plasticity and metastasis. *Nat. Rev. Mol. Cell Biol.* **2003**, *4*, 657–665. [CrossRef] [PubMed]
15. Kalluri, R.; Weinberg, R.A. The basics of epithelial-mesenchymal transition. *J. Clin. Investig.* **2009**, *119*, 1420–1428. [CrossRef] [PubMed]
16. Ye, X.; Weinberg, R.A. Epithelial-mesenchymal plasticity: A central regulator of cancer progression. *Trends Cell Biol.* **2015**, *25*, 675–686. [CrossRef] [PubMed]
17. Neve, R.M.; Chin, K.; Fridlyand, J.; Yeh, J.; Baehner, F.L.; Fevr, T.; Clark, L.; Bayani, N.; Coppe, J.P.; Tong, F.; et al. A collection of breast cancer cell lines for the study of functionally distinct cancer subtypes. *Cancer Cell* **2006**, *10*, 515–527. [CrossRef] [PubMed]
18. Lamouille, S.; Subramanyam, D.; Blelloch, R.; Derynck, R. Regulation of epithelial-mesenchymal and mesenchymal-epithelial transitions by microRNAs. *Curr. Opin. Cell Biol.* **2013**, *25*, 200–207. [CrossRef] [PubMed]
19. De Craene, B.; Berx, G. Regulatory networks defining EMT during cancer initiation and progression. *Nat. Rev. Cancer* **2013**, *13*, 97–110. [CrossRef]

20. Wei, S.C.; Fattet, L.; Tsai, J.H.; Guo, Y.; Pai, V.H.; Majeski, H.E.; Chen, A.C.; Sah, R.L.; Taylor, S.S.; Engler, A.J.; et al. Matrix stiffness drives epithelial-mesenchymal transition and tumour metastasis through a twist1-g3bp2 mechanotransduction pathway. *Nat. Cell Biol.* **2015**, *17*, 678–688. [CrossRef] [PubMed]
21. Hong, S.M.; Li, A.; Olino, K.; Wolfgang, C.L.; Herman, J.M.; Schulick, R.D.; Iacobuzio-Donahue, C.; Hruban, R.H.; Goggins, M. Loss of e-cadherin expression and outcome among patients with resectable pancreatic adenocarcinomas. *Mod. Pathol.* **2011**, *24*, 1237–1247. [CrossRef] [PubMed]
22. Horne, H.N.; Sherman, M.E.; Garcia-Closas, M.; Pharoah, P.D.; Blows, F.M.; Yang, X.R.; Hewitt, S.M.; Conway, C.M.; Lissowska, J.; Brinton, L.A.; et al. Breast cancer susceptibility risk associations and heterogeneity by e-cadherin tumor tissue expression. *Breast Cancer Res. Treat.* **2014**, *143*, 181–187. [CrossRef] [PubMed]
23. Yang, Y.L.; Chen, M.W.; Xian, L. Prognostic and clinicopathological significance of downregulated e-cadherin expression in patients with non-small cell lung cancer (NSCLC): A meta-analysis. *PLoS ONE* **2014**, *9*, e99763. [CrossRef] [PubMed]
24. Christou, N.; Perraud, A.; Blondy, S.; Jauberteau, M.O.; Battu, S.; Mathonnet, M. E-cadherin: A potential biomarker of colorectal cancer prognosis. *Oncol. Lett.* **2017**, *13*, 4571–4576. [CrossRef] [PubMed]
25. Canel, M.; Serrels, A.; Frame, M.C.; Brunton, V.G. E-cadherin-integrin crosstalk in cancer invasion and metastasis. *J. Cell Sci.* **2013**, *126*, 393–401. [CrossRef] [PubMed]
26. Peinado, H.; Olmeda, D.; Cano, A. Snail, zeb and bhlh factors in tumour progression: An alliance against the epithelial phenotype? *Nat. Rev. Cancer* **2007**, *7*, 415–428. [CrossRef] [PubMed]
27. Lamouille, S.; Xu, J.; Derynck, R. Molecular mechanisms of epithelial-mesenchymal transition. *Nat. Rev. Mol. Cell Biol.* **2014**, *15*, 178–196. [CrossRef]
28. Onder, T.T.; Gupta, P.B.; Mani, S.A.; Yang, J.; Lander, E.S.; Weinberg, R.A. Loss of e-cadherin promotes metastasis via multiple downstream transcriptional pathways. *Cancer Res.* **2008**, *68*, 3645–3654. [CrossRef] [PubMed]
29. Khalil, A.A.; Ilina, O.; Gritsenko, P.G.; Bult, P.; Span, P.N.; Friedl, P. Collective invasion in ductal and lobular breast cancer associates with distant metastasis. *Clin. Exp. Metastasis* **2017**, *34*, 421–429. [CrossRef] [PubMed]
30. de Beco, S.; Gueudry, C.; Amblard, F.; Coscoy, S. Endocytosis is required for e-cadherin redistribution at mature adherens junctions. *Proc. Natl. Acad. Sci. USA* **2009**, *106*, 7010–7015. [CrossRef]
31. Hong, S.; Troyanovsky, R.B.; Troyanovsky, S.M. Spontaneous assembly and active disassembly balance adherens junction homeostasis. *Proc. Natl. Acad. Sci. USA* **2010**, *107*, 3528–3533. [CrossRef] [PubMed]
32. Aiello, N.M.; Maddipati, R.; Norgard, R.J.; Balli, D.; Li, J.; Yuan, S.; Yamazoe, T.; Black, T.; Sahmoud, A.; Furth, E.E.; et al. Emt subtype influences epithelial plasticity and mode of cell migration. *Dev. Cell* **2018**, *45*, 681–695. [CrossRef] [PubMed]
33. Huang, R.Y.; Guilford, P.; Thiery, J.P. Early events in cell adhesion and polarity during epithelial-mesenchymal transition. *J. Cell Sci.* **2012**, *125*, 4417–4422. [CrossRef] [PubMed]
34. Thiery, J.P.; Sleeman, J.P. Complex networks orchestrate epithelial-mesenchymal transitions. *Nat. Rev. Mol. Cell Biol.* **2006**, *7*, 131–142. [CrossRef]
35. Moreno-Bueno, G.; Portillo, F.; Cano, A. Transcriptional regulation of cell polarity in emt and cancer. *Oncogene* **2008**, *27*, 6958–6969. [CrossRef] [PubMed]
36. Yilmaz, M.; Christofori, G. Emt, the cytoskeleton, and cancer cell invasion. *Cancer Metastasis Rev.* **2009**, *28*, 15–33. [CrossRef] [PubMed]
37. Philippar, U.; Roussos, E.T.; Oser, M.; Yamaguchi, H.; Kim, H.D.; Giampieri, S.; Wang, Y.; Goswami, S.; Wyckoff, J.B.; Lauffenburger, D.A.; et al. A mena invasion isoform potentiates EGF-induced carcinoma cell invasion and metastasis. *Dev. Cell* **2008**, *15*, 813–828. [CrossRef]
38. Shin, S.; Buel, G.R.; Nagiec, M.J.; Han, M.J.; Roux, P.P.; Blenis, J.; Yoon, S.O. Erk2 regulates epithelial-to-mesenchymal plasticity through dock10-dependent rac1/foxo1 activation. *Proc. Natl. Acad. Sci. USA* **2019**, *116*, 2967–2976. [CrossRef]
39. Pastushenko, I.; Brisebarre, A.; Sifrim, A.; Fioramonti, M.; Revenco, T.; Boumahdi, S.; Van Keymeulen, A.; Brown, D.; Moers, V.; Lemaire, S.; et al. Identification of the tumour transition states occurring during emt. *Nature* **2018**, *556*, 463–468. [CrossRef]
40. Nieberler, M.; Reuning, U.; Reichart, F.; Notni, J.; Wester, H.J.; Schwaiger, M.; Weinmuller, M.; Rader, A.; Steiger, K.; Kessler, H. Exploring the role of RGD-recognizing integrins in cancer. *Cancers* **2017**, *9*, 116. [CrossRef]

41. Yamaguchi, H.; Wyckoff, J.; Condeelis, J. Cell migration in tumors. *Curr. Opin. Cell Biol.* **2005**, *17*, 559–564. [CrossRef] [PubMed]
42. Nistico, P.; Bissell, M.J.; Radisky, D.C. Epithelial-mesenchymal transition: General principles and pathological relevance with special emphasis on the role of matrix metalloproteinases. *Cold Spring Harb. Perspect. Biol.* **2012**, *4*. [CrossRef] [PubMed]
43. Yoshida, T.; Akatsuka, T.; Imanaka-Yoshida, K. Tenascin-c and integrins in cancer. *Cell Adh. Migr.* **2015**, *9*, 96–104. [CrossRef] [PubMed]
44. Topalovski, M.; Brekken, R.A. Matrix control of pancreatic cancer: New insights into fibronectin signaling. *Cancer Lett.* **2016**, *381*, 252–258. [CrossRef] [PubMed]
45. Friedl, P.; Alexander, S. Cancer invasion and the microenvironment: Plasticity and reciprocity. *Cell* **2011**, *147*, 992–1009. [CrossRef] [PubMed]
46. Sanz-Moreno, V.; Marshall, C.J. The plasticity of cytoskeletal dynamics underlying neoplastic cell migration. *Curr. Opin. Cell Biol.* **2010**, *22*, 690–696. [CrossRef] [PubMed]
47. Yamada, K.M.; Cukierman, E. Modeling tissue morphogenesis and cancer in 3d. *Cell* **2007**, *130*, 601–610. [CrossRef]
48. Sahai, E.; Marshall, C.J. Differing modes of tumour cell invasion have distinct requirements for rho/rock signalling and extracellular proteolysis. *Nat. Cell Biol.* **2003**, *5*, 711–719. [CrossRef]
49. Wolf, K.; Mazo, I.; Leung, H.; Engelke, K.; von Andrian, U.H.; Deryugina, E.I.; Strongin, A.Y.; Brocker, E.B.; Friedl, P. Compensation mechanism in tumor cell migration: Mesenchymal-amoeboid transition after blocking of pericellular proteolysis. *J. Cell Biol.* **2003**, *160*, 267–277. [CrossRef]
50. Beerling, E.; Seinstra, D.; de Wit, E.; Kester, L.; van der Velden, D.; Maynard, C.; Schafer, R.; van Diest, P.; Voest, E.; van Oudenaarden, A.; et al. Plasticity between epithelial and mesenchymal states unlinks emt from metastasis-enhancing stem cell capacity. *Cell Rep.* **2016**, *14*, 2281–2288. [CrossRef]
51. Zhao, Z.; Zhu, X.; Cui, K.; Mancuso, J.; Federley, R.; Fischer, K.; Teng, G.J.; Mittal, V.; Gao, D.; Zhao, H.; et al. In vivo visualization and characterization of epithelial-mesenchymal transition in breast tumors. *Cancer Res.* **2016**, *76*, 2094–2104. [CrossRef]
52. Shamir, E.R.; Pappalardo, E.; Jorgens, D.M.; Coutinho, K.; Tsai, W.T.; Aziz, K.; Auer, M.; Tran, P.T.; Bader, J.S.; Ewald, A.J. Twist1-induced dissemination preserves epithelial identity and requires e-cadherin. *J. Cell Biol.* **2014**, *204*, 839–856. [CrossRef]
53. Shamir, E.R.; Coutinho, K.; Georgess, D.; Auer, M.; Ewald, A.J. Twist1-positive epithelial cells retain adhesive and proliferative capacity throughout dissemination. *Biol. Open* **2016**, *5*, 1216–1228. [CrossRef]
54. Ilina, O.; Campanello, L.; Gritsenko, P.G.; Vullings, M.; Wang, C.; Bult, P.; Losert, W.; Friedl, P. Intravital microscopy of collective invasion plasticity in breast cancer. *Dis. Model. Mech.* **2018**, *11*. [CrossRef]
55. Giampieri, S.; Manning, C.; Hooper, S.; Jones, L.; Hill, C.S.; Sahai, E. Localized and reversible tgfbeta signalling switches breast cancer cells from cohesive to single cell motility. *Nat. Cell Biol.* **2009**, *11*, 1287–1296. [CrossRef]
56. Lehmann, S.; Te Boekhorst, V.; Odenthal, J.; Bianchi, R.; van Helvert, S.; Ikenberg, K.; Ilina, O.; Stoma, S.; Xandry, J.; Jiang, L.; et al. Hypoxia induces a hif-1-dependent transition from collective-to-amoeboid dissemination in epithelial cancer cells. *Curr. Biol.* **2017**, *27*, 392–400. [CrossRef]
57. Condeelis, J.; Segall, J.E. Intravital imaging of cell movement in tumours. *Nat. Rev. Cancer* **2003**, *3*, 921–930. [CrossRef]
58. Cheung, K.J.; Ewald, A.J. Illuminating breast cancer invasion: Diverse roles for cell–cell interactions. *Curr. Opin. Cell Biol.* **2014**, *30*, 99–111. [CrossRef]
59. Friedl, P.; Gilmour, D. Collective cell migration in morphogenesis, regeneration and cancer. *Nat. Rev. Mol. Cell Biol.* **2009**, *10*, 445–457. [CrossRef]
60. Yu, X.; Zech, T.; McDonald, L.; Gonzalez, E.G.; Li, A.; Macpherson, I.; Schwarz, J.P.; Spence, H.; Futo, K.; Timpson, P.; et al. N-wasp coordinates the delivery and f-actin-mediated capture of mt1-mmp at invasive pseudopods. *J. Cell Biol.* **2012**, *199*, 527–544. [CrossRef]
61. Stuelten, C.H.; Parent, C.A.; Montell, D.J. Cell motility in cancer invasion and metastasis: Insights from simple model organisms. *Nat. Rev. Cancer* **2018**, *18*, 296–312. [CrossRef]
62. Wolf, K.; Wu, Y.I.; Liu, Y.; Geiger, J.; Tam, E.; Overall, C.; Stack, M.S.; Friedl, P. Multi-step pericellular proteolysis controls the transition from individual to collective cancer cell invasion. *Nat. Cell Biol.* **2007**, *9*, 893–904. [CrossRef]

63. Bronsert, P.; Enderle-Ammour, K.; Bader, M.; Timme, S.; Kuehs, M.; Csanadi, A.; Kayser, G.; Kohler, I.; Bausch, D.; Hoeppner, J.; et al. Cancer cell invasion and EMT marker expression: A three-dimensional study of the human cancer-host interface. *J. Pathol.* **2014**, *234*, 410–422. [CrossRef]
64. Hegerfeldt, Y.; Tusch, M.; Brocker, E.B.; Friedl, P. Collective cell movement in primary melanoma explants: Plasticity of cell–cell interaction, beta1-integrin function, and migration strategies. *Cancer Res.* **2002**, *62*, 2125–2130.
65. Nguyen-Ngoc, K.V.; Cheung, K.J.; Brenot, A.; Shamir, E.R.; Gray, R.S.; Hines, W.C.; Yaswen, P.; Werb, Z.; Ewald, A.J. Ecm microenvironment regulates collective migration and local dissemination in normal and malignant mammary epithelium. *Proc. Natl. Acad. Sci. USA* **2012**, *109*, 2595–2604. [CrossRef]
66. Alexander, S.; Koehl, G.E.; Hirschberg, M.; Geissler, E.K.; Friedl, P. Dynamic imaging of cancer growth and invasion: A modified skin-fold chamber model. *Histochem. Cell Biol.* **2008**, *130*, 1147–1154. [CrossRef]
67. Friedl, P.; Locker, J.; Sahai, E.; Segall, J.E. Classifying collective cancer cell invasion. *Nat. Cell Biol.* **2012**, *14*, 777–783. [CrossRef]
68. Westcott, J.M.; Prechtl, A.M.; Maine, E.A.; Dang, T.T.; Esparza, M.A.; Sun, H.; Zhou, Y.; Xie, Y.; Pearson, G.W. An epigenetically distinct breast cancer cell subpopulation promotes collective invasion. *J. Clin. Investig.* **2015**, *125*, 1927–1943. [CrossRef]
69. Konen, J.; Summerbell, E.; Dwivedi, B.; Galior, K.; Hou, Y.; Rusnak, L.; Chen, A.; Saltz, J.; Zhou, W.; Boise, L.H.; et al. Image-guided genomics of phenotypically heterogeneous populations reveals vascular signalling during symbiotic collective cancer invasion. *Nat. Commun.* **2017**, *8*, 15078. [CrossRef]
70. Dang, T.T.; Prechtl, A.M.; Pearson, G.W. Breast cancer subtype-specific interactions with the microenvironment dictate mechanisms of invasion. *Cancer Res.* **2011**, *71*, 6857–6866. [CrossRef]
71. Labernadie, A.; Kato, T.; Brugues, A.; Serra-Picamal, X.; Derzsi, S.; Arwert, E.; Weston, A.; Gonzalez-Tarrago, V.; Elosegui-Artola, A.; Albertazzi, L.; et al. A mechanically active heterotypic e-cadherin/n-cadherin adhesion enables fibroblasts to drive cancer cell invasion. *Nat. Cell Biol.* **2017**, *19*, 224–237. [CrossRef]
72. Celia-Terrassa, T.; Kang, Y. Distinctive properties of metastasis-initiating cells. *Genes Dev.* **2016**, *30*, 892–908. [CrossRef]
73. Gadea, G.; Sanz-Moreno, V.; Self, A.; Godi, A.; Marshall, C.J. Dock10-mediated cdc42 activation is necessary for amoeboid invasion of melanoma cells. *Curr. Biol.* **2008**, *18*, 1456–1465. [CrossRef]
74. Zeltz, C.; Gullberg, D. The integrin-collagen connection—A glue for tissue repair? *J. Cell Sci.* **2016**, *129*, 653–664. [CrossRef]
75. Teckchandani, A.; Mulkearns, E.E.; Randolph, T.W.; Toida, N.; Cooper, J.A. The clathrin adaptor dab2 recruits eh domain scaffold proteins to regulate integrin beta1 endocytosis. *Mol. Biol. Cell* **2012**, *23*, 2905–2916. [CrossRef]
76. Eckert, M.A.; Lwin, T.M.; Chang, A.T.; Kim, J.; Danis, E.; Ohno-Machado, L.; Yang, J. Twist1-induced invadopodia formation promotes tumor metastasis. *Cancer Cell* **2011**, *19*, 372–386. [CrossRef]
77. Maeda, M.; Johnson, K.R.; Wheelock, M.J. Cadherin switching: Essential for behavioral but not morphological changes during an epithelium-to-mesenchyme transition. *J. Cell Sci.* **2005**, *118*, 873–887. [CrossRef]
78. Li, C.F.; Chen, J.Y.; Ho, Y.H.; Hsu, W.H.; Wu, L.C.; Lan, H.Y.; Hsu, D.S.; Tai, S.K.; Chang, Y.C.; Yang, M.H. Snail-induced claudin-11 prompts collective migration for tumour progression. *Nat. Cell Biol.* **2019**, *21*, 251–262. [CrossRef]
79. Jolly, M.K.; Somarelli, J.A.; Sheth, M.; Biddle, A.; Tripathi, S.C.; Armstrong, A.J.; Hanash, S.M.; Bapat, S.A.; Rangarajan, A.; Levine, H. Hybrid epithelial/mesenchymal phenotypes promote metastasis and therapy resistance across carcinomas. *Pharmacol. Ther.* **2019**, *194*, 161–184. [CrossRef]
80. Gaggioli, C.; Hooper, S.; Hidalgo-Carcedo, C.; Grosse, R.; Marshall, J.F.; Harrington, K.; Sahai, E. Fibroblast-led collective invasion of carcinoma cells with differing roles for rhogtpases in leading and following cells. *Nat. Cell Biol.* **2007**, *9*, 1392–1400. [CrossRef]
81. Pearson, G.W.; Hunter, T. Real-time imaging reveals that noninvasive mammary epithelial acini can contain motile cells. *J. Cell Biol.* **2007**, *179*, 1555–1567. [CrossRef]
82. Schliekelman, M.J.; Taguchi, A.; Zhu, J.; Dai, X.; Rodriguez, J.; Celiktas, M.; Zhang, Q.; Chin, A.; Wong, C.H.; Wang, H.; et al. Molecular portraits of epithelial, mesenchymal and hybrid states in lung adenocarcinoma and their relevance to survival. *Cancer Res.* **2015**. [CrossRef]
83. Cheung, K.J.; Gabrielson, E.; Werb, Z.; Ewald, A.J. Collective invasion in breast cancer requires a conserved basal epithelial program. *Cell* **2013**, *155*, 1639–1651. [CrossRef]

84. Dang, T.T.; Westcott, J.M.; Maine, E.A.; Kanchwala, M.; Xing, C.; Pearson, G.W. Deltanp63alpha induces the expression of fat2 and slug to promote tumor invasion. *Oncotarget* **2016**, *7*, 28592–28611. [CrossRef]
85. Dang, T.T.; Esparza, M.A.; Maine, E.A.; Westcott, J.M.; Pearson, G.W. Deltanp63alpha promotes breast cancer cell motility through the selective activation of components of the epithelial-to-mesenchymal transition program. *Cancer Res.* **2015**, *75*, 3925–3935. [CrossRef]
86. Jolly, M.K.; Tripathi, S.C.; Jia, D.; Mooney, S.M.; Celiktas, M.; Hanash, S.M.; Mani, S.A.; Pienta, K.J.; Ben-Jacob, E.; Levine, H. Stability of the hybrid epithelial/mesenchymal phenotype. *Oncotarget* **2016**, *7*, 27067–27084. [CrossRef]
87. Lu, M.; Jolly, M.K.; Levine, H.; Onuchic, J.N.; Ben-Jacob, E. Microrna-based regulation of epithelial-hybrid-mesenchymal fate determination. *Proc. Natl. Acad. Sci. USA* **2013**, *110*, 18144–18149. [CrossRef]
88. Ye, X.; Tam, W.L.; Shibue, T.; Kaygusuz, Y.; Reinhardt, F.; Ng Eaton, E.; Weinberg, R.A. Distinct emt programs control normal mammary stem cells and tumour-initiating cells. *Nature* **2015**, *525*, 256–260. [CrossRef]
89. Rios, A.C.; Capaldo, B.D.; Vaillant, F.; Pal, B.; van Ineveld, R.; Dawson, C.A.; Chen, Y.; Nolan, E.; Fu, N.Y.; Group, D.; et al. Intraclonal plasticity in mammary tumors revealed through large-scale single-cell resolution 3d imaging. *Cancer Cell* **2019**, *35*, 618–632. [CrossRef]
90. Celia-Terrassa, T.; Meca-Cortes, O.; Mateo, F.; Martinez de Paz, A.; Rubio, N.; Arnal-Estape, A.; Ell, B.J.; Bermudo, R.; Diaz, A.; Guerra-Rebollo, M.; et al. Epithelial-mesenchymal transition can suppress major attributes of human epithelial tumor-initiating cells. *J. Clin. Investig.* **2012**, *122*, 1849–1868. [CrossRef]
91. Celia-Terrassa, T.; Bastian, C.; Liu, D.D.; Ell, B.; Aiello, N.M.; Wei, Y.; Zamalloa, J.; Blanco, A.M.; Hang, X.; Kunisky, D.; et al. Hysteresis control of epithelial-mesenchymal transition dynamics conveys a distinct program with enhanced metastatic ability. *Nat. Commun.* **2018**, *9*, 5005. [CrossRef]
92. Calbo, J.; van Montfort, E.; Proost, N.; van Drunen, E.; Beverloo, H.B.; Meuwissen, R.; Berns, A. A functional role for tumor cell heterogeneity in a mouse model of small cell lung cancer. *Cancer Cell* **2011**, *19*, 244–256. [CrossRef]
93. Neelakantan, D.; Zhou, H.; Oliphant, M.U.J.; Zhang, X.; Simon, L.M.; Henke, D.M.; Shaw, C.A.; Wu, M.F.; Hilsenbeck, S.G.; White, L.D.; et al. EMT cells increase breast cancer metastasis via paracrine gli activation in neighbouring tumour cells. *Nat. Commun.* **2017**, *8*, 15773. [CrossRef]
94. Husemann, Y.; Geigl, J.B.; Schubert, F.; Musiani, P.; Meyer, M.; Burghart, E.; Forni, G.; Eils, R.; Fehm, T.; Riethmuller, G.; et al. Systemic spread is an early step in breast cancer. *Cancer Cell* **2008**, *13*, 58–68. [CrossRef]
95. Rhim, A.D.; Mirek, E.T.; Aiello, N.M.; Maitra, A.; Bailey, J.M.; McAllister, F.; Reichert, M.; Beatty, G.L.; Rustgi, A.K.; Vonderheide, R.H.; et al. Emt and dissemination precede pancreatic tumor formation. *Cell* **2012**, *148*, 349–361. [CrossRef]
96. Harper, K.L.; Sosa, M.S.; Entenberg, D.; Hosseini, H.; Cheung, J.F.; Nobre, R.; Avivar-Valderas, A.; Nagi, C.; Girnius, N.; Davis, R.J.; et al. Mechanism of early dissemination and metastasis in HER2(+) mammary cancer. *Nature* **2016**, *540*, 588–592. [CrossRef]
97. Hosseini, H.; Obradovic, M.M.S.; Hoffmann, M.; Harper, K.L.; Sosa, M.S.; Werner-Klein, M.; Nanduri, L.K.; Werno, C.; Ehrl, C.; Maneck, M.; et al. Early dissemination seeds metastasis in breast cancer. *Nature* **2016**, *540*, 552–558. [CrossRef]
98. Rhim, A.D.; Thege, F.I.; Santana, S.M.; Lannin, T.B.; Saha, T.N.; Tsai, S.; Maggs, L.R.; Kochman, M.L.; Ginsberg, G.G.; Lieb, J.G.; et al. Detection of circulating pancreas epithelial cells in patients with pancreatic cystic lesions. *Gastroenterology* **2014**, *146*, 647–651. [CrossRef]
99. Casasent, A.K.; Schalck, A.; Gao, R.; Sei, E.; Long, A.; Pangburn, W.; Casasent, T.; Meric-Bernstam, F.; Edgerton, M.E.; Navin, N.E. Multiclonal invasion in breast tumors identified by topographic single cell sequencing. *Cell* **2018**, *172*, 205–217. [CrossRef]
100. Reichert, M.; Bakir, B.; Moreira, L.; Pitarresi, J.R.; Feldmann, K.; Simon, L.; Suzuki, K.; Maddipati, R.; Rhim, A.D.; Schlitter, A.M.; et al. Regulation of epithelial plasticity determines metastatic organotropism in pancreatic cancer. *Dev. Cell* **2018**, *45*, 696–711. [CrossRef]
101. Aceto, N.; Bardia, A.; Miyamoto, D.T.; Donaldson, M.C.; Wittner, B.S.; Spencer, J.A.; Yu, M.; Pely, A.; Engstrom, A.; Zhu, H.; et al. Circulating tumor cell clusters are oligoclonal precursors of breast cancer metastasis. *Cell* **2014**, *158*, 1110–1122. [CrossRef]
102. Cheung, K.J.; Padmanaban, V.; Silvestri, V.; Schipper, K.; Cohen, J.D.; Fairchild, A.N.; Gorin, M.A.; Verdone, J.E.; Pienta, K.J.; Bader, J.S.; et al. Polyclonal breast cancer metastases arise from collective dissemination of keratin 14-expressing tumor cell clusters. *Proc. Natl. Acad. Sci. USA* **2016**, *113*, 854–863. [CrossRef]

103. Tsai, J.H.; Donaher, J.L.; Murphy, D.A.; Chau, S.; Yang, J. Spatiotemporal regulation of epithelial-mesenchymal transition is essential for squamous cell carcinoma metastasis. *Cancer Cell* **2012**, *22*, 725–736. [CrossRef]
104. Ocana, O.H.; Corcoles, R.; Fabra, A.; Moreno-Bueno, G.; Acloque, H.; Vega, S.; Barrallo-Gimeno, A.; Cano, A.; Nieto, M.A. Metastatic colonization requires the repression of the epithelial-mesenchymal transition inducer PRRX1. *Cancer Cell* **2012**, *22*, 709–724. [CrossRef]
105. Robinson, D.R.; Wu, Y.M.; Lonigro, R.J.; Vats, P.; Cobain, E.; Everett, J.; Cao, X.; Rabban, E.; Kumar-Sinha, C.; Raymond, V.; et al. Integrative clinical genomics of metastatic cancer. *Nature* **2017**, *548*, 297–303. [CrossRef]
106. Castano, Z.; San Juan, B.P.; Spiegel, A.; Pant, A.; DeCristo, M.J.; Laszewski, T.; Ubellacker, J.M.; Janssen, S.R.; Dongre, A.; Reinhardt, F.; et al. Il-1beta inflammatory response driven by primary breast cancer prevents metastasis-initiating cell colonization. *Nat. Cell Biol.* **2018**, *20*, 1084–1097. [CrossRef]
107. Jolly, M.K.; Mani, S.A.; Levine, H. Hybrid epithelial/mesenchymal phenotype(s): The 'fittest' for metastasis? *Biochim. Biophys. Acta Rev. Cancer* **2018**, *1870*, 151–157. [CrossRef]
108. Pastushenko, I.; Blanpain, C. EMT transition states during tumor progression and metastasis. *Trends Cell Biol.* **2019**, *29*, 212–226. [CrossRef]
109. Tam, W.L.; Weinberg, R.A. The epigenetics of epithelial-mesenchymal plasticity in cancer. *Nat. Med.* **2013**, *19*, 1438–1449. [CrossRef]
110. Fischer, K.R.; Durrans, A.; Lee, S.; Sheng, J.; Li, F.; Wong, S.T.; Choi, H.; El Rayes, T.; Ryu, S.; Troeger, J.; et al. Epithelial-to-mesenchymal transition is not required for lung metastasis but contributes to chemoresistance. *Nature* **2015**, *527*, 472–476. [CrossRef]
111. Zheng, X.; Carstens, J.L.; Kim, J.; Scheible, M.; Kaye, J.; Sugimoto, H.; Wu, C.C.; LeBleu, V.S.; Kalluri, R. Epithelial-to-mesenchymal transition is dispensable for metastasis but induces chemoresistance in pancreatic cancer. *Nature* **2015**, *527*, 525–530. [CrossRef]
112. Aiello, N.M.; Brabletz, T.; Kang, Y.; Nieto, M.A.; Weinberg, R.A.; Stanger, B.Z. Upholding a role for EMT in pancreatic cancer metastasis. *Nature* **2017**, *547*, 7–8. [CrossRef]
113. Ye, X.; Brabletz, T.; Kang, Y.; Longmore, G.D.; Nieto, M.A.; Stanger, B.Z.; Yang, J.; Weinberg, R.A. Upholding a role for emt in breast cancer metastasis. *Nature* **2017**, *547*, 1–3. [CrossRef]

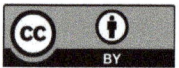

© 2019 by the author. Licensee MDPI, Basel, Switzerland. This article is an open access article distributed under the terms and conditions of the Creative Commons Attribution (CC BY) license (http://creativecommons.org/licenses/by/4.0/).

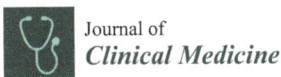

Review

# Consequences of EMT-Driven Changes in the Immune Microenvironment of Breast Cancer and Therapeutic Response of Cancer Cells

Snahlata Singh [1] and Rumela Chakrabarti [1,*]

Department of Biomedical Sciences, School of Veterinary Medicine, University of Pennsylvania, Philadelphia, PA 19104, USA; snsingh@vet.upenn.edu
* Correspondence: rumela@vet.upenn.edu; Tel.: +215-746-1873; Fax: +215-573-5186

Received: 9 April 2019; Accepted: 4 May 2019; Published: 9 May 2019

**Abstract:** Epithelial-to-mesenchymal transition (EMT) is a process through which epithelial cells lose their epithelial characteristics and cell–cell contact, thus increasing their invasive potential. In addition to its well-known roles in embryonic development, wound healing, and regeneration, EMT plays an important role in tumor progression and metastatic invasion. In breast cancer, EMT both increases the migratory capacity and invasive potential of tumor cells, and initiates protumorigenic alterations in the tumor microenvironment (TME). In particular, recent evidence has linked increased expression of EMT markers such as TWIST1 and MMPs in breast tumors with increased immune infiltration in the TME. These immune cells then provide cues that promote immune evasion by tumor cells, which is associated with enhanced tumor progression and metastasis. In the current review, we will summarize the current knowledge of the role of EMT in the biology of different subtypes of breast cancer. We will further explore the correlation between genetic switches leading to EMT and EMT-induced alterations within the TME that drive tumor growth and metastasis, as well as their possible effect on therapeutic response in breast cancer.

**Keywords:** breast cancer; subtypes; EMT; TWIST; MMPs; immune cells; TME; therapy resistance

## 1. Introduction

Breast cancer is a highly complex disease that has been classified into several subtypes based on morphological, immunohistochemical, and phenotypic characteristics of the tumor. The most commonly used classification is based on the presence or absence of hormone receptors. Breast cancers expressing estrogen (ER), progesterone (PR), and herceptin (HER2) receptors are termed hormone receptive while those that lack all three receptors are classified as hormone refractory or triple-negative breast cancer (TNBC) [1,2]. Such heterogeneity complicates choice of treatment options and highlights the critical need to study breast cancer in a subtype-specific manner.

Like other cancers, breast cancer is initiated by transformation of normal cells to cancerous ones. Following this transformation, epithelial-to-mesenchymal transition (EMT) plays an important role in enabling epithelial cells to acquire mesenchymal features and gain invasive potential [3–5], thereby driving cancer progression. During EMT, epithelial cells lose polarity and adhesive junctions that maintain cell–cell contact and undergo transformation to mesenchymal cells. Conversely, during mesenchymal-to-epithelial transformation (MET), tumor cells reacquire their epithelial characteristics and obtain cell–cell contact. MET is an essential step for tumor cells during colonization at the metastatic site [6–8]. EMT drives many developmental processes and is frequently observed in cancers, including breast cancer. EMT in the early stages of carcinogenesis is brought about by a switch in expression patterns of crucial genes, thereby initiating a cascade of cellular, molecular, and morphological changes in cells [3–5]. In addition to the dramatic effect of EMT on tumor cells, it brings a massive change in the dynamic landscape of the tumor microenvironment (TME). At the early stages of transformation, cytokines/chemokines secreted from tumor cells attract various stromal and immune cells to the TME [9,10]. These immune cells in turn provide a niche that facilitates tumor progression, invasion, and metastasis. Studies in the last decade have shown that immune cells in the TME determine the clinical outcome of the disease as well as the response of the tumor to chemo and immune therapy [11–15].

In this review, we will summarize the changes in gene expression during EMT leading to recruitment of immune cells in the TME that in turn facilitate progression, invasion, and metastasis of breast cancer. As breast cancer is notoriously heterogeneous and therapeutic regimen is decided according to the breast cancer subtype, we will focus on the role of EMT in different subtypes of breast cancer. We will also compile findings from studies describing how EMT-mediated changes in the immune landscape of the TME determine the therapeutic response of tumors.

## 2. Breast Cancer Subtypes and Their Association with EMT

As per the most recent molecular classification, breast cancer can be divided into the following subtypes: luminal A and B, HER2 positive, basal-like, and claudin-low. Luminal A and B breast cancers are generally ERα-positive. Luminal B tumors show higher expression of Ki67 and are therefore highly proliferative and associated with a worse prognosis [16,17]. HER2-positive tumors express the oncogene ERBB2 on their membrane [18,19]. Basal-like tumors show high expression of basal cell markers and basal cytokeratins [20,21]. Claudin-low tumors are high in stem-cell-associated processes and display high expression of genes involved in EMT [22,23]. Basal-like and claudin-low subtypes usually lack all of the characterized hormone receptors such as ER, PR, and HER2 and are categorized as triple-negative breast cancer (TNBC).

Breast cancer cells arise from mammary epithelial cells that undergo various transcriptional, morphological, and biochemical changes, including EMT, that contribute to tumorigenesis. Normal mammary epithelial cells undergo EMT, a process that occurs in three distinctive phases, each bearing a distinct cassette of EMT-activating transcription factors (TFs). In the first phase, cells lose their polarity and acquire mesenchymal markers such as vimentin and fibronectin. After morphological changes, a switch in gene expression from epithelial-expressed E-CADHERIN to mesenchymal-expressed N-CADHERIN occurs that is mediated by ZEB1 and SNAIL and is maintained by GOOSECOID and FOXC2. During the third phase of EMT, mesenchymal cells acquire phenotypic and functional cancer stem cell (CSC) properties (CD44$^{high}$CD24$^{low}$, invasive, and tumorsphere-forming abilities) [24]. Acquisition of mesenchymal properties by tumor cells is associated with an upregulation of EMT transcriptional inducers such as TWIST1/2, SNAI2/SLUG, and ZEB1 [25–28]. Physiological regulators such as Notch receptors and ligands, along with Wnt ligands, can induce EMT in mammary epithelial cells. Notch and Wnt factors are also important for different steps of breast cancer initiation and progression [29–33]. In addition, EMT in normal mammary epithelial cells can be induced by overexpression of the apoptosis regulator B-cell lymphoma/leukemia gene 2 (BCL2), highlighting a novel role of BCL2 in EMT [34]. Sarrio et al. showed that the nontumorigenic basal cell lines MCF10A, MCF10-2A, and MCF12A contain an epithelial subpopulation which is epithelial cell adhesion molecule (EPCAM)-positive and spontaneously generates EPCAM negative mesenchymal cells through EMT that exhibit CSC (CD44$^{high}$CD24$^{low}$) properties, as they are capable of forming tumorspheres and have increased invasive potential [25]. Consequently, it was suggested that EMT can increase the heterogeneity of the stem cell population in normal breast tissue, with a subset of epithelial cells displaying normal stem-cell-like features and a mesenchymal subset exhibiting CSC features that may contribute to tumor initiation and early dissemination.

### 2.1. Luminal A and B Breast Cancers and EMT

Tumors of the luminal A subtype are observed in the majority of breast cancer patients and both luminal subtypes A and B express ERα. Although estrogen signaling is necessary for breast tumor growth [35], the ERα signaling pathway can inhibit EMT [36,37], raising the intriguing possibility that ERα expression could be responsible for the better prognosis of luminal A and B patients as compared to TNBC patients. Mechanistically, Ye et al. showed that ERα prevents EMT through repression of SLUG, either by directly decreasing its transcription or by repressing the nuclear coreceptor which binds to the SLUG promoter, thereby increasing expression of E-CADHERIN [36]. In a similar study, Wang et al. reported that ERα inhibits EMT by inhibiting RELB-dependent BCL2 expression in luminal breast cancer cell lines [37]. Alternatively, another study showed that ERα suppresses BM1 and therefore promotes stemness and EMT in breast cancer cells [38]. It will be interesting to determine how ERα signaling promotes these distinct functions in breast cancer cells and how these events are regulated in future experiments.

Extrinsic factors, like the multipotent cytokine transforming growth factor β (TGF-β) stimulates EMT in breast cancers [39] and mechanistically, TGF-β stimulation is associated with upregulation of SNAIL, TWIST, ZEB1/2 in luminal A and B breast cancer cell lines [40–42]. TGF-β-induced EMT activates EGFR-, IGF1R-, and MAPK-dependent ERα signaling and promotes antiestrogen resistance [43]. Similar to the TGF-β pathway, the MEK–ERK pathway represses ESE1, a member of the ETS transcription factor family, resulting in upregulation of ETS1-regulated ZEBs. Therefore, activation of MEK–ERK positively correlates with an EMT phenotype in the luminal subtype of breast cancer [44,45]. Finally, in the luminal cancer cell line MCF7, VEGFR expression positively correlates with expression of SNAIL and N-CADHERIN, key regulators of EMT [46]. These studies suggest that while ERα can prevent EMT, environmental stimuli such as TGF-β and activators of the MEK–ERK pathway can promote EMT in luminal cancer, indicating that the final outcome depends on a balance between these pathways.

## 2.2. HER2-Positive Breast Cancer and EMT

Similar to luminal subtypes of breast cancer, HER2-positive breast cancers also undergo TGF-β-dependent EMT. Chihara et al. showed that the TGF-β–SMAD3 pathway is critical for EMT in HER2-positive cancers [47]. Analysis of signaling pathways influencing TGF-β expression in HER2-positive tumors revealed that silencing of AXL, a receptor tyrosine kinase that correlates with poor survival in HER2-positive patients, in a patient-derived xenograft reduces TGF-β, thereby impairing invasion [48]. Notably, HER2 directly regulates the production of TGF-β and activation of TGF-β/SMAD3 signaling [49]. This HER2/EGFR signaling controls the switch from a cell proliferative function for TGF-β to promotion of cell migration [50], therefore making it a central player in the functional consequences of EMT in HER2-positive tumors.

Along with TGF-β/SMAD3 signaling, upregulation of transcription factors SLUG and TWIST1 plays an important role in EMT in this breast cancer subtype. In HER2-positive breast cancer cell lines, MDA-MB-453 and BT474, Carpenter et al. showed that activation of AKT signaling upregulates SLUG expression [51]. However, clinical studies in which patients were categorized based on surface marker expressions showed that HER2-positive patients do not exhibit strong nuclear expression of SLUG [52], highlighting the need for further careful investigation. TWIST1, a known regulator of EMT, is highly phosphorylated on Serine 68 residue in HER2-positive invasive ductal carcinomas, thereby stabilizing the protein and promoting breast cancer invasiveness [53]. In addition, overexpression of HER2 in MCF7 luminal cells increased the expression of breast tumor kinase (Btk)/protein tyrosine kinase 6 (PTK-6) receptors, thereby augmenting EMT and invasive potential [54].

These studies collectively establish the role of TGF-β-associated pathways along with TWIST and SLUG genes in mediating EMT in HER2-positive breast cancer. Further studies are needed to identify novel pathways and mechanisms behind EMT in HER2-positive breast cancer.

## 2.3. TNBC or Basal-Like, Claudin-Low Breast Cancer and EMT

TNBCs are the most aggressive subtype of breast cancer, with limited therapeutic options due to their lack of hormone-responsive receptors. Based on their molecular characteristics, TNBC can be further divided into different subtypes such as PAM50, Vanderbilt, Baylor, and French [55]. In addition, TNBCs can be classified into four categories; basal-like, mesenchymal, immunomodulatory, and luminal androgen receptor (AR)-positive subtypes [56]. In the basal-like subtype of TNBC, cell cycle and DNA damage response pathways are highly activated, so these tumors are often treated with platinum drugs and ADP-ribose polymerase (PARP) inhibitors that target these pathways [57–59]. Genome analysis of mesenchymal TNBC tumors shows high expression of gene clusters involved in growth factor signaling, such as PI3K/AKT, along with an increase in EMT gene signatures. Accordingly, these tumors are susceptible to mTOR inhibitors and eribulin mesylate, which is an inhibitor of EMT [60]. Immunomodulatory TNBCs are enriched in gene pathways related to immune cell signaling associated with immune cell recruitment, as well as signal transduction such as NFκB and JAK/STAT pathways. Thus, in patients with immunomodulatory TNBC, immune checkpoint inhibitors have yielded promising results [61,62]. Luminal androgen receptor (AR)-positive subtype tumors have high levels of androgen-associated signaling and are therefore responsive to androgen receptor blockade [63].

EMT-related factors that have been widely described in TNBC are Notch and Hedgehog, TGF-β, and WNTs. High Notch expression in tumor samples from TNBC patients correlates with poor survival [64]. NUMB, an evolutionary conserved protein important for cell fate determination, antagonizes Notch signaling to prevent EMT in TNBC [65]. JAGGED1, a Notch ligand, can activate Notch signaling to induce EMT through upregulation of SLUG, which in turn represses the expression of E-CADHERIN [66]. Another recent study has shown that the Notch receptor NOTCH3 is important for TNBC breast cancer growth [67]. Moreover, reports show that NOTCH1 and NOTCH4 represent potential biomarkers in TNBC due to their high expression [68]. However, their connection to EMT in breast cancer is not very clear and further studies are needed to confirm the involvement of Notch signaling at the level of each receptor and ligands for EMT in TNBC. Like the Notch pathway, the Hedgehog pathway is crucial for embryonic development and stem cell renewal, and has also been associated with EMT in breast cancer. Hedgehog signaling activates three glioma-associated oncogenes, GLI1, 2, and 3. By employing a high-throughput screen, Colavito et al. have identified GLI1 as a critical determinant of EMT in breast cancer cell lines [69]. Activation of GLI1 is also associated with hypoxia-induced EMT and invasive potential of MDA-MB-231 TNBC cells [70]. Other Hedgehog signaling factors like SHH, PTCH1, and GLI2 are overexpressed in breast cancer, but their connection to EMT is not well established in breast cancer [71,72].

As in other types of breast cancer, TGF-β-mediated regulation of N-CADHERIN, BCL2, and CYCLIN D1 determines EMT and stemness in MDA-MB-231 TNBC cells [73]. In addition, musculoaponeurotic fibrosarcoma (MAF) oncogene family protein K (MAFK) induces EMT in a TGF-β-dependent manner in TNBC cell lines [74]. These studies suggest that TGF-β could be a universal master regulator of EMT in tumor cells. The functional importance of EMT in tumor progression was further demonstrated by addition of selective inhibitors of inducible nitric oxide synthase (iNOS), an enzyme associated with poor prognosis in TNBC patients. These inhibitors limited migration and self-renewal properties of TNBC cells along with reducing the levels of EMT transcription factors such as SNAIL, SLUG, TWIST1, and ZEB1 [75]. Interestingly, targeting β3 integrins using nanoparticles-based siRNA inhibited EMT and metastasis in TNBC tumors by attenuating TGF-β signaling [76]. Thus, TGF-β is connected to EMT either directly or indirectly promoting breast cancer progression.

Aberrant Wnt signaling is a characteristic of TNBC, with both canonical and noncanonical pathways implicated in TNBC tumorigenesis and metastasis [77,78]. Enrichment of Wnt/β-catenin signaling is evident in TNBC and is associated with poor clinical outcome within this subtype [78]. Earlier studies from our group showed that ΔNP63, a transcription factor, upregulates FZD7, a Wnt receptor, thereby increasing Wnt signaling and EMT in normal mammary stem cells and basal subtype of breast cancer [77]. Along with Wnt activators, GSK3β, a canonical Wnt pathway inhibitor, plays an important role in EMT in TNBC cells. A recent study shows that GSK3β is a potential therapeutic target for TNBCs and suggests that GSK3β inhibitors could serve as selective inhibitors of EMT and CSC function in the treatment of a subset of aggressive TNBC with more mesenchymal cells [79]. Another recent study shows that WNT10B, a noncanonical ligand, is important for EMT and CSC-like phenotypes in TNBC in a preclinical mouse model [80]. Together, these studies highlight that EMT is an integral part of multiple subsets of breast cancer. It can be regulated by diverse cell signaling mechanisms, and therapeutic targeting of EMT pathway may be beneficial, even in breast cancer subtypes that are notoriously treatment-resistant. We have summarized various genes and pathways responsible for EMT in different breast cancer subtypes in Table 1.

**Table 1.** Table shows genes and pathways involved in mediating EMT in different subtypes of breast.

| Breast Cancer Subtypes | Genes Involved | Signaling Pathways Involved | References |
|---|---|---|---|
| Luminal A and B | SLUG, BCL2, BM1, TGF-β, TWIST, ZEB1/2, ETS1, VEGFR | ERα signaling, TGF-β signaling, EGFR-, IGFR-, and MAPK-dependent, MEK–ERK | [36–46] |
| HER2-positive | TGF-β, TWIST1, PTK-6 | TGF-β signaling, AKT signaling, HER2/EGFR signaling | [47–50,52–54] |
| TNBC (Basal and Claudin-Low) | TGF-β, GLI1, SNAIL, SLUG, TWIST1, ZEB1, ΔNP63, GSK3β | PI3K/AKT, Notch signaling, Hedgehog signaling, Wnt signaling | [59,63–79] |

## 3. EMT Shapes the TME

Multiple studies demonstrate that EMT is associated with increased dissemination and metastasis of tumor cells to other organs [26,81,82]. In part, this is due to the ability of tumor cells undergoing EMT to modulate the TME. Dvorak H.F. in 1986 in his highly cited article, "Tumors: wounds that do not heal: Similarities between tumor stromal generation and wound healing", explains how phenomena that occur within tumor stroma are similar to processes underway at a wound site [83]. Later studies by Coussens et al. suggested that precancerous cells are identified as a "wound" by mast cells [84], and similar to wounds, high numbers of platelets are found at sites of tumorigenesis [83,84]. Coussens and Hanahan went on to describe tumor growth as a biphasic event [85]. In the first phase, the body treats the tumor site as a wound and tumor growth is promoted by stromal cells. In the second phase, the tumor takes control of proinflammatory cytokines and shapes the TME to further support cancer growth and metastasis. Similar observations are seen in breast cancer where the tumor growth is aided by the TME and at the same time the TME confers proinvasive features to the tumor cells [86].

Based on these observations, it is critical to understand the transcriptional events within the tumor that have a subsequent impact on TME function, thereby influencing tumor progression. RUNX3, a member of the RUNX family of transcription factors, is frequently connected to breast cancer [87]. The immune suppressive role of RUNX3 has been reported in breast tumors via regulation of Tregs. A recent report found that RUNX3 binds to the promoter of FOXP3 and increases Treg population in the tumor microenvironment, which is associated with the progression of breast tumors [88]. However, RUNX3 has also been indicated as a tumor suppressor in breast cancer, which needs further careful evaluation [87]. Similar to RUNX3, the transcription factor GATA3 inhibits breast cancer progression and metastasis by altering the TME [89,90]. Furthermore, overexpression of members of the ETS family of transcription factors can promote increased numbers of immune cells in the TME to drive tumor progression. For example, complete deletion of ETS2 from epithelial and stromal cells in breast tumors leads to early hyperplastic growth and tumor formation by affecting MMP-3 and MMP-9 in macrophages in TME [91,92]. We have reported that ELF5, another member of the ETS family, suppresses EMT and metastasis of TNBC cells [93]. In an unpublished work from our lab, we have seen that loss of ELF5 in a preclinical TNBC mouse model not only enhances tumor growth and metastasis, but also leads to increased numbers of immune cells in the TME. Previously, we had shown that another transcription factor, ΔNP63, promotes stem cell activity in basal tumors [77] and that its expression positively correlates with EMT in basal tumors [77]. Recently, we showed that overexpression of ΔNP63 induces tumor cell production of CXCL2 and CCL22, chemokines responsible for recruitment of MDSCs and enhancing growth and metastasis of basal tumors [94]. P53, a tumor suppressor, regulates miRNAs to inhibit EMT and stem cells by regulation [95]. In a separate study, p53 levels were associated with increased numbers of lymphocytes in basal breast cancer [96]. These studies suggest that transcription factors intrinsic to tumors are important in shaping the TME. For a comprehensive understanding of how cancer cell intrinsic mechanisms such as transcription factors and other genes shape tumor immune microenvironment, please refer to the recent extensive review [97].

Preparation of tumor in premetastatic niches also involves modulation of the extracellular matrix (ECM). Matrix metalloproteinases (MMPs) are a group of 23 enzymes, 17 of which are secreted and 6 are membrane-bound. MMPs are implicated in modification of the ECM, leading to tumor development, migration, and invasion. MMP-3 or MMP-7 overexpression in the mammary epithelium generates premalignant lesions and spontaneous tumor formation [98,99]. On the contrary, MMP-11 knockout mice treated with the carcinogen 7,12-dimethylbenzanthracene (DMBA) develop fewer tumors than control [100]. While epithelial cells can produce MMPs that promote protumorigenic changes in the ECM, a few reports suggest that epithelial cells undergoing EMT can also give rise to myofibroblasts and stromal-like cells that are an essential part of tumor stroma [101,102]. These myofibroblasts produce additional MMPs to assist tumor growth and invasion [103–105].

In addition to modulating ECM at the site of tumor generation, epithelial cells undergoing EMT secrete soluble factors and cytokines to create an inflammatory environment for recruitment of lymphocytes, leucocytes, and other immune cells. Two of the well-studied cytokines produced by tumor cells are Interleukin 6 (IL-6) and IL-8. IL-6 is overexpressed in multiple cancers including breast cancer [106,107] and high expression levels correlate with poor clinical outcomes in cancer patients [108]. IL-6 promotes tumorigenesis in a cancer cell autonomous manner as well as by influencing the differentiation of immune cells [109,110], including B cells, T cells, and myeloid cells, and by promoting immunoglobulin production by B cells. Circulating IL-6 levels correlate with worsening prognosis in metastatic breast cancer patients and also correlate with the extent of the disease [111]. In breast cancer, IL-6 on tumor cells has been shown to induce EMT by repressing E-CADHERIN via STAT3 activation [112]. In another study involving multiple breast cancer subsets, IL-6 has been shown to increase cancer stem cell properties of tumor cells via EMT [113]. IL-6 levels also correlate to increased number of MDSCs, tumor-associated neutrophils (TANs), regulatory T cells (Tregs) in many cancers including breast cancer, suggesting that the consequent immune-suppressive environment contributes to cancer evasion [114]. Dominguez et al. reported that neutralization of IL-8 in TNBCs not only reduces their mesenchymalization but also reduces the number of polymorphonuclear MDSCs (PMN-MDSCs). This suggests that IL-8 both promotes EMT in tumors and recruits immune cells involved in creating an immunosuppressive TME for progression and metastasis of tumor cells [115]. Together, these studies suggest that soluble factors and chemokines secreted by epithelial cells undergoing EMT play a critical role in restructuring the ECM and immune landscape to support tumor proliferation, progression, and metastasis.

## 4. Regulation of EMT by Immune Cells in TME

As detailed above, soluble factors released by cells undergoing EMT create an inflammatory milieu that promotes recruitment of immune cells to the site of tumorigenesis. These immune cells infiltrate the TME and assist tumor growth. In this subsection, we will highlight how different immune cells like macrophages, MDSCs, NK, and Tregs promote EMT and tumor progression in breast cancer.

Macrophages are monocytes that can be differentiated into M1 (antitumorigenic) and M2 (protumorigenic) phenotypes [116]. Recruitment of monocytes to the TME through stimuli such as CCL2/monocyte chemoattractant protein 1 (MCP-1) or colony-stimulating factor 1 (CSF-1) is well studied [117–119]. Stimulation of such monocytes with IL-4/IL-13, IL-10, or TGF-β leads to generation of M2 macrophages [120] or TAMs which facilitate tumor angiogenesis and immune suppression, invasion, and metastasis by limiting the ability of CD8$^+$ cytotoxic T cells. Macrophages are thought to promote early dissemination of cancer, angiogenesis, and metastasis by enhancing CSC-like features in tumor cells through EMT [121,122]. Specifically, TAMs secrete proangiogenic factors such as VEGF, PDGF, TGF-β and MMPs, IL-6, and IL-1 to induce neovascularization and promote EMT [123–125]. Through modulation of the TME and ECM, TAMs provide a prometastatic environment for tumor cells. In ER-positive luminal cancer cells like MCF7 and T47D, secretory factors like MMP-9 promote invasive and migratory potential in cancer cells once they are cultured with macrophages [126]. Depletion of TAMs by anti-CSF1 antibody, which is a macrophage regulator, in a luminal breast cancer model leads to a reduction in tumor growth [127]. In this model, increased TAMs result in a TME rich in TGF-β, an inducer of EMT, and is associated with increased invasion by tumor cells. TAM numbers also correlate with EMT and low E-cadherin expression levels and can therefore be used as an unfavorable prognostic factor for TNBC [128]. These data suggest that TAMs may promote EMT in multiple breast subsets to promote tumor progression and metastasis. As such, defining the precise mechanisms regulating the differentiation of TAMs from infiltrating macrophages in breast cancer may provide crucial insight for therapeutic intervention.

Myeloid-derived suppressor cells (MDSCs) contribute to invasion and metastasis of cancer in multiple ways, but their primary action is through suppression of the antitumor immune response [129]. Myeloid cells infiltrating into the TME during initial stages of tumorigenesis differentiate into MDSCs in the chronic proinflammatory environment of the TME. Indeed, activated T cells secrete IFN-γ, which plays a crucial role in differentiation of MDSCs from myeloid cells [130,131]. These activated MDSCs express CD40 and PD-L1, which suppress the antitumor response of T cells [132,133]. Additionally, MDSCs produce Prostaglandins E2 that amplify MDSC populations in the TME [134]. Indoleamine 2,3-dioxygenase (IDO) is often expressed on tumor cells and are responsible for recruitment of MDSCs in creating an immune-suppressive environment [135] via regulatory T cells (TRegs) which produce kynurenine in several cancers like melanoma [136]. This suggests that therapeutic targeting of IDO could be one of the central regulators of immune suppression. Similar correlation between IDO and MDSC has been observed in metastatic breast cancer patients [137]. Future studies delineating the molecular mechanism of IDO-mediated recruitment of MDSCs in breast cancer may provide innovative therapeutic strategies.

In addition to the immune suppressive property of MDSCs, recent studies show a novel nonimmunologic function of MDSCs in increasing CSCs in breast cancer, which in turn makes the tumor cells more invasive and metastatic [138–140]. Our study showed that PMN MDSCs are higher in the basal subset of TNBC and are recruited in a ΔNP63-dependent manner [94]. In return, these MDSC secrete prometastatic factors that increase EMT gene signatures and CSC gene signatures in the TNBC cells, making them more invasive and metastatic. In another recent example using the 4T1 TNBC mouse model, it was shown that CXCR2$^+$ MDSCs induces cancer cell EMT by IL-6 and these CXCR2$^+$ MDSCs promotes T cell exhaustion, suggesting that CXCR2$^+$ MDSCs may be a potential therapeutic target of TNBC [141]. Interestingly, MDSCs differentiate to tumor-associated macrophages in tumors, which are often more immune suppressive and support cancer stem cell properties. Together, MDSC and TAMs promote EMT and metastasis of breast cancer [142]. Thus, understanding the molecular mechanism of this differentiation step is integral to development of novel drugs targeting these immune-suppressive cells in breast cancer.

NK cells are classically known to induce antitumor immune responses [143,144]. However, multiple recent reports suggest that they may also promote tumor progression and metastasis in cancers in part by regulating EMT [145–147]. IL-18, present in the TME, can upregulate PD-1 expression on NK cells, resulting in an immune suppressive phenotype [148]. NK cells residing in tumors have a reduced antibody-dependent, cell-mediated cytotoxicity (ADCC) potential, thus limiting their antitumor activity [149,150]. Interestingly, tumor cells expressing Cell Adhesion Molecule 1 (CADM1), a cell adhesion molecule directly induced by the EMT-promoting TGF-β pathway [151], are susceptible to NK cell-mediated cytotoxicity [152]. In a cohort of breast cancer patients, CADM1 expression correlated with improved patient survival [153]. While these studies point towards a strong association between NK cell function and EMT in tumors, further investigation on their role in tumorigenesis is required.

T cells are a critical regulatory factor in tumor biology. CD8+ cytotoxic T cells secrete antitumor cytokines such as TNFα and IFN-γ that restrict the growth and metastasis of tumors [154–156].

However, CD8+ T cells within the TME frequently exhibit an "exhausted" phenotype due to overexposure to tumor antigens and/or the presence of immune suppressive antigens on tumor cells. Exhausted T cells neither produce antitumor cytokines nor undergo proliferation, thus restricting their antitumor activities [157]. In addition, FoxP3+ Tregs help tumor cells grow and metastasize through production of protumorigenic cytokines and expression of immunomodulatory receptors that suppress immune response and facilitate tumor growth [158]. Moreover, Tregs promote β-catenin-mediated EMT during radiation-induced pulmonary fibrosis [159], however, the molecular mechanism is not clear. In this regard, in our unpublished study, we have observed high levels of Treg infiltration in a preclinical murine model of TNBC undergoing EMT. Our future studies will establish the molecular mechanisms behind the association of Tregs and EMT in TNBC. Together, these reports collectively highlight that immune cells in the TME recruited during early stages of EMT additionally assist tumor cells in their proliferation, invasion, and metastasis in breast cancer.

## 5. EMT, TME, and Therapeutic Resistance of Tumor Cells

Resistance to therapy is one of the biggest challenges in tumor biology and was initially identified in the early 1990s in breast cancer cells [160]. EMT was implicated in conferring resistance to both conventional therapies such as radiation and chemotherapy and targeted therapies like the estrogen antagonists, Tamoxifen and Fulvestrant or cell cycle inhibitors, each used in specific subtypes of breast cancer. However, in recent years, immunotherapy has gained momentum. Under this section, we will discuss the effects of an EMT-driven protumorigenic TME on different therapeutic options, primarily focusing on chemo and immunotherapy resistance.

### 5.1. Chemotherapy

The response to chemotherapeutic drugs in breast cancer varies from patient to patient. Various groups have studied the correlation between the degree of response and immune cells present in the TME. Denkert C et al. 2010 showed that tumor-associated lymphocytes are an independent predictor of anthracycline/taxane response in breast cancer patients [161]. It is worth noting that these tumor-infiltrating lymphocytes could also promote EMT in multiple ways [162], further supporting the premise that the response to anthracycline/taxane could be dependent on EMT in tumor cells. In support, a recent study by Salvagno et al. demonstrated that targeting macrophages that are directly linked to EMT in tumors enhances the chemotherapeutic response of spontaneous mammary tumors [163]. In addition, Ladoire et al. observed that prior to neoadjuvant chemotherapy, patients display increased numbers of CD3-, CD8-, and FOXP3-positive cells [164]. However, patients who responded to therapy had significantly fewer FOXP3-positive cells than did nonresponders, in whom FOXP3-positive cells remained high. The authors concluded that high CD8+ and low FOXP3+ staining predicts a better response to neoadjuvant therapy in breast cancer. In contrast, other studies suggest that TNFα secreted by CD8+ cells through sphingosine kinase mediates tamoxifen resistance in MCF7 cells [165,166]. Therefore, correlation of CD8+ cells secreting TNFα and tamoxifen response needs further evaluation.

A potential role for MDSC-mediated increases in CSCs in chemoresistance has also been noted. Specifically, Montero et al. observed that the number of circulating MDSCs in breast cancer patients increase upon Doxorubicin-cyclophosphamide chemotherapy [167]. As MDSCs promote EMT in tumor cells, the consequent increase in CSC-like properties [139,168] could be responsible for decreased efficacy of Doxorubicin-cyclophosphamide in breast cancer patients. Together, these studies suggest that drug resistance to chemotherapy is linked to altered immune cells and cancer cells which needs to be studied in depth for better development of drugs against resistance.

Similar to chemotherapy, several monoclonal antibodies targeting immune cells such as Tregs (CD25 antibody) have shown some success in preclinical models, however, their function as monotherapy in established patient tumors is limited [169]. Moreover, antiangiogenic therapy with antibodies against vascular endothelial growth factor (VEGF) has not proven effective in patients with many tumor types, including breast cancer. VEGF has been shown to involve T cell development and therefore has been suggested to be connected to tumor-induced immune suppression [170]. It is recently shown that such resistance could be due to VEGF-mediated activation of IL-6 involving tumor microenvironment [171]. Trastuzumab, an FDA-approved anti-HER2 antibody, shows a 35% response rate in metastatic breast cancer patients, however, exact mechanisms of action are still unknown. It is believed that Trastuzumab alters signaling activation of immune effector mechanisms. It would be interesting to determine if such resistance is due to involvement of EMT, tumor microenvironment, and immune cells [172].

*5.2. Immunotherapy*

TNBC tumors, which lack known hormone receptors, are insensitive to hormone-based therapies and are often resistant to chemo and radiotherapy. However, these tumors are highly immunogenic and therefore immunotherapy for treatment of TNBC may be particularly useful. Checkpoint inhibitors such as PD-1 (Nivolumab, Pembrolizumab), PD-L1 (Atezolizumab, Avelumab), and CTLA4 (Ipilimumab) block the immunomodulatory pathways between tumor cells and immune cells that assist in immune evasion and are currently in clinical trials. PD-L1 expression varies from 20% to 50% in all types of breast cancer subtypes [173,174] and is higher in TNBC patients as compared to non-TNBC [174,175]. Accordingly, variable responses to checkpoint-based therapy could be dependent on expression levels of PD-L1 ligand on tumor cells. PD-L1 expression in EMT-activated breast cancer cells depends on the EMT-TF (ZEB1). Specifically, Noman et al. showed that mutual regulatory loop exists between two processes orchestrated by ZEB1, which functions as a transcriptional repressor of miR-200 that is able to activate the EMT program and as an activator of PD-L1 expression in tumor cells, leading to CD8$^+$ T cells immunosuppression [176]. A similar correlation between PD-L1 and ZEB1 expression was found in nonsmall cell lung carcinoma (NSCLC) [177]. In NSCLC, patients with circulating tumor cells (CTCs) positive for PD-L1 were resistant to Nivolumab while those with PD-L1-negative CTCs were responsive [178,179]. Notably, these PD-L1-positive CTCs showed EMT features, identifying EMT as a predictive biomarker for response towards checkpoint inhibitors in breast, NSCLC, and other tumor types. Additionally, these results provide a novel preclinical rationale to explore EMT inhibitors as adjuvants to boost immunotherapeutic responses in subgroups of patients in whom malignant progression is driven by EMT-promoting transcription factors.

Checkpoint inhibitors in combination with chemotherapy drugs increase the rate of complete clinical response in several cancers including breast cancer. Pembrolizumab added to a neoadjuvant regimen consisting of cisplatin and doxorubicin increased the response of patients (NCT01042379) and similar observations have been observed with anti-PDL1 and anti-CTLA4 drugs. A combinatorial approach of more than one checkpoint inhibitor with chemotherapy for treatment of breast cancer patients is currently underway in clinical trial (NCT01928394). Along with designing combinatorial strategies of checkpoint inhibitors and chemotherapeutic drugs, researchers are also trying to inhibit immune cells such as T cells and M1 macrophages along with treatment with checkpoint blockers as potential strategies to overcome resistance to checkpoint inhibitors observed in some patients [180,181]. Together, these studies reveal that immune cells in the TME have a significant impact on the response of patients to different drugs, and suggest that regulation of EMT in tumor cells may provide a way to influence the immune landscape to increase therapeutic response.

## 6. Conclusions

In this review, we have summarized the factors that determine EMT in different breast cancer subtypes and highlighted studies revealing how epithelial cancer cells undergoing EMT modulate the TME to promote tumorigenesis and enhance recruitment of immune cells. Notably, immune cell recruitment further enhances the ability of tumor cells to undergo EMT, thereby assisting in their tumor progression, invasion, and metastasis. Finally, we highlighted how immune cells and stromal components in TME determine the chemotherapeutic and immunotherapeutic response of patients. Resistance to checkpoint inhibitor-based immunotherapy can be answered through investigation of TME components. Blockade of their migration or recruitment into the tumor site may result in better immunotherapeutic response. The recruitment of immune cells into the tumor site is dependent on EMT in tumor cells. Thus future studies identifying novel combination therapies targeting immune cells in TME and tumor cells undergoing EMT will improve prognosis for breast cancer patients.

In a nutshell, a pictorial representation of the circuit between neoplastic mammary epithelial cells to mesenchymal cells and recruitment of immune cells in TME and its overall impact on therapy is provided in Figure 1.

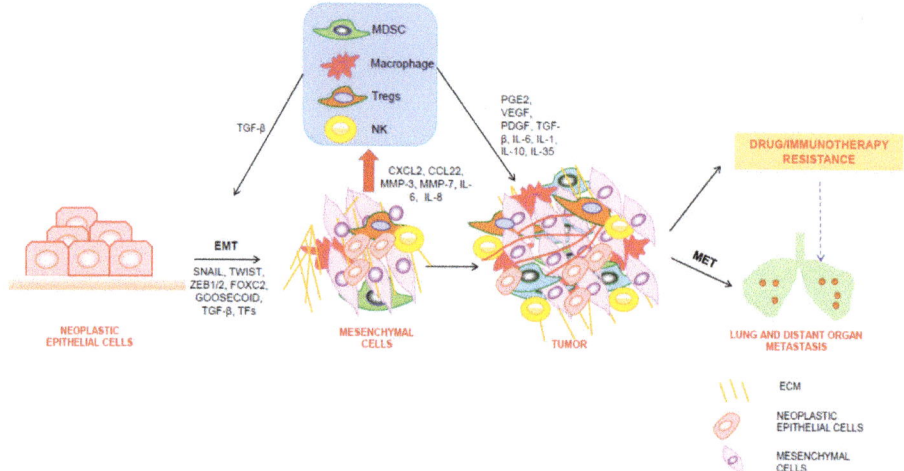

**Figure 1.** EMT, TME, and therapy. Neoplastic mammary epithelial cells undergoing transcriptional changes in key genes involved in EMT are transformed into mesenchymal cells. These mesenchymal cells secrete extracellular factors responsible for recruitment of immune cells and modulation of ECM. Recruited immune cells provide a proinflammatory milieu for growth of tumors by further secreting growth-promoting and prometastatic cytokines.

**Author Contributions:** Writing—review and editing, S.S. and R.C.; Visualization, S.S. and R.C.; supervision, S.S. and R.C.; project administration, S.S. and R.C.

**Acknowledgments:** We thank Leslie King, School of Veterinary Medicine, University of Pennsylvania for critical inputs on the review and helpful discussions.

**Conflicts of Interest:** The authors declare no conflict of interest.

## References

1. Desmedt, C.; Haibe-Kains, B.; Wirapati, P.; Buyse, M.; Larsimont, D.; Bontempi, G.; Delorenzi, M.; Piccart, M.; Sotiriou, C. Biological processes associated with breast cancer clinical outcome depend on the molecular subtypes. *Clin. Cancer Res.* **2008**, *14*, 5158–5165. [CrossRef]
2. Rouzier, R.; Perou, C.M.; Symmans, W.F.; Ibrahim, N.; Cristofanilli, M.; Anderson, K.; Hess, K.R.; Stec, J.; Ayers, M.; Wagner, P.; et al. Breast cancer molecular subtypes respond differently to preoperative chemotherapy. *Clin. Cancer Res.* **2005**, *11*, 5678–5685. [CrossRef] [PubMed]
3. Kalluri, R.; Weinberg, R.A. The basics of epithelial-mesenchymal transition. *J. Clin. Investig.* **2009**, *119*, 1420–1428. [CrossRef]

4. Lamouille, S.; Xu, J.; Derynck, R. Molecular mechanisms of epithelial-mesenchymal transition. *Nat. Rev. Mol. Cell Biol.* **2014**, *15*, 178–196. [CrossRef]
5. Thiery, J.P.; Sleeman, J.P. Complex networks orchestrate epithelial-mesenchymal transitions. *Nat. Rev. Mol. Cell Biol.* **2006**, *7*, 131–142. [CrossRef] [PubMed]
6. Del Pozo Martin, Y.; Park, D.; Ramachandran, A.; Ombrato, L.; Calvo, F.; Chakravarty, P.; Spencer-Dene, B.; Derzsi, S.; Hill, C.S.; Sahai, E.; et al. Mesenchymal Cancer Cell-Stroma Crosstalk Promotes Niche Activation. Epithelial Reversion, and Metastatic Colonization. *Cell Rep.* **2015**, *13*, 2456–2469. [CrossRef] [PubMed]
7. Stankic, M.; Pavlovic, S.; Chin, Y.; Brogi, E.; Padua, D.; Norton, L.; Massague, J.; Benezra, R. TGF-beta-Id1 signaling opposes Twist1 and promotes metastatic colonization via a mesenchymal-to-epithelial transition. *Cell Rep.* **2013**, *5*, 1228–1242. [CrossRef] [PubMed]
8. Gunasinghe, N.P.; Wells, A.; Thompson, E.W.; Hugo, H.J. Mesenchymal-epithelial transition (MET) as a mechanism for metastatic colonisation in breast cancer. *Cancer Metastasis Rev.* **2012**, *31*, 469–478. [CrossRef] [PubMed]
9. Brenot, A.; Knolhoff, B.L.; DeNardo, D.G.; Longmore, G.D. SNAIL1 action in tumor cells influences macrophage polarization and metastasis in breast cancer through altered GM-CSF secretion. *Oncogenesis* **2018**, *7*, 32. [CrossRef] [PubMed]
10. Cortes, M.; Sanchez-Moral, L.; de Barrios, O.; Fernandez-Acenero, M.J.; Martinez-Campanario, M.C.; Esteve-Codina, A.; Darling, D.S.; Gyorffy, B.; Lawrence, T.; Dean, D.C.; et al. Tumor-associated macrophages (TAMs) depend on ZEB1 for their cancer-promoting roles. *EMBO J.* **2017**, *36*, 3336–3355. [CrossRef]
11. De Palma, M.; Lewis, C.E. Macrophage regulation of tumor responses to anticancer therapies. *Cancer Cell* **2013**, *23*, 277–286. [CrossRef]
12. Hanahan, D.; Coussens, L.M. Accessories to the crime: Functions of cells recruited to the tumor microenvironment. *Cancer Cell* **2012**, *21*, 309–322. [CrossRef] [PubMed]
13. Swartz, M.A.; Iida, N.; Roberts, E.W.; Sangaletti, S.; Wong, M.H.; Yull, F.E.; Coussens, L.M.; DeClerck, Y.A. Tumor microenvironment complexity: Emerging roles in cancer therapy. *Cancer Res.* **2012**, *72*, 2473–2480. [CrossRef]
14. Taube, J.M.; Klein, A.; Brahmer, J.R.; Xu, H.; Pan, X.; Kim, J.H.; Chen, L.; Pardoll, D.M.; Topalian, S.L.; Anders, R.A. Association of PD-1. PD-1 ligands, and other features of the tumor immune microenvironment with response to anti-PD-1 therapy. *Clin. Cancer Res.* **2014**, *20*, 5064–5074. [CrossRef] [PubMed]
15. Quail, D.F.; Joyce, J.A. Microenvironmental regulation of tumor progression and metastasis. *Nat. Med.* **2013**, *19*, 1423–1437. [CrossRef]
16. Yerushalmi, R.; Woods, R.; Ravdin, P.M.; Hayes, M.M.; Gelmon, K.A. Ki67 in breast cancer: Prognostic and predictive potential. *Lancet Oncol.* **2010**, *11*, 174–183. [CrossRef]
17. Cheang, M.C.; Chia, S.K.; Voduc, D.; Gao, D.; Leung, S.; Snider, J.; Watson, M.; Davies, S.; Bernard, P.S.; Parker, J.S.; et al. Ki67 index. HER2 status, and prognosis of patients with luminal B breast cancer. *J. Natl. Cancer Inst.* **2009**, *101*, 736–750. [CrossRef] [PubMed]
18. Agus, D.B.; Akita, R.W.; Fox, W.D.; Lewis, G.D.; Higgins, B.; Pisacane, P.I.; Lofgren, J.A.; Tindell, C.; Evans, D.P.; Maiese, K.; et al. Targeting ligand-activated ErbB2 signaling inhibits breast and prostate tumor growth. *Cancer Cell* **2002**, *2*, 127–137. [CrossRef]
19. Yu, D.; Hung, M.C. Overexpression of ErbB2 in cancer and ErbB2-targeting strategies. *Oncogene* **2000**, *19*, 6115–6121. [CrossRef] [PubMed]
20. Rakha, E.A.; Reis-Filho, J.S.; Ellis, I.O. Basal-like breast cancer: A critical review. *J. Clin. Oncol.* **2008**, *26*, 2568–2581. [CrossRef] [PubMed]
21. Yehiely, F.; Moyano, J.V.; Evans, J.R.; Nielsen, T.O.; Cryns, V.L. Deconstructing the molecular portrait of basal-like breast cancer. *Trends Mol. Med.* **2006**, *12*, 537–544. [CrossRef]
22. De Craene, B.; Berx, G. Regulatory networks defining EMT during cancer initiation and progression. *Nat. Rev. Cancer* **2013**, *13*, 97–110. [CrossRef] [PubMed]
23. Hennessy, B.T.; Gonzalez-Angulo, A.M.; Stemke-Hale, K.; Gilcrease, M.Z.; Krishnamurthy, S.; Lee, J.S.; Fridlyand, J.; Sahin, A.; Agarwal, R.; Joy, C.; et al. Characterization of a naturally occurring breast cancer subset enriched in epithelial-to-mesenchymal transition and stem cell characteristics. *Cancer Res.* **2009**, *69*, 4116–4124. [CrossRef]

24. Lindley, L.E.; Briegel, K.J. Molecular characterization of TGFbeta-induced epithelial-mesenchymal transition in normal finite lifespan human mammary epithelial cells. *Biochem. Biophys. Res. Commun.* **2010**, *399*, 659–664. [CrossRef] [PubMed]
25. Sarrio, D.; Franklin, C.K.; Mackay, A.; Reis-Filho, J.S.; Isacke, C.M. Epithelial and mesenchymal subpopulations within normal basal breast cell lines exhibit distinct stem cell/progenitor properties. *Stem Cells* **2012**, *30*, 292–303. [CrossRef]
26. Kang, Y.; Massague, J. Epithelial-mesenchymal transitions: Twist in development and metastasis. *Cell* **2004**, *118*, 277–279. [CrossRef] [PubMed]
27. Yang, J.; Mani, S.A.; Donaher, J.L.; Ramaswamy, S.; Itzykson, R.A.; Come, C.; Savagner, P.; Gitelman, I.; Richardson, A.; Weinberg, R.A. Twist, a master regulator of morphogenesis, plays an essential role in tumor metastasis. *Cell* **2004**, *117*, 927–939. [CrossRef] [PubMed]
28. Yang, J.; Weinberg, R.A. Epithelial-mesenchymal transition: At the crossroads of development and tumor metastasis. *Dev. Cell.* **2008**, *14*, 818–829. [CrossRef]
29. Braune, E.B.; Seshire, A.; Lendahl, U. Notch and Wnt Dysregulation and Its Relevance for Breast Cancer and Tumor Initiation. *Biomedicines* **2018**, *6*, 101. [CrossRef] [PubMed]
30. Cleary, A.S.; Leonard, T.L.; Gestl, S.A.; Gunther, E.J. Tumour cell heterogeneity maintained by cooperating subclones in Wnt-driven mammary cancers. *Nature* **2014**, *508*, 113–117. [CrossRef] [PubMed]
31. Cai, J.; Guan, H.; Fang, L.; Yang, Y.; Zhu, X.; Yuan, J.; Wu, J.; Li, M. MicroRNA-374a activates Wnt/beta-catenin signaling to promote breast cancer metastasis. *J. Clin. Investig.* **2013**, *123*, 566–579. [PubMed]
32. Kumar, S.; Srivastav, R.K.; Wilkes, D.W.; Ross, T.; Kim, S.; Kowalski, J.; Chatla, S.; Zhang, Q.; Nayak, A.; Guha, M.; et al. Estrogen-dependent DLL1-mediated Notch signaling promotes luminal breast cancer. *Oncogene* **2019**, *38*, 2092–2107. [CrossRef] [PubMed]
33. Yook, J.I.; Li, X.Y.; Ota, I.; Hu, C.; Kim, H.S.; Kim, N.H.; Cha, S.Y.; Ryu, J.K.; Choi, Y.J.; Kim, J.; et al. A Wnt-Axin2-GSK3beta cascade regulates Snail1 activity in breast cancer cells. *Nat. Cell Biol.* **2006**, *8*, 1398–1406. [CrossRef] [PubMed]
34. An, J.; Lv, J.; Li, A.; Qiao, J.; Fang, L.; Li, Z.; Li, B.; Zhao, W.; Chen, H.; Wang, L. Constitutive expression of Bcl-2 induces epithelial-Mesenchymal transition in mammary epithelial cells. *BMC Cancer* **2015**, *15*, 476. [CrossRef]
35. Reis-Filho, J.S.; Pusztai, L. Gene expression profiling in breast cancer: Classification. prognostication, and prediction. *Lancet* **2011**, *378*, 1812–1823. [CrossRef]
36. Ye, Y.; Xiao, Y.; Wang, W.; Yearsley, K.; Gao, J.X.; Shetuni, B.; Barsky, S.H. ERalpha signaling through slug regulates E-cadherin and EMT. *Oncogene* **2010**, *29*, 1451–1462. [CrossRef] [PubMed]
37. Wang, X.; Belguise, K.; Kersual, N.; Kirsch, K.H.; Mineva, N.D.; Galtier, F.; Chalbos, D.; Sonenshein, G.E. Oestrogen signalling inhibits invasive phenotype by repressing RelB and its target BCL2. *Nat. Cell Biol.* **2007**, *9*, 470–478. [CrossRef] [PubMed]
38. Wei, X.L.; Dou, X.W.; Bai, J.W.; Luo, X.R.; Qiu, S.Q.; Xi, D.D.; Huang, W.H.; Du, C.W.; Man, K.; Zhang, G.J. ERalpha inhibits epithelial-mesenchymal transition by suppressing Bmi1 in breast cancer. *Oncotarget* **2015**, *6*, 21704–21717. [CrossRef] [PubMed]
39. Massague, J. TGFbeta in Cancer. *Cell* **2008**, *134*, 215–230. [CrossRef]
40. Lehmann, W.; Mossmann, D.; Kleemann, J.; Mock, K.; Meisinger, C.; Brummer, T.; Herr, R.; Brabletz, S.; Stemmler, M.P.; Brabletz, T. ZEB1 turns into a transcriptional activator by interacting with YAP1 in aggressive cancer types. *Nat. Commun.* **2016**, *7*, 10498. [CrossRef]
41. Pang, M.F.; Georgoudaki, A.M.; Lambut, L.; Johansson, J.; Tabor, V.; Hagikura, K.; Jin, Y.; Jansson, M.; Alexander, J.S.; Nelson, C.M.; et al. TGF-beta1-induced EMT promotes targeted migration of breast cancer cells through the lymphatic system by the activation of CCR7/CCL21-mediated chemotaxis. *Oncogene* **2016**, *35*, 748–760. [CrossRef]
42. Peinado, H.; Quintanilla, M.; Cano, A. Transforming growth factor beta-1 induces snail transcription factor in epithelial cell lines: Mechanisms for epithelial mesenchymal transitions. *J. Biol. Chem.* **2003**, *278*, 21113–21123. [CrossRef]
43. Tian, M.; Schiemann, W.P. TGF-beta Stimulation of EMT Programs Elicits Non-genomic ER-alpha Activity and Anti-estrogen Resistance in Breast Cancer Cells. *J. Cancer Metastasis Treat.* **2017**, *3*, 150–160. [CrossRef] [PubMed]

44. Xie, L.; Law, B.K.; Chytil, A.M.; Brown, K.A.; Aakre, M.E.; Moses, H.L. Activation of the Erk pathway is required for TGF-beta1-induced EMT in vitro. *Neoplasia* **2004**, *6*, 603–610. [CrossRef]
45. Janda, E.; Lehmann, K.; Killisch, I.; Jechlinger, M.; Herzig, M.; Downward, J.; Beug, H.; Grunert, S. Ras and TGF[beta] cooperatively regulate epithelial cell plasticity and metastasis: Dissection of Ras signaling pathways. *J. Cell Biol.* **2002**, *156*, 299–313. [CrossRef]
46. Ning, Q.; Liu, C.; Hou, L.; Meng, M.; Zhang, X.; Luo, M.; Shao, S.; Zuo, X.; Zhao, X. Vascular endothelial growth factor receptor-1 activation promotes migration and invasion of breast cancer cells through epithelial-mesenchymal transition. *PLoS ONE* **2013**, *8*, e65217. [CrossRef] [PubMed]
47. Chihara, Y.; Shimoda, M.; Hori, A.; Ohara, A.; Naoi, Y.; Ikeda, J.I.; Kagara, N.; Tanei, T.; Shimomura, A.; Shimazu, K.; et al. A small-molecule inhibitor of SMAD3 attenuates resistance to anti-HER2 drugs in HER2-positive breast cancer cells. *Breast Cancer Res. Treat.* **2017**, *166*, 55–68. [CrossRef]
48. Goyette, M.A.; Duhamel, S.; Aubert, L.; Pelletier, A.; Savage, P.; Thibault, M.P.; Johnson, R.M.; Carmeliet, P.; Basik, M.; Gaboury, L.; et al. The Receptor Tyrosine Kinase AXL Is Required at Multiple Steps of the Metastatic Cascade during HER2-Positive Breast Cancer Progression. *Cell Rep.* **2018**, *23*, 1476–1490. [CrossRef]
49. Gupta, P.; Srivastava, S.K. HER2 mediated de novo production of TGFbeta leads to SNAIL driven epithelial-to-mesenchymal transition and metastasis of breast cancer. *Mol. Oncol.* **2014**, *8*, 1532–1547. [CrossRef] [PubMed]
50. Huang, F.; Shi, Q.; Li, Y.; Xu, L.; Xu, C.; Chen, F.; Wang, H.; Liao, H.; Chang, Z.; Liu, F.; et al. HER2/EGFR-AKT Signaling Switches TGFbeta from Inhibiting Cell Proliferation to Promoting Cell Migration in Breast Cancer. *Cancer Res.* **2018**, *78*, 6073–6085. [CrossRef]
51. Carpenter, R.L.; Paw, I.; Dewhirst, M.W.; Lo, H.W. Akt phosphorylates and activates HSF-1 independent of heat shock, leading to Slug overexpression and epithelial-mesenchymal transition (EMT) of HER2-overexpressing breast cancer cells. *Oncogene* **2015**, *34*, 546–557. [CrossRef]
52. Pomp, V.; Leo, C.; Mauracher, A.; Korol, D.; Guo, W.; Varga, Z. Differential expression of epithelial-mesenchymal transition and stem cell markers in intrinsic subtypes of breast cancer. *Breast Cancer Res. Treat.* **2015**, *154*, 45–55. [CrossRef]
53. Hong, J.; Zhou, J.; Fu, J.; He, T.; Qin, J.; Wang, L.; Liao, L.; Xu, J. Phosphorylation of serine 68 of Twist1 by MAPKs stabilizes Twist1 protein and promotes breast cancer cell invasiveness. *Cancer Res.* **2011**, *71*, 3980–3990. [CrossRef]
54. Ai, M.; Liang, K.; Lu, Y.; Qiu, S.; Fan, Z. Brk/PTK6 cooperates with HER2 and Src in regulating breast cancer cell survival and epithelial-to-mesenchymal transition. *Cancer Biol. Ther.* **2013**, *14*, 237–245. [CrossRef]
55. Ahn, S.G.; Kim, S.J.; Kim, C.; Jeong, J. Molecular Classification of Triple-Negative Breast Cancer. *J. Breast Cancer* **2016**, *19*, 223–230. [CrossRef]
56. Lehmann, B.D.; Bauer, J.A.; Chen, X.; Sanders, M.E.; Chakravarthy, A.B.; Shyr, Y.; Pietenpol, J.A. Identification of human triple-negative breast cancer subtypes and preclinical models for selection of targeted therapies. *J. Clin. Investig.* **2011**, *121*, 2750–2767. [CrossRef] [PubMed]
57. Ibrahim, Y.H.; Garcia-Garcia, C.; Serra, V.; He, L.; Torres-Lockhart, K.; Prat, A.; Anton, P.; Cozar, P.; Guzman, M.; Grueso, J.; et al. PI3K inhibition impairs BRCA1/2 expression and sensitizes BRCA-proficient triple-negative breast cancer to PARP inhibition. *Cancer Discov.* **2012**, *2*, 1036–1047. [CrossRef]
58. Chuang, H.C.; Kapuriya, N.; Kulp, S.K.; Chen, C.S.; Shapiro, C.L. Differential anti-proliferative activities of poly(ADP-ribose) polymerase (PARP) inhibitors in triple-negative breast cancer cells. *Breast Cancer Res Treat.* **2012**, *134*, 649–659. [CrossRef]
59. Anders, C.K.; Winer, E.P.; Ford, J.M.; Dent, R.; Silver, D.P.; Sledge, G.W.; Carey, L.A. Poly(ADP-Ribose) polymerase inhibition: "targeted" therapy for triple-negative breast cancer. *Clin. Cancer Res.* **2010**, *16*, 4702–4710. [CrossRef]
60. Yoshida, T.; Ozawa, Y.; Kimura, T.; Sato, Y.; Kuznetsov, G.; Xu, S.; Uesugi, M.; Agoulnik, S.; Taylor, N.; Funahashi, Y.; et al. Eribulin mesilate suppresses experimental metastasis of breast cancer cells by reversing phenotype from epithelial-mesenchymal transition (EMT) to mesenchymal-epithelial transition (MET) states. *Br. J. Cancer* **2014**, *110*, 1497–1505. [CrossRef] [PubMed]
61. Vikas, P.; Borcherding, N.; Zhang, W. The clinical promise of immunotherapy in triple-negative breast cancer. *Cancer Manag. Res.* **2018**, *10*, 6823–6833. [CrossRef] [PubMed]

62. Wang, X.; Qi, Y.; Kong, X.; Zhai, J.; Li, Y.; Song, Y.; Wang, J.; Feng, X.; Fang, Y. Immunological therapy: A novel thriving area for triple-negative breast cancer treatment. *Cancer Lett.* **2019**, *442*, 409–428. [CrossRef] [PubMed]
63. Gucalp, A.; Tolaney, S.; Isakoff, S.J.; Ingle, J.N.; Liu, M.C.; Carey, L.A.; Blackwell, K.; Rugo, H.; Nabell, L.; Forero, A.; et al. Phase II trial of bicalutamide in patients with androgen receptor-positive. estrogen receptor-negative metastatic Breast Cancer. *Clin. Cancer Res.* **2013**, *19*, 5505–5512. [CrossRef] [PubMed]
64. Mittal, S.; Sharma, A.; Balaji, S.A.; Gowda, M.C.; Dighe, R.R.; Kumar, R.V.; Rangarajan, A. Coordinate hyperactivation of Notch1 and Ras/MAPK pathways correlates with poor patient survival: Novel therapeutic strategy for aggressive breast cancers. *Mol. Cancer Ther.* **2014**, *13*, 3198–3209. [CrossRef] [PubMed]
65. Zhang, J.; Shao, X.; Sun, H.; Liu, K.; Ding, Z.; Chen, J.; Fang, L.; Su, W.; Hong, Y.; Li, H.; et al. NUMB negatively regulates the epithelial-mesenchymal transition of triple-negative breast cancer by antagonizing Notch signaling. *Oncotarget* **2016**, *7*, 61036–61053. [CrossRef]
66. Leong, K.G.; Niessen, K.; Kulic, I.; Raouf, A.; Eaves, C.; Pollet, I.; Karsan, A. Jagged1-mediated Notch activation induces epithelial-to-mesenchymal transition through Slug-induced repression of E-cadherin. *J. Exp. Med.* **2007**, *204*, 2935–2948. [CrossRef]
67. Choy, L.; Hagenbeek, T.J.; Solon, M.; French, D.; Finkle, D.; Shelton, A.; Venook, R.; Brauer, M.J.; Siebel, C.W. Constitutive NOTCH3 Signaling Promotes the Growth of Basal Breast Cancers. *Cancer Res.* **2017**, *77*, 1439–1452. [CrossRef] [PubMed]
68. Speiser, J.; Foreman, K.; Drinka, E.; Godellas, C.; Perez, C.; Salhadar, A.; Ersahin, C.; Rajan, P. Notch-1 and Notch-4 biomarker expression in triple-negative breast cancer. *Int. J. Surg. Pathol.* **2012**, *20*, 139–145. [CrossRef]
69. Colavito, S.A.; Zou, M.R.; Yan, Q.; Nguyen, D.X.; Stern, D.F. Significance of glioma-associated Oncogene homolog 1 (GLI1) expression in claudin-low breast cancer and crosstalk with the nuclear factor kappa-light-chain-enhancer of activated B cells (NFkappaB) pathway. *Breast Cancer Res.* **2014**, *16*, 444. [CrossRef]
70. Lei, J.; Fan, L.; Wei, G.; Chen, X.; Duan, W.; Xu, Q.; Sheng, W.; Wang, K.; Li, X. Gli-1 is crucial for hypoxia-induced epithelial-mesenchymal transition and invasion of breast cancer. *Tumour Biol.* **2015**, *36*, 3119–3126. [CrossRef] [PubMed]
71. Hui, M.; Cazet, A.; Nair, R.; Watkins, D.N.; O'Toole, S.A.; Swarbrick, A. The Hedgehog signalling pathway in breast development. carcinogenesis and cancer therapy. *Breast Cancer Res.* **2013**, *15*, 203. [CrossRef] [PubMed]
72. Woodward, W.A.; Chen, M.S.; Behbod, F.; Rosen, J.M. On mammary stem cells. *J. Cell Sci.* **2005**, *118*, 3585–3594. [CrossRef]
73. Xu, X.; Zhang, L.; He, X.; Zhang, P.; Sun, C.; Xu, X.; Lu, Y.; Li, F. TGF-beta plays a vital role in triple-negative breast cancer (TNBC) drug-resistance through regulating stemness, EMT and apoptosis. *Biochem. Biophys. Res. Commun.* **2018**, *502*, 160–165. [CrossRef] [PubMed]
74. Okita, Y.; Kimura, M.; Xie, R.; Chen, C.; Shen, L.T.; Kojima, Y.; Suzuki, H.; Muratani, M.; Saitoh, M.; Semba, K.; et al. The transcription factor MAFK induces EMT and malignant progression of triple-negative breast cancer cells through its target GPNMB. *Sci. Signal.* **2017**, *10*, eaak9397. [CrossRef] [PubMed]
75. Granados-Principal, S.; Liu, Y.; Guevara, M.L.; Blanco, E.; Choi, D.S.; Qian, W.; Patel, T.; Rodriguez, A.A.; Cusimano, J.; Weiss, H.L.; et al. Inhibition of iNOS as a novel effective targeted therapy against triple-negative breast cancer. *Breast Cancer Res.* **2015**, *17*, 25. [CrossRef] [PubMed]
76. Parvani, J.G.; Gujrati, M.D.; Mack, M.A.; Schiemann, W.P.; Lu, Z.R. Silencing beta3 Integrin by Targeted ECO/siRNA Nanoparticles Inhibits EMT and Metastasis of Triple-Negative Breast Cancer. *Cancer Res.* **2015**, *75*, 2316–2325. [CrossRef]
77. Chakrabarti, R.; Wei, Y.; Hwang, J.; Hang, X.; Andres Blanco, M.; Choudhury, A.; Tiede, B.; Romano, R.A.; DeCoste, C.; Mercatali, L.; et al. DeltaNp63 promotes stem cell activity in mammary gland development and basal-like breast cancer by enhancing Fzd7 expression and Wnt signalling. *Nat. Cell Biol.* **2014**, *16*, 1004–1015. [CrossRef] [PubMed]
78. Khramtsov, A.I.; Khramtsova, G.F.; Tretiakova, M.; Huo, D.; Olopade, O.I.; Goss, K.H. Wnt/beta-catenin pathway activation is enriched in basal-like breast cancers and predicts poor outcome. *Am. J. Pathol.* **2010**, *176*, 2911–2920. [CrossRef] [PubMed]

79. Vijay, G.V.; Zhao, N.; Den Hollander, P.; Toneff, M.J.; Joseph, R.; Pietila, M.; Taube, J.H.; Sarkar, T.R.; Ramirez-Pena, E.; Werden, S.J.; et al. GSK3beta regulates epithelial-mesenchymal transition and cancer stem cell properties in triple-negative breast cancer. *Breast Cancer Res.* **2019**, *21*, 37. [CrossRef] [PubMed]
80. El Ayachi, I.; Fatima, I.; Wend, P.; Alva-Ornelas, J.A.; Runke, S.; Kuenzinger, W.L.; Silva, J.; Silva, W.; Gray, J.K.; Lehr, S.; et al. The WNT10B Network Is Associated with Survival and Metastases in Chemoresistant Triple-Negative Breast Cancer. *Cancer Res.* **2019**, *79*, 982–993. [CrossRef]
81. Thiery, J.P.; Lim, C.T. Tumor dissemination: An EMT affair. *Cancer Cell* **2013**, *23*, 272–273. [CrossRef]
82. Yu, M.; Bardia, A.; Wittner, B.S.; Stott, S.L.; Smas, M.E.; Ting, D.T.; Isakoff, S.J.; Ciciliano, J.C.; Wells, M.N.; Shah, A.M.; et al. Circulating breast tumor cells exhibit dynamic changes in epithelial and mesenchymal composition. *Science* **2013**, *339*, 580–584. [CrossRef]
83. Dvorak, H.F. Tumors: Wounds that do not heal. Similarities between tumor stroma generation and wound healing. *N. Engl. J. Med.* **1986**, *315*, 1650–1659.
84. Coussens, L.M.; Werb, Z. Inflammation and cancer. *Nature* **2002**, *420*, 860–867. [CrossRef]
85. Coussens, L.M.; Raymond, W.W.; Bergers, G.; Laig-Webster, M.; Behrendtsen, O.; Werb, Z.; Caughey, G.H.; Hanahan, D. Inflammatory mast cells up-regulate angiogenesis during squamous epithelial carcinogenesis. *Genes Dev.* **1999**, *13*, 1382–1397. [CrossRef]
86. Bissell, M.J.; Hines, W.C. Why don't we get more cancer? A proposed role of the microenvironment in restraining cancer progression. *Nat. Med.* **2011**, *17*, 320–329. [CrossRef]
87. Chuang, L.S.; Ito, Y. RUNX3 is multifunctional in carcinogenesis of multiple solid tumors. *Oncogene* **2010**, *29*, 2605–2615. [CrossRef] [PubMed]
88. Manandhar, S.; Lee, Y.M. Emerging role of RUNX3 in the regulation of tumor microenvironment. *BMB Rep.* **2018**, *51*, 174–181. [CrossRef]
89. Chou, J.; Lin, J.H.; Brenot, A.; Kim, J.W.; Provot, S.; Werb, Z. GATA3 suppresses metastasis and modulates the tumour microenvironment by regulating microRNA-29b expression. *Nat. Cell Biol.* **2013**, *15*, 201–213. [CrossRef]
90. Kouros-Mehr, H.; Bechis, S.K.; Slorach, E.M.; Littlepage, L.E.; Egeblad, M.; Ewald, A.J.; Pai, S.Y.; Ho, I.C.; Werb, Z. GATA-3 links tumor differentiation and dissemination in a luminal breast cancer model. *Cancer Cell* **2008**, *13*, 141–152. [CrossRef]
91. Tynan, J.A.; Wen, F.; Muller, W.J.; Oshima, R.G. Ets2-dependent microenvironmental support of mouse mammary tumors. *Oncogene* **2005**, *24*, 6870–6876. [CrossRef] [PubMed]
92. Man, A.K.; Young, L.J.; Tynan, J.A.; Lesperance, J.; Egeblad, M.; Werb, Z.; Hauser, C.A.; Muller, W.J.; Cardiff, R.D.; Oshima, R.G. Ets2-dependent stromal regulation of mouse mammary tumors. *Mol. Cell Biol.* **2003**, *23*, 8614–8625. [CrossRef]
93. Chakrabarti, R.; Hwang, J.; Andres Blanco, M.; Wei, Y.; Lukacisin, M.; Romano, R.A.; Smalley, K.; Liu, S.; Yang, Q.; Ibrahim, T.; et al. Elf5 inhibits the epithelial-mesenchymal transition in mammary gland development and breast cancer metastasis by transcriptionally repressing Snail2. *Nat. Cell Biol.* **2012**, *14*, 1212–1222. [CrossRef]
94. Kumar, S.; Wilkes, D.W.; Samuel, N.; Blanco, M.A.; Nayak, A.; Alicea-Torres, K.; Gluck, C.; Sinha, S.; Gabrilovich, D.; Chakrabarti, R. DeltaNp63-driven recruitment of myeloid-derived suppressor cells promotes metastasis in triple-negative breast cancer. *J. Clin. Investig.* **2018**, *128*, 5095–5109. [CrossRef] [PubMed]
95. Chang, C.J.; Chao, C.H.; Xia, W.; Yang, J.Y.; Xiong, Y.; Li, C.W.; Yu, W.H.; Rehman, S.K.; Hsu, J.L.; Lee, H.H.; et al. p53 regulates epithelial-mesenchymal transition and stem cell properties through modulating miRNAs. *Nat. Cell Biol.* **2011**, *13*, 317–323. [CrossRef] [PubMed]
96. Quigley, D.; Silwal-Pandit, L.; Dannenfelser, R.; Langerod, A.; Vollan, H.K.; Vaske, C.; Siegel, J.U.; Troyanskaya, O.; Chin, S.F.; Caldas, C.; et al. Lymphocyte Invasion in IC10/Basal-Like Breast Tumors Is Associated with Wild-Type TP53. *Mol. Cancer Res.* **2015**, *13*, 493–501. [CrossRef] [PubMed]
97. Wellenstein, M.D.; de Visser, K.E. Cancer-Cell-Intrinsic Mechanisms Shaping the Tumor Immune Landscape. *Immunity* **2018**, *48*, 399–416. [CrossRef]
98. Ha, H.Y.; Moon, H.B.; Nam, M.S.; Lee, J.W.; Ryoo, Z.Y.; Lee, T.H.; Lee, K.K.; So, B.J.; Sato, H.; Seiki, M.; et al. Overexpression of membrane-type matrix metalloproteinase-1 gene induces mammary gland abnormalities and adenocarcinoma in transgenic mice. *Cancer Res.* **2001**, *61*, 984–990.

99. Sternlicht, M.D.; Lochter, A.; Sympson, C.J.; Huey, B.; Rougier, J.P.; Gray, J.W.; Pinkel, D.; Bissell, M.J.; Werb, Z. The stromal proteinase MMP3/stromelysin-1 promotes mammary carcinogenesis. *Cell* **1999**, *98*, 137–146. [CrossRef]
100. Masson, R.; Lefebvre, O.; Noel, A.; Fahime, M.E.; Chenard, M.P.; Wendling, C.; Kebers, F.; LeMeur, M.; Dierich, A.; Foidart, J.M.; et al. In vivo evidence that the stromelysin-3 metalloproteinase contributes in a paracrine manner to epithelial cell malignancy. *J. Cell Biol.* **1998**, *140*, 1535–1541. [CrossRef] [PubMed]
101. Li, J.H.; Wang, W.; Huang, X.R.; Oldfield, M.; Schmidt, A.M.; Cooper, M.E.; Lan, H.Y. Advanced glycation end products induce tubular epithelial-myofibroblast transition through the RAGE-ERK1/2 MAP kinase signaling pathway. *Am. J. Pathol.* **2004**, *164*, 1389–1397. [CrossRef]
102. Petersen, O.W.; Nielsen, H.L.; Gudjonsson, T.; Villadsen, R.; Rank, F.; Niebuhr, E.; Bissell, M.J.; Ronnov-Jessen, L. Epithelial to mesenchymal transition in human breast cancer can provide a nonmalignant stroma. *Am. J. Pathol.* **2003**, *162*, 391–402. [CrossRef]
103. Del Casar, J.M.; Gonzalez, L.O.; Alvarez, E.; Junquera, S.; Marin, L.; Gonzalez, L.; Bongera, M.; Vazquez, J.; Vizoso, F.J. Comparative analysis and clinical value of the expression of metalloproteases and their inhibitors by intratumor stromal fibroblasts and those at the invasive front of breast carcinomas. *Breast Cancer Res. Treat.* **2009**, *116*, 39–52. [CrossRef] [PubMed]
104. Vizoso, F.J.; Gonzalez, L.O.; Corte, M.D.; Rodriguez, J.C.; Vazquez, J.; Lamelas, M.L.; Junquera, S.; Merino, A.M.; Garcia-Muniz, J.L. Study of matrix metalloproteinases and their inhibitors in breast cancer. *Br. J. Cancer* **2007**, *96*, 903–911. [CrossRef]
105. Heppner, K.J.; Matrisian, L.M.; Jensen, R.A.; Rodgers, W.H. Expression of most matrix metalloproteinase family members in breast cancer represents a tumor-induced host response. *Am. J. Pathol.* **1996**, *149*, 273–282.
106. Chang, Q.; Bournazou, E.; Sansone, P.; Berishaj, M.; Gao, S.P.; Daly, L.; Wels, J.; Theilen, T.; Granitto, S.; Zhang, X.; et al. The IL-6/JAK/Stat3 feed-forward loop drives tumorigenesis and metastasis. *Neoplasia* **2013**, *15*, 848–862. [CrossRef]
107. Lesina, M.; Kurkowski, M.U.; Ludes, K.; Rose-John, S.; Treiber, M.; Kloppel, G.; Yoshimura, A.; Reindl, W.; Sipos, B.; Akira, S.; et al. Stat3/Socs3 activation by IL-6 transsignaling promotes progression of pancreatic intraepithelial Neoplasia and development of pancreatic cancer. *Cancer Cell* **2011**, *19*, 456–469. [CrossRef]
108. Lippitz, B.E. Cytokine patterns in patients with cancer: A systematic review. *Lancet Oncol.* **2013**, *14*, e218–e228. [CrossRef]
109. Zhou, L.; Ivanov, I.I.; Spolski, R.; Min, R.; Shenderov, K.; Egawa, T.; Levy, D.E.; Leonard, W.J.; Littman, D.R. IL-6 programs T(H)-17 cell differentiation by promoting sequential engagement of the IL-21 and IL-23 pathways. *Nat. Immunol.* **2007**, *8*, 967–974. [CrossRef]
110. Chomarat, P.; Banchereau, J.; Davoust, J.; Palucka, A.K. IL-6 switches the differentiation of monocytes from dendritic cells to macrophages. *Nat. Immunol.* **2000**, *1*, 510–514. [CrossRef] [PubMed]
111. Salgado, R.; Junius, S.; Benoy, I.; Van Dam, P.; Vermeulen, P.; Van Marck, E.; Huget, P.; Dirix, L.Y. Circulating interleukin-6 predicts survival in patients with metastatic breast cancer. *Int. J. Cancer* **2003**, *103*, 642–646. [CrossRef] [PubMed]
112. Sullivan, N.J.; Sasser, A.K.; Axel, A.E.; Vesuna, F.; Raman, V.; Ramirez, N.; Oberyszyn, T.M.; Hall, B.M. Interleukin-6 induces an epithelial-mesenchymal transition phenotype in human breast cancer cells. *Oncogene* **2009**, *28*, 2940–2947. [CrossRef]
113. Xie, G.; Yao, Q.; Liu, Y.; Du, S.; Liu, A.; Guo, Z.; Sun, A.; Ruan, J.; Chen, L.; Ye, C.; et al. IL-6-induced epithelial-mesenchymal transition promotes the generation of breast cancer stem-like cells analogous to mammosphere cultures. *Int. J. Oncol.* **2012**, *40*, 1171–1179.
114. Liu, Q.; Yu, S.; Li, A.; Xu, H.; Han, X.; Wu, K. Targeting interlukin-6 to relieve immunosuppression in tumor microenvironment. *Tumour Biol.* **2017**, *39*, 1010428317712445. [CrossRef]
115. Dominguez, C.; McCampbell, K.K.; David, J.M.; Palena, C. Neutralization of IL-8 decreases tumor PMN-MDSCs and reduces mesenchymalization of claudin-low triple-negative breast cancer. *JCI Insight.* **2017**. [CrossRef]
116. Qian, B.Z.; Pollard, J.W. Macrophage diversity enhances tumor progression and metastasis. *Cell* **2010**, *141*, 39–51. [CrossRef]
117. Yoshimura, T. The production of monocyte chemoattractant protein-1 (MCP-1)/CCL2 in tumor microenvironments. *Cytokine* **2017**, *98*, 71–78. [CrossRef]

118. Ding, J.; Guo, C.; Hu, P.; Chen, J.; Liu, Q.; Wu, X.; Cao, Y.; Wu, J. CSF1 is involved in breast cancer progression through inducing monocyte differentiation and homing. *Int. J. Oncol.* **2016**, *49*, 2064–2074. [CrossRef] [PubMed]
119. Condeelis, J.; Pollard, J.W. Macrophages: Obligate partners for tumor cell migration. invasion, and metastasis. *Cell* **2006**, *124*, 263–266. [CrossRef]
120. Georgoudaki, A.M.; Prokopec, K.E.; Boura, V.F.; Hellqvist, E.; Sohn, S.; Ostling, J.; Dahan, R.; Harris, R.A.; Rantalainen, M.; Klevebring, D.; et al. Reprogramming Tumor-Associated Macrophages by Antibody Targeting Inhibits Cancer Progression and Metastasis. *Cell Rep.* **2016**, *15*, 2000–2011. [CrossRef]
121. Linde, N.; Casanova-Acebes, M.; Sosa, M.S.; Mortha, A.; Rahman, A.; Farias, E.; Harper, K.; Tardio, E.; Reyes Torres, I.; Jones, J.; et al. Macrophages orchestrate breast cancer early dissemination and metastasis. *Nat. Commun.* **2018**, *9*, 21. [CrossRef] [PubMed]
122. Yang, M.; Ma, B.; Shao, H.; Clark, A.M.; Wells, A. Macrophage phenotypic subtypes diametrically regulate epithelial-mesenchymal plasticity in breast cancer cells. *BMC Cancer* **2016**, *16*, 419. [CrossRef]
123. Barbera-Guillem, E.; Nyhus, J.K.; Wolford, C.C.; Friece, C.R.; Sampsel, J.W. Vascular endothelial growth factor secretion by tumor-infiltrating macrophages essentially supports tumor angiogenesis. and IgG immune complexes potentiate the process. *Cancer Res.* **2002**, *62*, 7042–7049. [PubMed]
124. Muraoka, R.S.; Dumont, N.; Ritter, C.A.; Dugger, T.C.; Brantley, D.M.; Chen, J.; Easterly, E.; Roebuck, L.R.; Ryan, S.; Gotwals, P.J.; et al. Blockade of TGF-beta inhibits mammary tumor cell viability. migration, and metastases. *J. Clin. Investig.* **2002**, *109*, 1551–1559. [CrossRef] [PubMed]
125. Yu, Q.; Stamenkovic, I. Cell surface-localized matrix metalloproteinase-9 proteolytically activates TGF-beta and promotes tumor invasion and angiogenesis. *Genes Dev.* **2000**, *14*, 163–176. [PubMed]
126. Bednarczyk, R.B.; Tuli, N.Y.; Hanly, E.K.; Rahoma, G.B.; Maniyar, R.; Mittelman, A.; Geliebter, J.; Tiwari, R.K. Macrophage inflammatory factors promote epithelial-mesenchymal transition in breast cancer. *Oncotarget* **2018**, *9*, 24272–24282. [CrossRef]
127. Lin, E.Y.; Nguyen, A.V.; Russell, R.G.; Pollard, J.W. Colony-stimulating factor 1 promotes progression of mammary tumors to malignancy. *J. Exp. Med.* **2001**, *193*, 727–740. [CrossRef] [PubMed]
128. Zhang, W.J.; Wang, X.H.; Gao, S.T.; Chen, C.; Xu, X.Y.; Sun, Q.; Zhou, Z.H.; Wu, G.Z.; Yu, Q.; Xu, G.; et al. Tumor-associated macrophages correlate with phenomenon of epithelial-mesenchymal transition and contribute to poor prognosis in triple-negative breast cancer patients. *J. Surg. Res.* **2018**, *222*, 93–101. [CrossRef]
129. Veglia, F.; Perego, M.; Gabrilovich, D. Myeloid-derived suppressor cells coming of age. *Nat. Immunol.* **2018**, *19*, 108–119. [CrossRef]
130. Lindau, D.; Gielen, P.; Kroesen, M.; Wesseling, P.; Adema, G.J. The immunosuppressive tumour network: Myeloid-derived suppressor cells, regulatory T cells and natural killer T cells. *Immunology* **2013**, *138*, 105–115. [CrossRef]
131. Gabrilovich, D.I.; Nagaraj, S. Myeloid-derived suppressor cells as regulators of the immune system. *Nat. Rev. Immunol.* **2009**, *9*, 162–174. [CrossRef] [PubMed]
132. Noman, M.Z.; Desantis, G.; Janji, B.; Hasmim, M.; Karray, S.; Dessen, P.; Bronte, V.; Chouaib, S. PD-L1 is a novel direct target of HIF-1alpha. and its blockade under hypoxia enhanced MDSC-mediated T cell activation. *J. Exp. Med.* **2014**, *211*, 781–790. [CrossRef] [PubMed]
133. Huang, J.; Jochems, C.; Talaie, T.; Anderson, A.; Jales, A.; Tsang, K.Y.; Madan, R.A.; Gulley, J.L.; Schlom, J. Elevated serum soluble CD40 ligand in cancer patients may play an immunosuppressive role. *Blood* **2012**, *120*, 3030–3038. [CrossRef]
134. Sinha, P.; Clements, V.K.; Fulton, A.M.; Ostrand-Rosenberg, S. Prostaglandin E2 promotes tumor progression by inducing myeloid-derived suppressor cells. *Cancer Res.* **2007**, *67*, 4507–4513. [CrossRef]
135. Munn, D.H. Blocking IDO activity to enhance anti-tumor immunity. *Front Biosci.* **2012**, *4*, 734–745. [CrossRef]
136. Holmgaard, R.B.; Zamarin, D.; Li, Y.; Gasmi, B.; Munn, D.H.; Allison, J.P.; Merghoub, T.; Wolchok, J.D. Tumor-Expressed IDO Recruits and Activates MDSCs in a Treg-Dependent Manner. *Cell Rep.* **2015**, *13*, 412–424. [CrossRef]
137. Yu, J.; Du, W.; Yan, F.; Wang, Y.; Li, H.; Cao, S.; Yu, W.; Shen, C.; Liu, J.; Ren, X. Myeloid-derived suppressor cells suppress antitumor immune responses through IDO expression and correlate with lymph node metastasis in patients with breast cancer. *J. Immunol.* **2013**, *190*, 3783–3797. [CrossRef]

138. Cui, T.X.; Kryczek, I.; Zhao, L.; Zhao, E.; Kuick, R.; Roh, M.H.; Vatan, L.; Szeliga, W.; Mao, Y.; Thomas, D.G.; et al. Myeloid-derived suppressor cells enhance stemness of cancer cells by inducing microRNA101 and suppressing the corepressor CtBP2. *Immunity* **2013**, *39*, 611–621. [CrossRef]

139. Peng, D.; Tanikawa, T.; Li, W.; Zhao, L.; Vatan, L.; Szeliga, W.; Wan, S.; Wei, S.; Wang, Y.; Liu, Y.; et al. Myeloid-Derived Suppressor Cells Endow Stem-like Qualities to Breast Cancer Cells through IL6/STAT3 and NO/NOTCH Cross-talk Signaling. *Cancer Res.* **2016**, *76*, 3156–3165. [CrossRef]

140. Welte, T.; Kim, I.S.; Tian, L.; Gao, X.; Wang, H.; Li, J.; Holdman, X.B.; Herschkowitz, J.I.; Pond, A.; Xie, G.; et al. Oncogenic mTOR signalling recruits myeloid-derived suppressor cells to promote tumour initiation. *Nat. Cell Biol.* **2016**, *18*, 632–644. [CrossRef] [PubMed]

141. Zhu, H.; Gu, Y.; Xue, Y.; Yuan, M.; Cao, X.; Liu, Q. CXCR2(+) MDSCs promote breast cancer progression by inducing EMT and activated T cell exhaustion. *Oncotarget* **2017**, *8*, 114554–114567. [CrossRef] [PubMed]

142. Ugel, S.; De Sanctis, F.; Mandruzzato, S.; Bronte, V. Tumor-induced myeloid deviation: When myeloid-derived suppressor cells meet tumor-associated macrophages. *J. Clin. Investig.* **2015**, *125*, 3365–3376. [CrossRef]

143. Fessenden, T.B.; Duong, E.; Spranger, S. A team effort: Natural killer cells on the first leg of the tumor immunity relay race. *J. Immunother. Cancer* **2018**, *6*, 67. [CrossRef] [PubMed]

144. Vivier, E.; Tomasello, E.; Baratin, M.; Walzer, T.; Ugolini, S. Functions of natural killer cells. *Nat. Immunol.* **2008**, *9*, 503–510. [CrossRef] [PubMed]

145. Huergo-Zapico, L.; Parodi, M.; Cantoni, C.; Lavarello, C.; Fernandez-Martinez, J.L.; Petretto, A.; DeAndres-Galiana, E.J.; Balsamo, M.; Lopez-Soto, A.; Pietra, G.; et al. NK-cell Editing Mediates Epithelial-to-Mesenchymal Transition via Phenotypic and Proteomic Changes in Melanoma Cell Lines. *Cancer Res.* **2018**, *78*, 3913–3925. [CrossRef]

146. Levi, I.; Amsalem, H.; Nissan, A.; Darash-Yahana, M.; Peretz, T.; Mandelboim, O.; Rachmilewitz, J. Characterization of tumor infiltrating natural killer cell subset. *Oncotarget* **2015**, *6*, 13835–13843. [CrossRef] [PubMed]

147. Bruno, A.; Ferlazzo, G.; Albini, A.; Noonan, D.M. A think tank of TINK/TANKs: Tumor-infiltrating/tumor-associated natural killer cells in tumor progression and angiogenesis. *J. Natl. Cancer Inst.* **2014**, *106*, dju200. [CrossRef]

148. Park, I.H.; Yang, H.N.; Lee, K.J.; Kim, T.S.; Lee, E.S.; Jung, S.Y.; Kwon, Y.; Kong, S.Y. Tumor-derived IL-18 induces PD-1 expression on immunosuppressive NK cells in triple-negative breast cancer. *Oncotarget* **2017**, *8*, 32722–32730. [CrossRef] [PubMed]

149. Berrien-Elliott, M.M.; Romee, R.; Fehniger, T.A. Improving natural killer cell cancer immunotherapy. *Curr. Opin. Organ Transplant.* **2015**, *20*, 671–680. [CrossRef] [PubMed]

150. Imai, K.; Matsuyama, S.; Miyake, S.; Suga, K.; Nakachi, K. Natural cytotoxic activity of peripheral-blood lymphocytes and cancer incidence: An 11-year follow-up study of a general population. *Lancet* **2000**, *356*, 1795–1799. [CrossRef]

151. Johansson, J.; Tabor, V.; Wikell, A.; Jalkanen, S.; Fuxe, J. TGF-beta1-Induced Epithelial-Mesenchymal Transition Promotes Monocyte/Macrophage Properties in Breast Cancer Cells. *Front. Oncol.* **2015**, *5*, 3. [CrossRef] [PubMed]

152. Faraji, F.; Pang, Y.; Walker, R.C.; Nieves Borges, R.; Yang, L.; Hunter, K.W. Cadm1 is a metastasis susceptibility gene that suppresses metastasis by modifying tumor interaction with the cell-mediated immunity. *PLoS Genet.* **2012**, *8*, e1002926. [CrossRef] [PubMed]

153. Chockley, P.J.; Chen, J.; Chen, G.; Beer, D.G.; Standiford, T.J.; Keshamouni, V.G. Epithelial-mesenchymal transition leads to NK cell-mediated metastasis-specific immunosurveillance in lung cancer. *J. Clin. Investig.* **2018**, *128*, 1384–1396. [CrossRef] [PubMed]

154. Halle, S.; Halle, O.; Forster, R. Mechanisms and Dynamics of T Cell-Mediated Cytotoxicity In Vivo. *Trends Immunol.* **2017**, *38*, 432–443. [CrossRef] [PubMed]

155. Martinez-Lostao, L.; Anel, A.; Pardo, J. How Do Cytotoxic Lymphocytes Kill Cancer Cells? *Clin. Cancer Res.* **2015**, *21*, 5047–5056. [CrossRef] [PubMed]

156. Pluhar, G.E.; Pennell, C.A.; Olin, M.R. CD8(+) T Cell-Independent Immune-Mediated Mechanisms of Anti-Tumor Activity. *Crit. Rev. Immunol.* **2015**, *35*, 153–172. [CrossRef] [PubMed]

157. Chen, L.; Diao, L.; Yang, Y.; Yi, X.; Rodriguez, B.L.; Li, Y.; Villalobos, P.A.; Cascone, T.; Liu, X.; Tan, L.; et al. CD38-Mediated Immunosuppression as a Mechanism of Tumor Cell Escape from PD-1/PD-L1 Blockade. *Cancer Discov.* **2018**, *8*, 1156–1175. [CrossRef]

158. Takeuchi, Y.; Nishikawa, H. Roles of regulatory T cells in cancer immunity. *Int. Immunol.* **2016**, *28*, 401–409. [CrossRef]
159. Xiong, S.; Pan, X.; Xu, L.; Yang, Z.; Guo, R.; Gu, Y.; Li, R.; Wang, Q.; Xiao, F.; Du, L.; et al. Regulatory T Cells Promote beta-Catenin—Mediated Epithelium-to-Mesenchyme Transition During Radiation-Induced Pulmonary Fibrosis. *Int. J. Radiat. Oncol. Biol. Phys.* **2015**, *93*, 425–435. [CrossRef]
160. Sommers, C.L.; Heckford, S.E.; Skerker, J.M.; Worland, P.; Torri, J.A.; Thompson, E.W.; Byers, S.W.; Gelmann, E.P. Loss of epithelial markers and acquisition of vimentin expression in adriamycin- and vinblastine-resistant human breast cancer cell lines. *Cancer Res.* **1992**, *52*, 5190–5197.
161. Denkert, C.; Loibl, S.; Noske, A.; Roller, M.; Muller, B.M.; Komor, M.; Budczies, J.; Darb-Esfahani, S.; Kronenwett, R.; Hanusch, C.; et al. Tumor-associated lymphocytes as an independent predictor of response to neoadjuvant chemotherapy in breast cancer. *J. Clin. Oncol.* **2010**, *28*, 105–113. [CrossRef]
162. Chockley, P.J.; Keshamouni, V.G. Immunological Consequences of Epithelial-Mesenchymal Transition in Tumor Progression. *J. Immunol.* **2016**, *197*, 691–698. [CrossRef]
163. Salvagno, C.; Ciampricotti, M.; Tuit, S.; Hau, C.S.; van Weverwijk, A.; Coffelt, S.B.; Kersten, K.; Vrijland, K.; Kos, K.; Ulas, T.; et al. Therapeutic targeting of macrophages enhances chemotherapy efficacy by unleashing type I interferon response. *Nat. Cell Biol.* **2019**, *21*, 511–521. [CrossRef] [PubMed]
164. Ladoire, S.; Arnould, L.; Apetoh, L.; Coudert, B.; Martin, F.; Chauffert, B.; Fumoleau, P.; Ghiringhelli, F. Pathologic complete response to neoadjuvant chemotherapy of breast carcinoma is associated with the disappearance of tumor-infiltrating foxp3+ regulatory T cells. *Clin. Cancer Res.* **2008**, *14*, 2413–2420. [CrossRef]
165. Antoon, J.W.; White, M.D.; Burow, M.E.; Beckman, B.S. Dual inhibition of sphingosine kinase isoforms ablates TNF-induced drug resistance. *Oncol. Rep.* **2012**, *27*, 1779–1786. [PubMed]
166. Sukocheva, O.A. Expansion of Sphingosine Kinase and Sphingosine-1-Phosphate Receptor Function in Normal and Cancer Cells: From Membrane Restructuring to Mediation of Estrogen Signaling and Stem Cell Programming. *Int. J. Mol. Sci.* **2018**, *19*, 420. [CrossRef] [PubMed]
167. Diaz-Montero, C.M.; Salem, M.L.; Nishimura, M.I.; Garrett-Mayer, E.; Cole, D.J.; Montero, A.J. Increased circulating myeloid-derived suppressor cells correlate with clinical cancer stage, metastatic tumor burden, and doxorubicin-cyclophosphamide chemotherapy. *Cancer Immunol. Immunother.* **2009**, *58*, 49–59. [CrossRef] [PubMed]
168. Ouzounova, M.; Lee, E.; Piranlioglu, R.; El Andaloussi, A.; Kolhe, R.; Demirci, M.F.; Marasco, D.; Asm, I.; Chadli, A.; Hassan, K.A.; et al. Monocytic and granulocytic myeloid derived suppressor cells differentially regulate spatiotemporal tumour plasticity during metastatic cascade. *Nat. Commun.* **2017**, *8*, 14979. [CrossRef]
169. Arce Vargas, F.; Furness, A.J.S.; Solomon, I.; Joshi, K.; Mekkaoui, L.; Lesko, M.H.; Miranda Rota, E.; Dahan, R.; Georgiou, A.; Sledzinska, A.; et al. Fc-Optimized Anti-CD25 Depletes Tumor-Infiltrating Regulatory T Cells and Synergizes with PD-1 Blockade to Eradicate Established Tumors. *Immunity* **2017**, *46*, 577–586. [CrossRef]
170. Ohm, J.E.; Gabrilovich, D.I.; Sempowski, G.D.; Kisseleva, E.; Parman, K.S.; Nadaf, S.; Carbone, D.P. VEGF inhibits T-cell development and may contribute to tumor-induced immune suppression. *Blood* **2003**, *101*, 4878–4886. [CrossRef]
171. Incio, J.; Ligibel, J.A.; McManus, D.T.; Suboj, P.; Jung, K.; Kawaguchi, K.; Pinter, M.; Babykutty, S.; Chin, S.M.; Vardam, T.D.; et al. Obesity promotes resistance to anti-VEGF therapy in breast cancer by up-regulating IL-6 and potentially FGF-2. *Sci. Transl. Med.* **2018**, *10*. [CrossRef]
172. Luque-Cabal, M.; García-Teijido, P.; Fernández-Pérez, Y.; Sánchez-Lorenzo, L.; Palacio-Vázquez, I. Mechanisms Behind the Resistance to Trastuzumab in HER2-Amplified Breast Cancer and Strategies to Overcome It. *Clin. Med. Insights Oncol.* **2016**, *10*, 21–30. [CrossRef]
173. Barrett, M.T.; Lenkiewicz, E.; Malasi, S.; Basu, A.; Yearley, J.H.; Annamalai, L.; McCullough, A.E.; Kosiorek, H.E.; Narang, P.; Wilson Sayres, M.A.; et al. The association of genomic lesions and PD-1/PD-L1 expression in resected triple-negative breast cancers. *Breast Cancer Res.* **2018**, *20*, 71. [CrossRef]
174. Mittendorf, E.A.; Philips, A.V.; Meric-Bernstam, F.; Qiao, N.; Wu, Y.; Harrington, S.; Su, X.; Wang, Y.; Gonzalez-Angulo, A.M.; Akcakanat, A.; et al. PD-L1 expression in triple-negative breast cancer. *Cancer Immunol. Res.* **2014**, *2*, 361–370. [CrossRef]

175. Muenst, S.; Soysal, S.D.; Gao, F.; Obermann, E.C.; Oertli, D.; Gillanders, W.E. The presence of programmed death 1 (PD-1)-positive tumor-infiltrating lymphocytes is associated with poor prognosis in human breast cancer. *Breast Cancer Res. Treat.* **2013**, *139*, 667–676. [CrossRef]
176. Noman, M.Z.; Janji, B.; Abdou, A.; Hasmim, M.; Terry, S.; Tan, T.Z.; Mami-Chouaib, F.; Thiery, J.P.; Chouaib, S. The immune checkpoint ligand PD-L1 is upregulated in EMT-activated human breast cancer cells by a mechanism involving ZEB-1 and miR-200. *Oncoimmunology* **2017**, *6*, e1263412. [CrossRef] [PubMed]
177. Chen, L.; Gibbons, D.L.; Goswami, S.; Cortez, M.A.; Ahn, Y.H.; Byers, L.A.; Zhang, X.; Yi, X.; Dwyer, D.; Lin, W.; et al. Metastasis is regulated via microRNA-200/ZEB1 axis control of tumour cell PD-L1 expression and intratumoral immunosuppression. *Nat. Commun.* **2014**, *5*, 5241. [CrossRef] [PubMed]
178. Nicolazzo, C.; Raimondi, C.; Mancini, M.; Caponnetto, S.; Gradilone, A.; Gandini, O.; Mastromartino, M.; Del Bene, G.; Prete, A.; Longo, F.; et al. Monitoring PD-L1 positive circulating tumor cells in non-small cell lung cancer patients treated with the PD-1 inhibitor Nivolumab. *Sci. Rep.* **2016**, *6*, 31726. [CrossRef] [PubMed]
179. Raimondi, C.; Carpino, G.; Nicolazzo, C.; Gradilone, A.; Gianni, W.; Gelibter, A.; Gaudio, E.; Cortesi, E.; Gazzaniga, P. PD-L1 and epithelial-mesenchymal transition in circulating tumor cells from non-small cell lung cancer patients: A molecular shield to evade immune system? *Oncoimmunology* **2017**, *6*, e1315488. [CrossRef] [PubMed]
180. Cassetta, L.; Kitamura, T. Targeting Tumor-Associated Macrophages as a Potential Strategy to Enhance the Response to Immune Checkpoint Inhibitors. *Front. Cell Dev. Biol.* **2018**, *6*, 38. [CrossRef]
181. Janakiram, M.; Abadi, Y.M.; Sparano, J.A.; Zang, X. T cell coinhibition and immunotherapy in human breast cancer. *Discov. Med.* **2012**, *14*, 229–236. [PubMed]

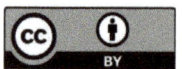

© 2019 by the authors. Licensee MDPI, Basel, Switzerland. This article is an open access article distributed under the terms and conditions of the Creative Commons Attribution (CC BY) license (http://creativecommons.org/licenses/by/4.0/).

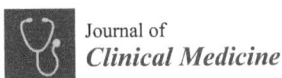 

*Review*

# UPR: An Upstream Signal to EMT Induction in Cancer

Patricia G. Santamaría [1,2,3,4], María J. Mazón [2,3], Pilar Eraso [1,2,3] and Francisco Portillo [1,2,3,4,*]

1. Departamento de Bioquímica, Universidad Autónoma de Madrid, 28029 Madrid, Spain; pgsantamaria@iib.uam.es (P.G.S.); peraso@iib.uam.es (P.E.)
2. Instituto de Investigaciones Biomédicas "Alberto Sols" CSIC-UAM, 28029 Madrid, Spain; mjmazon@iib.uam.es
3. IdiPAZ, 28029 Madrid, Spain
4. CIBERONC, 28029 Madrid, Spain
* Correspondence: francisco.portillo@uam.es; Tel.: +34-91-497-2732

Received: 27 March 2019; Accepted: 3 May 2019; Published: 8 May 2019

**Abstract:** The endoplasmic reticulum (ER) is the organelle where newly synthesized proteins enter the secretory pathway. Different physiological and pathological conditions may perturb the secretory capacity of cells and lead to the accumulation of misfolded and unfolded proteins. To relieve the produced stress, cells evoke an adaptive signalling network, the unfolded protein response (UPR), aimed at recovering protein homeostasis. Tumour cells must confront intrinsic and extrinsic pressures during cancer progression that produce a proteostasis imbalance and ER stress. To overcome this situation, tumour cells activate the UPR as a pro-survival mechanism. UPR activation has been documented in most types of human tumours and accumulating evidence supports a crucial role for UPR in the establishment, progression, metastasis and chemoresistance of tumours as well as its involvement in the acquisition of other hallmarks of cancer. In this review, we will analyse the role of UPR in cancer development highlighting the ability of tumours to exploit UPR signalling to promote epithelial-mesenchymal transition (EMT).

**Keywords:** epithelial-mesenchymal transition; endoplasmic reticulum stress; metastasis; plasticity; unfolded protein response

---

## 1. Introduction

The ER is responsible for a large number of metabolic processes, including folding and post-translational modification of secretory proteins. Cells must keep a balance between the protein synthetic load and their capacity to ensure that folding and post-translational modifications are correctly performed. Improper ER function causes misfolding of de novo synthesized proteins and their accumulation due to a stringent quality control. Proteins failing to pass this control are returned to the cytosol and targeted for degradation by the ER-associated degradation system (ERAD) [1,2]. Under some physiological or pathological conditions, the capacity of the ER protein maturation machinery may be overwhelmed, leading to the accumulation of unfolded or misfolded proteins, an event referred to as ER stress.

The UPR is an adaptive mechanism evolved to relieve the ER stress restoring the metabolic and protein folding efficiency of the ER [3]. Activation of the UPR is initiated by the stimulation of three stress sensors that reside in the ER membrane: protein kinase R-like ER kinase (PERK), inositol requiring enzyme 1α (IRE1) and activating transcription factor 6 (ATF6) (Figure 1). Stress sensing is mainly dependent on GRP78 (HSPA5), an ER resident chaperone also known as BiP. Under homeostatic conditions, GRP78 is bound to the ER luminal part of the three sensors preventing their activation. Upon ER stress, the dissociation of GRP78 from the UPR sensors allows their activation initiating downstream signalling pathways that will help cells to cope with ER stress. Activation of the UPR reduces unfolded protein load through several pro-survival mechanisms, including the reduction of protein translation to decrease the ER overload, increase in the degradation of misfolded proteins via the ERAD system, and upregulated transcription of a large number of target genes to facilitate correct secretory protein maturation. However, if ER stress is not adequately solved and homeostasis is not restored, UPR may lead to a persistent signal that rather than reinstating ER homeostasis drives cells to apoptosis [2]. UPR is thus a complex mechanism that includes adaptive pro-survival and also pro-apoptotic responses. All three ER stress sensors trigger downstream signalling pathways that control survival or death decisions.

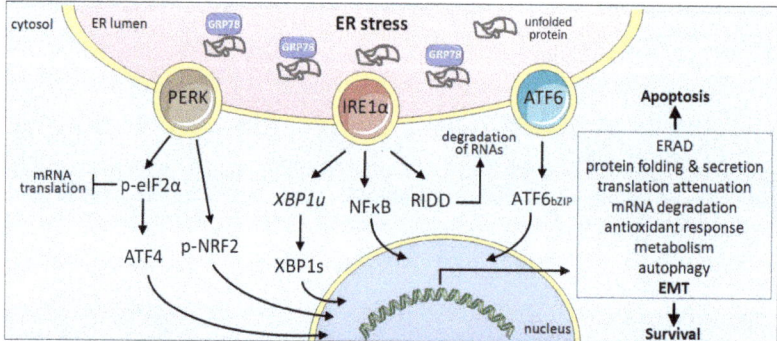

**Figure 1.** The UPR. The ER protein maturation capacity may be overwhelmed due to the action of several cell intrinsic and extrinsic factors, causing ER stress. The accumulation of unfolded proteins triggers the activation of the three ER-resident sensors responsible for UPR by sequestering GRP78. IRE1 mediates the unconventional splicing of the mRNA encoding XBP1 (XBP1u) rendering the functional transcription factor XBP1s and can activate NFκB signalling. IRE1 RNase degrades ER associated RNAs through RIDD (regulated IRE1-dependent decay). PERK phosphorylates eIF2α to inhibit global translation while promoting the translation of the transcription factor ATF4. PERK can also phosphorylate NRF2. ATF6 is exported from the ER to the Golgi apparatus, were the SP1 and SP2 proteases mediate the release of the bZIP domain (ATF6bZIP). In the nucleus, XBP1s, ATF4 and ATF6bZIP transcription factors trigger the expression of a large number of genes to help cells alleviate ER stress. Upon persistent ER stress, UPR favours apoptosis. Cancer cells exploit UPR signalling to promote survival under tumour-associated stress situations.

## 2. UPR Signalling Components

PERK is a type I transmembrane protein that, upon ER stress, dimerizes trans-autophosphorylates resulting in the activation of its kinase domain and the phosphorylation of eukaryotic translation initiation factor 2 alpha subunit (eIF2α) [4]. This phosphorylation transiently inhibits mRNA translation and attenuates global protein synthesis. This quick reduction of the ER overload relieves ER stress and has a pro-survival effect. Despite the overall reduction of protein synthesis, the phosphorylation of eIF2α allows the selective translation of a subset of UPR target proteins, including ATF4, a transcription factor that controls the expression of genes involved in protein folding, antioxidant response, amino acid metabolism and autophagy [5]. Active PERK also phosphorylates the nuclear factor erythroid related factor 2 (NRF2) which, upon translocation to the nucleus, controls the expression of anti-oxidant genes [6–8].

IRE1 is a type I transmembrane protein that contains two enzymatic activities on its cytosolic tail, a serine/threonine kinase and an endoribonuclease. In response to ER stress, IRE1 oligomerizes and trans-autophosphorylates undergoing a conformational change that activates its RNase domain. IRE1 RNase catalyses the unconventional splicing of an intron within XBP1 mRNA (XBP1u) shifting the XBP1 reading frame and producing a stable transcription factor known as XBP1s (thereafter XBP1) which promotes the transcription of genes involved in protein folding, ERAD, protein secretion and lipid synthesis [9–11]. Although IRE1 activity was first reported for its unconventional splicing activity, it is also involved in the degradation of ER-associated RNAs through a process known as RIDD (regulated IRE1-dependent decay) [12]. The molecular basis for the switch between RIDD and XBP1u mRNA splicing seems to be controlled by the oligomeric state of IRE1 [13–15]. Additionally, although less characterized, IRE1 activity also elicits the activation of the c-Jun N-terminal kinase (JNK) signalling [16].

ATF6 is a type II transmembrane protein that belongs to a family of transcription factors whose members contain a conserved bZIP domain on their cytosolic domain. Following ER stress ATF6 is transported from the ER to Golgi where it is cleaved by the proteases S1P and S2P [17]. The released ATF6 cytosolic domain (ATF6bZIP) translocates to the nucleus where it activates genes involved in ER quality control [18] and ERAD [19]. The cross-talk of ATF6 and XBP1 through heterodimerization further increases the scope of their target genes [2,20,21].

Several stresses both cell extrinsic and intrinsic may perturb the protein folding efficiency of the ER and lead to the accumulation of misfolded proteins, ER stress and UPR activation.

## 3. EMT: A Brief Update

EMT is a genetic and cellular programme that endows cells with mesenchymal features that ultimately facilitate motility (Figure 2) [22,23]. This reversible event was originally described while studying embryogenesis [24] and soon the EMT emerged as a crucial actor in tissue and organ development during morphogenesis and wound healing in adulthood [25]. EMT has since been linked to organ fibrosis and cancer, which is then referred to as pathological EMT [26]. In both physiological and pathological EMT, the expression of EMT transcription factors (EMT-TFs) launches a complex cellular programme that results in the loss of epithelial apical-basal cell polarity towards different degrees of mesenchymal morphology [27,28]. Essentially, the activation of EMT-TFs promotes a gene expression switch from genes involved in upholding epithelial cell polarity to genes responsible for the spindle-like morphology associated with mesenchymal features. These changes do not only relate to morphological traits, but also to the acquisition of several abilities that allow cells to move and invade nearby tissues [29].

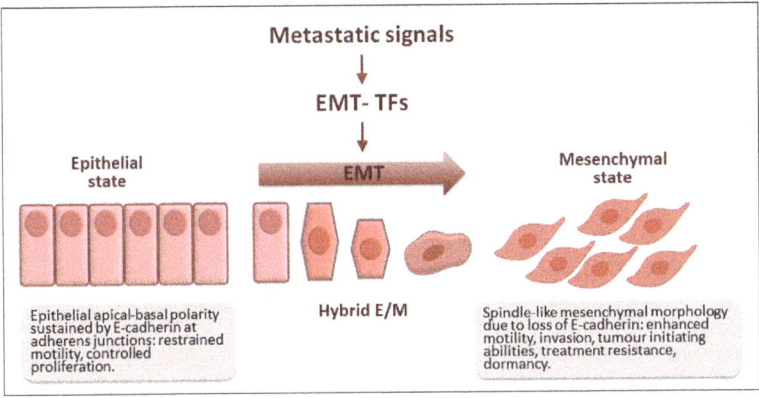

**Figure 2.** Epithelial-mesenchymal transition (EMT) in cancer progression. Different metastatic signals can activate one or more EMT-TFs which in turn trigger the EMT programme. During EMT, epithelial cells lose their apical-basal polarity and acquire mesenchymal traits that facilitate motility and contribute to the invasion-metastasis cascade. Some EMT-TFs directly control the expression of E-cadherin, whose functional loss is regarded as a hallmark of EMT. During EMT, hybrid epithelial/mesenchymal (E/M) states are also associated with tumour heterogeneity, tumour cell dissemination, cancer stem cell-like traits as well as immune evasion and resistance against conventional and targeted therapies.

It is nowadays well established that most carcinoma cells highjack the EMT programme to progress towards malignancy. In carcinomas, environmental cues and the exchange of signals among tumour cells and their microenvironment are mostly responsible for EMT implementation and the acquisition of mesenchymal traits and malignant progression. In fact, EMT is involved in the invasion-metastasis cascade, provides tumour-initiating abilities and contributes to the dormant state of disseminated tumour cells, cancer cell resistance to chemotherapy and immune evasion [22,23]. The core EMT-TFs responsible for implementing the EMT programme are the ZEB zinc finger TFs including ZEB1 and ZEB2, the zinc finger proteins belonging to the SNAIL family SNAI1 and SLUG (SNAI2), and the basic helix-loop-helix TFs TCF3, TWIST1 and TWIST2. These EMT-TFs can either bind directly to DNA or form transcriptional regulatory complexes to orchestrate the EMT by controlling the expression of numerous genes. ZEB, SNAIL, TCF3 and TWIST were originally described due to their ability to repress the invasion suppressor gene CDH1, encoding the cell adhesion protein E-cadherin [30], whose functional loss is considered a hallmark of EMT during carcinoma progression [31]. Hence, the transcription of EMT-TFs and their activity are tightly regulated by numerous layers and they act in distinct combinations to either activate or repress genes ultimately responsible for the features associated with a mesenchymal-like state during carcinoma progression [22,32]. Cell intrinsic and extrinsic signalling control the EMT programme by impinging on the expression and activity of the EMT-TFs and other cell-specific cofactors that act, in common or in non-redundant networks, to regulate the cellular plasticity associated with each particular context [22,29]. The reversion to the epithelial state through the mesenchymal-epithelial transition (MET) is responsible for metastatic outgrowth after tumour cell dissemination [33,34], characterized by the re-expression of epithelial markers and repression of mesenchymal traits [35]. Still poorly understood, MET regulation is most likely controlled by the shutdown of the aforementioned EMT-TFs, although signalling from the metastatic microenvironment may impinge on intracellular pathways to alter gene expression [23].

In cancer, increasing evidence indicates that the full implementation of the EMT programme, as defined in in vitro cellular models upon expression of an EMT-TF, would be a rare event. Besides, cells in different intermediate morphological states ranging from partially epithelial to quasi-mesenchymal are more likely to occur and be responsible for implementing different steps during tumour progression. Carcinoma cells undergoing EMT would thus show hybrid features and express a mixture of epithelial and mesenchymal markers, whereas incompletely losing their epithelial cell polarity. Indeed, these cells displaying partial EMT states have been documented in human cancers and are thought to be particularly plastic. These plastic EMT cells, while able to degrade and invade the surrounding stroma, may also, have given the signalling context, acquire stem cell-like traits, and become refractory to therapy and immune surveillance [22,27,36]. Moreover, these hybrid EMT cells are linked to increased metastatic potential in different mouse models of cancer, as well as in human tumours [27,37]. EMT was linked to breast cancer cell stemness [38,39] and its characteristic plasticity is now being related to cancer stem cell-like properties in different human tumours [27]. Cancer stem cells are also responsible for the appearance of tumour recurrence establishing a link between EMT and chemoresistance mechanisms, whereas tumour cells undergoing EMT have been shown to express immunosuppressive and immunoevasive molecules to avoid attack by the innate and adaptive immune systems in cancer mouse models [23].

Therefore, EMT endows subpopulations of cancer cells with a highly dynamic morphological plasticity tied to context-dependent functional abilities that facilitate malignant progression (Figure 2).

## 4. ER Stressors, UPR and EMT

Cancer cells are subjected to numerous intracellular and extracellular stresses that disturb ER homeostasis provoking ER stress and thus, UPR activation (Figure 1). During cancer progression the tumours acquire different biological properties including sustaining proliferative signalling, evading growth suppressors, resisting cell death, enabling replicative immortality, inducing angiogenesis, and activating invasion and metastasis. All of these biological properties constitute the so-called Hallmarks of Cancer [40]. In addition, to support the increased metabolic demand and the environmental pressure, cancer cells need to reprogramme their secretory functions to secrete metalloproteases, growth factors or cytokines that will facilitate tumour invasion and progression. Activation of the UPR influences this secretory switch [41]. Current evidence suggests that UPR activation favours tumour progression through the modulation of some of the Cancer Hallmarks [42]. One of the hallmarks powered by UPR signalling is the activation of the invasion-metastasis cascade, in which EMT plays a central role, as mentioned above [41,43–48]. Although a few reports suggest that EMT can in some instances result in UPR activation [49,50], the information is still scarce and this issue will not be addressed herein.

We will next describe the ER stressors that provoke UPR activation; linking how defined UPR signals modulate EMT (Figure 3).

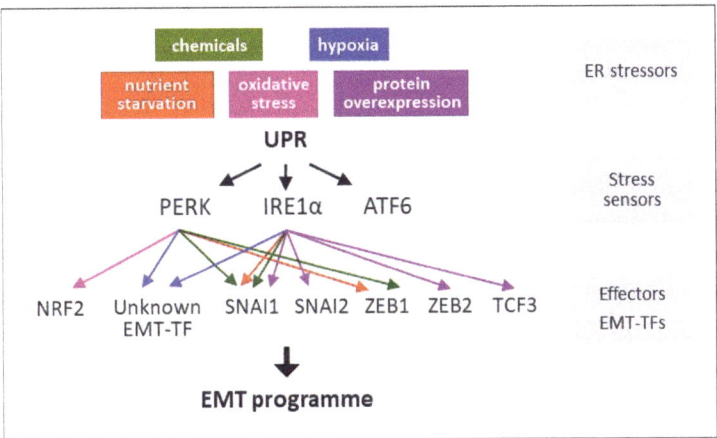

**Figure 3.** UPR signalling and EMT in cancer. In response to diverse ER stressors, UPR signalling is activated to relieve the stress and favour survival. In some tumours, the ER stress sensors and signalling players PERK and IRE1 are proposed to modulate EMT by impinging on particular EMT-TFs. Through the implementation of EMT, UPR can contribute to the progression and recurrence of tumours upon treatment. Thus, ER stress and UPR components can be exploited as plausible targets for anti-cancer therapy.

*4.1. Cell Extrinsic Stressors*

4.1.1. Chemicals

The UPR has been extensively studied in vitro by treating cells with chemical stressors such as thapsigargin, dithiothreitol or tunicamycin, which disturb calcium homeostasis, redox equilibrium or N-glycan synthesis, respectively. These drugs activate non-specifically the three arms of the UPR [51]. Also, ER stress can often be attributed to drug-induced adverse effects caused by numerous anti-cancer drugs used by present pharmacology such as bortezomib, cisplatin and doxorubicin, which impact the PERK and/or IRE1 branches of the UPR in different ways [52,53]. Recently, research efforts aimed at looking for IRE1 and PERK inhibitors as possible anti-tumoral drugs have intensified. In this sense, MKC8866 (IRE1 inhibitor) and ISRIB (p-eIF2α inhibitor), were shown to decrease breast cancer cell proliferation and promote tumour regression in patient-derived xenografts (PDX) from metastatic prostate cancer tumours, respectively [54,55].

EMT induction after UPR activation was first observed in vitro in rat alveolar epithelia cell lines upon treatment with the classical ER stressors tunicamycin and thapsigargin [56,57]. In both cases, activation of the IRE1 branch of the UPR leads to EMT in a SMAD2/3 and Src-dependent fashion although the underlying molecular mechanism was not analysed. These observations were further confirmed in vivo in a rat model of bleomycin-induced pulmonary fibrosis in which the analysis of bleomycin-treated animals revealed increased expression of IRE1-XBP1, mesenchymal cell markers, and the concomitant downregulation of epithelial cell markers [58]. These studies also showed that the promotion of EMT by XBP1 was dependent on SNAI1 expression in alveolar epithelia cell lines [58] (Figure 3).

The number of chemical stressors inducing EMT after UPR activation has been expanded by the recent finding that chemotherapeutic drugs activate ER stress and ultimately EMT [59]. Treatment of lung adenocarcinoma cell lines with cisplatin, cytarabine, doxorubicin, gemcitabine, vinorelbine or pemetrexed activate the PERK branch of the UPR which, in turn, induces EMT through the upregulation of SNAI1 and ZEB1 gene expression as well as EMT-like changes in several tissues in mice [59] (Figure 3).

4.1.2. Hypoxia

Hypoxia compromises ER protein folding leading to the activation of the UPR [43] whereas it is also a known inducer of EMT in solid tumours [60].

Hypoxia activates the PERK arm of the UPR to promote metastasis in human cervical tumoral cells [61]. Hypoxic stress, through activated PERK, produces a rapid inhibition of protein translation due to the transient phosphorylation of eIF2$\alpha$ and the preferred translation of a subset of transcripts including ATF4 [5] (Figure 3). IRE1 has also been involved in facilitating cell survival under hypoxic conditions since XBP1-deficient cells exhibited reduced survival in vitro as compared with their wild-type counterparts when exposed to hypoxic environment [62]. Work in triple negative breast cancer (TNBC) cells [63] points to an interaction between XBP1 and hypoxia-inducing factor 1$\alpha$ (HIF1$\alpha$) that form a transcriptional complex to promote efficient transcription of HIF1$\alpha$ target genes. By sustaining HIF1$\alpha$ transcriptional program, the IRE1-XBP1 arm of the UPR supports survival during hypoxia and sustains tumour growth [64] (Figure 3).

One consequence of the activation of the UPR in hypoxic tumours is an increase in autophagy. Through the liberation of amino-acids from long-lived proteins and the removal of damaged organelles, autophagy exerts a cytoprotective effect and helps cells to survive [43]. Both the PERK and IRE1 branches of the UPR participate in this survival mechanism. In several human cancer cell lines, hypoxia increased transcription of the essential autophagy genes microtubule-associated protein 1 light chain 3beta (LC3) and autophagy-related gene 5 (ATG5) through the activation of PERK [65]. Also, activation of IRE1 during the hypoxia-induced ER stress increases tumour cell tolerance to hypoxia [62] (Figure 3).

Activation of the UPR also plays a role in tumour adaptation to hypoxic stress by promoting angiogenesis. Angiogenesis is regulated by the secretion of soluble factors such as VEGF-A. Several examples implicate the IRE1-XBP1 axis in this process. In TNBC, XBP1 expression is required for HIF1$\alpha$-mediated VEGF-A production and vessel formation under hypoxia, and xenografts derived from cells transfected with XBP1 shRNA displayed reduced angiogenesis [63]. Also, IRE1$^{-/-}$ mouse embryo fibroblasts decreased the production of VEGF-A after ER stress [66]. In addition to IRE1, PERK signalling has also been involved in the upregulation of angiogenic factors. Xenografts derived from PERK KO cells showed delayed growth and the tumours presented reduced blood vessel formation [67]. More recently, it was shown that the PERK arm of the UPR controls the induction of angiogenic factors and that ATF4 itself binds to the promoter of VEGF-A [66,68].

The information about the axis hypoxia-UPR-EMT is still scarce, however several recent findings suggest that such a relationship exists. Gastric cancer cells under hypoxic conditions suffer EMT and the PERK and ATF6 arms of the UPR are activated. Moreover, knockout of PERK, ATF4 or ATF6 hinders the induction of EMT by hypoxia [69]. In TNBC, we have already mentioned that XBP1 drives tumorigenesis by assembling a transcriptional complex with HIF1$\alpha$ [63]. Perhaps the high metastatic potential of this subtype of breast cancer could be related to a positive action of HIF1$\alpha$-XBP1 on EMT, whose occurrence in TNBC is well established [70]. Finally, the hypoxic activation of the PERK-eIF2$\alpha$

arm in human cervix cancer cells mentioned above was shown to upregulate LAMP3, a putative metastasis-promoting gene, which promotes both the migratory phenotype and the development of lymph node metastases suggesting the possibility of EMT occurrence [61].

4.1.3. Nutrient Starvation

Intimately related with the insufficient vascularization of the tumour is the nutrient stress starvation suffered by tumour cells. The UPR participates in the rewiring of tumour metabolism by selectively activating catabolic pathways—we have already mentioned the induction of autophagy—but also biosynthetic pathways. In human tumour tissues, and several tumour cell lines, blocking UPR by silencing PERK or ATF4 significantly reduces the production of angiogenesis mediators induced by glucose deprivation [68]. Recently, oncogenic KRAS has been identified as a key regulator of the transcriptional response to nutrient deprivation in non-small cell lung cancer and ATF4, as a key transcription factor regulated by KRAS to support amino acid homeostasis. Through the regulation of ATF4, KRAS controls amino acid uptake and asparagine biosynthesis [71]. In addition to ATF4 signalling, IRE1 pathway activation of XBP1 controls the hexosamine biosynthetic pathway to generate substrates for protein glycosylation [72], and, in complex with HIF1$\alpha$, activates a transcriptional programme to upregulate glycolytic enzymes and glucose transport [63].

Another recently published study has described that the availability of asparagine controls metastasis in breast cancer, at least in part through the modulation of EMT. Limiting asparagine by asparagine dietary restriction or by knocking down asparagine synthetase reduces the metastatic capacity of the primary tumour and, by contrast, an increase in dietary asparagine or enforced asparagine synthetase expression promotes metastatic progression. Interestingly, asparagine synthetase is a target of the PERK-eIF2$\alpha$-ATF4 branch of the UPR and ATF4 knockdown mimics the phenotype caused by asparagine synthetase knockdown [73]. One plausible interpretation of these findings could be that asparagine starvation triggers activation of the PERK-eIF2$\alpha$-ATF4 branch which in turn could upregulate asparagine synthetase gene expression and, thus, EMT (Figure 3).

Cancer cells and melanoma in particular require an exogenous supply of glutamine since it is commonly depleted in tumours. Interestingly, it has been recently demonstrated that glutamine starvation is responsible for an upregulation of ATF4 in melanoma cells [74]. In this study, the authors demonstrate that glutamine limitation promotes an ATF4 dependent repression of MITF, considered a melanocyte lineage differentiation gene. MITF downregulation in response to stress is then associated with enhanced invasion, upregulation of ZEB1 and downregulation of SNAI2, hallmarks of EMT-associated reprogramming in late-stage melanoma [75] (Figure 3).

Deprivation of essential amino acids also causes activation of the UPR but, in this case, the arms activated are the IRE1 and ATF6 [76]. In this study, the induction of EMT was not analysed, however, based on the mentioned role of XBP1 in upregulating SNAI1, starvation of essential amino acids could result in stress inducing the UPR and subsequently EMT. Glucose starvation also promotes EMT [77] but whether this EMT induction is a consequence of the expected UPR activation due to limited glucose availability is nowadays not known. Finally, a recent review discusses the evidences linking starvation-induced ER stress to invasiveness and cancer progression [78]. In tumours, besides nutrient limitation and hypoxia, other cell extrinsic or intrinsic cues would be able to trigger a translational reprogramming through eIF2$\alpha$ phosphorylation, which in turn would promote an invasive phenotype [78].

*4.2. Cell Intrinsic Stressors*

4.2.1. Oncogenes

Malignant transformation by the activation of oncogenes is associated with an increased cell proliferation that imposes severe pressures on cellular processes such as an excessive demand for protein synthesis in the ER. When the folding capacity of the ER is exceeded, cancer cells trigger the UPR activating PERK, IRE1 and/or ATF6-dependent signalling pathways as shown in different types of cancer (Figure 1) [79–82]. The metabolic reset imposed by the oncogenic transformation establishes a complex interplay within the cancer cell among the different stress responses to promote cell survival and metastatic expansion. In some cases, UPR induction is clearly linked with a malignant phenotype and aggressiveness, as shown by XBP1 overexpression in human multiple myeloma [83], and overactivation of PERK-ATF4 in MYC-induced lymphomas [79], breast cancers [84] and colorectal adenocarcinomas [85]. Recent work with RAS-induced mouse primary tumours points to a complex role of IRE1 signalling. In mouse keratinocytes, RAS transformation promotes IRE1 activation and XBP1 splicing through the action of both ER stress and RAS-activated MEK-ERK signalling pathways, resulting in enhanced proliferation. However, following this initial proliferative response, keratinocytes stop growing and enter senescence prematurely. Senescence occurs in parallel with the dampening of the ER stress response and an increase in IRE1 supported by MEK-ERK signalling, indicating that in keratinocytes expressing oncogenic RAS, reduction of ER stress accelerates senescence dependent on IRE1-RIDD activity [82]. These results suggest that the type and the stage of the tumour may have an influence on the outcome of UPR activation either pro-survival or anti-tumorigenic.

In conclusion, the activation of the UPR upon oncogenic signalling is well documented but, in these cases, activation of the UPR pro-survival response is apparently unrelated to EMT induction.

4.2.2. Oxidative Stress

Tumour cells accumulate increased levels of reactive oxygen species (ROS) that lead to the general phenomenon of oxidative stress. ROS are produced intracellularly by both enzymatic and non-enzymatic reactions in different cellular compartments during cell growth [86]. Cancer cells have much higher levels of ROS than normal cells [87] and, additionally, activation of PERK due to hypoxia results in upregulation of ER-oxidase ERO1α [88] to facilitate the oxidative protein folding in the ER. In fact, a correlation between the levels of ERO1α and poor prognosis in breast cancer patients has been reported [89]. Oxidative protein folding brings about, on the other hand, an increase in ROS production that may aggravate cellular stress. Therefore, activation of the UPR upon exposure to oxidative stress is an adaptive mechanism to preserve cell function and survival although persistent oxidative stress ultimately initiates apoptotic cascades [90].

This protective function of the UPR against oxidative stress has an important impact during the first steps of tumour invasion, when an abnormal activation of EMT causes tumour cell detachment and acquisition of an invasive and migratory phenotype. In this situation, PERK activation favours survival upon ECM detachment [91] and alleviates the oxidative stress concomitant to the loss of matrix attachment contributing also to metastasis in in vivo models [92] (Figure 3).

Cumulative data suggest that oxidative stress governs several phases of tumour progression [93] including EMT, as revealed by the finding that overexpression of NOX1, a NADPH oxidase that generates ROS, induces EMT [94]. Cancer cells upregulate multiple antioxidant systems to overcome the negative effect of oxidative stress [95]. As mentioned above, one of the defence mechanisms activated by oxidative stress is the PERK-eIF2α-ATF4 arm of the UPR [90,96], which in turn upregulates NRF2, a master regulator of the antioxidant response [97]. A direct link among oxidative stress, UPR and EMT is suggested by the recent finding that NRF2 promotes EMT in cancer cell lines [98,99] (Figure 3).

4.2.3. Alterations in UPR Signalling Components

Different studies support a role for proteostasis imbalance in cancer development raising the possibility that alterations in the UPR itself may contribute to tumorigenesis [46,100]. Constitutive activation of UPR signalling components has been reported in various types of human cancers such as breast tumours, hepatocellular carcinomas or gastric tumours [101]. Overexpression of GRP78 is indicative of a more aggressive phenotype since it is overexpressed with higher frequency in high-grade estrogen-receptor-negative tumours than in low-grade estrogen-receptors-positive tumours [102] in line with the idea that UPR activation may play a protective role against apoptosis in tumour cells. In contrast, in lung adenocarcinoma a higher overall survival was shown for those patients displaying high expression of IRE1 [103].

Sequencing the genome of different types of human cancers exposed somatic mutations in IRE1. In fact, ERN1, the gene coding for IRE1, was found to rank fifth among all the genes coding for human protein kinases carrying driver mutations across various human cancers [104]. In a recent review [44], the authors describe the cancer-associated mutations identified in the three UPR stress sensors. Missense mutations are equally present in the three cases, silent mutations and in-frame deletions or insertions are enriched in IRE1 while nonsense mutations are more frequent in ATF6. Interestingly, the authors emphasize that not all somatic mutations are equally present in every cancer type but rather it appears to be some preferences, with IRE1 mutations being predominant in cancers from the nervous system, whereas gastrointestinal cancers are enriched in ATF6 and IRE1 mutations and urologic and lung cancers in ATF6 and PERK mutations. Unfortunately, the biological impact of these mutations on the expression, activity or stability of the ER sensors or, more importantly, on the tumour phenotype is still unknown in most cases. Significant advance has been reported in the case of some IRE1 mutations. In human cancer tissue samples of glioblastoma multiforme (GBM) two missense mutations (S769F and P336L) and one stop mutation (Q780stop) have been identified in IRE1 [104,105]. Very recently, the sequencing of additional GBM samples revealed a new somatic mutation in a less conserved amino acid (A414T) [106]. The authors analysed the differential impact of the IRE1 variants, expressed in a glioblastoma cell line, on their kinase and RNase activities and how they affected the cell phenotype, downstream signalling and gene expression profile. Together with the in vivo data of tumour development after expression of the IRE1 variants, the study demonstrates that mutations affecting IRE1 activity determine the development of GBM tumours [106]. While the IRE1-XBP1 splicing activity favours angiogenesis and higher expression of migration/invasion markers, IRE1-RIDD activity promotes attenuation of both responses in tumour cells, pointing to antagonistic roles of the two signalling outputs in GBM progression.

Nevertheless, although mutations in the distinct components of the UPR are present on different tumour types, knowledge on their role in cancer biology is still very limited.

4.2.4. Protein Overexpression

Overexpression of individual proteins, not necessarily involved in signalling pathways driving tumour progression, can also provoke UPR activation and subsequent EMT induction.

One early report showed that enhanced expression of the protease inhibitor SERPINB3 promotes tumorigenesis and EMT via the PERK and ATF6 arms of the UPR which lead to NFκB activation and subsequent expression of the pro-tumorigenic cytokine IL6 [107].

More recently, it has been reported that the overexpression of LOXL2 also causes UPR activation and subsequent EMT induction [108]. LOXL2 is a secreted enzyme involved in covalent inter and intramolecular crosslinking of the extracellular matrix components but its involvement in intracellular processes and tumorigenesis has been increasingly postulated [109]. LOXL2 is retained within the ER when it is endogenously or ectopically overexpressed. In the ER, LOXL2 interacts with GRP78 which in turn activates the IRE1-XBP1 and PERK-eIF2α arms of the UPR [108]. Furthermore, the processed form of XBP1 is shown to bind to the promoters of *SNAI1*, *SNAI2*, *TCF3* and *ZEB2* activating their expression [108] (Figure 3). Interestingly, IRE1 inhibition hampers the upregulation of these EMT-TFs and blocks LOXL2 ability to induce a full EMT program [108]. Remarkably, in human tumours with overexpression of LOXL2, the protein is accumulated in structures that are compatible with an ER location and this subcellular localization pattern correlates with poor prognosis of squamous cell carcinomas and distant metastasis of basal breast carcinomas [110,111].

## 5. UPR and EMT Footprint in Human Tumours

The information reviewed above relative to the cooperation between the UPR and EMT during tumour progression comes mainly from data derived from experiments performed using cell lines and mouse models. Concerning clinical samples, thorough reviews have recently addressed the evidences of ER stress in human tumours by examining the expression levels of UPR signalling components [41,81]. As a matter of fact, UPR components have been detected in samples from brain, breast, colorectal, kidney, liver, lung, and pancreatic cancer patients and their overexpression has been mostly correlated with worse prognosis [41,81]. In B-cell hematological malignancies, the IRE1-XBP1 arm is essential due to the B-cell inherent secretory phenotype and GRP78 and/or XBP1 upregulation is associated with poorer outcome in leukaemia, lymphoma and multiple myeloma [81].

There are few studies to date that analyse in human cancer biopsies markers of EMT along with UPR activation markers. These studies would help to elucidate the prognostic value of both programmes in terms of patient outcome, therapy choice and/or treatment response. Recent works addressing both UPR and EMT pathways in clinical samples are summarized in Table 1. Some of these studies characterize the underlying molecular mechanisms in cellular models mostly supporting that UPR activation precedes EMT in tumour progression.

**Table 1.** Studies analysing UPR and EMT in clinical samples and/or primary derived cell lines.

| Type of Cancer | UPR Activation | EMT Footprint | Source | Prognosis | Reference |
|---|---|---|---|---|---|
| Breast cancer | active PERK (ATF4 target genes) | EMT gene signature | human breast cancer datasets | NA | [49] |
|  | active PERK (ATF4 target genes) | EMT gene signature | human breast cancer datasets | increased metastasis | [112] |
| Colon cancer | active PERK (ATF4 target genes) | EMT gene signature | human colon cancer datasets | NA | [49] |
| Colorectal carcinoma | IRE1 | E-cad, N-cad | CRC tumour tissues and CRC cell lines | shorter overall survival | [113] |
|  | GRP78 | β-catenin | CRC tumour tissues | NA | [50] |
| Gastric cancer | active PERK (ATF4 target genes) | EMT gene signature | human gastric cancer datasets | NA | [49] |
| Glioblastoma | IRE1/XBP1 axis | VIM, ZEB1, TGFβ2 | human GBM cancer datasets and primary derived GBM cell lines | shorter overall survival, increased tumour aggressiveness | [106] |
| Hepatocellular carcinoma | XBP1 | VIM, E-cad | HCC tumour tissue | increased tumour size, increased metastasis | [114] |
| Lung cancer | active PERK (ATF4 target genes) | EMT gene signature | human cancer datasets | NA | [49] |
|  | IRE1, PERK | ZEB1, SNAI2, SNAI1 | LAC tumours | NA | [115] |

CRC: colorectal carcinoma; GBM: glioblastoma; HCC: hepatocellular carcinoma; LAC: Lung adenocarcinoma; NA: not analysed.

In this regard, the expression of an EMT signature is strongly correlated with ATF4 expression in datasets covering breast, colon, gastric, lung, and metastatic sites from patient tumour samples [49]. In colorectal carcinoma, there is an association of GRP78 and nuclear β-catenin staining at the invasive front of a small cohort of tumour tissues samples, suggestive of ER stress and EMT [50]. Also in colorectal carcinoma, higher IRE1 expression in patient samples is associated with lower overall survival and the molecular mechanism proposed is the activation of EMT by IRE1 [113]. Additionally, in hepatocellular carcinoma, the detection of XBP1 in tumour samples positively correlates with vimentin and negatively with E-cadherin [114]. In the case of glioblastoma, higher activity of the IRE1-XBP1 axis correlates with shorter patient survival, considerable tumour infiltration by immune cells and increased tumour angiogenesis and invasive properties. These tumour characteristics are associated with increased expression of EMT-related markers in primary derived glioblastoma cell lines [106]. In breast cancer, an EMT signature is the most relevant feature in tumours showing

PERK activation [112]. The authors propose that the transcription factor CREB3L1, downstream of PERK, promotes metastasis particularly in those tumours showing activated PERK signalling and an EMT signature [112]. Lastly, in lung adenocarcinoma tumours, ER stress proteins such as IRE1 and PERK co-express with EMT markers in lung tumour samples compared to matched normal adjacent tissues [115].

A direct connection between ER stress and UPR activation with malignancy has been formally established in different cancer settings [41,46,47,81]. In many occasions, the authors did not directly address the role played by EMT in tumour progression even when UPR signalling was linked to increased invasion or other EMT-related roles. This was the case in TNBC [63], glioblastoma [116], pancreatic ductal adenocarcinoma [117] or esophageal squamous cell carcinoma [118]. The opposite scenario, analysis of UPR activation in tumours with EMT-related markers, is even less common despite the central role of ER stress signalling in cancer progression [43,81]. Moreover, the biological significance of EMT in tumour development has been long debated by pathologists partly due to the transient nature of EMT and the spectrum of EMT phenotypic states involved in different steps of the invasion-metastasis cascade, which limits the detection of EMT in clinical samples [23,27]. Additionally, data obtained from analyses such as next-generation sequencing or proteomic and transcriptomic profiling in tumour biopsies derive from heterogeneous tissues samples. This fact hinders the contribution of particular cell subpopulations bearing ER stress and different degrees of mesenchymal features. Besides, the key influence of tumour microenvironment signalling on sustaining UPR and EMT cannot be disregarded.

## 6. UPR and Therapeutic Opportunities

Cancer cells undergoing UPR activation and prone to EMT may sustain malignant progression since they are able to migrate and invade, display tumour-initiating properties and resilience in foreign microenvironments while they become skilled to evade drug therapy and immune surveillance. Nevertheless, the UPR can also be a pro-apoptotic signalling pathway. When cells are subjected to a chronic ER stress or cannot resolve the stress, the UPR directs the cells to apoptosis [2]. This fact constitutes a therapeutic opportunity in the treatment of cancer. In this sense, some new drugs provoking ER stress have shown their potential in pre-clinical models. An example is matrine that suppresses prostate cancer aggressiveness by inhibiting EMT and activating the UPR [119]. Acriflavine, an antibiotic with several anticancer effects, has been shown to interfere with EMT and ATF4 dependent UPR activation in pancreatic cancer cell lines restoring sensitivity to cytotoxic drugs [120]. In breast cancer cell lines, AECHL-1, a triterpernoid, has been suggested as an anti-neoplastic agent by inducing ER stress and suppressing EMT [121]. Similarly, another alkaloid, sinomenine, prevents glioblastoma cell proliferation and invasion by triggering ER stress and EMT suppression [122]. Finally, the use of novel iron chelators has been proposed as a promising anti-cancer therapy by regulating ER stress signalling and inhibiting the EMT programme through the metastasis suppressor protein NDRG1 [123].

## 7. Conclusions and Perspectives

The involvement of ER stress and the activation of the UPR in cancer initiation and progression is now supported both by in vitro analyses and data from clinical samples [41,43,46,81]. Whether the UPR implication in cancer is mediated through EMT is still debated, although ER stress and EMT are both linked to similar hallmarks responsible for tumour progression. In this review, we have highlighted the ER stressors that activate the UPR and subsequently EMT, suggesting that the UPR may be an additional upstream signal for the induction of the EMT programme; this role of the UPR might well be dependent on the tumour type and/or the nature of the triggering stress (Figure 3). Probably, there is an underestimation of the actual UPR-EMT axis contribution to cancer. The understanding of these allied pathways and the hierarchy governing their signalling as well as the stromal cues that support their activation during tumour progression is far from complete. In order to improve the clinical management of cancer patients, the identification of specific markers for UPR and EMT status in cancer cell subpopulations within tumour biopsies possibly will aid in predicting tumour progression and therapy response.

In conclusion, the development of drugs targeting ER stress in particularly susceptible cells such as those in different EMT states might constitute a promising cancer therapy.

**Author Contributions:** All authors made substantial contributions to the conception, design and writing of the work and approved the submitted version. (Conceptualization, P.G.S., M.J.M., P.E. and F.P.; writing—original draft preparation, P.G.S., M.J.M., P.E. and F.P; review and editing, P.G.S., M.J.M., P.E. and F.P; funding acquisition, P.G.S. and F.P.).

**Funding:** This research was funded by the Spanish Ministerio de Economía y Competitividad (MICINN) (SAF2013-44739-R and SAF2016-76504-R, EU-FEDER funds), Instituto de Salud Carlos III (CIBERONC 16/12/00295, EU-FEDER funds), and Worldwide Cancer Research (AICR-12-1057 and WWCR-16-0295).

**Acknowledgments:** We thank Amparo Cano for valuable input and we apologize to all those colleagues whose important work has not been cited.

**Conflicts of Interest:** The authors declare no conflict of interest.

## References

1. Meusser, B.; Hirsch, C.; Jarosch, E.; Sommer, T. ERAD: The long road to destruction. *Nat. Cell Biol.* **2005**, *7*, 766–772. [CrossRef]
2. Hetz, C. The unfolded protein response: Controlling cell fate decisions under ER stress and beyond. *Nat. Rev. Mol. Cell Biol.* **2012**, *13*, 89–102. [CrossRef] [PubMed]
3. Ron, D.; Walter, P. Signal integration in the endoplasmic reticulum unfolded protein response. *Nat. Rev. Mol. Cell Biol.* **2007**, *8*, 519–529. [CrossRef]
4. Koumenis, C.; Naczki, C.; Koritzinsky, M.; Rastani, S.; Diehl, A.; Sonenberg, N.; Koromilas, A.; Wouters, B.G. Regulation of protein synthesis by hypoxia via activation of the endoplasmic reticulum kinase PERK and phosphorylation of the translation initiation factor eIF2alpha. *Mol. Cell. Biol.* **2002**, *22*, 7405–7416. [CrossRef]
5. Blais, J.D.; Filipenko, V.; Bi, M.; Harding, H.P.; Ron, D.; Koumenis, C.; Wouters, B.G.; Bell, J.C. Activating transcription factor 4 is translationally regulated by hypoxic stress. *Mol. Cell. Biol.* **2004**, *24*, 7469–7482. [CrossRef] [PubMed]
6. Cullinan, S.B.; Diehl, J.A. PERK-dependent activation of Nrf2 contributes to redox homeostasis and cell survival following endoplasmic reticulum stress. *J. Biol. Chem.* **2004**, *279*, 20108–20117. [CrossRef] [PubMed]
7. Cullinan, S.B.; Zhang, D.; Hannink, M.; Arvisais, E.; Kaufman, R.J.; Diehl, J.A. Nrf2 is a direct PERK substrate and effector of PERK-dependent cell survival. *Mol. Cell. Biol.* **2003**, *23*, 7198–7209. [CrossRef]
8. Del Vecchio, C.A.; Feng, Y.; Sokol, E.S.; Tillman, E.J.; Sanduja, S.; Reinhardt, F.; Gupta, P.B. De-differentiation confers multidrug resistance via noncanonical PERK-Nrf2 signaling. *PLoS Biol.* **2014**, *12*, e1001945. [CrossRef]
9. Lee, A.H.; Iwakoshi, N.N.; Glimcher, L.H. XBP-1 regulates a subset of endoplasmic reticulum resident chaperone genes in the unfolded protein response. *Mol. Cell. Biol.* **2003**, *23*, 7448–7459. [CrossRef]
10. Acosta-Alvear, D.; Zhou, Y.; Blais, A.; Tsikitis, M.; Lents, N.H.; Arias, C.; Lennon, C.J.; Kluger, Y.; Dynlacht, B.D. XBP1 controls diverse cell type- and condition-specific transcriptional regulatory networks. *Mol. Cell* **2007**, *27*, 53–66. [CrossRef]
11. Hetz, C.; Martinon, F.; Rodriguez, D.; Glimcher, L.H. The unfolded protein response: Integrating stress signals through the stress sensor IRE1alpha. *Physiol. Rev.* **2011**, *91*, 1219–1243. [CrossRef]
12. Hetz, C.; Chevet, E.; Oakes, S.A. Proteostasis control by the unfolded protein response. *Nat. Cell Biol.* **2015**, *17*, 829–838. [CrossRef]
13. Ghosh, R.; Wang, L.; Wang, E.S.; Perera, B.G.; Igbaria, A.; Morita, S.; Prado, K.; Thamsen, M.; Caswell, D.; Macias, H.; et al. Allosteric inhibition of the IRE1alpha RNase preserves cell viability and function during endoplasmic reticulum stress. *Cell* **2014**, *158*, 534–548. [CrossRef] [PubMed]
14. Tam, A.B.; Koong, A.C.; Niwa, M. Ire1 has distinct catalytic mechanisms for XBP1/HAC1 splicing and RIDD. *Cell Rep.* **2014**, *9*, 850–858. [CrossRef]
15. Han, D.; Lerner, A.G.; Vande Walle, L.; Upton, J.P.; Xu, W.; Hagen, A.; Backes, B.J.; Oakes, S.A.; Papa, F.R. IRE1alpha kinase activation modes control alternate endoribonuclease outputs to determine divergent cell fates. *Cell* **2009**, *138*, 562–575. [CrossRef]

16. Urano, F.; Wang, X.; Bertolotti, A.; Zhang, Y.; Chung, P.; Harding, H.P.; Ron, D. Coupling of stress in the ER to activation of JNK protein kinases by transmembrane protein kinase IRE1. *Science* **2000**, *287*, 664–666. [CrossRef] [PubMed]
17. Haze, K.; Yoshida, H.; Yanagi, H.; Yura, T.; Mori, K. Mammalian transcription factor ATF6 is synthesized as a transmembrane protein and activated by proteolysis in response to endoplasmic reticulum stress. *Mol. Biol. Cell* **1999**, *10*, 3787–3799. [CrossRef]
18. Adachi, Y.; Yamamoto, K.; Okada, T.; Yoshida, H.; Harada, A.; Mori, K. ATF6 is a transcription factor specializing in the regulation of quality control proteins in the endoplasmic reticulum. *Cell Struct. Funct.* **2008**, *33*, 75–89. [CrossRef]
19. Yoshida, H.; Haze, K.; Yanagi, H.; Yura, T.; Mori, K. Identification of the cis-acting endoplasmic reticulum stress response element responsible for transcriptional induction of mammalian glucose-regulated proteins. Involvement of basic leucine zipper transcription factors. *J. Biol. Chem.* **1998**, *273*, 33741–33749. [CrossRef] [PubMed]
20. Yamamoto, K.; Sato, T.; Matsui, T.; Sato, M.; Okada, T.; Yoshida, H.; Harada, A.; Mori, K. Transcriptional induction of mammalian ER quality control proteins is mediated by single or combined action of ATF6alpha and XBP1. *Dev. Cell* **2007**, *13*, 365–376. [CrossRef] [PubMed]
21. Shoulders, M.D.; Ryno, L.M.; Genereux, J.C.; Moresco, J.J.; Tu, P.G.; Wu, C.; Yates, J.R., 3rd; Su, A.I.; Kelly, J.W.; Wiseman, R.L. Stress-independent activation of XBP1s and/or ATF6 reveals three functionally diverse ER proteostasis environments. *Cell Rep.* **2013**, *3*, 1279–1292. [CrossRef]
22. Nieto, M.A.; Huang, R.Y.; Jackson, R.A.; Thiery, J.P. EMT: 2016. *Cell* **2016**, *166*, 21–45. [CrossRef]
23. Dongre, A.; Weinberg, R.A. New insights into the mechanisms of epithelial-mesenchymal transition and implications for cancer. *Nat. Rev. Mol. Cell Biol.* **2019**, *20*, 69–84. [CrossRef]
24. Hay, E.D. *Organization and Fine Structure of Epithelium and Mesenchyme in the Developing Chick Embryo*; Fleischmajer, R., Billingham, R.E., Eds.; Williams & Wilkins Co.: Baltimore, MD, USA, 1968; pp. 31–35.
25. Nieto, M.A. The ins and outs of the epithelial to mesenchymal transition in health and disease. *Annu. Rev. Cell Dev. Biol.* **2011**, *27*, 347–376. [CrossRef]
26. Thiery, J.P.; Acloque, H.; Huang, R.Y.; Nieto, M.A. Epithelial-mesenchymal transitions in development and disease. *Cell* **2009**, *139*, 871–890. [CrossRef]
27. Gupta, P.B.; Pastushenko, I.; Skibinski, A.; Blanpain, C.; Kuperwasser, C. Phenotypic Plasticity: Driver of Cancer Initiation, Progression, and Therapy Resistance. *Cell Stem Cell* **2019**, *24*, 65–78. [CrossRef]
28. Lamouille, S.; Xu, J.; Derynck, R. Molecular mechanisms of epithelial-mesenchymal transition. *Nat. Rev. Mol. Cell Biol.* **2014**, *15*, 178–196. [CrossRef]
29. Nieto, M.A.; Cano, A. The epithelial-mesenchymal transition under control: Global programs to regulate epithelial plasticity. *Semin. Cancer Biol.* **2012**, *22*, 361–368. [CrossRef]
30. Peinado, H.; Olmeda, D.; Cano, A. Snail, Zeb and bHLH factors in tumour progression: An alliance against the epithelial phenotype? *Nat. Rev. Cancer* **2007**, *7*, 415–428. [CrossRef]
31. Birchmeier, W.; Behrens, J. Cadherin expression in carcinomas: Role in the formation of cell junctions and the prevention of invasiveness. *Biochim. Biophys. Acta* **1994**, *1198*, 11–26. [CrossRef]
32. De Craene, B.; Berx, G. Regulatory networks defining EMT during cancer initiation and progression. *Nat. Rev. Cancer* **2013**, *13*, 97–110. [CrossRef]
33. Ocaña, O.H.; Corcoles, R.; Fabra, A.; Moreno-Bueno, G.; Acloque, H.; Vega, S.; Barrallo-Gimeno, A.; Cano, A.; Nieto, M.A. Metastatic colonization requires the repression of the epithelial-mesenchymal transition inducer Prrx1. *Cancer Cell* **2012**, *22*, 709–724. [CrossRef]
34. Stankic, M.; Pavlovic, S.; Chin, Y.; Brogi, E.; Padua, D.; Norton, L.; Massague, J.; Benezra, R. TGF-beta-Id1 signaling opposes Twist1 and promotes metastatic colonization via a mesenchymal-to-epithelial transition. *Cell Rep.* **2013**, *5*, 1228–1242. [CrossRef]
35. Lambert, A.W.; Pattabiraman, D.R.; Weinberg, R.A. Emerging Biological Principles of Metastasis. *Cell* **2017**, *168*, 670–691. [CrossRef]
36. Pastushenko, I.; Blanpain, C. EMT Transition States during Tumor Progression and Metastasis. *Trends Cell Biol.* **2019**, *29*, 212–226. [CrossRef] [PubMed]
37. Santamaria, P.G.; Moreno-Bueno, G.; Portillo, F.; Cano, A. EMT: Present and future in clinical oncology. *Mol. Oncol.* **2017**, *11*, 718–738. [CrossRef]

38. Mani, S.A.; Guo, W.; Liao, M.J.; Eaton, E.N.; Ayyanan, A.; Zhou, A.Y.; Brooks, M.; Reinhard, F.; Zhang, C.C.; Shipitsin, M.; et al. The epithelial-mesenchymal transition generates cells with properties of stem cells. *Cell* **2008**, *133*, 704–715. [CrossRef]
39. Morel, A.P.; Lievre, M.; Thomas, C.; Hinkal, G.; Ansieau, S.; Puisieux, A. Generation of breast cancer stem cells through epithelial-mesenchymal transition. *PLoS ONE* **2008**, *3*, e2888. [CrossRef] [PubMed]
40. Hanahan, D.; Weinberg, R.A. The hallmarks of cancer. *Cell* **2000**, *100*, 57–70. [CrossRef]
41. Avril, T.; Vauleon, E.; Chevet, E. Endoplasmic reticulum stress signaling and chemotherapy resistance in solid cancers. *Oncogenesis* **2017**, *6*, e373. [CrossRef]
42. Papaioannou, A.; Chevet, E. Driving Cancer Tumorigenesis and Metastasis Through UPR Signaling. *Curr. Top. Microbiol. Immunol.* **2018**, *414*, 159–192.
43. Clarke, H.J.; Chambers, J.E.; Liniker, E.; Marciniak, S.J. Endoplasmic reticulum stress in malignancy. *Cancer Cell* **2014**, *25*, 563–573. [CrossRef]
44. Chevet, E.; Hetz, C.; Samali, A. Endoplasmic reticulum stress-activated cell reprogramming in oncogenesis. *Cancer Discov.* **2015**, *5*, 586–597. [CrossRef]
45. Dejeans, N.; Barroso, K.; Fernandez-Zapico, M.E.; Samali, A.; Chevet, E. Novel roles of the unfolded protein response in the control of tumor development and aggressiveness. *Semin. Cancer Biol.* **2015**, *33*, 67–73. [CrossRef]
46. Urra, H.; Dufey, E.; Avril, T.; Chevet, E.; Hetz, C. Endoplasmic Reticulum Stress and the Hallmarks of Cancer. *Trends Cancer* **2016**, *2*, 252–262. [CrossRef]
47. Cubillos-Ruiz, J.R.; Bettigole, S.E.; Glimcher, L.H. Tumorigenic and Immunosuppressive Effects of Endoplasmic Reticulum Stress in Cancer. *Cell* **2017**, *168*, 692–706. [CrossRef]
48. Obacz, J.; Avril, T.; Le Reste, P.J.; Urra, H.; Quillien, V.; Hetz, C.; Chevet, E. Endoplasmic reticulum proteostasis in glioblastoma-From molecular mechanisms to therapeutic perspectives. *Sci. Signal.* **2017**, *10*, eaal2323. [CrossRef]
49. Feng, Y.X.; Sokol, E.S.; Del Vecchio, C.A.; Sanduja, S.; Claessen, J.H.; Proia, T.A.; Jin, D.X.; Reinhardt, F.; Ploegh, H.L.; Wang, Q.; et al. Epithelial-to-mesenchymal transition activates PERK-eIF2alpha and sensitizes cells to endoplasmic reticulum stress. *Cancer Discov.* **2014**, *4*, 702–715. [CrossRef] [PubMed]
50. Zeindl-Eberhart, E.; Brandl, L.; Liebmann, S.; Ormanns, S.; Scheel, S.K.; Brabletz, T.; Kirchner, T.; Jung, A. Epithelial-mesenchymal transition induces endoplasmic-reticulum-stress response in human colorectal tumor cells. *PLoS ONE* **2014**, *9*, e87386. [CrossRef] [PubMed]
51. Bergmann, T.J.; Fregno, I.; Fumagalli, F.; Rinaldi, A.; Bertoni, F.; Boersema, P.J.; Picotti, P.; Molinari, M. Chemical stresses fail to mimic the unfolded protein response resulting from luminal load with unfolded polypeptides. *J. Biol. Chem.* **2018**, *293*, 5600–5612. [CrossRef] [PubMed]
52. Mujtaba, T.; Dou, Q.P. Advances in the understanding of mechanisms and therapeutic use of bortezomib. *Discov. Med.* **2011**, *12*, 471–480.
53. Jiang, D.; Lynch, C.; Medeiros, B.C.; Liedtke, M.; Bam, R.; Tam, A.B.; Yang, Z.; Alagappan, M.; Abidi, P.; Le, Q.T.; et al. Identification of Doxorubicin as an Inhibitor of the IRE1alpha-XBP1 Axis of the Unfolded Protein Response. *Sci. Rep.* **2016**, *6*, 33353. [CrossRef]
54. Logue, S.E.; McGrath, E.P.; Cleary, P.; Greene, S.; Mnich, K.; Almanza, A.; Chevet, E.; Dwyer, R.M.; Oommen, A.; Legembre, P.; et al. Inhibition of IRE1 RNase activity modulates the tumor cell secretome and enhances response to chemotherapy. *Nat. Commun.* **2018**, *9*, 3267. [CrossRef]
55. Nguyen, H.G.; Conn, C.S.; Kye, Y.; Xue, L.; Forester, C.M.; Cowan, J.E.; Hsieh, A.C.; Cunningham, J.T.; Truillet, C.; Tameire, F.; et al. Development of a stress response therapy targeting aggressive prostate cancer. *Sci. Transl. Med.* **2018**, *10*, eaar2036. [CrossRef]
56. Tanjore, H.; Cheng, D.S.; Degryse, A.L.; Zoz, D.F.; Abdolrasulnia, R.; Lawson, W.E.; Blackwell, T.S. Alveolar epithelial cells undergo epithelial-to-mesenchymal transition in response to endoplasmic reticulum stress. *J. Biol. Chem.* **2011**, *286*, 30972–30980. [CrossRef]
57. Zhong, Q.; Zhou, B.; Ann, D.K.; Minoo, P.; Liu, Y.; Banfalvi, A.; Krishnaveni, M.S.; Dubourd, M.; Demaio, L.; Willis, B.C.; et al. Role of endoplasmic reticulum stress in epithelial-mesenchymal transition of alveolar epithelial cells: Effects of misfolded surfactant protein. *Am. J. Respir. Cell Mol. Biol.* **2011**, *45*, 498–509. [CrossRef]

58. Mo, X.T.; Zhou, W.C.; Cui, W.H.; Li, D.L.; Li, L.C.; Xu, L.; Zhao, P.; Gao, J. Inositol-requiring protein 1—X-box-binding protein 1 pathway promotes epithelial-mesenchymal transition via mediating snail expression in pulmonary fibrosis. *Int. J. Biochem. Cell Biol.* **2015**, *65*, 230–238. [CrossRef]
59. Shah, P.P.; Dupre, T.V.; Siskind, L.J.; Beverly, L.J. Common cytotoxic chemotherapeutics induce epithelial-mesenchymal transition (EMT) downstream of ER stress. *Oncotarget* **2017**, *8*, 22625–22639. [CrossRef]
60. Rankin, E.B.; Giaccia, A.J. Hypoxic control of metastasis. *Science* **2016**, *352*, 175–180. [CrossRef]
61. Mujcic, H.; Nagelkerke, A.; Rouschop, K.M.; Chung, S.; Chaudary, N.; Span, P.N.; Clarke, B.; Milosevic, M.; Sykes, J.; Hill, R.P.; et al. Hypoxic activation of the PERK/eIF2alpha arm of the unfolded protein response promotes metastasis through induction of LAMP3. *Clin. Cancer Res.* **2013**, *19*, 6126–6137. [CrossRef]
62. Romero-Ramirez, L.; Cao, H.; Nelson, D.; Hammond, E.; Lee, A.H.; Yoshida, H.; Mori, K.; Glimcher, L.H.; Denko, N.C.; Giaccia, A.J.; et al. XBP1 is essential for survival under hypoxic conditions and is required for tumor growth. *Cancer Res.* **2004**, *64*, 5943–5947. [CrossRef]
63. Chen, X.; Iliopoulos, D.; Zhang, Q.; Tang, Q.; Greenblatt, M.B.; Hatziapostolou, M.; Lim, E.; Tam, W.L.; Ni, M.; Chen, Y.; et al. XBP1 promotes triple-negative breast cancer by controlling the HIF1alpha pathway. *Nature* **2014**, *508*, 103–107. [CrossRef]
64. Madden, E.; Logue, S.E.; Healy, S.J.; Manie, S.; Samali, A. The role of the unfolded protein response in cancer progression: From oncogenesis to chemoresistance. *Biol. Cell* **2019**, *111*, 1–17. [CrossRef]
65. Rouschop, K.M.; van den Beucken, T.; Dubois, L.; Niessen, H.; Bussink, J.; Savelkouls, K.; Keulers, T.; Mujcic, H.; Landuyt, W.; Voncken, J.W.; et al. The unfolded protein response protects human tumor cells during hypoxia through regulation of the autophagy genes MAP1LC3B and ATG5. *J. Clin. Investig.* **2010**, *120*, 127–141. [CrossRef]
66. Ghosh, R.; Lipson, K.L.; Sargent, K.E.; Mercurio, A.M.; Hunt, J.S.; Ron, D.; Urano, F. Transcriptional regulation of VEGF-A by the unfolded protein response pathway. *PLoS ONE* **2010**, *5*, e9575. [CrossRef]
67. Blais, J.D.; Addison, C.L.; Edge, R.; Falls, T.; Zhao, H.; Wary, K.; Koumenis, C.; Harding, H.P.; Ron, D.; Holcik, M.; et al. Perk-dependent translational regulation promotes tumor cell adaptation and angiogenesis in response to hypoxic stress. *Mol. Cell. Biol.* **2006**, *26*, 9517–9532. [CrossRef]
68. Wang, Y.; Alam, G.N.; Ning, Y.; Visioli, F.; Dong, Z.; Nor, J.E.; Polverini, P.J. The unfolded protein response induces the angiogenic switch in human tumor cells through the PERK/ATF4 pathway. *Cancer Res.* **2012**, *72*, 5396–5406. [CrossRef]
69. Shen, X.; Xue, Y.; Si, Y.; Wang, Q.; Wang, Z.; Yuan, J.; Zhang, X. The unfolded protein response potentiates epithelial-to-mesenchymal transition (EMT) of gastric cancer cells under severe hypoxic conditions. *Med. Oncol.* **2015**, *32*, 447. [CrossRef]
70. Sarrio, D.; Rodriguez-Pinilla, S.M.; Hardisson, D.; Cano, A.; Moreno-Bueno, G.; Palacios, J. Epithelial-mesenchymal transition in breast cancer relates to the basal-like phenotype. *Cancer Res.* **2008**, *68*, 989–997. [CrossRef]
71. Gwinn, D.M.; Lee, A.G.; Briones-Martin-Del-Campo, M.; Conn, C.S.; Simpson, D.R.; Scott, A.I.; Le, A.; Cowan, T.M.; Ruggero, D.; Sweet-Cordero, E.A. Oncogenic KRAS Regulates Amino Acid Homeostasis and Asparagine Biosynthesis via ATF4 and Alters Sensitivity to L-Asparaginase. *Cancer Cell* **2018**, *33*, 91–107.e6. [CrossRef]
72. Wang, Z.V.; Deng, Y.; Gao, N.; Pedrozo, Z.; Li, D.L.; Morales, C.R.; Criollo, A.; Luo, X.; Tan, W.; Jiang, N.; et al. Spliced X-box binding protein 1 couples the unfolded protein response to hexosamine biosynthetic pathway. *Cell* **2014**, *156*, 1179–1192. [CrossRef] [PubMed]
73. Knott, S.R.V.; Wagenblast, E.; Khan, S.; Kim, S.Y.; Soto, M.; Wagner, M.; Turgeon, M.O.; Fish, L.; Erard, N.; Gable, A.L.; et al. Asparagine bioavailability governs metastasis in a model of breast cancer. *Nature* **2018**, *554*, 378–381. [CrossRef]
74. Falletta, P.; Sanchez-Del-Campo, L.; Chauhan, J.; Effern, M.; Kenyon, A.; Kershaw, C.J.; Siddaway, R.; Lisle, R.; Freter, R.; Daniels, M.J.; et al. Translation reprogramming is an evolutionarily conserved driver of phenotypic plasticity and therapeutic resistance in melanoma. *Genes Dev.* **2017**, *31*, 18–33. [CrossRef] [PubMed]
75. Caramel, J.; Papadogeorgakis, E.; Hill, L.; Browne, G.J.; Richard, G.; Wierinckx, A.; Saldanha, G.; Osborne, J.; Hutchinson, P.; Tse, G.; et al. A switch in the expression of embryonic EMT-inducers drives the development of malignant melanoma. *Cancer Cell* **2013**, *24*, 466–480. [CrossRef] [PubMed]

76. Bobak, Y.; Kurlishchuk, Y.; Vynnytska-Myronovska, B.; Grydzuk, O.; Shuvayeva, G.; Redowicz, M.J.; Kunz-Schughart, L.A.; Stasyk, O. Arginine deprivation induces endoplasmic reticulum stress in human solid cancer cells. *Int. J. Biochem. Cell Biol.* **2016**, *70*, 29–38. [CrossRef] [PubMed]
77. Liu, D.; Sun, L.; Qin, X.; Liu, T.; Zhang, S.; Liu, Y.; Li, S.; Guo, K. HSF1 promotes the inhibition of EMT-associated migration by low glucose via directly regulating Snail1 expression in HCC cells. *Discov. Med.* **2016**, *22*, 87–96.
78. Garcia-Jimenez, C.; Goding, C.R. Starvation and Pseudo-Starvation as Drivers of Cancer Metastasis through Translation Reprogramming. *Cell Metab.* **2019**, *29*, 254–267. [CrossRef]
79. Hart, L.S.; Cunningham, J.T.; Datta, T.; Dey, S.; Tameire, F.; Lehman, S.L.; Qiu, B.; Zhang, H.; Cerniglia, G.; Bi, M.; et al. ER stress-mediated autophagy promotes Myc-dependent transformation and tumor growth. *J. Clin. Investig.* **2012**, *122*, 4621–4634. [CrossRef]
80. Croft, A.; Tay, K.H.; Boyd, S.C.; Guo, S.T.; Jiang, C.C.; Lai, F.; Tseng, H.Y.; Jin, L.; Rizos, H.; Hersey, P.; et al. Oncogenic activation of MEK/ERK primes melanoma cells for adaptation to endoplasmic reticulum stress. *J. Investig. Dermatol.* **2014**, *134*, 488–497. [CrossRef]
81. Wang, M.; Kaufman, R.J. The impact of the endoplasmic reticulum protein-folding environment on cancer development. *Nat. Rev. Cancer* **2014**, *14*, 581–597. [CrossRef]
82. Blazanin, N.; Son, J.; Craig-Lucas, A.B.; John, C.L.; Breech, K.J.; Podolsky, M.A.; Glick, A.B. ER stress and distinct outputs of the IRE1alpha RNase control proliferation and senescence in response to oncogenic Ras. *Proc. Natl. Acad. Sci. USA* **2017**, *114*, 9900–9905. [CrossRef] [PubMed]
83. Carrasco, D.R.; Sukhdeo, K.; Protopopova, M.; Sinha, R.; Enos, M.; Carrasco, D.E.; Zheng, M.; Mani, M.; Henderson, J.; Pinkus, G.S.; et al. The differentiation and stress response factor XBP-1 drives multiple myeloma pathogenesis. *Cancer Cell* **2007**, *11*, 349–360. [CrossRef]
84. Fujimoto, T.; Onda, M.; Nagai, H.; Nagahata, T.; Ogawa, K.; Emi, M. Upregulation and overexpression of human X-box binding protein 1 (hXBP-1) gene in primary breast cancers. *Breast Cancer* **2003**, *10*, 301–306. [CrossRef]
85. Fujimoto, T.; Yoshimatsu, K.; Watanabe, K.; Yokomizo, H.; Otani, T.; Matsumoto, A.; Osawa, G.; Onda, M.; Ogawa, K. Overexpression of human X-box binding protein 1 (XBP-1) in colorectal adenomas and adenocarcinomas. *Anticancer Res.* **2007**, *27*, 127–131.
86. Dickinson, B.C.; Chang, C.J. Chemistry and biology of reactive oxygen species in signaling or stress responses. *Nat. Chem. Biol.* **2011**, *7*, 504–511. [CrossRef] [PubMed]
87. Trachootham, D.; Alexandre, J.; Huang, P. Targeting cancer cells by ROS-mediated mechanisms: A radical therapeutic approach? *Nat. Rev. Drug Discov.* **2009**, *8*, 579–591. [CrossRef]
88. Marciniak, S.J.; Yun, C.Y.; Oyadomari, S.; Novoa, I.; Zhang, Y.; Jungreis, R.; Nagata, K.; Harding, H.P.; Ron, D. CHOP induces death by promoting protein synthesis and oxidation in the stressed endoplasmic reticulum. *Genes Dev.* **2004**, *18*, 3066–3077. [CrossRef] [PubMed]
89. Kutomi, G.; Tamura, Y.; Tanaka, T.; Kajiwara, T.; Kukita, K.; Ohmura, T.; Shima, H.; Takamaru, T.; Satomi, F.; Suzuki, Y.; et al. Human endoplasmic reticulum oxidoreductin 1-alpha is a novel predictor for poor prognosis of breast cancer. *Cancer Sci.* **2013**, *104*, 1091–1096. [CrossRef]
90. Malhotra, J.D.; Kaufman, R.J. Endoplasmic reticulum stress and oxidative stress: A vicious cycle or a double-edged sword? *Antioxid. Redox Signal.* **2007**, *9*, 2277–2293. [CrossRef]
91. Avivar-Valderas, A.; Salas, E.; Bobrovnikova-Marjon, E.; Diehl, J.A.; Nagi, C.; Debnath, J.; Aguirre-Ghiso, J.A. PERK integrates autophagy and oxidative stress responses to promote survival during extracellular matrix detachment. *Mol. Cell. Biol.* **2011**, *31*, 3616–3629. [CrossRef]
92. Dey, S.; Sayers, C.M.; Verginadis, I.I.; Lehman, S.L.; Cheng, Y.; Cerniglia, G.J.; Tuttle, S.W.; Feldman, M.D.; Zhang, P.J.; Fuchs, S.Y.; et al. ATF4-dependent induction of heme oxygenase 1 prevents anoikis and promotes metastasis. *J. Clin. Investig.* **2015**, *125*, 2592–2608. [CrossRef]
93. Sabharwal, S.S.; Schumacker, P.T. Mitochondrial ROS in cancer: Initiators, amplifiers or an Achilles' heel? *Nat. Rev. Cancer* **2014**, *14*, 709–721. [CrossRef]
94. Liu, F.; Gomez Garcia, A.M.; Meyskens, F.L., Jr. NADPH oxidase 1 overexpression enhances invasion via matrix metalloproteinase-2 and epithelial-mesenchymal transition in melanoma cells. *J. Investig. Dermatol.* **2012**, *132*, 2033–2041. [CrossRef] [PubMed]

95. Harris, I.S.; Treloar, A.E.; Inoue, S.; Sasaki, M.; Gorrini, C.; Lee, K.C.; Yung, K.Y.; Brenner, D.; Knobbe-Thomsen, C.B.; Cox, M.A.; et al. Glutathione and thioredoxin antioxidant pathways synergize to drive cancer initiation and progression. *Cancer Cell* **2015**, *27*, 211–222. [CrossRef]
96. Bobrovnikova-Marjon, E.; Grigoriadou, C.; Pytel, D.; Zhang, F.; Ye, J.; Koumenis, C.; Cavener, D.; Diehl, J.A. PERK promotes cancer cell proliferation and tumor growth by limiting oxidative DNA damage. *Oncogene* **2010**, *29*, 3881–3895. [CrossRef]
97. Rojo de la Vega, M.; Chapman, E.; Zhang, D.D. NRF2 and the Hallmarks of Cancer. *Cancer Cell* **2018**, *34*, 21–43. [CrossRef] [PubMed]
98. Arfmann-Knubel, S.; Struck, B.; Genrich, G.; Helm, O.; Sipos, B.; Sebens, S.; Schafer, H. The Crosstalk between Nrf2 and TGF-beta1 in the Epithelial-Mesenchymal Transition of Pancreatic Duct Epithelial Cells. *PLoS ONE* **2015**, *10*, e0132978. [CrossRef]
99. Shen, H.; Yang, Y.; Xia, S.; Rao, B.; Zhang, J.; Wang, J. Blockage of Nrf2 suppresses the migration and invasion of esophageal squamous cell carcinoma cells in hypoxic microenvironment. *Dis. Esophagus* **2014**, *27*, 685–692. [CrossRef]
100. Hetz, C.; Chevet, E.; Harding, H.P. Targeting the unfolded protein response in disease. *Nat. Rev. Drug Discov.* **2013**, *12*, 703–719. [CrossRef]
101. Ma, Y.; Hendershot, L.M. The role of the unfolded protein response in tumour development: Friend or foe? *Nat. Rev. Cancer* **2004**, *4*, 966–977. [CrossRef] [PubMed]
102. Fernandez, P.M.; Tabbara, S.O.; Jacobs, L.K.; Manning, F.C.; Tsangaris, T.N.; Schwartz, A.M.; Kennedy, K.A.; Patierno, S.R. Overexpression of the glucose-regulated stress gene GRP78 in malignant but not benign human breast lesions. *Breast Cancer Res. Treat.* **2000**, *59*, 15–26. [CrossRef]
103. Sakatani, T.; Maemura, K.; Hiyama, N.; Amano, Y.; Watanabe, K.; Kage, H.; Fukayama, M.; Nakajima, J.; Yatomi, Y.; Nagase, T.; et al. High expression of IRE1 in lung adenocarcinoma is associated with a lower rate of recurrence. *Jpn. J. Clin. Oncol.* **2017**, *47*, 543–550. [CrossRef]
104. Greenman, C.; Stephens, P.; Smith, R.; Dalgliesh, G.L.; Hunter, C.; Bignell, G.; Davies, H.; Teague, J.; Butler, A.; Stevens, C.; et al. Patterns of somatic mutation in human cancer genomes. *Nature* **2007**, *446*, 153–158. [CrossRef] [PubMed]
105. Parsons, D.W.; Jones, S.; Zhang, X.; Lin, J.C.; Leary, R.J.; Angenendt, P.; Mankoo, P.; Carter, H.; Siu, I.M.; Gallia, G.L.; et al. An integrated genomic analysis of human glioblastoma multiforme. *Science* **2008**, *321*, 1807–1812. [CrossRef]
106. Lhomond, S.; Avril, T.; Dejeans, N.; Voutetakis, K.; Doultsinos, D.; McMahon, M.; Pineau, R.; Obacz, J.; Papadodima, O.; Jouan, F.; et al. Dual IRE1 RNase functions dictate glioblastoma development. *EMBO Mol. Med.* **2018**, *10*, e7929. [CrossRef]
107. Sheshadri, N.; Catanzaro, J.M.; Bott, A.J.; Sun, Y.; Ullman, E.; Chen, E.I.; Pan, J.A.; Wu, S.; Crawford, H.C.; Zhang, J.; et al. SCCA1/SERPINB3 promotes oncogenesis and epithelial-mesenchymal transition via the unfolded protein response and IL6 signaling. *Cancer Res.* **2014**, *74*, 6318–6329. [CrossRef]
108. Cuevas, E.P.; Eraso, P.; Mazon, M.J.; Santos, V.; Moreno-Bueno, G.; Cano, A.; Portillo, F. LOXL2 drives epithelial-mesenchymal transition via activation of IRE1-XBP1 signalling pathway. *Sci. Rep.* **2017**, *7*, 44988. [CrossRef] [PubMed]
109. Cano, A.; Santamaria, P.G.; Moreno-Bueno, G. LOXL2 in epithelial cell plasticity and tumor progression. *Future Oncol.* **2012**, *8*, 1095–1108. [CrossRef]
110. Peinado, H.; Moreno-Bueno, G.; Hardisson, D.; Perez-Gomez, E.; Santos, V.; Mendiola, M.; de Diego, J.I.; Nistal, M.; Quintanilla, M.; Portillo, F.; et al. Lysyl oxidase-like 2 as a new poor prognosis marker of squamous cell carcinomas. *Cancer Res.* **2008**, *68*, 4541–4550. [CrossRef]
111. Moreno-Bueno, G.; Salvador, F.; Martin, A.; Floristan, A.; Cuevas, E.P.; Santos, V.; Montes, A.; Morales, S.; Castilla, M.A.; Rojo-Sebastian, A.; et al. Lysyl oxidase-like 2 (LOXL2), a new regulator of cell polarity required for metastatic dissemination of basal-like breast carcinomas. *EMBO Mol. Med.* **2011**, *3*, 528–544. [CrossRef]
112. Feng, Y.X.; Jin, D.X.; Sokol, E.S.; Reinhardt, F.; Miller, D.H.; Gupta, P.B. Cancer-specific PERK signaling drives invasion and metastasis through CREB3L1. *Nat. Commun.* **2017**, *8*, 1079. [CrossRef] [PubMed]
113. Jin, C.; Jin, Z.; Chen, N.Z.; Lu, M.; Liu, C.B.; Hu, W.L.; Zheng, C.G. Activation of IRE1alpha-XBP1 pathway induces cell proliferation and invasion in colorectal carcinoma. *Biochem. Biophys. Res. Commun.* **2016**, *470*, 75–81. [CrossRef] [PubMed]

114. Wu, S.; Du, R.; Gao, C.; Kang, J.; Wen, J.; Sun, T. The role of XBP1s in the metastasis and prognosis of hepatocellular carcinoma. *Biochem. Biophys. Res. Commun.* **2018**, *500*, 530–537. [CrossRef] [PubMed]
115. Shah, P.P.; Beverly, L.J. Regulation of VCP/p97 demonstrates the critical balance between cell death and epithelial-mesenchymal transition (EMT) downstream of ER stress. *Oncotarget* **2015**, *6*, 17725–17737. [CrossRef]
116. Auf, G.; Jabouille, A.; Guerit, S.; Pineau, R.; Delugin, M.; Bouchecareilh, M.; Magnin, N.; Favereaux, A.; Maitre, M.; Gaiser, T.; et al. Inositol-requiring enzyme 1alpha is a key regulator of angiogenesis and invasion in malignant glioma. *Proc. Natl. Acad. Sci. USA* **2010**, *107*, 15553–15558. [CrossRef]
117. Niu, Z.; Wang, M.; Zhou, L.; Yao, L.; Liao, Q.; Zhao, Y. Elevated GRP78 expression is associated with poor prognosis in patients with pancreatic cancer. *Sci. Rep.* **2015**, *5*, 16067. [CrossRef]
118. Zhu, H.; Chen, X.; Chen, B.; Chen, B.; Song, W.; Sun, D.; Zhao, Y. Activating transcription factor 4 promotes esophageal squamous cell carcinoma invasion and metastasis in mice and is associated with poor prognosis in human patients. *PLoS ONE* **2014**, *9*, e103882. [CrossRef] [PubMed]
119. Chang, J.; Hu, S.; Wang, W.; Li, Y.; Zhi, W.; Lu, S.; Shi, Q.; Wang, Y.; Yang, Y. Matrine inhibits prostate cancer via activation of the unfolded protein response/endoplasmic reticulum stress signaling and reversal of epithelial to mesenchymal transition. *Mol. Med. Rep.* **2018**, *18*, 945–957. [CrossRef]
120. Dekervel, J.; Bulle, A.; Windmolders, P.; Lambrechts, D.; Van Cutsem, E.; Verslype, C.; van Pelt, J. Acriflavine Inhibits Acquired Drug Resistance by Blocking the Epithelial-to-Mesenchymal Transition and the Unfolded Protein Response. *Transl. Oncol.* **2017**, *10*, 59–69. [CrossRef]
121. Dasgupta, A.; Sawant, M.A.; Kavishwar, G.; Lavhale, M.; Sitasawad, S. AECHL-1 targets breast cancer progression via inhibition of metastasis, prevention of EMT and suppression of Cancer Stem Cell characteristics. *Sci. Rep.* **2016**, *6*, 38045. [CrossRef]
122. Jiang, Y.; Jiao, Y.; Liu, Y.; Zhang, M.; Wang, Z.; Li, Y.; Li, T.; Zhao, X.; Wang, D. Sinomenine Hydrochloride Inhibits the Metastasis of Human Glioblastoma Cells by Suppressing the Expression of Matrix Metalloproteinase-2/-9 and Reversing the Endogenous and Exogenous Epithelial-Mesenchymal Transition. *Int. J. Mol. Sci.* **2018**, *19*, 844. [CrossRef] [PubMed]
123. Lane, D.J.; Mills, T.M.; Shafie, N.H.; Merlot, A.M.; Saleh Moussa, R.; Kalinowski, D.S.; Kovacevic, Z.; Richardson, D.R. Expanding horizons in iron chelation and the treatment of cancer: Role of iron in the regulation of ER stress and the epithelial-mesenchymal transition. *Biochim. Biophys. Acta* **2014**, *1845*, 166–181. [CrossRef]

© 2019 by the authors. Licensee MDPI, Basel, Switzerland. This article is an open access article distributed under the terms and conditions of the Creative Commons Attribution (CC BY) license (http://creativecommons.org/licenses/by/4.0/).

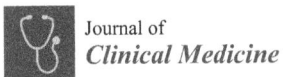

Review

# Epithelial to Mesenchymal Transition and Cell Biology of Molecular Regulation in Endometrial Carcinogenesis

Hsiao-Chen Chiu [1,2], Chia-Jung Li [3], Giou-Teng Yiang [4,5], Andy Po-Yi Tsai [6] and Meng-Yu Wu [4,5,*]

1. Department of Obstetrics and Gynecology, Taipei Tzu Chi Hospital, Buddhist Tzu Chi Medical Foundation, Taipei 231, Taiwan; 97311141@gms.tcu.edu.tw
2. Department of Obstetrics and Gynecology, School of Medicine, Tzu Chi University, Hualien 970, Taiwan
3. Department of Obstetrics and Gynecology, Kaohsiung Veterans General Hospital, Kaohsiung 813, Taiwan; nigel6761@gmail.com
4. Department of Emergency Medicine, Taipei Tzu Chi Hospital, Buddhist Tzu Chi Medical Foundation, New Taipei 231, Taiwan; gtyiang@gmail.com
5. Department of Emergency Medicine, School of Medicine, Tzu Chi University, Hualien 970, Taiwan
6. Department of Medical Research, Buddhist Tzu Chi General Hospital, Hualien 970, Taiwan; tandy@iu.edu
* Correspondence: skyshangrila@gmail.com; Tel.: +886-2-6628-9779 (ext. 42752)

Received: 22 February 2019; Accepted: 25 March 2019; Published: 30 March 2019

**Abstract:** Endometrial carcinogenesis is involved in several signaling pathways and it comprises multiple steps. The four major signaling pathways—PI3K/AKT, Ras/Raf/MEK/ERK, WNT/β-catenin, and vascular endothelial growth factor (VEGF)—are involved in tumor cell metabolism, growth, proliferation, survival, and angiogenesis. The genetic mutation and germline mitochondrial DNA mutations also impair cell proliferation, anti-apoptosis signaling, and epithelial–mesenchymal transition by several transcription factors, leading to endometrial carcinogenesis and distant metastasis. The PI3K/AKT pathway activates the ransforming growth factor beta (TGF-β)-mediated endothelial-to-mesenchymal transition (EMT) and it interacts with downstream signals to upregulate EMT-associated factors. Estrogen and progesterone signaling in EMT also play key roles in the prognosis of endometrial carcinogenesis. In this review article, we summarize the current clinical and basic research efforts regarding the detailed molecular regulation in endometrial carcinogenesis, especially in EMT, to provide novel targets for further anti-carcinogenesis treatment.

**Keywords:** endometrial cancer; epithelial-mesenchymal transition; AKT/PI3K; Ras/Raf/MEK/ERK; WNT/β-catenin

## 1. Introduction

Endometrial cancer is the most common neoplasm of the female genital tract. Its incidence and mortality rates are increasing. Endometrial carcinogenesis is a complex and multi-step process that features a slow progression from hyperplasia to endometrial cancer [1,2]. Several risk factors have been implicated and investigated, especially obesity and diabetes mellitus. As summarized by Sanderson et al. [3], the factors that contribute to endometrial carcinogenesis during estrogen stimulation include polycystic ovary syndrome (PCOS), obesity, perimenopause, functional tumor, and iatrogenic events. These conditions induce continuous estrogen stimulation that is unopposed by progesterone. Features of PCOS also include obesity and hyperinsulinemia, which also are important risk factors in endometrial carcinogenesis. Estrogen overstimulation was also associated with the phosphoinositide 3-kinase/protein kinase B (PI3K/AKT) pathway and the downstream mammalian target of rapamycin (mTOR) signaling to promote epithelial-mesenchymal transition (EMT), which occurs due to the inhibition of E-cadherin [4].

Genetic mutations also introduce several functional abnormalities and increased stress, which promote carcinogenesis. Kandoth et al. [5] collected and analyzed 373 high-grade endometrioid tumors. Mutations in *PTEN, CTNNB1, PIK3CA, ARID1A, KRAS,* and *ARID5B* were detected at high frequencies by array and sequencing analyses. *PTEN* and *KRAS* mutations in endometrial carcinoma may trigger the PI3K/AKT and mitogen-activated protein kinase/extracellular signal-activated kinase (MAPK/ERK) pathway. *PIK3CA* and *PIK3R1* mutations frequently occur with the *PTEN* mutation. *KRAS* and *CTNNB1* mutations are also involved in WNT signaling in endometrial carcinogenesis. Chang et al. [6] investigated genomic alterations in 14 tumor tissues from Taiwanese endometrial cancer patients. The authors reported nine potential driver genes (*MAPT, IL24, MCM6, TSC1, BIRC2, CIITA, DST, CASP8,* and *NOTCH2*) and 21 potential passenger genes (*ARMCX4, IGSF10, VPS13C, DCT, DNAH14, TLN1, ZNF605, ZSCAN29, MOCOS, CMYA5, PCDH17, UGT1A8, CYFIP2, MACF1, NUDT5, JAKMIP1, PCDHGB4, FAM178A, SNX6, IMP4,* and *PCMTD1*) and impaired cell functions that included cell proliferation, cell cycling, and death, via the mTOR, Wnt, MAPK, and vascular endothelial growth factor (VEGF) pathways. Gibson et al. [7] analyzed 98 tumor tissues using whole-exome sequencing. The mutation of *NRIP1*, which is an obligate cofactor of the estrogen receptor, accounted for 12.5% of the mutations.

However, detailed pathophysiology of endometrial cancer has remained unclear in clinical or basic studies. Many studies have focused on the molecular and cell biology on endometrial cancer, including the immune escape, local inflammation, mitochondria dysfunction, tumor cell proliferation, and cell death. These studies have informed novel approaches for the therapeutic strategies of endometrial cancer [8]. In this review, we present recent evidence and summarize the current concept of cell biology and molecular regulation of endometrial cancer. Our aim is to provide a strong foundation for the development of further therapeutic interventions.

## 2. Clinical Feature of Endometrial Carcinoma

Endometrial cancer is the seventh most common cancer globally, with increasing rates of incidence rate and mortality. An incidence of 24.7 per 100,000 women has been reported in Flanders and similar rates have been reported in other western European countries [9,10]. The typical presentation in endometrial cancer is abnormal uterine bleeding, especially in postmenopausal women. Abnormal uterine bleeding has been reported in about 60% of endometrial cancer patients [11,12] In some cases, due to atypical presentation the endocervical cavity anomaly may delay the diagnosis of endometrial cancer [13]. Other incidental findings of endometrial cancer may be obtained from cervical cytology or image findings. In cervical cytology analysis, adenocarcinoma was reported to arise from the cervix or endometrium, and further survey is necessary [14,15]. The presence of atypical glandular cells and endometrial cells in high risk patients is a hint to physicians to assess the endometrial neoplasm. In an update, Sanderson et al. [3] described the necessity for initial management of endometrial hyperplasia in abnormal uterine bleeding cases. In an atypical hyperplasia (AH) group, total hysterectomy with or without bilateral salpingo-oophorectomy (BSO) was suggested. If fertility is an issue or for patients in whom surgery is contraindicated, knowledge regarding the risk factors that are present is important in the control of estrogen stimulation. The Levonorgestrel-releasing intrauterine system (LNG-IUS) is the first-line therapy for these patients. In the endometrial hyperplasia without atypia group (EH), addressing the risk factors has also been suggested as a first step. Endometrial biopsy every six months in EH and three months in AH is prudent. The results are divided into three groups: regression, persistence, and prognosis. In regression cases, the continuation of LNG-IUS for five years was suggested, and oral progestogen may stop after six months. In the persistence group, 12 months of medical treatment was suggested in EH patients. Total hysterectomy with BSO was advised in AH patients with persistence and progression in pathological reports [16].

Transvaginal ultrasound (TVU) is an effective and noninvasive method in assessing the thickness and the characteristics of endometrium. The sensitivity and specificity of TVU with a cut-off of 5 mm were reported as 80.5% and 85.7% [17,18]. Computed tomography (CT) is an alternative tool to assess huge tumors in the pelvis [19]. However, the resolution of soft tissue by CT is lower when compared to magnetic resonance imaging (MRI). MRI can provide detailed information regarding tumor invasion and lymphadenopathy in endometrial cancer patients [20]. Preoperative staging via preoperative assessments, including TVU, CT for lung and liver, and MRI for retroperitoneal lymph nodes, is necessary for physicians to detect early stage or advanced disease [21,22]. In advanced disease, laparotomy, which prevents port-site metastasis, or palliative treatment, may be suitable for these patients [23]. However, endometrial cancer is a surgically staged disease, which comprises myometrial and intra-abdominal invasion. The International Federation of Gynecology and Obstetrics (FIGO) staging system is based on the myometrial and intra-abdominal invasion, such as the involvement of uterine serosa, adnexa, ascites, and intra-abdominal lymph nodes, to predict the mortality rate (Table 1). Previous studies reported that the FIGO staging system significantly reflected the five-year survival rate, with rates of 85% for stage I, 93% for stage IA, 90% for stage IB, 75% for stage II, 45% for stage III, and 25% for stage IV [24,25].

**Table 1.** TNM and International Federation of Gynecology and Obstetrics (FIGO) staging scoring system of endometrial cancer.

| When T | When N | When M | FIGO Stage |
| --- | --- | --- | --- |
| T1 | N0 | M0 | I |
| T1a | N0 | M0 | IA |
| T1b | N0 | M0 | IB |
| T2 | N0 | M0 | II |
| T3 | N0 | M0 | III |
| T3a | N0 | M0 | IIIA |
| T3b | N0 | M0 | IIIB |
| T1-3 | N1/N1mi/N1a | M0 | IIIC1 |
| T1-3 | N2/N2mi/N2a | M0 | IIIC2 |
| T4 | Any N | M0 | IVA |
| Any T | Any N | M1 | IVB |

T: Extent of the primary tumor, N: Involved regional lymph nodes, M: Distant metastasis, N1mi/N2mi: nodal micrometastases.

According to the clinicopathologic features, endometrial cancer is divided into two major types. Type 1 endometrial carcinomas include low-grade endometrioid endometrial carcinomas (FIGO grades 1 and 2), which accounted for the majority of cases (80% in one study [26]). Estrogen, from endometrial hyperplasia to the early stage induced these neoplasms. The prognosis is better than the prognosis for type 2 neoplasms, with FIGO grade 3 endometroid and nonendometrioid histologies that include serous, clear cell, mixed cell, and undifferentiated types. These type 2 neoplasms are not responsive to estrogen and they are associated with a poor prognosis. Endometrioid endometrial carcinoma can be induced by exposure to endogenous or exogenous estrogen, leading to abnormal endometrial proliferation, which causes endometrial adenocarcinoma. Several risk factors, including obesity and type 2 diabetes mellitus, reportedly promote the carcinogenesis of the endometrium. Genetic mutations, such as *PTEN, KRAS, ARID1A, PIK3CA,* and *CTNNB1* and microsatellite instability have been investigated [27]. These mutations and stress induced downstream pathways promote carcinogenesis [28]. Type 2 endometrial cancers, such as serous, clear cell carcinomas, and carcinosarcomas, are not associated with estrogen stimuli induced by different mechanisms. Mutations of p53 are commonly involved in the disease [29–31]. The detailed pathogenesis of endometrial carcinoma is still not well understood. Some of the mechanisms that have been implicated in the pathogenesis of endometrial carcinoma are considered in the following sections.

## 3. Signaling Pathways in Endometrial Carcinogenesis

Endometrial carcinogenesis involves several signaling pathways that promote cell proliferation and facilitate the escape from the immune system and apoptosis signaling [32–34]. Several major pathways that were identified in endometrial cancer,, such as hypoxia-inducible factor 1 alpha (HIF-1α)/VEGF, PI3K/AKT/mTOR, Ras/Raf/MEK/ERK, Wnt/β-catenin, and Insulin/Insulin growth factor-1 (IGF-I) signaling pathways (Figure 1). Detailed knowledge regarding these signaling pathways is necessary to understand the pathophysiology of carcinogenesis for the development of novel targeted endometrial cancer therapies.

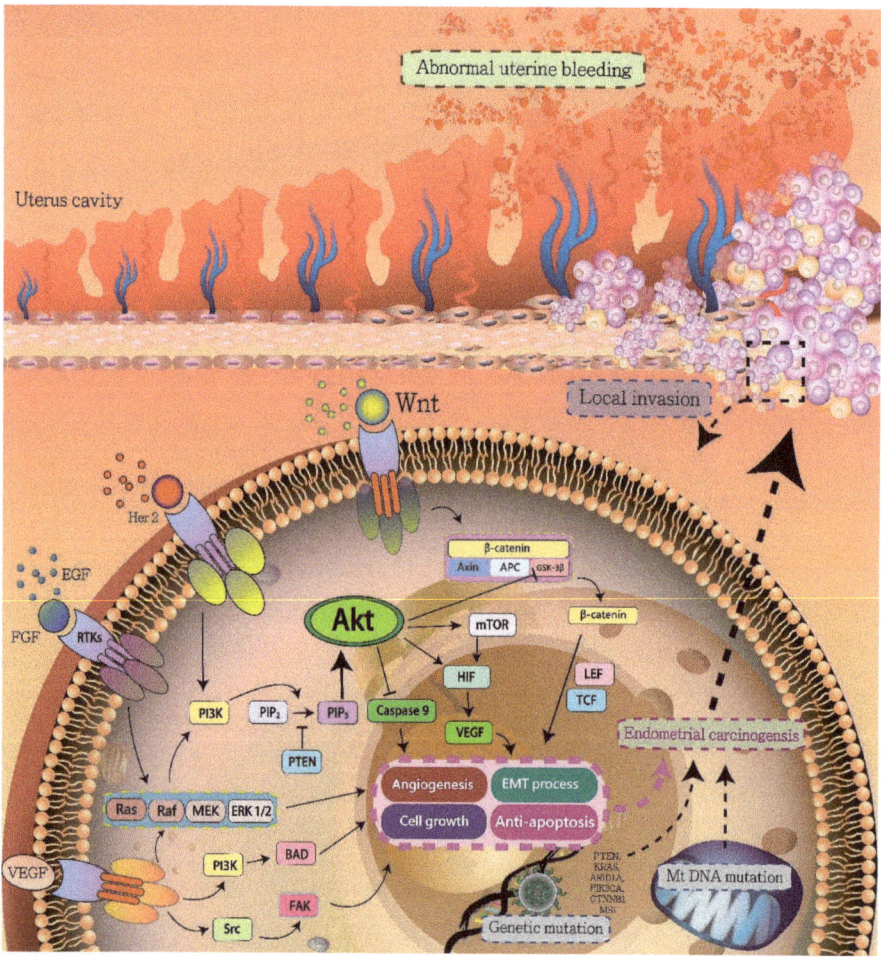

**Figure 1.** Schematic drawing presents the detail signaling pathways of endometrial carcinogenesis. The genes mutations and imbalance of estrogen and progesterone may triggered the several pathways, including Ras/Raf/MEK/ERK signaling pathway, Wnt/β-catenin signaling pathway, AKT/PI3K Pathway, vascular endothelial growth factor (VEGF) pathway, and mtDNA mutation, involved in carcinogenesis to induce cell proliferation, angiogenesis, epithelial-mesenchymal transition, and anti-apoptosis effect, promoting the cancer cell to local invasion and distant metastasis.

## 3.1. HIF-1α/VEGF Axis

Hypoxia is an important microenvironment in tumor growth and malignant progression. Hypoxia triggers the transcription of key genes for cell adaptation, including those that are important in angiogenesis and neovascularization, to increase oxygen availability, local invasion, and distant metastasis to escape from hypoxia and for metabolic reprogramming to adapt to hypoxia [35,36]. Hypoxia was initially commonly described in solid tumors, but further studies showed that hypoxia-inducible factor (HIF) is also involved in endometrial carcinogenesis [37–39]. The tumor has been associated with hypoxia, which stabilizes HIF-1α, which is a transcriptional activator of various genes, to upregulate VEGF levels and promote vascular growth and tumor progression. In a hypoxic environment, the stable form of HIF-1α acquires transactivation activity via the lowered activity of prolyl and asparagine dioxygenases. HIF-1α translocates to form a heterodimer with HIF-1β. HIF-1 induces the transcription of various genes by binding with HIF-responsive elements (Figure 1) [40]. VEGF is one of the important genes that is involved in endometrial carcinogenesis [41]. The VEGF levels are high and microvessel proliferation (MVP) is extensive in poorly differentiated, advanced, and metastatic endometrial cancer specimens. This clinical feature also reveals an important role for increased angiogenesis in the progression of endometrial cancer [42]. Endometrial cancer is a hypoxic tumor that occurs in endometrial epithelial tissue in peri-menopausal and postmenopausal women. In an anoxic environment, endometrial cancer cells form a new vascular system, which is an important mechanism in the adaptation to hypoxia [37,43].

VEGF is a key cell growth factor that stimulates tumor blood vessel growth [44]. Endometrial cancer is crucial in the expression of VEGF during the formation of new tumor blood vessels. However, HIF-1 directly regulates the increased expression of VEGF [45,46]. The regulation mechanism and clinical application of VEGF in endometrial cancer have become important topics of study [40]. In addition, estrogen may activate the nuclear factor-kappa B pathway by activating the PI3K/AKT pathway to produce VEGF factor, which in turn promotes the proliferation and migration of endometrial cancer cells [47,48]. PI3K/mTOR pathway inhibitors can sensitize endometrial cancer to radiation therapy by inhibiting HIF-1a/VEGF signaling (Figure 1) [49].

Angiogenesis plays a vital role in the pathological development of tumors. Due to the sustained action of VEGF, a large number of new blood vessels can be produced in the progression of endometrial cancer. The new blood vessels not only provide the tumor tissue with the nutrients necessary for growth, but they also remove metabolic products [50,51]. As a major regulator of neovascularization in endometrial cancer, HIF-1 directly regulates the expression of VEGF at the gene level. HIF-1α and VEGF are also closely related to early lymphatic metastasis of endometrial cancer [52]. Clinical pathological analysis has confirmed that lymphangiogenesis and lymphatic metastasis are early events in the dissemination of most solid tumors [53,54]. VEGF induces tumor lymph angiogenesis and it is an important cause of tumor cell metastasis through the lymphatic system [55]. In endometrial cancer tissues, the lower the degree of differentiation and the later the stage, the stronger is the positive expression rate of HIF-1α and the positive correlation with VEGF expression, suggesting that HIF-1α promotes angiogenesis by the regulation of the target gene, VEGF [56,57].

## 3.2. PI3K/AKT Pathway

The PI3K/AKT signaling pathway is a central regulator in endometrial carcinogenesis. The pathway connects intracellular and extracellular signaling [58]. The PI3K/AKT pathway reportedly mediates cell metabolism, growth, proliferation, survival, and angiogenesis [59]. In endometrial carcinogenesis progress, environmental stress and molecular alterations that result from growth factors, cytokines, insulin, and other factors induce PI3K signals by binding to the cell membrane receptors. The binding activates PI3K, which is then transformed to phosphatidylinositol 4,5-bisphosphate (PIP2), phosphatidylinositol 3,4,5-trisphosphate (PIP3), and phosphoinositide-dependent kinase 1 (PDK1). PDK1 phosphorylates the AKT protein [57,60], which inactivates the tuberous sclerosis complex (TSC) complex, which in turn leads to the downstream activation of mTORC1 [61]. The mTOR pathway was reported to activate endometrial carcinogenesis. In addition, signaling by receptor tyrosine kinases (RTKs) also induces the activation of the Ras/Raf/MEK/ERK signaling pathway (Figure 1) [62,63]. This pathway induces cell growth, proliferation, survival, and angiogenesis. The high frequency of the mutation of PIK3CA, a key gene that encodes the PI3K alpha subunit, has been described in endometrial cancer [64–66]. PTEN mutations are also frequently observed and they are present in up to 50% of endometrial cancers, followed by mutations of PIK3CA (30%) and K-Ras (20%) [64]. Mutations in PTEN may dysregulate PI3K/AKT/mTOR activation to inhibit apoptosis-related factors and activate anti-apoptotic factors, promoting endometrial carcinogenesis [67,68].

### 3.3. Ras/Raf/MEK/ERK Signaling Pathway

Multiple steps comprise the Ras/Raf/MEK/ERK signaling pathway. The pathway regulates cell proliferation and differentiation [69]. The signaling cascade is activated by several upstream signaling sources, which include genetic alterations, growth factors, cytokines, interleukin, and mitogen. These factors may interact with membranous receptors, such as RTKs, in endometrial cancer [70]. The activated Ras protein interacts with RAF to promote RAF phosphorylation and activate MEK. The activated MEK phosphorylates MAPK, which is also known as ERK [71]. MARK regulates cell proliferation and differentiation by mediating apoptosis signaling and cell cycle progression due to its interaction with the p53 pathway (Figure 1). In endometrial cancer, Ras/Raf/MEK/ERK signaling is often activated by the overexpression of receptors [72]. The mutation of the K-RAS gene, which encodes a small GTPase superfamily protein, has been frequently observed in 20% of endometrial cancers [64,73]. In addition, a similar mutation rate of K-RAS was noted in endometrial hyperplasia, when compared to endometrial carcinomas. The K-RAS mutations were as early events and were significantly associated with endometrial carcinogenesis [74].

### 3.4. Wnt/β-Catenin Signaling Pathway

The Wnt/β-catenin signaling pathway is divided into two major pathway types—the canonical (β-catenin dependent pathway) and the non-canonical pathway (Wnt/JNK or Wnt/calcium pathway)—which regulate several aspects of cell biology, including embryogenesis, cell differentiation, proliferation, and tumorigenesis [59]. Along with the Wnt ligand, Wnt interacts with the Frizzled family of proteins to inhibit the complex of APC/AXIN/CK1/GSK3β, which mediates the stabilization of β-catenin, and then it activates the translocation of β-catenin to the nucleus [75–77]. In the nucleus, β-catenin interacts with the T-cell factor/lymphoid enhancer-binding factor (TCF/LEF) family of transcription factors. This interaction preludes gene transcription that promotes cell proliferation and survival. In the non-canonical Wnt pathway, Wnt mediates the release of calcium and calmodulin by binding to the Frizzled receptors [78]. The non-canonical and canonical pathways interact with each other. Crosstalk and overlapping Wnt signaling pathways are features of the Wnt network theory [79]. The Wnt/β-catenin signaling is important in endometrial hyperplasia and cancer (Figure 1). Mutations in the gene encoding β-catenin gene mutations produced an accumulation of β-catenin in 38% of endometrial carcinoma cases in one study, and immunohistochemistry subsequently demonstrated the nuclear accumulation of β-catenin in 12–31% of the endometrial cancer cases examined [80,81]. The overexpression of Wnt pathway components, such as Wnt7a, has been correlated with advanced tumor progression and poor prognosis in endometrial cancer [82–84]. Progesterone and estrogen are also involved in Wnt signaling and they regulate the endometrial cycle [85]. These two hormones establish a dynamic balance that regulates the menstrual cycle. During the first two weeks of the menstrual cycle, the release of large amounts of estradiol from the cells triggers an increase in the levels of the endometrial estrogen receptor (ERα). The ER signaling promotes PI3K/AKT, MAPK, and Wnt signaling, which induce endometrial proliferation via the transcription of the downstream target genes [86–89]. During the late stage of the menstrual cycle, the release of progesterone by the corpus luteum inhibits estradiol control of the proliferation of endometrial cells. Endometrial carcinogenesis features an imbalance of the amounts of progesterone and estrogen. The overexpressed estrogen binds to ER-α, ER-β, and G protein-coupled estrogen receptor (GPR) 30, which triggers the over-transactivation of numerous growth-promoting genes, including epidermal growth factor (EGF), IGF-1, VEGF, and fibroblast growth factor (FGF). The over-activity leads to tumorigenesis. The dysfunction of progesterone in endometrial cancer has been reported [90]. In Ishikawa cells, progesterone may activate the expression of Dickkopf1 (DKK1) and Forkhead box protein O1 (FOXO1) to inhibit Wnt signaling [85]. Small interfering RNA-mediated knockdown of DKK1 and FOXO1 and immunohistochemical analysis have shown similar results and confirmed that progesterone inhibits Wnt signaling in endometrial hyperplasia and endometrial carcinogenesis. In stage I endometrial cancer, the expression of DKK1 and FOXO1 may be reduced due to poorly differentiated ER-α and the progesterone receptor (PR).

*3.5. Insulin/IGF-I Signaling Pathway*

Insulin/IGF-I activates the P13K/AKT signaling pathway through the tyrosine kinase receptor. This promotes downstream cyclinD1 expression and cell proliferation [91]. The observations that streptozotocin can reduce the circulating insulin levels in obese mice, and that the pro-proliferative effect of estrogen is significantly reduced, favor the suggestion that insulin may increase the estrogen sensitivity of the endometrial cells [92]. The changes in endometrial estrogen sensitivity may be associated with estrogen receptor levels. IGF-I can upregulate the expression of the G protein-coupled estrogen receptor (GPER) in endometrial cancer cells and promote cell migration and proliferation [93]. In addition, the IGF-I receptor can be overexpressed in endometrial proliferative lesions and tumor suppressor genes, and PTEN deficiency has been associated with a frequent incidence of endometrial proliferative lesions [94]. The collective findings indicate that the insulin/IGF-I signal can cooperate with other signals to play a role in promoting cancer.

## 4. Epithelial-Mesenchymal Transition (EMT) Signaling Pathways in Endometrial Carcinoma

*4.1. Classification of EMT*

EMT is an important process, in which epithelial cells lose their cell–cell contacts and adopt a mesenchymal-like property that features cytoskeleton remodeling and migratory activity [63]. EMT is important in embryonic development and tissue repair [95]. There are three types of EMT. Type 1 is responsible for embryogenesis and organ development. Cells can differentiate to form different types of secondary epithelial tissues [96]. Type 2 is induced by inflammation and fibrosis for tissue regeneration and organ fibrosis. In carcinogenesis, type 3 EMT reportedly explains the transformation of secondary epithelial cells into cancer cells and the resulting local invasion and distant metastasis [97,98]. Epithelial cell transformation to invasive cancer cells is a complex and multi-stage process. Initially, the polarity of epithelial cells is lost, leading to cell detachment from the basement membrane due to the changes of extracellular matrix (ECM) interactions [99]. EMT is involved in the tumor growth phase and the progression to metastatic cancer. The EMT signaling pathways may be activated by several cytokines or growth factors from the local microenvironment, followed by the interaction with transforming growth factor beta (TGF-β), bone morphogenetic protein, Wnt/β-catenin pathway, Notch, Hedgehog, and RTKs [100,101]. The involvement of EMT in the carcinogenesis process in endometrial cancer was recently demonstrated, which involved E-cadherin loss or the induction of its repressors. Other gynecologic cancers also feature the involvement of the EMT pathway [102].

*4.2. Effect of Tumor Microenvironment on TGF-β-Mediated EMT*

Normal cells and cancer cells respond differently to transforming growth factor beta (TGF-β) in different ECMs [103]. TGF-β regulates the activation of cancer-associated fibroblasts (CAF) around cells and myofibroblasts. CAFs secrete numerous pro-tumorigenic cytokines that include interleukin-6 (IL-6), which can be isolated from endometrial cancer tissues and promote cell proliferation [104]. CAFs are also involved in endometrial carcinogenesis due to their secretion of IL-6, IL-8, MCP-1, CCL5, and RANTES to promote cancer progression [105]. Subramaniam et al. [106] described the primary culture of CAFs that was obtained from human endometrial cancer tissues by antibody-conjugated magnetic bead isolation. The CAFs displayed specific effects that triggered endometrial cancer cell proliferation, as compared to fibroblasts that were cultured from benign endometrial hyperplasia tissues. The CAFs induced the proliferation of endometrial cancer cells by the SDF-1α/CXCR4 axis, which activated the PI3K/AKT and MAPK/ERK signaling pathways via paracrine hormone (Figure 1). The effect also promoted matrix metalloproteinase 2 (MMP-2) and MMP-9 secretion via autocrine the hormone [107]. The mTOR signaling was reported in CAF-mediated cell proliferation and it was confirmed by the use of the mTOR inhibitor rapamycin [106,108]. These results were not found in normal endometrial fibroblasts. When these cells were activated, they can synthesize and secrete a variety of growth factors, chemokines, and ECM proteins, which can promote the carcinogenesis of the adjacent epithelial cells [99,106,109]. In vitro experiments have demonstrated that these cells can be induced to exhibit cancer-like structures by selectively blocking the expression of type II TGF-β receptor (TβR-II) in prostate and gastric mesenchymal fibroblasts [110]. By inhibiting the activation of CAF, TGF-β can exert a tumor suppressor effect. The loss of the TGF-β signal in CAFs is an environmental factor that promotes the carcinogenesis and metastasis of CAFs.

### 4.3. Transcriptional Regulators in TGF-β and EMT

The EMT pathway is triggered by several transcription factors in different signaling pathways. TGF-β is the major factor that leads to EMT via SMAD-mediated and non-SMAD signaling. Both endometrial cancer and stromal cells produce high levels of TGF-β and they may recruit TGF-β secreting cells, including macrophages and neutrophils [111]. The release of TGF-β from epithelial cancer cells can also regulate the microenvironment of the tumor mass via an autocrine or paracrine [112]. TGF-β binding to membrane receptors activates SMAD2/3 to bind SMAD4 and form the SMAD complex [100]. By promoting EMT, this complex is involved in the regulation of transcription following its translocation into the nucleus (Figure 1) [113]. TGF-β has several roles in the EMT process, which include the activation of epithelial proteins expression via EMT transcription factors, reducing the expression of the epithelial splicing regulatory proteins, and increasing the activity of non-SMAD signaling pathways, including the PI3K/AKT pathway for translational regulation, partitioning defective 6 (PAR6) complex for cell junction dissolution, and the activity of RHOA, RAC, and CDC42 for cytoskeletal changes. In endometrial carcinogenesis, the imbalance of TGF-β signaling at the early stages is a key signal, which causes abnormal proliferation of the endometrium [114]. In a microarray gene expression analysis study, TGF-β1 induced EMT signaling to promote an invasive phenotype in HEC-1A and RL95-2 cells [113]. After administration of the TGF-β1 inhibitor, SB-431542, the endometrial carcinoma invasion was controlled and precluded [113,115]. Additionally, the overexpression of microsatellite instability dominant-negative RII (DNRII) blocked TGF-β signaling in human endometrial carcinoma HEC-1-A cells, which significantly inhibited cell proliferation and growth and stimulated apoptosis. The DNRII cells also showed more epithelial features and they were reduced in their capacity to migrate, invade, and metastasize, when compared to the control group [115].

TGF-β signaling has two major functions—the activation of SMAD signaling and non-SMAD pathways. Several non-SMAD signaling pathways have been implicated in the response to the full EMT process, including the PI3K/AKT, Ras/Raf/MEK/ERK, and Wnt/β-catenin signaling pathways (Figure 1) [116,117]. TGF-β interacts with the TGF-β receptor type I membrane receptor to phosphorylate the adaptor protein SRC homology 2 domain-containing-transforming A (SHCA). The phosphorylation leads to the activation of the Ras/Raf/MEK/ERK signaling pathway via the growth factor receptor-bound protein 2 (GRB2) and son of sevenless (SOS). TGF-β signaling also promotes the p38 and JNK activation by tumor necrosis factor receptor-associated factor 6 (TRAF6) to process EMT signaling. TGF-β signaling and several growth factors, such as VEGF, EGF, FGF, and hepatocyte growth factor, via RTKs induce the Ras/Raf/MEK/ERK signaling pathway. Wnt signaling is activated, which results in the release of β-catenin into the nucleus by the inhibition of glycogen synthase kinase-3β (GSK3β). β-catenin interacts with LEF and TCF, leading to the EMT process. Other signaling pathways, including the Notch and Hedgehog pathways, also promotes EMT in endometrial carcinogenesis by the induction of SNAIL1 expression, which leads to decreased local levels of E-cadherin. EMT promoted by SNAIL, and zinc-finger E-box-binding (ZEB) and basic helix–loop–helix (bHLH) transcription factors cause the downregulation of epithelial marker genes and the establishment of a mesenchymal phenotype. In endometrial cancer, a decreased level of E-cadherin was reported in 19.5% of G1, 40.8% of G2, and 72.7% of G3 of endometrial cancer [118] with an elevation of Snail and Slug nuclear expression. In addition, clinical outcomes, such as histological type, FIGO stage, local invasion, and cytology, have been strongly associated with the expression of E-cadherin and Snail, which significantly reflect the EMT status, and are prognostic factors in endometrial cancer [118].

*4.4. Estrogen Signaling in EMT*

Estrogen signaling is an important prognostic marker that reflects the resistance to hormonal therapies in endometrial cancer. Non-genomic and genomic responses may trigger the estrogen signaling pathways [119]. In the genomic pathway, estrogen directly binds estrogen receptor alpha (ERα) to form the ER-E complex. After dimerization, the ER-E complex may directly mediate gene expression or interact with transcription factors to regulate gene expression [120]. In the non-genomic pathway, the ER-E complex forms in the membrane, where it binds the proto-oncogene tyrosine-protein kinase Src. This triggers calcium release and induces the protein kinase A (PKA) pathway. PKA signaling regulates the expression of estrogen-responsive genes through the activation of transcription factors. These genetic expressions promote cell proliferation. ERα also closely regulates progesterone signaling. Mohammed et al. [121] described that the progesterone receptor is an ERα-induced target gene that also modulates ERα behavior. The PR-A and PR-B ligands can inhibit estradiol-stimulated ER activity to control the progression of endometrial cancer [122]. Estrogen also induces another non-transcriptional regulation pathway to over-activate the PI3K/AKT pathway. The in vitro results confirmed that the PI3K/AKT signal pathway is activated in Ishikawa cells via an ER-dependent pathway and in HEC-1A cells via an ER-independent pathway [123]. Estrogen stimulation in type I and II endometrial cancer has also been associated with the PI3K/AKT pathway via the binding to p85/p110 [124]. Downstream of the PI3K signaling pathway activates mTOR signaling, leading to the transcription of Snail 1/2 and Twist and the promotion of EMT via the inhibition of E-cadherin [4]. Poor estrogen signaling expression has been correlated with an advanced phenotype, especially in type II endometrial carcinoma [4]. In addition, the reduced expression of estrogen signaling has been associated with the increased expression of multiple EMT markers, including Snail1/2, Twist, and ZEB 1/2. Blocking Akt signaling by PI3K inhibitors may provide a new target in endometrial cancer.

GPER is a protein that is encoded by the GPER gene. The protein binds to estradiol with high affinity as the third estrogen receptor [125]. The binding of estrogen to GPER activates adenylyl cyclase to induce the activation of MMP and trigger the heparan bound EGF. These factors form the membrane-localized GPER-1, which promotes MAPK and PI3K signaling. Immunohistochemical studies have significantly associated GPER-1 expression with progression of female reproductive cancer. In the HEC50 endometrial cancer cell line, estrogen signaling is activated through GPER to induce the downstream PI3K/AKT pathway [126]. This pathway promotes the EMT process and induces high-grade invasive endometrial cancer.

*4.5. Progesterone Signaling in EMT*

The expression of PRs has been reported as a key factor that is associated with prognosis and drug-resistance of endometrial cancer [127,128] The well-differentiated endometrial cancer usually presented with PR, which may maintain the effect of hormone therapy, such as medroxyprogesterone acetate. When the expression of PR is lost, the target for hormone therapy is also lost, which is a negative prognostic factor. This type endometrial cancer usually progresses to a more advanced and invasive phenotype. The effect of hormone therapy may only be successful in 15–20% of cases of invasive phenotype endometrial cancer [129,130]. In endometrial cancer, the loss of the expression of progesterone signaling may trigger the EMT and diminish T-cell infiltration [131]. Several signaling pathways have been identified in progesterone modulated cell lines, including EGF, IL-6, PDGF, TGF-β, VEGF, and Wnt/β-catenin signaling, which mediate gene expression that is associated with the progressive and non-progressive phenotypes. A strong link between progesterone and the TGF-β signaling pathway has been reported in many studies. The increased expression of TGF-β triggers endometrial cancer that features a poor survival rate. Progesterone has a chemoprotective effect in endometrial cancer by impairing TGF-β signaling. In vitro, progesterone significantly decreased TGF-β signaling 72 h after treatment in Ishikawa cells [117]. In the same study, progesterone also effectively inhibited endometrial cancer cell viability and invasion during the increased expression of E-cadherin. Thus, the progesterone signaling in endometrial cancer may be critical in stimulating immunosurveillance and inhibition of EMT [131].

## 5. Conclusions

In the present article, we have summarized the clinical and basic research that has been focused on the detailed molecular regulation of endometrial carcinogenesis. The PI3K/AKT pathway mediates cell metabolism, growth, proliferation, survival, and angiogenesis. It also activates Ras/Raf/MEK/ERK signaling, which in turn regulates cell proliferation and differentiation. The Wnt/β-catenin signaling pathway is also involved in endometrial carcinogenesis by regulating cell proliferation. These major signaling pathways collectively promote EMT by triggering several transcription factors. The epithelial cells lose cell–cell contacts and adopt a mesenchymal-like property, with cytoskeleton remodeling and migratory activity via the EMT process, which promotes endometrial carcinogenesis and distant metastasis. The mutations of mtDNA, especially germline mutations, are associated with tumorigenesis. The detailed mechanism of mtDNA mutation-involved in endometrial cancer is still unclear. These concepts are worthy of investigation to provide novel targets in the development of efficacious therapeutic interventions.

**Funding:** This study was funded by grants from Taipei Tzu Chi Hospital (TCRD-TPE-108-5, TCRD-TPE-108-7).

**Conflicts of Interest:** The authors declare no conflict of interest.

## References

1. Braun, M.M.; Overbeek-Wager, E.A.; Grumbo, R.J. Diagnosis and Management of Endometrial Cancer. *Am. Fam. Phys.* **2016**, *93*, 468–474.
2. Sorosky, J.I. Endometrial cancer. *Obstet. Gynecol.* **2012**, *120*, 383–397. [CrossRef]
3. Sanderson, P.A.; Critchley, H.O.; Williams, A.R.; Arends, M.J.; Saunders, P.T. New concepts for an old problem: The diagnosis of endometrial hyperplasia. *Hum. Reprod. Update* **2017**, *23*, 232–254. [CrossRef] [PubMed]
4. Wik, E.; Raeder, M.B.; Krakstad, C.; Trovik, J.; Birkeland, E.; Hoivik, E.A.; Mjos, S.; Werner, H.M.; Mannelqvist, M.; Stefansson, I.M.; et al. Lack of estrogen receptor-alpha is associated with epithelial-mesenchymal transition and PI3K alterations in endometrial carcinoma. *Clin. Cancer Res.* **2013**, *19*, 1094–1105. [CrossRef] [PubMed]
5. Kandoth, C.; Schultz, N.; Cherniack, A.D.; Akbani, R.; Liu, Y.; Shen, H.; Robertson, A.G.; Pashtan, I.; Shen, R.; Benz, C.C.; et al. Integrated genomic characterization of endometrial carcinoma. *Nature* **2013**, *497*, 67–73.
6. Chang, Y.S.; Huang, H.D.; Yeh, K.T.; Chang, J.G. Identification of novel mutations in endometrial cancer patients by whole-exome sequencing. *Int. J. Oncol.* **2017**, *50*, 1778–1784. [CrossRef] [PubMed]
7. Gibson, W.J.; Hoivik, E.A.; Halle, M.K.; Taylor-Weiner, A.; Cherniack, A.D.; Berg, A.; Holst, F.; Zack, T.I.; Werner, H.M.; Staby, K.M.; et al. The genomic landscape and evolution of endometrial carcinoma progression and abdominopelvic metastasis. *Nat. Genet.* **2016**, *48*, 848–855. [CrossRef]

8. Lee, Y.C.; Lheureux, S.; Oza, A.M. Treatment strategies for endometrial cancer: Current practice and perspective. *Curr. Opin. Obstet. Gynecol.* **2017**, *29*, 47–58. [CrossRef] [PubMed]
9. Parkin, D.M.; Pisani, P.; Ferlay, J. Global cancer statistics. *Cancer J. Clin.* **1999**, *49*, 33–64. [CrossRef]
10. Amant, F.; Moerman, P.; Neven, P.; Timmerman, D.; Van Limbergen, E.; Vergote, I. Endometrial cancer. *Lancet* **2005**, *366*, 491–505. [CrossRef]
11. Kimura, T.; Kamiura, S.; Yamamoto, T.; Seino-Noda, H.; Ohira, H.; Saji, F. Abnormal uterine bleeding and prognosis of endometrial cancer. *Int. J. Gynaecol. Obstet.* **2004**, *85*, 145–150. [CrossRef] [PubMed]
12. Seebacher, V.; Schmid, M.; Polterauer, S.; Hefler-Frischmuth, K.; Leipold, H.; Concin, N.; Reinthaller, A.; Hefler, L. The presence of postmenopausal bleeding as prognostic parameter in patients with endometrial cancer: A retrospective multi-center study. *Bmc Cancer* **2009**, *9*, 460. [CrossRef]
13. Wu, M.-Y.; Ding, D.-C.; Chu, T.-Y.; Hong, M.-K. Endocervical Cavity Anomaly Mimicking the Uterine Cavity and Delaying Diagnosis of Endometrial Adenocarcinoma: A Case Report. *Reports* **2018**, *1*, 5. [CrossRef]
14. Gupta, D. Clinical Behavior and Treatment of Endometrial Cancer. *Adv. Exp. Med. Biol.* **2017**, *943*, 47–74.
15. McAlpine, J.N.; Temkin, S.M.; Mackay, H.J. Endometrial cancer: Not your grandmother's cancer. *Cancer* **2016**, *122*, 2787–2798. [CrossRef] [PubMed]
16. MacKintosh, M.L.; Derbyshire, A.E.; McVey, R.J.; Bolton, J.; Nickkho-Amiry, M.; Higgins, C.L.; Kamieniorz, M.; Pemberton, P.W.; Kirmani, B.H.; Ahmed, B.; et al. The impact of obesity and bariatric surgery on circulating and tissue biomarkers of endometrial cancer risk. *Int. J. Cancer* **2019**, *144*, 641–650. [CrossRef] [PubMed]
17. Jacobs, I.; Gentry-Maharaj, A.; Burnell, M.; Manchanda, R.; Singh, N.; Sharma, A.; Ryan, A.; Seif, M.W.; Amso, N.N.; Turner, G.; et al. Sensitivity of transvaginal ultrasound screening for endometrial cancer in postmenopausal women: A case-control study within the UKCTOCS cohort. *Lancet. Oncol.* **2011**, *12*, 38–48. [CrossRef]
18. Steiner, E.; Juhasz-Bösz, I.; Emons, G.; Kölbl, H.; Kimmig, R.; Mallmann, P. Transvaginal Ultrasound for Endometrial Carcinoma Screening—Current Evidence-based Data. *Geburtshlfe Frauenheilkd.* **2012**, *72*, 1088–1091. [CrossRef]
19. Bagaria, M.; Shields, E.; Bakkum-Gamez, J.N. Novel approaches to early detection of endometrial cancer. *Curr. Opin. Obstet. Gynecol.* **2017**, *29*, 40–46. [CrossRef]
20. Connor, J.P.; Andrews, J.I.; Anderson, B.; Buller, R.E. Computed tomography in endometrial carcinoma. *Obstet. Gynecol.* **2000**, *95*, 692–696.
21. Kitson, S.J.; Lindsay, J.; Sivalingam, V.N.; Lunt, M.; Ryan, N.A.J.; Edmondson, R.J.; Rutter, M.K.; Crosbie, E.J. The unrecognized burden of cardiovascular risk factors in women newly diagnosed with endometrial cancer: A prospective case control study. *Gynecol. Oncol.* **2018**, *148*, 154–160. [CrossRef]
22. Winterhoff, B.; Konecny, G.E. Targeting fibroblast growth factor pathways in endometrial cancer. *Curr. Probl. Cancer* **2017**, *41*, 37–47. [CrossRef] [PubMed]
23. Colombo, N.; Creutzberg, C.; Amant, F.; Bosse, T.; Gonzalez-Martin, A.; Ledermann, J.; Marth, C.; Nout, R.; Querleu, D.; Mirza, M.R.; et al. ESMO-ESGO-ESTRO Consensus Conference on Endometrial Cancer: Diagnosis, treatment and follow-up. *Ann. Oncol.* **2016**, *27*, 16–41. [CrossRef] [PubMed]
24. Grigsby, P.W.; Perez, C.A.; Kuten, A.; Simpson, J.R.; Garcia, D.M.; Camel, H.M.; Kao, M.S.; Galakatos, A.E. Clinical stage I endometrial cancer: Prognostic factors for local control and distant metastasis and implications of the new FIGO surgical staging system. *Int. J. Radiat. Oncol. Biol. Phys.* **1992**, *22*, 905–911. [CrossRef]
25. Morrow, C.P.; Bundy, B.N.; Kurman, R.J.; Creasman, W.T.; Heller, P.; Homesley, H.D.; Graham, J.E. Relationship between surgical-pathological risk factors and outcome in clinical stage I and II carcinoma of the endometrium: A Gynecologic Oncology Group study. *Gynecol. Oncol.* **1991**, *40*, 55–65. [CrossRef]
26. Lu, Z.; Chen, J. Introduction of WHO classification of tumours of female reproductive organs, fourth edition. *Chin. J. Pathol.* **2014**, *43*, 649–650.
27. Cuevas, D.; Valls, J.; Gatius, S.; Roman-Canal, B.; Estaran, E.; Dorca, E.; Santacana, M.; Vaquero, M.; Eritja, N.; Velasco, A.; et al. Targeted sequencing with a customized panel to assess histological typing in endometrial carcinoma. *Virchows Arch. Int. J. Pathol.* **2019**. [CrossRef]
28. Huang, H.N.; Lin, M.C.; Tseng, L.H.; Chiang, Y.C.; Lin, L.I.; Lin, Y.F.; Huang, H.Y.; Kuo, K.T. Ovarian and endometrial endometrioid adenocarcinomas have distinct profiles of microsatellite instability, PTEN expression, and ARID1A expression. *Histopathology* **2015**, *66*, 517–528. [CrossRef]

29. Rambau, P.F.; McIntyre, J.B.; Taylor, J.; Lee, S.; Ogilvie, T.; Sienko, A.; Morris, D.; Duggan, M.A.; McCluggage, W.G.; Kobel, M. Morphologic Reproducibility, Genotyping, and Immunohistochemical Profiling Do Not Support a Category of Seromucinous Carcinoma of the Ovary. *Am. J. Surg. Pathol.* **2017**, *41*, 685–695. [CrossRef] [PubMed]
30. Stelloo, E.; Bosse, T.; Nout, R.A.; MacKay, H.J.; Church, D.N.; Nijman, H.W.; Leary, A.; Edmondson, R.J.; Powell, M.E.; Crosbie, E.J.; et al. Refining prognosis and identifying targetable pathways for high-risk endometrial cancer; a TransPORTEC initiative. *Mod. Pathol.* **2015**, *28*, 836–844. [CrossRef]
31. Teer, J.K.; Yoder, S.; Gjyshi, A.; Nicosia, S.V.; Zhang, C.; Monteiro, A.N.A. Mutational heterogeneity in non-serous ovarian cancers. *Sci. Rep.* **2017**, *7*, 9728. [CrossRef]
32. McConechy, M.K.; Ding, J.; Cheang, M.C.; Wiegand, K.; Senz, J.; Tone, A.; Yang, W.; Prentice, L.; Tse, K.; Zeng, T.; et al. Use of mutation profiles to refine the classification of endometrial carcinomas. *J. Pathol.* **2012**, *228*, 20–30. [CrossRef]
33. McConechy, M.K.; Ding, J.; Senz, J.; Yang, W.; Melnyk, N.; Tone, A.A.; Prentice, L.M.; Wiegand, K.C.; McAlpine, J.N.; Shah, S.P.; et al. Ovarian and endometrial endometrioid carcinomas have distinct CTNNB1 and PTEN mutation profiles. *Mod. Pathol.* **2014**, *27*, 128–134. [CrossRef] [PubMed]
34. O'Hara, A.J.; Bell, D.W. The genomics and genetics of endometrial cancer. *Adv. Genom. Genet.* **2012**, *2012*, 33–47.
35. Harada, H.; Kizaka-Kondoh, S.; Li, G.; Itasaka, S.; Shibuya, K.; Inoue, M.; Hiraoka, M. Significance of HIF-1-active cells in angiogenesis and radioresistance. *Oncogene* **2007**, *26*, 7508–7516. [CrossRef] [PubMed]
36. Semenza, G.L. Targeting HIF-1 for cancer therapy. *Nat. Rev. Cancer* **2003**, *3*, 721–732. [CrossRef]
37. Berg, A.; Fasmer, K.E.; Mauland, K.K.; Ytre-Hauge, S.; Hoivik, E.A.; Husby, J.A.; Tangen, I.L.; Trovik, J.; Halle, M.K.; Woie, K.; et al. Tissue and imaging biomarkers for hypoxia predict poor outcome in endometrial cancer. *Oncotarget* **2016**, *7*, 69844–69856. [CrossRef]
38. Kato, H.; Inoue, T.; Asanoma, K.; Nishimura, C.; Matsuda, T.; Wake, N. Induction of human endometrial cancer cell senescence through modulation of HIF-1alpha activity by EGLN1. *Int. J. Cancer* **2006**, *118*, 1144–1153. [CrossRef]
39. Seeber, L.M.; Horree, N.; van der Groep, P.; van der Wall, E.; Verheijen, R.H.; van Diest, P.J. Necrosis related HIF-1alpha expression predicts prognosis in patients with endometrioid endometrial carcinoma. *BMC Cancer* **2010**, *10*, 307. [CrossRef]
40. Koyasu, S.; Kobayashi, M.; Goto, Y.; Hiraoka, M.; Harada, H. Regulatory mechanisms of hypoxia-inducible factor 1 activity: Two decades of knowledge. *Cancer Sci.* **2018**, *109*, 560–571. [CrossRef] [PubMed]
41. Seeber, L.M.; Zweemer, R.P.; Verheijen, R.H.; van Diest, P.J. Hypoxia-inducible factor-1 as a therapeutic target in endometrial cancer management. *Obstet. Gynecol. Int.* **2010**, *2010*, 580971. [CrossRef]
42. Sivridis, E. Angiogenesis and endometrial cancer. *Anticancer Res.* **2001**, *21*, 4383–4388.
43. Liu, H.; Zhang, Z.; Xiong, W.; Zhang, L.; Xiong, Y.; Li, N.; He, H.; Du, Y.; Liu, Y. Hypoxia-inducible factor-1alpha promotes endometrial stromal cells migration and invasion by upregulating autophagy in endometriosis. *Reproduction* **2017**, *153*, 809–820. [CrossRef]
44. De Palma, M.; Biziato, D.; Petrova, T.V. Microenvironmental regulation of tumour angiogenesis. *Nat. Rev. Cancer* **2017**, *17*, 457–474. [CrossRef]
45. Pugh, C.W.; Ratcliffe, P.J. Regulation of angiogenesis by hypoxia: Role of the HIF system. *Nat. Med.* **2003**, *9*, 677–684. [CrossRef]
46. Krock, B.L.; Skuli, N.; Simon, M.C. Hypoxia-induced angiogenesis: Good and evil. *Genes Cancer* **2011**, *2*, 1117–1133. [CrossRef]
47. Gordon, L.K.; Kiyohara, M.; Fu, M.; Braun, J.; Dhawan, P.; Chan, A.; Goodglick, L.; Wadehra, M. EMP2 regulates angiogenesis in endometrial cancer cells through induction of VEGF. *Oncogene* **2013**, *32*, 5369–5376. [CrossRef]
48. Ge, Q.L.; Liu, S.H.; Ai, Z.H.; Tao, M.F.; Ma, L.; Wen, S.Y.; Dai, M.; Liu, F.; Liu, H.S.; Jiang, R.Z.; et al. RelB/NF-kappaB links cell cycle transition and apoptosis to endometrioid adenocarcinoma tumorigenesis. *Cell Death Dis.* **2016**, *7*, e2402. [CrossRef] [PubMed]
49. Miyasaka, A.; Oda, K.; Ikeda, Y.; Sone, K.; Fukuda, T.; Inaba, K.; Makii, C.; Enomoto, A.; Hosoya, N.; Tanikawa, M.; et al. PI3K/mTOR pathway inhibition overcomes radioresistance via suppression of the HIF1-alpha/VEGF pathway in endometrial cancer. *Gynecol. Oncol.* **2015**, *138*, 174–180. [CrossRef] [PubMed]

50. Kotowicz, B.; Fuksiewicz, M.; Jonska-Gmyrek, J.; Berezowska, A.; Radziszewski, J.; Bidzinski, M.; Kowalska, M. Clinical significance of pretreatment serum levels of VEGF and its receptors, IL- 8, and their prognostic value in type I and II endometrial cancer patients. *PLoS ONE* **2017**, *12*, e0184576. [CrossRef]
51. Mahecha, A.M.; Wang, H. The influence of vascular endothelial growth factor-A and matrix metalloproteinase-2 and -9 in angiogenesis, metastasis, and prognosis of endometrial cancer. *Oncotargets Ther.* **2017**, *10*, 4617–4624. [CrossRef]
52. Horree, N.; van Diest, P.J.; van der Groep, P.; Sie-Go, D.M.; Heintz, A.P. Hypoxia and angiogenesis in endometrioid endometrial carcinogenesis. *Cell. Oncol.* **2007**, *29*, 219–227.
53. Sahoo, S.S.; Tanwar, P.S. VEGF-mTOR signaling links obesity and endometrial cancer. *Oncoscience* **2018**, *5*, 150–151.
54. Zhang, J.; Song, H.; Lu, Y.; Chen, H.; Jiang, S.; Li, L. Effects of estradiol on VEGF and bFGF by Akt in endometrial cancer cells are mediated through the NF-kappaB pathway. *Oncol. Rep.* **2016**, *36*, 705–714. [CrossRef]
55. Donoghue, J.F.; Lederman, F.L.; Susil, B.J.; Rogers, P.A. Lymphangiogenesis of normal endometrium and endometrial adenocarcinoma. *Hum. Reprod.* **2007**, *22*, 1705–1713. [CrossRef] [PubMed]
56. Papa, A.; Zaccarelli, E.; Caruso, D.; Vici, P.; Benedetti Panici, P.; Tomao, F. Targeting angiogenesis in endometrial cancer—New agents for tailored treatments. *Exp. Opin. Investig. Drugs* **2016**, *25*, 31–49. [CrossRef]
57. Sahoo, S.S.; Lombard, J.M.; Ius, Y.; O'Sullivan, R.; Wood, L.G.; Nahar, P.; Jaaback, K.; Tanwar, P.S. Adipose-Derived VEGF-mTOR Signaling Promotes Endometrial Hyperplasia and Cancer: Implications for Obese Women. *Mol. Cancer Res.* **2018**, *16*, 309–321. [CrossRef]
58. Bian, X.; Gao, J.; Luo, F.; Rui, C.; Zheng, T.; Wang, D.; Wang, Y.; Roberts, T.M.; Liu, P.; Zhao, J.J.; et al. PTEN deficiency sensitizes endometrioid endometrial cancer to compound PARP-PI3K inhibition but not PARP inhibition as monotherapy. *Oncogene* **2018**, *37*, 341–351. [CrossRef] [PubMed]
59. Markowska, A.; Pawałowska, M.; Lubin, J.; Markowska, J. Signalling pathways in endometrial cancer. *Contemp. Oncol.* **2014**, *18*, 143–148.
60. Philip, C.A.; Laskov, I.; Beauchamp, M.C.; Marques, M.; Amin, O.; Bitharas, J.; Kessous, R.; Kogan, L.; Baloch, T.; Gotlieb, W.H.; et al. Inhibition of PI3K-AKT-mTOR pathway sensitizes endometrial cancer cell lines to PARP inhibitors. *BMC Cancer* **2017**, *17*, 638. [CrossRef] [PubMed]
61. Hagiwara, A.; Cornu, M.; Cybulski, N.; Polak, P.; Betz, C.; Trapani, F.; Terracciano, L.; Heim, M.H.; Ruegg, M.A.; Hall, M.N. Hepatic mTORC2 activates glycolysis and lipogenesis through Akt, glucokinase, and SREBP1c. *Cell Metab.* **2012**, *15*, 725–738. [CrossRef] [PubMed]
62. Chen, J.; Zhao, K.N.; Li, R.; Shao, R.; Chen, C. Activation of PI3K/Akt/mTOR pathway and dual inhibitors of PI3K and mTOR in endometrial cancer. *Curr. Med. Chem.* **2014**, *21*, 3070–3080. [CrossRef] [PubMed]
63. Dong, P.; Konno, Y.; Watari, H.; Hosaka, M.; Noguchi, M.; Sakuragi, N. The impact of microRNA-mediated PI3K/AKT signaling on epithelial-mesenchymal transition and cancer stemness in endometrial cancer. *J. Transl. Med.* **2014**, *12*, 231. [CrossRef] [PubMed]
64. Oda, K. Targeting Ras-PI3K/mTOR pathway and the predictive biomarkers in endometrial cancer. *Gan Kagaku Ryoho. Cancer Chemother.* **2011**, *38*, 1084–1087.
65. Salvesen, H.B.; Carter, S.L.; Mannelqvist, M.; Dutt, A.; Getz, G.; Stefansson, I.M.; Raeder, M.B.; Sos, M.L.; Engelsen, I.B.; Trovik, J.; et al. Integrated genomic profiling of endometrial carcinoma associates aggressive tumors with indicators of PI3 kinase activation. *Proc. Natl. Acad. Sci. USA* **2009**, *106*, 4834–4839. [CrossRef]
66. Dedes, K.J.; Wetterskog, D.; Ashworth, A.; Kaye, S.B.; Reis-Filho, J.S. Emerging therapeutic targets in endometrial cancer. *Nat. Rev. Clin. Oncol.* **2011**, *8*, 261–271. [CrossRef]
67. Risinger, J.I.; Hayes, K.; Maxwell, G.L.; Carney, M.E.; Dodge, R.K.; Barrett, J.C.; Berchuck, A. PTEN mutation in endometrial cancers is associated with favorable clinical and pathologic characteristics. *Clin. Cancer Res.* **1998**, *4*, 3005–3010.
68. Levine, D.A.; Cancer Genome Atlas Research Network. Integrated genomic characterization of endometrial carcinoma. *Nature* **2013**, *497*, 67.
69. Eritja, N.; Yeramian, A.; Chen, B.J.; Llobet-Navas, D.; Ortega, E.; Colas, E.; Abal, M.; Dolcet, X.; Reventos, J.; Matias-Guiu, X. Endometrial Carcinoma: Specific Targeted Pathways. *Adv. Exp. Med. Biol.* **2017**, *943*, 149–207.

70. Wang, L.E.; Ma, H.; Hale, K.S.; Yin, M.; Meyer, L.A.; Liu, H.; Li, J.; Lu, K.H.; Hennessy, B.T.; Li, X.; et al. Roles of genetic variants in the PI3K and RAS/RAF pathways in susceptibility to endometrial cancer and clinical outcomes. *J. Cancer Res. Clin. Oncol.* **2012**, *138*, 377–385. [CrossRef]
71. Wu, Y.L.; Maachani, U.B.; Schweitzer, M.; Singh, R.; Wang, M.; Chang, R.; Souweidane, M.M. Dual Inhibition of PI3K/AKT and MEK/ERK Pathways Induces Synergistic Antitumor Effects in Diffuse Intrinsic Pontine Glioma Cells. *Transl. Oncol.* **2017**, *10*, 221–228. [CrossRef] [PubMed]
72. Hoshino, R.; Chatani, Y.; Yamori, T.; Tsuruo, T.; Oka, H.; Yoshida, O.; Shimada, Y.; Ari-i, S.; Wada, H.; Fujimoto, J.; et al. Constitutive activation of the 41-/43-kDa mitogen-activated protein kinase signaling pathway in human tumors. *Oncogene* **1999**, *18*, 813. [CrossRef] [PubMed]
73. Alexander-Sefre, F.; Salvesen, H.B.; Ryan, A.; Singh, N.; Akslen, L.A.; MacDonald, N.; Wilbanks, G.; Jacobs, I.J. Molecular assessment of depth of myometrial invasion in stage I endometrial cancer: A model based on K-ras mutation analysis. *Gynecol. Oncol.* **2003**, *91*, 218–225. [CrossRef]
74. Dobrzycka, B.; Terlikowski, S.J.; Mazurek, A.; Kowalczuk, O.; Niklińska, W.; Chyczewski, L.; Kulikowski, M. Mutations of the KRAS Oncogene in Endometrial Hyperplasia and Carcinoma. *Folia Histochem Cytobiol.* **2009**, *47*, 65–68. [CrossRef]
75. Yang, Y. Wnt signaling in development and disease. *Cell Biosci.* **2012**, *2*, 14. [CrossRef] [PubMed]
76. Kestler Hans, A.; Kühl, M. From individual Wnt pathways towards a Wnt signalling network. *Philos. Trans. R. Soc. B Biol. Sci.* **2008**, *363*, 1333–1347. [CrossRef] [PubMed]
77. Hurley, R.L.; Anderson, K.A.; Franzone, J.M.; Kemp, B.E.; Means, A.R.; Witters, L.A. The $Ca^{2+}$/calmodulin-dependent protein kinase kinases are AMP-activated protein kinase kinases. *J. Biol. Chem.* **2005**, *280*, 29060–29066. [CrossRef] [PubMed]
78. Dellinger, T.H.; Planutis, K.; Tewari, K.S.; Holcombe, R.F. Role of canonical Wnt signaling in endometrial carcinogenesis. *Expert Rev. Anticancer Ther.* **2012**, *12*, 51–62. [CrossRef] [PubMed]
79. Coopes, A.; Henry, C.E.; Llamosas, E.; Ford, C.E. An update of Wnt signalling in endometrial cancer and its potential as a therapeutic target. *Endocr. Relat. Cancer* **2018**. [CrossRef] [PubMed]
80. Fukuchi, T.; Sakamoto, M.; Tsuda, H.; Maruyama, K.; Nozawa, S.; Hirohashi, S. Beta-catenin mutation in carcinoma of the uterine endometrium. *Cancer Res.* **1998**, *58*, 3526–3528. [PubMed]
81. Saegusa, M.; Hashimura, M.; Yoshida, T.; Okayasu, I. Beta- Catenin mutations and aberrant nuclear expression during endometrial tumorigenesis. *Br. J. Cancer* **2001**, *84*, 209–217. [CrossRef]
82. Liu, Y.; Meng, F.; Xu, Y.; Yang, S.; Xiao, M.; Chen, X.; Lou, G. Overexpression of Wnt7a is associated with tumor progression and unfavorable prognosis in endometrial cancer. *Int. J. Gynecol. Cancer* **2013**, *23*, 304–311. [CrossRef] [PubMed]
83. Liu, N.; Gu, B.; Liu, N.; Nie, X.; Zhang, B.; Zhou, X.; Deng, M. Wnt/β-Catenin Pathway Regulates Cementogenic Differentiation of Adipose Tissue-Deprived Stem Cells in Dental Follicle Cell-Conditioned Medium. *PLoS ONE* **2014**, *9*, e93364. [CrossRef] [PubMed]
84. Liu, J.; Pan, S.; Hsieh, M.H.; Ng, N.; Sun, F.; Wang, T.; Kasibhatla, S.; Schuller, A.G.; Li, A.G.; Cheng, D.; et al. Targeting Wnt-driven cancer through the inhibition of Porcupine by LGK974. *Proc. Natl. Acad. Sci. USA* **2013**, *110*, 20224–20229. [CrossRef]
85. Wang, Y.; Hanifi-Moghaddam, P.; Hanekamp, E.E.; Kloosterboer, H.J.; Franken, P.; Veldscholte, J.; van Doorn, H.C.; Ewing, P.C.; Kim, J.J.; Grootegoed, J.A.; et al. Progesterone Inhibition of Wnt/β-Catenin Signaling in Normal Endometrium and Endometrial Cancer. *Clin. Cancer Res.* **2009**, *15*, 5784–5793. [CrossRef] [PubMed]
86. Wang, Y.; van der Zee, M.; Fodde, R.; Blok, L.J. Wnt/B-catenin and sex hormone signaling in endometrial homeostasis and cancer. *Oncotarget* **2010**, *1*, 674–684.
87. Zhao, E.; Mu, Q. Phytoestrogen biological actions on Mammalian reproductive system and cancer growth. *Sci. Pharm.* **2011**, *79*, 1–20. [CrossRef]
88. Hong, K.; Choi, Y. Role of estrogen and RAS signaling in repeated implantation failure. *BMB Rep.* **2018**, *51*, 225–229. [CrossRef]
89. Yaşar, P.; Ayaz, G.; User, S.D.; Güpür, G.; Muyan, M. Molecular mechanism of estrogen-estrogen receptor signaling. *Reprod. Med. Biol.* **2017**, *16*, 4–20. [CrossRef]
90. Kim, J.J.; Kurita, T.; Bulun, S.E. Progesterone action in endometrial cancer, endometriosis, uterine fibroids, and breast cancer. *Endocr. Rev.* **2013**, *34*, 130–162. [CrossRef] [PubMed]

91. De Marco, P.; Cirillo, F.; Vivacqua, A.; Malaguarnera, R.; Belfiore, A.; Maggiolini, M. Novel Aspects Concerning the Functional Cross-Talk between the Insulin/IGF-I System and Estrogen Signaling in Cancer Cells. *Front. Endocrinol.* **2015**, *6*, 30. [CrossRef] [PubMed]
92. Zhang, Q.; Celestino, J.; Schmandt, R.; McCampbell, A.S.; Urbauer, D.L.; Meyer, L.A.; Burzawa, J.K.; Huang, M.; Yates, M.S.; Iglesias, D.; et al. Chemopreventive effects of metformin on obesity-associated endometrial proliferation. *Am. J. Obs. Gynecol.* **2013**, *209*, 24e1–24e12. [CrossRef]
93. De Marco, P.; Bartella, V.; Vivacqua, A.; Lappano, R.; Santolla, M.F.; Morcavallo, A.; Pezzi, V.; Belfiore, A.; Maggiolini, M. Insulin-like growth factor-I regulates GPER expression and function in cancer cells. *Oncogene* **2013**, *32*, 678–688. [CrossRef] [PubMed]
94. McCampbell, A.S.; Broaddus, R.R.; Loose, D.S.; Davies, P.J. Overexpression of the insulin-like growth factor I receptor and activation of the AKT pathway in hyperplastic endometrium. *Clin. Cancer Res.* **2006**, *12*, 6373–6378. [CrossRef]
95. Laskov, I.; Abou-Nader, P.; Amin, O.; Philip, C.A.; Beauchamp, M.C.; Yasmeen, A.; Gotlieb, W.H. Metformin Increases E-cadherin in Tumors of Diabetic Patients With Endometrial Cancer and Suppresses Epithelial-Mesenchymal Transition in Endometrial Cancer Cell Lines. *Int. J. Gynecol. Cancer* **2016**, *26*, 1213–1221. [CrossRef] [PubMed]
96. Kent, C.N.; Guttilla Reed, I.K. Regulation of epithelial-mesenchymal transition in endometrial cancer: Connecting PI3K, estrogen signaling, and microRNAs. *Clin. Transl. Oncol.* **2016**, *18*, 1056–1061. [CrossRef] [PubMed]
97. Kalluri, R.; Weinberg, R.A. The basics of epithelial-mesenchymal transition. *J. Clin. Investig.* **2009**, *119*, 1420–1428. [CrossRef] [PubMed]
98. Lamouille, S.; Xu, J.; Derynck, R. Molecular mechanisms of epithelial-mesenchymal transition. *Nat. Rev. Mol. Cell Biol.* **2014**, *15*, 178–196. [CrossRef]
99. Makker, A.; Goel, M.M. Tumor progression, metastasis, and modulators of epithelial-mesenchymal transition in endometrioid endometrial carcinoma: An update. *Endocr. Relat. Cancer* **2016**, *23*, R85–R111. [CrossRef]
100. Colas, E.; Pedrola, N.; Devis, L.; Ertekin, T.; Campoy, I.; Martinez, E.; Llaurado, M.; Rigau, M.; Olivan, M.; Garcia, M.; et al. The EMT signaling pathways in endometrial carcinoma. *Clin. Transl. Oncol.* **2012**, *14*, 715–720. [CrossRef]
101. Gonzalez, D.M.; Medici, D. Signaling mechanisms of the epithelial-mesenchymal transition. *Sci. Signal.* **2014**, *7*, re8. [CrossRef]
102. Chiu, H.-C.; Wu, M.-Y.; Li, C.-H.; Huang, S.-C.; Yiang, G.-T.; Yen, H.-S.; Liu, W.-L.; Li, C.-J.; Kao, W.-Y. Epithelial-Mesenchymal Transition with Malignant Transformation Leading Multiple Metastasis from Disseminated Peritoneal Leiomyomatosis. *J. Clin. Med.* **2018**, *7*, 207. [CrossRef] [PubMed]
103. Wendt, M.K.; Tian, M.; Schiemann, W.P. Deconstructing the mechanisms and consequences of TGF-beta-induced EMT during cancer progression. *Cell Tissue Res.* **2012**, *347*, 85–101. [CrossRef] [PubMed]
104. Subramaniam, K.S.; Omar, I.S.; Kwong, S.C.; Mohamed, Z.; Woo, Y.L.; Mat Adenan, N.A.; Chung, I. Cancer-associated fibroblasts promote endometrial cancer growth via activation of interleukin-6/STAT-3/c-Myc pathway. *Am. J. Cancer Res.* **2016**, *6*, 200–213.
105. Sahoo, S.S.; Zhang, X.D.; Hondermarck, H.; Tanwar, P.S. The Emerging Role of the Microenvironment in Endometrial Cancer. *Cancers* **2018**, *10*, 408. [CrossRef] [PubMed]
106. Subramaniam, K.S.; Tham, S.T.; Mohamed, Z.; Woo, Y.L.; Mat Adenan, N.A.; Chung, I. Cancer-associated fibroblasts promote proliferation of endometrial cancer cells. *PLoS ONE* **2013**, *8*, e68923. [CrossRef]
107. Teng, F.; Tian, W.Y.; Wang, Y.M.; Zhang, Y.F.; Guo, F.; Zhao, J.; Gao, C.; Xue, F.X. Cancer-associated fibroblasts promote the progression of endometrial cancer via the SDF-1/CXCR4 axis. *J. Hematol. Oncol.* **2016**, *9*, 8. [CrossRef] [PubMed]
108. Franco, O.E.; Shaw, A.K.; Strand, D.W.; Hayward, S.W. Cancer associated fibroblasts in cancer pathogenesis. *Semin. Cell Dev. Biol.* **2010**, *21*, 33–39. [CrossRef] [PubMed]
109. Wang, X.; Zhang, W.; Sun, X.; Lin, Y.; Chen, W. Cancer-associated fibroblasts induce epithelial-mesenchymal transition through secreted cytokines in endometrial cancer cells. *Oncol. Lett.* **2018**, *15*, 5694–5702. [CrossRef]
110. Bhowmick, N.A.; Chytil, A.; Plieth, D.; Gorska, A.E.; Dumont, N.; Shappell, S.; Washington, M.K.; Neilson, E.G.; Moses, H.L. TGF-beta signaling in fibroblasts modulates the oncogenic potential of adjacent epithelia. *Science* **2004**, *303*, 848–851. [CrossRef]

111. Papageorgis, P.; Stylianopoulos, T. Role of TGFβ in regulation of the tumor microenvironment and drug delivery (review). *Int. J. Oncol.* **2015**, *46*, 933–943. [CrossRef]
112. Derynck, R.; Akhurst, R.J.; Balmain, A. TGF-beta signaling in tumor suppression and cancer progression. *Nat. Genet.* **2001**, *29*, 117–129. [CrossRef] [PubMed]
113. Muinelo-Romay, L.; Colas, E.; Barbazan, J.; Alonso-Alconada, L.; Alonso-Nocelo, M.; Bouso, M.; Curiel, T.; Cueva, J.; Anido, U.; Forteza, J.; et al. High-risk endometrial carcinoma profiling identifies TGF-beta1 as a key factor in the initiation of tumor invasion. *Mol. Cancer Ther.* **2011**, *10*, 1357–1366. [CrossRef]
114. Parekh, T.V.; Gama, P.; Wen, X.; Demopoulos, R.; Munger, J.S.; Carcangiu, M.L.; Reiss, M.; Gold, L.I. Transforming growth factor beta signaling is disabled early in human endometrial carcinogenesis concomitant with loss of growth inhibition. *Cancer Res.* **2002**, *62*, 2778–2790.
115. Lei, X.; Wang, L.; Yang, J.; Sun, L.Z. TGFbeta signaling supports survival and metastasis of endometrial cancer cells. *Cancer Manag. Res.* **2009**, *2009*, 15–24.
116. Yu, L.; Hu, R.; Sullivan, C.; Swanson, R.J.; Oehninger, S.; Sun, Y.P.; Bocca, S. MFGE8 regulates TGF-beta-induced epithelial mesenchymal transition in endometrial epithelial cells in vitro. *Reproduction* **2016**, *152*, 225–233. [CrossRef] [PubMed]
117. Bokhari, A.A.; Lee, L.R.; Raboteau, D.; Hamilton, C.A.; Maxwell, G.L.; Rodriguez, G.C.; Syed, V. Progesterone inhibits endometrial cancer invasiveness by inhibiting the TGFbeta pathway. *Cancer Prev. Res.* **2014**, *7*, 1045–1055. [CrossRef]
118. Tanaka, Y.; Terai, Y.; Kawaguchi, H.; Fujiwara, S.; Yoo, S.; Tsunetoh, S.; Takai, M.; Kanemura, M.; Tanabe, A.; Ohmichi, M. Prognostic impact of EMT (epithelial-mesenchymal-transition)-related protein expression in endometrial cancer. *Cancer Biol. Ther.* **2013**, *14*, 13–19. [CrossRef] [PubMed]
119. Marino, M.; Galluzzo, P.; Ascenzi, P. Estrogen signaling multiple pathways to impact gene transcription. *Curr. Genom.* **2006**, *7*, 497–508. [CrossRef]
120. Pietras, R.J.; Márquez-Garbán, D.C. Membrane-Associated Estrogen Receptor Signaling Pathways in Human Cancers. *Clin. Cancer Res.* **2007**, *13*, 4672–4676. [CrossRef] [PubMed]
121. Mohammed, H.; Russell, I.A.; Stark, R.; Rueda, O.M.; Hickey, T.E.; Tarulli, G.A.; Serandour, A.A.; Birrell, S.N.; Bruna, A.; Saadi, A.; et al. Progesterone receptor modulates ERα action in breast cancer. *Nature* **2015**, *523*, 313. [CrossRef] [PubMed]
122. Yang, S.; Thiel, K.W.; Leslie, K.K. Progesterone: The ultimate endometrial tumor suppressor. *Trends Endocrinol. Metab.* **2011**, *22*, 145–152. [CrossRef] [PubMed]
123. Guo, R.X.; Wei, L.H.; Tu, Z.; Sun, P.M.; Wang, J.L.; Zhao, D.; Li, X.P.; Tang, J.M. 17 beta-estradiol activates PI3K/Akt signaling pathway by estrogen receptor (ER)-dependent and ER-independent mechanisms in endometrial cancer cells. *J. Steroid Biochem. Mol. Biol.* **2006**, *99*, 9–18. [CrossRef] [PubMed]
124. Hou, X.; Zhao, M.; Wang, T.; Zhang, G. Upregulation of estrogen receptor mediates migration, invasion and proliferation of endometrial carcinoma cells by regulating the PI3K/AKT/mTOR pathway. *Oncol. Rep.* **2014**, *31*, 1175–1182. [CrossRef]
125. Revankar, C.M.; Mitchell, H.D.; Field, A.S.; Burai, R.; Corona, C.; Ramesh, C.; Sklar, L.A.; Arterburn, J.B.; Prossnitz, E.R. Synthetic Estrogen Derivatives Demonstrate the Functionality of Intracellular GPR30. *ACS Chem. Biol.* **2007**, *2*, 536–544. [CrossRef] [PubMed]
126. Petrie, W.K.; Dennis, M.K.; Hu, C.; Dai, D.; Arterburn, J.B.; Smith, H.O.; Hathaway, H.J.; Prossnitz, E.R. G protein-coupled estrogen receptor-selective ligands modulate endometrial tumor growth. *Obstet. Gynecol. Int.* **2013**, *2013*, 472720. [CrossRef]
127. Ehrlich, C.E.; Young, P.C.; Stehman, F.B.; Sutton, G.P.; Alford, W.M. Steroid receptors and clinical outcome in patients with adenocarcinoma of the endometrium. *Am. J. Obstet. Gynecol.* **1988**, *158*, 796–807. [CrossRef]
128. Jeon, Y.T.; Park, I.A.; Kim, Y.B.; Kim, J.W.; Park, N.H.; Kang, S.B.; Lee, H.P.; Song, Y.S. Steroid receptor expressions in endometrial cancer: Clinical significance and epidemiological implication. *Cancer Lett.* **2006**, *239*, 198–204. [CrossRef]
129. Thigpen, J.T.; Brady, M.F.; Alvarez, R.D.; Adelson, M.D.; Homesley, H.D.; Manetta, A.; Soper, J.T.; Given, F.T. Oral medroxyprogesterone acetate in the treatment of advanced or recurrent endometrial carcinoma: A dose-response study by the Gynecologic Oncology Group. *J. Clin. Oncol.* **1999**, *17*, 1736–1744. [CrossRef]

130. Hanekamp, E.E.; Kuhne, E.C.; Smid-Koopman, E.; de Ruiter, P.E.; Chadha-Ajwani, S.; Brinkmann, A.O.; Burger, C.W.; Grootegoed, J.A.; Huikeshoven, F.J.; Blok, L.J. Loss of progesterone receptor may lead to an invasive phenotype in human endometrial cancer. *Eur. J. Cancer* **2002**, *38*, S71–S72. [CrossRef]
131. Van der Horst, P.H.; Wang, Y.; Vandenput, I.; Kuhne, L.C.; Ewing, P.C.; van Ijcken, W.F.; van der Zee, M.; Amant, F.; Burger, C.W.; Blok, L.J. Progesterone inhibits epithelial-to-mesenchymal transition in endometrial cancer. *PLoS ONE* **2012**, *7*, e30840. [CrossRef] [PubMed]

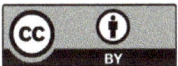

© 2019 by the authors. Licensee MDPI, Basel, Switzerland. This article is an open access article distributed under the terms and conditions of the Creative Commons Attribution (CC BY) license (http://creativecommons.org/licenses/by/4.0/).

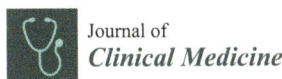 

*Review*

# Exosome-Mediated Signaling in Epithelial to Mesenchymal Transition and Tumor Progression

Alice Conigliaro [1,*,†] and Carla Cicchini [2,*,†]

1 Dipartimento di Biopatologia e Biotecnologie Mediche, University of Palermo, 90100 Palermo, Italy
2 Dipartimento di Medicina Molecolare, Sapienza University of Rome, 00161 Rome, Italy
* Correspondence: alice.conigliaro@unipa.it (A.C.); carla.cicchini@uniroma1.it (C.C.)
† These authors contributed equally to this work.

Received: 16 November 2018; Accepted: 21 December 2018; Published: 27 December 2018

**Abstract:** Growing evidence points to exosomes as key mediators of cell–cell communication, by transferring their specific cargo (e.g., proteins, lipids, DNA and RNA molecules) from producing to receiving cells. In cancer, the regulation of the exosome-mediated intercellular communication may be reshaped, inducing relevant changes in gene expression of recipient cells in addition to microenvironment alterations. Notably, exosomes may deliver signals able to induce the transdifferentiation process known as Epithelial-to-Mesenchymal Transition (EMT). In this review, we summarize recent findings on the role of exosomes in tumor progression and EMT, highlighting current knowledge on exosome-mediated intercellular communication in tumor-niche establishment, migration, invasion, and metastasis processes. This body of evidence suggests the relevance of taking into account exosome-mediated signaling and its multifaceted aspects to develop innovative anti-tumoral therapeutic approaches.

**Keywords:** tumor niche; Epithelial–Mesenchymal plasticity; cancer-derived exosomes; extracellular vesicles; metastasis

## 1. Introduction

The lipid-bilayer extracellular vesicles (EVs) include at least three main classes of vesicles that differ in dimension, biogenesis and biophysical properties: exosomes, microvesicles, and apoptotic bodies. Here, we focused on exosomes, small vesicles with an average diameter from 30 to 200 nm that originate inside the Multi Vesicular Bodies (MVBs) and are released by the parental cell after MVB fusion with plasma membrane.

Although exosomes were first identified as garbage disposal [1,2], current knowledge highlights the direct role of these vesicles in governing physiological and pathological conditions by transferring information from producing to receiving cells. Exosomes, indeed, may signal in autocrine but, most importantly, in paracrine and endocrine manner, being taken up by neighboring cells or carried to distant sites. Thus, they assure the horizontal transfer of specific bioactive molecules (including proteins, lipids, RNAs, and DNA [3]) from donor to recipient cells.

Exosomes are ordinarily released by different cell types [4]. They have been identified in various body fluids (including semen, blood, urine, cerebrospinal fluid, and milk) and their role is strongly associated with the cytotype of the producing cells. For example, exosomes participating in supporting immune response [5] and, as vesicles secreted by cells of the nervous system, have been found to coordinate myelin membrane biogenesis, neuronal development, transmission and regeneration [6–8]. Interestingly, several studies recently reviewed by Guay and Reguazzi [9], pointed to the involvement of exosomes in a "new endocrinology", being mediators of the crosstalk between metabolic organs.

Despite the exosome role in homeostasis maintenance and physiology, the most recent intensive investigation was focused on the involvement of these EVs in pathological processes. Particularly in cancer, the regulation of the exosome-mediated intercellular communication may be reshaped. Exosomes, indeed, may carry messages from transformed to healthy cells or to other cells in the tumor or they may signal in an autocrine manner back to the producing tumor cell, thus allowing relevant changes in recipient cells behavior and microenvironment alterations. Notably, exosomes may deliver signals able to induce an Epithelial-to-Mesenchymal Transition (EMT), a transdifferentiation process that underlines tumor dissemination.

In this review, we focus our interest on the role of exosomes during the EMT process in tumor progression. Starting with an overview on the molecular composition of these vesicles, with a focus on their emerging heterogeneity, we highlight current knowledge on the exosome-mediated intercellular communication in tumor niche establishment, migration, invasion, and metastasis processes.

This body of evidence suggests the relevance of taking into account exosome-mediated signaling and its multifaceted aspects to develop innovative anti-tumoral therapeutic approaches.

## 2. Exosome Heterogeneity and Cargo Composition

Exosomes are generally characterized by markers such as tetraspanins (e.g., CD63 [10]) and heat shock proteins (HSP70 and HSP90 [11]) while their biogenesis involves the endosomal sorting complex required for transport (ESCRT; [12]), Rab proteins [13], syndecan-syntenin-Alix [14], and others. Despite that, the improvement in the technologies adopted for exosomes isolation and characterization highlighted that, even if originating within the MVBs and presenting common markers, exosomes may show physical and chemical differences. Therefore, for a better comprehension of the variety and the apparent discrepancy of current literature reports, we should consider that exosomes may exhibit per se heterogeneity, both in physiological and in pathological conditions.

With respect to exosome features, Kowal and collaborators [15] demonstrated by a quantitative proteomic analysis, that high-speed ultracentrifugation, considered the gold-standard purification method for exosomes, allows the isolation of four different populations, among which, only two are associated with the endosomal pathway, and can be further separated for the different expression/enrichment in tetraspanin Cluster of Differentiation (CD) 63, CD81, and/or CD9. Interestingly, Willms et al. [16] demonstrated that several cell types release two major subpopulations of exosomes with distinct molecular compositions and biological properties. At least two different types of exosomes have been recovered from saliva, differing in size and content in term of proteins and RNAs [17,18]. Furthermore, the Lotvall group proved that human mast cells release two distinct exosome families that, separated by floatation on a density gradient, present "substantial" differences in RNA species content as demonstrated by microarray and Next Generation Sequencing (NGS). Interestingly, while RNA from Low Density exosome correlated with cellular mRNA, High Density exosomes were enriched in non-coding RNA (ncRNA). Moreover, differences in RNA signatures and protein patterns led the authors to hypothesize about possible different exosome biogenesis pathways [19].

Exosomes with different protein composition and surface markers have been identified after flotation onto sucrose gradient by Bobrie et al. [20]. These authors reported that high-speed ultracentrifugation co-purified vesicles bearing the endosomal tetraspanin CD63 together with smaller vesicles which exposed the CD9 tetraspanin and the peripheral membrane-associated protein Mfge8. Most interestingly, the discovery that Rab27a, a small GTPase known to be involved in exosome secretion, is required for the release of the only CD63 positive exosomes, enforcing the hypothesis that heterogeneity comes from different molecular mechanisms of formation and secretion of exosomes.

With respect to cargo molecules, exosomes embed several macromolecules e.g., lipids, metabolites, nucleic acids and proteins (the complete lists of exosome embedded macromolecules can be found on ExoCarta [21] or Vesiclepedia [22]. Cargo molecules depend on the cell of origin, the change in response to physiological and pathological conditions [23] and maintain their biological function when transferred to the receiving cells, impacting their fate [24]. Nucleic acid analysis revealed, inside exosomes, an abundance of RNA families that, protected from RNases by lipoprotein envelop, maintain their functions. Notably, specific subsets of miRNAs appear to preferentially localize to exosomes [25–27] and, as demonstrated by Pegtel at al. [28], exosome-mediated miRNAs delivery directly modulates specific targets once in the cytoplasm of receiving cells. Even if numerically less abundant than small RNAs, long non-coding RNAs (lncRNAs) have been found in exosomes released by different cell types, specifically by tumor cells, thus representing new specific tumor markers [29–31]. However, further studies are required to fully understand the effects induced by non-coding RNAs in target cells, specifically concerning lncRNAs, whose pleiotropic roles make them protagonists in the control of gene expression from epigenetics to miRNAs inhibition. Concerning this, two interesting manuscripts from the Lorico group [32,33] demonstrated that internalized exosomes, or part of these, can directly reach the nucleus of receiving cells. These data initiate interest on all of the compounds that, transported by the exosomes, have a nuclear biological activity (e.g., transcription factors, histone modification enzymes, and lncRNAs).

Deeper investigations are required also to characterize the loading of specific macromolecules. The study of miRNA-motifs mediated loading are so far limited to a few reports that identified specific RNA-binding-proteins and some miRNA consensus sequences mediating the process [34–36]. While the mechanisms of selective loading of RNAs, as well as proteins, in exosomes are still poorly understood, it is conceivable that pH [37] and hypoxia [38] may affect both the entity of the release and the sorting of a specific content. The lack of standardized well-characterized methods to isolate, purify, and quantify the exosomes further limits the study of their content as cell signature.

The high variability of exosome-induced effects is also determined by the type of interactions occurring between exosomes and target cells that, as recently reviewed in [39], are governed by numerous factors. Depending on their origin, exosomes have been found to interact preferentially with specific cell types, and this interaction seems to be strongly conditioned by the integrins exposed on the exosome surface [40]. It is conceivable that an extensive proteomic analysis of adhesion proteins, such as extracellular matrix proteins (e.g., fibronectin and laminin) and tetraspanins might help to predict exosome-cell interactions but we lack efficient protocols for the isolation of outer membrane proteins only.

Once in touch with target cells, the strategy used to transform these are multiple. First, exosomes may activate receiving cells from the outside, through a ligand/receptor interaction and subsequent activation of downstream pathways.

Paradigmatic is the immune tolerance induced by several cancer cells through exosomes, which express death signals as the PD-L1 (programmed death-ligand 1) or Fas Ligand, and systemically induce apoptosis in receiving T cells and Natural Killer (NK) cells [41,42]. Ligand/receptor interaction have a role also in exosome migration around the body as recently demonstrated for CCR7 (CC-chemokine receptor 7) that, exposed on the Dendritic Cell exosomes, contributes to both their migration on spleen and the induction of inflammation [43]. Exosomes expressing the amphiregulin (AREG), isolated from several tumor cells, have been found able to activate the Epidermal Growth Factor Receptor (EGFR) in receiving cells thus affecting the bone marrow microenvironment [44] or promoting bone metastases [45]. Finally, several groups demonstrated a regulation of the Transforming Growth Factor (TGF)β pathway mediated by membrane-bound molecules [46,47] or (GPI)-anchored cell surface glycoprotein [48].

In most cases, the interaction with cellular receptors drives exosome internalization. Receptors or proteins located on the EV surface participate in fusion, endocytosis or phagocytosis with subsequent release of the exosome content in the receiving cells.

## 3. EMT Associated with Tumor Progression: The Role of Exosomes

EMT is a physiological or pathological transdifferentiation process in which epithelial cells lose their cell-cell contacts and apicobasal polarity and acquire mesenchymal properties, coupled to the ability to migrate and to invade the surrounding tissues. EMT is crucial in organogenesis, development, wound healing and regeneration but it is aberrantly activated in tumor progression and metastasis (for review, [49]). EMT, indeed, allows in situ differentiated cells to acquire the ability to migrate out of the primary tumor, invading basement membrane and entering the vasculature. Transitional tumor cells exit from circulation and migrate into the tissue parenchyma in potentially secondary tumor sites. In this process of colonization of target tissues by metastatic cells (as well as during morphogenesis), the shift toward a mesenchymal state is often reversed by an inverse Mesenchymal-to-Epithelial Transition (MET). The MET occurs in different microenvironments and it is necessary to support the reacquisition of epithelial features to seed metastasis [50,51].

EMT/MET plasticity implies a profound reprogramming of gene expression mainly orchestrated by specific "master" transcription factors, known as EMT-inducing transcription factors (EMT-TFs; i.e., ZEB1; SIP1/ZEB2; Twist1; Twist2; E12/E47; Tbx3; the Snail family members Snail2 (Slug), Snail3 (Smuc) and, in particular, Snail1 (Snail) [52–56]. The EMT-TFs primarily act as repressors of the epithelial genes and may guide the recruitment of the epigenetic machinery to the chromatin context, thus allowing the proper regulation of gene expression [57,58].

Rather than a simple shift between two alternative states (i.e., the mesenchymal and the epithelial phenotype), the current view is that the EMT/MET implies multiple and dynamic transdifferentiation states. This greater flexibility may result in a "partial EMT" or in the co-presence of epithelial and mesenchymal traits, as in the hybrid "metastable" features identified in several tumors [59–61] and attributed to a stem phenotype [62–65]. The complexity of the EMT/MET phenotypes reflects the complexity of the regulatory circuitries that, beyond the transcriptional control, also involve several ncRNAs, including miRNAs (e.g., miR-200 family or miR-34) [66–68] or lncRNAs (e.g., HOTAIR) [57]. Notably, transitional tumor cells need to be continuously reprogrammed to adapt to different microenvironments and to ensure tumor growth and metastasis [69–71].

Exosome composition profoundly differs between untransformed and transformed cells [72–74] and increasing evidence suggests that tumor-derived exosomes (TDEs), as well as exosomes from tumor associated cells in the microenvironment (TME), exert a key role in the regulation of tumor growth and survival as well as tumor invasion, angiogenesis, and metastasis.

Notably, TDEs may carry pro-EMT cargoes that include EMT inducer molecules, e.g., TGF-β, Hypoxia-inducible factor (HIF)1α, β-catenin or miRNAs, such as miR-23a. All this content is able to (i) confer mesenchymal properties to epithelial cells, (ii) promote the initiation phase of the epithelial tumor metastasis (when in situ tumor cells migrate out of the primary tumor, invading basement membrane and entering the vasculature) and (iii) guarantee tumor-microenvironment cross-talk [75–80] (Figure 1A,B).

It is conceivable that a fine tuning of the EMT plasticity may result in the capacity by the cell to export specific bioactive molecules and, vice versa, the exosome-mediated signaling may impact on the EMT/MET dynamics. Coherently, exosomes from transitional cells exert a role in the regulation of tumor niche, migration, invasion, and metastasis.

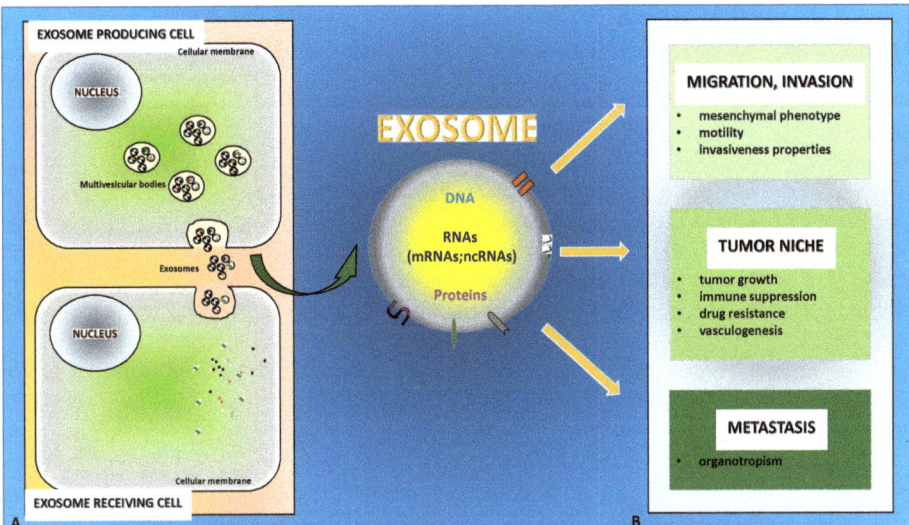

**Figure 1.** The role of exosomes in Epithelial-to-Mesenchymal Transition (EMT) and tumor progression is depicted. (**A**) Exosomes originate from the multivesicular bodies that release them by fusing with the cellular membrane. (**B**) Exosome cargo content of DNA, RNA (including ncRNA) and proteins specifically mediates cell–cell communication in EMT and in the associated tumor progression to promote different outcomes.

## 3.1. Exosomes in Tumor Niche

In primary tumor, exosomes contribute to the definition of tumor niche by promoting tumor growth (despite nutrient deprivation and stress condition), immune suppression and drug resistance, and enhancing vasculogenesis.

Cell growth can be stimulated by cytokines that, loaded in TDEs, are then transported to closer tumor cells; Raimondo et al. demonstrated that exosomes released by chronic myeloid leukemia cells promoted tumor cell growth and inhibited apoptosis by activating TGFβ receptor [46]. Moreover, TDEs can induce proliferation of adjacent cells by non-coding RNA-mediated signaling e.g., the miR-27 in gastric cancer exosomes [81] and the lncRNA c-Myc-Upregulated (MYU) in prostate cancer exosomes [82]. Meanwhile, paracrine stimulation of tumor cell proliferation is induced by cancer associate fibroblasts (CAFs). These cells are pivotal players in the tumor microenvironment by stimulating Cancer Stem Cells maintenance and EMT [83]. Interestingly, exosomes released by tumor cells may activate resident fibroblasts inducing CAFs [81,84]. In bladder cancer, Ringuette et al. showed that CAF activation is mainly due to the induction of TGFβ/Small Mothers Against Decapentaplegic (SMAD) pathway resulting from the transport of TGFβ by TDEs [84]. Furthermore, in gastric cancer an important contribute to fibroblasts activation is due to the exosome mediated transport of miR-27a [81].

The contribution of CAF released exosomes to tumor growth is supported by studies investigating CAF proteome and transcriptome that identified a huge number of molecules with pro tumorigenic activity [85,86]. Interestingly, Zhang and colleagues underlined the possibility that exosomes may carry both pro- and anti-tumor factors. These authors, in fact, by comparing miRNA sequencing of exosomes derived from CAFs and exosomes secreted by fibroblasts from HCC (Hepatocellular Carcinoma) patients, demonstrated that CAF-derived exosomes stimulate cell proliferation lacking protective elements such as the miR-320a that, on the contrary, is transported by NF-exo and is able to inhibit HCC growth through MAPK targeting [87].

TDEs may also contribute to acidification of the tumor microenvironment by modulating stromal cell metabolism. Recently, it was demonstrated that human melanoma-derived exosomes, once internalized by dermal fibroblasts, promote aerobic glycolysis and downregulate oxidative phosphorylation [88]. Meanwhile, the Nagrath group elegantly demonstrated that exosomes from CAFs downregulate mitochondrial activity and increase glycolysis. Furthermore, intra-exosome metabolomic analyses showed that exosomes contain metabolites, amino acids, and lipids, "which can fuel the metabolic activity of the recipient cells" [89].

Finally, as mentioned above, exosomes indirectly support tumor growth by favoring immune escape in different ways; they inactivate T cells or induce their apoptosis by cell surface interaction or after internalization [90–92]. With respect to immunomodulatory properties, TDEs exposing CD39 and CD37 on their surface can mediate T-cell suppression by extracellular adenosine production [93]. Meanwhile it was shown that the internalization by Kupffer cells of pancreatic ductal adenocarcinoma TDEs induced fibronectin production, thus promoting the gathering of bone marrow-derived macrophages and neutrophils and leading to liver pre-metastatic niche formation [94].

A key component of tumor microenvironment is the vascular network that supports tumor growth; several extracellular mechanisms take part in endothelial cell stimulation, among these TDEs contribute to modulating both angiogenesis and vascular permeability [95].

It is of note that the ability to promote angiogenesis has been mainly attributed to exosomes isolated from tumor initiating cells (TICs). In renal cell carcinoma and hepatocellular carcinoma for example, only CD105+ and CD90+ cells respectively, release exosomes able to stimulate production and release of the Vascular Endothelial Growth Factor (VEGF); TIC derived exosomes, once engulfed in endothelial cells, activate the VEGF autocrine loop through the delivery of different ncRNAs [31,96]. Recently, Sun et al. demonstrated pro-angiogenetic activity also in exosomes from Glioma stem cells, that stimulate endothelial cell motility by activating a miR-21/VEGF/Vascular Endothelial Growth Factor Receptor (VEGFR) 2 signal pathway [97]. In addition, exosomes can directly stimulate endothelial cell VEGF receptor through the delivery of 90-kDa VEGF (VEGF90k), which was found to interact with Hsp90 in extracellular vesicles [98].

Several observations correlate hypoxia, exosomes, and neo angiogenesis stimulation. Low oxygen partial pressure, a common characteristic of all types of cancer, induces activation and nuclear translocation of the transcription factor HIF1 that, inside the nucleus, interacts with several co-factors to induce the up regulation of a huge number of genes whose coordinated expression drives tumor cells to a most aggressive phenotype [99]. Among the HIF target is the VEGF. Evidence collected in past years demonstrated that hypoxia stimulates production and release of exosomes [100] that, in turn participate in promotion of tumor neo-angiogenesis as described by ref. [101] and enclosed references.

Although VEGF signaling is the best-validated pathway in angiogenesis, the refractoriness to anti-VEGF therapies in several cancers highlighted the involvement of VEGF-independent strategies in promoting tumor angiogenesis [102]. An interesting study performed by Tang et al. [103] demonstrated that exosomes, released by ovarian cancer cells, participate in cleavage and delivery of soluble E-cadherin that once delivered on endothelial cell surface, interacts with VE-cadherin and induces activation of β-catenin and Nuclear Factor kappa-light-chain-enhancer of activated B cells (NF-κB) signaling, resulting in endothelial cell migration, and tube formation in vitro and in vivo.

*3.2. Exosomes in Migration, Invasion, and Metastasis*

A body of evidence points to the role of exosome-triggered EMT in the inception of high metastatic potential that correlates with high motility and increased invasiveness. Exosomes from cancer cells were found to be able to activate intracellular pathways by transporting specific proteins such as phosphorylated tyrosine kinases receptor (RTKs) [104]. Exosomes from muscle-invasive bladder cancer induced a decrease in E-cadherin expression and enhanced migration and invasion of uroepithelial cells [79]. Similarly, exosomes from highly metastatic lung cancer cells induced an EMT associated with migration, invasion, and proliferation in recipient human bronchial epithelial cells [105]. Furthermore, exosomes secreted by highly metastatic MHCC97H hepatocarcinoma (HCC) cells conferred the ability to migrate and give invasiveness properties to low metastatic HCC cells by inducing EMT via

MAPK/Extracellular signal-Regulated Kinase (ERK) signaling pathway activation [106]. Finally, human breast and colorectal cancer cells released full-length, signaling-competent EGFR ligands, i.e., amphiregulin, able to increase the invasiveness of recipient cancer cells [107].

Harris et al. investigated the role of exosomes released from different breast cancer cells, modeling different stages of metastasis. They showed that tumor cells of increasing metastatic potential are able to secrete exosomes with protein signatures different in identity and abundance; these exosomes increased cell migration proportionally, with exosomes from high-metastatic potential cells able to induce the greatest degree of cell movement [108]. Interestingly, xenograft tumor cell motility studies in the chorioallantoic membrane (CAM) of chick embryos revealed a key role of exosome secretion for the directional migration of fibrosarcoma cells. These vesicles, indeed, carry extracellular matrix (ECM) molecules promoting adhesion assembly [109].

Furthermore, Schillaci et al. [110] recently demonstrated that exosomes released by metastatic colon cancer cell lines affected tumor behavior promoting a more aggressive phenotype. They found that metastatic amoeboid cells (SW620) release exosomes that are enriched in Thrombin, activating RhoA/Rho-associated protein kinase (ROCK) pathway in receiving cells. This activation induces migration and invasion in primary tumor cells while, in endothelial cells, causes VE-cadherin delocalization and junction disruption.

Concerning exosomal lncRNAs, a role for BCAR4 (breast cancer anti-estrogen resistance 4) has been suggested in colorectal cancer development [111] while HOTAIR (Hox antisense intergenic RNA) was found overexpressed in bladder cancer patients and correlated with the invasiveness of the tumor [30]. Notably, HOTAIR has a key functional role in promoting EMT in different cell types [57,112,113].

With respect to TMEs, Luga et al. demonstrated that CD81-positive CAF-released exosomes induced in breast cancer cells the release of Wnt11 that, in an autocrine manner, promoted the activation of Planar Cell Polarity (PCP) [114]. Meanwhile, Condorelli's group attributed the induction of EMT in breast cancer to three different miRNAs (miRs-21, -378e, and -143), delivered by CAF-derived exosomes [115]. These observations enforced the idea that cellular transformation, induced by exosome uptake, must be mediated by multiple biological compounds that converge on the same molecular pathways. Li and collaborators demonstrated that ovarian CAF-derived exosomes were enriched in TGFβ1 that may induce an EMT and an aggressive phenotype in ovarian cancer cells lines [116]. More recently, Zhao and colleagues demonstrated that human umbilical cord mesenchymal stem cells-derived conditioned medium was able to induce migration and invasion capability in A549 lung cancer cells by activating TGFβ-related pathways [117].

The ability to migrate and invade surrounding tissues can be enhanced by hypoxia-induced exosomes by shuttling different molecules. Firstly, exosomes released in hypoxia may contain hypoxia-inducible factors (HIFs), able to trigger EMT in recipient cells [78]. Coherently, Ramteke and colleagues showed that hypoxia-induced exosomes increased the invasiveness of prostate cancer cells by promoting the loss of E-cadherin [118]. Furthermore, exosome-mediated mechanisms to promote migration and invasiveness by tumor cells in hypoxia may involve lncRNAs, such as UCA1 in bladder cancer cells [119] or the lncRNA-regulator of reprogramming (RoR) in HCC [120], as well as specific miRNAs, e.g., miR-21 in oral squamous cell carcinoma [94] or miR-23a in lung cancer [121].

Interestingly, Zhou and colleagues reported that exosomes secreted by cervical squamous cell carcinoma (CSCC) cells may shuttle miR-221-3p, targeting vasohibin1 (VASH1), to human lymphatic endothelial cells (HLECs). This promotes migration in vitro as well as lymphangiogenesis and lymph node metastasis in vivo [122].

The role of TDEs is not limited to the primary tumor site and their ability to cross long distances within the body makes exosomes a suitable vehicle to trace the way of tumor metastases. TDEs promote the organotropism of metastatic tumors and contribute to pre-metastatic niche formation by showing "avidity" for specific recipient cells [11,40,94]. Notably, Hoshino and colleagues showed that the exosomal integrins guide the exosomes to specific secondary sites. Furthermore, exosomes from lung-, liver- and brain-tropic tumor cells preferentially fuse with lung fibroblasts and epithelial cells, liver Kupffer cells, and brain endothelial cells [40].

## 4. Conclusions and Perspectives

EMT exerts a key role in tumor progression and exosomes, released by transitional cells, transport specific signaling molecules to promote invasion, migration, metastasis, and microenvironment changes, able to sustain tumor growth and dissemination. In fact, the horizontally transferred TDE specific content promotes the acquisition by tumor cells of mesenchymal markers and increases cell motility, associated with a more aggressive phenotype. Furthermore, exosome cargo impacts on tumor niche establishment and regulates the tropism of metastasis (Tables 1 and 2). Therefore, the identification of molecules (mRNA, ncRNAs, proteins) specifically enriched in exosomes from different tumor stages may represent an efficient real-time staging of tumor evolution or response to therapy, also in patients differing in gender or age. Notably, EVs may be isolated from body fluids, and several RNA and protein molecules have already been identified as potential diagnostic and prognostic biomarkers of different tumor types or different stages of the same tumor. Interestingly, the study of the secretome of HCC cells overexpressing the master transcriptional factor Slug, and exhibiting a partial EMT phenotype, showed the enrichment in exosomes of Fibronectin 1 (FN1), collagen type II alpha 1 (COL2A1), and fibrinogen gamma chain (FGG); therefore, these proteins may represent useful and non-invasive biomarkers associated with partial transitional cells [123]. Notably, a partial EMT may characterize circulating tumor cells (CTCs) that pose a metastatic risk for patients [124].

**Table 1.** Summary of recent evidence on exosome signaling molecules and their effects on tumor progression.

| Exosome-Mediated Effect | Producing Cell | Specific TDE Content and Mechanism of Action | Reference |
|---|---|---|---|
| Tumor cell proliferation | Prostate cancer cells | lncRNAc-Myc Upregulated (MYU)-mediated upregulation of c-Myc by competitively binding miR-184 | [82] |
| | Hypoxic bladder cancer cells | lncRNA-UCA (unknown mechanism) | [119] |
| | Hypoxic hepatocellular carcinoma cells | lncRoR-induced hypoxic responses (by downregulation of miR-145 and upregulation of Hypoxia-inducible factor 1 (HIF1) | [120] |
| | CAF from Human Oral Tongue Squamous Cell Carcinoma | MFAP5 (Microfibril Associated Protein 5)-induced activation of mitogen-activated protein kinase (MAPK) and AKT | [85] |
| | CAF from Hepatocellular carcinoma | MAPK activation by negative regulation of miR-320a | [87] |
| | CAF from pancreatic ductal adenocarcinomas | Snail and microRNA-146a upregulation | [125] |
| EMT and metastasis of tumor cells | Bladder cancer cells Colon cancer cell lines | RhoA/ROCK (Rho-associated protein kinase) signaling pathway activation and acquisition of migratory capacity | [79,110] |
| | Epstein-Barr-Virus EBV infected Nasopharyngeal carcinoma (NPC) | HIF1 upregulation | [78] |
| | metastatic melanoma cells | MET induced pro-vasculogenic and metastatic effects | [11] |
| | Hypoxic cancer cells | Activation of Epithelial-to-Mesenchymal Transition (EMT) genes in receiving cells | [101] and enclosed references |
| | Lung cancer cells | vimentin | [105] |
| | Hepatocellular carcinoma cells | MAPK/ERK (Extracellular signal-Regulated Kinase) signalling activation (unknown mechanism) | [106] |
| | High aggressive breast cancer | proteins involved in metastasis and invasion | [108] |
| | Prostate cancer cells | metalloproteinases induction and targeting of adherens junction proteins | [118] |
| | Hypoxic bladder cancer | lncRNA-UCA1 (Urothelial Cancer Associated 1) (mechanism of action unspecified) | [119] |
| | Metastatic breast cancer | miR-10b targeting HOXD10 (HomeoboxD10) | [126] |

Table 1. Cont.

| Exosome-Mediated Effect | Producing Cell | Specific TDE Content and Mechanism of Action | Reference |
|---|---|---|---|
| | CAF from Human Oral Tongue Squamous Cell Carcinoma | MFAP5 activation of MAPK and AKT | [85] |
| | CAF from Hepatocellular carcinoma | MAPK activation | [87] |
| | CAF from breast cancer | EMT activation by miRs -21, miR-378 and miR-143 | [115] |
| | CAF from ovarian cancer | TGF (Transforming Growth Factor) β1-induced EMT | [116] |
| | Mesenchymal stem cells | TGFβ1 activation of Smad2/3, Akt/GSK (Glycogen synthase kinase)-3β/β-catenin, NF-κB (Nuclear Factor kappa-light-chain-enhancer of activated B cells), ERK (Extracellular signal-Regulated Kinase), JNK (c-Jun N-terminal kinase and p38 MAPK (mitogen-activated protein kinase) | [117] |

Table 2. Summary of recent evidence on exosome signaling molecules and their effects in the tumor microenvironment.

| Tumor Microenvironment Modification | Producing Cell | Specific Content and Mechanism of Action | Reference |
|---|---|---|---|
| CAF activation | Gastric cancer cells | miR-27a-mediated downregulation of CSRP2 (cysteine and glycine rich protein 2) | [81] |
| | Bladder cancer cells | TGFβ-induced SMAD (small mothers against decapentaplegic) activation | [84] |
| | Pancreatic ductal adenocarcinomas | Stellate cells activation and induction of a pro-inflammatory milieu. (unknown mechanism) | [94] |
| | Prostate cancer cells | Induction of TGF-β2, TNF1α (Tumor necrosis factor1 α), IL6 (Interleukin 6), TSG101 (Tumor susceptibility gene 101), Akt, ILK1 (Integrin-linked kinase1) and β-catenin. | [118] |
| Angiogenesis and vascular permeability | Cancer Stem Cells from Hepatocellular Carcinoma | lncRNA H19-mediated VEGF (Vascular endothelial growth factor) induction | [31] |
| | Metastatic breast cancer | miR-105 targeting of ZO-1 | [95] |
| | Glioma stem cells | miR21-mediated induction of VEGF pathway. | [97] |
| | Hypoxic cancer cells | Upregulation of miR-135-b, miR-23a, miR-210, miR-494 and Wnt pathway activation. | [101] and enclosed references |
| | Ovarian cancer | E-cadherin-mediated activation of β-catenin and NFκB (Nuclear Factor kappa-light-chain-enhancer of activated B cells) signaling | [103] |
| | Cervical squamous cell carcinoma | miR-221-3p-mediated activation of the ERK (Extracellular signal-Regulated Kinase)/AKT pathway | [122] |
| Immunomodulation | Head and neck squamous cell carcinoma | Receptor–ligand interactions regulating gene expression in T cells | [90] |
| | Melanoma cells | miR-690 induction of mitochondrial apoptotic pathway in CD4+ T cells | [91] |
| | Several cancer cells | miRNAs regulation | [92] and enclosed references |
| | Lung adenocarcinoma, hepatocellular carcinoma, breast carcinoma | Monocyte recruitment and Generation of Tumor Associated Macrofages | [104] |
| | Hypoxic lung cancer | miR-103a-mediated targeting of PTEN (Phosphatase and tensin homolog) and activation of Tumor Associated Macrofages | [120] |
| Chemoresistence and Cancer Stem Cell stimulation | CAF from colon rectal cancer | Wnt3a induction of WNT signalling activation in CSC (Cancer Stem Cells) | [127] |
| | CAF from breast cancer | miR-21, miR-378e and mir-143-mediated Cancer Stem Cells maintenance | [113] |
| | Renal cell carcinoma | lncRNA ARSR-mediated chemoresistance via competitively binding of miR-34/miR-449. | [128] |
| Metabolism modulation | Melanoma cells | miR-155 and miR-210-mediated promotion of glycolysis and inhibition of oxidative phosphorylation. | [88] |
| | CAF from prostate cancer and from pancreatic cancer | Metabolites inhibiting mitochondrial oxidative phosphorylation and increasing glycolysis. | [89] |

All further efforts in the study of biomarkers would have a great impact particularly on early diagnosis, considering that the development of non-invasive diagnostic tools currently represents a major challenge. Moreover, an optimization of exosome isolation protocols is required to better disclose the functional role of specific exosome cargo molecules. The isolation of exosomes with high purity and quality is still difficult and the demonstrated heterogeneity of exosomes further impairs the isolation efficiency; all these aspects represent a limitation, particularly for the study of low copy number molecule species, such as lncRNAs.

A deep understanding of mechanisms controlling the loading of specific molecules in exosomes is also needed. This field of study is to be considered still at infancy even if some mechanisms of sequence-specific miRNA sorting (by EXO- and hEXO-motifs) and specific heterogeneous nuclear ribonucleoproteins (hnRNPA2B1 and hnRNPQ) involved in the recognition of these signals, have been recently identified [34,35]. Interestingly, the sorting of lncRNA ARSR in exosomes by renal cancer cells also involves hnRNPA2B1 [128]; furthermore, a "zipcode" in the mRNAs may control their selective loading [129]. All of this evidence suggests common regulative mechanisms, at least for RNA loading, and opens the way towards possible innovative therapeutic strategies oriented to the selective modulation of RNA exosomal cargo by engineering signaling sequences. Other approaches could aim to interfere with, or promote, the in vivo sorting of these vesicles. The use of specific inhibitors, targeting key regulators of both exosome biogenesis and release, could be a suitable approach. For example, the release of EVs by primary hepatocytes and Huh7 cells may be reduced by inactivating mediators of the DR5 signaling pathway or ROCK1 inhibition. Interestingly, the ROCK1 inhibitor *fasudil* reduced serum levels of EVs in nonalcoholic steatohepatitis (NASH) mice and this reduction was associated with decreased liver injury, inflammation, and fibrosis [130]. The drug GW4869 was efficiently used to inhibit exosome biogenesis by interfering with sphingomyelinase function [125,126]. The release of exosomes was shown to be influenced by calcium and the monensin drug was found able to affect exosome biogenesis [131]. Further studies are still necessary to investigate the effective translational application of these protocols.

Remarkably, exosomes show low immunogenicity, high biocompatibility, and high efficacy of delivery. Considering all these features, they might be engineered to convey molecules of interest and achieve targeted therapeutic intervention. For a recent example, paclitaxel-loaded exosomes, modified to improve circulation time, were shown to selectively deliver the drug to target cancer cells and increase the survival rate of lung cancer patients [132].

Finally, an in-depth understanding of exosome cargo composition and functional role in EMT associated with tumor progression would pave the way for innovative therapeutic opportunities. In particular, further studies must be focused on the characterization and potential engineering in vivo and/or ex vivo of exosomes from EMT cells. The plasticity of transitional cells might, indeed, imply a fine-tuning regulation of the loading machinery that, in turn, might be mirrored by the great complexity of exosome cargoes.

**Author Contributions:** Both authors made substantial contributions to the conception and design of the work and approved the submitted version (Conceptualization, A.C. and C.C.; Writing—Original Draft Preparation, Review and Editing, A.C. and C.C.; Funding Acquisition, A.C. and C.C.).

**Funding:** Sapienza University of Rome RM116154BE5E14B2; AIRC (Italian Association for Cancer Research) MFAG 2017-ID. 19982 project–P.I. Conigliaro Alice.

**Acknowledgments:** We thank F. Citarella for critical revision of the manuscript.

**Conflicts of Interest:** The authors declare no conflict of interest.

## References

1. Johnstone, R.M.; Adam, M.; Hammond, J.R.; Orr, L.; Turbide, C. Vesicle formation during reticulocyte maturation. Association of plasma membrane activities with released vesicles (exosomes). *J. Biol. Chem.* **1987**, *262*, 9412–9420. [PubMed]

2. Pan, B.T.; Johnstone, R.M. Fate of the transferrin receptor during maturation of sheep reticulocytes in vitro: Selective externalization of the receptor. *Cell* **1983**, *33*, 967–978. [CrossRef]
3. Thierry, A.R.; El Messaoudi, S.; Gahan, P.B.; Anker, P.; Stroun, M. Origins, structures, and functions of circulating DNA in oncology. *Cancer Metastasis Rev.* **2016**, *35*, 347–376. [CrossRef]
4. Mittelbrunn, M.; Sanchez-Madrid, F. Intercellular communication: Diverse structures for exchange of genetic information. *Nat. Rev. Mol. Cell Biol.* **2012**, *13*, 328–335. [CrossRef]
5. Robbins, P.D.; Morelli, A.E. Regulation of immune responses by extracellular vesicles. *Nat. Rev. Immunol.* **2014**, *14*, 195–208. [CrossRef]
6. Bakhti, M.; Winter, C.; Simons, M. Inhibition of myelin membrane sheath formation by oligodendrocyte-derived exosome-like vesicles. *J. Biol. Chem.* **2011**, *286*, 787–796. [CrossRef] [PubMed]
7. Fruhbeis, C.; Frohlich, D.; Kuo, W.P.; Amphornrat, J.; Thilemann, S.; Saab, A.S.; Kirchhoff, F.; Mobius, W.; Goebbels, S.; Nave, K.A.; et al. Neurotransmitter-triggered transfer of exosomes mediates oligodendrocyte-neuron communication. *PLoS Biol.* **2013**, *11*, e1001604. [CrossRef] [PubMed]
8. Lopez-Verrilli, M.A.; Picou, F.; Court, F.A. Schwann cell-derived exosomes enhance axonal regeneration in the peripheral nervous system. *Glia* **2013**, *61*, 1795–1806. [CrossRef] [PubMed]
9. Guay, C.; Regazzi, R. Exosomes as new players in metabolic organ cross-talk. *Diabetes Obes. Metab.* **2017**, *19* (Suppl. 1), 137–146. [CrossRef] [PubMed]
10. Logozzi, M.; De Milito, A.; Lugini, L.; Borghi, M.; Calabro, L.; Spada, M.; Perdicchio, M.; Marino, M.L.; Federici, C.; Iessi, E.; et al. High levels of exosomes expressing CD63 and caveolin-1 in plasma of melanoma patients. *PLoS ONE* **2009**, *4*, e5219. [CrossRef]
11. Peinado, H.; Aleckovic, M.; Lavotshkin, S.; Matei, I.; Costa-Silva, B.; Moreno-Bueno, G.; Hergueta-Redondo, M.; Williams, C.; Garcia-Santos, G.; Ghajar, C.; et al. Melanoma exosomes educate bone marrow progenitor cells toward a pro-metastatic phenotype through MET. *Nat. Med.* **2012**, *18*, 883–891. [CrossRef] [PubMed]
12. Colombo, M.; Moita, C.; van Niel, G.; Kowal, J.; Vigneron, J.; Benaroch, P.; Manel, N.; Moita, L.F.; Thery, C.; Raposo, G. Analysis of ESCRT functions in exosome biogenesis, composition and secretion highlights the heterogeneity of extracellular vesicles. *J. Cell Sci.* **2013**, *126*, 5553–5565. [CrossRef] [PubMed]
13. Ostrowski, M.; Carmo, N.B.; Krumeich, S.; Fanget, I.; Raposo, G.; Savina, A.; Moita, C.F.; Schauer, K.; Hume, A.N.; Freitas, R.P.; et al. Rab27a and Rab27b control different steps of the exosome secretion pathway. *Nat. Cell Biol.* **2010**, *12*, 19–30. [CrossRef] [PubMed]
14. Baietti, M.F.; Zhang, Z.; Mortier, E.; Melchior, A.; Degeest, G.; Geeraerts, A.; Ivarsson, Y.; Depoortere, F.; Coomans, C.; Vermeiren, E.; et al. Syndecan-syntenin-ALIX regulates the biogenesis of exosomes. *Nat. Cell Biol.* **2012**, *14*, 677–685. [CrossRef]
15. Kowal, J.; Arras, G.; Colombo, M.; Jouve, M.; Morath, J.P.; Primdal-Bengtson, B.; Dingli, F.; Loew, D.; Tkach, M.; Thery, C. Proteomic comparison defines novel markers to characterize heterogeneous populations of extracellular vesicle subtypes. *Proc. Natl. Acad. Sci. USA* **2016**, *113*, E968–E977. [CrossRef]
16. Willms, E.; Johansson, H.J.; Mager, I.; Lee, Y.; Blomberg, K.E.; Sadik, M.; Alaarg, A.; Smith, C.I.; Lehtio, J.; El Andaloussi, S.; et al. Cells release subpopulations of exosomes with distinct molecular and biological properties. *Sci. Rep.* **2016**, *6*, 22519. [CrossRef] [PubMed]
17. Ogawa, Y.; Miura, Y.; Harazono, A.; Kanai-Azuma, M.; Akimoto, Y.; Kawakami, H.; Yamaguchi, T.; Toda, T.; Endo, T.; Tsubuki, M.; et al. Proteomic analysis of two types of exosomes in human whole saliva. *Biol. Pharm. Bull.* **2011**, *34*, 13–23. [CrossRef]
18. Ogawa, Y.; Taketomi, Y.; Murakami, M.; Tsujimoto, M.; Yanoshita, R. Small RNA transcriptomes of two types of exosomes in human whole saliva determined by next generation sequencing. *Biol. Pharm. Bull.* **2013**, *36*, 66–75. [CrossRef] [PubMed]
19. Lasser, C.; Shelke, G.V.; Yeri, A.; Kim, D.K.; Crescitelli, R.; Raimondo, S.; Sjostrand, M.; Gho, Y.S.; van Keuren Jensen, K.; Lotvall, J. Two distinct extracellular RNA signatures released by a single cell type identified by microarray and next-generation sequencing. *RNA Biol.* **2017**, *14*, 58–72. [CrossRef] [PubMed]
20. Bobrie, A.; Colombo, M.; Krumeich, S.; Raposo, G.; Thery, C. Diverse subpopulations of vesicles secreted by different intracellular mechanisms are present in exosome preparations obtained by differential ultracentrifugation. *J. Extracell. Ves.* **2012**, *1*, 18397. [CrossRef] [PubMed]
21. ExoCarta. Available online: http://www.exocarta.org (accessed on 24 December 2018).
22. Vesiclepedia. Available online: http://www.microvesicles.org (accessed on 24 December 2018).

23. Skog, J.; Wurdinger, T.; van Rijn, S.; Meijer, D.H.; Gainche, L.; Sena-Esteves, M.; Curry, W.T., Jr.; Carter, B.S.; Krichevsky, A.M.; Breakefield, X.O. Glioblastoma microvesicles transport RNA and proteins that promote tumour growth and provide diagnostic biomarkers. *Nat. Cell Biol.* **2008**, *10*, 1470–1476. [CrossRef] [PubMed]
24. Conigliaro, A.; Fontana, S.; Raimondo, S.; Alessandro, R. Exosomes: Nanocarriers of Biological Messages. *Adv. Exp. Med. Biol.* **2017**, *998*, 23–43. [PubMed]
25. Nolte-'t Hoen, E.N.; Buermans, H.P.; Waasdorp, M.; Stoorvogel, W.; Wauben, M.H.; 't Hoen, P.A. Deep sequencing of RNA from immune cell-derived vesicles uncovers the selective incorporation of small non-coding RNA biotypes with potential regulatory functions. *Nucleic Acids Res.* **2012**, *40*, 9272–9285. [CrossRef] [PubMed]
26. Mittelbrunn, M.; Gutierrez-Vazquez, C.; Villarroya-Beltri, C.; Gonzalez, S.; Sanchez-Cabo, F.; Gonzalez, M.A.; Bernad, A.; Sanchez-Madrid, F. Unidirectional transfer of microRNA-loaded exosomes from T cells to antigen-presenting cells. *Nat. Commun.* **2011**, *2*, 282. [CrossRef] [PubMed]
27. Valadi, H.; Ekstrom, K.; Bossios, A.; Sjostrand, M.; Lee, J.J.; Lotvall, J.O. Exosome-mediated transfer of mRNAs and microRNAs is a novel mechanism of genetic exchange between cells. *Nat. Cell Biol.* **2007**, *9*, 654–659. [CrossRef] [PubMed]
28. Pegtel, D.M.; Cosmopoulos, K.; Thorley-Lawson, D.A.; van Eijndhoven, M.A.; Hopmans, E.S.; Lindenberg, J.L.; de Gruijl, T.D.; Wurdinger, T.; Middeldorp, J.M. Functional delivery of viral miRNAs via exosomes. *Proc. Natl. Acad. Sci. USA* **2010**, *107*, 6328–6333. [CrossRef]
29. Zhang, J.; Liu, S.C.; Luo, X.H.; Tao, G.X.; Guan, M.; Yuan, H.; Hu, D.K. Exosomal Long Noncoding RNAs are Differentially Expressed in the Cervicovaginal Lavage Samples of Cervical Cancer Patients. *J. Clin. Lab. Anal.* **2016**, *30*, 1116–1121. [CrossRef]
30. Berrondo, C.; Flax, J.; Kucherov, V.; Siebert, A.; Osinski, T.; Rosenberg, A.; Fucile, C.; Richheimer, S.; Beckham, C.J. Expression of the Long Non-Coding RNA HOTAIR Correlates with Disease Progression in Bladder Cancer and Is Contained in Bladder Cancer Patient Urinary Exosomes. *PLoS ONE* **2016**, *11*, e0147236. [CrossRef]
31. Conigliaro, A.; Costa, V.; Lo Dico, A.; Saieva, L.; Buccheri, S.; Dieli, F.; Manno, M.; Raccosta, S.; Mancone, C.; Tripodi, M.; et al. CD90+ liver cancer cells modulate endothelial cell phenotype through the release of exosomes containing H19 lncRNA. *Mol. Cancer* **2015**, *14*, 155. [CrossRef]
32. Santos, M.F.; Rappa, G.; Karbanova, J.; Kurth, T.; Corbeil, D.; Lorico, A. VAMP-associated protein-A and oxysterol-binding protein-related protein 3 promote the entry of late endosomes into the nucleoplasmic reticulum. *J. Biol. Chem.* **2018**, *293*, 13834–13848. [CrossRef]
33. Rappa, G.; Santos, M.F.; Green, T.M.; Karbanova, J.; Hassler, J.; Bai, Y.; Barsky, S.H.; Corbeil, D.; Lorico, A. Nuclear transport of cancer extracellular vesicle-derived biomaterials through nuclear envelope invagination-associated late endosomes. *Oncotarget* **2017**, *8*, 14443–14461. [CrossRef] [PubMed]
34. Santangelo, L.; Giurato, G.; Cicchini, C.; Montaldo, C.; Mancone, C.; Tarallo, R.; Battistelli, C.; Alonzi, T.; Weisz, A.; Tripodi, M. The RNA-Binding Protein SYNCRIP Is a Component of the Hepatocyte Exosomal Machinery Controlling MicroRNA Sorting. *Cell Rep.* **2016**, *17*, 799–808. [CrossRef] [PubMed]
35. Villarroya-Beltri, C.; Gutierrez-Vazquez, C.; Sanchez-Cabo, F.; Perez-Hernandez, D.; Vazquez, J.; Martin-Cofreces, N.; Martinez-Herrera, D.J.; Pascual-Montano, A.; Mittelbrunn, M.; Sanchez-Madrid, F. Sumoylated hnRNPA2B1 controls the sorting of miRNAs into exosomes through binding to specific motifs. *Nat. Commun.* **2013**, *4*, 2980. [CrossRef]
36. Hobor, F.; Dallmann, A.; Ball, N.J.; Cicchini, C.; Battistelli, C.; Ogrodowicz, R.W.; Christodoulou, E.; Martin, S.R.; Castello, A.; Tripodi, M.; et al. A cryptic RNA-binding domain mediates Syncrip recognition and exosomal partitioning of miRNA targets. *Nat. Commun.* **2018**, *9*, 831. [CrossRef] [PubMed]
37. Parolini, I.; Federici, C.; Raggi, C.; Lugini, L.; Palleschi, S.; De Milito, A.; Coscia, C.; Iessi, E.; Logozzi, M.; Molinari, A.; et al. Microenvironmental pH is a key factor for exosome traffic in tumor cells. *J. Biol. Chem.* **2009**, *284*, 34211–34222. [CrossRef]
38. Kucharzewska, P.; Christianson, H.C.; Welch, J.E.; Svensson, K.J.; Fredlund, E.; Ringner, M.; Morgelin, M.; Bourseau-Guilmain, E.; Bengzon, J.; Belting, M. Exosomes reflect the hypoxic status of glioma cells and mediate hypoxia-dependent activation of vascular cells during tumor development. *Proc. Natl. Acad. Sci. USA* **2013**, *110*, 7312–7317. [CrossRef] [PubMed]
39. French, K.C.; Antonyak, M.A.; Cerione, R.A. Extracellular vesicle docking at the cellular port: Extracellular vesicle binding and uptake. *Semin. Cell Dev. Biol.* **2017**, *67*, 48–55. [CrossRef] [PubMed]

40. Hoshino, A.; Costa-Silva, B.; Shen, T.L.; Rodrigues, G.; Hashimoto, A.; Tesic Mark, M.; Molina, H.; Kohsaka, S.; Di Giannatale, A.; Ceder, S.; et al. Tumour exosome integrins determine organotropic metastasis. *Nature* **2015**, *527*, 329–335. [CrossRef]
41. Chen, G.; Huang, A.C.; Zhang, W.; Zhang, G.; Wu, M.; Xu, W.; Yu, Z.; Yang, J.; Wang, B.; Sun, H.; et al. Exosomal PD-L1 contributes to immunosuppression and is associated with anti-PD-1 response. *Nature* **2018**, *560*, 382–386. [CrossRef]
42. Lugini, L.; Cecchetti, S.; Huber, V.; Luciani, F.; Macchia, G.; Spadaro, F.; Paris, L.; Abalsamo, L.; Colone, M.; Molinari, A.; et al. Immune surveillance properties of human NK cell-derived exosomes. *J. Immunol.* **2012**, *189*, 2833–2842. [CrossRef]
43. Wei, G.; Jie, Y.; Haibo, L.; Chaoneng, W.; Dong, H.; Jianbing, Z.; Junjie, G.; Leilei, M.; Hongtao, S.; Yunzeng, Z.; et al. Dendritic cells derived exosomes migration to spleen and induction of inflammation are regulated by CCR7. *Sci. Rep.* **2017**, *7*, 42996. [CrossRef] [PubMed]
44. Corrado, C.; Saieva, L.; Raimondo, S.; Santoro, A.; De Leo, G.; Alessandro, R. Chronic myelogenous leukaemia exosomes modulate bone marrow microenvironment through activation of epidermal growth factor receptor. *J. Cell. Mol. Med.* **2016**, *20*, 1829–1839. [CrossRef] [PubMed]
45. Taverna, S.; Pucci, M.; Giallombardo, M.; Di Bella, M.A.; Santarpia, M.; Reclusa, P.; Gil-Bazo, I.; Rolfo, C.; Alessandro, R. Amphiregulin contained in NSCLC-exosomes induces osteoclast differentiation through the activation of EGFR pathway. *Sci. Rep.* **2017**, *7*, 3170. [CrossRef]
46. Raimondo, S.; Saieva, L.; Corrado, C.; Fontana, S.; Flugy, A.; Rizzo, A.; De Leo, G.; Alessandro, R. Chronic myeloid leukemia-derived exosomes promote tumor growth through an autocrine mechanism. *Cell Commun. Signal.* **2015**, *13*, 8. [CrossRef] [PubMed]
47. Yu, L.; Yang, F.; Jiang, L.; Chen, Y.; Wang, K.; Xu, F.; Wei, Y.; Cao, X.; Wang, J.; Cai, Z. Exosomes with membrane-associated TGF-beta1 from gene-modified dendritic cells inhibit murine EAE independently of MHC restriction. *Eur. J. Immunol.* **2013**, *43*, 2461–2472. [CrossRef] [PubMed]
48. Sakakura, H.; Mii, S.; Hagiwara, S.; Kato, T.; Yamamoto, N.; Hibi, H.; Takahashi, M.; Murakumo, Y. CD109 is a component of exosome secreted from cultured cells. *Biochem. Biophys. Res. Commun.* **2016**, *469*, 816–822. [CrossRef] [PubMed]
49. Nieto, M.A.; Huang, R.Y.; Jackson, R.A.; Thiery, J.P. Emt: 2016. *Cell* **2016**, *166*, 21–45. [CrossRef]
50. Brabletz, T.; Jung, A.; Reu, S.; Porzner, M.; Hlubek, F.; Kunz-Schughart, L.A.; Knuechel, R.; Kirchner, T. Variable beta-catenin expression in colorectal cancers indicates tumor progression driven by the tumor environment. *Proc. Natl. Acad. Sci. USA* **2001**, *98*, 10356–10361. [CrossRef]
51. Dahl, U.; Sjodin, A.; Larue, L.; Radice, G.L.; Cajander, S.; Takeichi, M.; Kemler, R.; Semb, H. Genetic dissection of cadherin function during nephrogenesis. *Mol. Cell. Biol.* **2002**, *22*, 1474–1487. [CrossRef]
52. Perez-Moreno, M.A.; Locascio, A.; Rodrigo, I.; Dhondt, G.; Portillo, F.; Nieto, M.A.; Cano, A. A new role for E12/E47 in the repression of E-cadherin expression and epithelial-mesenchymal transitions. *J. Biol. Chem.* **2001**, *276*, 27424–27431. [CrossRef]
53. Nieto, M.A. The snail superfamily of zinc-finger transcription factors. *Nat. Rev. Mol. Cell Biol.* **2002**, *3*, 155–166. [CrossRef] [PubMed]
54. Yang, J.; Mani, S.A.; Donaher, J.L.; Ramaswamy, S.; Itzykson, R.A.; Come, C.; Savagner, P.; Gitelman, I.; Richardson, A.; Weinberg, R.A. Twist, a master regulator of morphogenesis, plays an essential role in tumor metastasis. *Cell* **2004**, *117*, 927–939. [CrossRef] [PubMed]
55. Rodriguez, M.; Aladowicz, E.; Lanfrancone, L.; Goding, C.R. Tbx3 represses E-cadherin expression and enhances melanoma invasiveness. *Cancer Res.* **2008**, *68*, 7872–7881. [CrossRef] [PubMed]
56. Peinado, H.; Olmeda, D.; Cano, A. Snail, Zeb and bHLH factors in tumour progression: An alliance against the epithelial phenotype? *Nat. Rev. Cancer* **2007**, *7*, 415–428. [CrossRef] [PubMed]
57. Battistelli, C.; Cicchini, C.; Santangelo, L.; Tramontano, A.; Grassi, L.; Gonzalez, F.J.; de Nonno, V.; Grassi, G.; Amicone, L.; Tripodi, M. The Snail repressor recruits EZH2 to specific genomic sites through the enrollment of the lncRNA HOTAIR in epithelial-to-mesenchymal transition. *Oncogene* **2017**, *36*, 942–955. [CrossRef]
58. Battistelli, C.; Tripodi, M.; Cicchini, C. Targeting of polycombs to DNA in EMT. *Oncotarget* **2017**, *8*, 57936–57937. [CrossRef] [PubMed]
59. Yu, M.; Bardia, A.; Wittner, B.S.; Stott, S.L.; Smas, M.E.; Ting, D.T.; Isakoff, S.J.; Ciciliano, J.C.; Wells, M.N.; Shah, A.M.; et al. Circulating breast tumor cells exhibit dynamic changes in epithelial and mesenchymal composition. *Science* **2013**, *339*, 580–584. [CrossRef] [PubMed]

60. Huang, R.Y.; Wong, M.K.; Tan, T.Z.; Kuay, K.T.; Ng, A.H.; Chung, V.Y.; Chu, Y.S.; Matsumura, N.; Lai, H.C.; Lee, Y.F.; et al. An EMT spectrum defines an anoikis-resistant and spheroidogenic intermediate mesenchymal state that is sensitive to e-cadherin restoration by a src-kinase inhibitor, saracatinib (AZD0530). *Cell Death Dis.* **2013**, *4*, e915. [CrossRef] [PubMed]
61. Schliekelman, M.J.; Taguchi, A.; Zhu, J.; Dai, X.; Rodriguez, J.; Celiktas, M.; Zhang, Q.; Chin, A.; Wong, C.H.; Wang, H.; et al. Molecular portraits of epithelial, mesenchymal, and hybrid States in lung adenocarcinoma and their relevance to survival. *Cancer Res.* **2015**, *75*, 1789–1800. [CrossRef] [PubMed]
62. Pastushenko, I.; Brisebarre, A.; Sifrim, A.; Fioramonti, M.; Revenco, T.; Boumahdi, S.; Van Keymeulen, A.; Brown, D.; Moers, V.; Lemaire, S.; et al. Identification of the tumour transition states occurring during EMT. *Nature* **2018**, *556*, 463–468. [CrossRef]
63. Ruscetti, M.; Quach, B.; Dadashian, E.L.; Mulholland, D.J.; Wu, H. Tracking and Functional Characterization of Epithelial-Mesenchymal Transition and Mesenchymal Tumor Cells during Prostate Cancer Metastasis. *Cancer Res.* **2015**, *75*, 2749–2759. [CrossRef] [PubMed]
64. Yamashita, N.; Tokunaga, E.; Iimori, M.; Inoue, Y.; Tanaka, K.; Kitao, H.; Saeki, H.; Oki, E.; Maehara, Y. Epithelial Paradox: Clinical Significance of Coexpression of E-cadherin and Vimentin With Regard to Invasion and Metastasis of Breast Cancer. *Clin. Breast Cancer* **2018**, *18*, e1003–e1009. [CrossRef] [PubMed]
65. Conigliaro, A.; Amicone, L.; Costa, V.; De Santis Puzzonia, M.; Mancone, C.; Sacchetti, B.; Cicchini, C.; Garibaldi, F.; Brenner, D.A.; Kisseleva, T.; et al. Evidence for a common progenitor of epithelial and mesenchymal components of the liver. *Cell Death Differ.* **2013**, *20*, 1116–1123. [CrossRef]
66. Garibaldi, F.; Cicchini, C.; Conigliaro, A.; Santangelo, L.; Cozzolino, A.M.; Grassi, G.; Marchetti, A.; Tripodi, M.; Amicone, L. An epistatic mini-circuitry between the transcription factors Snail and HNF4alpha controls liver stem cell and hepatocyte features exhorting opposite regulation on stemness-inhibiting microRNAs. *Cell Death Differ.* **2012**, *19*, 937–946. [CrossRef]
67. Diaz-Lopez, A.; Moreno-Bueno, G.; Cano, A. Role of microRNA in epithelial to mesenchymal transition and metastasis and clinical perspectives. *Cancer Manag. Res.* **2014**, *6*, 205–216. [PubMed]
68. Costa, V.; Lo Dico, A.; Rizzo, A.; Rajata, F.; Tripodi, M.; Alessandro, R.; Conigliaro, A. MiR-675-5p supports hypoxia induced epithelial to mesenchymal transition in colon cancer cells. *Oncotarget* **2017**, *8*, 24292–24302. [CrossRef]
69. Jolly, M.K.; Tripathi, S.C.; Jia, D.; Mooney, S.M.; Celiktas, M.; Hanash, S.M.; Mani, S.A.; Pienta, K.J.; Ben-Jacob, E.; Levine, H. Stability of the hybrid epithelial/mesenchymal phenotype. *Oncotarget* **2016**, *7*, 27067–27084. [CrossRef]
70. Lu, M.; Jolly, M.K.; Levine, H.; Onuchic, J.N.; Ben-Jacob, E. MicroRNA-based regulation of epithelial-hybrid-mesenchymal fate determination. *Proc. Natl. Acad. Sci. USA* **2013**, *110*, 18144–18149. [CrossRef]
71. Tian, X.J.; Zhang, H.; Xing, J. Coupled reversible and irreversible bistable switches underlying TGFbeta-induced epithelial to mesenchymal transition. *Biophys. J.* **2013**, *105*, 1079–1089. [CrossRef]
72. Kalluri, R. The biology and function of exosomes in cancer. *J. Clin. Investig.* **2016**, *126*, 1208–1215. [CrossRef]
73. Green, T.M.; Alpaugh, M.L.; Barsky, S.H.; Rappa, G.; Lorico, A. Breast Cancer-Derived Extracellular Vesicles: Characterization and Contribution to the Metastatic Phenotype. *Biomed. Res. Int.* **2015**, *2015*, 634865. [CrossRef]
74. Cesi, G.; Walbrecq, G.; Margue, C.; Kreis, S. Transferring intercellular signals and traits between cancer cells: Extracellular vesicles as "homing pigeons". *Cell Commun. Signal.* **2016**, *14*, 13. [CrossRef] [PubMed]
75. You, Y.; Shan, Y.; Chen, J.; Yue, H.; You, B.; Shi, S.; Li, X.; Cao, X. Matrix metalloproteinase 13-containing exosomes promote nasopharyngeal carcinoma metastasis. *Cancer Sci.* **2015**, *106*, 1669–1677. [CrossRef] [PubMed]
76. Zomer, A.; Maynard, C.; Verweij, F.J.; Kamermans, A.; Schafer, R.; Beerling, E.; Schiffelers, R.M.; de Wit, E.; Berenguer, J.; Ellenbroek, S.I.; et al. In Vivo imaging reveals extracellular vesicle-mediated phenocopying of metastatic behavior. *Cell* **2015**, *161*, 1046–1057. [CrossRef] [PubMed]
77. Tang, M.K.; Wong, A.S. Exosomes: Emerging biomarkers and targets for ovarian cancer. *Cancer Lett.* **2015**, *367*, 26–33. [CrossRef]
78. Aga, M.; Bentz, G.L.; Raffa, S.; Torrisi, M.R.; Kondo, S.; Wakisaka, N.; Yoshizaki, T.; Pagano, J.S.; Shackelford, J. Exosomal HIF1alpha supports invasive potential of nasopharyngeal carcinoma-associated LMP1-positive exosomes. *Oncogene* **2014**, *33*, 4613–4622. [CrossRef] [PubMed]

79. Franzen, C.A.; Blackwell, R.H.; Todorovic, V.; Greco, K.A.; Foreman, K.E.; Flanigan, R.C.; Kuo, P.C.; Gupta, G.N. Urothelial cells undergo epithelial-to-mesenchymal transition after exposure to muscle invasive bladder cancer exosomes. *Oncogenesis* **2015**, *4*, e163. [CrossRef] [PubMed]
80. Jeppesen, D.K.; Nawrocki, A.; Jensen, S.G.; Thorsen, K.; Whitehead, B.; Howard, K.A.; Dyrskjot, L.; Orntoft, T.F.; Larsen, M.R.; Ostenfeld, M.S. Quantitative proteomics of fractionated membrane and lumen exosome proteins from isogenic metastatic and nonmetastatic bladder cancer cells reveal differential expression of EMT factors. *Proteomics* **2014**, *14*, 699–712. [CrossRef]
81. Wang, J.; Guan, X.; Zhang, Y.; Ge, S.; Zhang, L.; Li, H.; Wang, X.; Liu, R.; Ning, T.; Deng, T.; et al. Exosomal miR-27a Derived from Gastric Cancer Cells Regulates the Transformation of Fibroblasts into Cancer-Associated Fibroblasts. *Cell. Physiol. Biochem.* **2018**, *49*, 869–883. [CrossRef] [PubMed]
82. Wang, J.; Yang, X.; Li, R.; Wang, L.; Gu, Y.; Zhao, Y.; Huang, K.H.; Cheng, T.; Yuan, Y.; Gao, S. Long non-coding RNA MYU promotes prostate cancer proliferation by mediating the miR-184/c-Myc axis. *Oncol. Rep.* **2018**, *40*, 2814–2825. [CrossRef]
83. Kalluri, R.; Zeisberg, M. Fibroblasts in cancer. *Nat. Rev. Cancer* **2006**, *6*, 392–401. [CrossRef] [PubMed]
84. Ringuette Goulet, C.; Bernard, G.; Tremblay, S.; Chabaud, S.; Bolduc, S.; Pouliot, F. Exosomes Induce Fibroblast Differentiation into Cancer-Associated Fibroblasts through TGFbeta Signaling. *Mol. Cancer Res.* **2018**, *16*, 1196–1204. [CrossRef] [PubMed]
85. Principe, S.; Mejia-Guerrero, S.; Ignatchenko, V.; Sinha, A.; Ignatchenko, A.; Shi, W.; Pereira, K.; Su, S.; Huang, S.H.; O'Sullivan, B.; et al. Proteomic Analysis of Cancer-Associated Fibroblasts Reveals a Paracrine Role for MFAP5 in Human Oral Tongue Squamous Cell. Carcinoma. *J. Proteome Res.* **2018**, *17*, 2045–2059. [CrossRef] [PubMed]
86. Herrera, M.; Llorens, C.; Rodriguez, M.; Herrera, A.; Ramos, R.; Gil, B.; Candia, A.; Larriba, M.J.; Garre, P.; Earl, J.; et al. Differential distribution and enrichment of non-coding RNAs in exosomes from normal and Cancer-associated fibroblasts in colorectal cancer. *Mol. Cancer* **2018**, *17*, 114. [CrossRef]
87. Zhang, Z.; Li, X.; Sun, W.; Yue, S.; Yang, J.; Li, J.; Ma, B.; Wang, J.; Yang, X.; Pu, M.; et al. Loss of exosomal miR-320a from cancer-associated fibroblasts contributes to HCC proliferation and metastasis. *Cancer Lett.* **2017**, *397*, 33–42. [CrossRef] [PubMed]
88. La Shu, S.; Yang, Y.; Allen, C.L.; Maguire, O.; Minderman, H.; Sen, A.; Ciesielski, M.J.; Collins, K.A.; Bush, P.J.; Singh, P.; et al. Metabolic reprogramming of stromal fibroblasts by melanoma exosome microRNA favours a pre-metastatic microenvironment. *Sci. Rep.* **2018**, *8*, 12905. [CrossRef]
89. Zhao, H.; Yang, L.; Baddour, J.; Achreja, A.; Bernard, V.; Moss, T.; Marini, J.C.; Tudawe, T.; Seviour, E.G.; et al. Tumor microenvironment derived exosomes pleiotropically modulate cancer cell metabolism. *Elife* **2016**, *5*, e10250. [CrossRef] [PubMed]
90. Muller, L.; Mitsuhashi, M.; Simms, P.; Gooding, W.E.; Whiteside, T.L. Tumor-derived exosomes regulate expression of immune function-related genes in human T cell subsets. *Sci. Rep.* **2016**, *6*, 20254. [CrossRef]
91. Zhou, J.; Yang, Y.; Wang, W.; Zhang, Y.; Chen, Z.; Hao, C.; Zhang, J. Melanoma-released exosomes directly activate the mitochondrial apoptotic pathway of CD4(+) T cells through their microRNA cargo. *Exp. Cell Res.* **2018**, *371*, 364–371. [CrossRef]
92. Hirschberger, S.; Hinske, L.C.; Kreth, S. MiRNAs: Dynamic regulators of immune cell functions in inflammation and cancer. *Cancer Lett.* **2018**, *431*, 11–21. [CrossRef]
93. Clayton, A.; Al-Taei, S.; Webber, J.; Mason, M.D.; Tabi, Z. Cancer exosomes express CD39 and CD73, which suppress T cells through adenosine production. *J. Immunol.* **2011**, *187*, 676–683. [CrossRef] [PubMed]
94. Costa-Silva, B.; Aiello, N.M.; Ocean, A.J.; Singh, S.; Zhang, H.; Thakur, B.K.; Becker, A.; Hoshino, A.; Mark, M.T.; Molina, H.; et al. Pancreatic cancer exosomes initiate pre-metastatic niche formation in the liver. *Nat. Cell Biol.* **2015**, *17*, 816–826. [CrossRef] [PubMed]
95. Zhou, W.; Fong, M.Y.; Min, Y.; Somlo, G.; Liu, L.; Palomares, M.R.; Yu, Y.; Chow, A.; O'Connor, S.T.; Chin, A.R.; et al. Cancer-secreted miR-105 destroys vascular endothelial barriers to promote metastasis. *Cancer Cell* **2014**, *25*, 501–515. [CrossRef] [PubMed]
96. Grange, C.; Tapparo, M.; Collino, F.; Vitillo, L.; Damasco, C.; Deregibus, M.C.; Tetta, C.; Bussolati, B.; Camussi, G. Microvesicles released from human renal cancer stem cells stimulate angiogenesis and formation of lung premetastatic niche. *Cancer Res.* **2011**, *71*, 5346–5356. [CrossRef] [PubMed]

97. Sun, X.; Ma, X.; Wang, J.; Zhao, Y.; Wang, Y.; Bihl, J.C.; Chen, Y.; Jiang, C. Glioma stem cells-derived exosomes promote the angiogenic ability of endothelial cells through miR-21/VEGF signal. *Oncotarget* **2017**, *8*, 36137–36148. [CrossRef] [PubMed]
98. Takasugi, M.; Okada, R.; Takahashi, A.; Virya Chen, D.; Watanabe, S.; Hara, E. Small extracellular vesicles secreted from senescent cells promote cancer cell proliferation through EphA2. *Nat. Commun.* **2017**, *8*, 15729. [CrossRef]
99. Petrova, V.; Annicchiarico-Petruzzelli, M.; Melino, G.; Amelio, I. The hypoxic tumour microenvironment. *Oncogenesis* **2018**, *7*, 10. [CrossRef]
100. Zhang, W.; Zhou, X.; Yao, Q.; Liu, Y.; Zhang, H.; Dong, Z. HIF-1-mediated production of exosomes during hypoxia is protective in renal tubular cells. *Am. J. Physiol. Ren. Physiol.* **2017**, *313*, F906–F913. [CrossRef]
101. Shao, C.; Yang, F.; Miao, S.; Liu, W.; Wang, C.; Shu, Y.; Shen, H. Role of hypoxia-induced exosomes in tumor biology. *Mol. Cancer* **2018**, *17*, 120. [CrossRef]
102. Dey, N.; De, P.; Brian, L.J. Evading anti-angiogenic therapy: Resistance to anti-angiogenic therapy in solid tumors. *Am. J. Transl. Res.* **2015**, *7*, 1675–1698. [CrossRef]
103. Tang, M.K.S.; Yue, P.Y.K.; Ip, P.P.; Huang, R.L.; Lai, H.C.; Cheung, A.N.Y.; Tse, K.Y.; Ngan, H.Y.S.; Wong, A.S.T. Soluble E-cadherin promotes tumor angiogenesis and localizes to exosome surface. *Nat. Commun.* **2018**, *9*, 2270. [CrossRef] [PubMed]
104. Song, X.; Ding, Y.; Liu, G.; Yang, X.; Zhao, R.; Zhang, Y.; Zhao, X.; Anderson, G.J.; Nie, G. Cancer Cell-derived Exosomes Induce Mitogen-activated Protein Kinase-dependent Monocyte Survival by Transport. of Functional Receptor Tyrosine Kinases. *J. Biol. Chem.* **2016**, *291*, 8453–8464. [CrossRef] [PubMed]
105. Rahman, M.A.; Barger, J.F.; Lovat, F.; Gao, M.; Otterson, G.A.; Nana-Sinkam, P. Lung cancer exosomes as drivers of epithelial mesenchymal transition. *Oncotarget* **2016**, *7*, 54852–54866. [CrossRef] [PubMed]
106. Chen, L.; Guo, P.; He, Y.; Chen, Z.; Chen, L.; Luo, Y.; Qi, L.; Liu, Y.; Wu, Q.; Cui, Y.; et al. HCC-derived exosomes elicit HCC progression and recurrence by epithelial-mesenchymal transition through MAPK/ERK signalling pathway. *Cell Death Dis.* **2018**, *9*, 513. [CrossRef] [PubMed]
107. Higginbotham, J.N.; Demory Beckler, M.; Gephart, J.D.; Franklin, J.L.; Bogatcheva, G.; Kremers, G.J.; Piston, D.W.; Ayers, G.D.; McConnell, R.E.; Tyska, M.J.; et al. Amphiregulin exosomes increase cancer cell invasion. *Curr. Biol.* **2011**, *21*, 779–786. [CrossRef] [PubMed]
108. Harris, D.A.; Patel, S.H.; Gucek, M.; Hendrix, A.; Westbroek, W.; Taraska, J.W. Exosomes released from breast cancer carcinomas stimulate cell movement. *PLoS ONE* **2015**, *10*, e0117495. [CrossRef] [PubMed]
109. Sung, B.H.; Ketova, T.; Hoshino, D.; Zijlstra, A.; Weaver, A.M. Directional cell movement through tissues is controlled by exosome secretion. *Nat. Commun.* **2015**, *6*, 7164. [CrossRef]
110. Schillaci, O.; Fontana, S.; Monteleone, F.; Taverna, S.; Di Bella, M.A.; Di Vizio, D.; Alessandro, R. Exosomes from metastatic cancer cells transfer amoeboid phenotype to non-metastatic cells and increase endothelial permeability: Their emerging role in tumor heterogeneity. *Sci. Rep.* **2017**, *7*, 4711. [CrossRef]
111. Dong, L.; Lin, W.; Qi, P.; Xu, M.D.; Wu, X.; Ni, S.; Huang, D.; Weng, W.W.; Tan, C.; Sheng, W.; et al. Circulating Long RNAs in Serum Extracellular Vesicles: Their Characterization and Potential Application as Biomarkers for Diagnosis of Colorectal Cancer. *Cancer Epidemiol. Biomarkers Prev.* **2016**, *25*, 1158–1166. [CrossRef]
112. Battistelli, C.; Sabarese, G.; Santangelo, L.; Montaldo, C.; Gonzalez, F.J.; Tripodi, M.; Cicchini, C. The lncRNA HOTAIR transcription is controlled by HNF4alpha-induced chromatin topology modulation. *Cell Death Differ.* **2018**. [CrossRef]
113. Amicone, L.; Citarella, F.; Cicchini, C. Epigenetic regulation in hepatocellular carcinoma requires long noncoding RNAs. *Biomed. Res. Int.* **2015**, *2015*, 473942. [CrossRef] [PubMed]
114. Luga, V.; Zhang, L.; Viloria-Petit, A.M.; Ogunjimi, A.A.; Inanlou, M.R.; Chiu, E.; Buchanan, M.; Hosein, A.N.; Basik, M.; Wrana, J.L. Exosomes mediate stromal mobilization of autocrine Wnt-PCP signaling in breast cancer cell migration. *Cell* **2012**, *151*, 1542–1556. [CrossRef] [PubMed]
115. Donnarumma, E.; Fiore, D.; Nappa, M.; Roscigno, G.; Adamo, A.; Iaboni, M.; Russo, V.; Affinito, A.; Puoti, I.; Quintavalle, C.; et al. Cancer-associated fibroblasts release exosomal microRNAs that dictate an aggressive phenotype in breast cancer. *Oncotarget* **2017**, *8*, 19592–19608. [CrossRef] [PubMed]
116. Li, W.; Zhang, X.; Wang, J.; Li, M.; Cao, C.; Tan, J.; Ma, D.; Gao, Q. TGFbeta1 in fibroblasts-derived exosomes promotes epithelial-mesenchymal transition of ovarian cancer cells. *Oncotarget* **2017**, *8*, 96035–96047.

117. Zhao, X.; Wu, X.; Qian, M.; Song, Y.; Wu, D.; Zhang, W. Knockdown of TGF-beta1 expression in human umbilical cord mesenchymal stem cells reverts their exosome-mediated EMT promoting effect on lung cancer cells. *Cancer Lett.* **2018**, *428*, 34–44. [CrossRef] [PubMed]
118. Ramteke, A.; Ting, H.; Agarwal, C.; Mateen, S.; Somasagara, R.; Hussain, A.; Graner, M.; Frederick, B.; Agarwal, R.; Deep, G. Exosomes secreted under hypoxia enhance invasiveness and stemness of prostate cancer cells by targeting adherens junction molecules. *Mol. Carcinog.* **2015**, *54*, 554–565. [CrossRef]
119. Xue, M.; Chen, W.; Xiang, A.; Wang, R.; Chen, H.; Pan, J.; Pang, H.; An, H.; Wang, X.; Hou, H.; et al. Hypoxic exosomes facilitate bladder tumor growth and development through transferring long non-coding RNA-UCA1. *Mol. Cancer* **2017**, *16*, 143. [CrossRef]
120. Takahashi, K.; Yan, I.K.; Haga, H.; Patel, T. Modulation of hypoxia-signaling pathways by extracellular linc-RoR. *J. Cell Sci.* **2014**, *127*, 1585–1594. [CrossRef]
121. Hsu, Y.L.; Hung, J.Y.; Chang, W.A.; Jian, S.F.; Lin, Y.S.; Pan, Y.C.; Wu, C.Y.; Kuo, P.L. Hypoxic Lung-Cancer-Derived Extracellular Vesicle MicroRNA-103a Increases the Oncogenic Effects of Macrophages by Targeting PTEN. *Mol. Ther.* **2018**, *26*, 568–581. [CrossRef]
122. Zhou, C.F.; Ma, J.; Huang, L.; Yi, H.Y.; Zhang, Y.M.; Wu, X.G.; Yan, R.M.; Liang, L.; Zhong, M.; Yu, Y.H.; et al. Cervical squamous cell carcinoma-secreted exosomal miR-221-3p promotes lymphangiogenesis and lymphatic metastasis by targeting VASH1. *Oncogene* **2018**. [CrossRef]
123. Karaosmanoglu, O.; Banerjee, S.; Sivas, H. Identification of biomarkers associated with partial epithelial to mesenchymal transition in the secretome of slug over-expressing hepatocellular carcinoma cells. *Cell. Oncol.* **2018**, *41*, 439–453. [CrossRef] [PubMed]
124. Grosse-Wilde, A.; Fouquier d'Herouel, A.; McIntosh, E.; Ertaylan, G.; Skupin, A.; Kuestner, R.E.; del Sol, A.; Walters, K.A.; Huang, S. Stemness of the hybrid Epithelial/Mesenchymal State in Breast Cancer and Its Association with Poor Survival. *PLoS ONE* **2015**, *10*, e0126522. [CrossRef] [PubMed]
125. Richards, K.E.; Zeleniak, A.E.; Fishel, M.L.; Wu, J.; Littlepage, L.E.; Hill, R. Cancer-associated fibroblast exosomes regulate survival and proliferation of pancreatic cancer cells. *Oncogene* **2017**, *36*, 1770–1778. [CrossRef] [PubMed]
126. Singh, R.; Pochampally, R.; Watabe, K.; Lu, Z.; Mo, Y.Y. Exosome-mediated transfer of miR-10b promotes cell invasion in breast cancer. *Mol. Cancer* **2014**, *13*, 256. [CrossRef] [PubMed]
127. Hu, Y.; Yan, C.; Mu, L.; Huang, K.; Li, X.; Tao, D.; Wu, Y.; Qin, J. Fibroblast-Derived Exosomes Contribute to Chemoresistance through Priming Cancer Stem Cells in Colorectal Cancer. *PLoS ONE* **2015**, *10*, e0125625. [CrossRef] [PubMed]
128. Qu, L.; Ding, J.; Chen, C.; Wu, Z.J.; Liu, B.; Gao, Y.; Chen, W.; Liu, F.; Sun, W.; Li, X.F.; et al. Exosome-Transmitted lncARSR Promotes Sunitinib Resistance in Renal Cancer by Acting as a Competing Endogenous RNA. *Cancer Cell* **2016**, *29*, 653–668. [CrossRef]
129. Bolukbasi, M.F.; Mizrak, A.; Ozdener, G.B.; Madlener, S.; Strobel, T.; Erkan, E.P.; Fan, J.B.; Breakefield, X.O.; Saydam, O. miR-1289 and "Zipcode"-like Sequence Enrich. mRNAs in Microvesicles. *Mol. Ther. Nucleic Acids* **2012**, *1*, e10. [CrossRef]
130. Hirsova, P.; Ibrahim, S.H.; Krishnan, A.; Verma, V.K.; Bronk, S.F.; Werneburg, N.W.; Charlton, M.R.; Shah, V.H.; Malhi, H.; Gores, G.J. Lipid-Induced Signaling Causes Release of Inflammatory Extracellular Vesicles From Hepatocytes. *Gastroenterology* **2016**, *150*, 956–967. [CrossRef] [PubMed]
131. Savina, A.; Furlan, M.; Vidal, M.; Colombo, M.I. Exosome release is regulated by a calcium-dependent mechanism in K562 cells. *J. Biol. Chem.* **2003**, *278*, 20083–20090. [CrossRef]
132. Kim, M.S.; Haney, M.J.; Zhao, Y.; Yuan, D.; Deygen, I.; Klyachko, N.L.; Kabanov, A.V.; Batrakova, E.V. Engineering macrophage-derived exosomes for targeted paclitaxel delivery to pulmonary metastases: In vitro and in vivo evaluations. *Nanomedicine* **2018**, *14*, 195–204. [CrossRef]

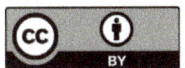

© 2018 by the authors. Licensee MDPI, Basel, Switzerland. This article is an open access article distributed under the terms and conditions of the Creative Commons Attribution (CC BY) license (http://creativecommons.org/licenses/by/4.0/).

MDPI
St. Alban-Anlage 66
4052 Basel
Switzerland
Tel. +41 61 683 77 34
Fax +41 61 302 89 18
www.mdpi.com

*Journal of Clinical Medicine* Editorial Office
E-mail: jcm@mdpi.com
www.mdpi.com/journal/jcm

www.ingramcontent.com/pod-product-compliance
Lightning Source LLC
LaVergne TN
LVHW070128100526
838202LV00016B/2248